Diseases of the temporomandibular apparatus

A MULTIDISCIPLINARY APPROACH

Diseases of the temporomandibular apparatus

A MULTIDISCIPLINARY APPROACH

Edited and with contributions by

DOUGLAS H. MORGAN, D.D.S.

Diplomate, American Board of Ambulatory Anesthesia; Fellow, American Dental Society of Anesthesiology; Member, Southern California Academy of Oral Pathology; Founding Director, TMJ Clinic, White Memorial Medical Center, Los Angeles; President, The Temporomandibular Joint Research Foundation, La Crescenta; Attending Oral Surgeon, University of California at Irvine Medical Center, Irvine; Fellow, American Academy of Craniomandibular Disorders and International College of Craniomandibular Orthopedics; Former Lecturer, Department of Oral Medicine, Loma Linda University School of Dentistry, Loma Linda, California

LELAND R. HOUSE, M.D.

Diplomate, American Board of Otolaryngology; Chairman, Department of Otolaryngology and Head and Neck Surgery, White Memorial Medical Center, Los Angeles; Professor, Otolaryngology Section, Department of Surgery, Loma Linda University School of Medicine, Loma Linda; President, White Memorial Otolaryngology Foundation, Inc.; Clinical Professor, Department of Otolaryngology, University of Southern California School of Medicine, Los Angeles, California

WILLIAM P. HALL, M.D.

Diplomate, American Board of Otolaryngology and Head and Neck Surgery; Vice-President, White Memorial Otolaryngology Foundation, Inc.; Associate Professor, Otolaryngology Section, Department of Surgery, Loma Linda University School of Medicine, Loma Linda, California

S. JAMES VAMVAS, D.D.S., F.A.C.D.

Former Trustee, American Association of Oral and Maxillofacial Surgeons; Fellow, American Dental Society of Anesthesiology; Cofounder, Southern California Academy of Oral Pathology; Senior Oral Surgeon, Saint Francis Hospital of Lynwood, Lynwood, and Mission and Community Hospitals, Huntington Park; Consulting Staff, White Memorial Medical Center, Los Angeles, California

SECOND EDITION

With **1196** *illustrations*

The C. V. Mosby Company

ST. LOUIS • TORONTO • LONDON 1982

MOSBY

A TRADITION OF PUBLISHING EXCELLENCE

Editor: Eugenia A. Klein
Assistant editor: Kathryn H. Falk
Book design: Jeanne Bush
Cover design: Diane Beasley
Production: Carolyn Biby, Margaret B. Bridenbaugh

SECOND EDITION

Printed in the United States of America

The C.V. Mosby Company
11830 Westline Industrial Drive, St. Louis, Missouri 63141

Library of Congress Cataloging in Publication Data

Main entry under title:

Diseases of the temporomandibular apparatus.

Includes bibliographies and index.
1. Temporomandibular joint—Diseases. I. Morgan, Douglas H. [DNLM: 1. Temporomandibular joint syndrome. WU 140 D611]
RK470.D57 1982 617'.522 81-16819
ISBN 0-8016-3492-X AACR2

C/CB/B 9 8 7 6 5 4 3 2 1 02/C/290

Contributors

S. KENDRICK CRANDALL, D.D.S.

Private practice, Anaheim; Former Instructor, TMJ Clinic, White Memorial Medical Center, Los Angeles, California

DONALD C. CURNUTTE, D.D.S.

Associate Clinical Professor and Chairman, Occlusion Section, Restorative Department, University of Southern California School of Dentistry, Los Angeles, California

LAWRENCE D. DAY, D.D.S., M.S.

Associate Professor, Department of Oral Surgery, and Chairman, Section of Pain Control, Loma Linda University School of Dentistry, Loma Linda, California

DONALD E. DOYLE, M.D.

Staff member, Cedars-Sinai Medical Center, Los Angeles, California

CARL B. ERMSHAR, Jr., M.D.

Diplomate, American Board of Otolaryngology; Instructor, Department of Otolaryngology and Head and Neck Surgery, White Memorial Medical Center, Los Angeles; Clinical Instructor, Otolaryngology Section, Department of Surgery, Loma Linda University School of Medicine, Loma Linda, California

MARTIN E. FRANKEL, D.M.D., M.D.S.

Chief, Craniofacial Dysfunction Center, North Shore University Hospital; Chief, Craniofacial Dysfunction Center, Department of Otolaryngology, New York Eye and Ear Infirmary, New York, New York; Member, Omicron Kappa Upsilon, Robert R. Andrews Research Society, and American Equilibration Society; Fellow, American Academy of Craniomandibular Disorders, International College of Dentists, and International College of Craniomandibular Orthopedics; Territorial Consultant, U.S. Virgin Islands

JAMES F. GARRY, D.D.S., F.A.S.C.D., F.I.C.D.

Pedodontist; Chief of Dental Staff, Fullerton Community Hospital; Former President, American Endodontic Society; Fellow, American Endodontic Society, International College of Oral Implantology, American Society of Dentistry for Children, and International College of Dentists; Private practice, Fullerton, California

JOHN R.J. GAWLEY, D.D.S., M.S.

Diplomate, American Board of Orthodontics; Private practice, Alhambra, California

DAVID J. GOODFRIEND, D.D.S.

Research Appointee, Dental Department, and Director, Edward C. Kirk Dental Research, University of Pennsylvania, Philadelphia, Pennsylvania; Honorary Fellow in Otolaryngology; Life Affiliate Member, American Medical Association

BARBARA J. GREENE, M.F.T.

Myofunctional Therapist, Oral Muscle Retraining Center, Camarillo, California

MURRAY GROSSAN, M.D.

Diplomate, American Board of Otolaryngology; Member, Biofeedback Research Society and American Association for the Study of Headaches; Private practice, Los Angeles, California

WILLIAM P. HALL, M.D.

Diplomate, American Board of Otolaryngology and Head and Neck Surgery; Vice-President, White Memorial Otolaryngology Foundation, Inc.; Associate Professor, Otolaryngology Section, Department of Surgery, Loma Linda University School of Medicine, Loma Linda, California

CHARLES D. HASSE, D.D.S.

Private practice, Irvine; Attending Oral and Maxillofacial Surgeon, Western Medical Center, Santa Ana, and Hoag Memorial Presbyterian Hospital, Newport Beach; Consultant, Orofacial Deformities Panel, Children's Hospital of Orange County; Assistant Professor, Department of Surgery, Charles R. Drew Postgraduate School of Medicine; Fellow, International College of Craniomandibular Orthopedics, International Congress of Oral Implantologists, and Southern California Academy of Oral Pathology; Former Chief Resident, Oral and Maxillofacial Surgery, Veterans Administration Medical Center, Long Beach, and University of California at Irvine Medical Center, Irvine, California

LELAND R. HOUSE, M.D.

Diplomate, American Board of Otolaryngology; Chairman, Department of Otolaryngology and Head and Neck Surgery, White Memorial Medical Center, Los Angeles; Professor, Otolaryngology Section, Department of Surgery, Loma Linda University School of Medicine, Loma Linda; President, White Memorial Otolaryngology Foundation, Inc.; Clinical Professor, Department of Otolaryngology, University of Southern California School of Medicine, Los Angeles, California

ROBERT A. JAMES, D.D.S., M.S.

Associate Professor, Department of Restorative Dentistry, Loma Linda University School of Dentistry, Loma Linda, California

BERNARD JANKELSON, D.M.D.

Diplomate, American Board of Prosthodontics; F.I.C.D.; F.A.C.P.; F.I.C.C.M.O. (F. International College of Craniomandibular Orthopedics); A.A.C.D. (American Academy of Craniomandibular Disorders); Director of Research, Departments of Basic Science Research, Instrumentation Research and Development, and Applied Clinical Research, Myo-Tronics Research, Inc., Seattle, Washington

PETER J. JANNETTA, M.D.

Professor and Chairman, Department of Neurosurgery, University of Pittsburgh, Pittsburgh, Pennsylvania

WARREN L. JONES, M.D., Ph.D.

Diplomate, American Board of Psychiatry and Neurology; Training Analyst, Southern California Psychoanalytic Institute; Psychiatric Consultant, Student Health Department of the California Institute of Technology, Pasadena, California

EUEL KING, D.D.S.

Fellow, International College of Craniomandibular Orthopedics; Director, Temporomandibular Joint Clinic, Division of the White Memorial Otolaryngology Foundation, Inc.; Member, San Gabriel Valley Dental Society, Los Angeles, California

ROGER A. MARUM, Ph.D.

Private practice, psychology, La Canada, Flintridge, California

VICTOR W. MINTZ, D.D.S.

Assistant Clinical Professor, Department of Fixed Prosthodontics, University of California; Consultant to Headache Research Clinic, Department of Neurology, School of Medicine, and Former Director, Temporomandibular Joint Clinic, School of Dentistry, University of California at Los Angeles; Consultant, U.S. Veterans Administration Hospitals at Sepulveda, Wadsworth, and Brentwood, Los Angeles, California; Diplomate, American Board of Prosthodontics; Fellow, American College of Prosthodontics; Member, American Prosthodontic Society, American Equilibration Society, and Federation of Prosthodontic Organizations

DOUGLAS H. MORGAN, D.D.S.

Diplomate, American Board of Ambulatory Anesthesia; Fellow, American Dental Society of Anesthesiology; Member, Southern California Academy of Oral Pathology; Founding Director, TMJ Clinic, White Memorial Medical Center, Los Angeles; President, The Temporomandibular Joint Research Foundation, La Crescenta; Attending Oral Surgeon, University of California at Irvine Medical Center, Irvine; Fellow, American Academy of Craniomandibular Disorders and International College of Craniomandibular Orthopedics; Former Lecturer, Department of Oral Medicine, Loma Linda University School of Dentistry, Loma Linda, California

RICHARD B. OLIVER, D.D.S.

Private practive, La Palma; Clinical Instructor, TMJ Clinic, White Memorial Medical Center, Los Angeles, California

YALE S. PALCHICK, D.D.S., F.A.G.D.

Postgraduate Adjunct Lecturer, University of Pittsburgh, Pittsburgh, Pennsylvania; Guest Lecturer, University of Detroit, Detroit, Michigan; Guest Lecturer, Case Western Reserve University, Cleveland; Visiting Professor, Ohio State University, Department of Physical Medicine, Columbus; Consulting Staff, Akron City Hospital, Akron, Ohio

ROBERT J. PESHEK, D.D.S.

Clinical Instructor, TMJ Clinic, White Memorial Medical Center, Los Angeles; Director of the Peshek Dental and Nutritional Research Clinic, Riverside, California

NORMAN M. POKRAS, D.D.S., M.S.D.

Diplomate, American Board of Oral Surgery; Private practice, Long Beach, California

HARRY QUINT, Jr., D.D.S., F.A.C.D., F.I.C.D.

Professor, Department of Community Dentistry, University of Southern California School of Dentistry, Los Angeles, California

J. RONALD RICH, M.D., F.A.C.S.

Diplomate, American Board of Neurological Surgery; Private practice, Los Angeles, California

LAWRENCE M. ROSEN, M.D.

Diplomate, American Board of Radiology and American Board of Nuclear Medicine; Associate Clinical Professor, Department of Radiology, University of California at Irvine School of Medicine, Irvine; Associate Radiologist, St. Francis Hospital of Lynwood, Lynwood, California

WILLIAM S. SEIBLY, D.D.S., Ph.D.

Assistant Professor, Department of Restorative Dentistry, Loma Linda University School of Dentistry, Loma Linda, California

ERIC PAUL SHABER, D.D.S.

Chief, Division of Oral and Maxillofacial Surgery, and Director, Maxillofacial Pain Unit, Veterans Administration Medical Center; Assistant Professor, Department of Oral and Maxillofacial Surgery, University of California, San Francisco, California

RICHARD S. SHEPPARD, D.D.S.

Founding member of Holistic Dental Association; President, Bio-Perceptions, Inc., Carlsbad, California

CARY B. SIMONDS, D.D.S., M.S.

Private practice, oral and maxillofacial surgery, Marysville, California

DOUGLAS F. SNOW, D.D.S., F.A.C.D., F.A.G.D.

Private practice, North Hollywood, California

S. JAMES VAMVAS, D.D.S., F.A.C.D.

Former Trustee, American Association of Oral and Maxillofacial Surgeons; Fellow, American Dental Society of Anesthesiology; Cofounder, Southern California Academy of Oral Pathology; Senior Oral Surgeon, Saint Francis Hospital of Lynwood, Lynwood, and Mission and Community Hospitals, Huntington Park; Consulting Staff, White Memorial Medical Center, Los Angeles, California

EUGENE P. WAGNER, D.D.S., F.A.C.D.

Clinical Instructor, TMJ Clinic, White Memorial Medical Center, Los Angeles; Private practice, Monterey Park, California

EDWIN J. ZINMAN, D.D.S., J.D.

Former Lecturer, Department of Periodontics, University of California at San Francisco School of Dentistry; Attorney-at-Law, San Francisco, California

To our wives

Adrienne Atwood Morgan

Billie Gay Hall

Antonia Vamvas

whose unfailing support and understanding of time away from family activities enabled us to complete this work

To my daughter

Darleen Hemmerlin, D.D.S.

for her interest in scientific dentistry

Foreword

The inquiring mind will find this book a rich pasture of information about the diagnosis and management of the diverse problems that affect the entire masticatory apparatus. Disorders of the temporomandibular joint, its capsule, disc, and ligaments, the adjacent bony structures, dentition, orofacial soft tissues, and the muscles of mastication, as well as related muscles of the neck, are discussed in detail. Neural modulation of pain perception and of motor, sensory, and autonomic function is considered. The muscular, or myofascial, trigger-point features of the pain-dysfunction syndrome are an important inclusion in this second edition, since without the muscles there can be no movement or function of the temporomandibular joint.

This book is a practical reference for those professionals in dentistry and medicine who deal with the common and complex problems of the temporomandibular apparatus. A team effort has succeeded in coordinating data from both the basic sciences and clinical research, which enlarges our understanding of the mechanisms that underlie the patient's signs and symptoms and his or her attitudes toward them. Each contributor has brought special knowledge to bear on the recent factual and conceptual advances that make this volume necessary and valuable.

Janet Travell, M.D.

Preface

It has been over 4 years since the first edition of this book was published and distributed to members of the professions. During this period there has been increased interest relating to the area of the temporomandibular apparatus, a region also described as the craniomandibular area. Both designations are valid and will be used frequently in the years ahead.

Originally it was estimated that over 20% of the average population have symptoms relating to the temporomandibular apparatus at one time or another. This percentage now has increased to over 50%, since more and more symptoms are being connected with this craniomandibular, or temporomandibular, area.

It is interesting to note that this TMJ syndrome was earlier named after James Costen, an otolaryngologist who wrote of its various symptoms in the early 1930s. Dr. Costen had been influenced by David J. Goodfriend of Philadelphia. We feel honored that this same Dr. Goodfriend, for this second edition, has contributed an epilogue of historical and scientific significance.

Just prior to the publication of our first edition the second edition of Nathan Allen Shore's *TMJ Dysfunction and Occlusal Equilibration* came into print. Dr. Shore's first edition and an earlier published book by Dr. Laszlo were the first two books that attempted to cover the TMJ field in its entirety. Shortly after our first edition was published, another outstanding book was produced by Harold Gelb, furthering the approach of interdisciplinary treatment strategies.

Since the first edition of this text more significant information and techniques have emerged. We are indebted to the outstanding new work of Bernard Jankelson, who has developed scientific measuring devices for the jaw joint, muscle, and mandibular function with the Mandibular Kinesiograph and the Myo-Monitor. In the field of radiology many new techniques are being utilized. Clyde Wilkes has done much good work with arthrography, as have William McCarty and William Farrar with their inferior joint space arthrograms. Donald Blaschke, recently of the Radiology Department of the University of California at Los Angeles, has used laminagraphy with his work in superior and inferior joint space arthrography. He has produced much helpful information. William Murphy, from the Radiology Department, Washington University School of Medicine, St. Louis, has greatly improved magnification techniques of TMJ x-ray films using transcranial lateral oblique procedures. To complement the improvement in transcranial lateral oblique procedures, several companies—the Rinn Corporation, the Denar Corporation, and Ron McCormack Enterprises—now manufacture head-holding devices to take these radiographs, which can be done in the office. In addition to these individual developments, two new organizations have been formed to increase education and understanding in the craniomandibular-orthopedic field: the American Academy of Craniomandibular Disorders and the International College of Craniomandibular Orthopedics.

We would like to express particular appreciation and respect for the pioneering work of Janet Travell. As will be remembered, it was Dr. Travell who enabled the then Senator John F. Kennedy to throw away his crutches and continue an active life, an achievement in large part resulting from her knowledge, understanding, and research in physical medicine. Dr. Travell's work is acknowledged extensively in this book by those authors who discuss the myofascial pain-dysfunction syndrome. A forthcoming book written by Dr. Travell and David G. Simons, entitled *Myofascial Pain and Dysfunction: The Trigger Point Manual,* will set the standard for future treatment of musculoskeletal problems.

Work in the area of the temporomandibular apparatus is particularly fascinating because it is not limited to any one discipline in either dentistry or medicine but rather encompasses every discipline of both these professions. As dental caries becomes less of a primary concern, the dentist has greater motivation to expand his or her understanding and knowledge into the field of the temporomandibular apparatus. There are literally millions of people suffering from these problems who currently have nowhere to go. The dentist of the future will use basic dental skills plus increased knowledge to help these people while working more closely with medical colleagues. We are beginning to realize that such a minute thing as a high filling may have a disastrous effect on the entire body. Dentists and physicians working closely together will bring great benefits to their patients. The field of the temporomandibular apparatus effectively breaks down the artificial barriers that have existed between medicine and dentistry. No longer can dentists afford to look on themselves as being in a limited field, in which their treatment has little or no effect on the rest of the human structure.

The material in this book represents over 20 years of our working in this field as well as a major attempt to gather the latest material that has come to our attention since the first edition. In some chapters there has been minimal change, but most have had major revisions with new material. Some chapters have been reluctantly omitted so that newer material could be introduced. Even more than the first edition, this new text should be of particular interest to the general dentist, orthodontist, pedodontist, prosthodontist, and oral and maxillofacial surgeon in the dental professions; and in the medical field, to the otolaryngologist, head and neck surgeon, radiologist, neurologist, neurosurgeon, plastic surgeon, psychiatrist, and orthopedist. We always emphasize the team approach, although an individual patient may be effectively treated by a single modality. But it has been our firm observation throughout the years that most individuals receive the greatest help through a combination of treatment modalities applied in an organized fashion.

In the preparation of this manuscript, as in the first edition, we are most grateful to Patsy Clay, who has done an outstanding job again in coordinating the work of the various contributors, as well as assisting in the initial editing and working with the various authors. Dan Slotten has again contributed his superb artwork for this edition with many new drawings. Bill Watson has once again provided the photography.

We wish to thank the White Memorial Otolaryngology Foundation, Inc., and its executive board members, who include Dr. Leland R. House, President; Dr. William P. Hall, Vice-President; and Dr. George Gay, Secretary, for the help they have given us in regard to the TMJ work, as well as for sponsoring, with the TMJ Research Foundation, the annual courses that are given to both dentists and physicians in the TMJ field. We wish to thank the Board of Directors of the TMJ Research Foundation, which includes Arthur L. Neff, Sidney Adair, Robert Baker, Mary Gaston, Adrienne Morgan, William Ivers, Robert Van Aiken, Thomas Wright, Lawrence Burr, and Catherine Stover. We also would like to thank members of the Medical and Dental Advisory Board of the TMJ Research Foundation, who include Drs. Leland R. House, William P. Hall, S. James Vamvas, Carlton Williams, Edward Furstman, and Richard Bing.

The field of the temporomandibular apparatus, we believe, will bring forth a new specialty in the future encompassing both the dental and medical components. This is an ambitious project with ramifications that will be of great value for humankind.

The longest journey starts with one step. The first step has been taken.

Douglas H. Morgan, D.D.S.
Leland R. House, M.D.
William P. Hall, M.D.
S. James Vamvas, D.D.S., F.A.C.D.

Contents

PART ONE
GROWTH AND DEVELOPMENT

1 Embryology and evolution, 3
Donald E. Doyle, M.D.

2 Anatomy and neuroanatomy, 8
Carl B. Ermshar, Jr., M.D.

3 Skeletal muscle, 26
Eric Paul Shaber, D.D.S.

4 Early iatrogenic orofacial muscle, skeletal, and TMJ dysfunction, 35
James F. Garry, D.D.S., F.A.S.C.D., F.I.C.D.

PART TWO
DIAGNOSIS

5 History taking, 73
Lawrence D. Day, D.D.S., M.S.

6 Initial examination, 82
Douglas F. Snow, D.D.S., F.A.C.D., F.A.G.D.

7 The role of occlusion in diagnosis and treatment planning, 117
Donald C. Curnutte, D.D.S.

8 Radiographic procedures, 132
Lawrence M. Rosen, M.D., and **Douglas H. Morgan, D.D.S.**

9 Interpretation of radiographs, 166
Douglas H. Morgan, D.D.S.

10 Differential diagnosis of TMJ disease, 211
S. James Vamvas, D.D.S., F.A.C.D.

11 The ear, nose, and throat, 224
Leland R. House, M.D., and **William P. Hall, M.D.**

12 The orthopedic influence, 232
Victor W. Mintz, D.D.S.

13 Psychogenic factors contributing to the etiology and symptoms of temporomandibular joint pain-dysfunction syndrome, 236
Roger A. Marum, Ph.D.

PART THREE
TREATMENT

14 Gnathological treatment, 245
William S. Seibly, D.D.S., Ph.D., and **Robert A. James, D.D.S., M.S.**

15 Splints, 265
Eugene P. Wagner, D.D.S., F.A.C.D., S. Kendrick Crandall, D.D.S., and **Richard B. Oliver, D.D.S.**

16 Considerations in the treatment of muscle spasm, 278
Eric Paul Shaber, D.D.S.

17 Treatment of muscle spasm, 300
Yale S. Palchick, D.D.S., F.A.G.D.

18 Biofeedback, 327
Murray Grossan, M.D.

19 Acupuncture, 335
Harry Quint, Jr., D.D.S., F.A.C.D., F.I.C.D.

20 Electrical acupoint therapy for temporomandibular joint–myofacial pain, 340
Robert J. Peshek, D.D.S.

21 Pharmacological methods, 350
William P. Hall, M.D.

22 Surgery of the temporomandibular joint, 355
Douglas H. Morgan, D.D.S., Leland R. House, M.D., William P. Hall, M.D., and **S. James Vamvas, D.D.S., F.A.C.D.**

23 Treatment of fractures and ankylosis, 443
Cary B. Simonds, D.D.S., M.S., with case histories by **Douglas H. Morgan, D.D.S.**

24 Oral myofunctional therapy, 461
Barbara J. Greene, M.F.T., and **Richard S. Sheppard, D.D.S.**

25 Psychological treatment, 486
Warren L. Jones, M.D., Ph.D.

PART FOUR
DEVELOPING AREAS

26 Kinesiology, 497
Euel King, D.D.S.

27 Orthodontic considerations in temporomandibular joint dysfunction: some highlights, 500
John R.J. Gawley, D.D.S., M.S.

28 Interrelationship of myofacial pain syndrome, temporomandibular joint dysfunction, and orthodontics, 512
Martin E. Frankel, D.M.D., M.D.S.

29 Orthognathic surgery, 526
Charles D. Hasse, D.D.S., and **Douglas H. Morgan, D.D.S.**

30 Neurosurgical treatment of facial pain, 557
J. Ronald Rich, M.D., F.A.C.S.

31 Microvascular decompression in the treatment of trigeminal neuralgia, 580
Peter J. Jannetta, M.D.

32 Modern diagnosis and management of musculoskeletal dysfunctions of the head and neck, 591
Bernard Jankelson, D.M.D.

33 Legal aspects, 600
Edwin J. Zinman, D.D.S., J.D.

34 Prevention of disease, 616
Norman M. Pokras, D.D.S., M.S.D.

Epilogue

The temporomandibular joints in dentistry and dental medicine, 621
David J. Goodfriend, D.D.S.

Vertigo attributable to dental and temporomandibular joint causes, 625
Herbert T. Kelly, M.D., F.A.C.P., and **David J. Goodfriend, D.D.S.**

PART ONE

GROWTH AND DEVELOPMENT

1 Embryology and evolution

DONALD E. DOYLE, M.D.

The jaw joint holds a particularly interesting and peculiar position, historically, in the development of the vertebrates, of which humans are thought to be currently the highest form. To be classified as a complete vertebrate, a creature must have developed not only a backbone but also biting jaws. A mammal is distinguished from all other forms of vertebrate animals by the relationship of its jaw-ear structure.[3] Perhaps even more significant to vertebrate evolution is the fact that the first true diarthrodial joint developed at the jaw. Definitive diarthrodial joints (eudiarthrodial joints) probably were developed first in the common ancestors of bony fishes and may have been part of the mechanism that differentiated the Gnathostomata from the Agnatha.[4]

Gnathostomes were the first jawed vertebrates, and the Agnatha were vertebrates without jaws. The Agnatha are thought to be the basic ground plan for the vertebrates, which developed with the evolution of the Gnathostomes. Therefore it may be said that the jaws lead the way in joint evolution.

THE MAMMALIAN JAW

There are several morphological features that mark the mammalian jaw and distinguish it from those of mammal-like reptiles as well as from those of other lower orders. Among these is the fact that the lower jaw is made of just one bone, known as the *mandible*. It is homologous with the dentary bone of reptiles, and, like that bone, all the lower teeth are attached here. The lower jaw is joined to the skull by a dentary-squamosal articulation, the squamosa being that part of the temporal bone which forms the upper part of the temporomandibular joint. The direct counterpart of the jaw joint of the reptile (the articular-quadrate joint) has no part in jaw support in the mammalian skull. These two bones (articular = malleus; quadrate = incus) are the ossicles of the middle ear of the mammalian skull.[3] Thus the jaw joint of reptiles is still present in mammals, but it has a decidedly new function.

The evolution of the lower jaw from a series of bones to a single bone is significant in that this form obviously provides a stronger and more rigid unit. This was necessary as the jaw became more important for biting efficiency. As the upper limbs developed, the function of prehension was no longer essential for the jaw; thus there was a need for greater efficiency in the mouth.

The biomechanics of the temporomandibular joint are affected in another way by the evolution of humans as upright animals. An animal that is basically horizontally oriented can accommodate a simple hinged joint. That joint swings widely downward because there is nothing below it, and the neck and body stream directly backward away from the head. Vertically oriented animals, such as humans, have their neck running downward in close relationship to the posterior aspect of the mandible. The important conduits such as the esophagus and trachea are in front of this axis. Because the rear margin of the jaw would strike the rather large mastoid process, a simple hinge would not be possible in this upright animal. With full function its symphysis would forcibly compress the trachea and esophagus against the hard vertebral column. However, add to the hingelike rotation of the joint a forward and downward sliding of the condyles on their respective articular eminences, and the jaw can open widely and at the same time be brought away from impinging on the structure of the neck, which is so vital. Even a primate as close to humans as the baboon cannot open its mouth widely without first swinging its head up and backward, which is in actuality placing the head in a horizontal relationship to the vertebral column.[3]

GROSS ANATOMY

A discussion of an anatomical entity, such as a functioning joint, requires consideration not only of the joint itself but also of the various attachments and encircling tissues. From the most basic viewpoint a study of the temporomandibular joint must deal separately with the embryology of the temporal bone and that of the mandible.

The anatomy of the area is described in Chapter 2. However, the basic elements of the temporomandibular joint are listed here, with comments to the degree that seems appropriate.

The bony elements are, of course, the mandibular condyle, the mandibular fossa, and the temporal bone. The muscular attachments to the temporal bone that are involved in the functioning of the joint are the masseter and temporal muscles. Although there are several other muscles that have origins on the temporal bone, they do not act directly in joint function. The muscles of mastication that have origins or insertions on the mandible are the masseter, temporal, external (lateral) pterygoid, and internal (medial) pterygoid muscles. No true joint exists without ligamenture that provides the necessary biomechanical struts and hinges. For the temporomandibular joint these ligaments are the articular capsule, the sphenomandibular, the temporomandibular, the stylomandibular, and the articular disc. In addition, there are two synovial membranes, one above and one below the articular disc.

The synovial membranes begin immediately at the edge of the articular covering. One segment runs along the bone to the limit of the joint space and then reflects back on the inner surface of the fibrous capsule with various degrees of thickness and laxity, depending on the amount of movement in that area of the joint. The disc is a special interarticular meniscus, which is interposed between the fibrocartilaginous coverings of the surfaces of the synovial membranes. It is tough but thin and is a fibrous plate with a few cartilaginous cells. It is attached all around to the fibrous capsule. The disc itself heretofore has been considered not to be covered by the synovial membrane; however, recent histological studies indicate that there is a synovial covering around the disc.[7] The disc receives fibers of the external pterygoid muscle, which attach near its anteromedial margin.

EMBRYOLOGICAL DEVELOPMENT

Despite the relatively large size of both the temporal and mandibular bones, this discussion centers around a fraction of their combined masses. According to Baume[1] the structures of the temporomandibular articulation have been found to originate from two different blastemas. They are situated at a relatively large distance from one another and grow at different rates. They are, respectively, the condylar blastema and the temporal blastema. The first evolves to contribute to the formation of the condylar cartilage, the aponeurosis of the external pterygoid muscle, the disc, and the capsular elements of the lower joint. The second develops into the articular structures of the upper level.

The condylar blastema forms at the distal end of the primordium of the mandible, or dentary. The dentary begins to ossify in the symphyseal integument at about the seventh week of fetal life at approximately the 19-mm stage of fetal development. By the time the 22-mm stage, or eighth week, is reached, a significant amount of bone has been laid down in a platelike form lateral to Meckel's cartilage. Meckel's cartilage extends from the midline to the developing chin to the developing middle ear. Remember that, phylogenetically, the developing middle ear in the primate, and especially the human, was the initial jaw joint of the vertebrates. It is here in the middle ear region that the malleus and probably the incus develop as posterior extensions of Meckel's cartilage (Fig. 1-1).

The intermediate portion of Meckel's cartilage disappears, but its sheath remains to persist in the formation of the anterior malleolar ligament and the sphenomandibular ligament.

When the embryo has reached the 24-mm stage, the pterygoid and masseter muscles have differentiated. At the superior border of the external pterygoid muscle and just mesial to the masseter muscle there is a layer of mesenchyme. It is this bulk of mesenchymal tissue which is the anlage of the articular disc. It is separated from the blastema of the zygomatic process of the temporal bone by an area with few cells that eventually develops into the superior joint cavity.[6] It should be pointed out, as a matter of interest, that at the 28-mm stage the middle ear ossicles are fully formed in true cartilage, and the malleus is continuous with Meckel's cartilage. The articular disc and external pterygoid tendons also are attached to the malleus.

The condylar cartilage becomes an evident structure by the eleventh week. It is located at the upper end of the posterior border of the developing mandible. As the condyle continues to grow, its articular surface changes shape. In the 30-mm embryo its articular surface faces directly lateral.[6] It is parallel to the articular disc as well as to the articular surface of the zygomatic process of the temporal bone. The condylar cartilage shapes the articulating surface of the condyle in a hemisphere by the 50-mm stage of embryonic development. At the same stage the articular disc has flattened, and the plane of the articular surfaces has undertaken a shift of 45 degrees. The joint cavities have not completely formed yet, and the disc and the condyle are not in contact with the temporal bone.

At the 55-mm stage the condylar head produces an osseous head, which matures into condylar cartilage by the 65-mm stage, according to Baume.[1] This condylar cartilage begins ossification at the 85-mm stage, after which it is the growth center of the mandible. It is during this period that joint cavity formation becomes evident as the loose connective tissue on either side of the

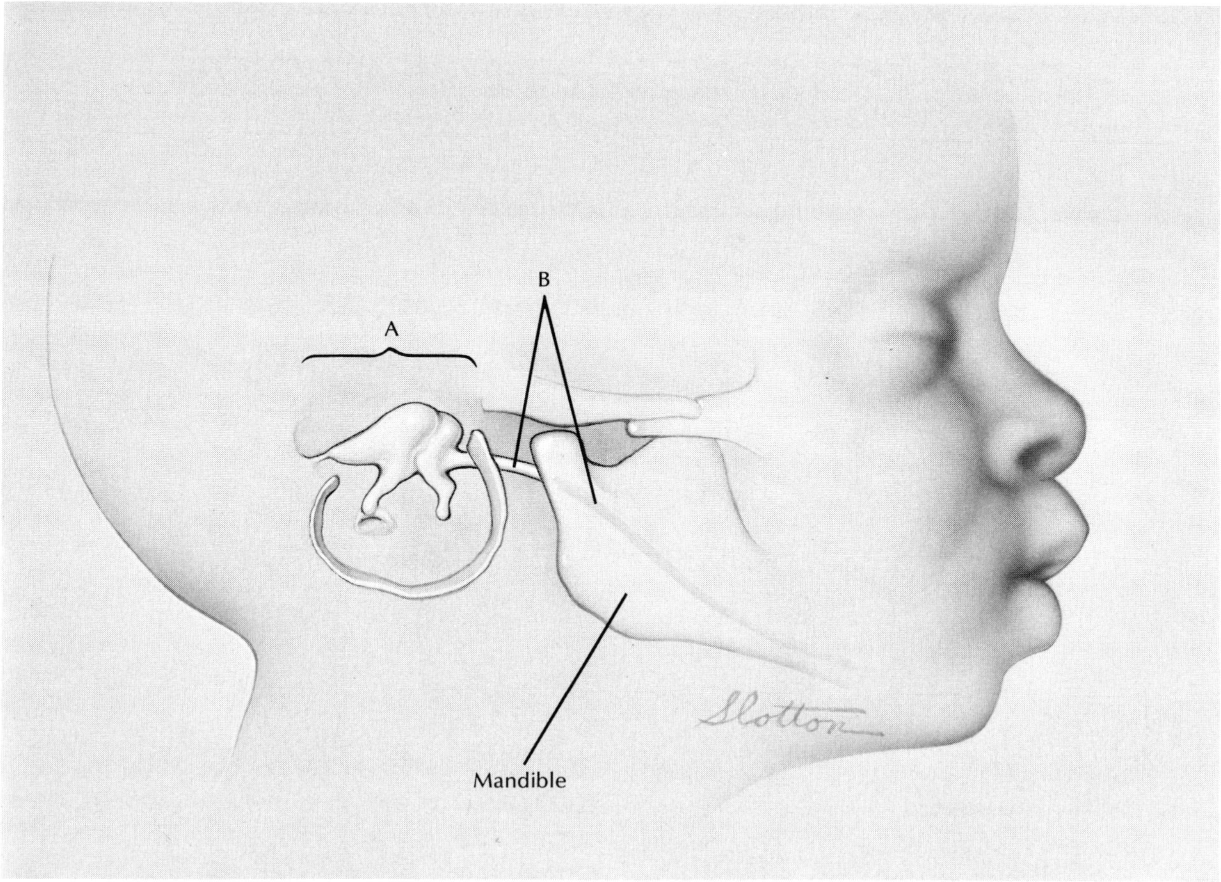

Fig. 1-1. Relationship of developing mandible to middle ear, *A*, in reference to Meckel's cartilage, *B*.

future articular disc becomes less dense. The inferior portion of the joint cavity begins to take on the appearance of a distinct cleft.

About the time the embryo has reached 13 weeks of development, the lower joint cavity is fairly well formed around the superior surface of the mandibular condyle. The upper part of the joint cavity is also becoming a distinct entity during this period. By the time the fifteenth week of fetal development has been reached, the vascular mesenchyme of the condylar cartilage can be seen breaking down. Both joint cavities are formed by this stage. Differentiation continues anteriorly to arrive at a point of full articulation at the 155-mm stage, and all elements of the joint are fully formed at the 190-mm stage. As Baume[1] points out, full differentiation of all articular elements by the fourth fetal month is in keeping with a general embryogenetic law that all vital organs are formed by this stage.

JOINT INNERVATION

Development of the innervation of the joint has been described by Kitamura.[5] The joint is innervated by branches of the auriculotemporal nerve, masseter nerve, and the posterior deep temporal nerve, which are all branches of the mandibular portion of the trigeminal nerve. From the fourth fetal month nerve fibers may be observed in the articular capsule. They appear to reach the articular disc at about the fifth month. At the sixth month the widest distribution over the condyle and within the disc may be seen. At this point in fetal development there begins a diminution in the number and distribution of the nerve fibers, with localization occurring at the joint margin. Most of the nerve endings of the fetal temporomandibular joint are free nerve endings, with a few encapsulated ones around the joint. The nerve fibers in the capsule innervate the synovial membrane of the joint as well.

In the evolution of the temporomandibular joint, from vertebrates through primates, DuBrul[2] points out that the key relationship between jaw and ear dysfunctions lies in the embryological development of the neural patterns of the temporomandibular joint. He has demonstrated that the nerve to the internal pterygoid muscle also sends a branch to the tensor tympani muscle, which moves the malleus. The malleus develops from the proximal end of Meckel's cartilage, and it is

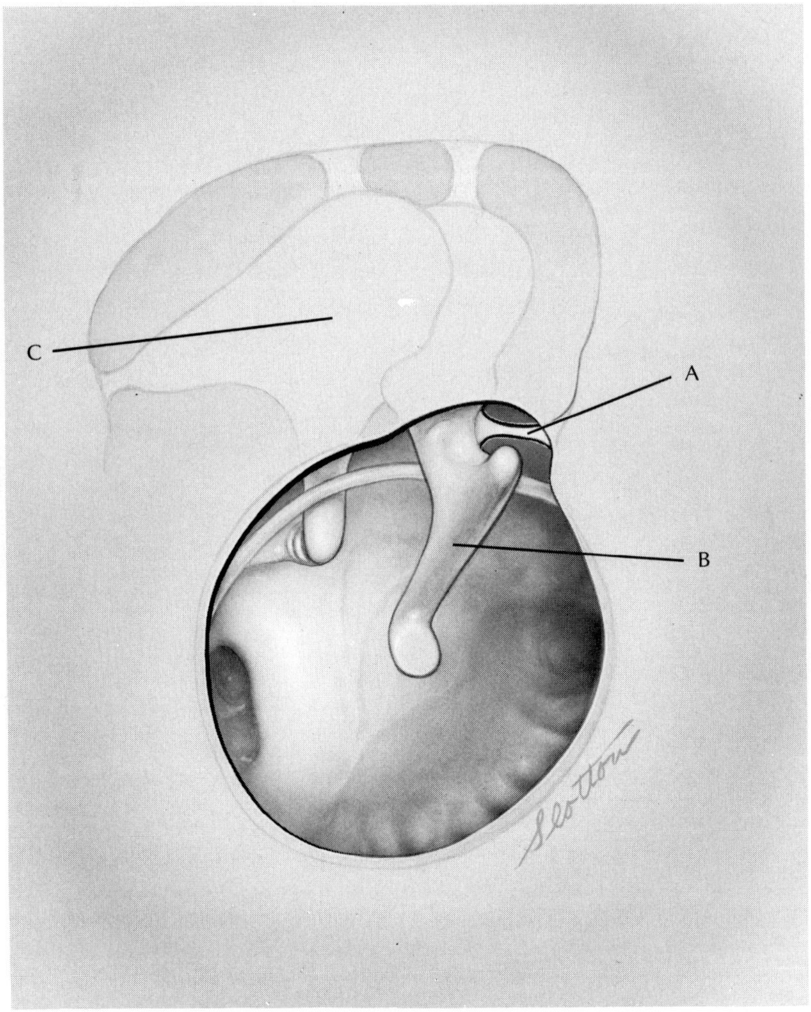

Fig. 1-2. Structures of middle ear that develop from Meckel's cartilage: anterior malleolar ligament, *A*, malleus, *B*, and incus, *C*.

worthwhile to reiterate that the malleus develops from the articular bone of the old jaw joint of reptiles. The nerve of Meckel's cartilage and of the first branchial arch is the trigeminal nerve. It is the belief of many, including DuBrul, that the disturbances in neuromuscular-joint coordination emanate from the central nervous system. He[3] states unequivocally that "Herein lies the key to the relationship between jaw and ear dysfunctions sometimes plaguing modern man along with the deterioration of other parts of the jaw and dental apparatus."

No direct conclusions are made from this brief discussion of temporomandibular joint embryology; however, there are certain important and diagnostically salient facts that should be underscored. The nerve of the human dentition is also the innervating source of the temporomandibular joint, including those muscles which surround it and attach on it. Furthermore, Meckel's cartilage is the forerunner of the mandible, as it is enveloped by membrane bone, and of the middle ear structures—the malleus, the anterior malleolar ligament, and possibly the incus (Fig. 1-2).

CONCLUSION

This brief discourse on the evolution and embryology of the temporomandibular joint is primarily academic; however, some practical, clinical notions inevitably arise. Most noteworthy, perhaps, is the fact that the present middle ear and its important structures, which are significant to the sensory function of hearing, are phylogenetic elements of the primitive jaw joint. Also, a neurological connection between these middle ear structures and the muscles of mastication, which are intimately involved with the temporomandibular joint, is well documented.

Present theories that attempt to explain the multitudinous and extremely disturbing symptoms of patients who have temporomandibular joint function problems are dealt with in other chapters. Those interested in an in-depth discussion of the evolution of the temporomandibular joint from the Agnatha through the primates should refer to the monumental and extremely valuable works by E. Lloyd DuBrul.

REFERENCES

1. Baume, L.J.: Embryogenesis of the human temporomandibular joint, Science **138**:904, 1962.
2. DuBrul, E.L.: Embryological development of the temporomandibular joint. In Sarnat, B.G.: The temporomandibular joint, ed. 2, Springfield, Ill., 1964, Charles C Thomas, Publisher.
3. DuBrul, E.L.: Evolution of the temporomandibular joint. In Sarnat, B.G.: The temporomandibular joint, ed. 2, Springfield, Ill., 1964, Charles C Thomas, Publisher.
4. Haines, R.W.: Eudiarthroidal joints in fishes, J. Anat. (London) **77**:12, 1942.
5. Kitamura, H.: Development of temporomandibular joint innervation, Bull. Tokyo Med. Dent. Univ. **21**:83, 1974.
6. Levy, B.M.: Embryological development of the temporomandibular joint. In Sarnat, B.G.: The temporomandibular joint, ed. 2, Springfield, Ill., 1964, Charles C Thomas, Publisher.
7. Morgan, D.H.: Personal communication, 1977.

2 Anatomy and neuroanatomy

CARL B. ERMSHAR, Jr., M.D.

The normal temporomandibular joint is a finely balanced structure with a high degree of anatomical precision. Functional integrity is related to the harmony of the joint movements themselves as well as to the interaction of surrounding structures.

An understanding of functionally pathological conditions requires a knowledge of the basic anatomical and functional relationships of normal temporomandibular joints.

THE JOINT PROPER

The temporomandibular joint is located between the mandibular fossa (glenoid fossa), in the inferior surface of the temporal bone, and the condylar process of the mandibular bone. The external ear canal is just posterior to the joint. The glenoid fossa is concave and generally oval. The articular eminence is anterior, and the posterior glenoid process of the temporal bone is posterior (Fig. 2-1). There is no fibrocartilage in the

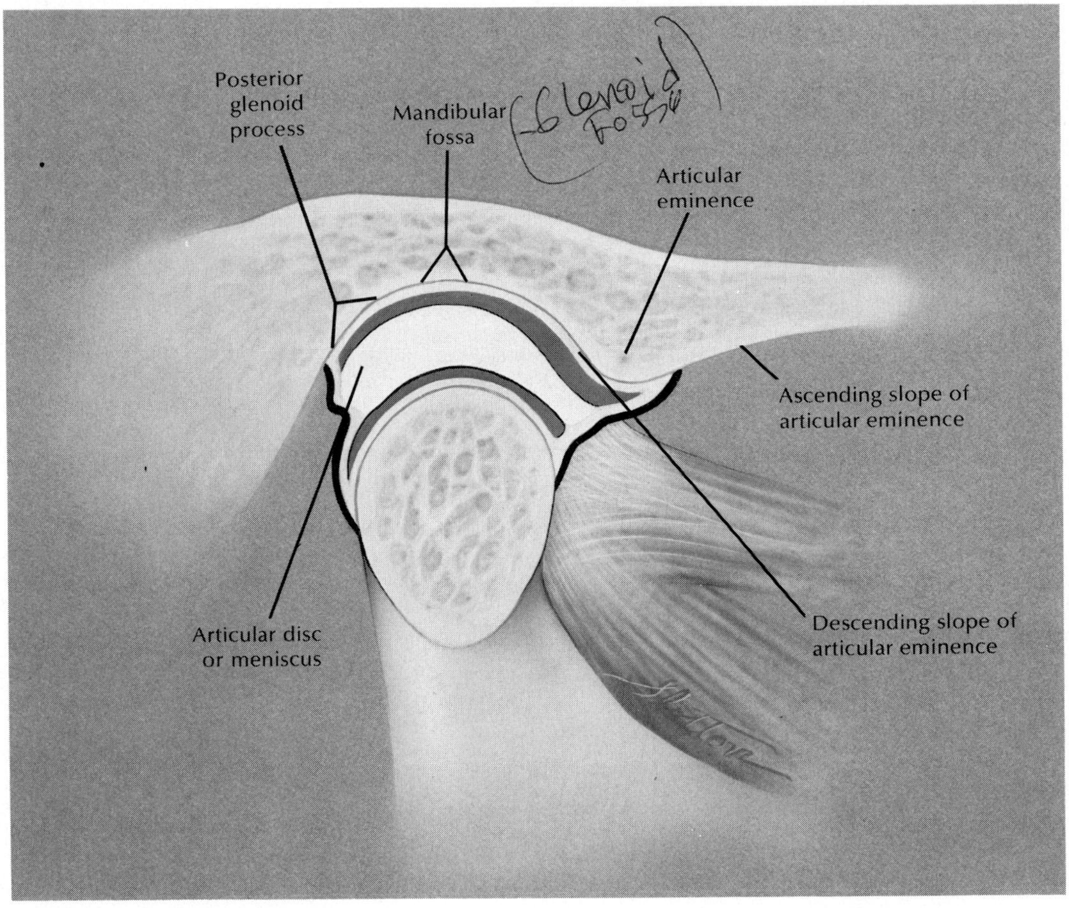

Fig. 2-1. Schematic representation of structures of temporomandibular joint, closed position.

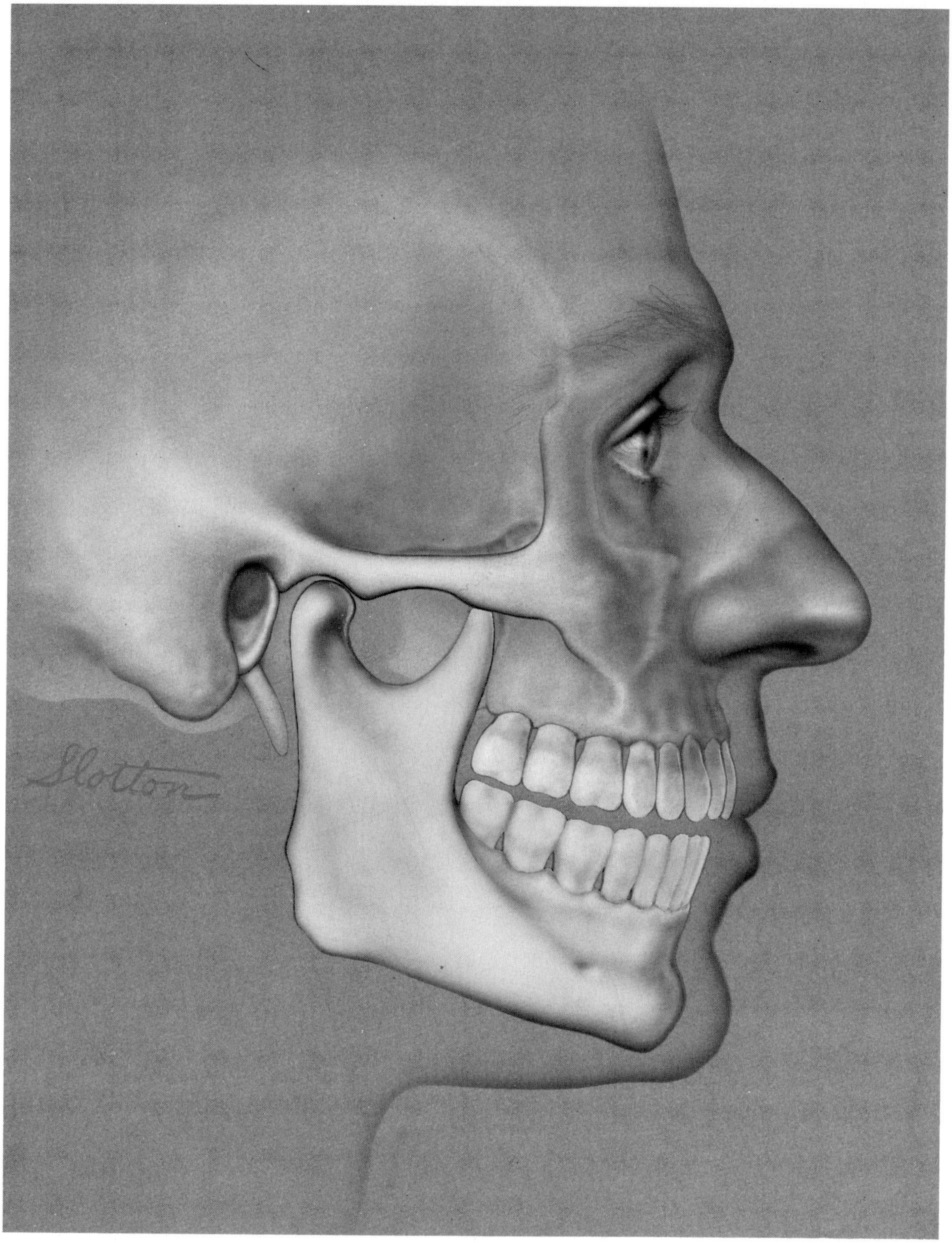

Fig. 2-1, cont'd. For legend see opposite page.

posterior portion of the glenoid fossa. The remainder of the glenoid fossa, condylar head, and articular eminence is covered by fibrocartilage. The mandibular condyle is about 15 to 20 mm long and 8 to 10 mm thick. The long axis is at right angles to the plane of the mandibular ramus.

The articulation of the axial skeleton includes the temporomandibular joints as well as the intervertebral joints. The temporomandibular joint differs from other joints of the body in several ways. A functionally unique feature is the unusual combination of a gliding movement and a ginglymus, or hinge, movement of the joint. The temporomandibular joints cannot act independently; they move simultaneously when they are functionally intact. Another difference is that the articular surfaces are covered by avascular fibrous tissue rather than the usual hyaline cartilage.

LIGAMENTOUS STRUCTURES

The ligamentous structures in and around the temporomandibular joint include (1) the articular disc (articular meniscus, interarticular fibrocartilage), (2) the synovial membranes, (3) the articular capsule (capsular ligament), (4) the temporomandibular ligament (lateral ligament), (5) the sphenomandibular ligament (internal ligament), and (6) the stylomandibular ligament.

The *articular disc* lies between the condyle of the mandible and the mandibular fossa (Figs. 2-1 and 2-2). It is concavoconvex on its superior surface to accommodate the form of the mandibular fossa and articular tubercle (articular eminence). The inferior surface is concave over the condyle. The outer edges are connected with the articular capsule ligament. The disc divides the joint into two cavities.

The *synovial membranes* line the two cavities above and below the articular disc (Figs. 2-1 and 2-2). The upper cavity is the larger of the two.

The *articular capsule* is attached to the circumference of the mandibular fossa and extends downward to attach to the neck of the condyle of the mandible (Figs. 2-3 and 2-4). It consists of a thin, loose envelope.

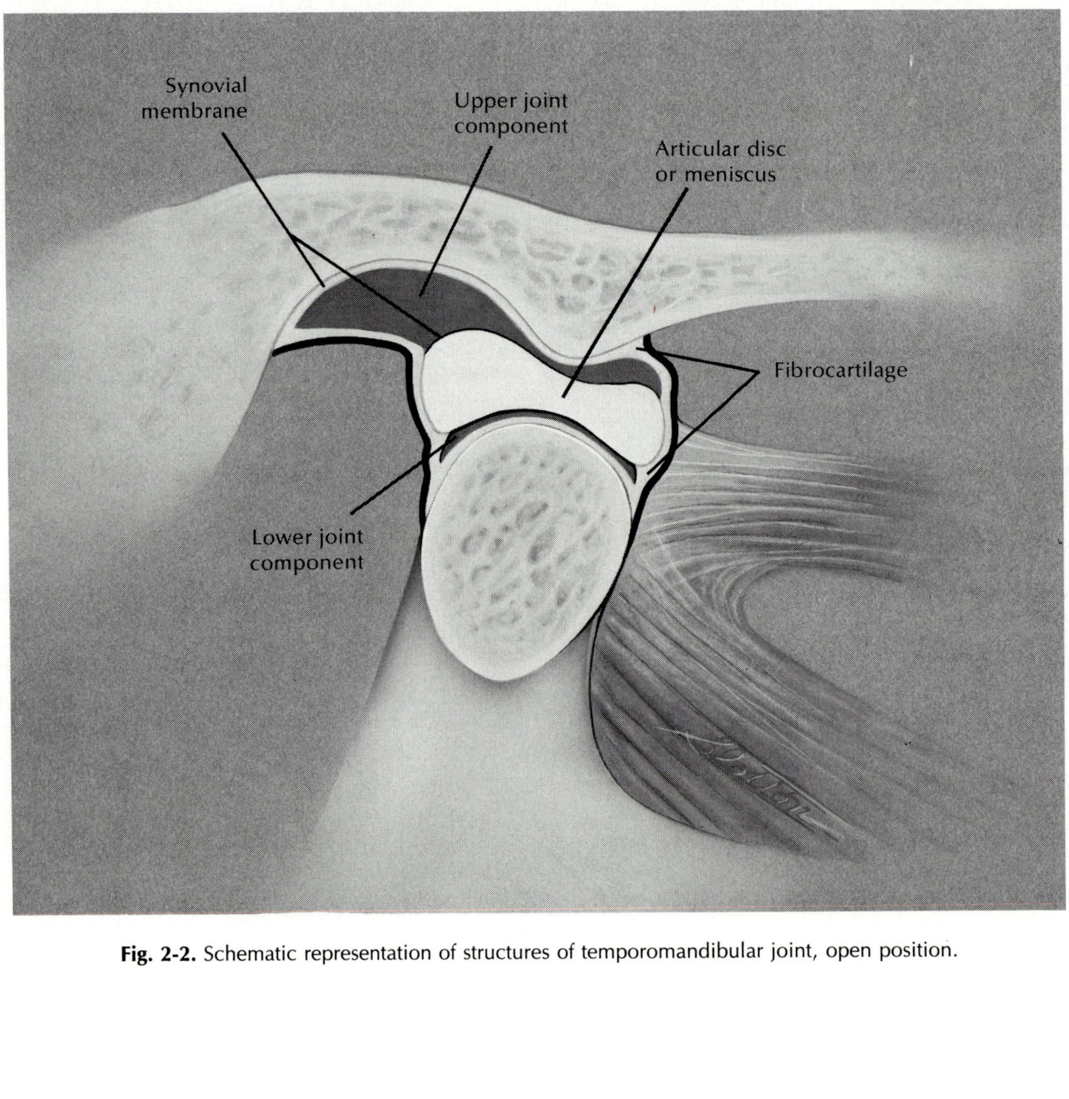

Fig. 2-2. Schematic representation of structures of temporomandibular joint, open position.

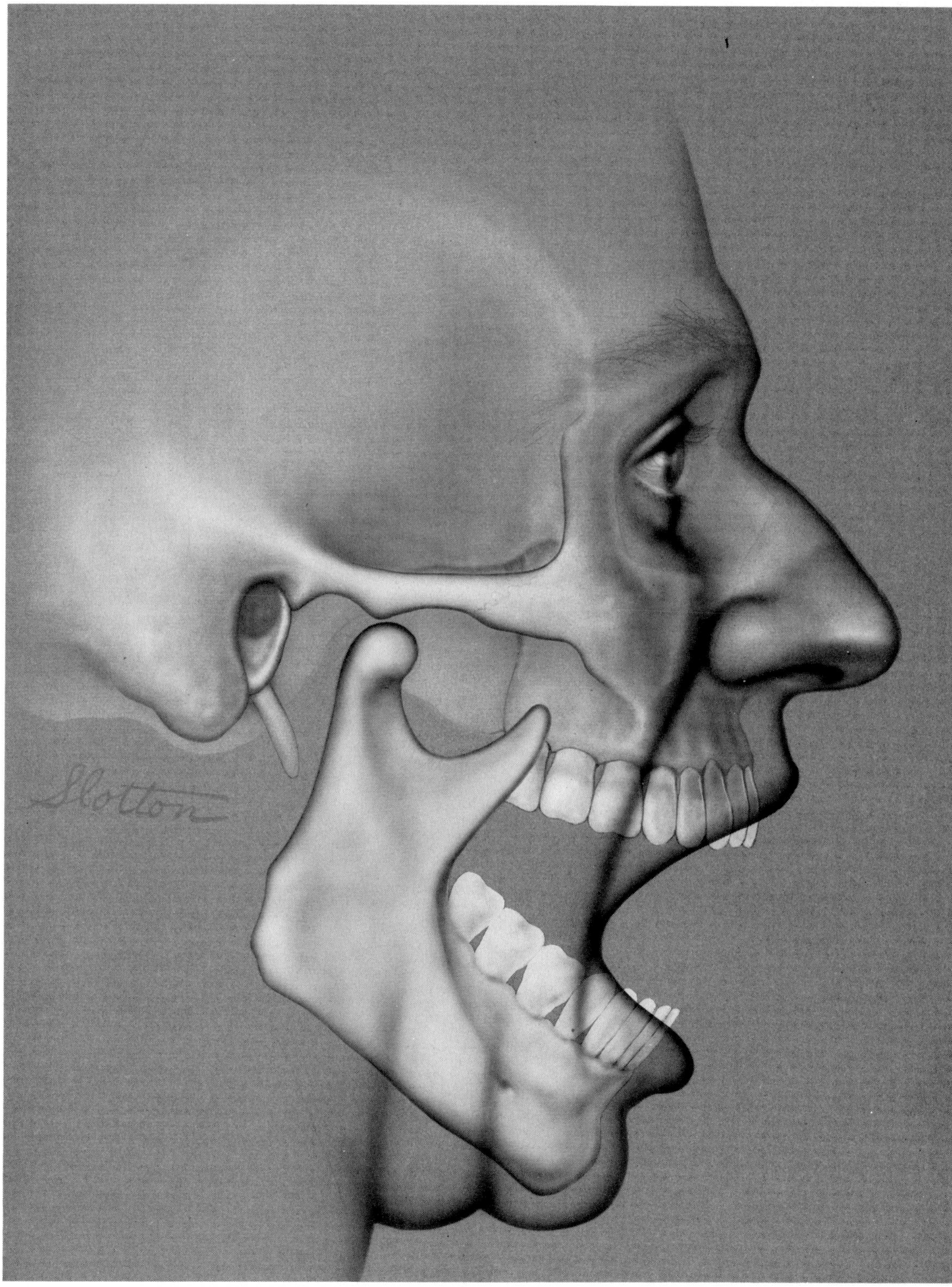

Fig. 2-2, cont'd. For legend see opposite page.

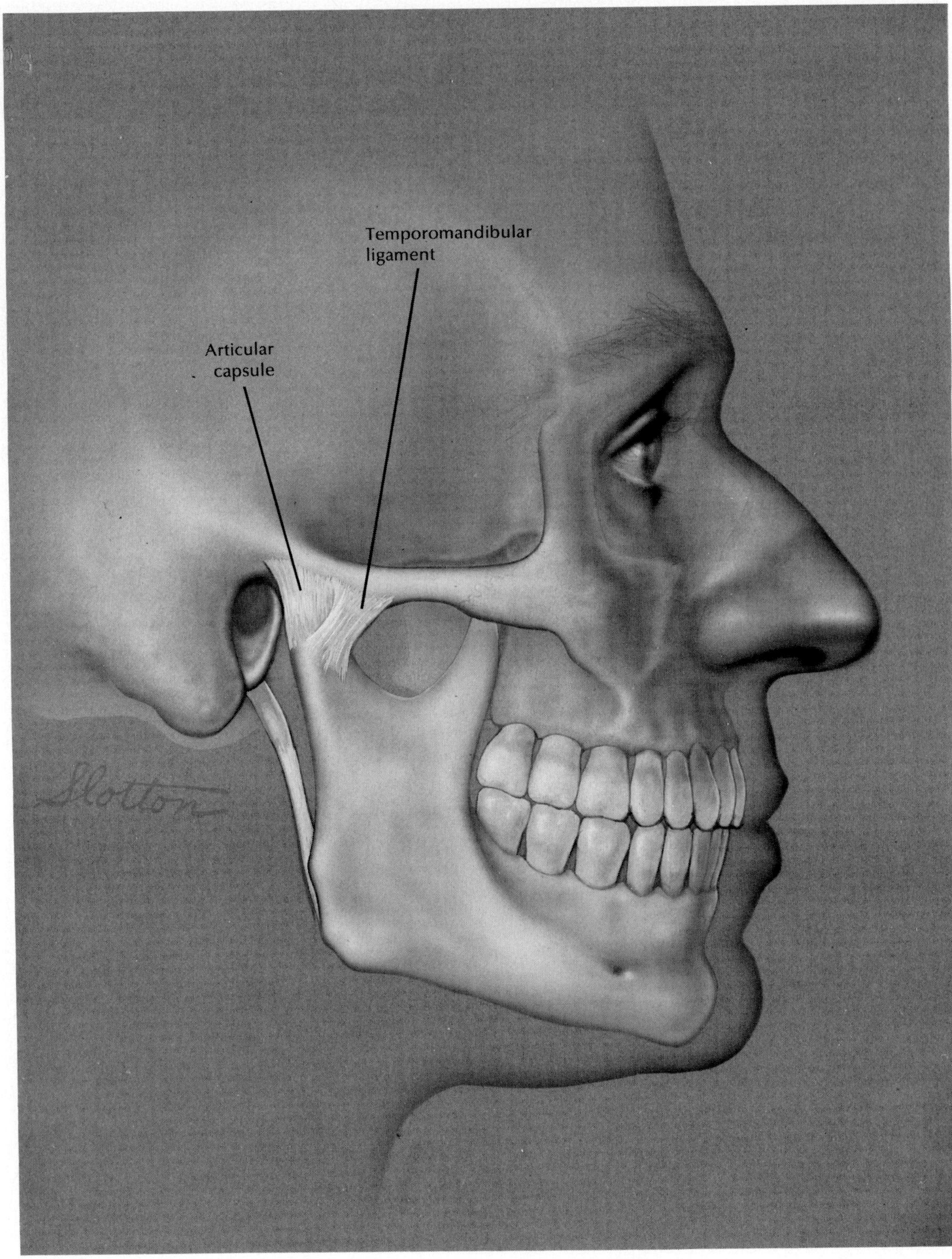

Fig. 2-3. Temporomandibular ligaments and capsule.

The *temporomandibular ligament* is attached in a superior position from the lateral surface of the zygomatic arch and articular eminence to the lateral surface and posterior border of the neck of the mandible in the inferior position. This ligament strengthens the joint and prevents extensive forward and backward lateral movement (Fig. 2-3).

The *sphenomandibular ligament* is a flat, thin band from the spine of the sphenoid to the lingula of the mandible at the mandibular foramen (Fig. 2-4). The external pterygoid muscle is lateral to this ligament. The maxillary vessels pass inferiorly between the neck of the mandible and lateral to the sphenomandibular ligament. The internal pterygoid muscle is associated with its medial surface.

The *stylomandibular ligament* is considered an accessory ligament and passes from the styloid process to the angle and posterior portion of the ramus of the mandible. This ligament separates the masseter muscle and the internal pterygoid muscle (Fig. 2-4).

The *mandibular-malleolar ligament* is not described in the anatomy textbooks but is demonstrated by Pinto[6] and others. This ligament of fibroelastic tissue with ligamentous qualities was found connecting the neck and anterior process of the malleus to the medioposterosuperior partof the capsule, the interarticular disc, and

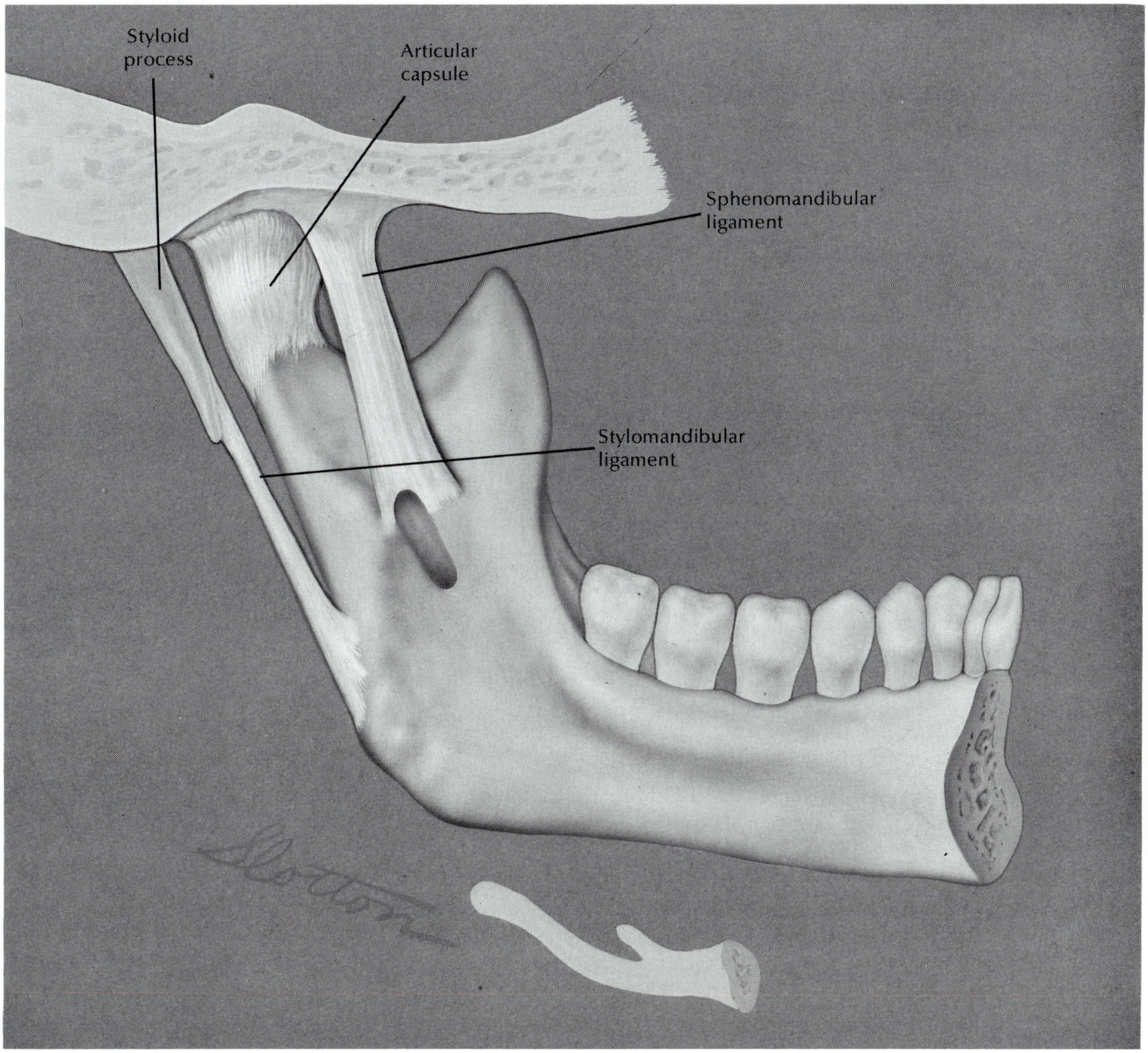

Fig. 2-4. Stylomandibular and sphenomandibular ligaments.

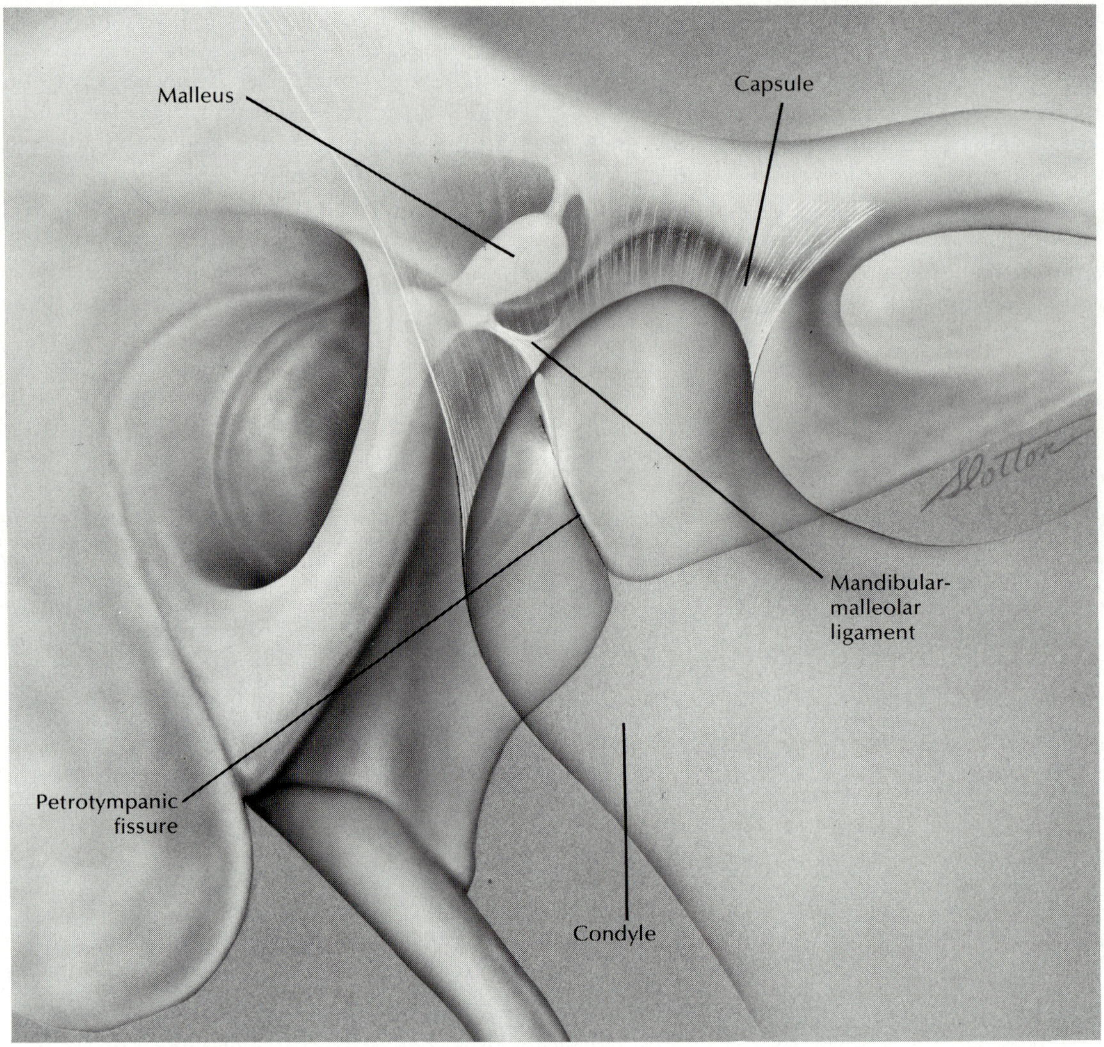

Fib. 2-5. Mandibular-malleolar ligament. (Modified from Pinto, O.: J. Prosthet. Dent. **12:**95, 1962.)

the sphenomandibular ligament. Other studies[3] have shown the embryological stage of this tiny ligament in common origin with the malleus and incus. This tiny anatomical interassociation of the joint apparatus and middle ear may well explain many of the middle ear complaints described by Costen[2] and others in the presence of temporomandibular dysfunction (Fig. 2-5).

MANDIBULAR MUSCULATURE

Primary muscles of mastication

The primary muscles of mastication are (1) the temporal, (2) the masseter, (3) the medial, or internal, pterygoid, and (4) the lateral, or external, pterygoid.

The *temporal* muscle (Figs. 2-6, 2-9, and 2-10) arises from the whole of the temporal fossa and deep surface of the temporal fascia. The broad, radiating muscle fibers converge as they descend, becoming tendinous, passing deeply to the zygomatic arch, and inserting into the medial surface, apex, and anterior border of the coronoid process of the mandible.

Action: Closes the jaws; the posterior portion retracts the mandible

Nerves: Anterior and posterior deep temporal nerves from the mandibular division of the trigeminal nerve

The *masseter* muscle (Figs. 2-7 and 2-10) is a thick, quadrilateral muscle composed of two bellies—the deep and the superficial. The superficial portion arises from the lower border of the zygomatic arch and the zygomatic process of the maxilla. Its fibers pass inferiorly and posteriorly to be inserted into the angle and inferior half of the lateral surface of the ramus of the mandible. The smaller, deep portion arises from the posterior third of the inferior border and medial surface

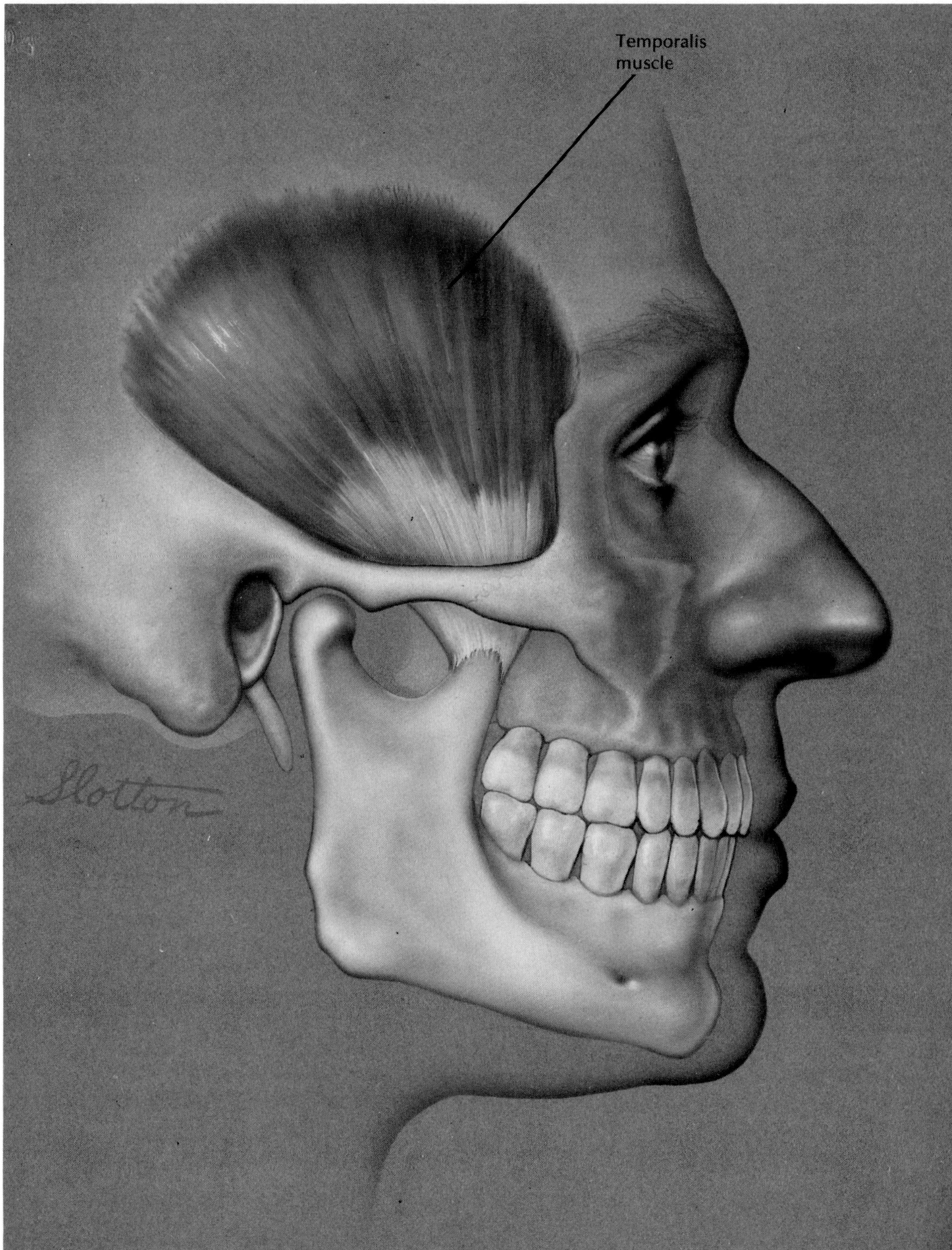

Fig. 2-6. Temporalis muscle.

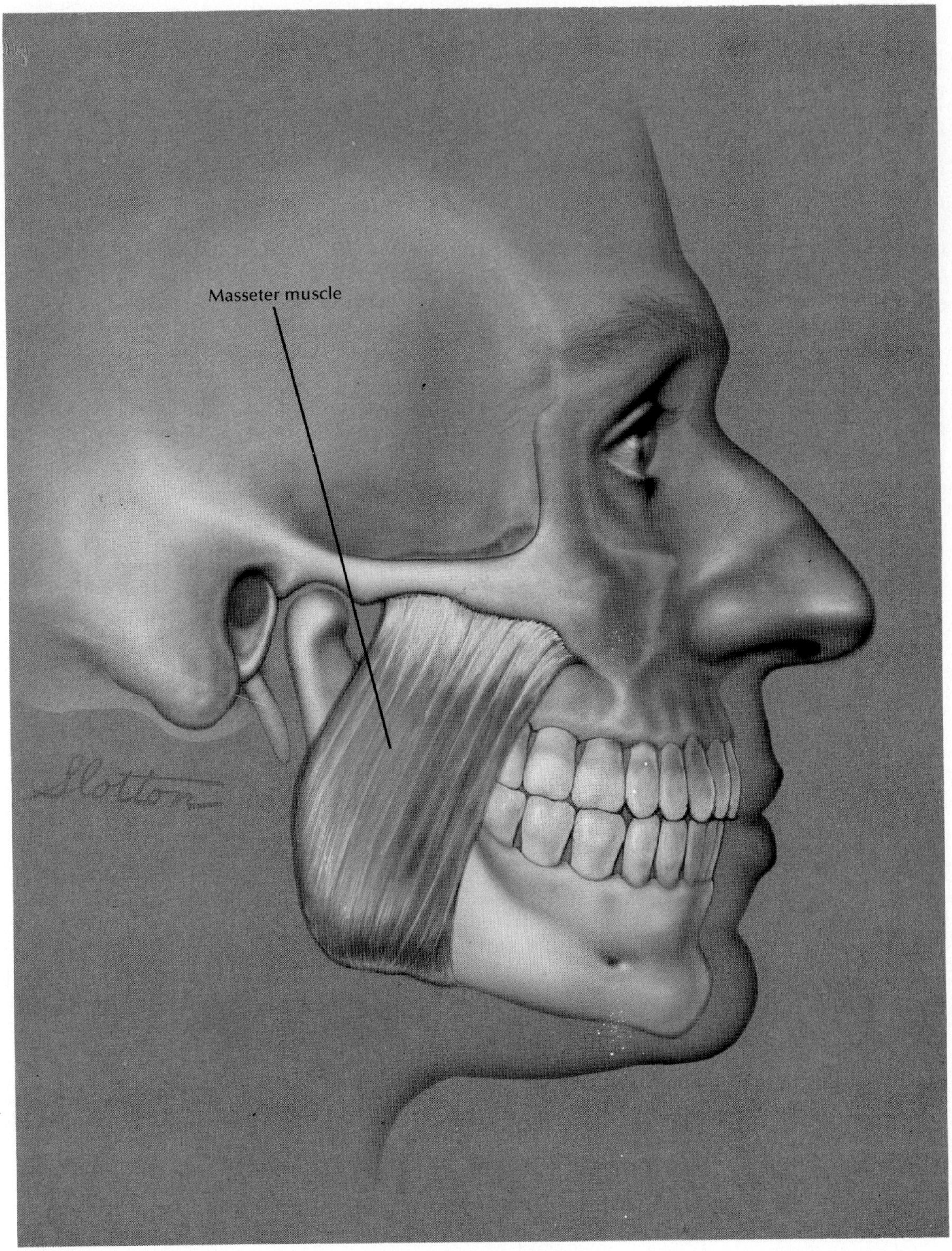

Fig. 2-7. Masseter muscle.

of the zygomatic arch and passes anteriorly and inferiorly to be inserted onto the lateral surface of the coronoid process and superior half of the ramus.

Action: Closes the jaws
Nerves: Masseteric nerve from the mandibular division of trigeminal nerve

The *internal (medial) pterygoid* muscle is a thick, quadrilateral muscle (Figs. 2-8 and 2-9). It arises from the medial surface of the lateral pterygoid plate and the pyramidal process of the palatine bone. A small belly arises from the lateral surfaces of the pyramidal process of the palatine and tuberosity of the maxilla. The fibers pass laterally, posteriorly, and inferiorly and insert into the inferior and posterior part of the medial surface of the ramus and angle of the mandible. The maxillary vessels, the inferior alveolar vessels and nerves, and the lingual nerve pass between the mandible and internal pterygoid muscle along the superior portion.

Action: Closes jaws
Nerves: Internal pterygoid nerve from the mandibular division of the trigeminal nerve

The *external (lateral) pterygoid* muscle is a thick, short, conical muscle extending horizontally between the infratemporal fossa and the condyle of the mandible. There are two bellies (Figs. 2-8 and 2-9). The upper head arises from the inferior part of the lateral surface of the great wing of the sphenoid and from the infratemporal crest. The lower head arises from the lateral surface of the lateral pterygoid plate. The fibers pass horizontally and insert into a depression on the anterior portion of the neck of the condyle and into the anterior margin of the articular disc.

Action: Opens the jaws; protrudes the mandible, moves the mandible from side to side
Nerves: External pterygoid nerve from the mandibular division of the trigeminal nerve

Accessory muscles of mastication

The accessory muscles of mastication include the following:

1. Suprahyoid group
    a. Digastric muscle (anterior and posterior belly)
    b. Mylohyoid muscle
    c. Geniohyoid muscle
    d. Stylohyoid muscle
2. Infrahyoid group
3. Platysma

The *digastric* muscle has two bellies (Figs. 2-9 and 2-11). The anterior belly arises from the digastric fossa of the minor side of the lower border of the mandible close to the symphysis. The posterior belly arises from the mastoid notch of the temporal bone. Both bellies descend toward the hyoid bone and are united by an intermediate tendon, which is connected to the hyoid bone by a loop of fibrous tissue.

Action: Aids in opening the jaw; elevates the hyoid bone
Nerves: Posterior belly supplied by the facial nerve (VII); anterior belly supplied by the mylohyoid branch of the interior alveolar nerve (V)

The *mylohyoid* muscle (Figs. 2-9 and 2-12) arises from the whole length of the mylohyoid line of the mandible from the symphysis to the last molar tooth. The fibers pass downward, and some meet in the median raphe; some attach directly on the hyoid bone. It makes up the floor of the mouth.

Action: Depresses the mandible when the hyoid is fixed and elevates the hyoid bone when the mandible is fixed
Nerves: Mylohyoid branch of the inferior alveolar nerve (V)

The *geniohyoid* muscle is a narrow muscle that lies adjacent to the midline and agove the mylohyoid muscle (Figs. 2-9 and 2-12). It arises from the genial tubercle of the symphysis of the mandible and inserts on the anterior surface of the hyoid bone.

Action: Depresses mandible when hyoid bone is fixed; elevates hyoid bone and tongue
Nerves: Hypoglossal nerve

The *stylohyoid* muscle (Fig. 2-11) arises from the syloid process of the temporal bone and inserts on the body of the hyoid bone. It is nearly parallel to the posterior belly of the digastric muscle.

Action: Draws the hyoid bone upward and backward
Nerves: Branch of the facial nerve (VII)

The *infrahyoid group* of muscles (Fig. 2-11) includes the stenohyoid, thyrohyoid, and omohyoid. These muscles act together to steady or depress the hyoid bone and therefore allow the suprahoid group to act on the mandible.

The *platysma* muscle is a large, thin muscle arising from the upper pectoral and deltoid regions. These fibers pass upward, covering the neck. The anterior fibers connect with the muscles around the lower lip. The posterior fibers insert into the mandible and skin of the lower part of the face.

Action: Depresses the lower jaw and lip
Nerves: Cervical branches of the facial nerve (VII)

Muscle group actions

Jaw closing. The mandibular elevators (closing the jaw) include the coordinated function of the masseter, temporal, and medial pterygoid muscles (Fig. 2-13). The smooth function of these muscles is essential for proper occlusion of the teeth.

Text continued on p. 24.

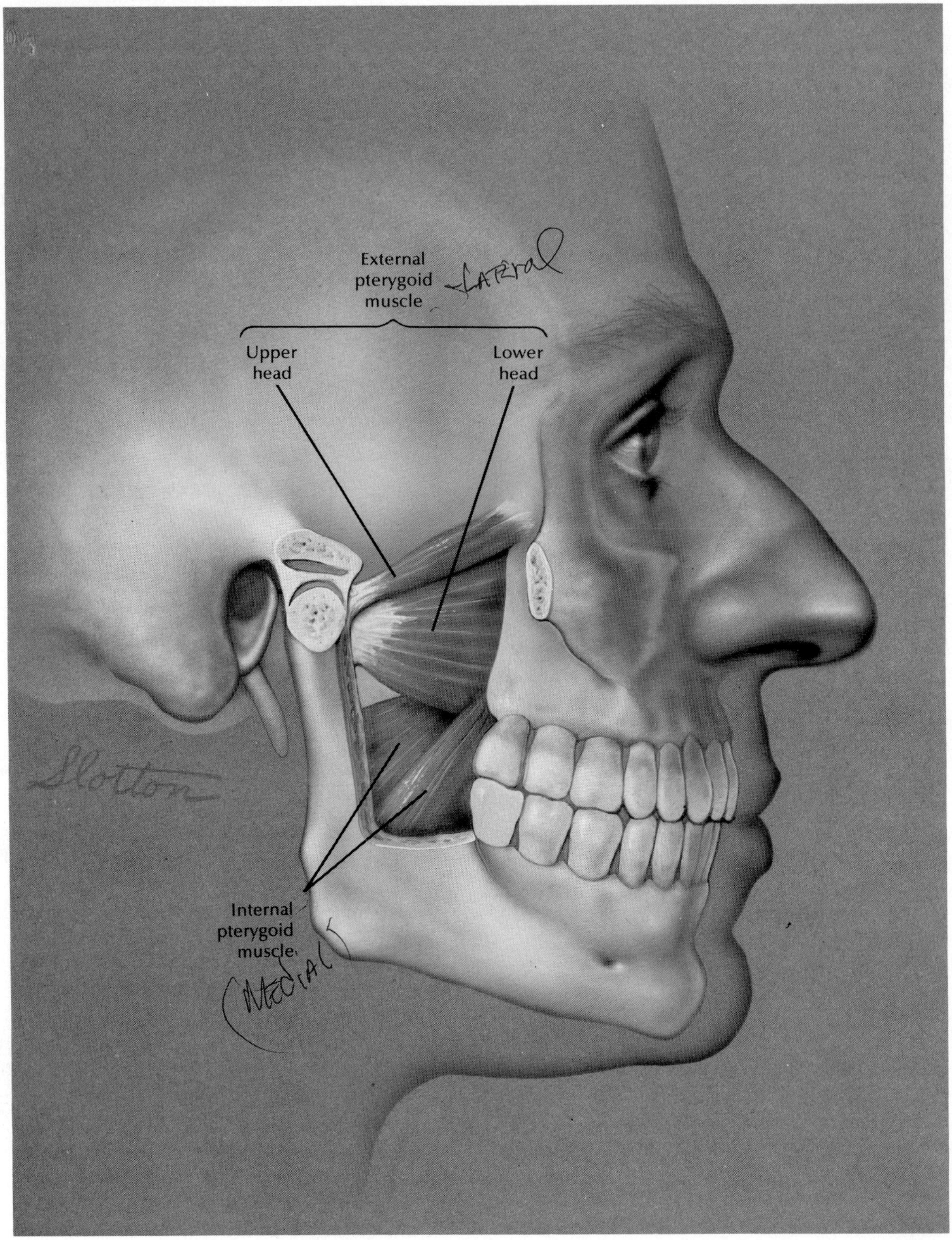

Fig. 2-8. Internal and external pterygoid muscles.

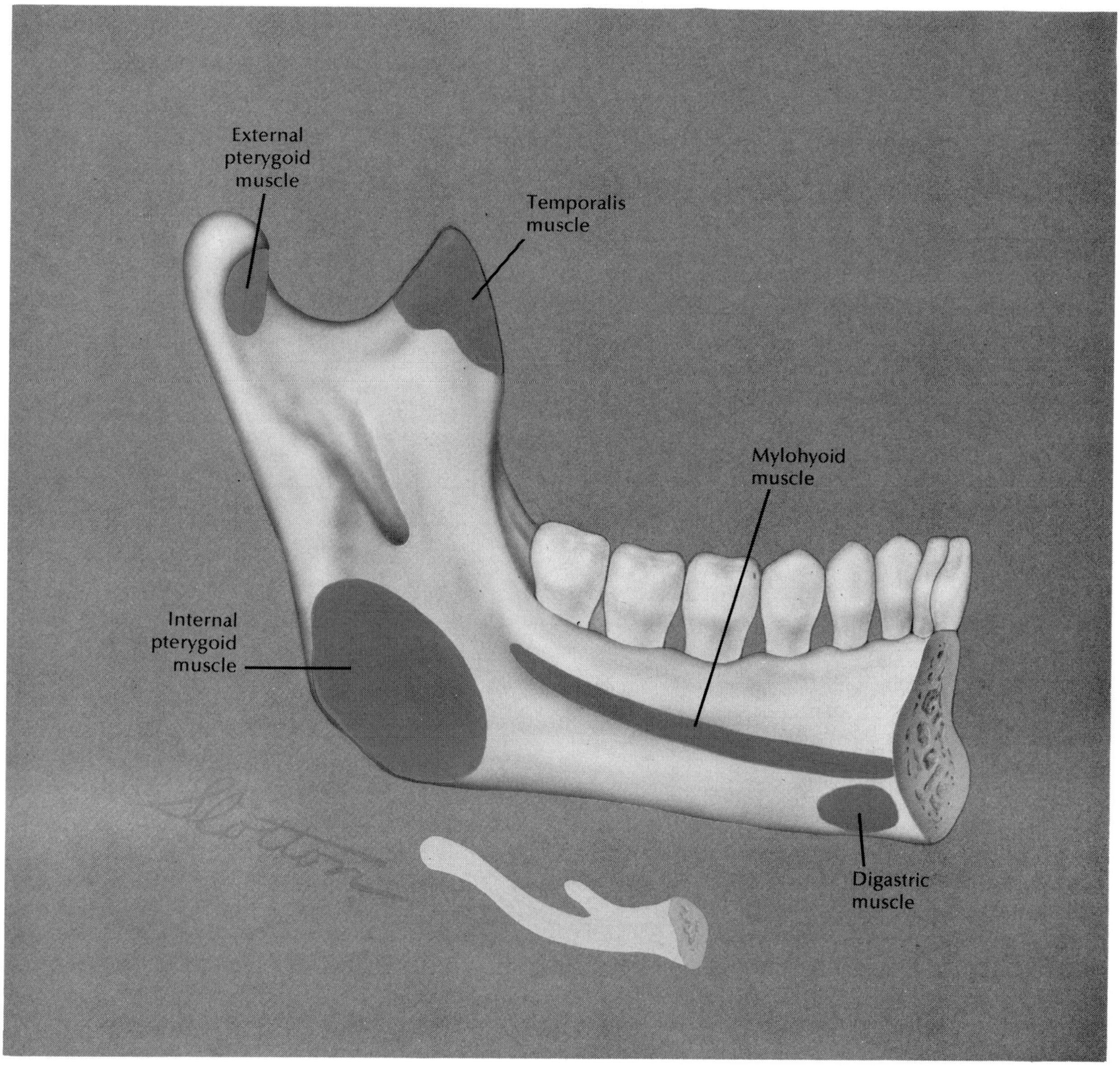

Fig. 2-9. Attachments of mandibular muscles, medial aspect.

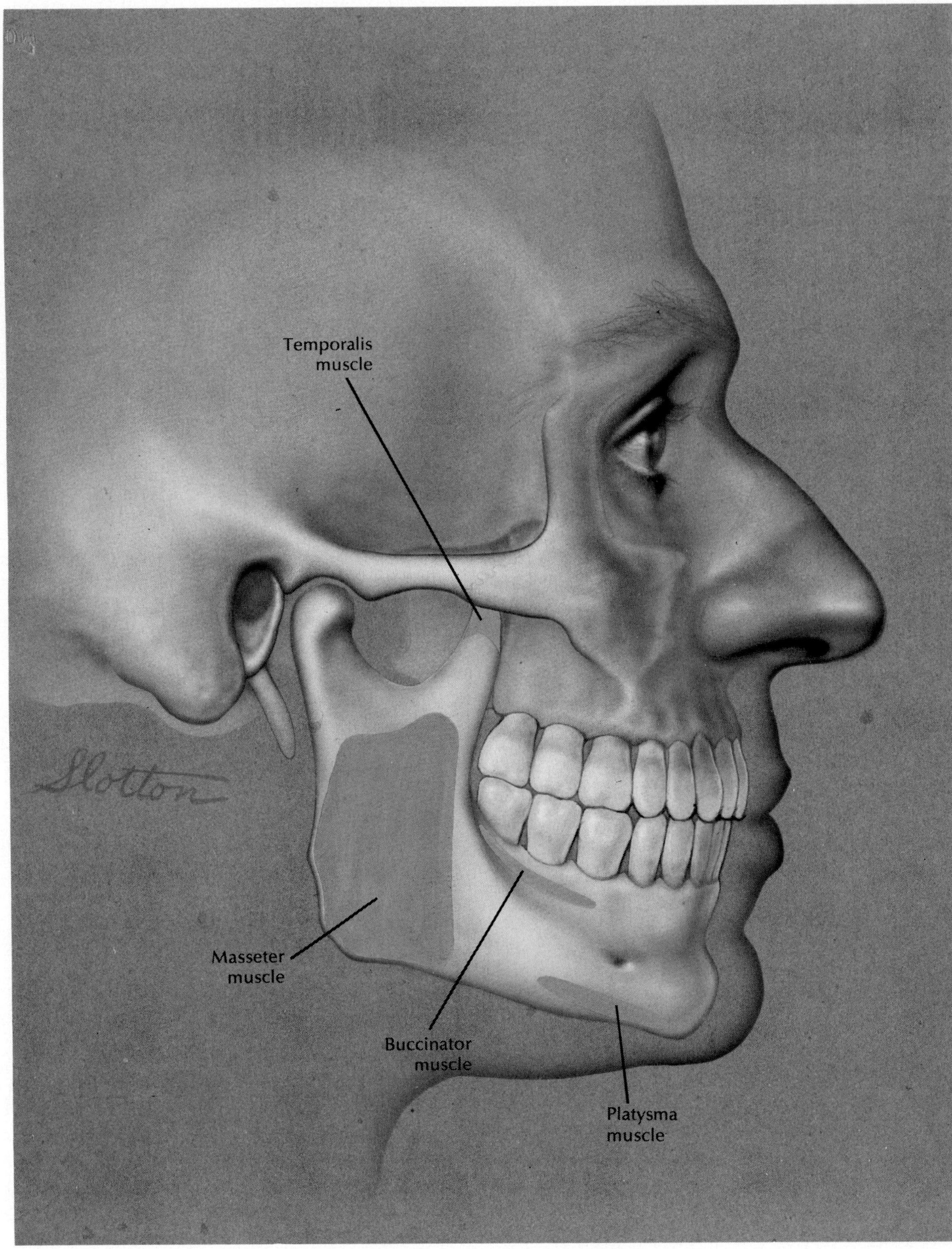

Fig. 2-10. Attachments of mandibular muscles, lateral aspect.

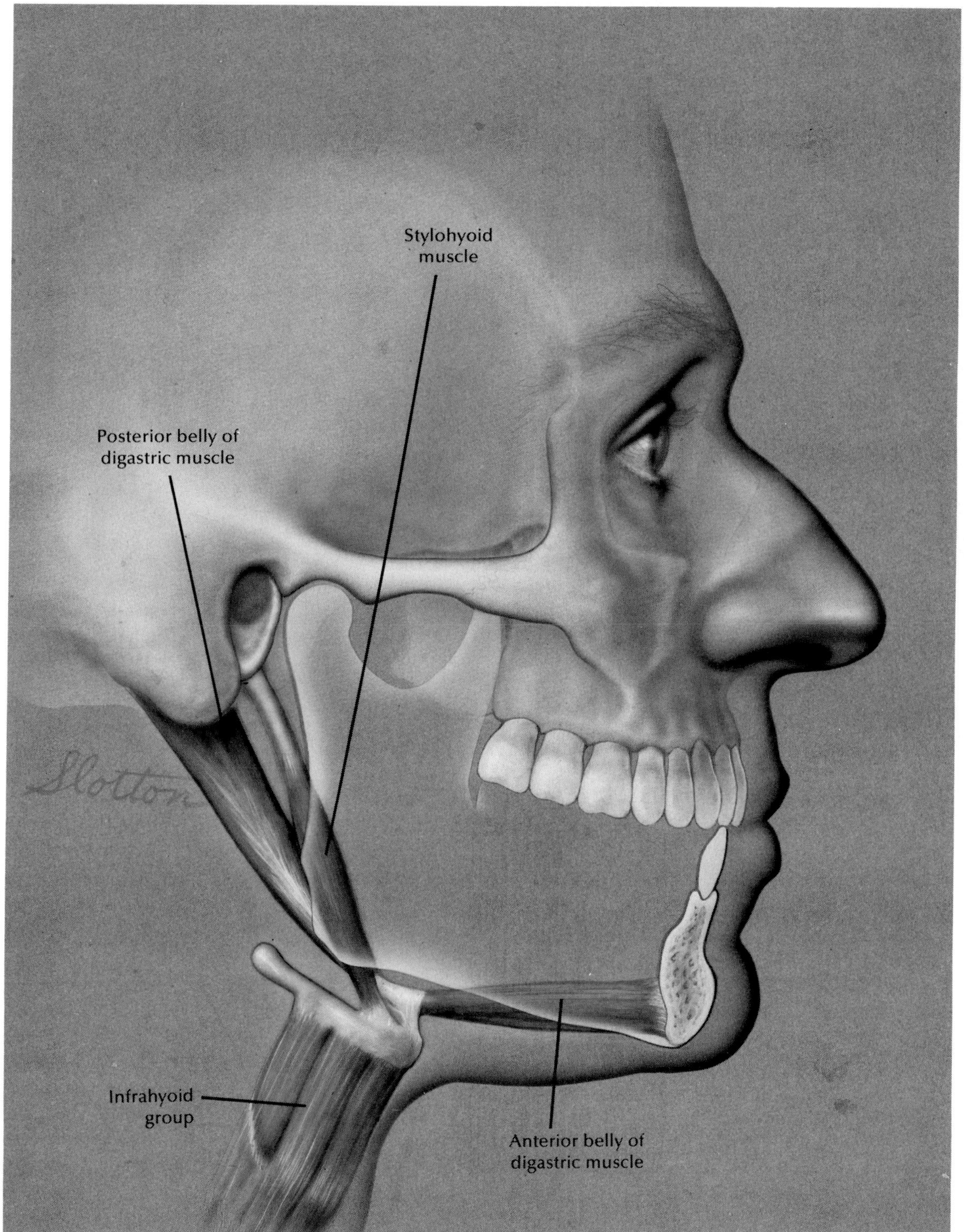

Fig. 2-11. Digastric muscle.

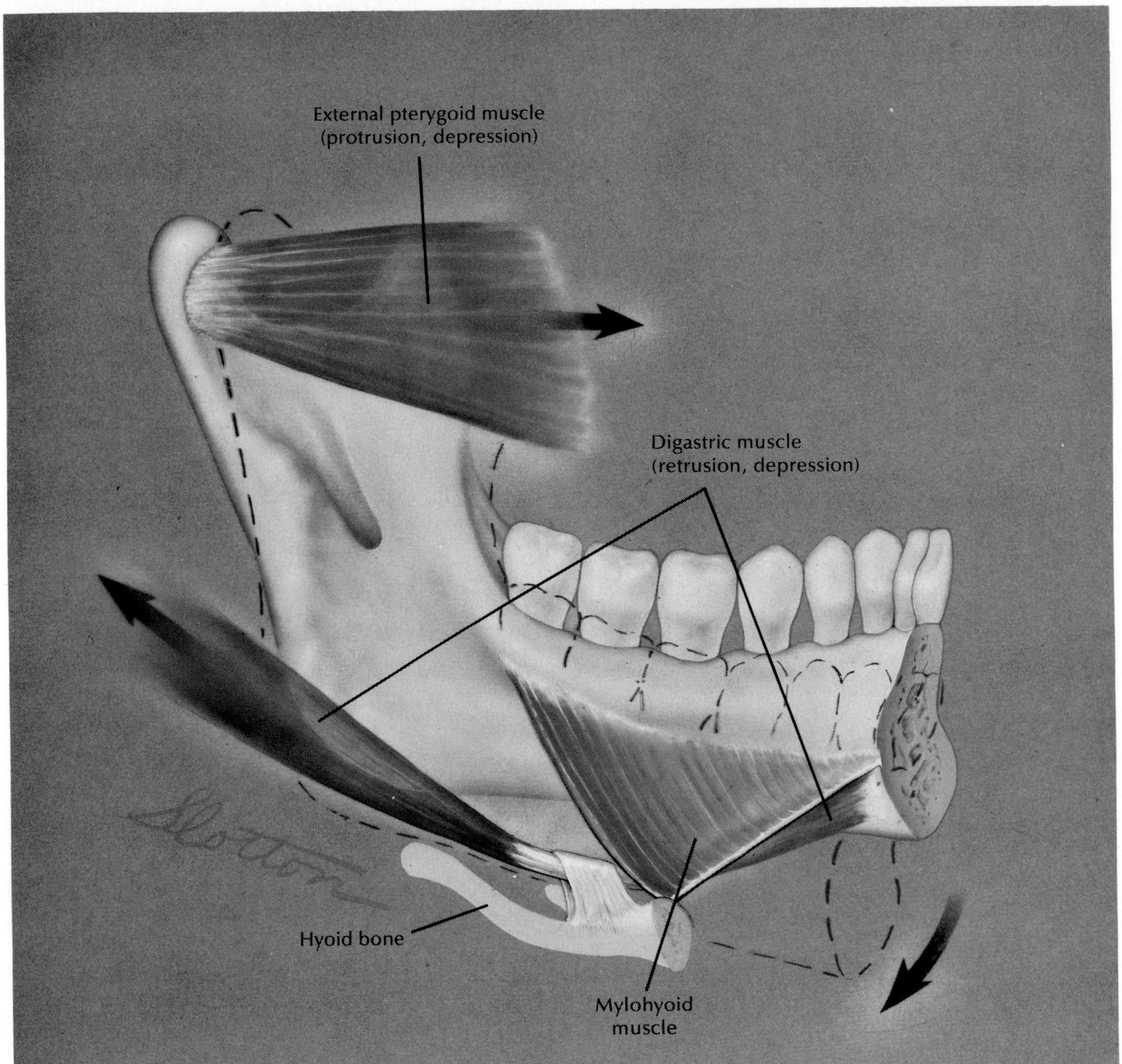

Fig. 2-12. Muscle group action.

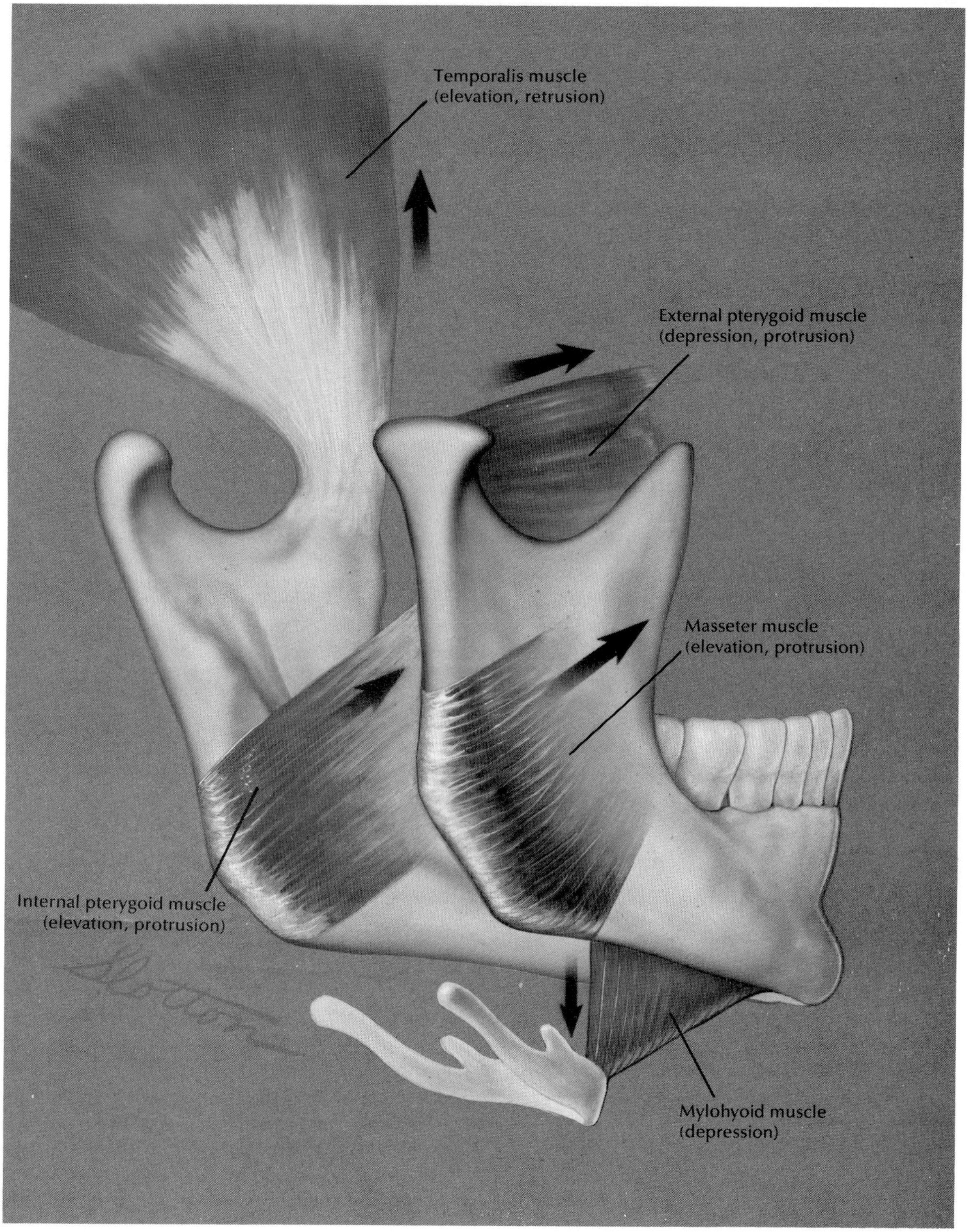

Fig. 2-13. Muscle group action.

Jaw opening. The mandibular depressors include the activity of the external pterygoid and the suprahyoid muscles. The inferior head of the external pterygoid is the main muscle used in opening the mouth. The superior head of the external pterygoid pulls the articular disc forward, creating the gliding joint activity. The digastric muscle also plays a major role in opening the mouth (Figs. 2-12 and 2-13).

The digastric, mylohyoid, geniohyoid, and stylohyoid muscles also act in mandibular movement by initiating and assisting opening of the jaw. These belong to the suprahyoid group of muscles. The infrahyoid muscles participate by fixing the hyoid bone, enabling the suprahyoid muscle group to exert a downward pull on the mandible (Figs. 2-11 to 2-13).

Protrusion and retrusion. Protrusion of the mandible is performed by the masseter, internal pterygoid, and the external pterygoid. Retrusion is accomplished by the temporal and digastric muscles (Figs. 2-12 and 2-13).

Summary. These functional relationships are summarized in the accompanying diagram.

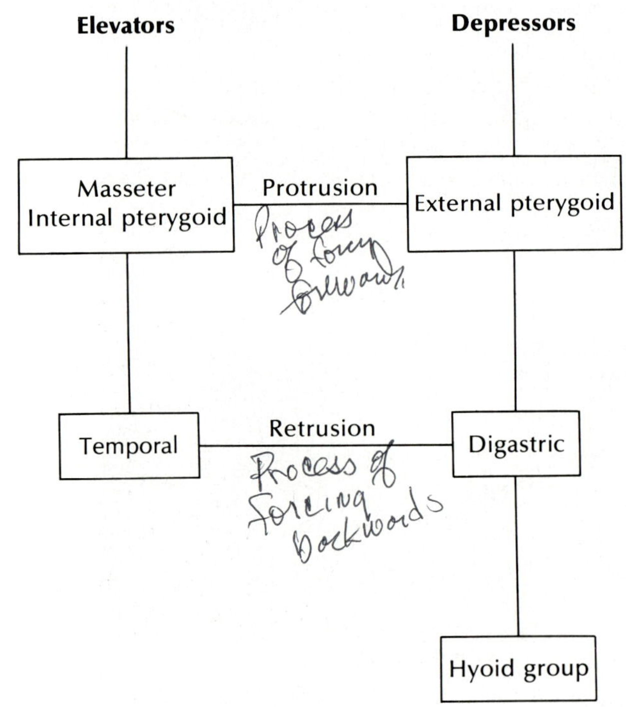

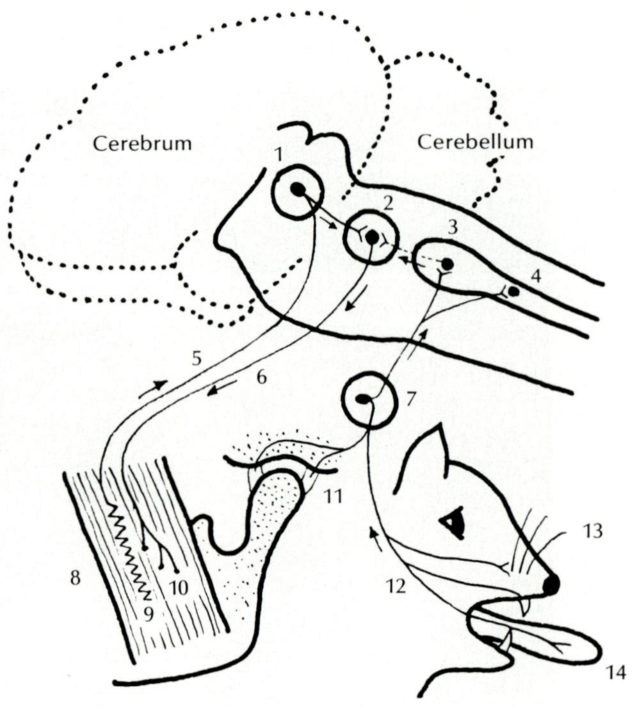

Fig. 2-14. Schematic diagram of jaw muscle reflex system. *1,* Mesencephalic trigeminal nucleus; *2,* trigeminal motor nucleus; *3,* trigeminal main sensory nucleus; *4,* trigeminal spinal sensory nucleus; *5,* muscle afferent; *6,* trigeminal motor nerve; *7,* semilunar ganglion; *8,* jaw muscle; *9,* muscle spindle; *10,* motor end-plate; *11,* temporomandibular joint; *12,* trigeminal sensory nerve; *13,* whisker; *14,* tongue. (From Kawamura, Y.: In Schwartz, L., and Chayes, C., editors: Facial pain and mandibular dysfunction, Philadelphia, 1968, W.B. Saunders Co.)

RELATED NERVES OF THE TMJ

It has been shown by Schmid[7] and Clark[1] that the nerve distribution of the TMJ includes branches of the mandibular division of the fifth cranial nerve, fibers of the facial nerve, and autonomic fibers of the otic ganglion. The *auriculotemporal nerve* leaves the main trunk of the mandibular division soon after exiting the skull through the foramen ovale. This nerve sends several branches around the joing capsule. The terminal portion ends in the skin of the temple area. The *masseteric nerve* has been shown to send some fibers to the discotemporal part and the disc region of the capsule. A small branch of the *posterior deep temporal nerve* also shares in the nerve supply to the joint.

Schmid[7] also demonstrated a connection with the *otic ganglion,* which sends autonomic fibers to the joint on the inner side of the capsule. The same investigator found free nerve endings (some of them bushlike) and encapsulated corpuscles of the Golgi-Mazzoni type in and around the joint.

The trigeminal nerve transmits most of the sensory information regarding the mandibular-oral reflexes. The reflex mechanism consists of a sense organ (receptor), an afferent neuron, one or more synapses in the brain or spinal cord, an efferent neuron, and an effector organ such as muscle. The trigeminal afferent sensory neurons from the joint and mouth pass to the trigeminal

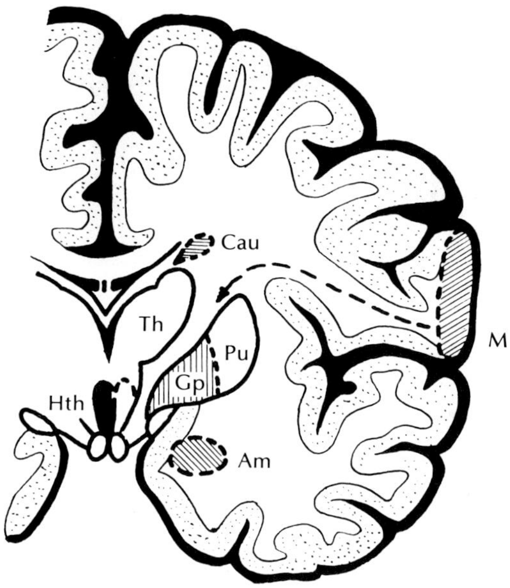

Fig. 2-15. Brain structures controlling jaw movement. *Am,* Amygdaloid nucleus; *Cau,* caudate nucleus; *Gp,* globus pallidus; *Hth,* hypothalamus; *M,* cortical jaw motor area; *Pu,* putamen; *Th,* thalamus. (From Kawamura, Y.: In Schwartz, L., and Chayes, C., editors: Facial pain and mandibular dysfunction, Philadelphia, 1968, W.B. Saunders Co.)

sensory nuclei of the medulla or trigeminal spiral sensory nucleus. Afferent sensory neurons from the mandibular muscles pass to the mesencephalic trigeminal nucleus. The efferent neurons then leave the trigeminal motor nucleus in the pons and travel by way of the mandibular nerve (third division of the trigeminal nerve) to the effector organ[4] (Fig. 2-14).

Volitional control of mandibular movement is mediated by the higher brain centers. These areas of control are the cortical jaw motor area, amygdaloid nucleus, caudate nucleus, globus pallidus, hypothalamus, thalamus, putamen, and the cerebellum[4] (Fig. 2-15). The cortical jaw areas represent a large area of the motor cortex, which allows rather skilled movements of the jaw, lips, and tongue.[5]

REFERENCES

1. Clark, W.E.LeG.: The tissues of the body, Oxford, England, 1946, Claredon Press.
2. Costen, J.: Syndrome of ear and sinus symptoms dependent upon disturbed function of the temporomandibular joint, Ann. Otol. Rhinol. Laryngol. **43**:1, 1934.
3. Debrul, E.L.: Embryological development of the temporomandibular joint. In Sarnet, B.G.: The temporomandibular joint, ed. 2, Springfield, Ill., 1964, Charles C Thomas, Publisher.
4. Kawamura, Y.: Mandibular movement: normal anatomy and physiology and clinical dysfunction. In Schwartz, L., and Chayes, C., editors: Facial pain and mandibular dysfunction, Philadelphia, 1968, W.B. Saunders Co.
5. Penfield, W., and Boldrey, E.: Somatic motor and sensory representation in cerebral cortex of man as studied by electrical stimulation, Brain **60**:389, 1937.
6. Pinto, O.: A new structure related to the temporomandibular joint and the middle ear, J. Prosthet. Dent. **12**(1):95, 1962.
7. Schmid, F.: On the nerve distribution of the temporomandibular joint capsule, Oral Surg. **28**:63, 1969.

3 Skeletal muscle

ERIC PAUL SHABER, D.D.S.

The single most evident clinical common denominator associated with temporomandibular joint disease is the presence of muscular spasm. This muscular spasm can cause pain, dysfunction, or both. The implication that muscular spasm can cause disorders of the TMJ need no longer be subtle; the literature is replete with confirmatory data, teaching us that the temporomandibular joint acts and reacts in delicate interplay with its affiliated musculature.

A book of this scope would be remiss to diminish the importance of muscular biophysiology in the total kinetics of the gnathostomatic apparatus. This chapter is presented to build a sound framework based on integrated basic sciences from which a scientific rationale for therapy may be structured.

CONTRACTING TISSUES

Apart from the trivial movements caused by cilia and flagellae, all motion in and of the body is the result of contraction in muscle cells. The delicate finger movements of a surgeon, a beat of the heart, the expulsion of a fetus, and the constriction and dilation of the pupil illustrate the variety of these movements. Muscle must have the accommodating ability to vary the speed, power, and extent of contraction. Some muscular tissues are under somatic control, whereas others are dominated by the autonomic nervous system or circulating hormones. Some tissues contract only when stimulated by their nerve, whereas others have inherent rhythmicity. The main differences lie in the shape, size, and content of the muscle cells themselves. In most mammals, including humans, skeletal muscle accounts for about half the body weight, contains more than half the body water, and has an extracellular fluid content that is about one and a half times the volume of the blood plasma. When mild exercise is undertaken, such as walking 4 miles per hour, the oxygen consumption can increase to between five and six times the basal level. When contractile tissues are subjected to measured stress, pathological conditions, or subtle physiological alterations, the nutrient demand becomes enormous. Thus the pattern of energy metabolism in the body is almost entirely determined by skeletal (striated) muscle.[4]

MOTOR UNIT

The motor unit is the physiological unit of reflex and willed contraction in mammalian skeletal muscle. The motor unit, by definition, consists of the motor neuron, its axonal extensions, the myoneural junction, and the basic muscle fibers. Under normal conditions this unit behaves in an all-or-none manner, such that an impulse in the motor nerve fiber produces an effectively synchronous contraction of all the muscle fibers it supplies. Conversely, each striated muscle fiber responds once and only once to each impulse passing down the motor nerve. The resultant contraction is thus the sum of the mechanical responses of the component muscle fibers.

This normally noted response in muscle is not particularly consistent in some muscular disorders. Given abnormal conditions, the motor unit may be fractionated in that only some of the muscle fibers supplied by a single nerve fiber respond to the nervous impulse. Furthermore, the number of muscle fibers responding may fluctuate with time and circumstance. Under such pathological conditions it is inappropriate to consider the motor unit activity, and therefore, attention must be directed to the more elemental structural component, that is, the muscle fiber.[6]

MUSCLE FIBER

A muscle fiber is any of the many cylindrical multinucleated cells that are bound together within a connective tissue framework to form the complete skeletal muscle. The length of the fiber may vary from several millimeters to centimeters, and its diameter from 10 to 100 μm, depending on the animal species and the particular muscle. Each fiber is bounded by a membrane

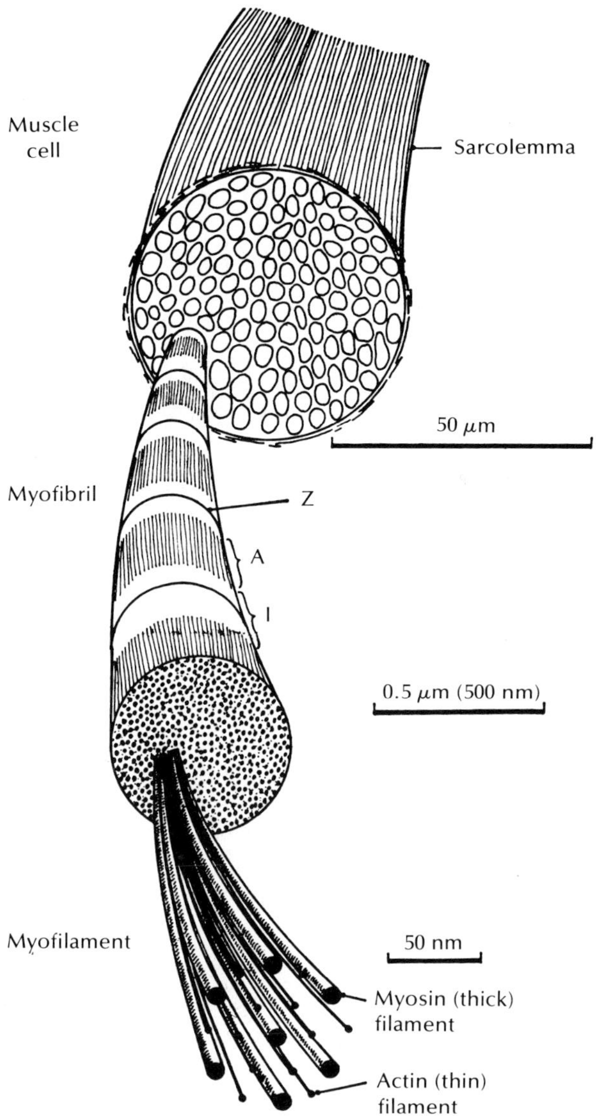

Fig. 3-1. Arrangement of myofilaments and myofibrils in skeletal muscle fiber. (From Passmore, R., and Robson, J., editors: A companion to medical students, vol. 1, Oxford, England, 1968, Blackwell Scientific Publications, Ltd.)

system referred to as the *sarcolemma*. Along the sarcolemma there is a region adapted for functional contact with a motor nerve called the *myoneural (end-plate) junction*.

The major portion of the cell volume is occupied by a highly ordered fibrillar contractile system designed for unidirectional shortening during contraction (actin-myosin complex). Superimposed on the contractile components are two tubular networks—the sarcoplasmic reticulum and the T system—which play an important role in the activation and subsequent deactivation of the contractile elements. In addition to these highly specialized structures, the sarcoplasm (cytoplasm) of the muscle fiber contains organelles common to other cells (that is, mitochondria, Golgi apparatus, lipid droplets, lipofuscin, glycogen granules, and ribosomes).

Because of the orderly arrangement of the myofibrillar components within the muscle fiber, there is an appearance of transverse banding (striations) (Fig. 3-1). These striations permit muscle fibers to be divided and studied in structural subunits called *sarcomeres*. A sarcomere is delineated by two adjacent Z lines, within whose limits there is an orderly array of the two major contractile proteins—actin and myosin. Each of these proteins is arranged in filaments and is associated with other less abundant, but functionally important, proteins. The myosin filaments are arranged longitudinally within the central portion of the cylindrical sarcomere, and actin filaments, which also are arranged longitudinally and radiate from both sides of the Z lines, interdigitate with them. Although certain circumstances remain obscure, it is now almost certain that the shortening produced during muscular contraction is achieved by a sliding of the actin filaments between the myosin filaments (Fig. 3-2), a mechanism that results in a net shortening of the sarcomere, while the lengths of the individual filaments remain unchanged (Huxley's *ratchet theory*)[6] (Fig. 3-3).

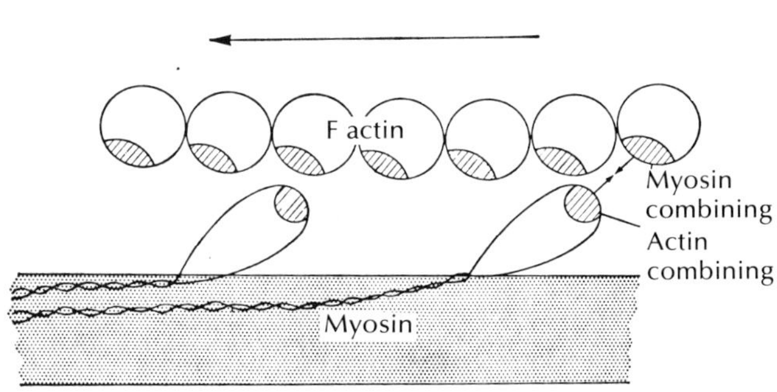

Fig. 3-2. Interaction of myosin and actin. (From Passmore, R., and Robson, J., editors: A companion to medical students, vol. 1, Oxford, England, 1968, Blackwell Scientific Publications, Ltd.)

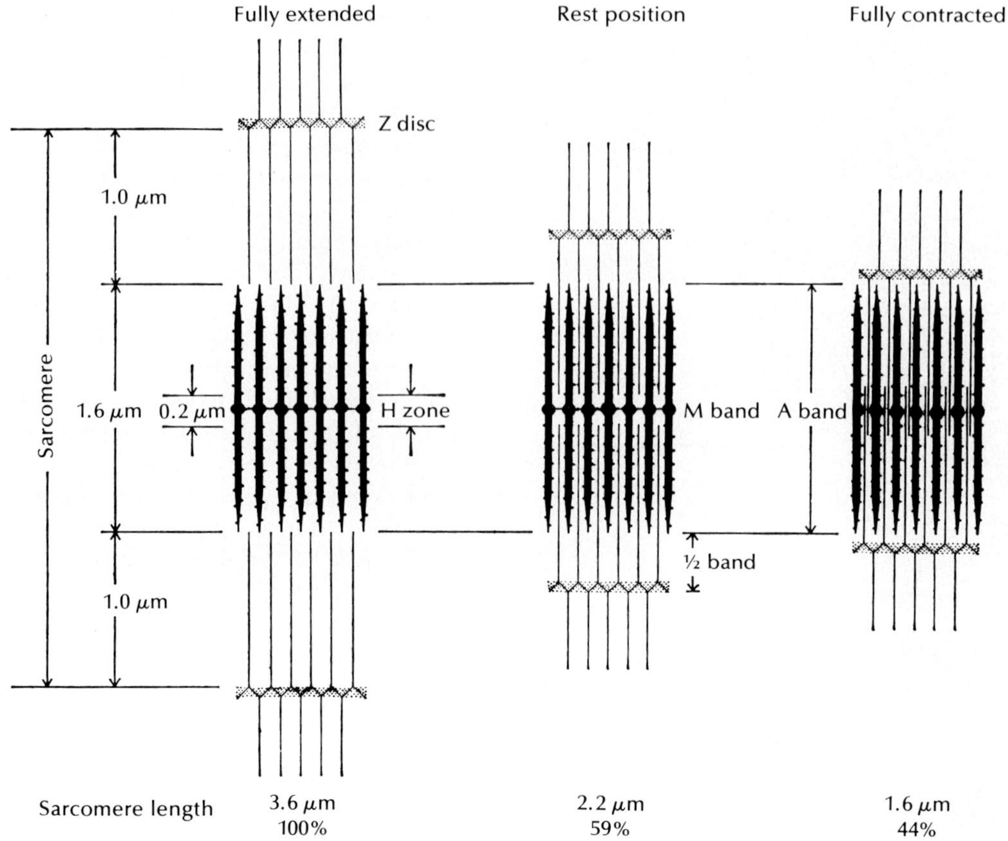

Fig. 3-3. Arrangement of myofilaments in myofibril. Note zonal relationships and uniformity of length of myofilaments. (From Passmore, R., and Robson, J., editors: A companion to medical students, vol. 1, Oxford, England, 1968, Blackwell Scientific Publications, Ltd.)

CONTRACTILE PROTEINS

Contraction in mammalian striated muscle depends on the interactions between four proteins: actin and myosin (the contractile proteins) and tropomyosin and troponin (the regulatory proteins).

Actin and myosin are the essential elements of the contractile machinery. An in vitro system formed from these two proteins can convert chemical energy to mechanical work. These proteins are able to perform this mechanochemical transduction through the release of chemical energy as a property of their molecular combination. This complex can hydrolyze adenosine triphosphate (ATP) and thus act as an adenosine triphosphatase (ATPase) enzyme capable of releasing high-energy particles that can initiate contraction (Fig. 3-4).

Myosin is a large (about 500,000 daltons), highly asymmetrical protein that makes up the thick filament of the sarcomere. The elongated myosin molecule resembles a tadpole with a long, thin tail (light meromyosin) and a globular head (heavy meromyosin) that contains two main types of low–molecular weight subunits. The tails of the myosin molecule constitute the backbone of the thick filament. This thick filamentous conformation provides considerable rigidity to the structure. The cross-bridges contain the light subunits of myosin and can be shown to include both the ATPase and actin-binding moieties of the molecules. Through their interaction with actin in the thin filament, the myosin cross-bridges are able to convert chemical energy derived from ATP hydrolysis into mechanical work. During relaxation a shift in the orientation of the cross-bridges, which is coupled to ATP hydrolysis, effects the generation of both tension and motion.

Actin, the second of the contractile proteins, is a simpler globular molecule. Each actin monomer is slightly ovoid and has a molecular weight of about 45,000 daltons. Actin monomers readily aggregate to form the double helical polymer that makes up the essential structure of the thin filament of the sarcomere. The role of actin in muscular contraction can be demonstrated and studied in vitro. Here, actin accelerates myosin ATPase activity and participates in a complex physiochemical interaction with the myosin cross-bridges that can generate tension and motion. The es-

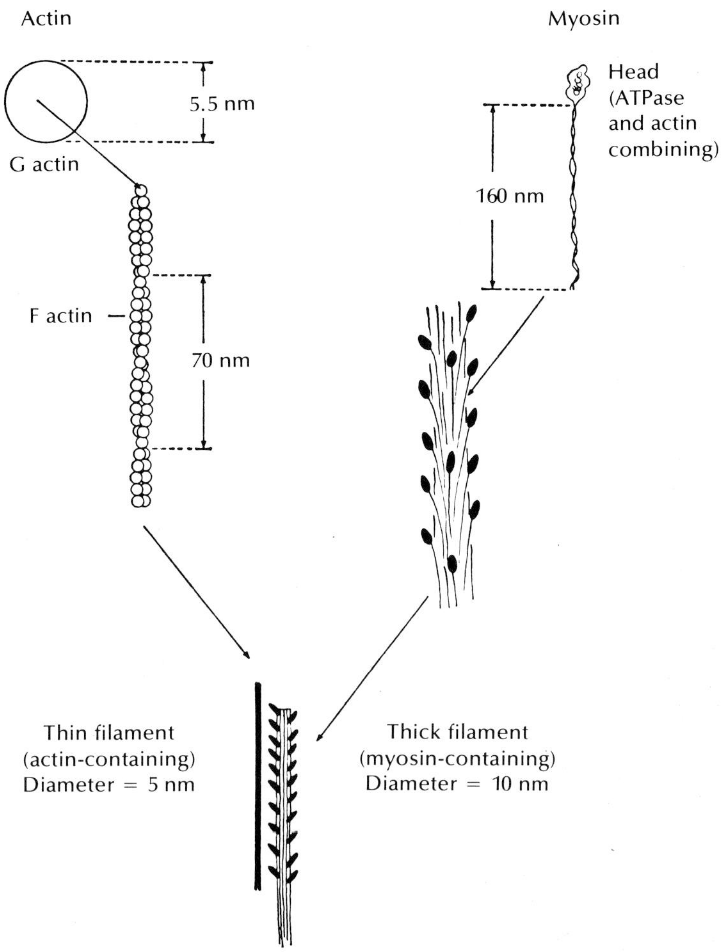

Fig. 3-4. Molecular structure of contractile proteins. (From Passmore, R., and Robson, J., editors: A companion to medical students, vol. 1, Oxford, England, 1968, Blackwell Scientific Publications, Ltd.)

sential property of muscle—mechanochemical transduction—therefore can be shown to arise from the interactions of the two contractile proteins.

Tropomyosin and troponin, the regulatory proteins of the contractile apparatus, are found in association with the actin in the thin filament of the sarcomere. Tropomyosin is like the tail of the myosin molecule and has a molecular weight of 70,000 daltons. The gross asymmetry of the tropomyosin has complex actions on the contractile process, the most important of which is its ability to control the interactions between actin and myosin.

Troponin, the fourth of the major proteins in the contractile apparatus, consists of at least three distinct peptide chains. One of these chains, troponin C, contains high-affinity calcium-binding sites. The other two troponin compounds—troponin I (which, along with tropomyosin, inhibits interaction between actin and myosin) and troponin T (which binds the other components of troponin to tropomyosin)—complete a complex control system that permits calcium to control the contractile process. All the troponin components are relatively small, having molecular weights between 18,000 and 35,000 daltons. Although a full and thorough description of the complex interactions between the four regulatory proteins (tropomyosin and troponin I, C, and T) is not yet possible, one property that is of considerable importance to the present discussion is their remarkable ability to recognize the arrival of calcium as the signal that initiates the interactions between actin and myosin, thereby triggering contraction and terminating the contractile process when calcium is removed from the cytosome. It is imperative to note that calcium is not itself an activator, but rather it is an initiator of the contractile process by its releasing an inhibition of the process that is affected by the tropomyosin-torponin complex.

A characterization of the contractile tissues is de-

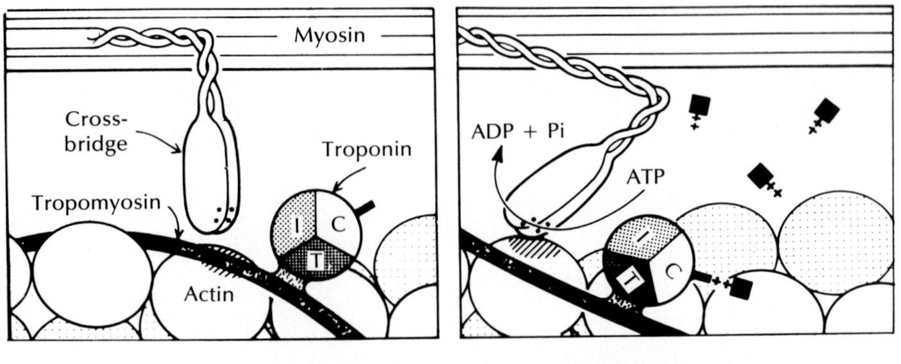

Fig. 3-5. Contraction results from interaction between thick filament (myosin) and thin filament (actin, tropomyosin, and troponin complex). Tension develops, and shortening occurs when myosin cross-bridges of thick filament interact with actin of thin filament. (From Katz, A.M.: N. Engl. J. Med. **293:**1184, 1975. Reprinted by permission.)

picted by the tubular system, with contractile proteins, regulatory proteins, and calcium as the fine muscular machinery and ATP operating as the specialized fuel this machinery requires for proper function (Fig. 3-5).

MUSCLE CELL MEMBRANE

The muscle cell membrane, with its complex pattern of polysaccharide, mucoprotein, and lipoprotein, separates aqueous solutions having the same total osmotic pressure but radically different compositions. The extracellular fluid has high concentrations of sodium (Na^+) and chloride (Cl^-) and a low concentration of potassium (K^+). On the other hand, the intracellular fluid is rich in K^+ and protein, but its content of Na^+ and Cl^- ions is low. Many other substances also are dissolved in the aqueous phases, but Na^+, K^+, and possibly Cl^- are the main ions carrying appreciable currents through the membrane. This unequal distribution of inorganic ions across the muscle fiber membrane gives rise to an electrical potential difference (about 90 mV, inside negative) between the interior of the cell and its environment.

The maintenance of these concentration differences depends mainly on the net movement of ions against their electrochemical potential gradients. These, in turn, develop because of the structure of the membrane (which is such that it allows the diffusion of ions at only a minute fraction of the rate at which they diffuse through water) and because the cell can use metabolically derived energy to actively transport Na^+ out of it and K^+ into it. The demonstration that muscle cells lose K^+ and Na^+ on stimulation and that these exchanges reverse concentrations during the recovery period suggests that there must be a "pump" located in the fiber membrane, which can pump out Na^+ and pump in the K^+ to reestablish membrane potential difference. It is generally agreed that this process requires the expenditure of energy, which must be supplied by cellular metabolism (ATP synthesis).

It appears evident that cellular metabolism and the synthesis of high-energy compounds are essential for muscular function and membrane stability. If cellular metabolism is deranged, a decrease in the concentration of high-energy compounds would be expected with concomitant changes in the biochemical nature of the cellular by-products.

ENERGY METABOLISM

The biochemical scheme by which energy is derived from cells is infinitely complex. High-energy compounds are essential for the body's enzymatic reactions. ATP is present everywhere in the cytoplasm and nucleoplasm of all cells; essentially all the physiological mechanisms that require energy for operation obtain this directly from the stored ATP. In turn, under ideal conditions the food in the cells is gradually oxidized, and the released energy is used to reform the ATP, thus always maintaining a supply of this substance. All these energy transfers take place by means of coupled reactions. ATP frequently has been referred to as the *energy currency of the body*, which can be gained and spent again and again.[1]

All the energy foods—carbohydrates, fats, proteins—can be oxidized with oxygen in the cells, and in this process certain amounts of energy are released. Certain foods (carbohydrates) enzymatically affected in the presence of oxygen can liberate fantastically greater quantities of free energy. For instance, the amount of energy liberated by the oxidation of 1 mole of glucose (180 g glucose) is 686,000 calories, whereas when forced to metabolize anaerobically, this same mole of glucose generates only 16,000 calories; that is, it generates calories at about 2% efficiency.

The principal energy food is the carbohydrate, and

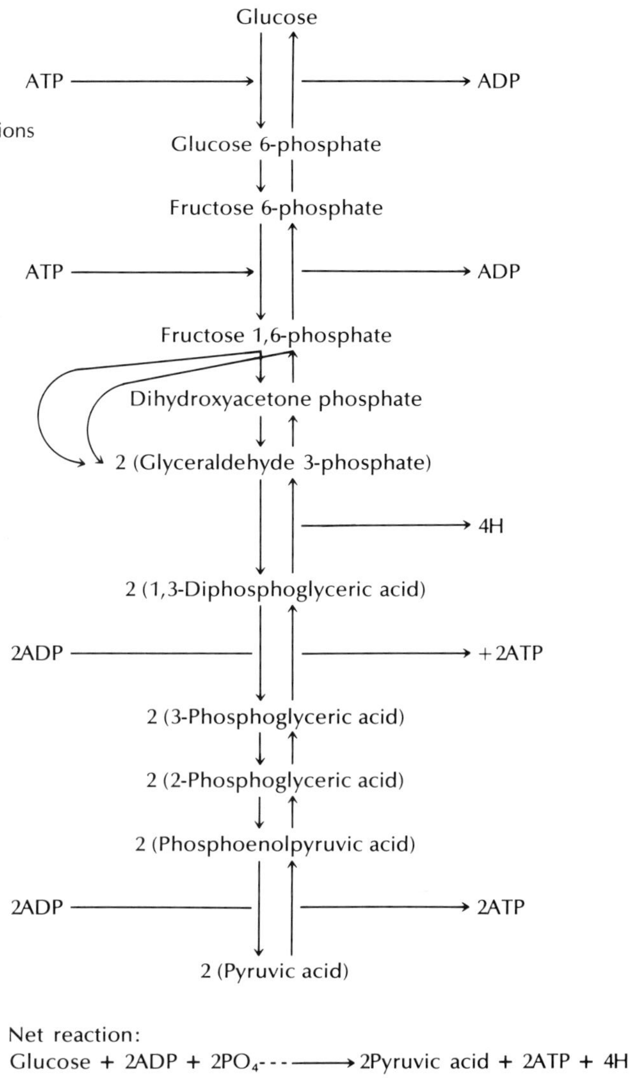

Fig. 3-6. Sequence of chemical reactions responsible for glycolysis.

at least 99% of *all* carbohydrates used by the body are used for the purpose of energy (ATP) production. Breakdown of this carbohydrate to the simple glucose molecule and subsequent enzymatic reactions in the presence of oxygen give the highest yield of energy compounds. Since complete oxidation of 1 gram-mole of glucose releases 686,000 calories of energy, and only 8000 calories of energy are required to form 1 gram-mole of ATP, it would be extremely wasteful of energy for glucose to decompose all the way to water and carbon dioxide at once while forming only a single ATP molecule. Fortunately cells contain extensive series of different protein enzymes that cause the glucose molecule to split a little at a time in many successive steps, with its energy released in small packets to form one molecule of ATP at a time, forming a total of 38 moles of ATP for each mole of glucose used by the cells.

Again, the chemistry by which the glucose molecule is progressively dissected and its energy released to form ATP is grossly complex. The following discussion is a simplistic view of these reactions.

Glycolysis and the formation of pyruvic acid

Glycolysis is by far the most important means by which energy is released from the glucose molecule. Glycolysis is the splitting of the glucose molecule to form two molecules of pyruvic acid. Fig. 3-6 shows the sequence of chemical reactions responsible for glycolysis.

Conversion of pyruvic acid to acetyl coenzyme A

The next stage in degradation of glucose is conversion of the two pyruvic acid molecules into two mole-

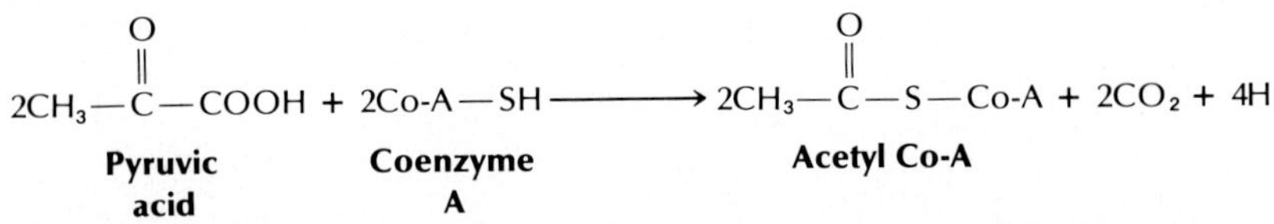

Fig. 3-7. Reaction by which pyruvic acid is converted to acetyl coenzyme A.

cules of acetyl coenzyme A (acetyl Co-A) in accordance with the reaction shown in Fig. 3-7.

Citric acid cycle

The third stage, known as the citric acid cycle, tricarboxylic acid cycle, or Krebs cycle, is a series of chemical reactions in which the acetyl portion of the acetyl Co-A is degraded to carbon dioxide and hydrogen atoms. The reaction begins with oxaloacetic acid, and then at the bottom of the chain of reactions oxaloacetic acid is once again formed; thus the cycle can continue over and over again. Fig. 3-8 shows the chemical reactions of the citric acid cycle.

Oxidation of hydrogen atoms by the oxidative enzymes

The chemical processes of oxidative phosphorylation, showing ionization of hydrogen and oxygen formation of water and ATP, are seen in Fig. 3-9.

Conclusions

Despite all the complexities of the previously described reactions, pitifully small amounts of ATP are formed during all these processes. Instead about 90% of the final amount of ATP is formed during subsequent oxidation of the 16 hydrogen atoms that are released during these earlier stages of glucose degradation. Indeed the principal function of all these earlier stages is to make the hydrogen of the glucose molecule available in a form that can be used for oxidation.

It is evident that the factors determining muscular contractility and viability are too varied to be discussed in depth. Pathological conditions can result from anything that disrupts the motor unit, the muscle fiber, the molecular proteins, or the biochemistry of the contractile system.

GENESIS OF MYOSPASM

Armed with the scientific evidence that ATP is required for both contraction and relaxation of skeletal muscle, it now can be understood how prolonged and/or strong contractions can lead to a state of muscle fatigue and subsequent muscle spasm. Simplistically, this condition results from an inability of the contractile and metabolic processes of the muscle fibers to continue supplying the same work output. The nerve continues

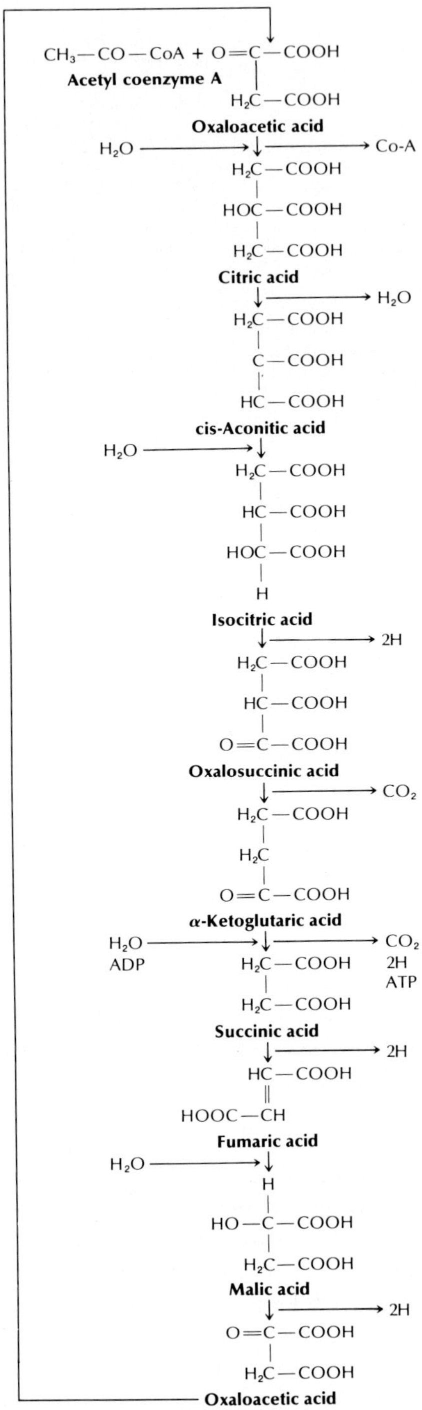

Net reaction per molecule of glucose:
$2\text{Acetyl Co-A} + 6H_2O + 2ADP \quad 4CO_2 + 16H + 2\text{Co-A} + 2ATP$

Fig. 3-8. Citric acid cycle.

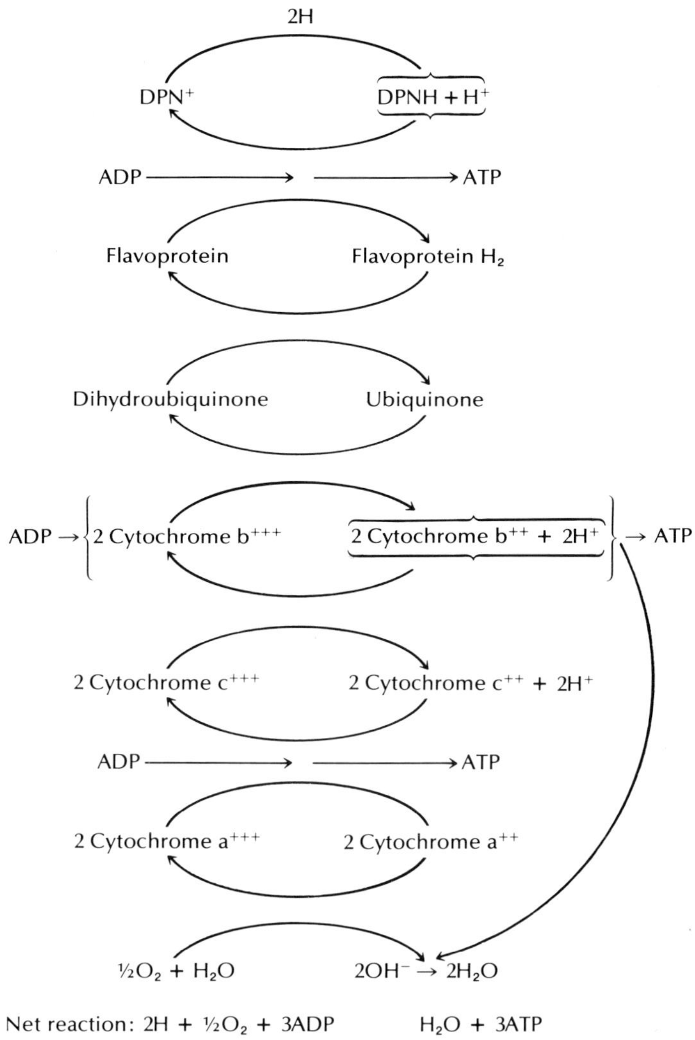

Fig. 3-9. Oxidation of hydrogen atoms by oxidative enzymes.

to function properly, the nerve impulses pass normally through the neuromuscular junction into the muscle fiber, and even normal action potentials spread over the muscle fibers. However, the contraction becomes weaker and weaker because of depletion of energy supplies in the muscles themselves. Interruption of blood flow through a contracting muscle leads to almost complete muscle fatigue in a minute or more because of obvious loss of nutrient supply (oxygen).

If a muscle becomes fatigued to an extreme extent, it is likely to become continually contracted, remaining contracted and rigid for many minutes even without an action potential as a stimulus. This is called *physiological (hemostatic) contracture of muscle*. It is believed to result from a peculiar feature of the contractile process itself. As was pointed out earlier, ATP is required to make actin and myosin separate during the process of muscle relaxation. Otherwise the myosin and actin filaments will continue to be attracted to each other. In extreme degrees of muscle fatigue essentially all the ATP has been depleted, thus accounting for the rigid binding of actin and myosin filaments.

Simultaneously, as this molecular derangement continues, biochemical and anatomical processes compound the pathological condition within the skeletal muscle. Again, when muscle fibers are subjected to noxious stimulation (emotional, mechanical, infectious, metabolic, nutritional, or more likely a combination of several of these stresses), they react by developing spasm and shortening.[5] Intially the ensuing shortening of the musculature is physiological. If the stimuli producing the spasm of the entire muscle may ensue. On the other hand, if the insulting mechanism is low grade or chronic, only a portion of the muscular fibers may

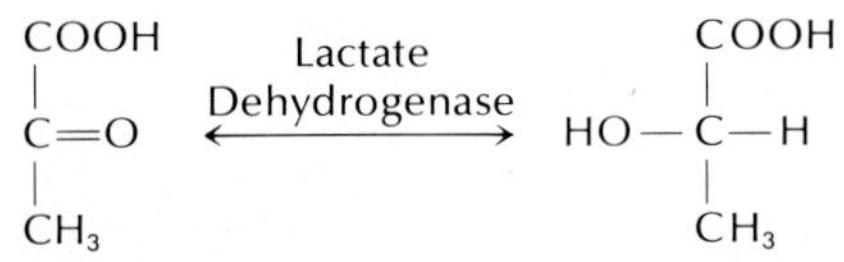

Pyruvate **Lactate**

Fig. 3-10. Anaerobic metabolism. When cell is forced to produce ATP anaerobically, there is marked decrease in cellular efficiency, with concomitant production of possible spasmogenic by-products.

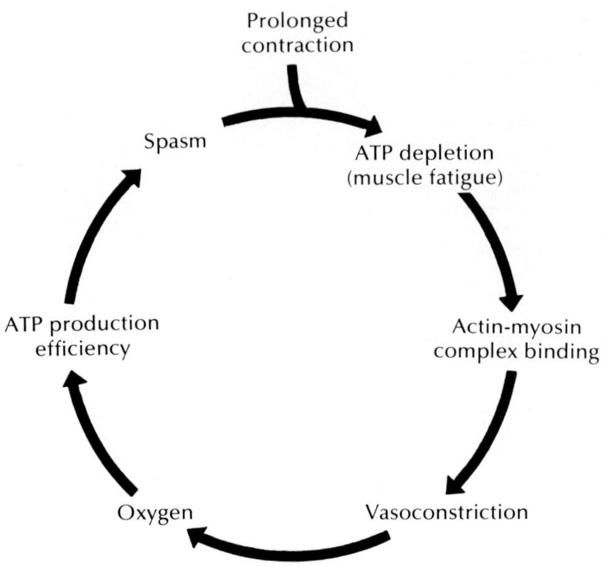

Fig. 3-11. Pain-spasm-pain cycle. Biochemical and molecular cycle resulting in decrease in cellular efficiency with subsequent perpetuation of myofibrillar spasm.

become spastic. A localized area of spastic skeletal muscle fibers is called a *trigger zone*. By definition, this trigger zone is a small, hypersensitive area from which afferent impulses bombard the central nervous system and give rise to *referred pain*, that is a predictable anatomical pathway of pain symptoms manifested at some distance from the associated trigger zone. When the trigger zone continuously forwards high-intensity volleys to the central nervous system, vasoconstriction can be noted in the area of spasm.

It follows that an area of spastic musculature secondarily involved with vasoconstriction will respond with a progression of sequential physiological responses (Fig. 3-10). This area of muscle which is being poorly perfused will be forced, as all ischemic tissue must, to metabolize anerobically, thereby negating the efficiency of the previously reviewed enzymatic reactions—glycolysis with subsequent oxidation of the hydrogen ions and formation of ATP.

This anaerobic metabolism causes the accumulation of possible spasm-inducing agents, most notable of which is lactic acid. The buildup of noxious metabolites within muscle substance becomes, in and of itself, a significant stimulus capable of perpetuating spasm and causing pain even after the elimination of the prime cause. Thus a vicious deteriorative biochemical cycle is begun. In summation, this constant biochemical cycle results in the production of spasmogenic agents while decreasing the efficiency of the cells to produce high-energy phosphate compounds that can facilitate muscular relaxation. This creates a perpetuation of spasm with pain referral and a pattern classically known as the *pain-spasm-pain cycle* (Fig. 3-11).

REFERENCES

1. Guyton, A.C., editor: Textbook of medical physiology, ed. 4, Philadelphia, 1971, W.B. Saunders Co.
2. Katz, A.M.: Congestive heart failure: role of altered myocardial cellular control, N. Engl. J. Med. **293**:1184, 1975.
3. Katz, A.M.: Contractile proteins. In Galanger, A.J., editor: The mammalian myocardium, New York, 1974, John Wiley & Sons, Inc.
4. Passmore, R., and Robson, J., editors: A companion to medical students, vol. 1, Oxford, England, 1968, Blackwell Scientific Publications, Ltd.
5. Travell, J., and Rinzler, S.: The myofascial genesis of pain, Postgrad. Med. **11**:425, 1952.
6. Walton, J., editor: Disorders of voluntary muscle, ed. 3, Edinburgh, 1974, Churchill Livingstone.

4 Early iatrogenic orofacial muscle, skeletal, and TMJ dysfunction

JAMES F. GARRY, D.D.S., F.A.S.C.D., F.I.C.D.

The concept that the mandible is a free-floating anatomical bony structure, positioned in its relationship to the maxilla by neuromuscular proprioception, has not been fully understood by most of our colleagues in the dental profession. To further complicate the relationship of the maxilla to the mandible, there are teeth in these bony structures with cusps and fossae that should occlude in a neuromuscular centric occlusion. Muscle force vectors are acting constantly on teeth, and an imbalance between intraoral and extraoral muscular patterns will move teeth, causing an abnormal maxillomandibular relationship because of proprioceptive occlusal accomodation, resulting in a predisposition to TMJ dysfunction. There arises the question, then, of when we should begin to concern ourselves with the possibility of orofacial muscle imbalance.

PRENATAL GESTATION AND SUCKING

Prenatal studies[6] have documented that the human fetus begins to swallow at approximately 12 weeks of gestation. Taste receptors are present at this time, so for at least 28 weeks the gustatory system is exposed to chemicals in the amniotic fluid. Chemicals present in amniotic fluid include glucose, fructose, lactic, pyruvic, and citric acids, fatty acids, phospholipids, creatinine, urea, uric acid, amino acids, polypeptides, proteins, and salts.[16] The composition of the amniotic fluid changes periodically during gestation. Large volumes of amniotic fluid, ranging from 200 to 760 ml/day, are swallowed by the fetus in the last third of gestation.[2] It is interesting to note that the fetus is responsible for gradual short-term changes in amniotic fluid composition by urinating into the fluid. The volume ranges from 173 to 677 ml/day.[23]

The peripheral and central taste system develops in the presence of changing, low concentrations of a variety of chemicals. Intrauterine environment may influence the formation of neural connections in the taste system. Perhaps prolonged fetal exposure to low levels of chemicals in the amniotic fluid explains why some prenatal thumb- and/or finger-sucking occurs. The fetus's autonomic sucking reflex possibly is stimulated by the altered nutritional composition of amniotic fluid.

The proximity of the hand to the oral cavity in a developing fetus is such that the thumb can readily enter the mouth, thus enabling a premature sucking reflex to occur when nutritional needs stimulate the autonomic nervous system (Figs. 4-1 and 4-2). However, *prenatal sucking is the exception, not the rule.*

SUCKING REFLEX (POST PARTUM)

The neonatal sucking reflex is an autonomic reflex that enables an infant to extract nutrients from a breast or artificial nipple. This reflex is clinically evidenced immediately post partum. The infant's tongue undulates anteriorly and posteriorly, attempting to suck on any object thrust into the oral cavity. The sucking reflex is normal and essential to sustain life; however, one must consider what Nature had intended the infant to suck—a finger, an object, or a breast. This issue may seem superfluous, yet many dentists state that thumb- or finger-sucking is not harmful to a child if stopped by 4 or 5 years of age. Nothing could be further from the truth unless one qualifies this statement (Fig. 4-3).

Any object placed in the oral cavity on which an infant sucks, other than the breast, can act as an orthodontic appliance, depending on the force, intensity, direction, and duration of the sucking. The reason is obvious. For humans to survive, they have had to adapt to their environment, which results in evolutionary changes in their physiology to best procreate the species. Our present form and function has been the result of environmental changes. The human breast and milk have developed genetically to give an infant the neces-

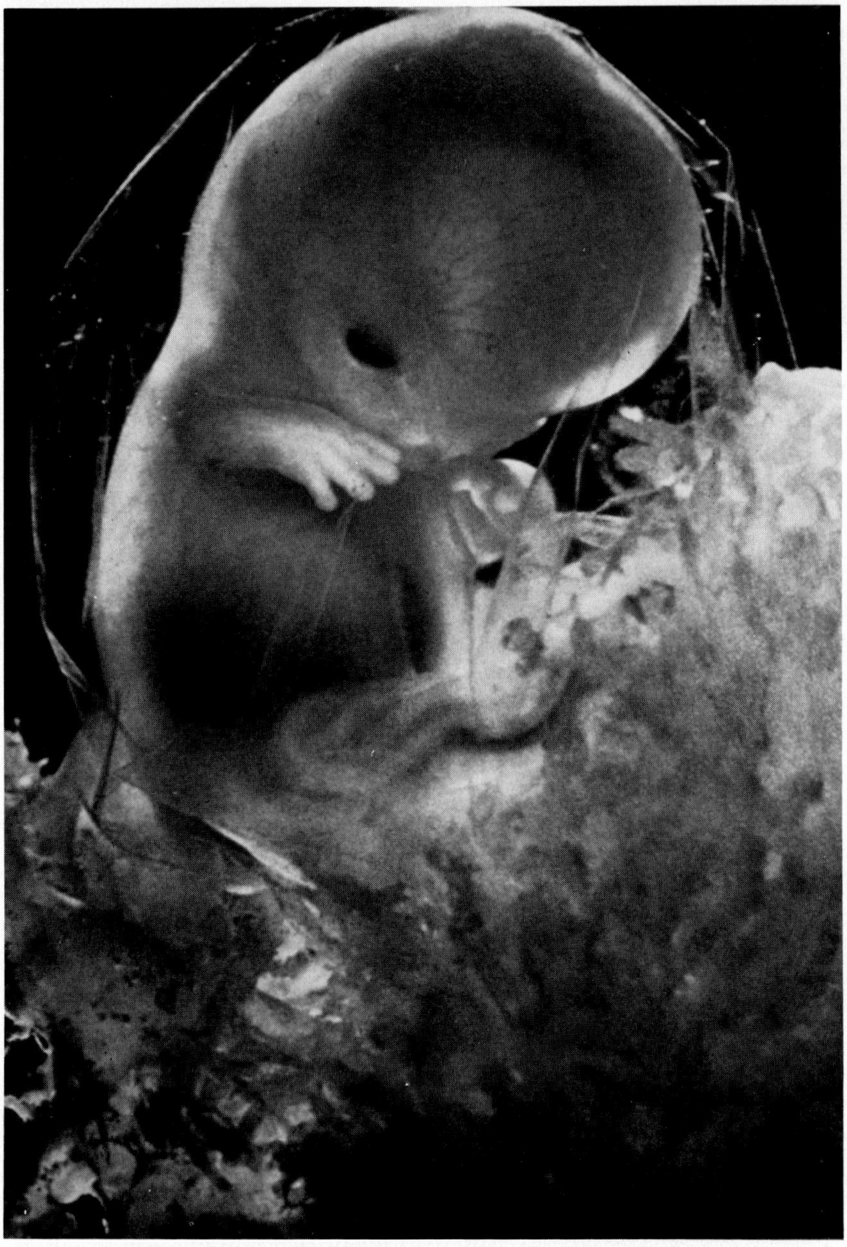

Fig. 4-1. Hand of developing fetus approximates the oral cavity.

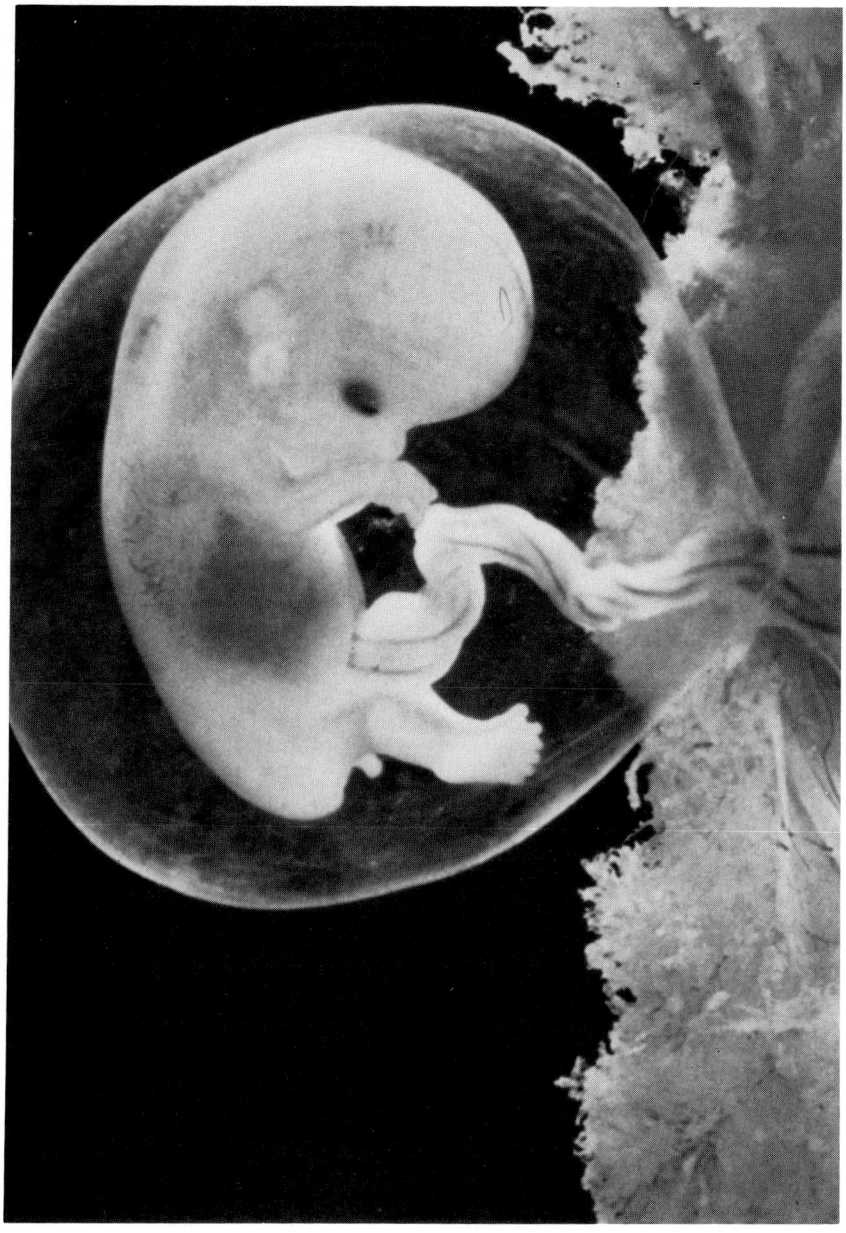

Fig. 4-2. As appendages develop, prenatal sucking may occur because of stimulation of sucking reflex.

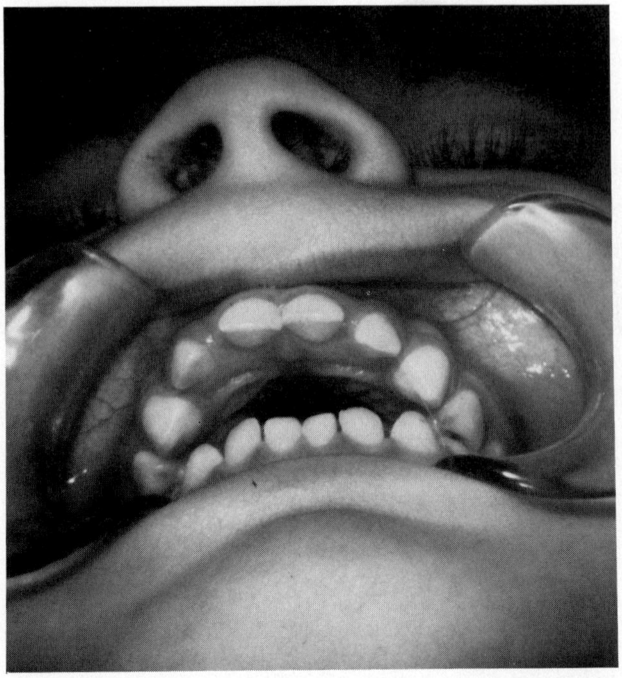

Fig. 4-3. A 2½-year-old thumb-sucker with Class II, division 1 malocclusion, high V-shaped palatal vault, speech defect with sibilant sounds, open-mouth habitus, and predisposition to anterior fracture, avulsion, and TMJ disorientation.

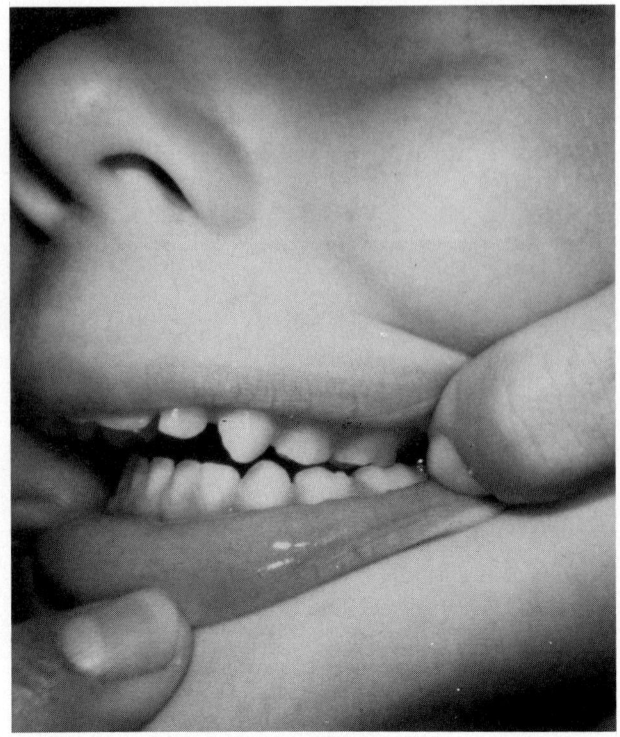

Fig. 4-4. A 2-year 8-month-old thumb-sucker with Class II, division 1 malocclusion, cross-bite, open bite (second primary molars only teeth occluding in centric), microrhinic dysplasia (restricted nasal passage because premaxilla is rotated upward with concomitant upward tilt of nose), mouth-breathing habitus, and an abnormal orientation of condyle to glenoid fossa.

sary nutrients and most advantageous orofacial muscle balance. Changing this environment potentiates a change in form and function.

Appendage sucking

When an infant does not satisfy the sucking reflex and/or nutritional needs are not met, he or she will attempt to satisfy this autonomic requirement by sucking on any object or appendage that approximates the oral cavity (rooting reflex). The hand of a newborn infant is continually raised to the mouth, and when there is a compulsive need to suck and/or a nutritional need, the infant will begin to suck on the tiny fist, thumb, or finger. Since so many experts have stated that the act of sucking is normal and healthy, we look on the act with little concern, often commenting "Isn't that cute," or "He is so contented and happy." I cannot disagree with the fact that these children are content and even tranquilized to some extent. However, it is essential that the dentist be aware of the fact that sucking an appendage or an object has the potential for creating malocclusions if continued during and after the eruption of deciduous as well as permanent teeth—and malocclusions potentiate TMJ dysfunction. Note the malocclusion created by a child less than 3 years old because of chronic thumb-sucking (Fig. 4-4). This child has created a Class II malocclusion, constricted maxillary arch, high palatal vault, potential for avulsion and/or fractured anteriors, hypotonicity of the extraoral musculature, an inability to develop proper sibilant sounds, an open lip posture, a mouth-breathing habitus, and a tongue thrust. This type of malocclusion is seldom seen in healthy, breast-fed children who suck nothing other than the breast. I reemphasize: any object placed into the oral cavity other than the breast has the potential for creating malocclusion with a resultant TMJ dysfunction.

Children who do not suck their appendages or conventional pacifiers do not suffer from malcontent and usually have better facial features and better tonal quality[3] and adapt to their environment with less harassment.

A dentist cannot determine a predisposition to malocclusion simply by observing a child who sucks an object other than the breast. Therefore it is the dentist's duty to inform colleagues and patients of the damage that could result from noxious habits. There are children who are passive suckers and do not create a malocclusion, but rather than take the risk that a child may not be a passive sucker, it is far better to control the habit.

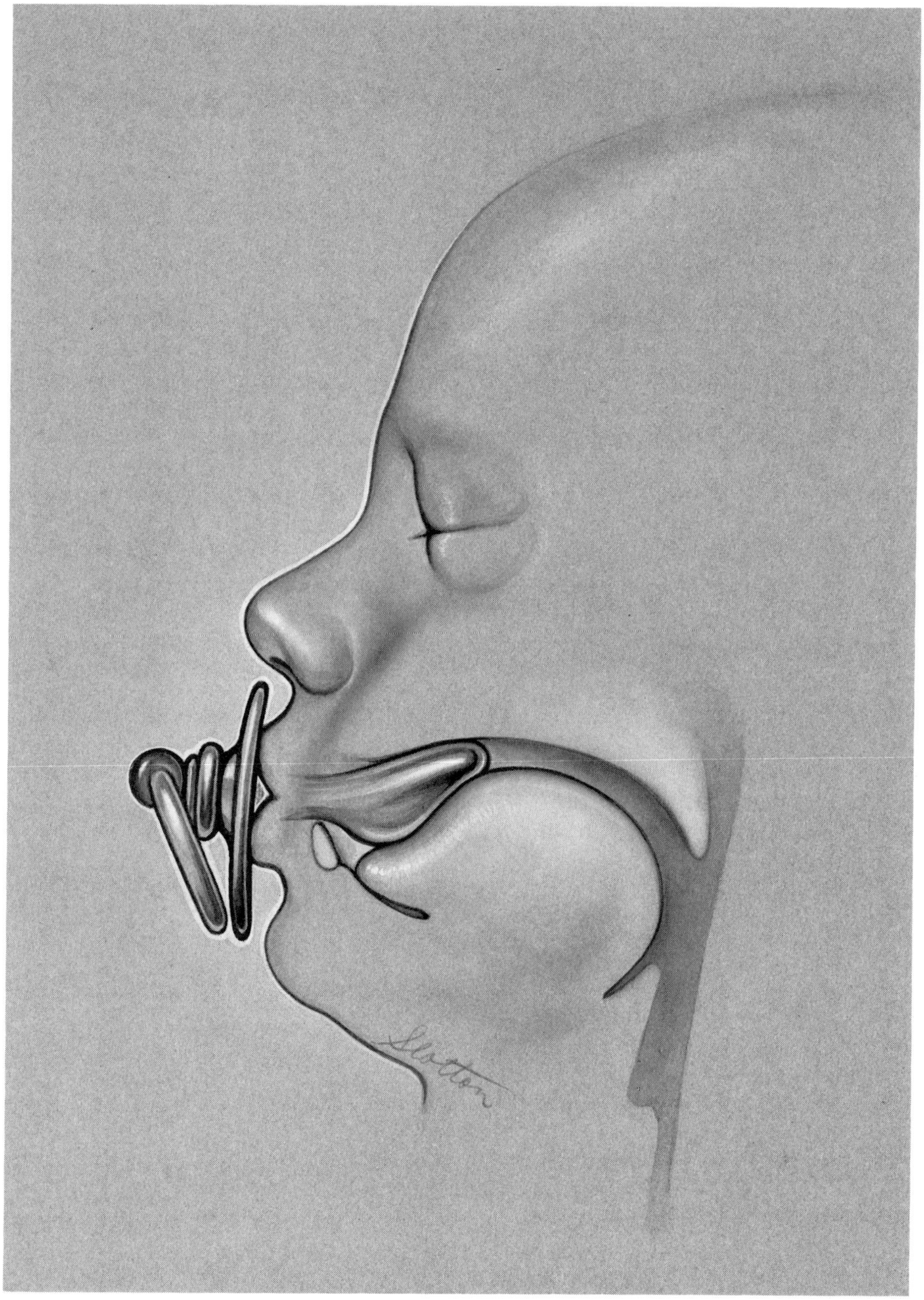

Fig. 4-5. Nuk exerciser conforms to normal palatal and arch form, positions tongue beneath the baglet, and allows lateral borders of tongue to expand and offset extraoral pressures during sucking.

Once a noxious habit begins, it is extremely difficult to terminate (ask any smoker). The habit becomes addictive and truly satisfying. If the habit is prevented immediately post partum, it can be controlled. Do not allow the hand or its appendages to enter the mouth uncovered. If necessary, the sleeve of an infant's gown can be tied beyond the hand, allowing freedom of movement but preventing suction because of an inability to form a seal through the garment. If the habit never starts, it will never be missed; ask any nonsmoker.

To prevent infant anxiety from the emotional need to suck, simply allow the infant to suck on the most physiologically perfect nipple known to us—the human breast. If the infant is not satisfied and appears to have a desire to suck after feeding, place a Nuk exerciser in the mouth, and satisfaction is immediate (Fig. 4-5). Do not attempt to use a standard pacifier, since it could distort the orofacial musculature, and the child will not accept a Nuk exerciser subsequently.

Nuk exerciser

There are two orthodontic Nuk exercising units: a small primary exerciser and a larger secondary exerciser. Although they differ in size, both are identical in form and function (Fig. 4-6). The primary exerciser is a supplement to be used in conjunction with the Nuk nipple or breast. The objective is to use normal sucking and oral desires more beneficially by channeling this activity through the exerciser to stimulate healthier growth and development. The secondary (larger) exerciser can be used after the first $1^1/_2$ years, if necessary.

During sucking and oral activities the baglet flattens and expands readily under the action of the baby's tongue. The top or palatal portion is designed broad and curved to conform to the normal palatal and arch form. The bottom or lingual portion of the baglet is concave, positioning the tongue beneath the baglet during swallowing. This is in contrast to the conventional pacifier or finger, which encourages the tongue to wrap around the object.

Like the nipple, the exerciser has two anterior inclined planes that allow the lateral borders of the tongue to expand and offset the extraoral pressures during sucking. The flat passage encourages the child to close the lips and to obtain full closure of the posterior elements of the jaw without compromising the anterior gum pads (Fig. 4-7).

Continuous use of an exerciser after deciduous teeth erupt occasionally has resulted in an anterior open bite comparable to that of a child with poor tongue repose. The resultant degree of malocclusion is far less than with conventional pacifiers.

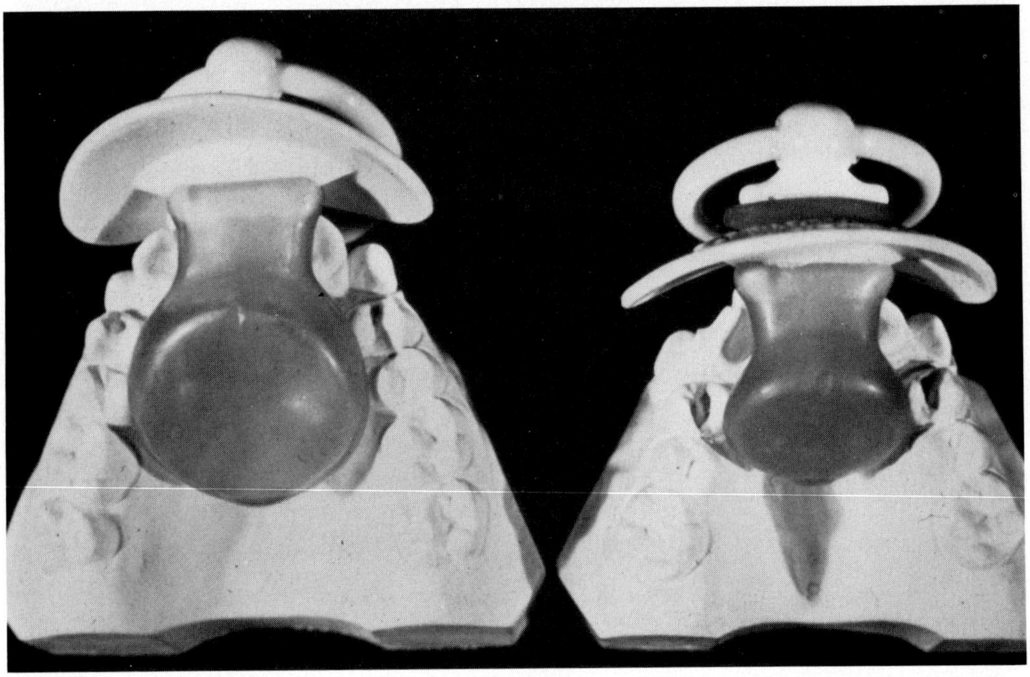

Fig. 4-6. Primary (smaller) Nuk exerciser is recommended for use from birth until approximately $1^1/_2$ years of age. Secondary (larger) exerciser is recommended for use after approximately $1^1/_2$ years of age, if necessary.

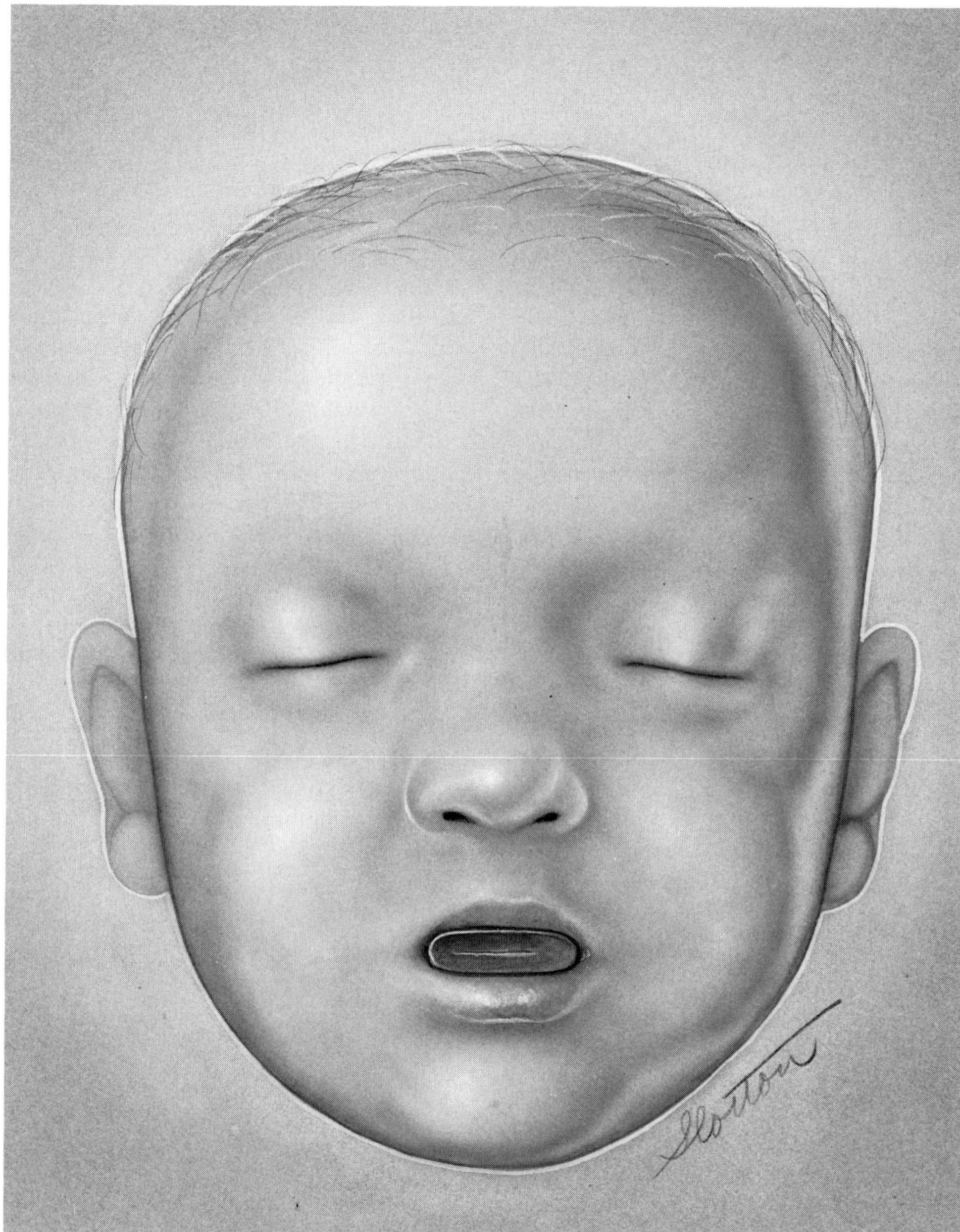

Fig. 4-7. Flat passage of Nuk exerciser encourages child to close lips to obtain full closure of posterior elements of jaw and enables normal anteroposterior movement of mandible, as in nursing. It allows lips to flatten to more normal configuration.

BREAST FEEDING

The value of breast feeding has not been properly stressed by the dental profession as a deterrent to malocclusion. Many dentists are not aware of the fact that human milk (1) is more digestible than cow's milk, (2) has antibodies which protect the infant from upper respiratory tract allergies and bacterial infection, (3) supplies necessary nutrition, (4) reduced mortality in the first few months, and (5) reduces the chance of contamination. Additionally, breast feeding is emotionally satisfying to both mother and baby, and the orofacial muscles during nursing are physiologically balanced to best adapt to the postnatal environment.

A study in 1963 by Najera[21] of St. Louis University confirmed that breast-fed children show excellent, more desirable facial features than do bottle-fed children. There is a definite relationship between orofacial form and function and the way the infant is fed.

Breast feeding requires much more physical energy than is expended during conventional, artificial feeding. As a rule, an infant who nurses 20 to 30 minutes at each feeding will display less need to satisfy the sucking reflex. One common mistake made by many nursing mothers is allowing an infant to fall asleep on the breast after 5 or 10 minutes of nursing. Gently shaking or tickling the infant under the chin will awaken him or her pleasantly, and nursing will continue. The mother should alternate breasts since this allows equal stimulation of milk production in each breast during nursing.

The mother should hold her infant in such a manner that the head is slightly elevated when lying down. If the baby lies on the right side, the mother should lie on her left side and nurse at the left breast (and vice versa). The head is elevated by placing the mother's arm under the infant's head. The best position to hold a nursing infant is upright rather than reclining (Fig. 4-8). Healthy swallowing in a reclining position is just as difficult for the baby as it is for the adult. The baby is apt to swallow improperly and react negatively to feelings of suffocation induced by the gravitation flow of milk. Nursing in a reclining position often causes milk to flow into the middle ear and may cause inflammation and possibly other pharyngeal complications. The infant will thrust the tongue forward to expel the milk and thereby prevent pooling in the pharyngeal region. Continued feeding in a reclining position may potentiate tongue thrust. When babies are held in upright positions they are encouraged to take the breast with the neck stretched and a forward stretching of the chin, which is most important for healthy orofacial development. Encourage all healthy expectant mothers to breast feed. If impossible, encourage breast massage followed by manual expression or a breast pump to extract milk for storage (Fig. 4-9). The nutritional value of

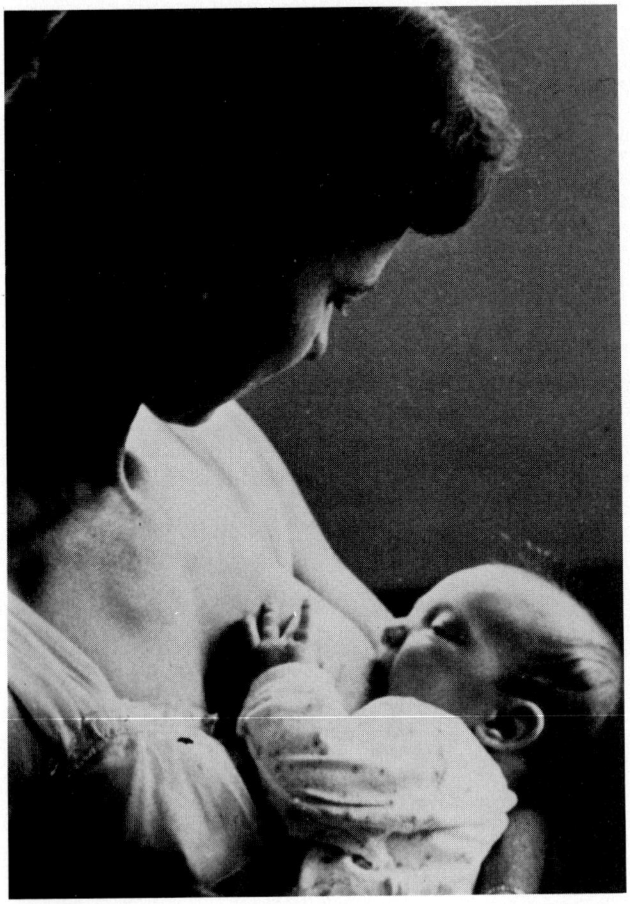

Fig. 4-8. Best position to hold a nursing infant is upright rather than reclining.

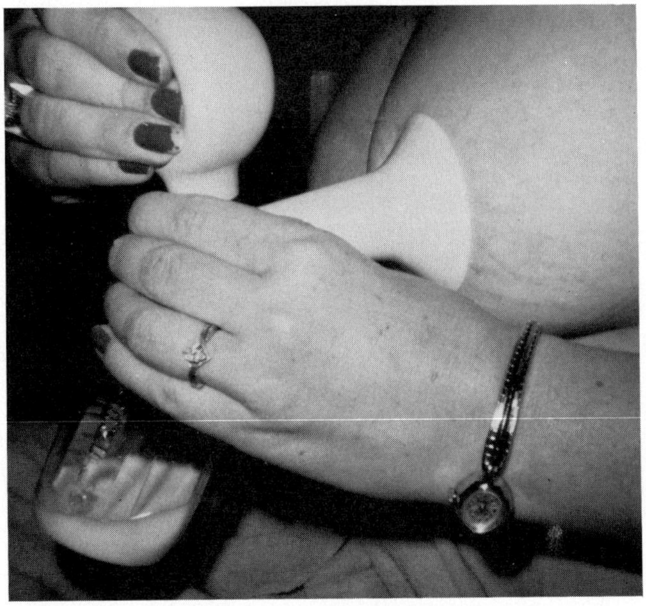

Fig. 4-9. Breast pump: working mother may use manual expression or breast pump to extract human milk for storage.

human milk as opposed to cow's milk or milk substitutes is irrefutable.

Value of human milk

Artificially fed infants have a greater overall incidence of allergies. Breast feeding should be recommended for infants whose immediate families have a history of allergy, since it minimizes the likelihood of allergy caused by foreign milk proteins. Cow's milk allergy is the most common allergy in infancy. The time of introduction of cow's milk may be related to the likelihood of allergy; therefore withholding cow's milk from the infant's diet during the first months of life may minimize the chance of allergic reaction to it.[8] Keep in mind that upper respiratory tract allergies occlude the nasal passages because of edema in the paranasal structures, resulting in mouth breathing and predisposition to malocclusion and TMJ dysfunction.

To motivate an expectant mother to breast feed, it is essential that the dentist understand the advantages. Commercial formulas superficially simulate mature human milk but are considerably different from colostrum, the thick yellow fluid that lactating women produce during the first 3 to 5 days post partum. Colostrum is a rich source of antibodies, particularly secretory immunoglobulin A (IgA), which work against allergies, and pathogens that enter through the gastrointestinal tract. None of these protective factors are found in formulas; and lysozyme, an antimicrobial enzyme, is present in appreciable quantities in human milk and may produce a bactericidal effect.[19]

A group of nitrogen-containing polysaccharides, the bifid factor, promotes the growth of Bifidobacterium flora characteristic of breast-fed children.[12] These bacteria (particularly *Lactobacillus bifidus*) produce acids that lower the pH of the intestinal tract. An acid environment inhibits growth of *Escherichia coli*, yeast, and *Shigella* organisms.[15]

Another substance in human milk that helps prevent microbial infections is protein lactoferrin. Lactoferrin inhibits the growth of staphylococci and *E. coli* by binding iron, which the bacteria need to proliferate.[4] In addition, human milk contains an antistaphylococcal factor that appears to be a fatty acid, although it has not been fully characterized.[12] Lactoperoxidase, which has been shown to act with other substances in combating streptococci, is also found in human milk.[9] The combined effect suggests that human milk is superior to any other milk for infants.

Milk substitutes contain cholesterol concentrations ranging from 1.5 to 3.3 mg/100 ml,[5,29] whereas human milk contains 20 mg/100 ml. The amount of cholesterol needed by infants has not been established, but according to several studies[13,25] infants may require a moderate amount of dietary cholesterol to establish mechanisms for proper metabolism of cholesterol in later life. Research findings[13,24] imply that low-cholesterol formulas may contribute to arteriosclerosis in later life.

There are additional biochemical differences that exist between human milk and formulas. Human milk contains a rich supply of nucleotides, which are involved in nucleic acid synthesis.[12] The fatty acid composition of human milk substitutes varies appreciably from that of human milk, and lipase, an enzyme that enhances availability of free fatty acids, is present in large quantities only in human milk.[12] An infant has difficulty digesting the protein casein and digests whey proteins with relative ease. In cow's milk there is twice the amount of casein as in human milk, and in human milk there is three times the amount of whey protein as in cow's milk. It is apparent why the child ingesting cow's milk suffers from intestinal constipation, whereas the breast-fed child has a loose stool.

There is 43 mg/L vitamin C in human milk and only 11 mg/L in cow's milk. Pasteurization and/or storage destroys the vitamin C in cow's milk. Scurvy is not evidenced in breast-fed children. Clearly, an infant on cow's milk and formula starts life with difficulty in adapting biochemically to the environment. Cow's milk is intended for calves, not humans. The effects of cow's milk require an abnormal nutritional adaptation for an infant, with a resultant allergic response in many infants. Edematous mucous membranes then occur in the nasal and paranasal cavities, and the mouth-breathing habitus is initiated, which if continued through childhood, leads to malocclusion and a predisposition to TMJ disorders. (See section on mouth breathing.)

Healthy mothers can nurse

Several suggestions have been offered by Applebaum[1] and have proven very successful in my practice. The expectant mother who wishes to breast feed should begin preparation at least 2 months before the infant is born. Manual expression (hand nursing) stimulates the nerve endings and releases more prolactin, which builds her colostrum supply and starts the flow of oxytocin, which acts on the myoepithelial cells and gradually sets off the flow of colostrum, thereby helping to keep the ducts free from obstruction. The result is a faster and more abundant milk supply.

The woman should not use soap on the nipples for at least 6 weeks prior to giving birth. Soap will wash away the sebaceous secretion that forms a protective coat. During nursing, tight bras accumulate moisture, no evaporation takes place, and the skin becomes sensitive. Mothers can toughen the area by exposing the nipple to air when indoors during the day. When a bra must be worn during the day, a breast shield is an ex-

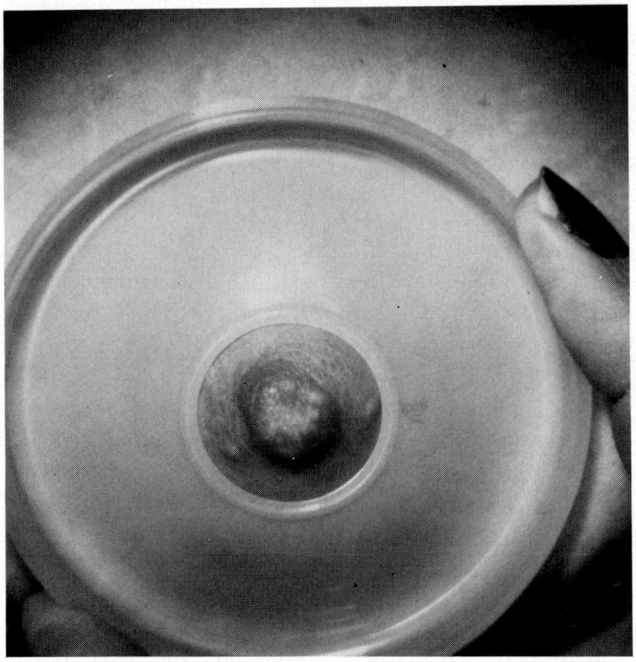

Fig. 4-10. Breast shields should be recommended to prevent sensitivity of human nipple from accumulation of moisture and lack of evaporation under a bra. NOTE: With separated shield, nipple is not confined against any material.

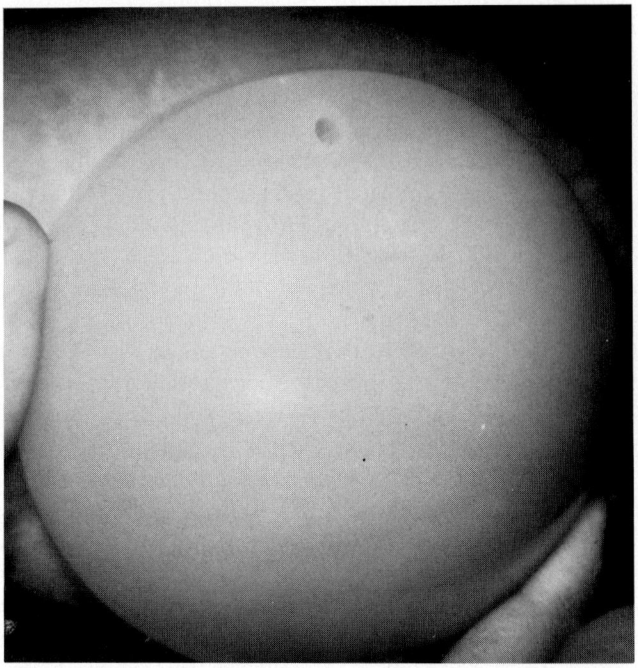

Fig. 4-11. Breast shield with ventilation channel at top to allow air to enter and circulate within shield. This toughens nipple.

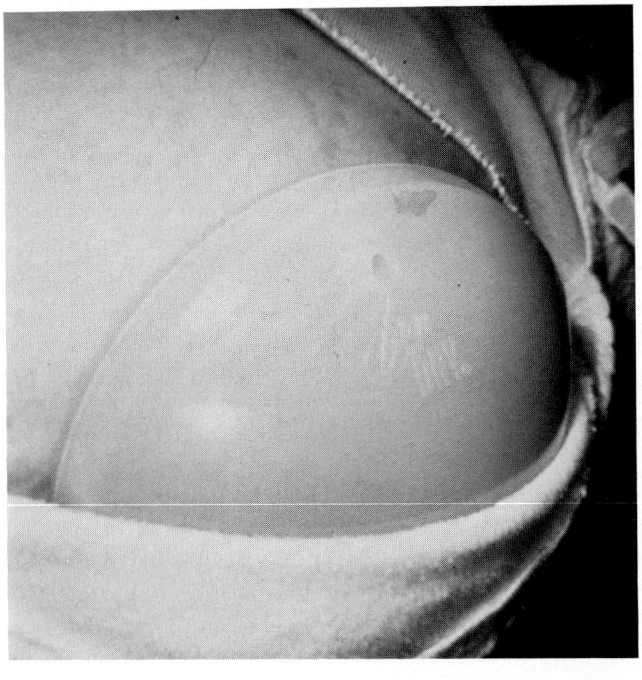

Fig. 4-12. Breast shield is worn under bra, and colostrum secreted during pregnancy and several days following delivery may be contained within shields.

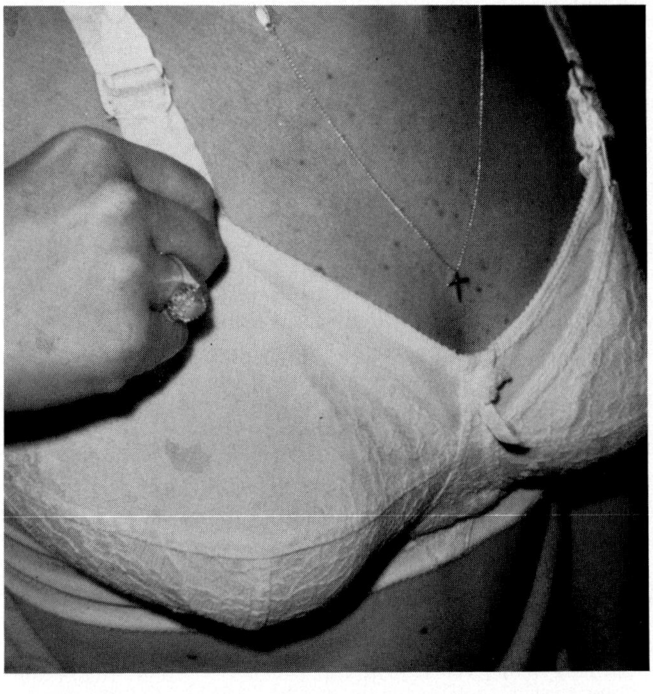

Fig. 4-13. Breast shields are not unsightly and stimulate evacuation of excess milk from breast. This relieves discomfort of swollen, engorged breasts.

cellent adjunct. The Free & Dry Breast Care Shield* collects the excess milk within the shield, and the milk will not penetrate the shield (Figs. 4-10 to 4-13). It applies gentle pressure around the nipples to help stimulate the evacuation of excess milk in the breasts and relieves the discomfort of swollen, engorged breasts. It is an aid in bringing forth inverted nipples for more comfortable and successful nursing.

Colostrum, secreted during pregnancy and for several days following delivery, may be contained within the shields, which are worn under the bra with the ventilation channel at the top to allow air to enter and circulate within the shield, which toughens the nipples. If nipples are sore or sensitive, Masse breast cream can be lightly massaged into the nipple and surrounding area.

When an expectant mother refuses to breast feed, after all the advantages have been discussed, recommend manual expression of milk, as described by Applebaum[1] in great detail. The breast pump is a second alternative with the advantage of having milk expressed directly into a bottle for storage.

SUBSTITUTES FOR BREAST FEEDING

Nuk Sager nipple

The Nuk Sager nipple is by no means an imitation of breast feeding, since Nature cannot be duplicated (Figs. 4-14 and 4-15). The Nuk nipple of today is not as pliable as the early version; however, it is the best physiological nipple on the market. The oral baglet is designed to broadly fit the anatomy of the baby's palate and inner arch. The nipple hole, being on top and toward the palate, distributes fluid over the palate and on top of the tongue and prolongs the time that milk is in the mouth. This enables digestion to initiate in the oral cavity rather than forcing unpredigested milk directly into the stomach. The tongue side of the baglet is cupped, causing the tongue to lie flatly under the Nuk Sager nipple and not around it, as with conventional nipples. The soft baglet has two inclined anterior guide planes or surfaces. These are designed to broadly and flatly contact important anterior elements of the upper and lower jaw during nursing. The conduit connecting the breast bulb and oral baglet is designed flat. The purpose of this is to encourage and enable the child to close the lips during nursing and to obtain full closure of the posterior elements of the jaw without negatively affecting the shape of the anterior gum pads. A further purpose of the flat passage is to encourage coordinated nasal breathing and create a seal at the corners of the mouth to reduce sucking and swallowing of air (which occurs with conventional nipples), thereby reducing the likelihood of colic. The upper part of the bulb is slightly in front of the lower part so the upper lip comes immediately in contact with it. Since the lower part of the bulb is slightly behind the upper, there is a slight freeway space opposite the lower lip that allows the baby to freely work the mandible forward and backward in an elliptical motion. Once a round nipple is used, it is very difficult to transfer the infant to a Nuk. Therefore, by starting the child on the Nuk, it will be accepted. The expectant parent should bring a Nuk nipple to the hospital and have it sterilized to be used as the initial nipple post partum.

It is important to boil the Nuk nipple approximately 5 minutes prior to use. The orifice will constrict and prevent a rapid flow of milk, thereby satisfying the sucking reflex. The color of the nipple will lighten without affecting the efficiency.

Conventional nipples

Humans have done a poor job in attempting to mimic the soft, supple, warm natural breast by creating a comparatively hard, round, rubber nipple that changes the configuration of the orofacial musculature compared with that of breast-fed infants (Figs. 4-16 and 4-17). Parents sometimes enlarge the orifice of conventional nipples, thereby reducing the energy exertion necessary to satisfy the infant's sucking reflex. In addition, large amounts of milk flow from the nipple, causing the infant to thrust the tongue forward to avoid drowning. The orifice of a nipple should never be enlarged unless no milk flow is evidenced. Clinically, a drowning infant will have milk draining from the corners of the mouth; this somewhat common *drowning phenomenon* initiates a tongue thrust response.

The configuration of a conventional nipple displaces the tongue from its normal breast-nursing posture. The tongue wraps around the nipple, and its dorsum is positioned away from the palate (Figs. 4-18 and 4-19). The results are an abnormal configuration of the intrinsic muscles of the tongue, which constricts its lateral borders, and an abnormal contraction of the infrahyoid and suprahyoid musculature, which are primarily concerned with swallowing, speech, and postural position. In many cases another result is a retained infantile swallow. In addition, the orbicularis oris muscle becomes distorted because of the nonphysiological form to which it must accommodate itself (Piccard's lip).

PATTERNS OF SWALLOWING

Infantile swallow (visceral)

An infant who is first attempting to suckle the breast may seem to turn the head away from the nipple. If one strokes the infant's cheek with the nipple, he or

Text continued on p. 50.

*Monterey Laboratories, Inc., Box 15129, Las Vegas, Nev. 89114.

A

B

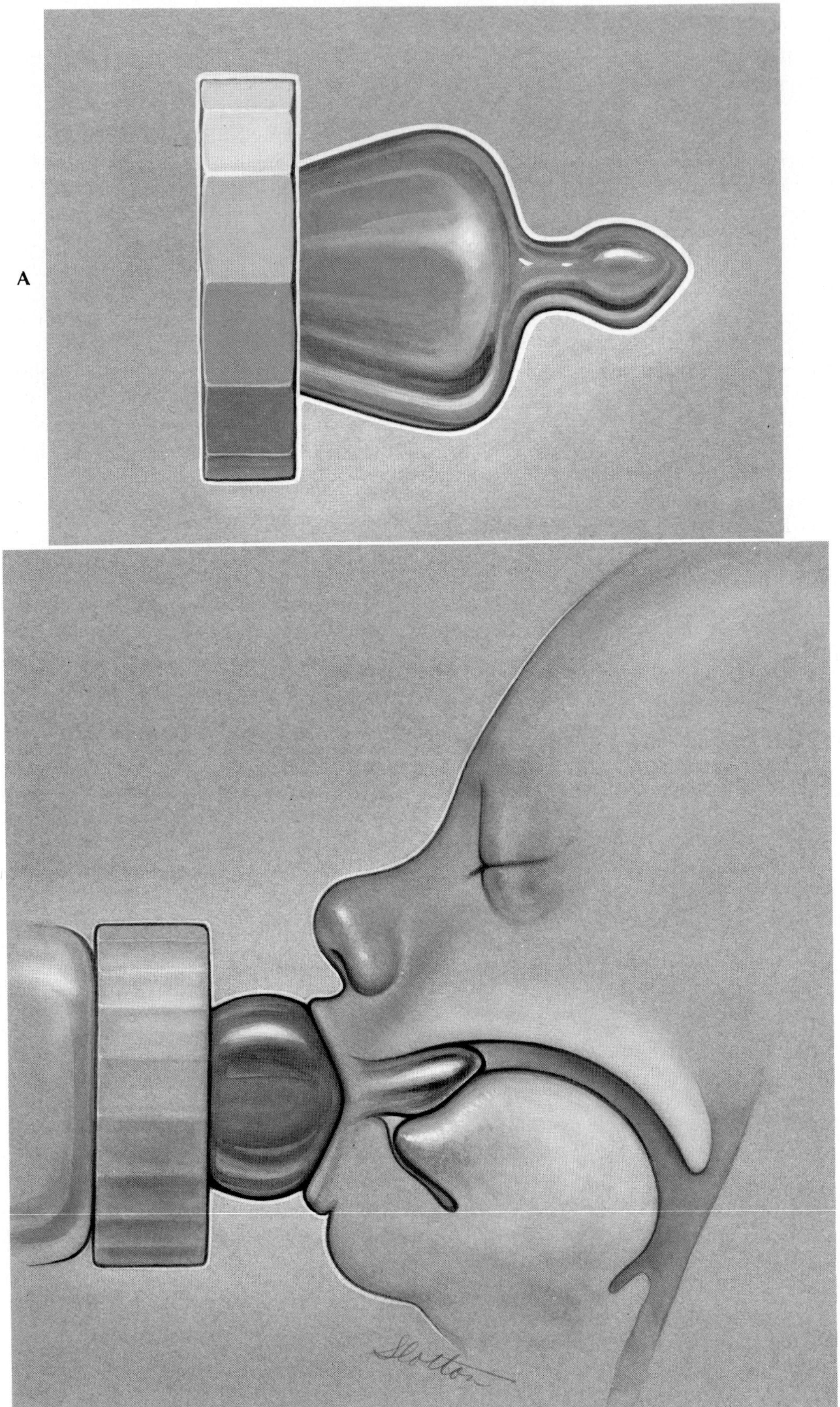

Fig. 4-14. A, Nuk Sager nipple. **B,** Oral baglet is designed to fit anatomy of baby's palate. Tongue lies flat under nipple and not around it. As with conventional nipples, it allows mandible to work forward and backward, as in nursing, and creates a seal at corner of mouth to prevent swallowing of air.

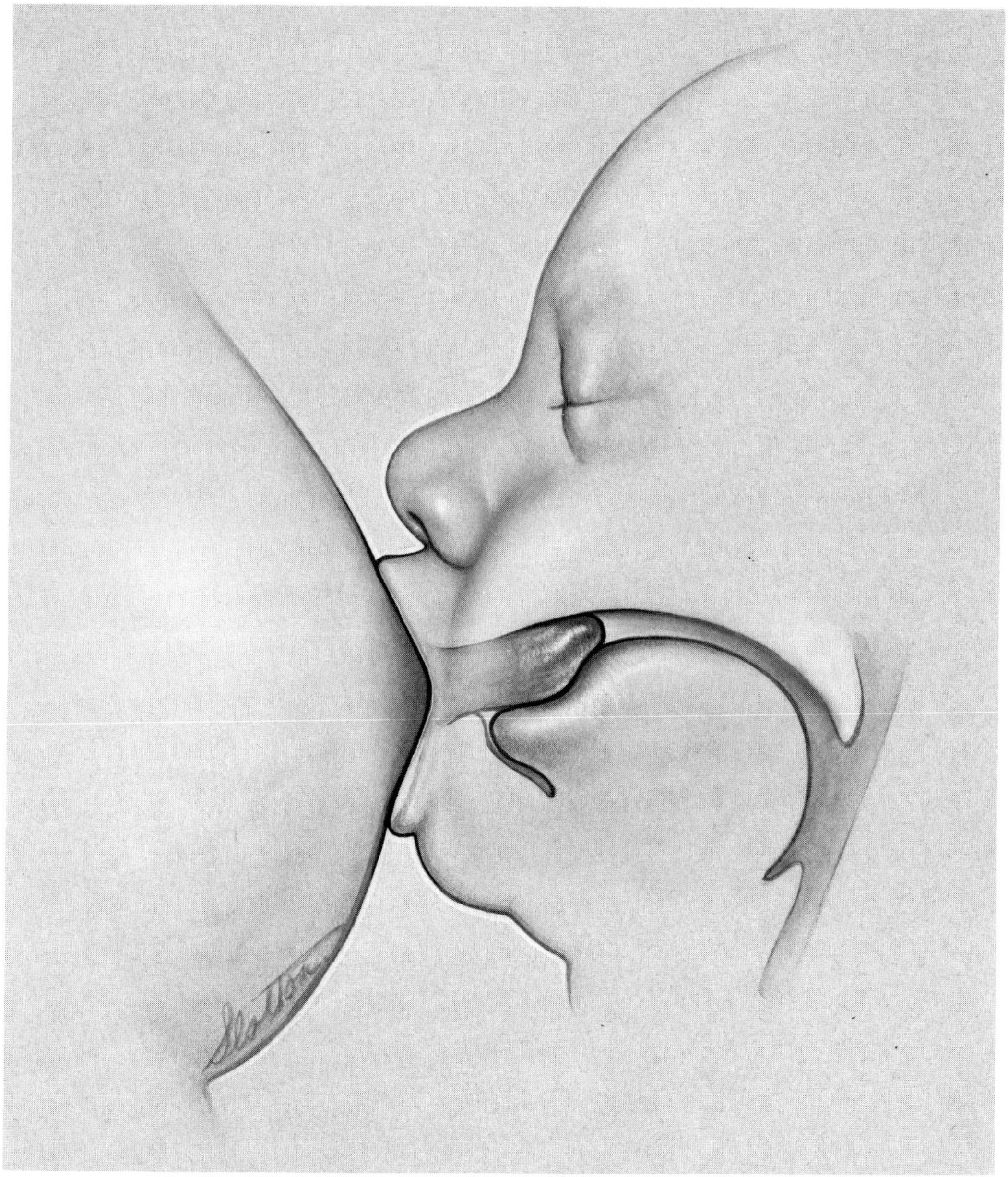

Fig. 4-15. Breast nipple: note similarity of tongue configuration between Nuk feeding and breast feeding. Action of mandible is also comparable. There is tight lip seal around the areola, and more energy is expended than during artificial feeding.

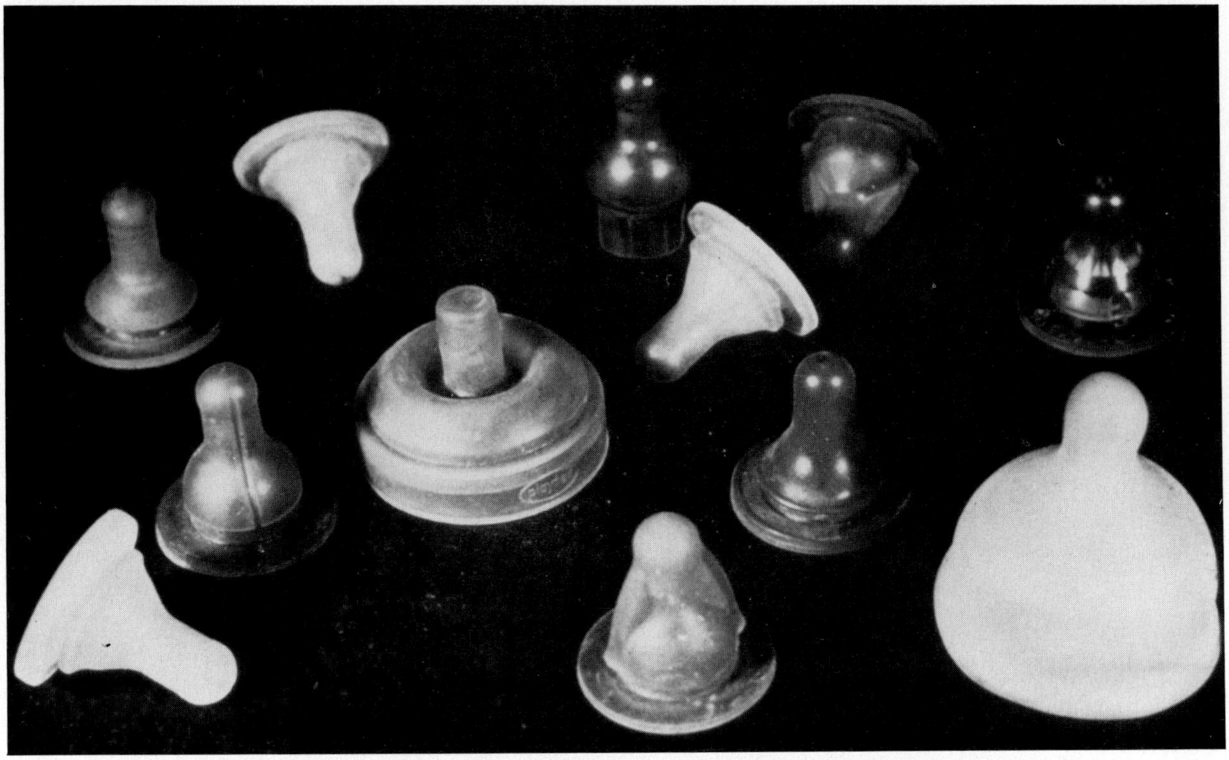

Fig. 4-16. Conventional nipples: society's contribution to orofacial muscle imbalance and predisposition to TMJ dysfunction. When compared with supple human breast, the round configuration and lack of flexibility distort extraoral and intraoral musculature and thereby alter infant's orofacial muscle function.

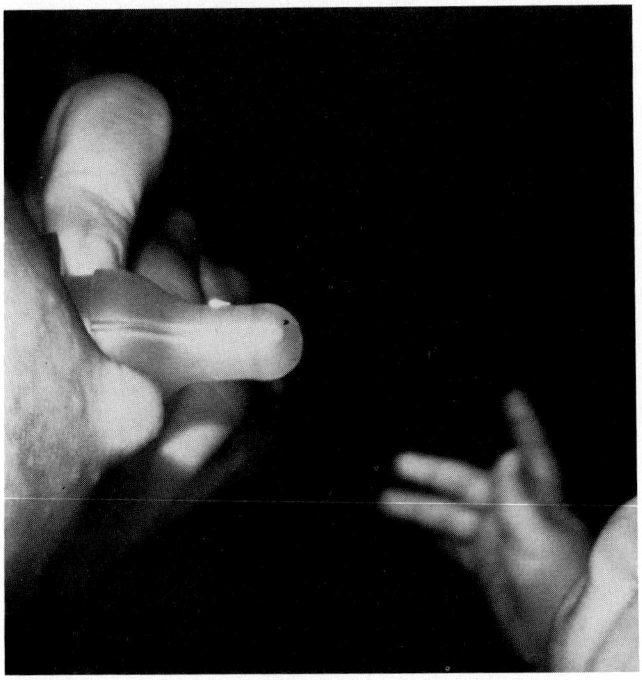

Fig. 4-17. Human nipple and artificial nipple: configuration of conventional nipple displaces tongue from its normal breast-feeding posture and distorts lips and tongue.

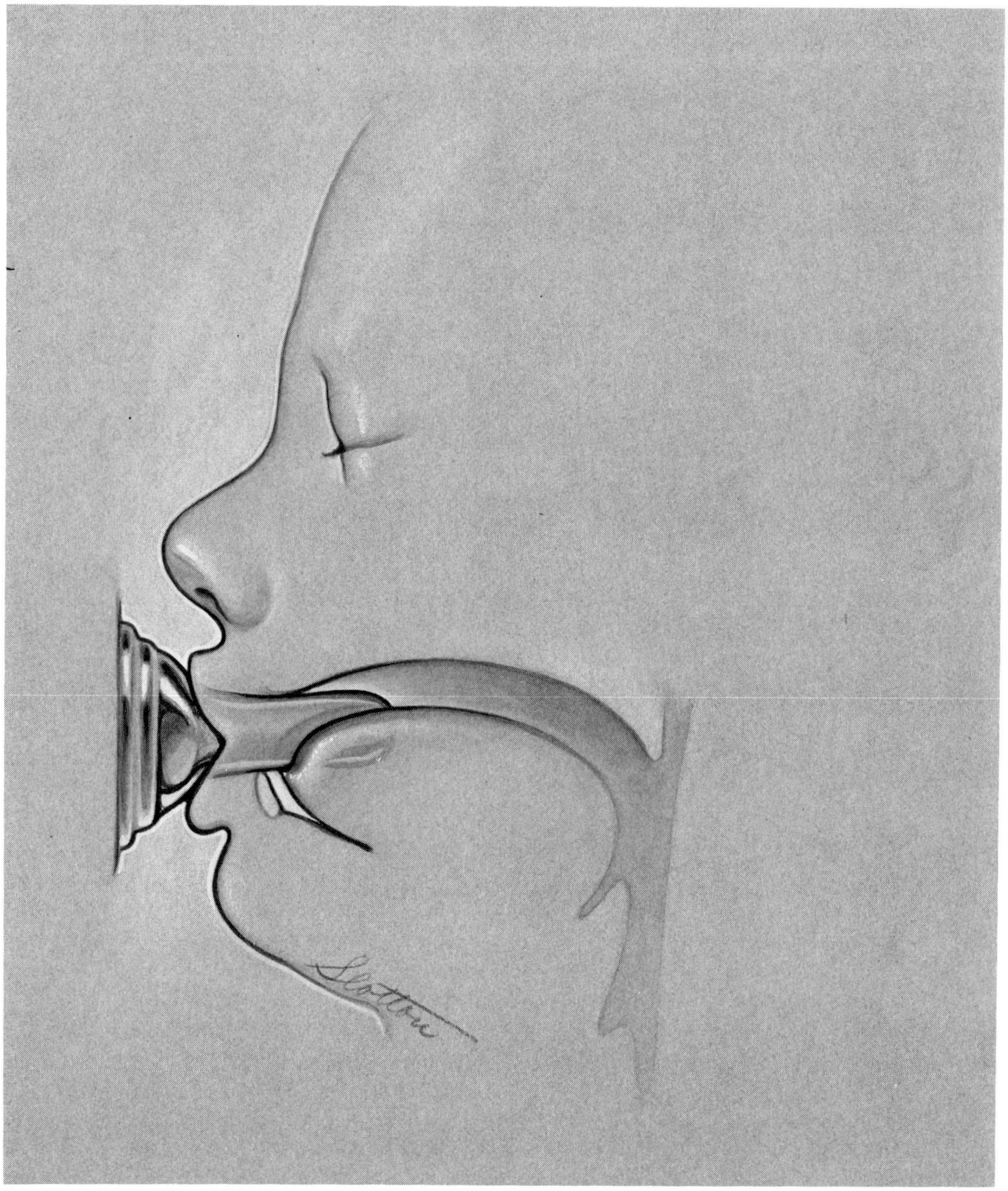

Fig. 4-18. Conventional nipple: tongue wraps around nipple, and its dorsum is positioned away from palate.

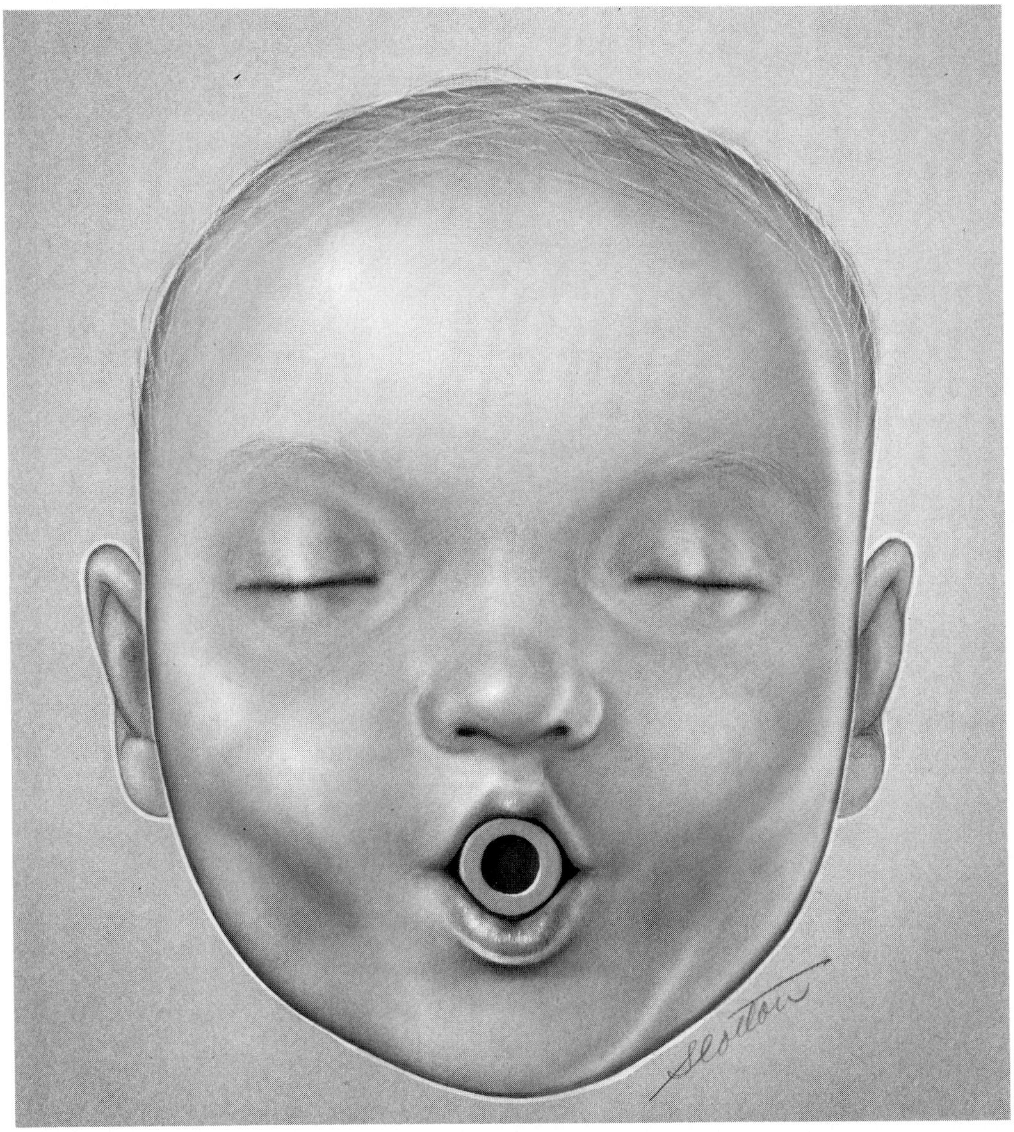

Fig. 4-19. Conventional nipple: there is no seal at corners of mouth, lips are not flat and become hypotonic, cheeks cave in, and tongue wraps around nipple rather than flattening, as in nursing.

she will automatically turn toward it. This is called the *rooting reflex*. The infant will employ the entire facial musculature while seeking food from the mother. Clinical observations of a nursing child reveal that the jaws are apart, the mandible stabilized forward by the tongue and facial muscles, with a tight seal around the areolar margin (Fig. 4-20), which is compressed between the tongue and gum pad while the tongue undulates anteroposteriorly along the areola. The nipple is drawn back well into the infant's mouth where it is compressed by suction against the hard palate by the tongue and cheek muscles. The milk will then flow from the high positive pressure of the breast into the negative pressure in the infant's mouth by *compression* and *suction*. After several nursing actions the milk accumulates on top of the tongue by sealing the posterior portion of the oral cavity between the soft palate and back of the tongue. Once the milk has accumulated, the infant will swallow the partially predigested milk.

The infantile swallow is characterized by a nursing plungerlike action of the tongue (tongue thrust), a perioral sphincter action to create a seal around the areola (pursed lips), and a mandibular thrust to fix the mandible forward against the mother's breast. The tongue lies over the gum pads, and the cheek pads flow between the posterior gum pads during nursing.

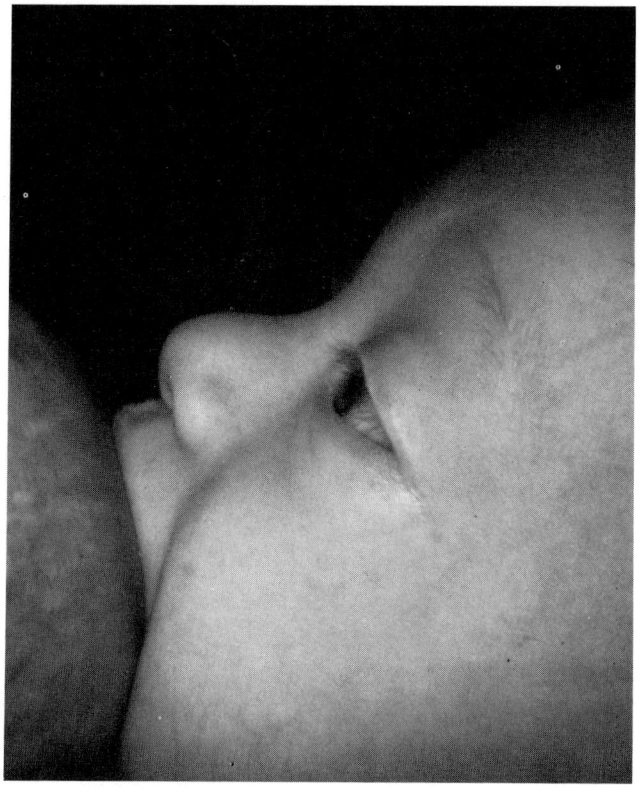

Fig. 4-20. Nursing child: jaws are apart, mandible moves anteroposteriorly in elliptical motion, tongue undulates anteroposteriorly along areola, lips create a seal, and by compression and suction milk flows from high positive pressure within breast to negative pressure in infant's mouth.

Transitional swallow

The only swallowing variation between an infant and a young child with a retained infantile swallow is that as maturation occurs the mandible is no longer stabilized forward by facial muscles. The glenoid fossa develops rapidly, and the condyle becomes oriented within the fossa because of rapid maturation of the muscles of mastication.

During the transitional stage between the infantile swallow and the mature swallow (which is usually the period when the infant is introduced to solid foods) the infant expels food with the tongue, forcing the parent to catch it with the feeding spoon. This unlearned reflex disappears as the child matures, provided there is no retention of noxious habits such as placing appendages or objects into the mouth, no chronic upper respiratory tract allergies, no chronic hypertrophied tonsils or adenoids, and no genetic orofacial deformities that continually displace the tongue, lips, and cheeks, creating abnormal force vectors against the palate and erupting dentition.

Mature swallowing pattern

The mature swallow evolves slowly. At birth the tongue is too large for the oral cavity and lies over the gum pads. There is no proprioception for its lateral borders because of lack of teeth. Slow transitional change in the swallowing pattern occurs when deciduous teeth begin to erupt. The tongue becomes contained within the framework of the dental arches by proprioception. The mandibular posture is no longer prognathous and is now controlled by the muscles of mastication rather than by facial muscles. Mature swallowing characteristics are evidenced at approximately $1^1/_2$ years of age, provided noxious habits have been controlled, there are no serious upper respiratory tract allergic manifestations such as chronic mouth breathing, and there are no chronic hypertrophied tonsils and/or adenoids.

If a mature swallow does not develop because of continued displacement of the tongue, lips, and cheeks, form and function are affected as a result of intraoral and extraoral muscle imbalance. The lips become weak and the tongue hypotonic, the teeth develop a malocclusion, and there is characteristic facial expression during the so-called abnormal swallow. The lips purse, the mentalis muscle overcontracts, and the cheeks cave in at the corners of the mouth (Figs. 4-21 to 4-24).

In a mature swallow there is no facial grimace such as pursed lips, the teeth occlude, and lateral borders of the tongue are confined within the dental arch. The tip

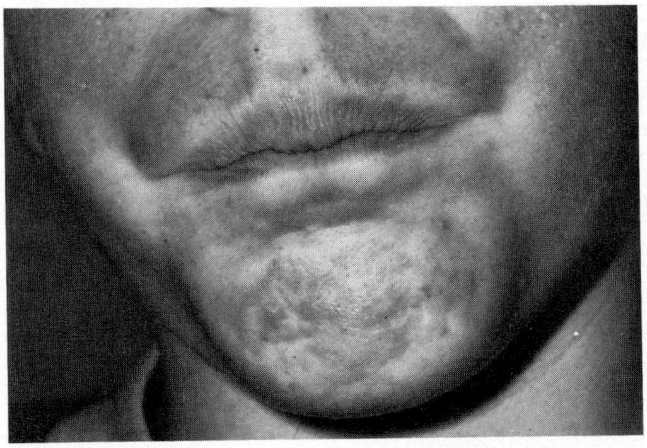

Fig. 4-21. Orofacial muscle imbalance (tongue thrust) involves overcontraction of mentalis muscle, pursed lips, and abnormal muscle force vectors at corners of mouth (modiolus) during swallowing.

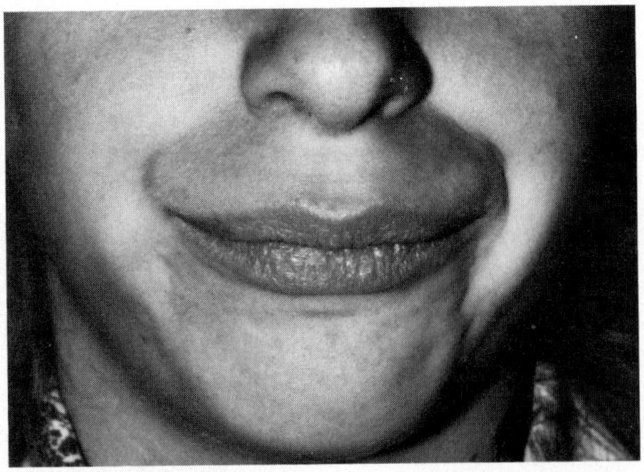

Fig. 4-22. Orofacial muscle imbalance: facial grimaces are similar in all tongue thrusters when swallowing.

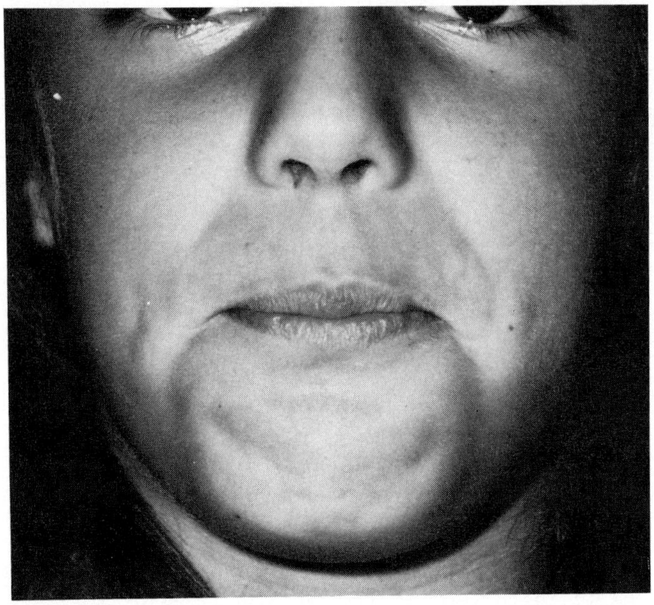

Fig. 4-23. Orofacial muscle imbalance: facial grimace occurs during swallowing. Mentalis muscle overcontracts to prevent tongue from thrusting through lips, thereby breaking lip seal required during swallowing.

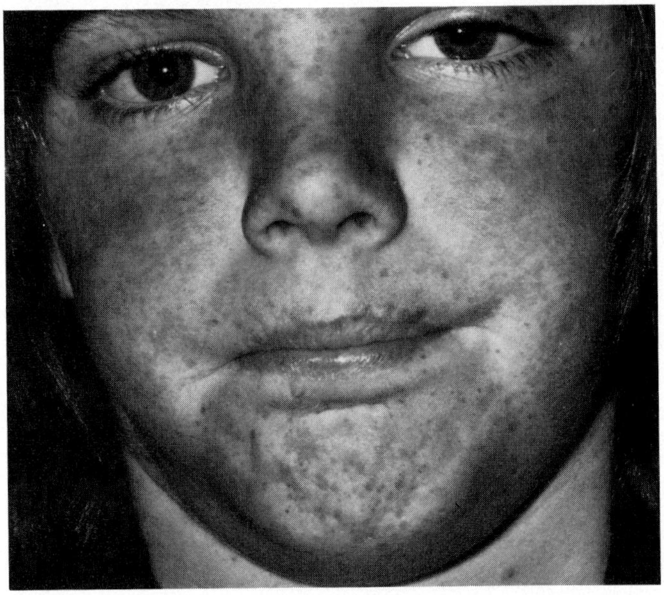

Fig. 4-24. Orofacial muscle imbalance: facial grimace force vectors and tongue force vectors create malocclusion and potentiate TMJ dysfunction.

of the tongue is held against the palate above and behind the incisors. Moyers' work[20] in the 1940s using electromyography to plot normal and abnormal muscle function is a classic study. His recordings indicated a difference between the use of facial muscles in the suckle swallow and their relative nonuse in the mature swallow. He concluded that the muscles of facial expression are active in support of the infantile swallow pattern but play only a minor role in the mature pattern.

Graber's study[10] on comparative muscle pressures during a normal swallow corroborate the conclusions of Moyers.[20] Only the external and internal pterygoid, middle temporal, and anterior and posterior masseter fibers show moderate activity. The remaining muscles, including the facial group, show only slight activity, whereas in an abnormal swallow there is a relatively large component of facial muscle activity and an altered pattern in the muscles of mastication.

EFFECTS OF MUSCLE IMBALANCE

When the terms *tongue thrust, deviate swallow, abnormal swallow, orofacial muscle imbalance,* and *retained infantile swallow* are used, the references usually are related to a clinical manifestation whereby the tongue protrudes anteriorly or laterally over the dentition during a swallow, the lips purse, and the mentalis muscle overcontracts. Clinically, the teeth may be intruded, crowded, or protruded with diastema, depending on where the tongue force vectors are directed. The tongue may act as an impeding force to eruption if its posture or repose is such that its lateral borders lie between the dentition. There may be an open bite anteriorly or posteriorly or a collapse of the maxillary and mandibular arches (See Figs. 4-31 and 4-32.)

Tongue repose is one of the most important etiological factors of orofacial muscle imbalance. Since constant light forces move teeth, it becomes clear why the relationship of the tongue influences tooth position.

An imbalance between extraoral and intraoral musculature will affect the position of deciduous as well as permanent teeth. The malposed teeth cause the mandible to accommodate for occlusion, thus initiating a predisposition to TMJ dysfunction. Every dental practitioner has seen conditions such as cross-bites, open bites, dental Class II malocclusions, pseudo–Class III malocclusions, lingually inclined mandibular incisors, and protruded maxillary incisors that have resulted from an imbalance of muscle forces initiated by noxious habits, upper respiratory tract allergic manifestations such as chronic mouth breathing, and/or chronic enlarged tonsils and adenoids. Skeletal or genetic malocclusions also can be complicated by orofacial muscle imbalance.

The maxillomandibular dentition is surrounded extraorally by a group of muscles that act in unison as a sphincter on the buccal and labial surfaces of teeth, creating force vectors that move teeth within the dental arch. Intraoral musculature should be in balance with extraoral musculature to maintain a stable dentition.

The shape of the buccal orifice and the posture of the lips are controlled by a complex assembly of muscular slips. These include elevators and retractors of the upper lip (levator labii superioris alaeque nasi, levator labii superioris, zygomaticus major and minor, levator anguli oris, and risorius), depressors, retractors, and elevators of the lower lip (depressor labii inferioris, depressor anguli oris, and mentalis), and a sphincter (orbicularis oris, buccinator, and superior constrictor of the pharynx). Some eight or nine muscles converge on each of the two angles of the mouth and interlace at a palpable nodular mass, the modiolus. This can be fixed in any given position by the combined action of the zygomaticus major, levator anguli oris, and the depressor anguli oris. These serve to fix the attachments of the orbicularis oris and buccinator in this area. To simplify the terminology for the combined action of all circumoropharyngeal muscles that create extraoral force vectors on the dentition, the term *buccinator mechanism* has been employed.

Buccinator mechanism

The term *buccinator mechanism* applies to a group of muscles consisting primarily of the buccinator, orbicularis oris, and superior constrictor of the pharynx. The buccinator is a thin quadrilateral muscle, occupying the interval between the maxilla and mandible in the cheek and attached to the alveolar process of the maxilla and mandible and behind to the anterior border of the pterygomandibular raphe, which separates the muscle from the superior constrictor of the pharynx. To complete the sphincter action, fibers of the buccinator converge anteriorly toward the angle of the mouth where the central fibers intersect each other, those from below being continuous with the upper segment of the orbicularis oris and those from above with the lower segment.

The buccinator mechanism therefore is a continuous band of muscles that act as an extraoral mold and support for the dental arch and contain the muscular tongue (Fig. 4-25). Any imbalance between the buccinator mechanism and the tongue will move teeth within the dental arch, creating predisposition to malocclusion and TMJ dysfunction. Only neuromuscular accommodation allows a patient to survive for years without adverse symptoms. However, the potential is always present when orofacial muscle imbalance exists.

Muscles of the tongue

When myofunctional therapy is employed to balance extraoral and intraoral force vectors on the dentition, the tongue musculature must balance with the buccinator mechanism.

The tongue is divided into right and left halves by a median fibrous septum and fixed below by the body of the hyoid. In each half there are two sets of muscles, extrinsic and intrinsic. Extrinsic muscles have attachments outside the tongue, and intrinsic muscles are contained within it.

The extrinsic muscles include the genioglossus, hyoglossus, styloglossus, chondroglossus, and palatoglossus. They protrude, depress, and raise the tongue upward and backward.

The intrinsic muscles are the superior and inferior longitudinal, the transverse, and the vertical. These muscles alter the shape of the tongue. The superior and inferior longitudinal muscles shorten the tongue, but in addition, the former turns the tip of the tongue up-

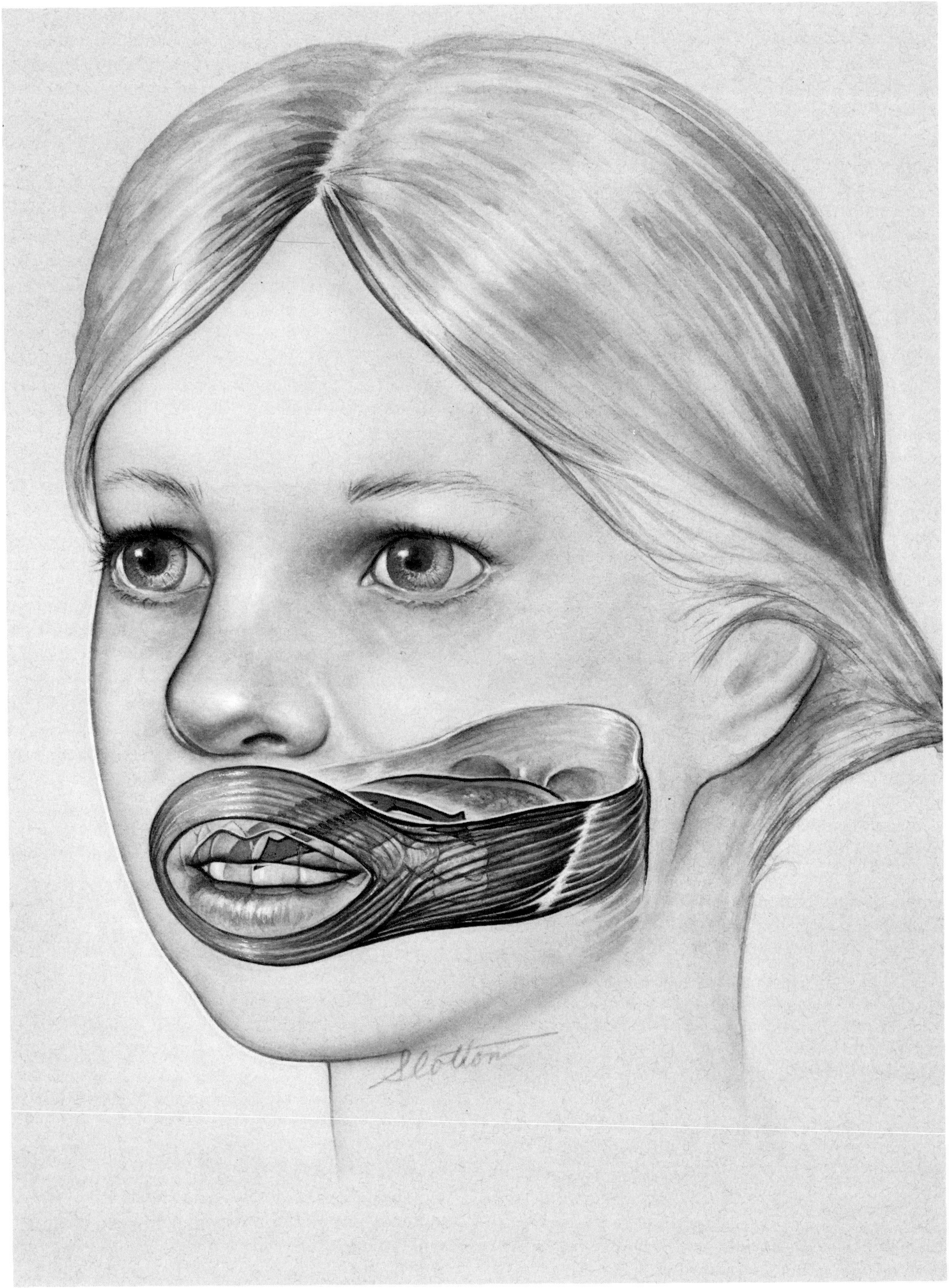

Fig. 4-25. Buccinator mechanism is continuous band of muscles (orbicularis oris, buccinator, and superior of the pharynx) that acts as extraoral mold and support for dental arch and contains muscular tongue.

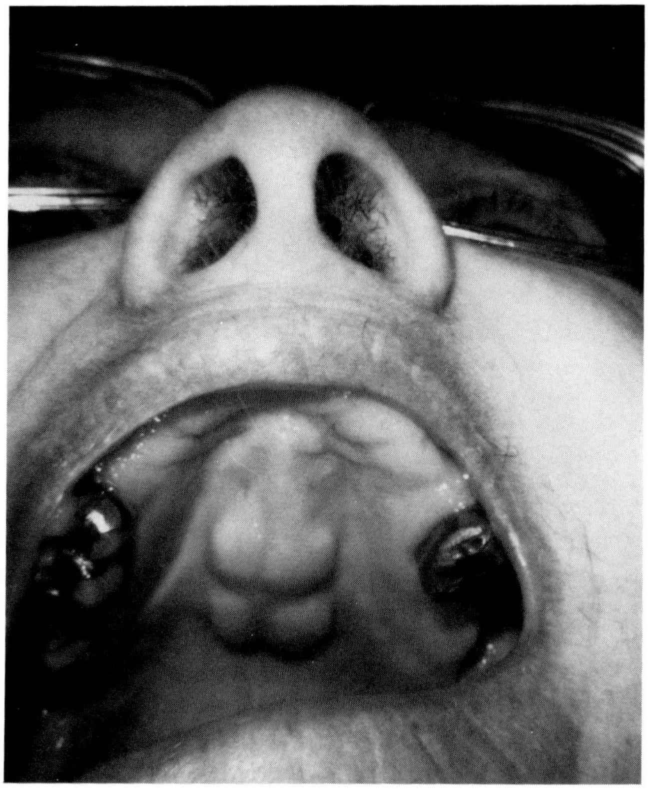

Fig. 4-26. Torus palatinus may create indentation of tongue corresponding to shape of torus. Fig. 4-28 shows the clinical result.

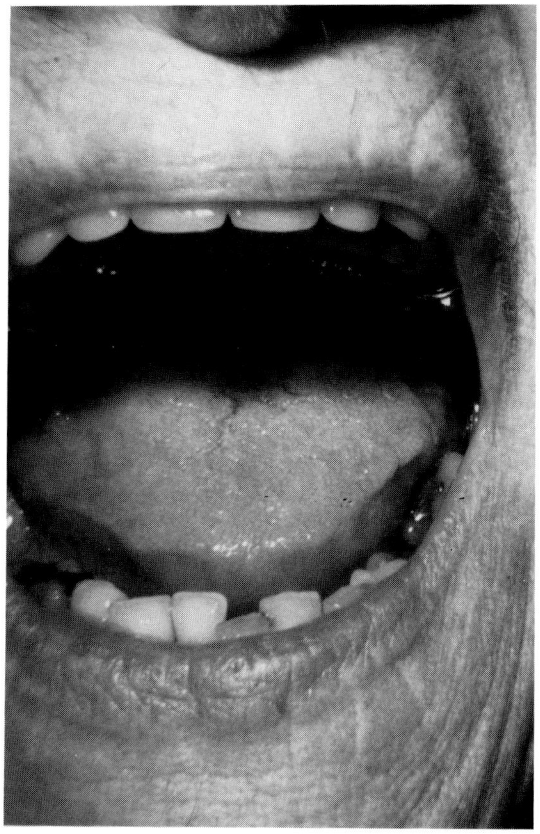

Fig. 4-27. Torus palatinus: note indentations on lower border of tongue caused by lingual version of posterior teeth created as tongue arched around torus palatinus. This will predispose patient to TMJ dysfunction.

ward, creating a concavity, and the latter pulls the tip downward and renders the dorsum convex. The transverse muscle narrows and elongates the tongue, and the vertical muscle flattens and broadens it.

As teeth erupt into the oral cavity, the lateral and anterior borders of the tongue are stimulated by proprioception to constrict and create light forces that balance teeth in a neutral position within the buccinator mechanism. When this delicate balance is altered, the dentition is altered. An extreme example is the patient without a tongue (aglossia). The entire maxillary and mandibular dentition collapses.

A small mouth with tight lips (microstomia) in combination with a very small tongue results in small dental arches and crowding of the teeth, even though the jaws are of normal size and relationship.[14] Harvold's animal experiments,[14] as well as clinical observations, have demonstrated that a reduction in tongue size is followed by a corresponding collapse of the dental arches. He also found that a plastic insert in the palatal vault produces an indentation of the tongue corresponding to the shape of the insert. This is comparable to a very large torus mandibularis, etc. will alter the configuration and and indentations of the lower border of the tongue caused by lingual version of posterior teeth created as the tongue arched around the torus palatinus (Figs. 4-26 and 4-27).

A torus mandibularis can also cause the tongue to deviate from its normal position by proprioception. The tongue will find an accommodative position by selective contraction of the intrinsic and extrinsic muscles, which may result in poor tongue repose and malposed teeth. If large bilateral mandibular tori are present, the tongue may deviate away from the larger torus, since the proprioceptive mechanism is stimulated to a greater degree at the primary point of contact (Figs. 4-28 and 4-29). Tori that are large should be removed surgically.

Muscles of the tongue will seek an accommodative position during a swallow by thrusting away from the primary stimulation (for example, enlarged tonsils), creating forces against the teeth that result in open bites, cross-bites, and/or protruding teeth (Fig. 4-30).

Continuous displacement of the tongue by an object, finger, thumb, tonsils, adenoids, torus palatinus,

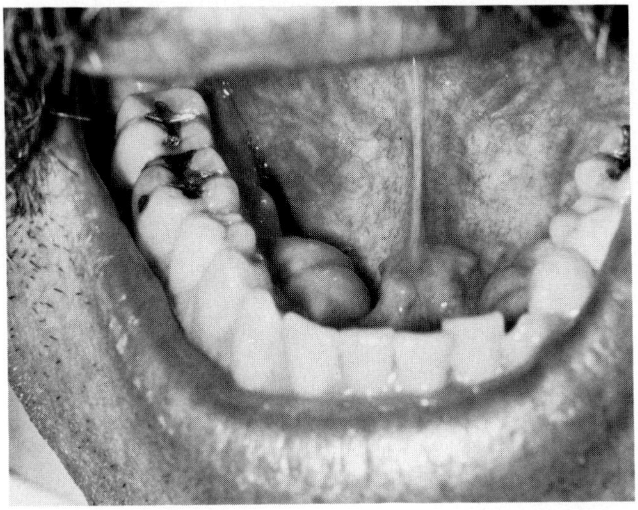

Fig. 4-28. Torus mandibularis: torus on patient's right is larger than on left. Therefore the tongue will find an accommodative position by selective contraction of intrinsic and extrinsic muscles.

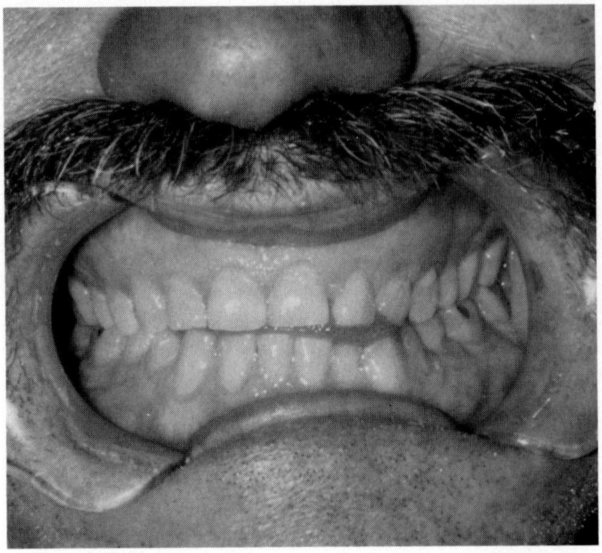

Fig. 4-29. Torus mandibularis: when patient (Fig. 4-28) was asked to close his mouth, tongue repose accommodated to left and anteriorly away from primary point of contact. Bite was open because of impeding force of tongue.

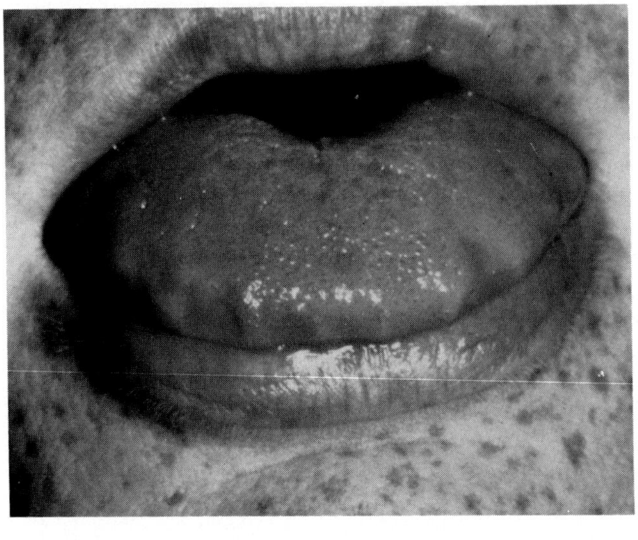

Fig. 4-30. Note tooth indentations on borders of tongue caused by accommodative position of tongue as a result of chronically enlarged tonsils. Continuous light forces move teeth. Therefore removal of tonsils and adenoids should be considered prior to orthodontia or TMJ orientation.

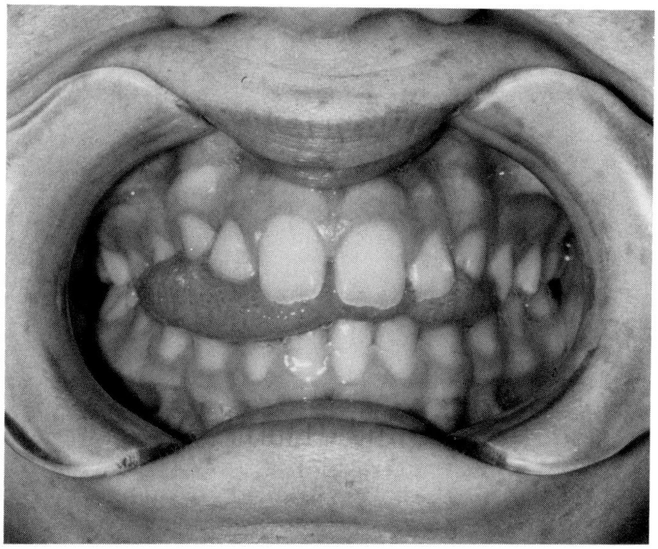

Fig. 4-31. Hypotonic tongue: continuous displacement of tongue will impede eruption of teeth wherever tongue protrudes. Myofunctional therapy and orthodontia can correct this pathologic condition. Posterior teeth are occluding.

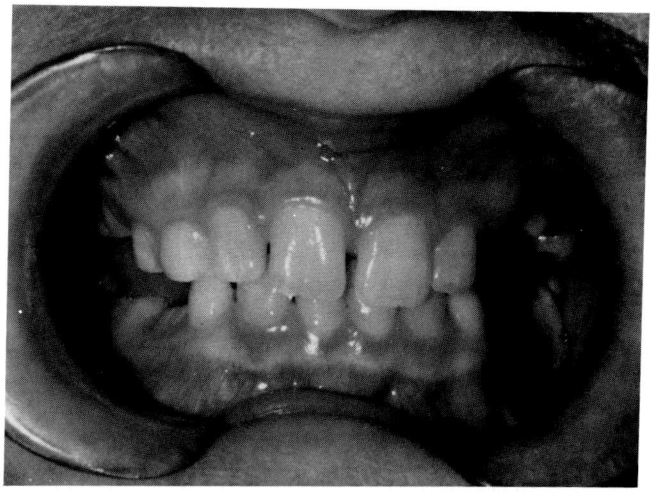

Fig. 4-32. Posterior open bite of patient as a result of tongue repose. Teeth are in occlusion.

torus mandibularis, etc. will alter the configuration and muscular pattern of the tongue, causing abnormal stresses on the dentition (Figs. 4-31 and 4-32).

Harvold[14] found that stimulation of the posterior part of the tongue makes it narrow and pointed, resulting in an open bite and a narrowing of the dental arches. This is comparable to the effect of chronically enlarged tonsils and adenoids. If a tonsil is enlarged unilaterally, the tongue will deviate away from the hypertrophied tonsil at its dorsum, forcing the tip of the tongue into a deviant orientation and distorting the dentition (Fig. 4-33). Bilateral chronic hypertrophy of the tonsils will force the tongue anteriorly and create an open bite in humans as well as in rhesus monkeys (Figs. 4-34 and 4-35). If there is a chronic hypertrophy of the tonsils and adenoids, the patient should have them removed before any orthodontic treatment or TMJ orientation is attempted.

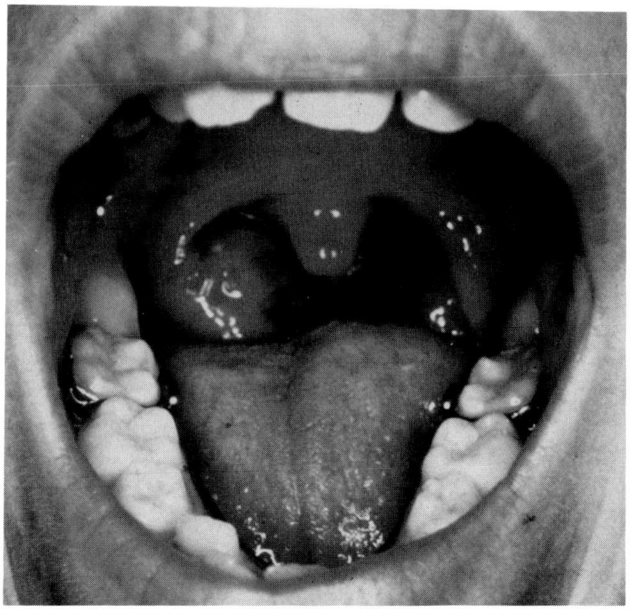

Fig. 4-33. Unilateral chronic hypertrophied tonsil: stimulation of posterior part of tongue makes it narrow and pointed. Tongue deviates away from hypertrophied tonsil at its dorsum, forcing tip of tongue into a deviant orientation, distorting dentition.

Ankyloglossia

The median plane of the tongue is connected to the floor of the mouth by the frenulum linguae. When the attachment of the frenulum approximates the tip of the tongue, a child is unable to protrude the tip of the tongue or raise the tip to the roof of the mouth when it is open. The term *tongue-tied* has been applied to this condition. In addition, the child may have a noticeable lisp during speech, especially with sibilant sounds.

The superior longitudinal muscle of the tongue is limited in function, since its action is restricted by an

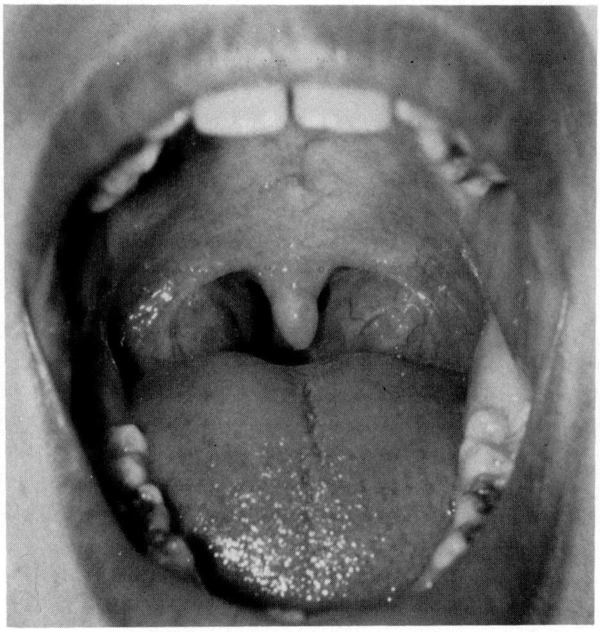

Fig. 4-34. Bilateral chronic hypertrophied tonsils will, by proprioception, force tongue anterior and create open bite.

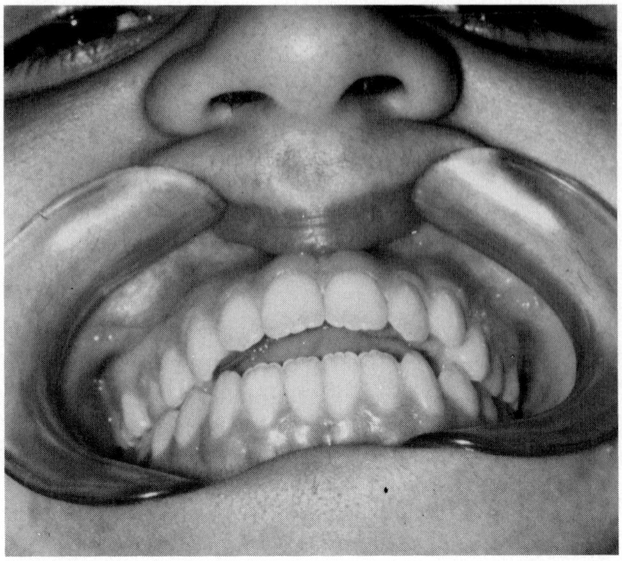

Fig. 4-35. Open bite resulting from continual anterior displacement of tongue.

inability to lift the tip of the tongue upward. The vertical muscles of the tongue become overactive as they flatten and broaden the tongue (Fig. 4-36).

When the tongue is confined within the dental arches, there is a tendency for the arches to expand as the tongue broadens. However, the tip of the tongue may create a dental or pseudo–Class III malocclusion if the tongue force vectors are directed against the lingual surfaces of the mandibular incisors. On the other hand, if the tongue is not confined within the dentition as it broadens and extrudes laterally over the dental arches, the arches will become narrow because of an imbalance between the intraoral and extraoral musculature.

When the tip of the tongue is held back from the lingual and incisal surfaces of the mandibular incisors, the incisors will extrude, resulting in a closed bite and maxillary protrusion.

An oral examination must include the tongue and its attachments. Have the patient open the mouth and lift the tip of the tongue to the palate. If limited movement is noted, a lingual frenectomy is recommended before attempting orthodontia or TMJ orientation.

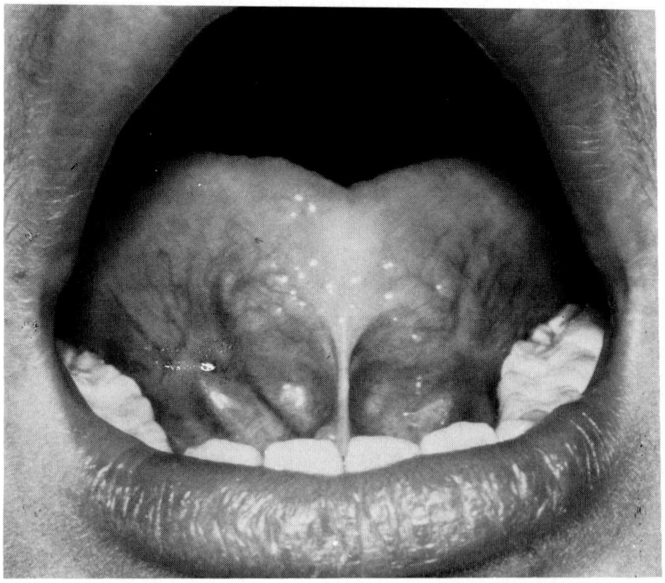

Fig. 4-36. Ankyloglossia: frenulum linguae attachment approximates tip of tongue, preventing normal tongue movement during speech and swallowing. If dental arch or speech is affected, frenectomy should be done.

Muscles of mastication

All masticatory movements are carried out primarily by six masticatory muscles: the external pterygoid, the internal pterygoid, the masseter, the temporal, the anterior belly of the digastric, and the geniohyoid. There are basically two kinds of movements resulting from the contraction of these muscles: translatory movement and rotary movement. Rotary movement is when the mandible turns on an axis. Translatory movement is when the entire body of the mandible moves in a straight line. The geniohyoid and both bellies of the digastric muscles rotate the mandible, and the condyles are brought forward by simultaneous contraction of both external pterygoids when the jaw opens. The direction of pull of the external pterygoids is forward, inward, and downward. The anterior belly of the digastric and geniohyoid muscles affects mandibular rotation by its posterior pull on the mandible. The opening muscles of the mandible therefore are the digastric, geniohyoid, and external pterygoid.

The three primary closing muscles are the masseter, temporal, and the internal pterygoid. These muscles exert a slightly anterior and superior pull on the mandible.

Muscles of mastication become more active as the child progresses from an infantile swallow to a mature swallow. However, when the infantile swallow is retained, there is a generalized weakening of the muscles of mastication. These muscles can be strengthened by myofunctional therapy exercises.

ALLERGIES

Allergies and mouth breathing

Allergies of the edematous mucous membranes of the paranasal cavity and sinuses occur early in infancy. Mouth breathing has been evidenced in infants allergic to cow's milk, as determined by a nasal smear that shows a 4+ eosinophilia.[17] Most mouth breathing in children is caused secondarily from obstruction of the nasal cavities by allergic edema of the mucous membranes.

The pterygoid plexus is a reservoir that receives veins which drain from the maxillae and the nasal and paranasal cavities. When allergic edema occurs because of the release of histamines, it interferes with venous drainage, causing distal venous congestion in the dental alveoli and surrounding tissues, with a resultant anoxia and acidosis (Fig. 4-37). The result may be premature exfoliation or retention of primary teeth and weakening of the containing musculature of the dental arch. Thus the predisposition to early orofacial dental deformities and TMJ dysfunction has been initiated. When the edematous nasal and paranasal mucous membranes restrict the airway, mouth breathing becomes a compensatory function (Figs. 4-38 and 4-39).

Mouth breathing may occur by anatomical blockage such as by enlarged turbinates and deviated septums. However, this is relatively insignificant in terms of numbers of mouth breathers and can be handled surgically in the vast majority of cases. In 1926 Duke[7] reported a 32% incidence of deviated nasal septums occurring in patients with chronic nasal allergy. The defect probably arises from the same factors that cause the oral and dentofacial abnormalities resulting from sensitization to cow's milk in infancy and from early feeding of adult-type foods containing synthetic ingredients.

Chronic mouth breathing

Chronic mouth breathing will result in malocclusion, since the lateral and anterior borders of the tongue are no longer confined within the dentition and therefore no longer offset the constant buccinator mechanism force vectors against the buccal and labial surfaces of the teeth. The primary etiology of chronic mouth breathing in children is upper respiratory tract allergies and/or enlarged tonsils and adenoids. The neurologically handicapped child usually has an open-mouth posture with poor tongue repose and malocclusion. By breathing through the mouth one can notice how the tongue no longer touches the lingual surfaces of the maxillary teeth. If this posture were chronic, one would develop a malocclusion, the tongue would no longer have teeth-stimulating proprioceptors, and intrinsic muscles of the tongue would become hypotonic. The primary muscles affected would be the transverse and vertical muscles. The tongue appears to enlarge as it fans out between the maxillary and mandibular arches, and occasionally the misnomer *macroglossia* is used, although I prefer the term *hypotonic tongue*. (See Fig. 4-31.)

As the maxillary arch constricts because of the buccinator mechanism, the hypotonic tongue appears enlarged, since it protrudes laterally beyond the narrowing maxillary arch. If one expands the arch, exercises the tongue, closes the lips, and balances the extraoral musculature, the tongue that once appeared enlarged will return to a normal configuration.

Recognizing the allergic child

It is possible to diagnose a child with allergic respiratory disorders before a history is taken when one becomes familiar with the various early physical manifestations.

As nasal and paranasal edema increases, many children develop bluishblack discolorations under the lower eyelids. This has been termed by Marks[17] as *allergic shiners*, caused by venous stasis in the areolar tissue of the lower orbitopalpebral grooves from pressure on veins by edematous allergic membranes (Fig. 4-40). Occasionally edema, or *bags*, develop under the lower eyelids. (See Figs. 4-38 and 4-39.) Often there is an open-mouth habitus caused by mouth breathing with pseudocheilosis, dry lips, rolled lower lip (bulbous lips) from hypotonicity of the circumoral musculature, long silky eyelashes, tearing in the eyes, high, arched V-shaped palate and hyperemia of the pharynx (Fig. 4-41), muddy injected conjunctivae (red eyes), radiating lines in the lower orbitopalpebral groove extending from the inner corner of the eye with downward slant and an upward swing (Dennie's sign), swollen interior of the nose (nasal polyps), hypertrophied lymphoid follicles,

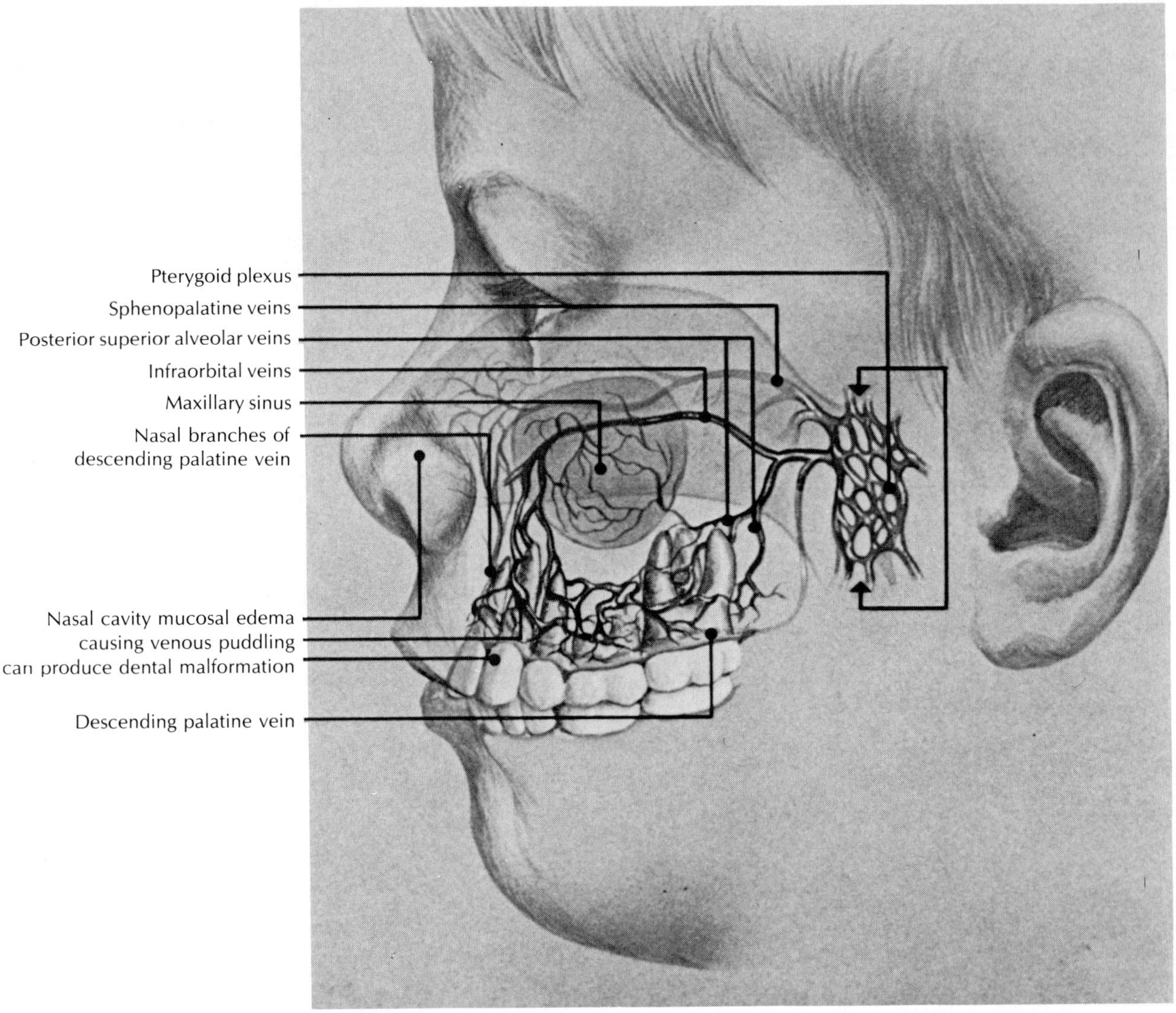

Fig. 4-37. Anatomy and pathogenesis of orofacial dental deformities secondary to allergic respiratory tract disease. (From Marks, M.B.: Stigmata of respiratory tract allergies, Kalamazoo, Mich., 1967, Scope Publication, Upjohn Co.)

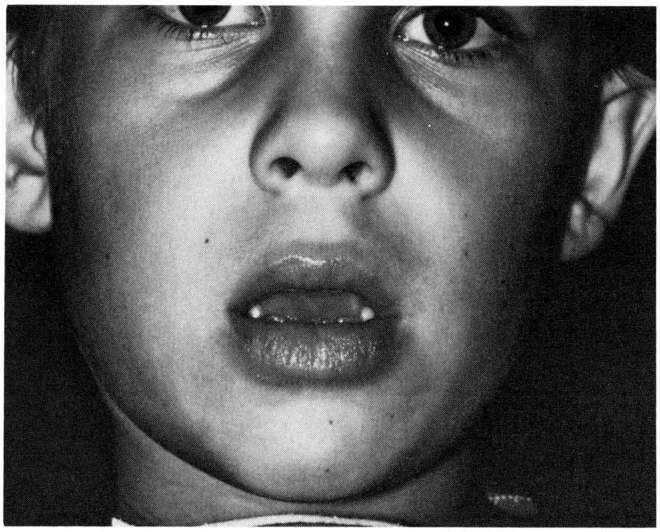

Fig. 4-38. Upper resipiratory tract allergies: edematous nasal and paranasal mucous membranes restrict airway, and mouth breathing is compensatory result. Characteristic picture of allergic child is mouth breathing (open-mouth habitus), dry large bulbous lips, allergic shiners, tearing from eyes, long silky eyelashes, and radiating lines in lower orbitopalpebral groove extending from the corner of eye with a downward slant and upward swing (Dennie's sign).

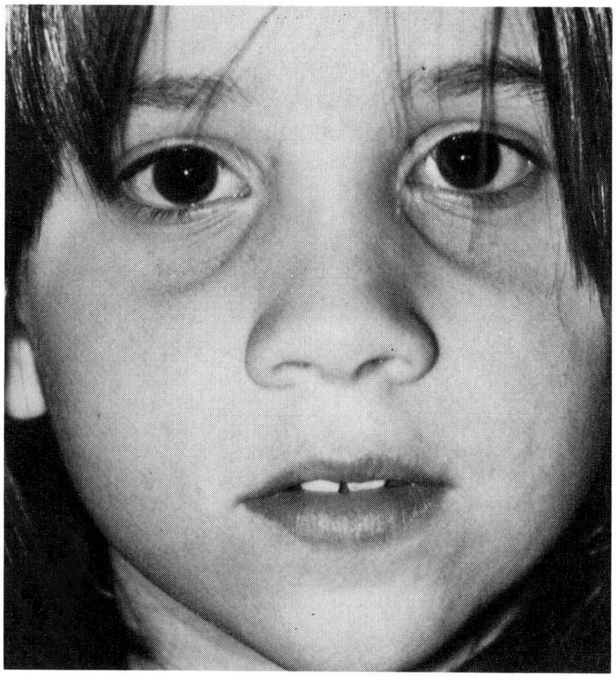

Fig. 4-39. Upper respiratory tract allergies manifest characteristic picture. Compare with Fig. 4-38.

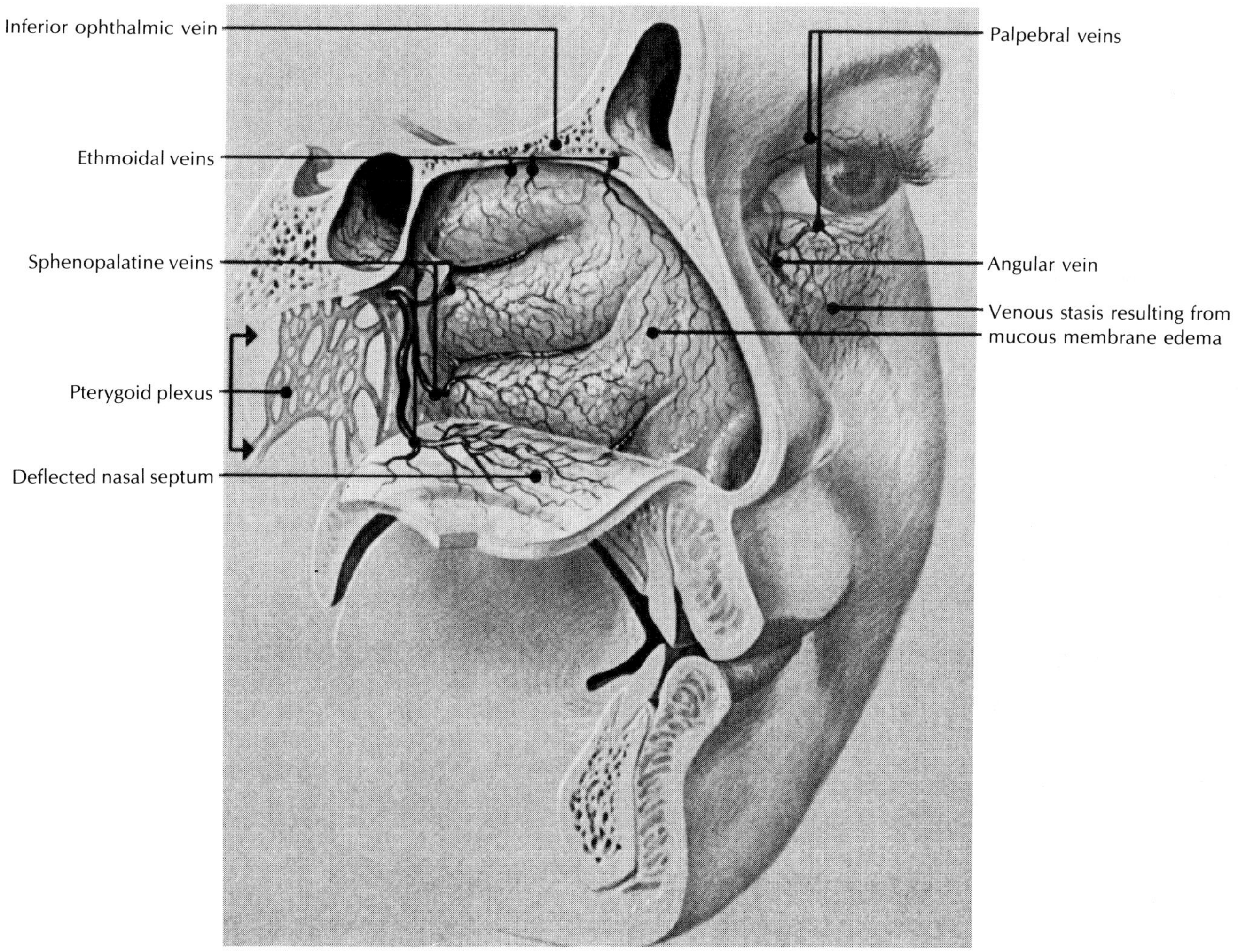

Fig. 4-40. Anatomy and pathogenesis of allergic shiner. (From Marks, M.B.: Stigmata of respiratory tract allergies, Kalamazoo, Mich., 1967, Scope Publication, Upjohn Co.)

migrating geographic tongue, gingivitis and/or hyperplasia of the gingiva because of dehydration, skin pruritus (itching), and papules with excoriated and crusted tops. One or a combination of these physical manifestations can enable the dentist to determine, with experience, whether a child has an allergic upper respiratory tract disorder.

A history of allergies should include whether there were any prenatal injuries or injuries during delivery. Such injuries may predispose the patient to mucous membrane sensitization and lead to servere nasal obstruction. Other signs are if the child is a chronic mouth breather or the parent hears snapping sounds when the child is asleep (tracheal clicks). These are caused by inspissated (thickened) secretion in the larynx and posterior laryngeal wall, which leads to inhibited swallowing reflexes at night. Thus postnasal secretions stagnate and cause constant clearing of the throat and/or a persistent cough. Older children may attempt to screen the oral cavity with their thumb, finger, or an object.

Allergies and bruxism. A study done by Marks[17] at the Pediatric Allergy Clinic in Jackson Memorial Hospital, Miami, indicated an increased incidence of bruxism in allergic children. Only 20% of nonallergic children were bruxists compared with 60% of allergic children. The dentist's orientation has been to explain the cause of bruxism as psychogenic because of local irritating factors, systemic factors, occupational factors, or a combination of these. Allergies as a cause of bruxism have been ignored or cursorily considered by dental experts.

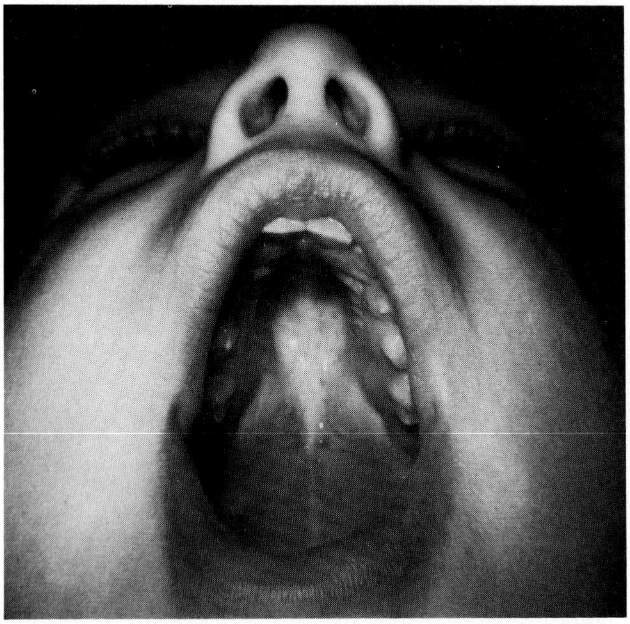

Fig. 4-41. Upper respiratory tract allergies result in mouth breathing, high arched V-shaped palate, hyperemia of pharynx, and collapse of dental arches.

Bruxism also can become a habit as an unconscious attempt to establish contact of a greater number of teeth. Many allergic children are hyperkinetic and brux to alleviate hypertension. Histamine release during stress may be the exciting agent. Nocturnal clenching and/or bruxing often allays symptoms of allergic itching or tickling of the palate and ears and aids in terminating episodes of sneezing and coughing. There is a high increase of negative pressure in the middle ear cavity with auditory tubuli dysfunction in allergic bruxists. Intermittent allergic edema of the mucosa in the eustachian tube and repetitive nocturnal bruxism may be initiated reflexly by increased negative or disturbed pressures in the tympanic cavities.[18]

Ordinarily the auditory tubes are held open during the waking hours by swallowing, chewing, yawning, and sneezing, thus normalizing the atmospheric pressure on both sides of the eardrum. During sleep most of these functions cease with the exception of the swallowing of saliva. It is believed that allergic children who are nocturnal bruxists have dryness of the oral cavity from mouth breathing and consequently have a lessened flow of saliva. The need for swallowing is thus diminished, enhancing the tendency to indulge in teeth grinding at night.[18] The bruxist with TMJ dysfunction may have chronic allergies, which must be considered in the overall treatment plan.

An astute clinician is aware that many children grow out of allergies. When a child is hypersensitive, metabolic changes in the affected areas interfere with normal growth and development. The most common dental manifestation is malocclusion caused by chronic mouth breathing as a result of upper respiratory tract edema. If the malocclusion is not treated, a neuromuscular imbalance between the mandible and maxilla will result. The patient may accomodate for many years, then suddenly develop myofacial pain-dysfunction. The clinician may find that the patient has been bruxing in an unconscious attempt to establish maximum cusp fossa centric occlusion.

The distressed adult patient may indicate that he or she has no allergies and, in most cases, is not aware of or does not recall childhood allergic manifestations. This does not rule out childhood allergies for bruxism in the adult patient. Leading allergists agree that bruxism is three times more predominant in allergic children than in nonallergic children. The resultant malocclusion creates a continuation of bruxism into adulthood after the patient has been hyposensitized unless neuromuscular centric occlusion is established.

The development of TMJ disorders, myofacial pain-dysfunction, and organic disorders of the TMJ does not occur overnight. A childhood malocclusion may not surface as a TMJ or myofacial pain-dysfunction syndrome until adulthood, leading researchers to faulty conclusions if based on self-reports or histories which indicate, on standard medical questionnaires, that the distressed bruxing adult patient is currently nonallergic.

Ears of the allergic child. The ears of the allergic child have many of the same symptoms as those of the TMJ patient. There are intermittent hearing difficulties, popping of the ears, feeling of fullness in the head, vertigo, and tinnitus caused by a release of histamine and other chemical mediators that cause vasodilation of the internal auditory artery and its branches, resulting in edema of the endolymphatic system.

Sense of smell and taste. Most allergic children who are chronic mouth breathers have a diminished sense of smell. Some are incapable of differentiating between the aroma of an apple and an orange until nasal breathing is restored. This may seem fundamental, since it is common knowledge that one must be able to breath through the nose to detect odors. Yet few dentists ask the patient to make a simple comparison between aromas when chronic mouth breathing is evidenced. Taste is dramatically improved when nasal breathing has been restored. Persons with severe colds frequently state that they have lost their sense of taste. However, on testing the taste sensation they are found to be completely normal.[11] This illustrates that much of what we call taste is actually smell. Odors from food that pass upward into the nasal antrum stimulate the olfactory system thousands of times in excess of the taste system.

Sounds of the allergic child. The sounds of an allergic child will vary according to the degree of upper respiratory tract disorder. As edema increases, the following symptoms often occur: nasal speech, air movement through the mouth, coughing spells followed by wheezing, constant clearing of the throat, frequent gulping, low-pitched froglike croaks from paranasal drainage, and smacking of the lips while eating.

POSTURAL CONSIDERATIONS

Although primarily recognized as a physician in the United States, Pierre Robin,[28] physician and stomatologist of Paris hospitals, is considered by many as one of the most important influences in the development of functional orthodontics. His first publications on the subject were as far back as 1902. In 1934 he presented a brief summary of *Pierre Robin's syndrome* and his work at the meeting of the Society of Dental Medicine and Surgery in Paris. Little did he dream that his description of the physical signs of glossoptosis is directly related to TMJ dysfunction. Glossoptosis is tongue pressure on the cervical portion of the spinal colum (Fig. 4-42). Posterior positioning of the tongue causes a

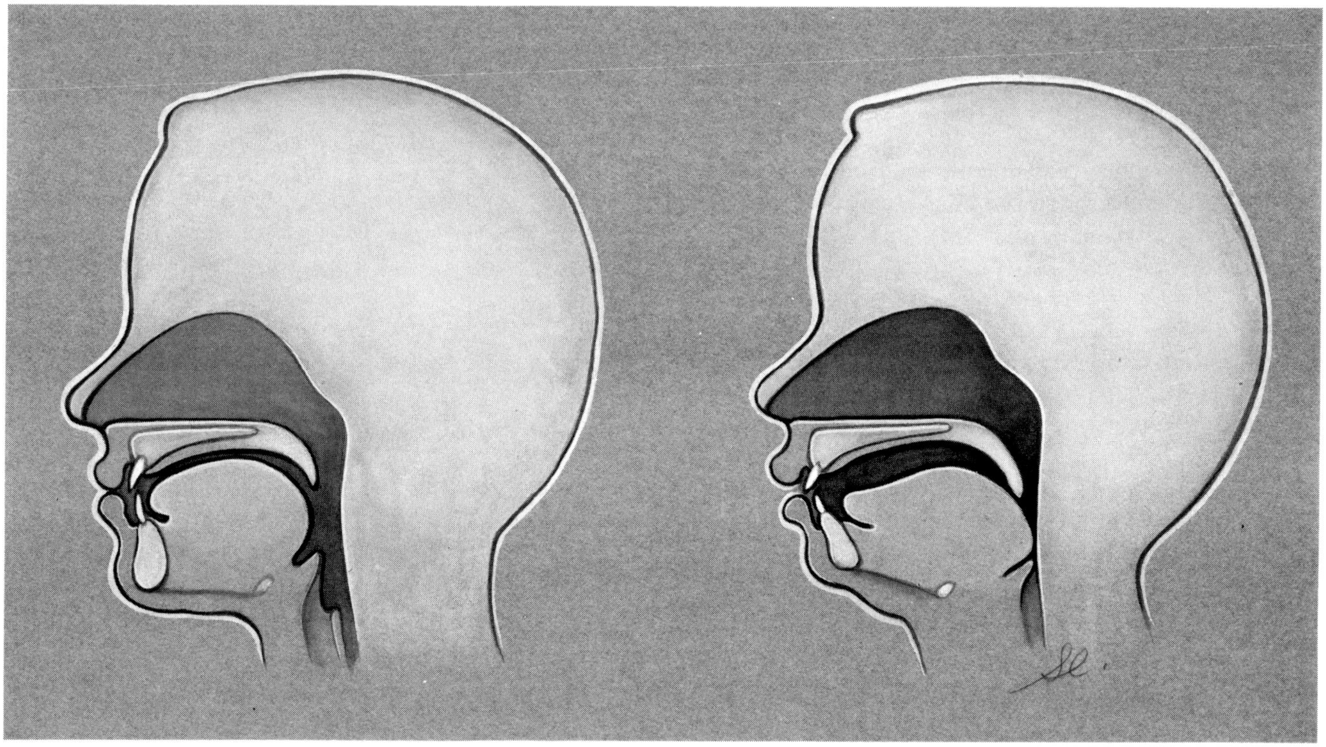

Fig. 4-42. *Left,* Normal child with straight profile, normal occluding dentition, and base of tongue away from spinal column. *Right,* Receding chin and slanted profile, Class II malocclusion with teeth protruding and lower dentition behind the upper, and base of tongue against spinal column (glossoptosis).

pressure on the glottis. This closes the latter if the mouth is shut. The airways to the nasopharyngeal space also are closed. Consequently children with glossoptosis are forced by anatomical environment to breath and eat with an open mouth. Keep in mind, that all chronic mouth breathers create a malocclusion and potential for TMJ dysfunction.

The more the tongue base presses against the spine, the more the nerve cords will be pressed together. This has a tendency to cause disturbances in the function of the blood circulation to the nerves and vessels of the cephalothoracic lymph channels. The obstruction of breathing and compression of the vital nerve cords cause disturbances in functional and psychological reactions.

Glossoptosis can be recognized by these symptoms: the head bends forward, the shoulders hang, the body seems bent and collapsed, the thighs appear excessively relaxed, and the facial expression is, in most cases, adenoidal (Fig. 4-43). The teeth of the upper jaw are forward with reference to those of the retrograde lower jaw. The mouth responds to the condition of the weak receding chin by hanging open during breathing. This predisposes the patient to malocclusion and TMJ dysfunction. The dull appearance of the patient combined with sloppy posture indicates deficient development. Such children seem physically and psychologically stunted in growth, since they constantly feel indisposed without being seriously ill.

Breast feeding is usually difficult and often impossible. This is usually attributed to the mother being a poor nurser. Proper breast feeding and breast preparation generally can overcome this nursing problem.

The height and weight curves are not satisfactory. The lungs, situated as they are in an excessively narrow chest, are usually deformed as a result of the pressure. With classic glossoptosis the rib cage is shaped like a keel. Also, the breastbone is collapsed regardless of whether the ribs are collapsed. Most of the other signs of rachitis also are present, and the lungs function badly with little or no air flow to the lung points and roots. This causes congestion and invites respiratory tract infections.

Robin[28] states, "The probable etiology of atresia of the jaws and its consequent glossoptosis is heterogenic between persons who belong to different morphological types." Since we are the result of such diverse hereditary mixtures, the concept of a "normal" facial and dental pattern is not truly realistic. Actually there are merely balanced relationships and unbalanced relationships, with infinite individual variations.

The posture of each child will vary to some degree. However, when a child exhibits the physical characteristics of glossoptosis, careful consideration of the medical history must be taken. The child may have chronic upper respiratory tract allergies or infection, enlarged tonsils and/or vegetative adenoids, open-mouth habitus, poor tongue repose, large bulbous hypotonic lips, etc. The child will usually exhibit a Class II, division 1 malocclusion.

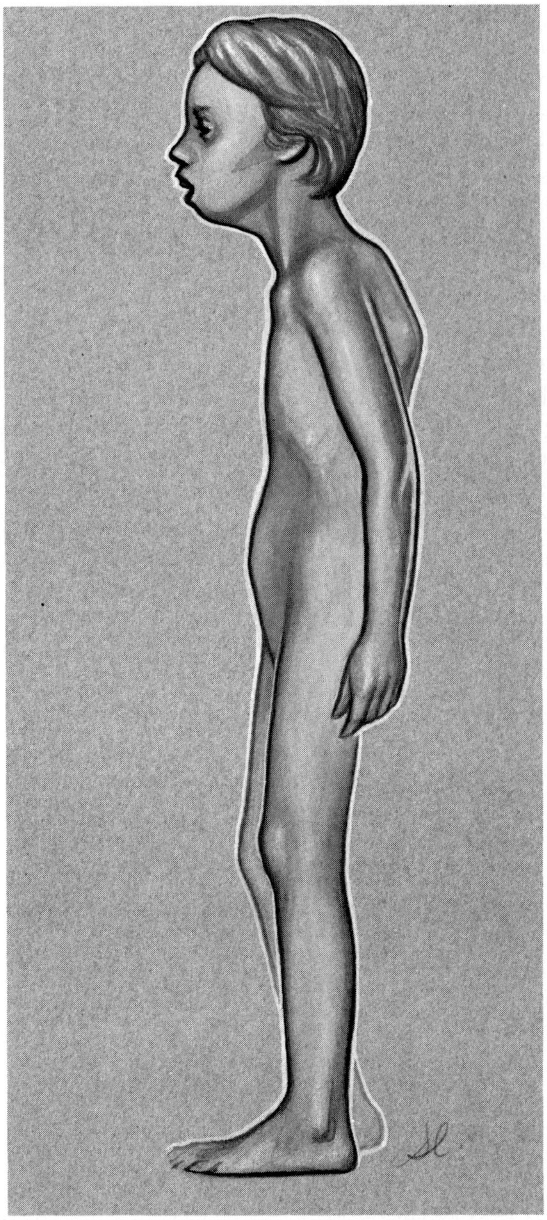

Fig. 4-43. Physical signs of glossoptosis: adenoidal facial expression, head bent forward, receding chin, hanging shoulders, body bent and collapsed, general tired appearance, and relaxed thighs.

While a child is standing, note whether the shoulders are level, the head is cocked to one side (mandibular torticollis), the spine appears straight, and the eyes are parallel and symmetrical. Many times TMJ dysfunction is accompanied by physical asymmetry. If postural asymmetry is noted, recommend that the parent consult with a physician. The orthopedist uses a variety of appliances to help establish functional balance and harmony of the upper and lower extremities. Growth divergencies can be corrected in many children. An orthopedist, working with a physical therapist, can use therapeutic exercises that will produce optimum physical conditioning for a given age. Dentists must understand that their role in establishing optimum maxillomandibular relations requires coordinated synchronization between the neuromuscular joint balance and postural consideration. Children must be diagnosed in a truly holistic fashion, taking into account environmental factors, physical health, mental health, socioeconomic status, age, and sex.

TMJ trauma in children

A blow to the mandible can create TMJ pain in infants and children that is usually transitory because of the resiliency of the anatomical structures involved. Soft foods should be recommended and chewing gum restricted for a period of 6 weeks to reduce stresses of mastication in the glenoid fossa. All erupted teeth should be examined for fractures and/or dislocation.

When children begin contact sports, mouth guards should be recommended to reduce traumatic displacement of the mandible and its condyles within the glenoid fossae.

An examination of a battered child should include palpation of both temporomandibular joints and preauricular and postauricular areas. Mobility of the mandible should be noted in opening, closing, protrusive, and lateral functions. This history could shed light on future TMJ dysfunction.

Low forceps deliveries may potentiate TMJ dysfunction by damaging the meniscus if the forceps compress the condylar preauricular area. A history should include any knowledge a parent may have regarding the mode of delivery. Fortunately an infant's injured tissues from a traumatic delivery regenerate rapidly, and the condition usually resolves itself.

Facial asymmetry in an infant may result from birth trauma, congenital deformity, infantile osteomyelitis, juvenile rheumatoid arthritis, untreated fractures, benign or malignant tumors, or orofacial muscle imbalances.

Cervical traction places abnormal stresses on the glenoid fossa. Extreme caution should be exercised when cervical traction is employed by a physician or therapist. The slightest complaint regarding pain or pressure in the fossa should be regarded as a serious warning of possible impending TMJ pain dysfunction. I prefer to use a mandibular neuromuscular splint prior to any cervical traction. The splint prevents distal, vertical, and lateral displacement of the mandible during traction.

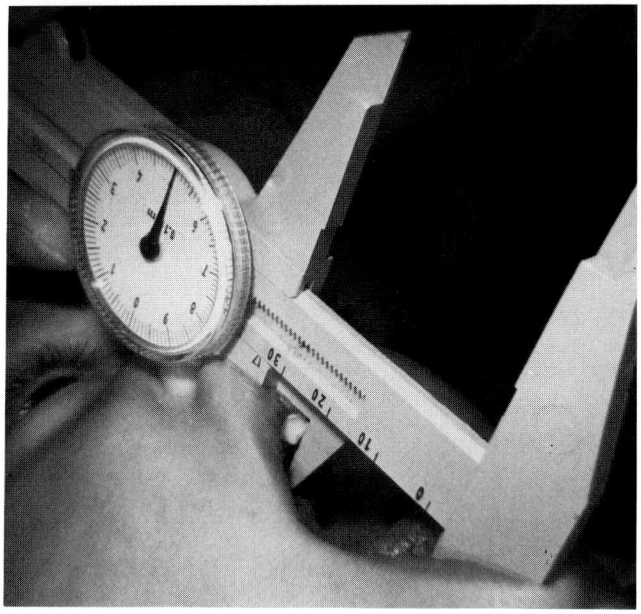

Fig. 4-44. Conscious unstrained vertical measurement is made prior to general anesthesia or heavy sedation and should not be exceeded while patient is unconscious.

Protracted mandibular displacement during nasal or oral intubation, bronchoscopy procedures, tonsillectomies, dental surgery, and extensive dental procedures potentiate TMJ dysfunction. A patient under general anesthesia cannot warn the dentist when the mandible has reached maximum opening and the pain threshold is reached. Caution should be employed when using mouth props or mouth-opening forceps (mouth gags) during in-office or hospital dental procedures.

Mandibular hyperextension can result in injury to the tissues in the condylar retrodistal pad with possible ligamentous involvement. The posterior attachment of the disc may be torn or even detached with concomitant masticatory muscle hypertrophy.

The dentist or physician who contemplates any invasive procedure into the oral cavity with the patient under general anesthesia or heavy sedation should determine the patient's maximum unstrained vertical (opening) measurement prior to administration of anesthesia or sedation. The measurement can be made between the incisal edges of the maxillary and mandibular centrals with a millimeter gauge and recorded on the patient's record (Figs. 4-44 and 4-45). If the unstrained vertical measurement is exceeded for a given procedure, it should be noted on the postsurgical record with an explanation of the necessity for exceeding the measure. This record would be extremely beneficial should TMJ symptoms occur postsurgically.

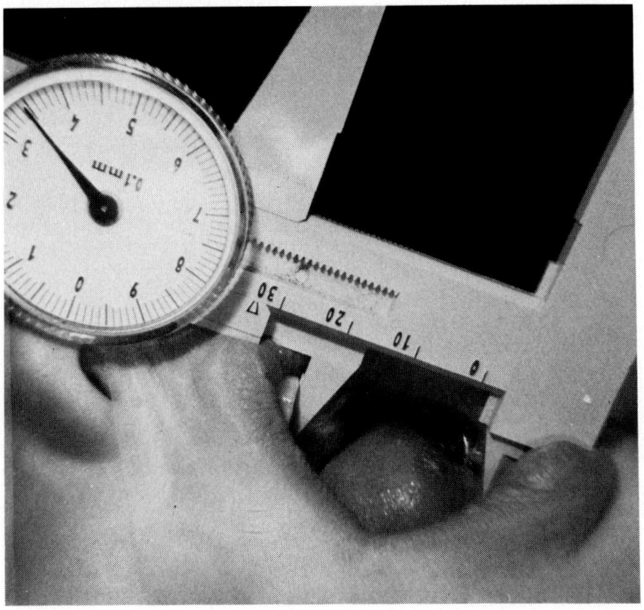

Fig. 4-45. Unconscious vertical measurement is made after patient is anesthetized or heavily sedated and should not exceed conscious unstrained vertical measurement.

Condylar trauma also may occur when posterior teeth are extracted because of the leverage action of forceps without adequate mandibular support to prevent traumatic impingement or jamming of the condyle in the glenoid fossa. This may also occur by overzealous placement of orthodontic bands that are difficult to adapt to a tooth. It is essential that the mandible recieve support whenever a procedure requires excessive force in any direction.

TMJ DYSFUNCTION IN CHILDREN

There has been no definitive method of determining the presence of TMJ dysfunction in children except in those with blatant condylar displacements, intracapsular pathological conditions, or condylar size discrepancies. Crepitus is rare in children. Occasionally popping of the disc is evidenced. The only consistent symptoms usually present are a headache and/or earache. It is common to misdiagnose these symptoms as merely an allergic manifestation resulting in chronic sinusitis.

Many attempts have been made to determine the position of a normal condyle in its relationship to the glenoid fossa by tomography. Ricketts[25-27] found that the space between the glenoid fossa and the condyle was 1.5 mm anterior, 2.5 mm superior, and 7.5 mm posterior to the center of the auditory meatus. Each patient was lying on the side on a sandbag; however, there was no provision to prevent the mandible from shifting while the tomograph was being taken as a result of gravitational forces. Stack and Funt[30] took tomographs through the right and left joints with teeth in occlusion. They found that the normal joint will appear to have the condylar heads located somewhat mesial and inferior to the center of the fossa. This has been my clinical impression.

Condylar displacement

Radiographically, the bony surface of the condyle, eminence, and roof of the fossa should appear smoothly contoured, intact, and well defined. The condyles should be symmetrically placed within their fossae. In symptomatic patients the condylar heads lack symmetry and usually are not positioned symmetrically within their fossae. The displacements commonly seen in symptomatic children are distal, mesial, and superior.

Distal displacement of condyle. Distal to the condylar head lies the petrotympanic fissure, which leads into the tympanic cavity; it contains the anterior ligament of the malleus, the anterior tympanic branch of the maxillary artery, and the chorda tympani nerve. The petrotympanic fissure is relatively wide open in children. When the condyle is displaced distally, pressure is created through the fissure to the middle ear, giving rise to symptoms such as tinnitus, roaring, vertigo, fullness, crepitus, earache, and weeping of the ear. Usually the cause of distal condylar displacement is an accommodative movement of the mandible to obtain maximum intercuspation in centric occlusion. It is common in children with a deep overbite whose front teeth initially touch, and proprioception shifts the mandible distally.

The posterior aspect of the TMJ capsule gives rise to the mandibular-malleolar ligament (Pinto's ligament),[22] which passes backward and upward to insert into the malleus and is a possible explanation for some of the auditory symptoms while chewing, biting, and swallowing. Distal condylar displacements change the tension on Pinto's ligament by creating a pull on the malleus, resulting in a change in ear sensations.

Mesial displacement of condyle. Mesial condylar displacement is normal during nursing, since the mandible is fixed forward by the facial muscles. The glenoid fossa is relatively flat at birth and produces a characteristic profile or configuration by the age of 2 (Figs. 4-46 and 4-47). Many children who develop a dental or skeletal Class II, division 1 malocclusion attempt to improve the unesthetic appearance by moving the mandible forward. In addition, the child must move the mandible forward to incise food, to create a lip seal during the swallow as the mentalis muscle contracts, and to create an adequate airway. The micrognathic and/or retrognathic mandible has a tendency to confine the tongue, occluding the nasopharyngeal airway. By moving the mandible forward, the child creates an airway, since the tongue concomitantly moves forward.

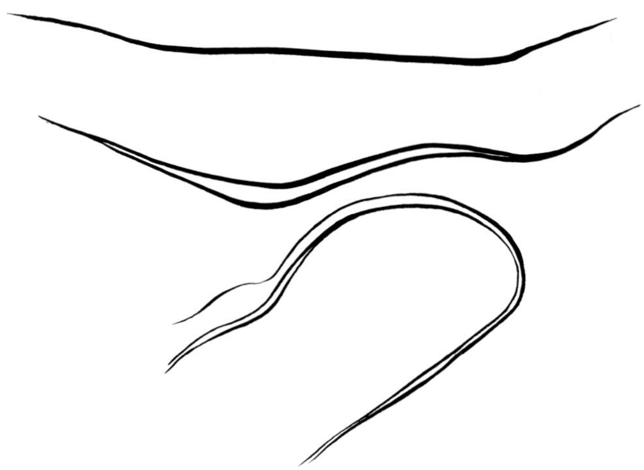

Fig. 4-46. Two-day-old child whose condylar tubercle is flat, condylar cartilage is thick, and osseous structure is highly trabecular. This enables infant to nurse by moving mandible anteroposteriorly in relatively straight luxating movement.

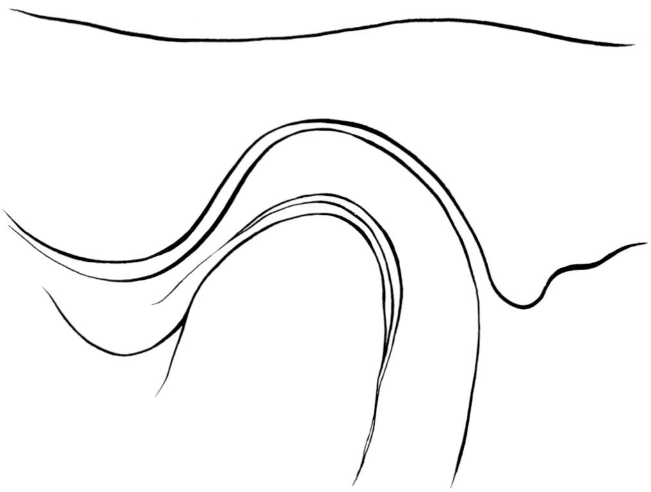

Fig. 4-47. Glenoid fossa of this 2-year-old child has achieved its characteristic profile with formation of primary dentition. During first 2 years abnormal condylar stresses can affect development and configuration of condylar head in glenoid fossa.

Pseudo–Class III malocclusions create bilateral mesial displacement of the condyles. The child will protrude the mandible forward to establish maximum posterior occlusion. The mandibular incisors, maxillary incisors, and canines contact prematurely in an attempt to occlude the molars. Proprioceptive reflex moves the mandible anteriorly, allowing the molars to occlude in a pseudo–Class III relationship. This should be corrected as soon as possible, since the anterior aspect of the condyle is displaced against the descending slope of the articular eminences.

Mesial displacement can range from 3 to 7 mm forward on the descending slope of the articular eminences. Continued forward displacement of the mandible will result in hypertonicity of protruding muscles, resulting in pain in the preauricular, postauricular, temporal, neck, and back areas. Positioning the mandible using a neuromuscular physiological splint will relieve the muscle spasms. If no treatment is instituted, the condylar head and/or eminences may resorb, creating an osteorthritic condition. Proper relocation of the condyles in the glenoid fossae allows a recontouring of the condyles and eminences in the growing child.[30]

To establish the proper relationship of the mandible to the maxilla, the fifth (trigeminal) nerve is gently pulsated (40 minutes) using a Myo-Monitor* to relax the muscles of mastication. During the pulsation the neuromuscular trajectory of the mandible can be traced on an oscilloscope (Kinesiograph) and recorded on film. When the recordings reveal a relaxed trajectory and an overclosure, the mandible is pulsated into a soft acrylic splint that is placed over the teeth until the acrylic hardens. The patient must be standing upright with the head and eyes looking forward at an eye-level object, and the arms must hang comfortalby by the side during pulsation into the splint. This reduces the error created by abnormal positioning of the head in its relationship to the neck and back. To understand how tilting the head affects occlusion, merely have the patient close the mandible until the teeth are in light contact. Then have the patient look up to the ceiling, and feel the occlusion change as the mandible moves distal. The reverse is true when the patient moves the head downward. The temporary splint is then removed from the mouth, and all excess acrylic is removed. The splint is then contoured, polished, and placed in the mouth to be worn continuously until TMJ symptoms subside.

Unilateral mesial and rotational condylar displacement. Most unilateral cross-bites in children are not truly unilateral. When the mandible is relaxed and properly positioned, it becomes apparent that the so-called unilateral cross-bite is bilateral or end to end. This causes the mandible to shift to one side to establish maximum occlusion. When deciduous canines prematurely contact, the mandible deviates laterally to avoid the interfering cusp and establish maximum posterior tooth contact. Lateral deviation (cross-bite) of the mandible will create condylar movement bilaterally. Lateral movement of the mandible displaces the condyle mesially on the opposite side than that to which the mandible deviates, with rotational displacement on the same side. Cross-bites should be corrected as soon as possible to avoid

*Myo-Tronics Research, 1404 Medical-Building, Seattle, Wash. 98101.

such condylar displacements and the possibility of TMJ dysfunction or unilateral condylar hyperplasia.

Condylar hyperplasia. The etiology of condylar hyperplasia is unknown. It may be hypothesized that the rate of condylar growth is affected by abnormal stresses within the condylar capsule and disc. The condyle, in its normal relationship to the glenoid fossa, is physiologically unstrained in the capsular area. However, any condylar displacement places stress on the capsular area, including the articular layer of the condyle. During the first 2 years of life the growth cartilage of the condyle is penetrated by vascularized connective tissue septa, whose function appears to be nourishment of the cartilage.[31]

Restricted blood supply to the growth cartilage because of a loss of dynamic equilibrium, triggered by condylar displacement, may alter cell proliferation with a resultant condylar hyperplasia and/or degenerative joint disease.

Superior condylar displacement. In young patients premature loss of posterior teeth, ankylosed molars, anodontia, and molars prematurely worn flat frequently create superior displacement of the condyle, compressing the meniscus. Muscles (such as masseter, internal pterygoid, and temporal) that elevate the mandible overcontract unless neuromuscular vertical measurement is restored, resulting in spasm and referred pain to the preauricular and postauricular areas. Posterior molars must be restored, missing teeth replaced, and ankylosed molars restored to a proper vertical measurement to avoid a predisposition to TMJ dysfunction.

Degenerative TMJ

TMJ degeneration has been evidenced as early as 7 years of age. The condylar head becomes flattened, and the eminence is not smooth. It results primarily in the Class II, division 1 patient who compensates the mandible by moving it forward. The condyles are compressed against the descending slope of the articular tubercle. Circulation is restricted, and the disc is diminished. Crepitus usually is not evident. The child suffers from generalized headaches and frequent earaches, which may continue throughout the learning years. The child often is diagnosed as a problem learner or malingerer. In the teens popping, clicking, earaches, and headaches are evidenced. Crepitus is more common in the 20s. Ear complaints such as roaring, vertigo, fullness, ringing, and slight hearing loss are more common in the 30s.

In addition to supplying the muscles of mastication, the trigeminal nerve supplies the tensor tympani, tensor veli palatini, and dilator tubae. When condylar displacement occurs, these muscles become stressed, and spasm results. A spastic tensor tympani muscle pulls the ossicular chain medially, the stapes protrude into the middle ear, and middle-ear pressure increases. Spastic tensor veli palatini and dilator tubae prevent the opening of the eustachian tube, resulting in a fullness and stuffiness in the middle ear.

Clinically, TMJ dysfunction creates a myriad of muscle imbalances, manifested in distant anatomical locations such as the spine. Unilateral spasms have been shown to cause curvature of the spine, unilateral depression of the shoulders, and torticollis (contraction of neck muscles causing the head to be twisted in an abnormal position), with a resultant loss of equilibrium and symptoms of vertigo, since the semicircular canals are no longer parallel to the floor.

A neuromuscular splint is an excellent diagnostic means to enable a dentist to position the mandible orthopedically in a three-dimensional relationship to the maxilla. If TMJ symptoms are subsequently relieved, the diagnosis is confirmed, and corrective procedures can be instituted.

SUMMARY

To understand a predisposition to TMJ dysfunction, it is essential that we have a thorough understanding of the etiology of abnormal force vectors that initiate tooth movement. Teeth seek a neutral position within a system of forces, and any imbalance between intraoral and extraoral musculature will move teeth. Although force systems change continuously during growth and development in response to stimuli from their environment, with careful clinical observation it is possible to assess the oral force system in a child.

Preventing TMJ dysfunction should begin immediately post partum by encouraging breast feeding. If impossible, recommend the Nuk nipple, supplemented by the Nuk exerciser when necessary. Appendage, object, and conventional pacifier sucking should be controlled immediately post partum.

If headaches, earaches, clicking, popping, or intracapsular pathological conditions are evidenced, a neuromuscular splint should be constructed to establish a normal maxillomandibular relationship. Most TMJ dysfunctions in children result from mesial, distal, and superior displacement of the mandible.

Coronoplasty (occlusal equilibration) should be recommended when interfering cusps displace the mandible. Care must be taken not to close the bite during coronoplasty, and the mandible must be neuromuscularly positioned in its relationship to the maxilla. A typodont Class I occlusion may not be the patient's neuromuscular centric. Proper use of a Myomonitor and Kinesiograph will enable a dentist to establish a neuromuscular centric and record the findings.

Treatment for TMJ dysfunction in children entails

an accurate diagnosis and a plan of treatment that may include neuromuscular splints, orthodontics, crowns, space maintainers, and/or coronoplasty.

ACKNOWLEDGMENT

Acknowledgment is made to Rocky Mountain/Orthodontics, which for years has been a leader in preventive orthodontics. Their promotion of the Nuk Sager system deserves our thanks and appreciation.

REFERENCES

1. Applebaum, R.M.: Abreast of the times, 1969, 7914 S.W. 104th St., Miami, Florida.
2. Astrom, K.E.: On the early development of the isocorte in fetal sheep. In Bernard, C.G., and Schade, J.P., editors: Progress in brain research, vol. 26, Development of neurology, New York, 1967, Elsevier.
3. Broad, F.: The effects of infant feeding on speech quality, N. Zealand Med. J. **76**:28, 1972.
4. Bullen, J.J., Rogers, H.J., and Leigh, L.: Iron binding proteins in milk and resistance to *Escherichia coli* infections in infants, Br. Med. J. **1**:75, 1972.
5. Citizens Committee on Nutrition: White paper on infant feeding, Washington, D.C., 1974, Center for Science in the Public Interest.
6. Davis, M.E., and Potter, E.L.: Intrauterine respiration of the human fetus, J.A.M.A. **131**:1194, 1946.
7. Duke, W.W.: Allergy, asthma, hayfever, urticaria and allied manifestations of reactions, ed. 2, St. Louis, 1926, The C.V. Mosby Co.
8. Glaser, J., and Johnstone, D.: Prophylaxis of allergic disease in the newborn, J.A.M.A. **153**:620, 1953.
9. Goldman, A.S., and Smith, C.W.: Host resistance factors in human milk, J. Pediatr. **82**:1082, 1973.
10. Graber, T.M.: The three m's; muscles, malformation and malocclusion, Am. J. Orthod. **49**:418, 1963.
11. Guyton, A.C.: Textbook of medical physiology, ed. 5, Phildelphia, 1976, W.B. Saunders Co.
12. György, P.: The uniqueness of human milk: biochemical aspects, Am. J. Clin. Nutr. **24**:970, 1971.
13. Hahn, P., and Kirby, L.: Immediate and late effects of premature weaning and feeding a high fat or high carbohydrate diet, J. Nutr. **103**:690, 1973.
14. Harvold, E.G.: The activator in interceptive orthodontics, St. Louis, 1974, The C.V. Mosby Co.
15. Hentges, D.J.: Influence of pH on the inhibitory activity of formic and acetic acids for *Shigella*, J. Bacteriol. **92**:2029, 1967.
16. Liley, A.W.: Disorders of amniotic fluid. In Assali, N.S.: Pathophysiology of gestation, vol. 2, Fetal placental disorders, New York, 1972, Academic Press, Inc.
17. Marks, M.: Stigmata of respiratory tract allergies, Kalamazoo, Michigan, 1967, Scope Publication, Upjohn Co.
18. Marks, M.: Bruxism in allergic children, Am. J. Orthod. **7**:48, 1980.
19. Miller, T.E.: Killing and lysis of gram negative bacteria through the synergistic effect of hydrogen peroxide, ascorbic acid and lysozyme, J. Bacteriol. **98**:949, 1969.
20. Moyers, R.E.: Handbook of orthondontics for the student and general practitioner, ed. 3, Chicago, 1973, Year Book Medical Publishers, Inc.
21. Najera, A.: A critical evaluation of early feeding procedures and their implication on oral-facial morpho-physiology and related factors, Master's thesis, St. Louis, 1963, St. Louis University School of Dentistry.
22. Pinto, O.F.: A new structure related to temporomandibular joint and middle ear, J. Prosthet. Dent. **12**:95, 1962.
23. Rankin, J.H.G., et al.: Measurement of fetal renal insulin clearance in the chronic sheep preparation, J. Appl. Physiol. **32**:129, 1972.
24. Reiser, R., and Sidelman, Z.: Control of serum cholesterol homeostasis by cholesterol in the milk of the suckling rat, J. Nutr. **102**:1009, 1972.
25. Ricketts, R.M.: Laminagraphy in diagnosis of TMJ disorders, J. Am. Dent. Assoc. **46**:620, 1953.
26. Ricketts, R.M.: Abnormal function of the TMJ, Am. J. Orthod. **41**:435, 1955.
27. Ricketts, R.M.: The role of cephalometrics in prosthetics diagnosis, J. Prosthet. Dent. **6**:488, 1956.
28. Robin, P.: A syndrome of facial pathology, Lecture before Society of Dental Medicine and Surgery, Paris, Jan. 8, 1934.
29. Schubert, W.K.: Fat, nutrition and diet in childhood, Am. J. Cardiol. **31**:581, 1973.
30. Stack, D., and Funt, L.: Temporomandibular joint dysfunctions in children, J. Pediatr. **3**:240, 1977.
31. Wright, D., and Moffett, B.: The postnatal development of the temporomandibular joint, Am. J. Anat. **141**:235, 1968.

PART TWO

DIAGNOSIS

5 History taking

LAWRENCE D. DAY, D.D.S., M.S.

THE HISTORY

The objectives of this chapter are (1) to present a history-taking form designed to obtain the needed information, and (2) to indicate the possible significance of each item of information recorded on the form.

Importance

Schwartz and Chayes[11] state:

> In evaluating a patient who presents symptoms that may be the result of a temporomandibular joint disorder, the most important single problem is that of obtaining a complete history. . . . In the systematic process of differential diagnosis, history alone can provide the answer to most mandibular dysfunction resulting from organic and traumatic disorders.

To help a patient, it seems a practitioner must know at least as much about the condition as the patient does. The principle of "never treat a stranger"[16] is especially important in TMJ patients. The necessary information can be readily obtained by having the patient write it on an appropriate form. A suggested form is included as the final section of this chapter. The number-letter combinations in parentheses in the text attempt to correlate subject matter with questions on the history form.

Method of obtaining the history

Some professionals prefer to use a plain sheet of paper and let patients tell their own story.[11] This, however, requires a certain skill to obtain all the necessary information without asking leading questions. Therefore in this chapter stress is placed on a suggested history form that can be used by almost any practitioner to obtain the needed facts in an organized sequence. Patients should be allowed to complete the form in a quiet place at their own rate before any in-depth discussion with the practitioner. This can save a lot of time for the practitioner and may be less stressful to the patient. It also may help identify some patients who "just want to talk to the doctor" and are frustrated by completing the form.

After the practitioner has reviewed the form (at a comfortable rate), all the pertinent facts may be reviewed in detail with the patient. As Sir William Osler said, "Listen to the patient; he is giving you the diagnosis."[11] Often when the patient hears the question read and hears the answer that was previously written, an offer to qualify it or to add more information will be made. Thus the practitioner will be able to add more detail by writing it directly on the form.

HISTORY OF PREVIOUS CARE

Patients with temporomandibular joint problems often have consulted many dentists or physicians, including neurologists, ear, nose, and throat specialists, orthopedists, psychiatrists, and chiropractors, in search of the cause and remedy for their problem. One should be aware of the practitioners they have seen, diagnoses made, treatment rendered, and results. This information should make it possible to avoid unnecessary discomfort for patients during the examination and to prevent repeating unsuccessful therapy. I believe that obtaining this information early on the form, before questioning patients personally, prevents possible indication of blame on any practitioner for what has been done or omitted.

PERTINENT MEDICAL HISTORY

If the patient has either osteoarthritis or rheumatoid *arthritis* in other joints (1a), the disease also may have affected the TMJ. However, the TMJ may be affected in the absence of arthritis in other parts of the body. In osteoarthritis of the TMJ the patient may have a grating noise (4c) or crepitus during function.

Infections in the ear such as otitis media or furuncle of the ear may result in tinnitus, a sensation of fullness in the ear, or limitation of mandibular opening (5a).[5] Infections such as parotitis, sinusitis, or tonsillitis may affect mandibular function.[5] Ear or sinus infections may exhibit many of the same symptoms as TMJ disorders and must be ruled out. Lymphadenopathy in the corresponding areas could result from any of these and also could be the cause of tenderness on palpation.

History of *blood vessel disease* is important in differential diagnoses because in periarteritis nodosa symptoms include intermittent myalgia, arthralgia, and peripheral neuritis.[2]

Headaches may be of the migraine type, which are generally associated with dilated extracranial blood vessels, or the tension type, which are associated with muscle spasm (1b). This same muscle spasm may cause the TMJ syndrome, so the relationship of the two should be analyzed. The pain from myospasm results primarily from muscle ischemia.[1] Any systemic disease affecting the muscles or blood vessels thus may be an important consideration.

Any type of *trauma* that may have affected the head and neck region, changing the positioning of the head and resulting in muscle strain and spasm, is important. Whiplash injury or other accidents, general anesthesia,[7] and cervical traction[13] are good examples of this type of trauma (1c, 5m). Certainly trauma that affected the condyles themselves or altered the occlusion in any way should receive consideration, since occlusal trauma is, according to some, "probably the most frequent cause of pain in the TMJ."[8]

Mandibular muscle atrophy occurs in neuropathy or myopathy. Myopathy may be caused by *nutritional* deficiencies (1d), hormonal disturbances, infections, or *metabolic disturbances*. A history of these or other metabolic diseases affecting bone, such as hyperparathyroidism, multiple myeloma, or Paget's disease, should be noted. In Paget's disease, for example, atypical facial neuralgia, osteoporosis, malocclusion, and painful oral lesions may be found; these could contribute to, or be confused with, TMJ symptoms.[11]

Any *medication* being taken or any *allergies* to medication (1e) should be known so that their effects on the patient and possible drug interactions can be considered. Allergy to metal rings (5q) would be important if a metal prosthesis were to be considered in treatment.

The *emotional state* of the patient (1g, 5k, m) may be important as a causative factor in the TMJ syndrome. Emotional stress may be manifested as clenching, bruxing, gum chewing, or nail biting that cause fatigue (5c-g), aggravate inflamed temporomandibular joints, or cause muscle spasm. Emotions such as agitation, fear, and hostility are also important in determining how patients will handle the additional stress of TMJ pain and how they will cooperate during therapy and respond to treatment. The emotional state may be evaluated by observation, inference, frank discussion (possible with some patients), and psychometric tests such as the Minnesota Multiphasic Personality Inventory (MMPI). This may be administered by the dental assistant but is evaluated by a psychologist or psychiatrist, who may furnish a written report or diagnostic impression and indicate whether further psychometric testing or interviewing is needed. (Only 2 of 24 patients [8%] studied by Woods[17] at the Orange County Medical Center received an MMPI diagnostic impression of "essentially within normal limits.") Another study[12] shows that the higher the MMPI scores (indicating greater degrees of depression, agitation, and anger), the less likely it is that conventional therapy will be successful in female patients.

CHIEF COMPLAINT

First, patients are asked to state their chief complaint, its duration, and whether it is unilateral or bilateral (2a-d).

Disorders of the masticatory system have two main symptoms—pain and dysfunction. Masticatory pain refers to that which emanates from the temporomandibular joints (arthralgia), from the masticatory muscles (myalgia), or from both. Masticatory dysfunction identifies itself as either interference or restriction of mandibular movement or acute malocclusion because of mandibular displacement. Proper interpretation of these symptoms is essential for accurate diagnosis.[4]

Pain

Pain is probably the most frequent chief complaint and is certainly the most pressing problem the patient has. A grouping of various problems by the quality of pain that is typical of them is given in the following list (3k-o):

1. *Sharp* (localized, superficial pain in general): Gingival, mucosal, and skin pain[3]; trigeminal neuralgia (shocklike)[11]; swelling or stretching of salivary gland; for example, early obstruction[11]
2. *Dull* (diffuse, deep pain in general): Myalgia and arthralgia[1]; sinusitis[11]; atypical facial pain[11]; vascular pain
3. *Aching:* Myalgia and arthralgia; sinusitis
4. *Burning:* Neuritis[11]
5. *Pulsating:* Vascular pain
6. *Spreading:* Deep pain
7. *Pressure, drawing, or pulling:* Atypical facial pain[11]
8. *Constant:* Sinusitis[11]; neuritis[3]; masticatory pain (may increase to severe with movement and stress; intensity and character may vary from day to day)[1]
9. *Intermittent:* Neuralgia
10. *Stops suddenly:* Neuralgia; masticatory pain when local anesthetic is injected into appropriate joint or tender muscles

11. *Stops gradually:* Myalgia and arthralgia if chronic and untreated; referred pain

Dysfunction

Mandibular dysfunction is a direct result of physical and/or emotional stress and is next to pain in frequency as the chief complaint.[11] There are four stress areas related to mandibular dysfunction: muscle status, occlusal status, emotional status, and joint status. Imbalance in the interrelationship of one or more of these states results in the pain-dysfunction syndrome. At different times during the last 40 years each of these had its turn at being considered the most important. At present emotional status seems to be the main predisposing factor to the pain dysfunction syndrome.[11] Dysfunction is usually described as:

1. *Restricted or deflected jaw movements* (opening, closing, protrusive or lateral excursion). Limitation of movement (4a) is the most common cause of a patient's seeking treatment for mandibular dysfunction. It is most frequently the result of muscle spasm but may have several other causes. Painful limitation is usually preceded by clicking, incoordination, and some symptoms of subluxation.[11]
2. *Noises* in the joint, which usually precede the painful limitation (4c, d). Clicking is bred by incoordination, which in turn probably is related to muscle dysfunction or increased muscle tension. Incoordination often leads to subluxation and rarely to dislocation. Dislocation occurs when muscle spasm locks one or both condylar heads forward of the articular eminences (4b). Subluxation is partial or incomplete dislocation and is described by patients as the jaw slipping or going out of place, locking briefly on occasion, and sometimes giving the feeling that the teeth do not "mesh" properly. It usually presents as a malocclusion that disappears with the relief of the causative muscle spasm.[11]
3. *Change in the bite* (4e).

Miscellaneous and associated complaints

Sore scalp, sore throat, throat pain on swallowing, burning pain down the side of the neck (3u, v), shoulder pain, and fullness or pressure in the ear, along with tinnitus and vertigo, are also among symptoms found in the TMJ syndrome.[10] Pain from any of these areas readily induces masticatory muscle spasm.[8] The patient may have a subjective sense of hearing loss, probably associated with ear noises (tinnitus [5a]), rather than a true loss of hearing.[5]

Vertigo and its associated neurological signs and symptoms (5b) may be caused by malocclusion. Patients with vertigo may have headache, dizziness, tinnitus, blurred vision, nausea, vomiting, and ataxia. Their symptoms may be aggravated by postural changes, and syncope may develop. The cause of this syndrome may be sudden movements of the footplate of the stapes.[11]

Some patients with hysterical face pain (primary atypical facial neuralgia) show evidence of TMJ dysfunction and muscle spasm as well (5h). These patients may have attacks of pain with vasomotor symptoms, flushing, edema, unilateral lacrimation (5k), and nasal swelling (5i). Many of them also complain of gastrointestinal symptoms such as anorexia, dysphagia, vomiting, and increased salivation (5j).[11]

LOCATION OF SYMPTOMS

Initial location

The location of dysfunction and especially pain should be determined as accurately as possible (3a-j). Attention first is given to the area where the patient feels the pain described under "Chief complaint." However, masticatory pain typically is not well localized. It occurs in and about the ear, frequently as a definite preauricular pain, but many times it is also felt diffusely throughout the face, teeth, jaws, and mouth. The discomfort may extend to the temple, orbit, entire mandibular area, floor of the mouth, and even sternocleidomastoid and trapezius muscle areas.[1] Because of this diffuse, spreading characteristic (3k, v), it is important to ask the patient where the pain was *first* noticed and any changes in location or character of the symptoms since then (5r).

Secondary locations

Arthralgia and myalgia are typical forms of deep pain and are the main components of masticatory pain. They present four definite behavioral characteristics.

1. The location of pain does not identify its source (3a-j).
2. The pain is rather steady but variable and has a dull, aching quality (3k).
3. The pain spreads by central excitation, so that soon the referred pain, secondary hyperalgesia, and painful muscle spasm in *otherwise normal* structures and muscles constitute the *main complaint* (2a-d).
4. The apprehension and alarm provoked are out of proportion to the true significance of the condition present (1g).

To further confuse the issue, the referred pain and secondary hyperalgesia (3k) may be felt superficially and be well localized, giving the patient (and practitioner) the definite impression of being the primary pain.[1]

CIRCUMSTANCES SURROUNDING ONSET OF SYMPTOMS

Gradual onset (2b) of dysfunction and pain is characteristic of the following:

1. *True arthopathy* (other than that caused by acute trauma), including rheumatoid arthritis, osteoarthritis (arthrosis), ankylosis, and capsular fibrosis.[3] Clenching (5c-g) predisposes the patient to disc interference, discitis, and degenerative changes.[3] Chewing habits, excessive movements, excessively hard chewing, gum chewing, nail and thread biting, mannerisms such as jaw thrusting, sleeping positions, and postural habits (3u, v) all contribute to degenerative changes in the discs and articular surfaces.[3]
2. *Contracture* of masticatory muscles results from prolonged shortening of the muscle or prior myositis (4a).[3]

Sudden onset (2b) of pain and dysfunction is usually caused by injury or muscle spasm and frequently is associated with specific events, including the following:

1. *Emotional upset* (5k, m) may cause jaw thrust, clenching (5c, d), or grinding. If the pain is more severe in the morning or causes awakening at night, the patient is doing it while sleeping. Increased pain in the afternoon or evening suggests daytime jaw habits that may be related to an activity (3p). Many patients will say exactly what difficult, nerve-wracking, or all-consuming activity makes them tense or tired, but few patients have come to relate the activity and pain consciously (5m).[1] Anxious, tense, and nervous patients are prone to have myospasm of the masticatory muscles with related facial pain.[1]
2. *Wide opening* occurring rapidly, such as in yawning, or continuous opening, such as for a long dental appointment (5m), may initiate pain and dysfunction by producing myospasm in susceptible individuals. The predisposition to muscle spasm may be either psychological or physiological.[11]
3. *Trauma* may be of the acute type such as a blow to the jaw, causing joint or muscle symptoms that are immediately evident.
4. *Dental treatment* (5m-o) resulting in rapid or extensive changes in occlusion through restoration, selective grinding, or use of an appliance may produce sudden pain by muscle spasm as with wide opening.[11] In some individuals even slight occlusal interference may induce proprioceptive interference, resulting in spasm and incoordination. It may also induce clenching and bruxism and by any of these routes cause pain and dysfunction.[3]
5. *Cervical traction*, used in treating whiplash and other cervical injuries (5m), may aggravate a primary temporomandibular arthropathy or cause a secondary one. Bite plates are recommended to stabilize the mandible and protect the joint from trauma during traction.[6]

COURSE OF SYMPTOMS

Progression of symptoms

A chronological progression of symptoms must be known, since both location and character of pain and degree of dysfunction may change with time in some conditions (5r). For example, in the myofascial pain-dysfunction (MFPD) syndrome, by the time there is limitation of jaw function, there is rarely clicking, but there is a history of clicking.[9] Some of the changes in the MFPD syndrome may be more readily visualized with the aid of the diagram in Fig. 5-1, modified from Laskin,[9] who used it to illustrate his logical psychophysiological theory.

Aggravating factors

From Fig. 5-1 it can be seen that emotional stress or physical stress of muscles (such as yawning, chewing, swallowing, brushing teeth, or moving the head, neck, or shoulders [3u]) could aggravate certain tense muscles or areas of hyperalgesia or touch trigger areas in trigeminal neuralgia. If patients relate that their symptoms are more severe in a certain environment, such as at home or at work, it may indicate the presence of a psychological problem with a personality or situation.

Relieving factors

Moist heat, resting the involved structures (3t), and decreasing tension by tranquilizers, muscle relaxants (3s), spacers (such as cotton rolls between the teeth to prevent premature contacts and feedback mechanisms), ethyl chloride spray (cold), or local anesthetic injections into areas of muscle spasm or tender joints can be helpful in diagnosing areas of primary pain as well as in bringing relief to the patient.

Typical symptom patterns

A history of *stiffness on awakening* with pain in function that gradually disappears with use and returns with fatigue at the end of the day suggests *osteoarthritis* (1a).[11]

The *sudden onset* (2b) of painful limited mandibular movement on awakening or after a yawn or wide bite (5m), with a previous history of clicking, suggests a sudden transition from the incoordination phase of the pain-dysfunction syndrome to the phase of *painful limitation* of function.[11] (My impression is that incoordination of the mandibular muscles is caused by emotional

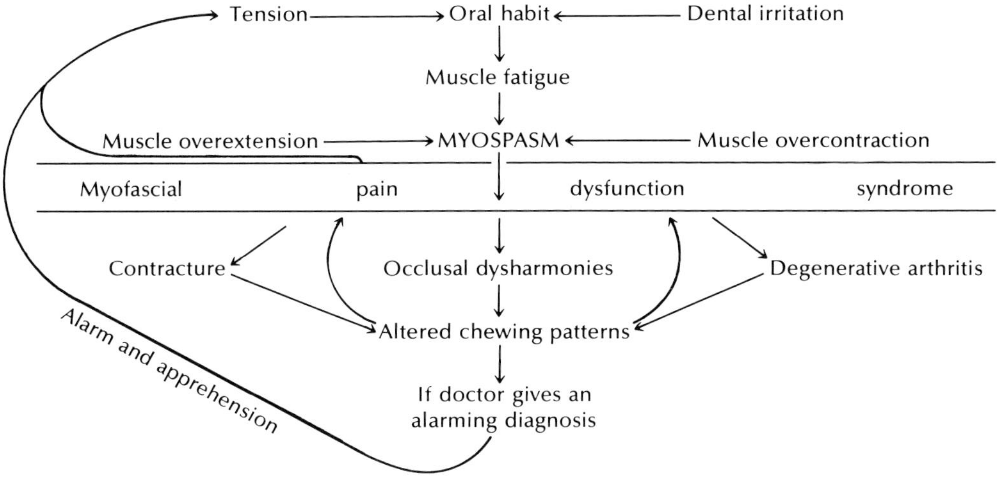

Fig. 5-1. Changes in the myofascial pain-dysfunction (MFPD) syndrome. (Modified from Laskin, D.M.: J. Am. Dent. Assoc. **79:**148, 1969.)

stress acting through the mechanism of increased muscle tension and resulting pain. Clicking is the most common symptom of incoordination. Such incoordination often leads to limitation.)

Contracture may be indicated by a report of painless limited mandibular movement which appeared so slowly (2b) that the patient has difficulty in describing its early stages, particularly if there were a prior history of clicking, subluxation or dislocation, and/or limited painful mandibular movement (4a-e).[11]

In arthritis initial symptoms are dysfunction and clicking. Only when *inflammation* is sufficient to cause deep pain are secondary myospasms produced (4a-e). Then it may mimic the MFPD syndrome.[4]

PERTINENT DENTAL HISTORY

The dental history pertinent to the MFPD syndrome includes the following:

1. The general condition of teeth and tissues and any changes in them. Pain from any pulpal or periodontal disease or exposed cementum may cause muscle spasm and referred pain, which must be differentiated from the MFPD syndrome.
2. The *bite relationship* with any inability to find a comfortable rest position or overclosure because of developmental anomaly or loss of posterior teeth (4e).
3. *Previous dental treatment,* including restorations, orthodontia (5n), extractions, or bite adjustments (5o), especially since they may have altered the occlusion and correlate with symptoms.
4. *Oral habits,* including clenching or playing with certain teeth, lip licking, tongue thrust, and lateral jaw thrust (5c-h). These are important in causing joint dysfunction and may be obvious on the first consultation, or they may nearly defy detection. A complete list of possible habits is too long to include here, but a few ideas to explore are the following[15]:
   a. Habitual eccentric occlusal relationships
   b. Sleeping habits (does the sleeping position move the mandible away from centric?)
   c. Cupping the chin in the hand or resting the head with the hand on the side of the face
   d. Pen or pencil chewing; pipe holding
   e. Instrument playing (violin, clarinet, saxophone, bugle, trumpet)
   f. Posture at work (holding the phone with the head, always turning or holding the head in one direction)
   g. Working under an air-conditioning duct
   h. Lip or lateral tongue biting
   i. Setting the teeth in an incisal or protrusive position to perform a task that requires strength or skill
   j. Jobs of unusual pressure or responsibility
5. The psychological significance of the oral area to the patient. This may be indicated by the degree of agitation or distress (1g) evinced during the discussion.

MISCELLANEOUS

"No specific set of questions is adequate,"[1] so it is always necessary to give the patient a chance to include anything else that the practitioner should know about him or her which might have an effect on the present problem (5s) or on the relationship of practitioner and patient.

PATIENT INFORMATION FORM

The patient information or personal history form is designed to obtain the needed information in a consistent sequence, at the patient's own rate, and without taking any unnecessary amount of the examiner's time. It has been adapted primarily from forms used by Nathan Allen Shore,[13] Douglas H. Morgan, and Weldon E. Bell.[3] It is admittedly long and may be discouraging to some patients if used in its entirety. However, it is designed to include most of the information that might be useful in most TMJ problems. Certainly more detailed questioning will be necessary once it has been determined which general grouping of symptoms or type of problems a certain patient has. Once the practitioner has gained adequate proficiency in dealing with TMJ patients, a blank piece of paper or a shorter form with written summary history, as used by Bell,[3] may be used.

PERSONAL HISTORY

Date ____________ No. ________

Name (Mr./Mrs./Miss) ________________________________
Last name First name Middle initial

Residence ________________________________ Tel. ____________
No. Street City State Zip code Area code

Occupation ________________ Firm's name ________________
If housewife, write "Housewife" Leave blank, if housewife

Firm's address ________________________________ Tel. ____________
No. Street City State Zip code

Date of birth ____________ Marital status ____________ Ages of children ____________

Spouse's name ________________________________
Last name First name Middle initial

Spouse's occupation ________________ Firm's name ________________

Firm's address ________________________________ Tel. ____________
No. Street City State Zip code

Whom may we thank for referring you to us? ________________________

Address ________________________________ Tel. ____________

Name of your regular physician ________________________

Address ________________________________ Tel. ____________

Name of your regular dentist ________________________

Address ________________________________ Tel. ____________

On the lines below please list any physicians, dentists, neurologists, ear, nose, and throat specialists, orthopedists, chiropractors, psychiatrists, or clinical teams you have consulted. Please also list their specialties. Briefly describe their diagnosis and treatment.

Dr. ________________ M.D./D.D.S. Specialty ________________

Address ________________________________ Tel. ____________
Area code

Diagnosis and treatment ________________________________

____

____

Dr. ________________ M.D./D.D.S. Specialty ________________

Address ________________________________ Tel. ____________
Area code

Diagnosis and treatment ________________________________

____

____

Dr. ______ M.D./D.D.S. Specialty ______
Address ______ Tel. ______
Area code
Diagnosis and treatment ______

Dr. ______ M.D./D.D.S. Specialty ______
Address ______ Tel. ______
Area code
Diagnosis and treatment ______

Dr. ______ M.D./D.D.S. Specialty ______
Address ______ Tel. ______
Area code
Diagnosis and treatment ______

Dr. ______ M.D./D.D.S. Specialty ______
Address ______ Tel. ______
Area code
Diagnosis and treatment ______

Please answer as many of the following questions as possible by circling the disease or symptom you have, its location, or "Yes" or "No." However, write freely on the discussion questions.

1. GENERAL HEALTH
   a. Have you had the following? Arthritis Osteoarthritis Rheumatoid arthritis Sinus infection Ear infection Swollen glands Blood vessel disease
   b. Do you have frequent headaches? What area of the head? ______ How long do they last? ______ Migraine? ______
   c. Have you ever had a severe blow to the head or had a whiplash injury? ______ What part of the head? ______ Date ______
   d. Have you ever suffered nutritional deficiencies? Yes No
   e. Do you regularly take any medication? Yes No Which? ______
      Are you allergic to any medication? Yes No Which? ______
   f. If you have any other current nondental physical problems or diseases, please describe them. ______
   g. If you have any emotional problems regarding your teeth or jaws, please describe them. ______
   h. Please indicate anything else about yourself that you suspect may be related to your condition. ______

2. CHIEF COMPLAINT
   a. What is the main problem that brings you here? ______
   b. Did this problem begin suddenly or gradually? (Circle one)
   c. How long have you been bothered by this problem? ______ Years ______ Months ______ Weeks ______ Days
   d. Do symptoms affect one or both sides? Right Left Both If both, which side seems most affected? ______

Continued.

PERSONAL HISTORY—cont'd

3. PAIN SYMPTOMS

Do you have *pain* in the following areas? Please circle R for right side or L for left side.

a. Joint R L
b. Ear R L
c. Upper teeth or jaw R L
d. Lower teeth or jaw R L
e. Tongue R L
f. Facial muscles R L
g. Eyes R L
h. Forehead R L
i. Neck R L
j. Shoulder R L
k. Circle kinds of pain you have.
Sharp Dull Aching Deep Superficial Burning Pulsating Spreading
l. Is the pain constant? Intermittent?
m. Does the pain last for a moment? Minutes? Hours? All day? Longer?
n. Does the pain start suddenly? Gradually?
o. Does the pain stop suddenly? Gradually?
p. What time of day or night is pain most severe? ______
q. How often do you have pain? ______
r. What is the longest period you have gone without pain? ______
______
s. What medication, if any, do you take to relieve pain?
______
t. Does rest increase or decrease pain? ______
u. Please describe any method of positioning the jaw or head that you have found for relieving pain. ______
______
v. Do any of the following normal daily activities cause pain? If yes, circle and indicate where you feel pain.
Yawning ______ Chewing ______ Swallowing ______ Speaking ______
Singing ______ Shouting ______ Brushing teeth ______ Moving head ______
Moving neck ______ Moving shoulders ______ Moving arms ______
Moving trunk ______

4. DYSFUNCTION

a. Can you open your mouth normally? Partially? Almost not at all?
b. Do you ever open so wide your mouth locks open? Yes No
c. Do you have any of these sounds in the joint?
Grating R L Clicking R L
Snapping R L Popping R L
d. If you have any of these problems, is it frequent? Occasional? Constant?
e. Have you noticed any change in your bite? Any change in your ability to chew?

5. MISCELLANEOUS AND ASSOCIATED COMPLAINTS AND QUESTIONS

a. In which ear do you ever notice a hearing change? R L Ringing (tinnitus) R L
Fullness, pressure, or blockage R L
b. Do you experience dizziness (vertigo)? Fainting? Nausea?
c. Are your jaws clenched or teeth sore when you awaken from sleep?
d. Do you grind your teeth (brux) when asleep? When awake?
e. Do you clench or grind your teeth during moments of concentration?
f. Do you chew gum? Frequently Moderately Seldom Never
g. Are your jaw muscles ever tired? When? ______
______
h. Do you have a jaw thrust habit or nervous twitch about the face (tic)?
Where? ______ When? ______
i. Does your face swell? What part? ______ When? ______

j. Have you ever noticed production of more saliva or less saliva?
k. Do tears form in your eyes for no apparent reason?
l. Is there anyone else in your family with a similar problem? Yes No If yes, explain. ______
m. Did the symptoms start after any of the following conditions?
Severe emotional upset Excessively large bite or yawn A blow on the jaw
Irregular or raised dental filling Prolonged or excessive opening during dental treatment
Traction for cervical arthritis or whiplash Accident General anesthesia
n. Have you had your teeth straightened (orthodontia)? Yes No
o. Have you had your bite adjusted by your dentist? Yes No
p. Have you had cortisone injections in jaws or face? Yes No
q. Are you sensitive to metal rings or earrings? Yes No
r. Please describe briefly any changes in location or character of symptoms since this problem began. ______

s. Please write any other pertinent information not covered above. ______

Finally, by referring back to the names of doctors, please answer:
6. Did any of their treatments make you feel better? If so, which helped the most? In what manner?
______

7. Did any of the treatments make you feel worse? Which ones? In what manner? ______

REFERENCES

1. Alling, C.C.: Facial pain, Philadelphia, 1968, Lea & Febiger.
2. Anderson, W.A.D., and Kissane, J.M.: Pathology, ed. 7, St. Louis, 1977, The C.V. Mosby Co.
3. Bell, W.E.: Synopsis: oral and facial pain and the temporomandibular joint, Dallas, 1967, W.E. Bell.
4. Bell, W.E.: Clinical diagnosis of the pain-dysfunction syndrome, J. Am. Dent. Assoc. **79**:157, 1969.
5. Burket, L.W.: Oral medicine diagnosis and treatment, ed. 6, Philadelphia, 1971, J.B. Lippincott Co.
6. Frankel, V.H.: Temporomandibular joint pain syndrome following deceleration injury to the cervical spine, J. Bone Joint Surg. **52**(A):4, 1970.
7. Kaye, L.B., Moran, J.H., and Fritz, M.E.: Statistical analysis of an urban population of 236 patients with head and neck pain, J. Periodontol. **50**:55, 1979.
8. Kerr, D.A., Ash, M.M., Jr., and Millard, H.D.: Oral diagnosis, ed. 4, St. Louis, 1974, The C.V. Mosby Co.
9. Laskin, D.M.: Etiology of the pain-dysfunction syndrome, J. Am. Dent. Assoc. **79**:148, 1969.
10. Norris, C.W., and Eakins, K.: Head and neck pain: temporomandibular joint syndrome, Laryngoscope **84**:1466, 1974.
11. Schwartz, L., and Chayes, C.M.: Facial pain and mandibular dysfunction, Philadelphia, 1968, W.B. Saunders Co.
12. Schwartz, R.A., Greene, C.S., and Laskin, D.M.: Personality characteristics of patients with myofascial pain-dysfunction (MPD) syndrome unresponsive to conventional therapy, J. Dent. Res. **58**:1435, 1979.
13. Shore, N.A.: Occlusal equilibration and temporomandibular joint dysfunction, Diseases of temporomandibular apparatus seminar syllabus, Los Angeles, 1974, TMJ Research Foundation and White Memorial Otolaryngology Foundation, Inc.
14. Shore, N.A., Schaefer, M.G., and Hoppenfeld, S.: Iatrogenic TMJ difficulty: cervical traction may be the etiology, J. Prosthet. Dent. **41**:541, 1979.
15. Snow, D.F.: Personal correspondence to Douglas H. Morgan, 1976.
16. Tarsitano, J.J.: Never treat a stranger, J. Am. Dent. Assoc. **73**:856, 1966.
17. Woods, W.: A screening psychological evaluation of patients with temporomandibular joint dysfunction, Masters thesis, Loma Linda, Calif., 1974, Loma Linda University.

6 Initial examination

DOUGLAS F. SNOW, D.D.S., F.A.C.D., F.A.G.D.

A great many chronic temporomandibular joint patients have spent years seeking relief from their pain. Histories disclose that the quest of patients seeking relief often takes them to several general practitioners and specialists in the public health field. Many extensive tests are performed and repeated in an attempt to reveal "the Great Imposter."[10] The electrocardiogram, the electroencephalogram, lumbar puncture, heart catheterization, neurological and psychiatric examinations, and many radiographs seem to the rule rather than the exception.

The fact that no satisfactory diagnosis has ever been made for their problem has led many to believe that they have an undiagnosed cancer or some terminal illness. To escape this unrelenting pain, some have attempted suicide, and many have considered it. It is because of this background that the health-care professional must exercise diligence in the examination and treatment of the patient.

ATTITUDE OF THE EXAMINER

The personality and deportment with the patient of the examiner during the initial examination are important. The examiner's manner should display an aura of confidence but not callousness, empathy but not sympathy. The apprehensive patient should be assured that the symptoms presented are not extraordinary if, indeed, they are not. An impatient examiner will not be successful treating diseases of the temporomandibular joint. When the examination is finished and the treatment plan is presented, the practitioner should promise to extend his or her best care, not a cure.

Because temporomandibular joint dysfunction is not a well-known disease, and because the symptoms may vary distinctly from one case to another, patients may not be perfectly candid in discussing their symptoms. The examiner must be alert to media other than the spoken word in gathering information to make a diagnosis. There is a tremendous amount of nonverbal information communicated between examiner and patient. An awareness of the possibilities and patterns in this area of study may disclose repressed or unrecognized attitudes of the patient.[1]

Proxemics (how a person reacts to the closeness of other people) should be considered. Does the invasion of what the patient considers personal territory alter the capability to give uncolored answers to questions? Physical behavior should reinforce what is being said verbally.[4] However, body movements can contradict the oral message. The seated position and eye contact can each divulge nonverbal cues as to the patient's real feelings.

Hand-to-nose gestures might represent a state of fear, and fist gestures could possibly indicate aggression. Fingers at the lips might suggest shame, and open hands dangling between the legs could signify feelings of frustration.

Nonverbal leakage also is revealed in a person's speech. For example, hesitant speech and speech that includes errors, incomplete sentences, and the repetition of words have been found to indicate anxiety and negative feelings.

Nonverbal communication may be an important consideration as one begins the clinical examinations.

QUALITIES OF THE NORMAL TEMPOROMANDIBULAR JOINT

The normal temporomandibular joint is one that displays an absence of the symptoms of noise, pain, and altered function. Noise is easy to detect, especially when a stethoscope is placed over a moving temporomandibular joint. The presence of pain is likewise simple to determine by merely questioning the patient. Altered function is the area that must be skillfully explored by a methodical dentist or physician. An understanding of altered function is best gained by reviewing normal relations or occlusal harmony.

The four major properties used to ascertain normal relations or occlusal harmony are (1) the presence of interocclusal clearance when the muscles relax, (2) terminal closure such that the clenched occlusal position does not require a shifting movement from the unclenched position of primary occlusal contact, (3) return from protrusive and lateral excursions with freedom from cuspal interference, and (4) proper muscle coordination.[2]

Certain structures should be noted that are located close to the temporomandibular joint. These structures will become more interesting when symptomatology is studied. Consider that the bone medial to the condyle is the temporal bone, which is the hardest bone in the head and which encloses the organs of hearing and balance.[14]

PATHOLOGICAL TEMPOROMANDIBULAR JOINT AND ITS SYMPTOMS

Pathological conditions of the temporomandibular joint arise when functional demands on the joint, its related musculature, and proximal tructures exceed their ability to adapt.[8] Many authc ties agree that the cause of temporomandibular joint pain is a combination of occlusal factors and stress factors.[3,7,12,19]

Following are symptoms of the temporomandibular dysfunction syndrome:

1. Pain and/or crepitus in the temporomandibular joint
2. Pain and /or tinnitus in the ear
3. Pain in the muscles of mastication, principally the masseter, temporal, and internal and external pterygoids
4. Pain in the muscles of support to the head, principally the trapezius, scalenius, and sternocleidomastoid
5. Pain in the temples, vertex, and occipital areas of the head
6. Pain on opening, yawning, or chewing
7. Reduced ability to open or close the mouth
8. Reduced ability to make excursive movements
9. Deviation of the jaw to one side on opening
10. Headache, neck aches, shoulder aches
11. Vertigo
12. Tic douloureux
13. Reduced hearing acuity
14. Uncomfortable occlusion or lack of a stable centric occlusion[5]

TEMPOROMANDIBULAR JOINT HISTORY FORM

An accurate diagnosis of temporomandibular joint dysfunction must begin with a complete history of the patient. This history may be handwritten from answers to verbal questions by the examiner. Probably a more complete history can be obtained by use of the temporomandibular history form, which is completed by the patient in the relative quiet of the reception room before being seen by the examining dentist.

The history form example shown and discussed in depth in Chapter 5 lists most of the important symptoms. It is an essential element of the initial examination.

FACIAL ASYMMETRY

As the dentist or physician begins the physical examination of the temporomandibular joint patient, first, attention is given to the symmetry of the face. At roughly an arm's length the practitioner visually compares the two sides of the face. Asking the patient to clench may help disclose any asymmetry. This condition usually will be noted in the area of the temporal muscle or along the body of the masseter to its insertion at the angle of the mandible.

Viewing the profile of the face will reveal the relative development of the skull, the face, and the mandible.[15] Asymmetry, if present, would disclose an unusual muscular activity. This would probably result from constrictures and muscle spasms caused by stress or by an occlusal interference and would not be associated with habitual unilateral mastication of food.

In cases of Class II malocclusions it is well to check facial symmetry with the occlusion. The patient may have two centric occlusions: a rather retruded relationship and a more anterior one, which has been assumed by the patient to improve the facial appearance. This is also known as a *Sunday bite*.

PALPATION

The joints

The joints can be palpated easily by placing the fingertips lightly over the temporomandibular joint area. The condyles should move smoothly in a forward and slightly downward arc when the mouth is opened. Any soreness or dissimilar morphology should be noted.

Next, place the tips of the little fingers in the external auditory canal, and pull the fingers forward gently. One can now feel the distal surfaces of the condyles. Ask the patient to move the jaw from side to side, and determine whether both condyles exhibit movement.

Place a stethoscope over a condyle, and ask the patient to open and close slowly several times, opening only to the point where he or she might begin to feel pain. Note and describe the presence or absence of noise, such as clicking, popping, or grating, in each joint. Repeat this test over the other condyle.

The muscles

Palpation of the muscles of mastication and of support to the head (Figs. 6-1 and 6-2) will be of great help in the clinical diagnosis of TMJ pathosis. Painful mas-

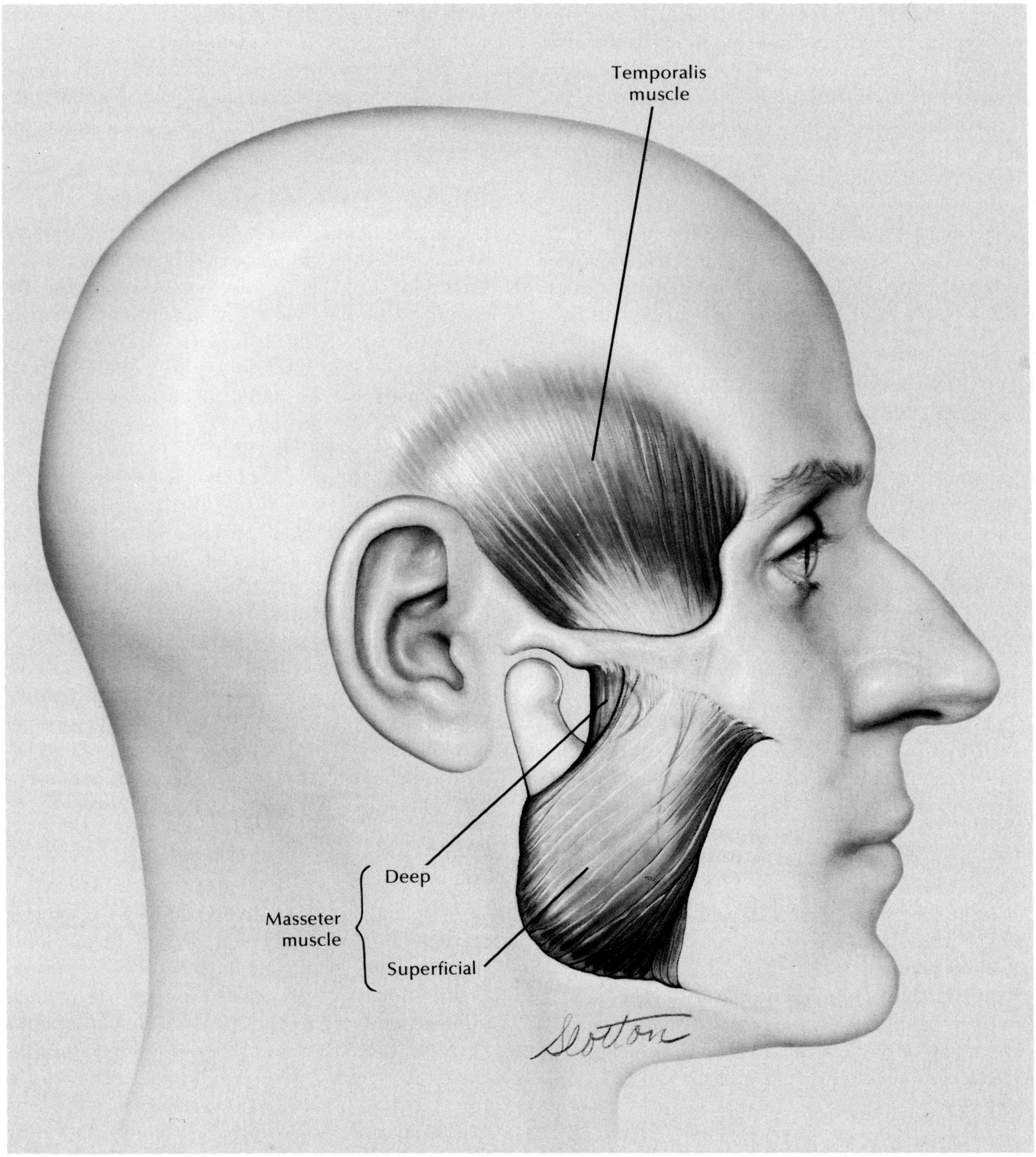

Fig. 6-1. Temporalis and deep and superficial masseter muscles.

seters and temporals would lead one to suspect that the patient had been bruxing or clenching. Pain in the external pterygoid might indicate a muscular adaptation to proprioceptive stimuli from interferences in the occlusion.

Where and how to palpate the muscles that are of concern in TMJ examination are covered in the TMJ examination form. Control of pain spasms in the musculature by Fluori-Methane spray or by procaine (Novocain) is covered in another chapter.

EXAMINATION OF THE OPENING MOVEMENT

Gait

Stand in front of the patient, and ask him or her to open and close the mouth. Have the patient vary the speed of the opening movement to bypass any accom-

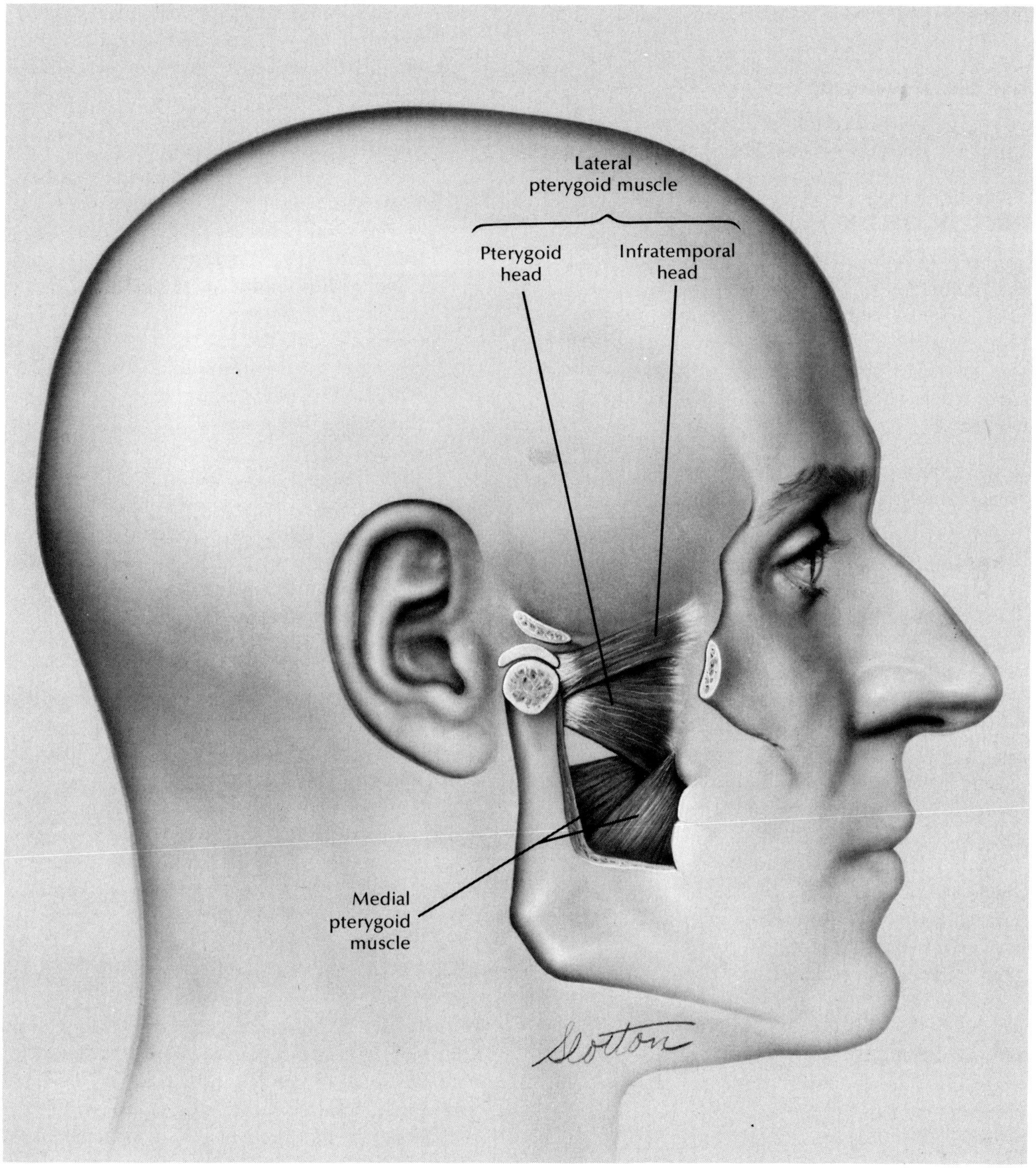

Fig. 6-2. Lateral pterygoid muscle (pterygoid and infratemporal heads) and medial pterygoid muscle.

modation he or she may have learned to assume. Watch the gait of the opening closely to determine whether it is smooth and continuous or asynchronous.

Restriction

Is the amount of opening restricted? With a Boley gauge, measure the maximum opening that the patient can make without pain. The normal opening for a male patient is 40 to 50 mm; the normal opening for a female patient is 35 to 45 mm.

Deviation

With the patient's teeth in a closed position examine the relationship of the lower (movable) to the upper (fixed) midline. Now have the patient open, and see if there is a deviation to one side. Measure the amount.

If it is excessive, check for arthritis, muscle spasm (internal pterygoid), or ankylosis.[17]

Protrusive and lateral excursions

Have the patient move into protrusive and both lateral excursions. Note variations in the ability to make these movements easily or not at all.

EXAMINATION OF THE MOUTH

Before the examiner becomes preoccupied with a detailed examination of the teeth, the whole mouth—the gums, cheeks, tongue, palate, and pharynx—should be methodically examined. It would be well for examiners to train themselves to follow the systematic oral cancer examination suggested by the American Cancer Society.

Oral cancer examination

External examination

1. In the initial confrontation examine the face for skin blemishes, moles, pigmentations, symmetry, and swellings.
2. Palpate preauricular, parotid, submental, and submaxillary chains of the head and the jugular and posterior cervical chains in the neck.
3. Palpate the temporomandibular joints with the mouth open and closed. Note tenderness, crepitus, and deviation.
4. Examine lips with mouth closed, then open. Note color, texture, and any surface irregularities.
5. Palpate the lips for induration.

Vestibule and tongue

1. Examine visually and by palpation the mandibular vestibule and frenum with the mouth partially open. Observe color, character, and swellings of the mucosa.
2. Examine the cheeks and Stenson's duct. Check all areas of buccal mucosa.
3. Examine the maxillary mucobuccal fold and frenum. Palpate the area.
4. Inspect the dorsum of the tongue at rest for swelling, ulceration, and coating and for variation in size, color, or texture.
5. With the patient's tongue protruded observe for tremor, asymmetry, or limitation of motion. Note variation in size, color, or texture.

Tongue and floor of the mouth

1. Wrap a 4 × 4-inch gauze around the tip of the protruded tongue. Lightly press a warm mirror against the uvula, and observe the base of the tongue and circumvallate papillae.
2. Move the tongue to the left, and retract the right cheek. Observe the entire lateral border of the tongue and its attachment to the floor of the mouth back to the anterior pillar. Swing the tongue to the right, and repeat examination of the left border.
3. Release the tongue, and instruct the patient to touch its tip to the palate. Observe the ventral surface, and note any varicosities and swellings. With the tongue still elevated, inspect the floor of the mouth for swellings or other abnormalities, and note Wharton's ducts, the sublingual ridge with openings of the sublingual ducts, and the lingual frenum.
4. Carefully palpate the entire tongue, including the base, for any induration.
5. Palpate the entire floor of the mouth. Identify the submaxillary gland.

Palate

1. With the patient's mouth wide open and head back, gently depress the base of the tongue with a tongue depressor or mirror. Inspect and then palpate the hard palate.
2. Observe and palpate the soft palate and uvula.

Fauces and pharynx

1. With the tongue still depressed, inspect both fauces (tonsillar area), the anterior pillars (glossopalatine arch), and the posterior pillars (pharyngopalatine arch). Instruct the patient to say, "Eh," which will expose a wide area of the oropharynx for inspection.
2. The nasopharynx may be examined by placing a mirror of suitable size behind the uvula. Tell the patient to breathe through the nose and mouth.[17]

The teeth

It is essential that one has a good full-mouth or Panorex radiograph so that one can make a complete examination. Note all pathological conditions disclosed in the radiographs, and plan to correct them if they are of a nature so as to conflict with the TMJ examination or subsequent treatment (for example, deep cavities, loose or abscessed teeth). Check suspicious-looking teeth with percussion and vitality tests. Deep cavities may need to be excavated and closed with sedative cements. Use fremitus to explore the presence and degree of tooth movement in dynamic function. Note and study open contacts, periodontal problems, occlusal flaring, missing teeth, fractured teeth, or fillings in relation to the occlusion.[16]

Make a visual examination of the coronal surfaces to discover any cracks or areas of unusual wear. Examine unusual wear on the incisal surfaces by bringing the worn areas into approximation. This is done by guiding the patient into a lateral, lateroprotrusive, or protrusive relationship so that the intimacy of the worn incisal areas is complete. Have the patient hold still in that position, and hand him or her a mirror. Most patients will declare that they never go into such a position, so point out that bruxing in this position is the only way that such unusual wear could be accomplished. Explain that an assumed habit, interferences in the occlusion, or subconscious tensions tensions are the cause of this unfortunate wear. Miller calls this daytime grinding *bruxomania*.[9]

The occlusion

The relationships of teeth should be studied and occlusal contacts checked with articulating ribbon, which, unlike articulating paper, marks only areas of actual tooth contact. The use of thin sheets of articulating wax, which adheres to the teeth while the patient chews food, allows habitual chewing habits to disclose any unusual occlusal contacts. It must be remembered that if the case under examination is one in which the musculature is distorted by spasms and contractures, the occlusal patterns will be different when the muscle problems are eliminated. Therefore all occlusal adjustments, except gross areas, are contraindicated at this time.

Check the intimacy of the occlusion of the posterior teeth with Mylar tape. The examiner should not be able to pull the tape free while the patient is biting on it. This is often a problem where a prosthesis is involved. If the prosthesis is faulty, it may have to be relined or remade to afford good occlusal contact. This is especially true when the occlusal surface is plastic. All such surfaces should be changed to porcelain or metal so that solid support to the occlusion in the posterior area of the mouth is ensured and so that wear will be commensurate with the wear of the natural teeth.

Examine areas of missing and extruded teeth. Are malposed teeth contributing to the occlusion are they out of contact, or are they an actual interference? Periodontally involved teeth with a poor prognosis should be removed. The intimacies and interaction of the articulation can be scientifically evaluated only by mounting good models on an adjustable articulator. The procedure for this is detailed at the end of this chapter.

RADIOGRAPHS

In the clinical examination of temporomandibular joint dysfunction syndrome, radiographs have an important diagnostic role. A complete treatise on this subject is found in Chapters 8 and 9.

NEUROLOGICAL EXAMINATION

An impairment of nervous stimulation (signal communication) by way of the cranial nerves to the brain or impairment of motor signals to various areas of the head and neck by way of the parasympathetic nervous system may be a complication of the TMJ dysfunction syndrome.

The cranial nerves are the peripheral nerves of the brain. They transmit input to the brain from the special sensors of sight, smell, hearing, and taste. They convey output to the voluntary muscles involved with the movements of the eyes, mouth, face, tongue, pharynx, and larynx. They are the major outlet for the parasympathetic nervous system.

The autonomic nervous system is composed of two parts, the sympathetic and the parasympathetic. The sympathetic system stimulates those activities mobilized during stress or emergency situations—otherwise called the *fight or flight* activities. For instance, it accelerates the rate and the force of the heartbeat, increases blood pressure, and directs blood flow to voluntary muscles. In contrast, the parasympathetic system acts to conserve and restore the energy reserves of the organism. It decreases the rate and the force of the heartbeat, decreases blood pressure, encourages digestion, and, finally, eliminates water and waste products.

However, these two systems are not antagonistic. Their actions are complementary and synergistic, and they act in concert to respond to the intensity of stress and emotional demands of the current situation.[11]

ORTHOPEDICS

Everyone assumes that the body is bilaterally symmetrical, but close inspection will show absolute symmetry to be a rarity. Inspection of the skeletal system is necessary to expose unilateral or aberrant relationships that could cause chronic muscle pains similar to those caused by true TMJ problems.

These relationships, if not properly treated, could cause a continuation of somatic pain even though the other causes of TMJ pain have been properly and satisfactorily treated. This, of course, would be discouraging to the patient and confounding to the practitioner.

DIET

A good diet is important, since a poor diet increases the probability of a slower than normal recovery from TMJ problems. When diet is mentioned, many patients will admit that they have adopted a diet which they know is not beneficial to them. Too often the pain of TMJ syndrome has compromised their diet to one of fast foods, quickly eaten, that supply very little valuable nutrition.

EMOTIONS

It has been found that stress will precipitate physical as well as emotional illness. The death rate of widows and widowers is 10 times higher during the first year of bereavement than for others their age. Divorced persons in the year following divorce have an illness rate 12 times higher than that of married persons. Up to 80% of physical illnesses seem to develop at a time when the victims feel helpless and hopeless. It is difficult for a patient to follow suggested treatment when emotions are telling him or her to scream, recoil, flee, rebel, argue, or cry.

We are interested here in the emotional disturbances caused by situational difficulty and by emotional irritation resulting from suppression of the fight or flight responses, which unsettle the glandular balance of the body. We must allow the patient a mental catharsis for these problems, since the very expression of these problems, bringing them to consciousness where they can be discussed with someone, is the first step in their solution.

Simple tests, discussed in Chapter 13, can disclose whether a patient should receive professional counseling or whether just a good listener can satisfy the needed emotional release by verbalization.

MYOFUNCTIONAL THERAPY

A complete discussion on myofunctional therapy is found in Chapter 24.

STUDY MODELS

Study models are invaluable in assessing all the variables and relationships of the dental occlusion. Margins of fillings may look fairly good in an oral examination but may appear faulty on a study model. Nuances in a pathological occlusion that defy detection in the mouth or in hand-held models are graphically revealed when good study models are gnathologically mounted on an adjustable articulator. The study models should be taken with the same care that would be devoted to a fine inlay. If *any* detail is missing, it may be that very area which holds the answer to the problem.

To properly examine the study casts, they should be dry and properly trimmed so that no parts of the casts are in contact except the teeth (that is, opposing areas of contacting gum must be relieved).

Hand-held models

Following are areas of interest to be studied on hand-held models:

1. Arch form, missing teeth
2. Rotated teeth, uneven marginal ridges
3. Trusions
4. Tipping
5. Versions
6. Diastemas
7. Tori
8. Positions of contact points
9. Erosions or abrasions
10. Plunger cusps
11. Degree of compensating curves (curves of Spee and Wilson)
12. Defective margins and surfaces (contours) of restorations
13. Functional and nonfunctional facets of wear[13,18]

Mounted models

In mounting casts on articulator it is necessary to record an arbitrary hinge axis first. The arbitrary measurement is used because abnormal conditions in the muscles of mastication have repositioned the condyle in an abnormal posture in the glenoid fossa.

The maxillary cast is mounted with a face-bow to the arbitrary hinge axis registration. The mandibular cast is mounted using a bite technique that allows no tooth-to-tooth contact and ensures a centric relation, or terminal hinge relationship. This is important because it is a reproducible (objective) relationship, not a subjective one.

When the cast is correctly mounted in this manner, the operator has the equivalent of the patient's teeth on a machine that reasonably duplicates all the movements as they are made by the patient. A complete horizontal envelope of motion is reproduced, and all excursions are demonstrable.

Mounted models will disclose the following:

1. The teeth whose interferences prevent the casts from closing in terminal hinge relation are easily identified by the use of dental articulating tape.
2. Visibility of the teeth and the articulation from all aspects is possible.
3. Discrepancies of arch relationship and tooth relationships are more readily visible.
4. There is no proprioceptor action to prevent the casts from contact in terminal hinge relationship.
5. Duplicate models mounted on the articulator in the identical manner used in mounting the original models can be used to correct interferences in the occlusion by cutting away the premature contacts.
6. The same duplicate models can be used and wax buildup techniques employed to correct tooth contours and alter the occlusal relationships to obtain a definite and stable articulation in terminal hinge relationship.
7. The final treatment plan for alteration of the occlusion is determined from information revealed by the mounted casts. Therefore the procedures suggested in paragraphs 5 and 6 should be done to make sure that the projected treatment is not impractical or totally impossible.

Text continued on p. 104.

A

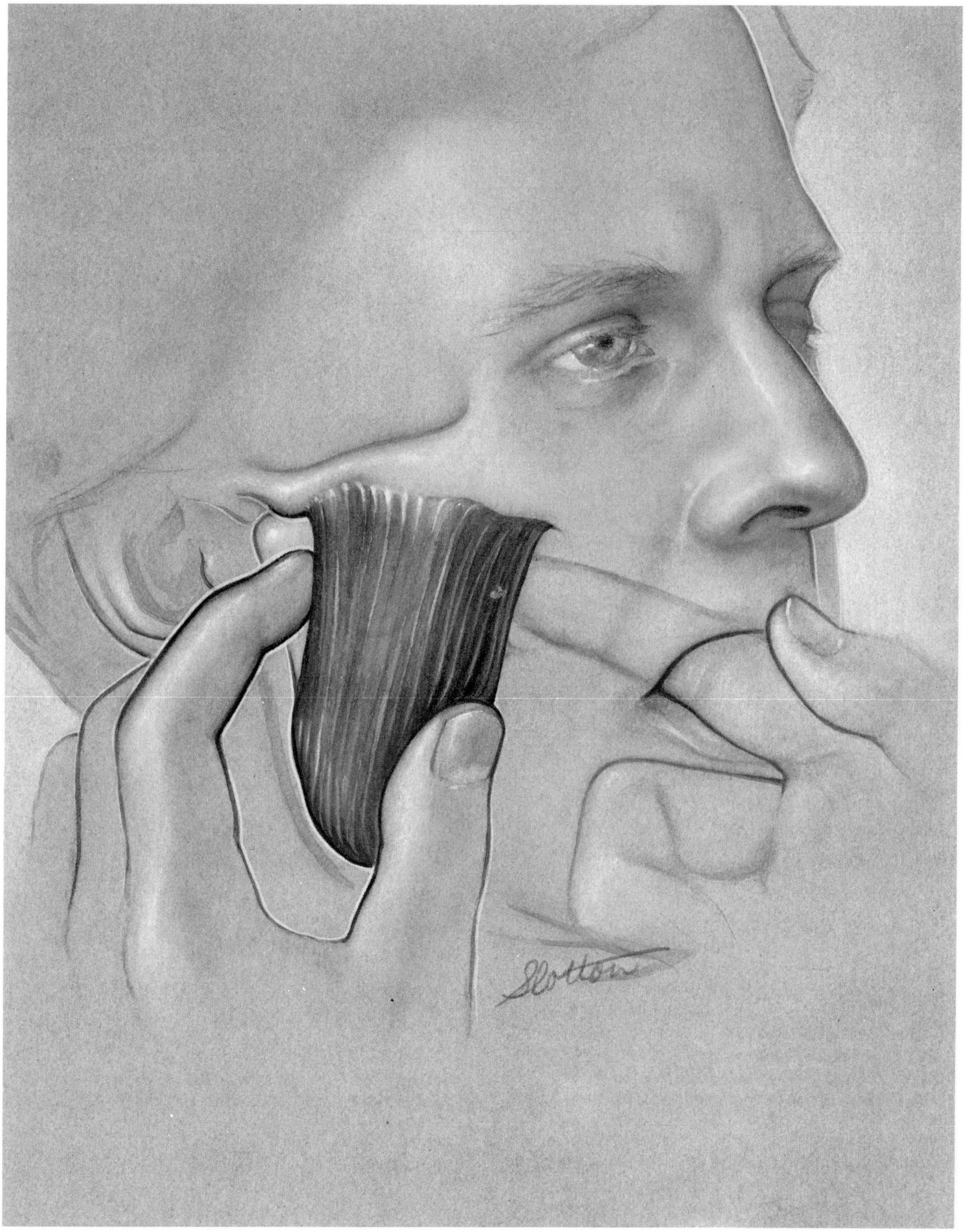

Fig. 6-3. A, Palpation of origin and body of masseter.
Continued.

B

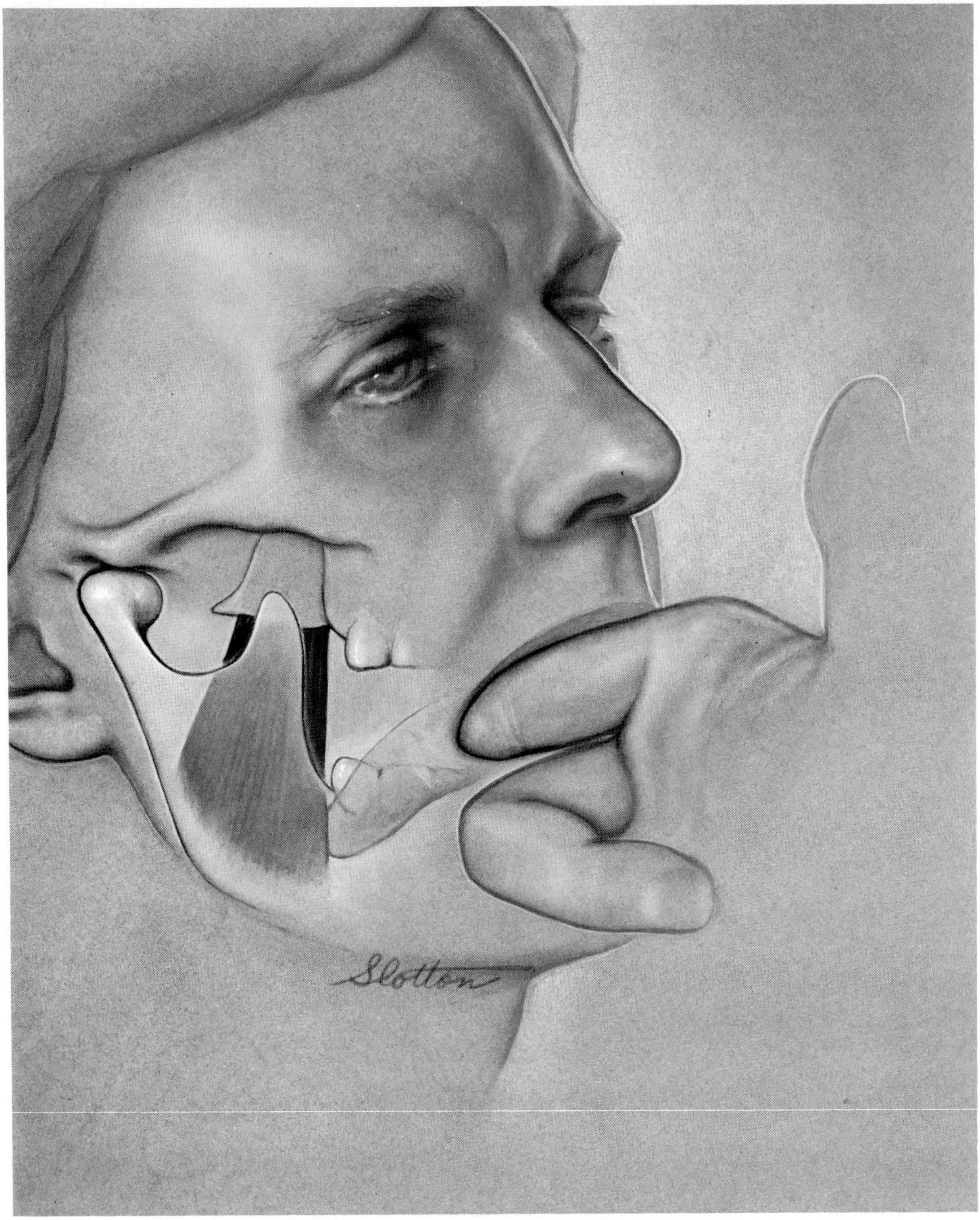

Fig. 6-3, cont'd. B, Palpation of insertion of internal pterygoid.

TMJ CLINICAL EXAMINATION FORM

Patient ______________________________ Date ____________

1. CHIEF COMPLAINT ______________________________
2. SYMPTOMS have been present for ________ months or ________ years.
3. CHRONOLOGY OF SYMPTOMS
   a.
   b.
   c.
4. FACIAL ASYMMETRY
   a. None
   b. Yes, asymmetry is {Perceptible / Obvious / Gross} on the {Right / or / Left} at {Temporal / or / Masseter areas}
5. PALPATION OF THE JOINTS

	Pain		
a. On TMJ palpation (teeth in rest position)	Right	Left	None
b. On TMJ palpation (teeth clenched)	Right,	Left	None
c. On digital examination of the auditory canal	Right	Left	None
d. During right lateral movement	Right	Left	None
e. During left lateral movement	Right	Left	None
f. Right condyle translation	Smooth	Grating	Asynchronous
g. Left condyle translation	Smooth	Grating	Asynchronous

6. PALPATION OF THE MUSCLES

	Pain		
a. Masseter			
(1) Origin: With the index finger intraorally, press laterally inside the cheek.	Right	Left	None
(2) Insertion: With the fingers extraorally, press medially down on the muscle to its insertion at the angle.	Right	Left	None
b. Internal pterygoid (both tests are made intraorally)			
(1) Origin: Press the index finger laterally just distal to the hamular process.	Right	Left	None
(2) Insertion: Trace muscle down medial side of ramus to its insertion; with the index finger press laterally inside the angle of the jaw.	Right	Left	None
c. External pterygoid			
Origin: Press the index finger medially behind tuberosity of the maxilla.	Right	Left	None

Continued.

C

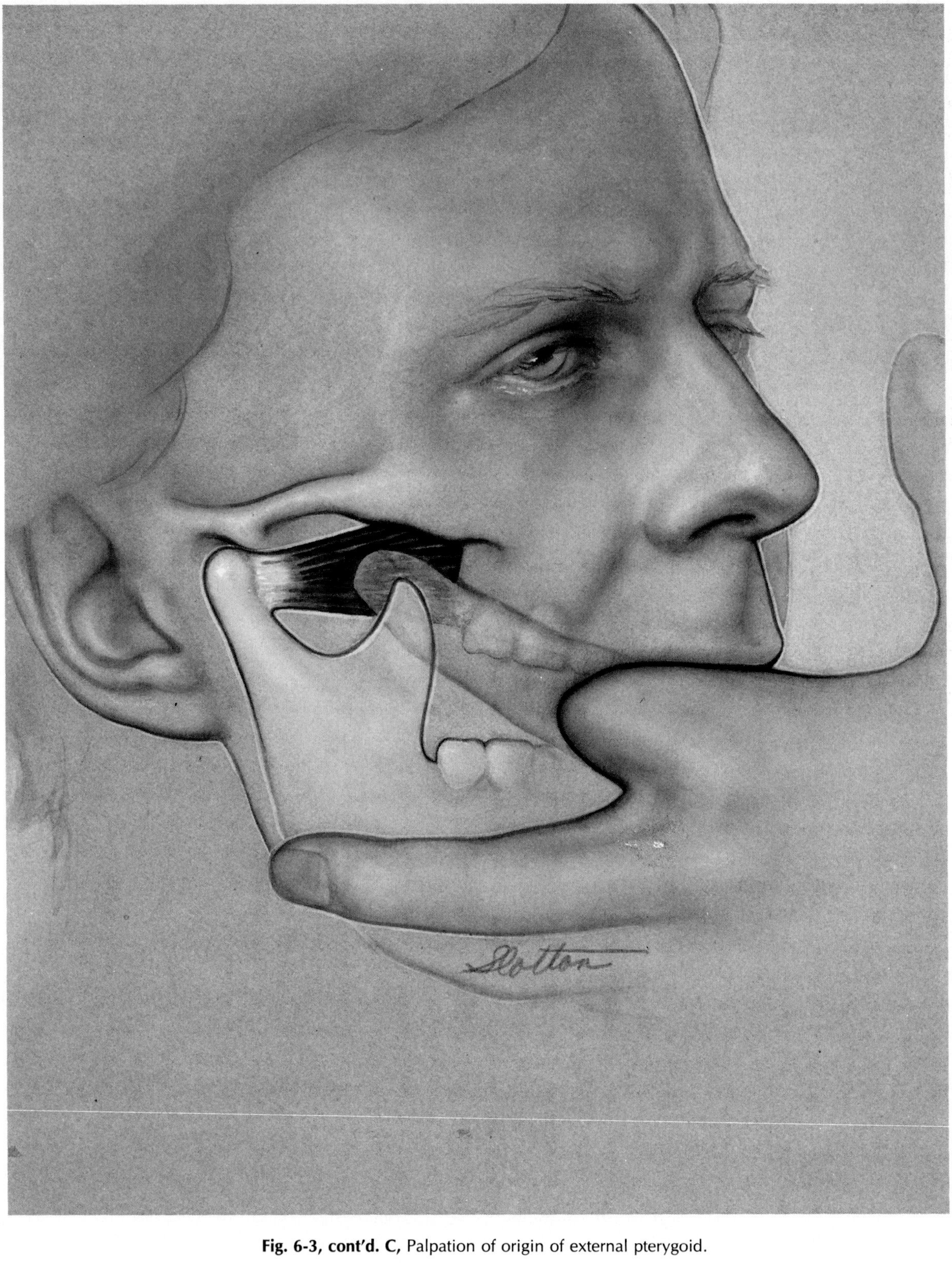

Fig. 6-3, cont'd. C, Palpation of origin of external pterygoid.

TMJ CLINICAL EXAMINATION FORM—cont'd

d. Temporal			
(1) Origin: Palpate each of the three muscle heads in the temporal fossa.	Right	Left	None
(2) Insertion: With the index finger intraorally, palpate the cheek laterally at the retromolar fossa.	Right	Left	None
e. Digastric			
(1) Anterior belly: At a point halfway between the angle of the mandible and the chin apply pressure extraorally in an upward and medial direction, intraoral pressure can also be applied simultaneously on the floor of the mouth.	Right	Left	None
(2) Posterior belly: Pressure is applied medially and upward, beginning just medial and distal to the angle of the mandible; the palpating finger falls between the angle of the mandible and the sternocleidomastoid muscle.	Right	Left	None
f. Sternocleidomastoid (roll head to the side being tested)			
(1) Origin: Pinch muscle at the sternum.	Right	Left	None
(2) Body: Pinch muscle at its midpoint.	Right	Left	None
(3) Insertion: Press on mastoid process.	Right	Left	None
g. Trapezius			
(1) Upper portion on neck	Right	Left	None
(2) Middle portion on shoulders	Right	Left	None
(3) Lower portion on middle back	Right	Left	None
h. Splenius capitis			
Press firmly in the depression between the insertion of the sternocleidomastoid and the origin of the trapezius.	Right	Left	None
7. PAIN IN THE HEAD AND NECK		*Pain*	
a. Vertex (check sternomastoid as a cause of referred pain)		Yes	None
b. Temporal (check temporal as a cause of referred pain)	Right	Left	None
c. Occiput (check posterior temporal, subscapular part of trapezius)	Right	Left	None
d. Neck (check sternomastoid, cleidomastoid, trapezius)	Right	Left	None
e. Cervical lymph glands	Right	Left	None
f. Maxillary sinus and face (check external pterygoid, sternomastoid, trapezius)	Right	Left	None

Continued.

D

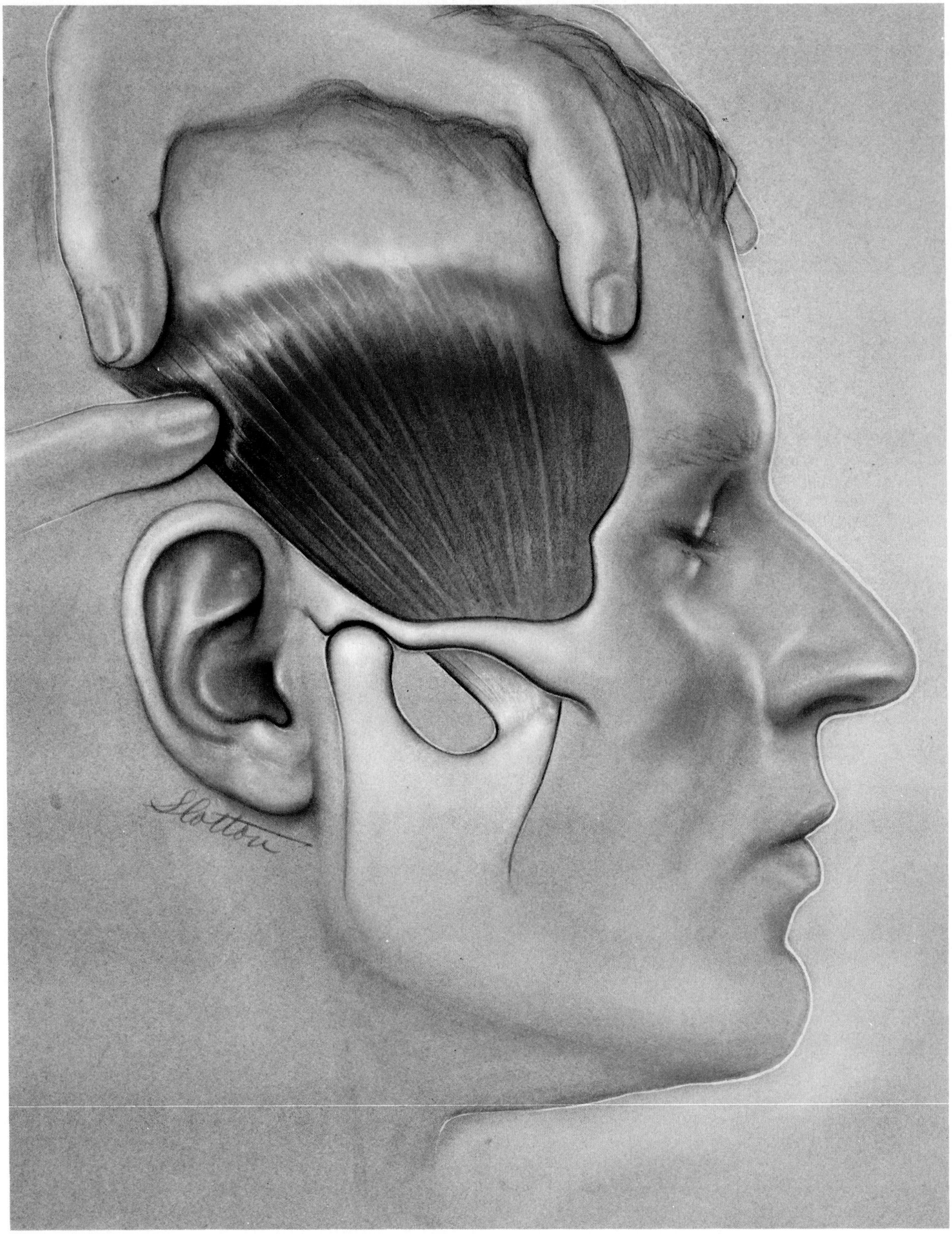

Fig. 6-3, cont'd. D, Palpation of temporal: anterior portion, middle portion, posterior portion.

TMJ CLINICAL EXAMINATION FORM—cont'd

g. Ear and middle ear (check deep masseter, sternomastoid) — Right Left None

h. Tongue and hard palate (check internal pterygoid) — Right Left None

i. Jaws and gums (check masseter, suprascapular part of trapezius) — Right Left None

Where?____________________

j. Teeth

(1) Upper
- Anteriors (check anterior fibers of temporal)
- Posteriors (check posterior fibers of temporal)

(2) Lower posteriors (check suprascapular and trapezius)

8. OPENING MOVEMENT

a. Maximum opening without pain ________ mm

b. Synchronous or Asynchronous on the Right or Left

c. Jaw deviates on opening to the — Right Left None

d. Jaw deviates first to the right, then left — Yes No

e. Jaw deviates first to the left, then right — Yes No

f. Jaw deviates laterally about ________ mm from midline of upper teeth

g. A right lateral excursion is demonstrable — Yes No

h. A left lateral excursion is demonstrable — Yes No

9. EXAMINATION OF THE SOFT TISSUES

a. External: Skin of the face, lymph chains, lips

b. Vestibule and tongue: Vestibule, cheeks, mucosa, gums, tongue

c. Tongue and floor of the mouth: Floor of the mouth, the base, lateral borders, and ventral surfaces of the tongue

d. Palate: Observe and palpate the hard and soft palate and uvula

e. Fauces and pharynx: Tonsils, anterior and posterior palatine arches, and nasopharynx

10. EXAMINATION OF THE TEETH

a. List areas requiring immediate attention (deep cavities, loose teeth, extractions). ________________

b. List areas of

(1) Periodontal problems (mobility) ________________

(2) Incisal and occlusal wear. Move the mandible slowly to position the worn maxillomandibular incisors in relationships that reveal whether the wear is caused by habitual eccentric bruxing; show this to the patient.

Continued.

E

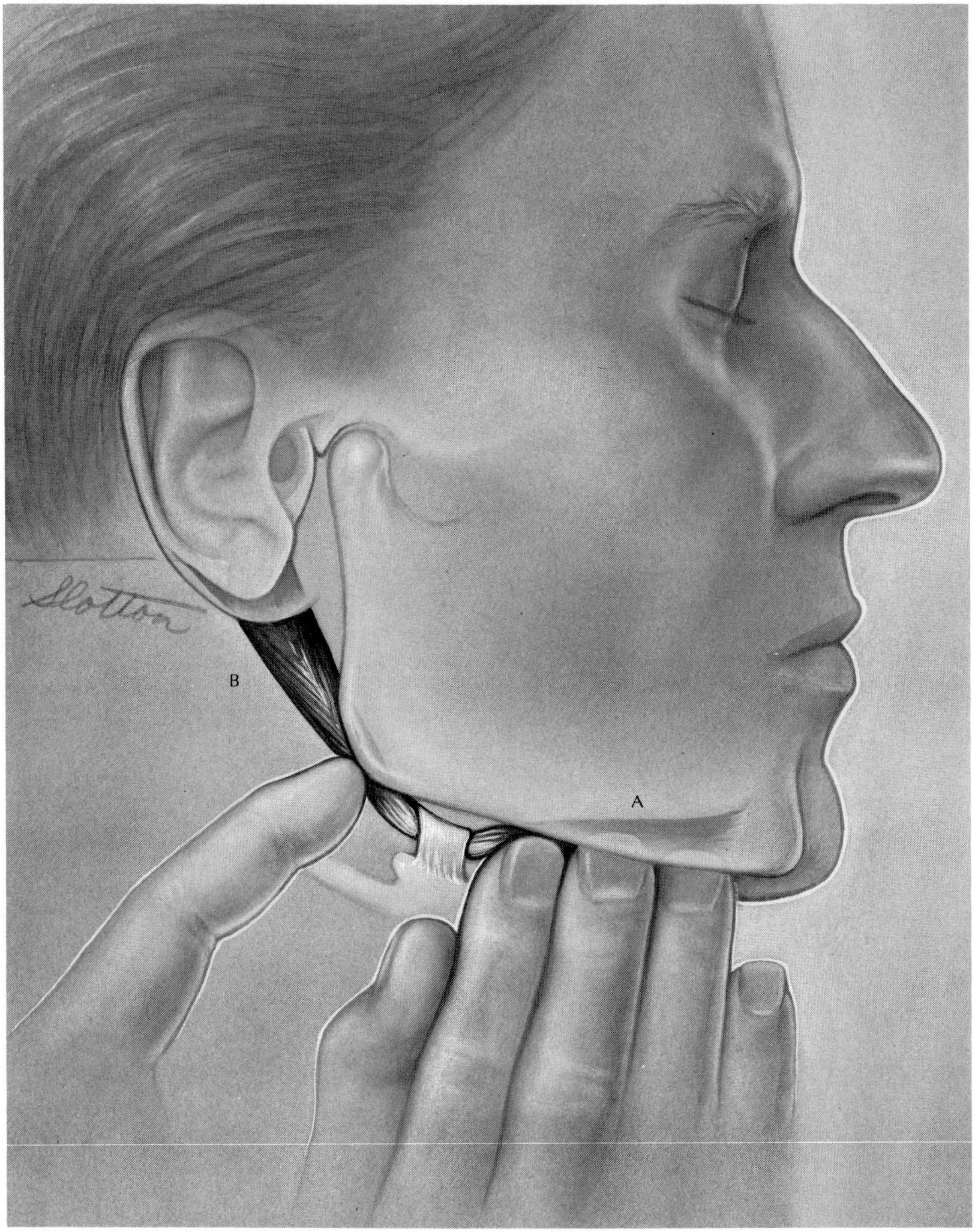

Fig. 6-3, cont'd. E, Palpation of digastric. *A,* Anterior belly; *B,* posterior belly.

TMJ CLINICAL EXAMINATION FORM—cont'd

11. EXAMINATION OF THE OCCLUSION

a. Anterior slide (centric relation to centric occlusion)		Yes	No	
b. Lateral slide (centric relation to centric occlusion)		Yes	No	
c. Distal slide (rest position to centric occlusion) (C1-II)		Yes	No	
d. Firm posterior support		Yes	No	No posterior teeth
e. Prosthesis satsifactory		Yes	No	No posterior prothesis
f. Canine protected occlusion	Right side	Yes	No	
(or group function)	Left side	Yes	No	
g. In right lateral				
(1) Working interferences are present		Yes	No	
(2) Balancing interferences are present		Yes	No	
h. In left lateral				
(1) Working interferences are present		Yes	No	
(2) Balancing interferences are present		Yes	No	

i. Bruxing or Clenching habits are Suspected or Admitted

j. Mark the occlusion by having patient bite in centric occlusion with articulating paper or ribbon between the teeth.

(1) Bilateral or Unilateral contacts show Evenly or Unevenly on premolars and molars	Yes	No
(2) Hyperocclusion on the anterior teeth	Yes	No

k. Fremitus of the teeth on closure? Numbers ________

l. Occlusion Class I II III

m. Vertical overbite ________ mm Horizontal overjet ________ mm

12. FULL MOUTH X-RAY FILMS

Property of ________________________________

a. Cavities requiring immediate attention ________________________________

b. Pathology (exposures, abscesses, cysts) ________________________________

c. Periodontia (widened periodontal space, occlusal flaring, loose teeth) ________________

13. TEMPOROMANDIBULAR JOINT X-RAY FILMS

Type of x-ray films ________________ Property of ________________

a. Condyle morphology	Right side	Normal	Abnormal
	Left side	Normal	Abnormal
b. Fossa morphology	Right side	Normal	Abnormal
	Left side	Normal	Abnormal
c. Eminence morphology	Right side	Normal	Abnormal
	Left side	Normal	Abnormal

Continued.

F

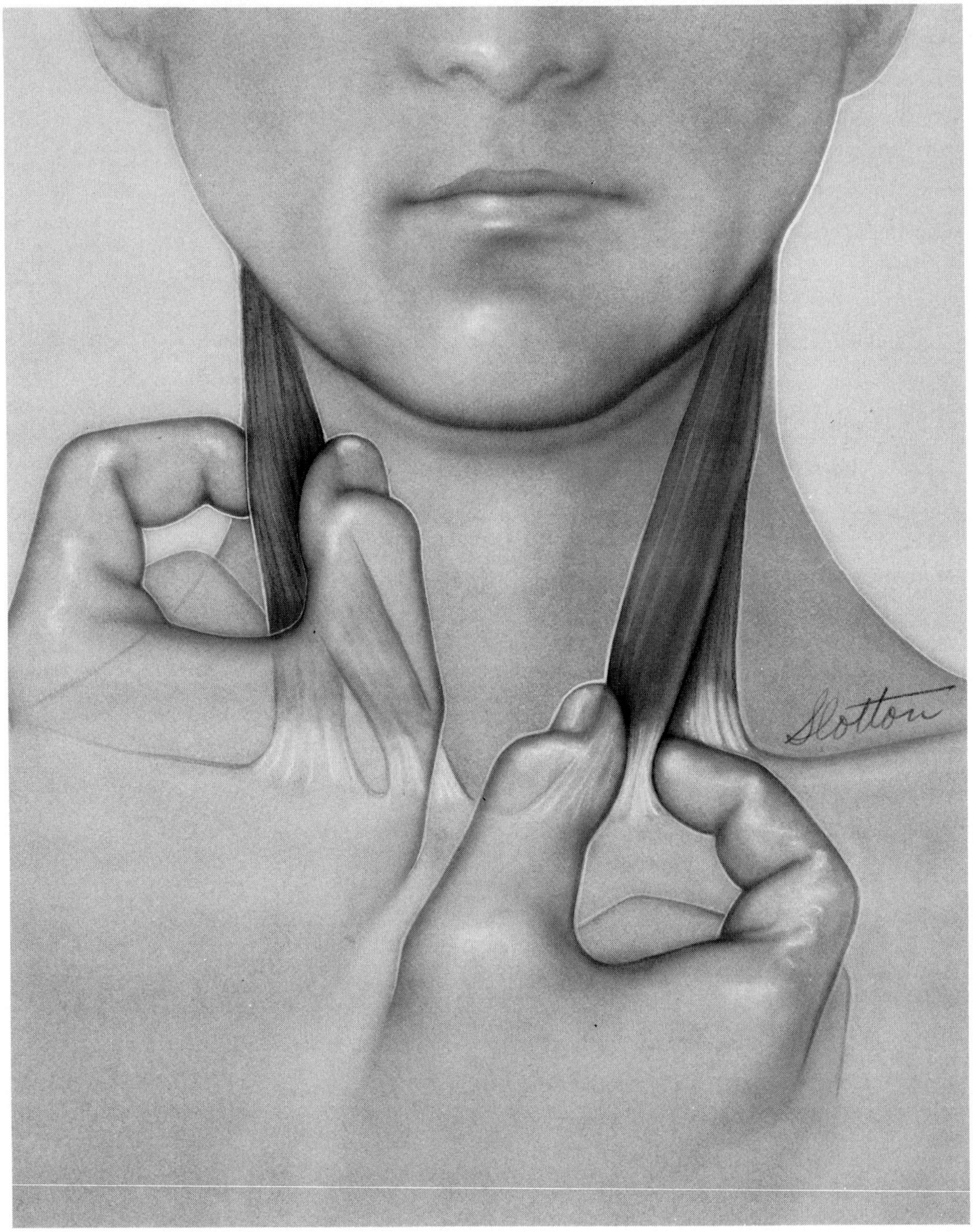

Fig. 6-3, cont'd. F, Palpation of sternocleidomastoid; right, origin; left, body.

TMJ CLINICAL EXAMINATION FORM—cont'd

d. Posture of condyle in the fossa*	Right side	Normal	Abnormal
	Left side	Normal	Abnormal
e. Condyle translates on the	Right side	Yes	No
	Left side	Yes	No
f. Evidence of neoplasms on the	Right side	Yes	No
	Left side	Yes	No
g. Evidence of osteoarthritis	Right side	Yes	No
	Left side	Yes	No

14. LIMITED NEUROLOGICAL EXAMINATION
   a. Optic nerve (II) (vision test)

      Cover the eye, and have the patient read something. Repeat for the other eye. Ask if vision is clear or if there are blind spots.
   b. Nerves III, IV, VI (supply movement to the eye and pupil reactions)
      (1) Pupils: Note size, equality, and iris reaction to light. Have patient follow your finger. Note conjugate (moving together) movement and nystagmus (rapid involuntary oscillation of the eyeballs).
      (2) Eyelids: Note any ptosis (drooping).
   c. Trigeminal nerve V (supplies sensation to the face and movement to the muscles of mastication)
      (1) Sensory: Test sensitivity of the thirds of the face (upper, middle, lower) with a wisp of cotton. Test bilaterally.
      (2) Motor: Check contraction of masseters and temporals.
   d. Facial nerve VII (supplies movement to muscles of facial expression and taste in anterior two thirds of the tongue)

      Test facial movement: ask patient to move eyebrows up, frown, show teeth, whistle, purse lips.
   e. Auditory nerve VIII (hearing, equilibrium)

      Test patient's ability to hear a watch tick.
   f. If test results leave you in doubt, refer patient for a full neurological examination.
15. ORTHOPEDICS (have the patient stand)†
   a. General posture   Erect   Slouch   Deviation
   b. Head equidistant from shoulders   Yes   No, the head is nearer the Right, Left shoulder
   c. Eyes and eyebrows level   Yes   No, the Right, Left is higher
   d. Shoulders level   Yes   No, the Right, Left shoulder is higher
   e. Spine Straight or Scoliosis
   f. Hips level   Yes   No, the Right, Left hip is higher
   g. Presence of lower back pain   Yes   No
   h. Legs of equal length   Yes   No, the Right, Left leg is longer

*Average measurements: (1) from the condyle to the eminence = 1.5 mm; (2) from the condyle to the top of the fossa = 2.5 mm; (3) from the condyle to the center of the auditory canal = 7.5 mm.
†From Gelb, H.: Personal communication, 1976.

Continued.

G

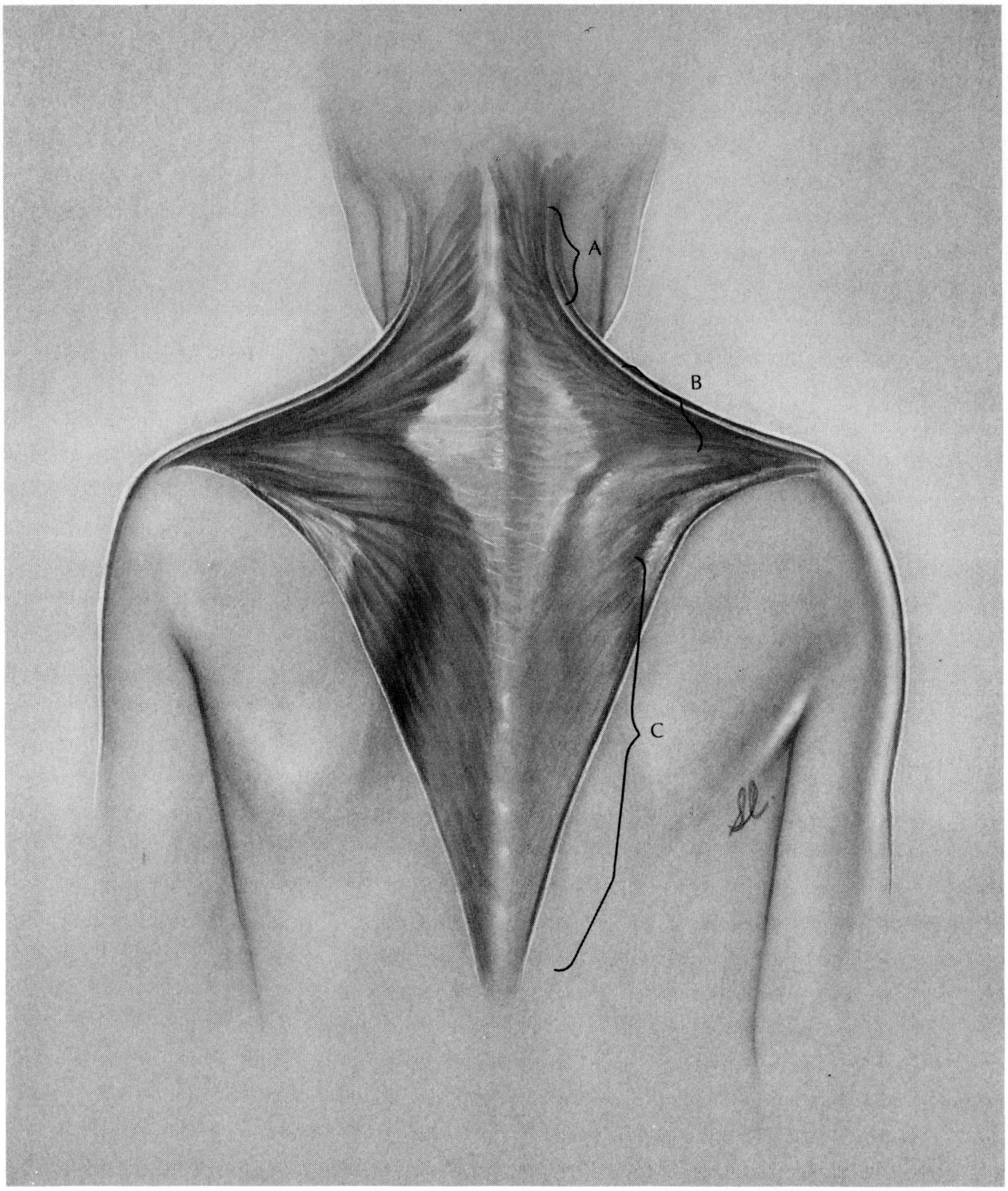

Fig. 6-3, cont'd. G, Palpation of trapezius. *A,* Upper fibers; *B,* middle fibers; *C,* lower fibers.

TMJ CLINICAL EXAMINATION FORM—cont'd

16. SEVEN RULES FOR HEALTH
    a. Three meals a day at regular intervals
    b. A good breakfast, daily
    c. No smoking
    d. Moderate exercise two or three times a week
    e. Six to seven hours sleep a night
    f. Moderate weight
    g. No alcohol, or only in moderation
    h. Additional health considerations
       (1) Ingestion of sugar: Excessive Average Slight
       (2) Vitamin supplements: Which? ________ None ________
       (3) Mineral supplements (especially calcium and magnesium): Which? ________ None ________
17. EMOTIONAL FACTORS (get patients to talk about themselves)
    a. Are you fatigued?
    b. Do you sleep well?
    c. Accident prone?
    d. Indigestion?
    e. Married? Happy?
    f. Job satisfy you?
    g. Children? At home?
    h. Are you depressed?
    i. Do your friends (or spouse) consider you a perfectionist?
    j. Spouse help you?
    k. Are you nervous?
18. PSYCHOLOGICAL CONSIDERATIONS
    Considering the answers to the previous set of questions and to your own estimation of the stability of this patient, should an MMPI test or a Cornell Medical Index test be made?
19. ORAL MYOFUNCTIONAL CONSIDERATIONS
    a. Lips
       (1) Normal ________ Flaccid ________ Compressed ________
       (2) Habitually open ________ Closed ________ Tense ________
       (3) Composed ________ Hyperactive ________
    b. Tongue
       (1) Rest position: Visible ________ Palatal ________ Floor of mouth ________
       Against dentition: Upper ________ Lower ________ Posterior ________
       (2) In speech: Lateral flaring ________ Between anterior teeth ________
       (3) Tongue frequently bitten? Habitually ________ Accidentally ________
       (4) Lateral pressure markings: Scalloping ________ Ridges ________

Continued.

H

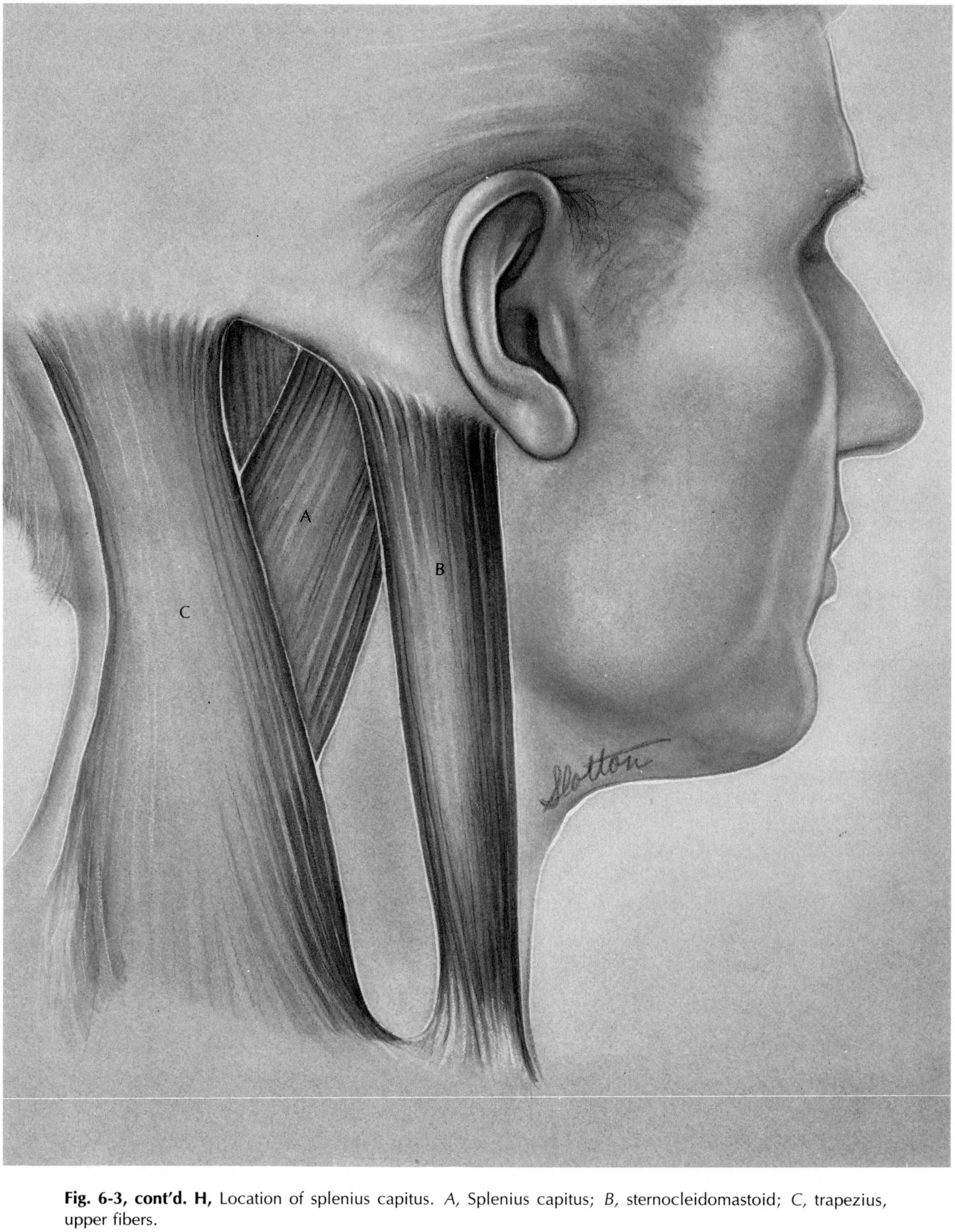

Fig. 6-3, cont'd. H, Location of splenius capitus. *A,* Splenius capitus; *B,* sternocleidomastoid; *C,* trapezius, upper fibers.

TMJ CLINICAL EXAMINATION FORM—cont'd

c. Swallow

(1) Swallow appears Easy ________ Difficult ________

(2) Is a change in head position necessary? Yes No

(3) Do the lips part during the swallow? Yes No

(4) Is there an obvious tightening of the facial muscles? Yes No

(5) Tongue position during the swallow

(a) On the rugae posterior to upper centrals ________ (normal)

(b) Against the maxillary anteriors ________

(c) Against the mandibular anteriors ________

(d) Separates the bite posteriorly ________

(e) Visible between the teeth anteriorly ________

d. NOXIOUS HOBBIES AND HABITS

(1) Musical instruments, for example, reed instruments, flute, violin

(2) Shooting guns

(3) Gum chewing

(4) Stomach sleeping

(5) Lip or cheek biting

(6) Fingernail biting

(7) Clenching or bruxing

(8) Holding telephone with shoulder

(9) Sweating

(10) Emotional instability

(11) Anterior teeth in eccentric relationships

(12) Working under an air-conditioning duct

(13) Cupping chin in hand and leaning on it

20. NOTES (on your first impression of this case)

21. PROJECTED TREATMENT PROGRAM (number treatments in projected order of importance)

None
Deprogrammer
Vapocoolant spray
Preventive counseling
Moist heat
Muscle exercises
Soft diet
Drug therapy
Removal of gross prematurities
Kinesiology
Transcutaneous nerve stimulation

Biofeedback training
Flat occlusal splint
Orthopedic occlusal splint
Articulation correction
Orthodontic consultation
Myofunctional consultation
Cranial osteopathic consultation
Medical consultation
Neurological consultation
Psychiatric consultation
Surgical consultation

TECHNIQUE FOR MOUNTING CASTS ON AN ADJUSTABLE ARTICULATOR FOR OCCLUSAL STUDY

Clinical phase

Model impressions and the face-bow

1. With the index finger, press impression material into the occlusal surfaces of the posterior teeth to achieve essential detail and bubble-free impressions (Fig. 6-4).
2. Take upper and lower impressions in this manner, and pour them in a good model stone. Trim the art portion of the casts.
3. On the patient mark the location of the anterior reference point, 43 mm superior to the incisal edge of the left maxillary central incisor, with the Denar reference plane marker* (Fig. 6-5).
4. Mark the location of the posterior reference point (the arbitrary terminal hinge axis point) with the Denar reference planemarker (Fig. 6-6).
5. Lute Sylver horseshoe wax laminated wafers† to the top and bottom of the bite fork. Soften the wax in warm water (Fig. 6-7).

*Denar Corp., Anaheim, Calif.
†Jac Son Co., Burbank, Calif.

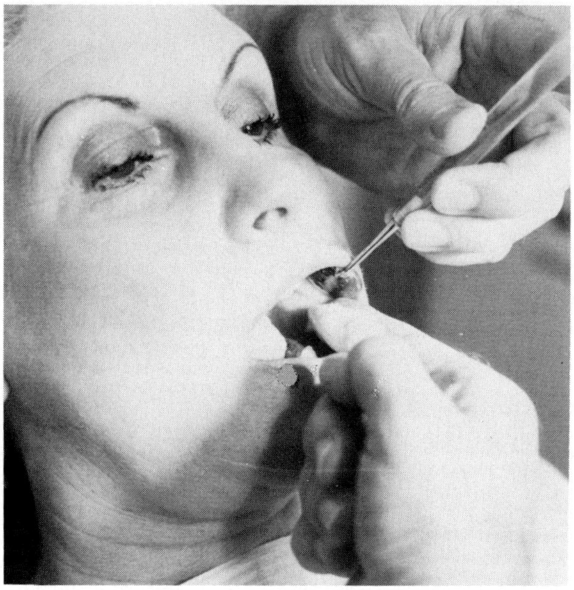

Fig. 6-4. Press alginate impression material onto occlusal surfaces before seating impression tray.

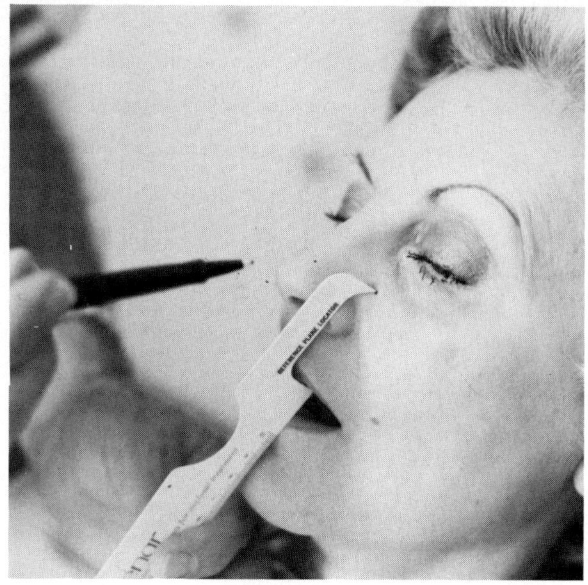

Fig. 6-5. Mark anterior reference point with small felt-tip pen.

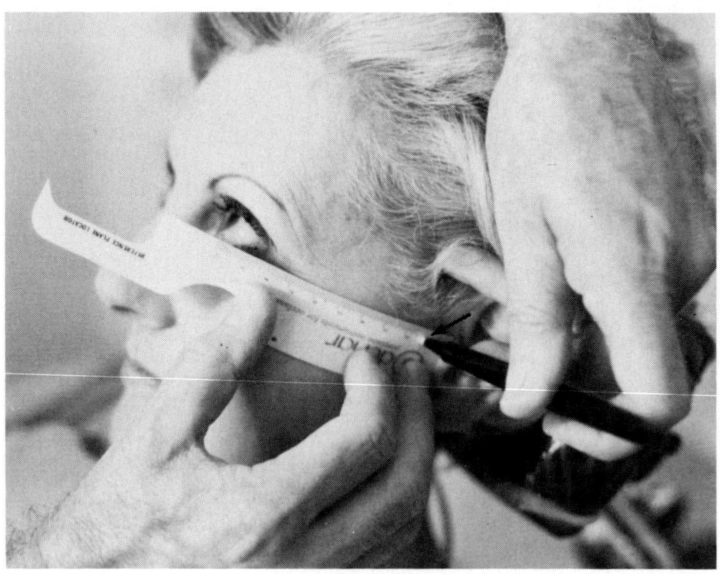

Fig. 6-6. Place Denar ruler along line connecting outer canthus of eye and tragus of ear to mark posterior reference point.

6. Press the bite fork and its top layer of wax onto the maxillary teeth hard enough to make indentations in the wax. Do not allow teeth to go through the wax into the bite fork (Fig. 6-8).
7. Bring the mandibular teeth up to make similar light indentations into the lower layer of wax (Fig. 6-9).
8. Remove the bite fork, and chill the wax in cold water.
9. Replace the bite fork, and have the patient bite hard enough to hold it steady.
10. Attach the face-bow anterior cross bar and side arms (Fig. 6-10).

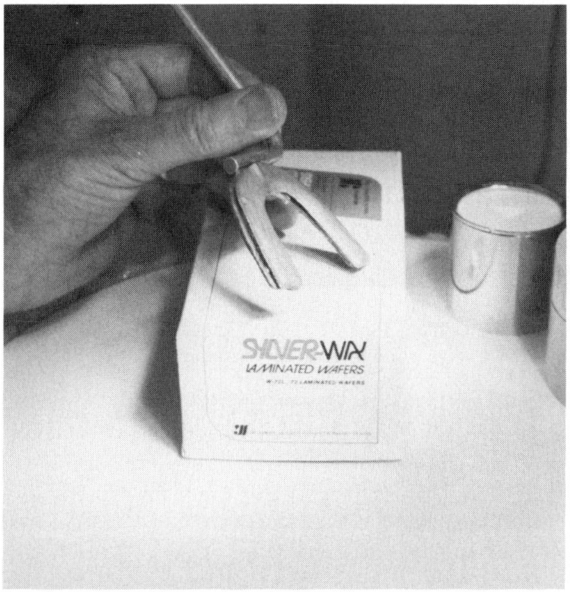

Fig. 6-7. Sylver-Wax wafers luted to top and bottom of bite fork.

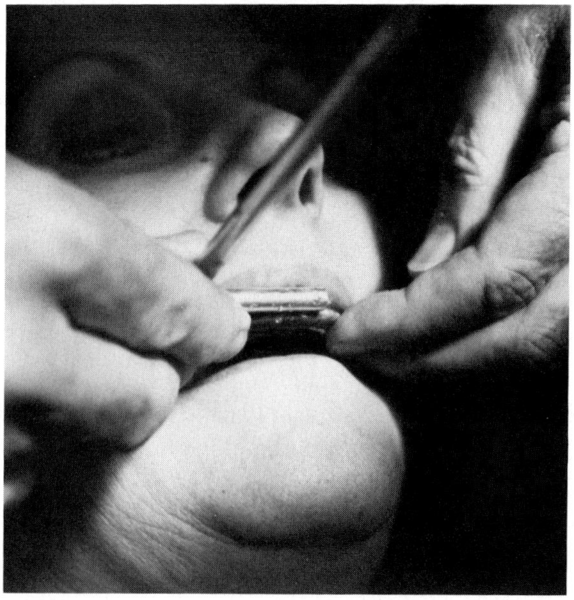

Fig. 6-8. Softened wax wafer is pressed up onto maxillary teeth.

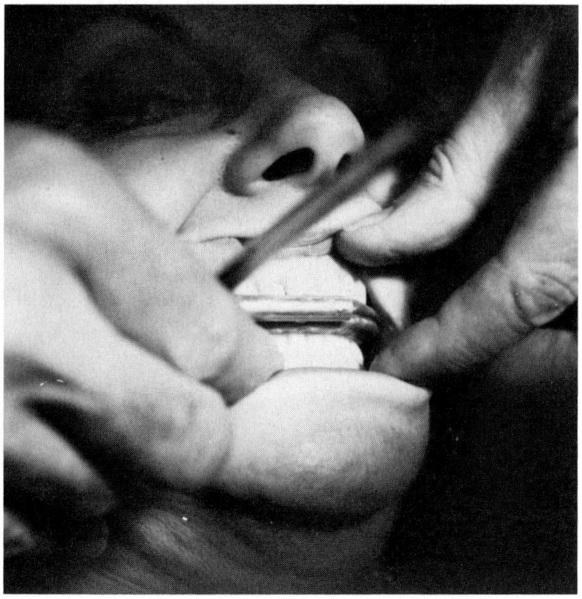

Fig. 6-9. Mandibular teeth are brought up into wax on bottom of bite fork.

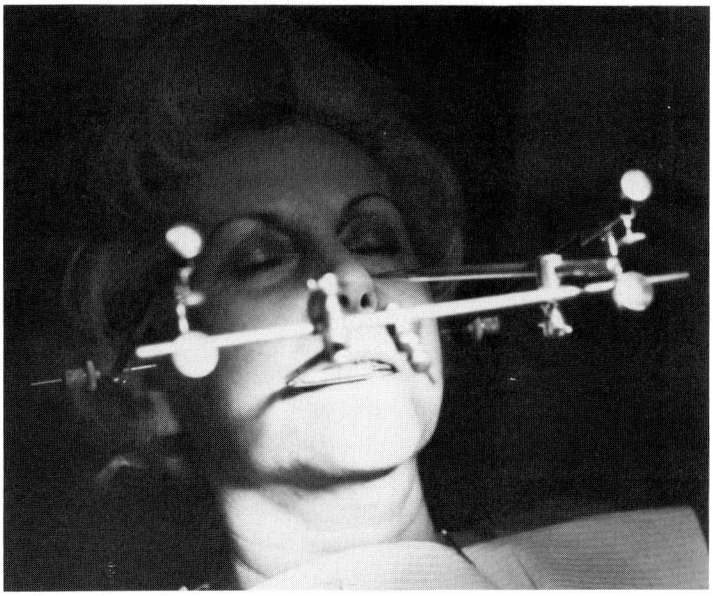

Fig. 6-10. Bite fork supporting face-bow.

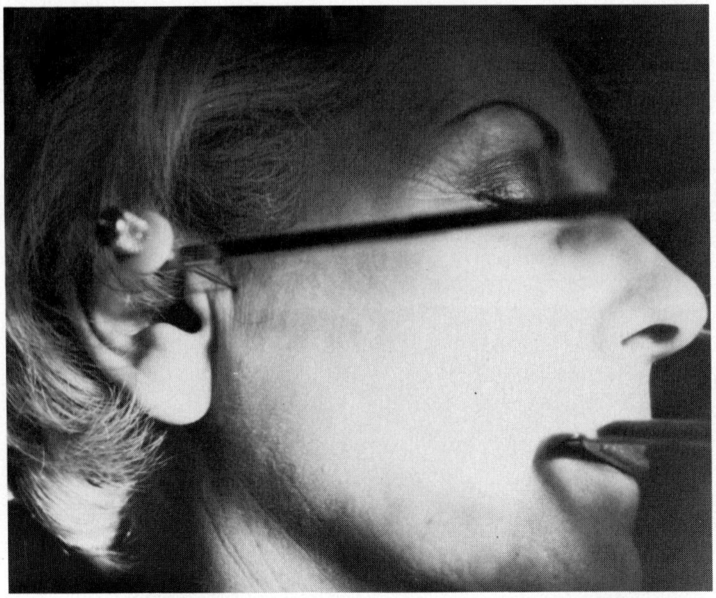

Fig. 6-11. Condyle marking pins centered in posterior reference point.

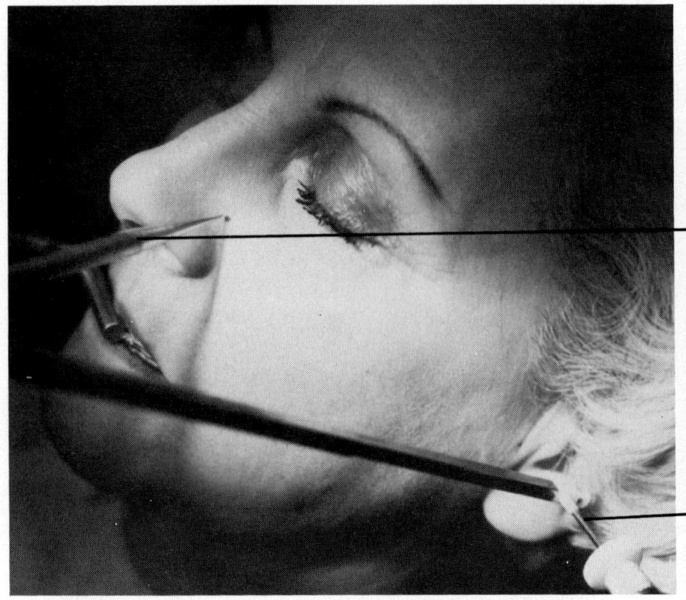

Fig. 6-12. *A,* Orbital marking rod centered over anterior reference point. *B,* Retracted condyle rotation marking pin.

11. Use the side-arm adjustments to center condyle marking pins over the hinge axis marks (step 4) (Fig. 6-11).
12. Attach the anterior reference plane rod. Retract the condyle rotation marking pins (Fig. 6-12).
13. Remove the complete face-bow assembly.
14. Secure the face-bow assembly on the mounting stand (Fig. 6-13).

Construction of the anterior jaw programmer. The function of the anterior jaw programmer is to bypass the proprioceptive impulses to the muscles of mastication and obtain a true terminal hinge registration. In cases of acute spastic contraction of the muscles of mastication the programmer may be used to deprogram those muscles and eliminate the painful spasticity within minutes, simply by preventing interdigitation of the teeth and moving the lower jaw into a terminal hinge relationship.

1. Make a small mix of tray acrylic to produce a cake $1 \times 1^{1}/_{2} \times {}^{1}/_{8}$ inch (Fig. 6-14).
2. Lubricate all anterior plastic fillings (labial and lingual) with petroleum jelly (Vaseline).
3. With moistened hands, adapt the cake to the lingual surfaces of the maxillary centrals and laterals and adjacent palate. Fold the anterior portion up to cover the incisal half of the labial surfaces (Fig. 6-15).
4. Remove the programmer, and dip it in a bowl of water to reduce heat of polymerization, then replace it in the mouth. Repeat until the plastic is firm, then set it aside to complete its set. Trim the programmer so that it extends to, but not beyond, the distal surfaces of the laterals (Fig. 6-16).

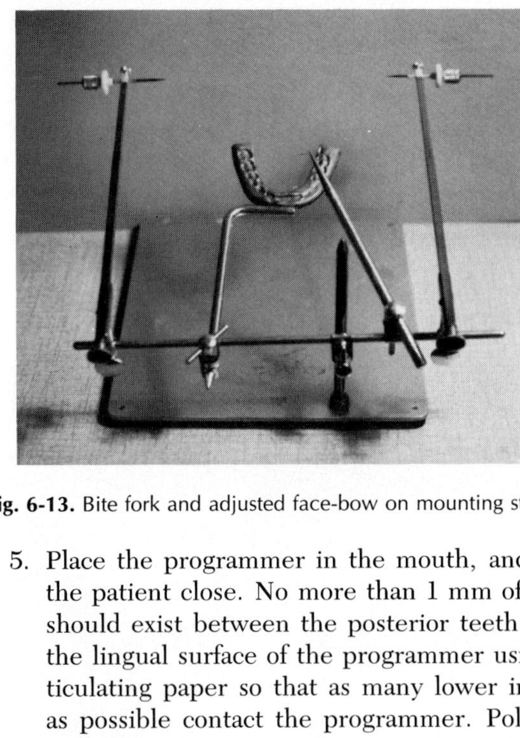

Fig. 6-13. Bite fork and adjusted face-bow on mounting stand.

5. Place the programmer in the mouth, and have the patient close. No more than 1 mm of space should exist between the posterior teeth. Trim the lingual surface of the programmer using articulating paper so that as many lower incisors as possible contact the programmer. Polish on a dental lathe (Fig. 6-17).
6. Place the thumb on the mental symphysis to provide positive direction of the jaw toward terminal hinge relation. Place the index finger under the left angle of the mandible, and place the second finger under the right angle of the mandible. The fingers provide support to the mandible and prevent subluxation when bites are being taken. This is called the *condyle support position* (Fig. 6-18).

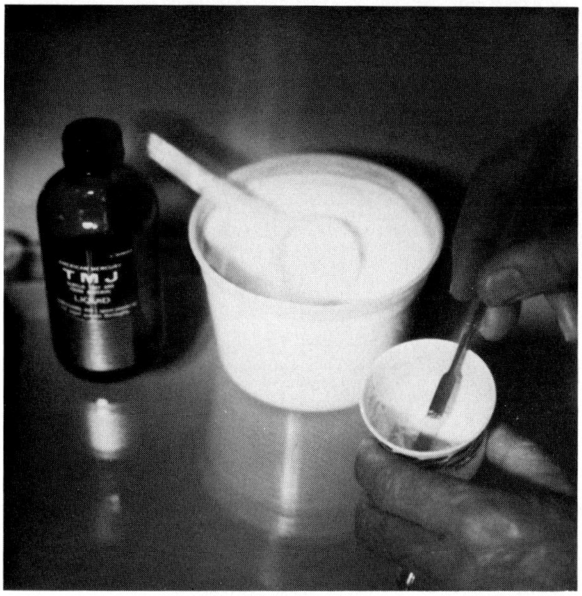

Fig. 6-14. Mix tray acrylic in wax-paper cup.

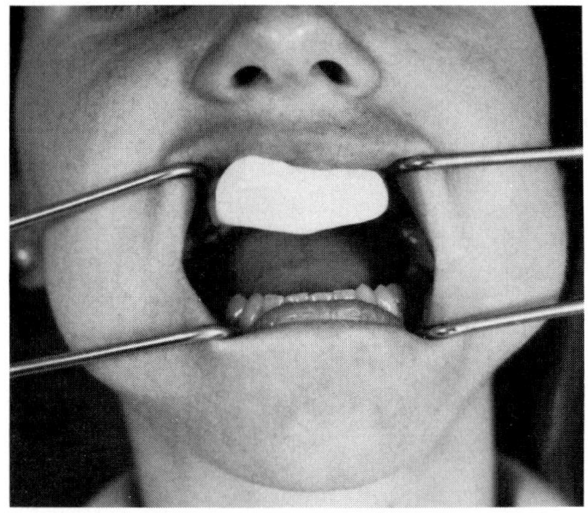

Fig. 6-15. Cake of acrylic pressed onto maxillary teeth.

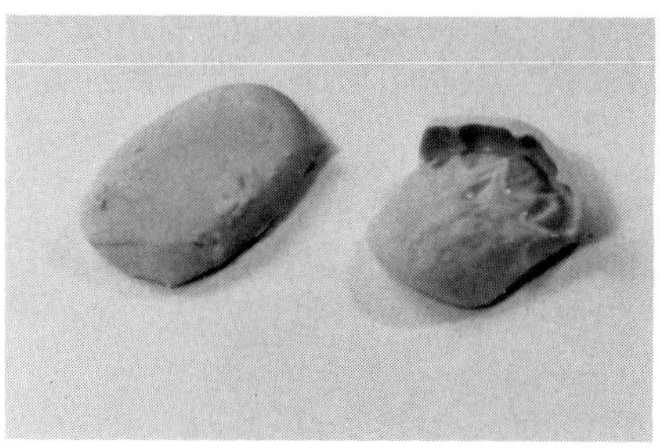

Fig. 6-16. Cake of acrylic before use, *left,* and after pressing it on maxillary teeth.

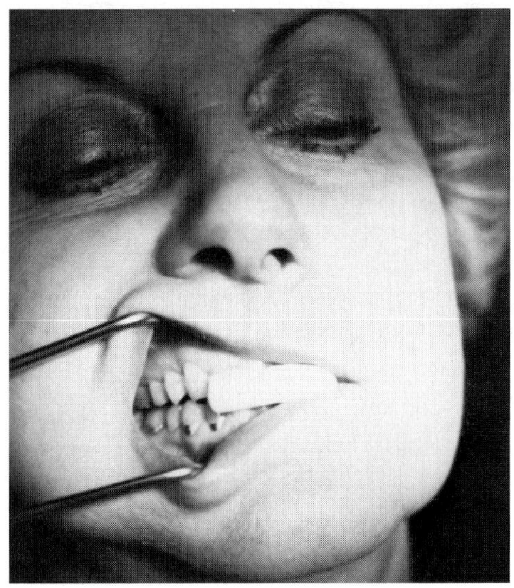

Fig. 6-17. Corrected and polished programmer in place.

A

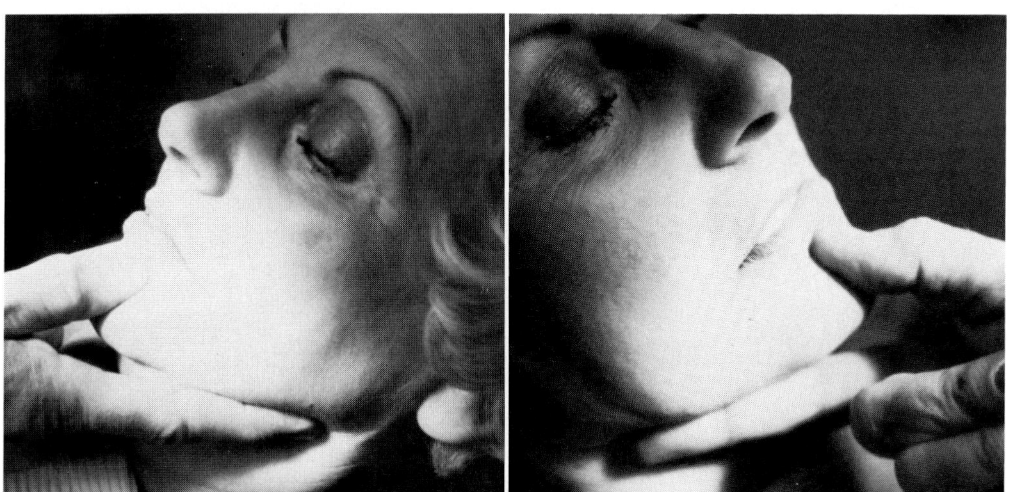

B

Fig 6-18. A, Condyle support position, left side. **B,** Condyle support position, right side.

7. With the programmer in place, ask the patient to slide the jaw forward and backward several times, using the condyle support position to guide the mandible. Make sure that there is no posterior occlusal contact during this excursion.
8. When you are certain that the condyles have reached their most retruded position (you may be able to feel them bump), use a sharp pencil held against the mandibular incisal teeth, and scribe a line on the adjacent acrylic programmer. Also mark the midline of the mandibular centrals (Fig. 6-19).
9. Verify these marks by repeated movements.
10. Make a mix of Coltoflax* following the directions of the manufacturer. Mix enough to make two ropes the diameter of a lead pencil and long enough to cover the occlusal surfaces of the posterior teeth *only* on each side of the arch (Fig. 6-20).

*Union Broach Co., New York, N.Y.

A 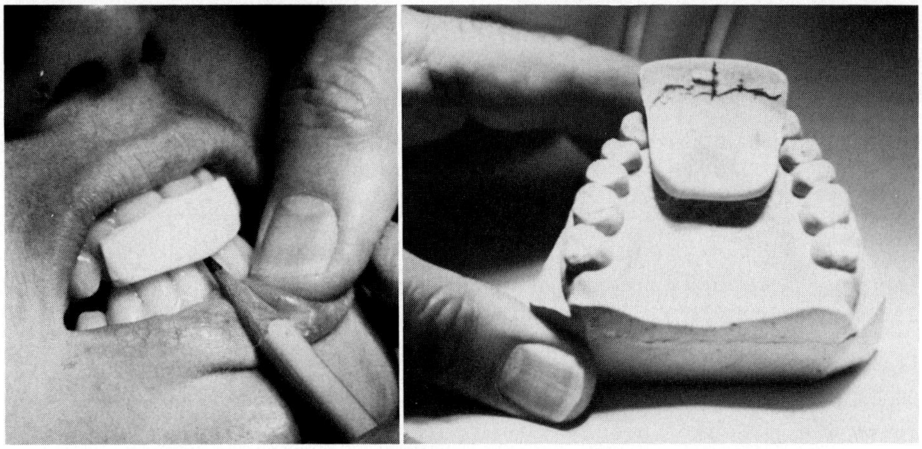 B

Fig. 6-19. A, Midline and outline of mandibular anterior teeth scribed on programmer. **B,** Programmer on maxillary model. Do not seat on model.

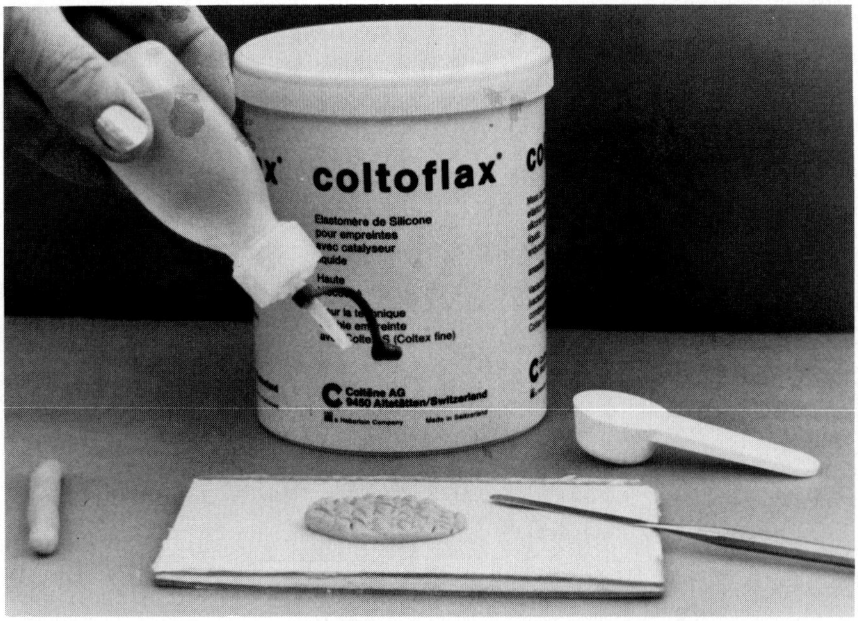

Fig 6-20. Drop liquid onto serrated Coltoflax patty for mixing.

11. Position both ropes of Coltoflax over the mandibular teeth on the right and left sides, respectively (Fig. 6-21).
12. With the anterior acrylic programmer in position, place your fingers in the condyle support position. Ask the patient to close easily. As the anterior teeth touch the programmer, support and guide the mandible into the terminal hinge position (Fig. 6-22). Continue to support the mandible until the Coltoflax reaches its set. Then check the accuracy of your registration by inspecting the pencil line previously scribed on the programmer (step 8) (Fig. 6-23).

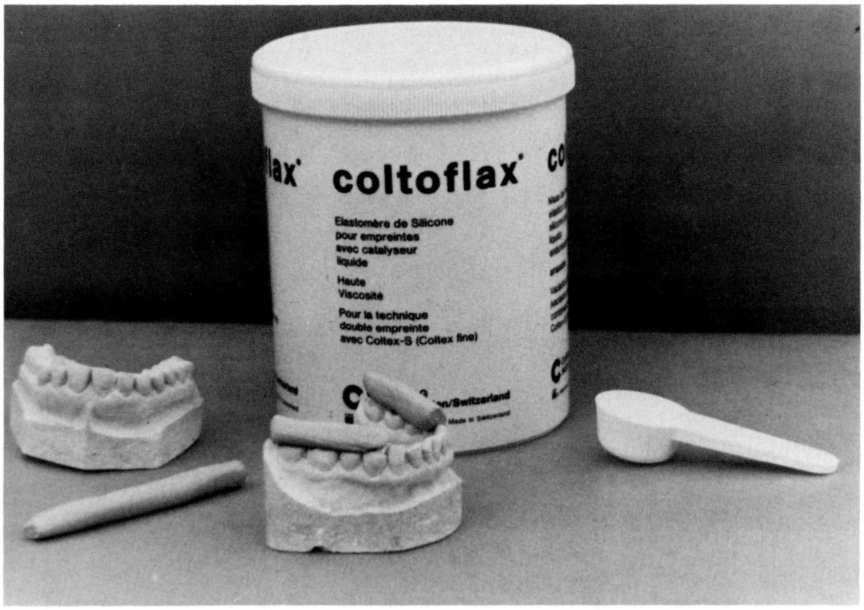

Fig 6-21. Coltoflax ropes cut in lengths to cover posterior teeth.

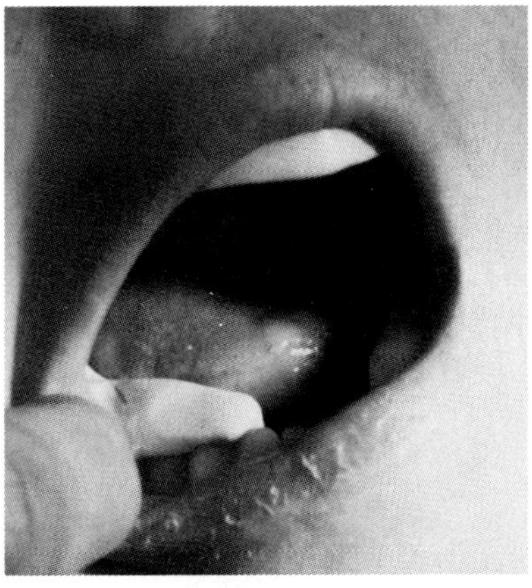

Fig. 6-22. Coltoflax ropes being placed over mandibular posterior teeth.

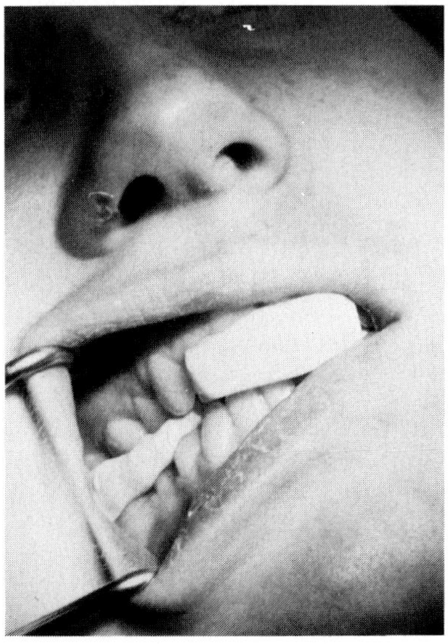

Fig. 6-23. Appearance of Coltoflax bite when patient bites on programmer.

13. Remove the programmer and the Coltoflax bites. With a sharp knife, trim the bite records so that only the indentations of the cuspal tips of the maxillary and mandibular teeth remain (Fig. 6-24).
14. The Coltoflax bites will be used later to relate the mandibular cast to the already mounted maxillary cast without using the programmer.

Protrusive registration

1. Prepare a half sheet of hard baseplate wax (Kerr No. 5 Set Up Wax).
2. Warm the wax and adapt it, making indentations in the wax of the incisal and occlusal surfaces of the maxillary cast (Fig. 6-25, *A*). With experience, one can adapt the wax directly to the maxillary teeth in the mouth and save an extra appointment (Fig. 6-25, *B*).
3. With scissors, trim away excess wax just lateral to the impressions of the buccal cusps and incisal edges, except in the canine areas, where small ears are left to be turned up against the labial surfaces. These help orient the wax tray as it is placed in the mouth (Fig. 6-26).
4. Place the wax tray on the maxillary teeth, and guide the mandible up into a 4– to 5–mm straight protrusive relationship. Have the mandibular incisors indent, but not penetrate, the wax covering the maxillary incisors (Fig. 6-27). NOTE: A protrusive record of less than 3 mm will not provide sufficient movement for an accurate articulator setting. More than 5 mm will cut off some of the curvature of the eminences (condyle guidance).
5. With the mandibular incisors in contact with the wax tray, retract the cheeks, and estimate the number of Aluwax (Bite and Impression Wax)* strips needed on each side to afford contact with the mandibular teeth (Fig. 6-27).
6. From warm sheets of Aluwax impression wax cut several strips $^{1}/_{4}$ inch (0.7 mm) wide and long enough to cover all the posterior teeth.
7. Lute enough of these strips to the mandibular side of the wax tray to afford indentations of the buccal cusps of the mandibular posterior teeth when the jaws are closed in a protrusive relationship (Fig. 6-28).
8. Flame the Aluwax only. Carry the wax tray to the mouth, and seat it on the maxillary teeth.

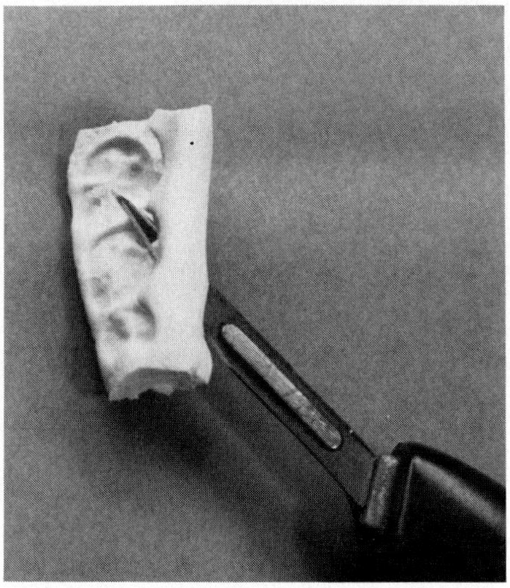

Fig. 6-24. Trim Coltoflax bites with Bard-Parker knife.

*Hickok Specialties Co., Grand Rapids, Mich.

A

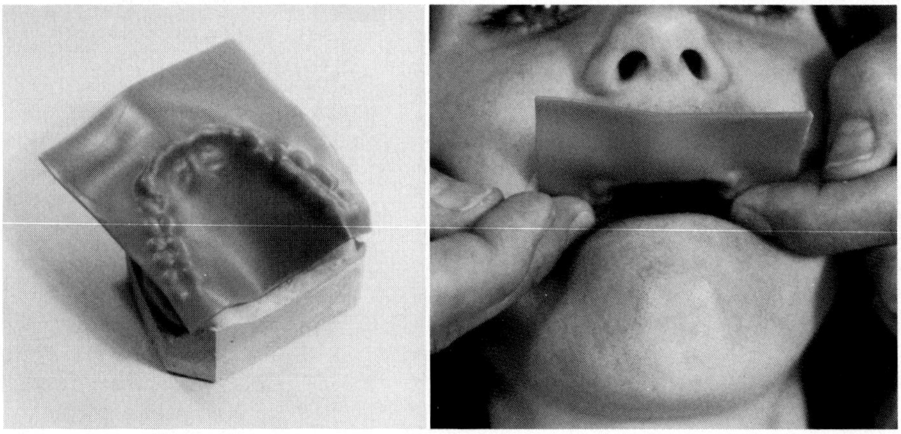

B

Fig. 6-25. A, Warmed sheet of baseplate wax adapted to cast of maxillary teeth. **B,** Warmed sheet of baseplate wax being adapted directly to maxillary teeth.

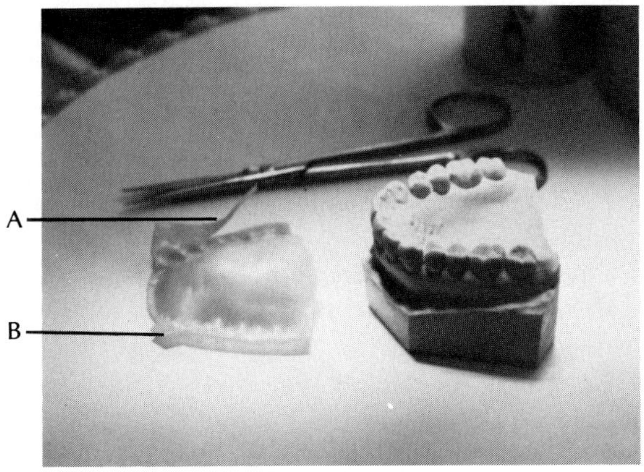

Fig. 6-26. Baseplate wax trimmed for use as wax tray. *A,* Excess wax was being trimmed. *B,* Ear left on to help orient wax tray.

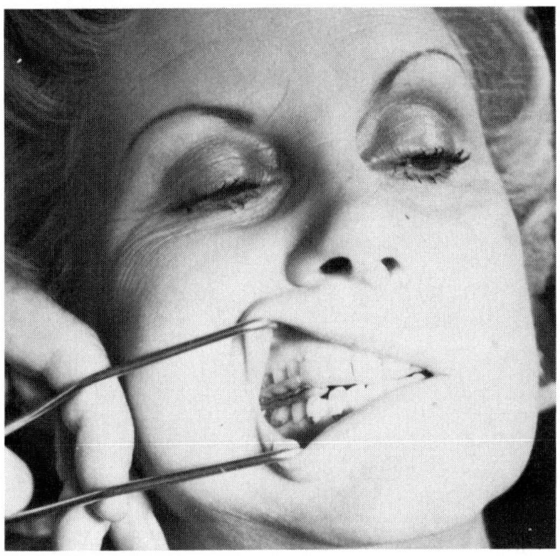

Fig. 6-27. Aluwax strips added to mandibular side of wax tray.

Ask the patient to slowly close, as you guide the mandible forward until the mandibular incisors touch the indentations that were previously made (step 4).

9. Remove the wax tray, and chill it. Inspect the indentations in the Aluwax, and cut away all wax except the indentations of the buccal cusps (Fig. 6-29).
10. Make a mix of zinc oxide paste (Plastopaste),* which has a setting time of a minute or less.
11. Place a *small* amount of the zinc oxide paste in the cuspal indentations in both sides of the wax tray.
12. Seat the wax tray in place on the maxillary teeth. Guide the mandible anteriorly, and have the patient slowly close into the incisal indentations previously made in step 4 (Fig. 6-30).

*Harry J. Bosworth Co., Chicago, Ill.

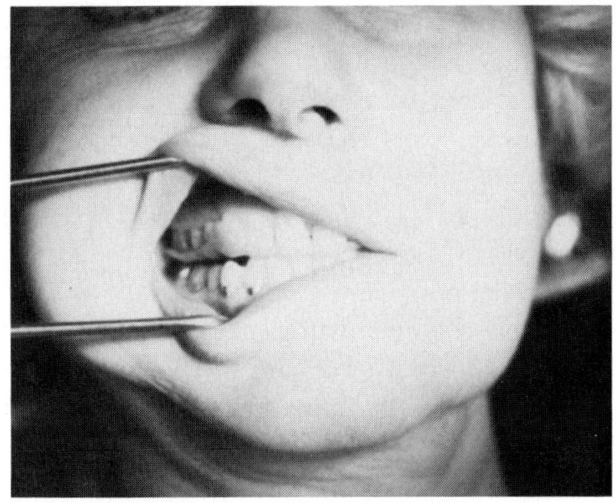

Fig. 6-28. Wax tray in position. Patient biting in protrusive relation.

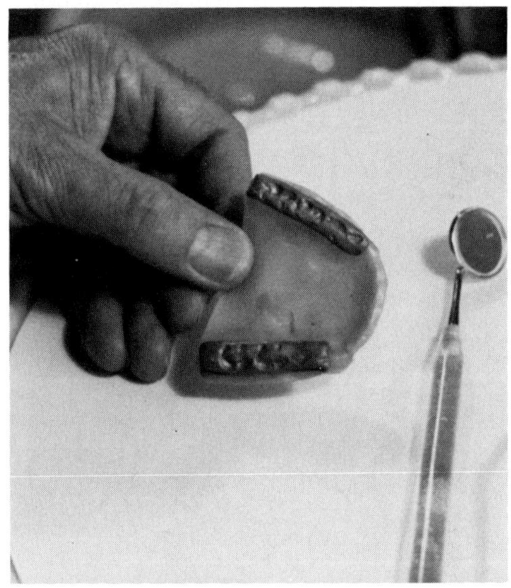

Fig. 6-29. Inspect Aluwax strips for indentations of lower buccal cusps only.

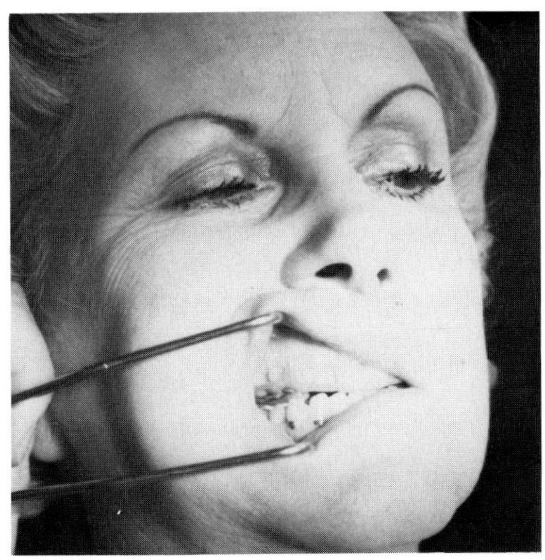

Fig 6-30. Zinc oxide paste corrected protrusive bite registration.

13. When the zinc oxide paste is dry, remove the wax tray and inspect it. If the past reproduces the grooves in the teeth, these areas must be cut away, leaving paste in the cuspal indentations only (Fig. 6-31). Dismiss the patient.

Laboratory phase

Cast mounting procedure

1. Position the articulator on the mounting stand. Attach the face-bow so that the hinge axis pins (Fig. 6-32, *A*) are pointing to the center of the condyles and the orbital indicator rod (Fig. 6-32, *B*) touches the orbital plane.
2. Place support under the bite fork, and position the maxillary cast on the top of the bite fork (Fig. 6-33).
3. Plaster the maxillary cast to the upper mounting ring.
4. Remove the articulator from the mounting stand.
5. Place a sheet of cast mounting paper between the lower mounting ring and the lower arm of the articulator.
6. Lengthen the incisal pin about 3 mm. This is done so that when the wax bite is removed and

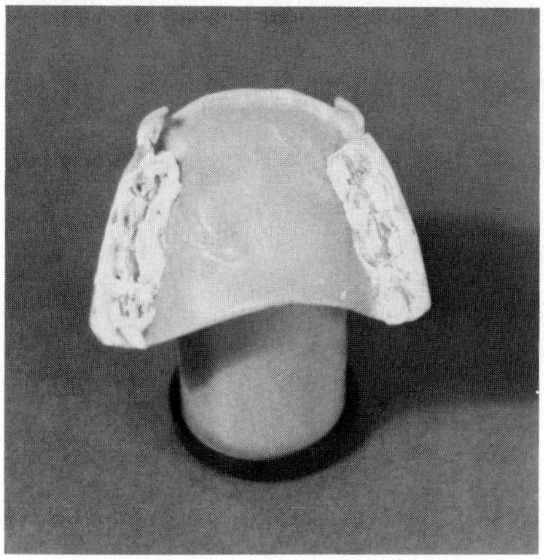

Fig. 6-31. Paste corrected cuspal indentations, upper and lower.

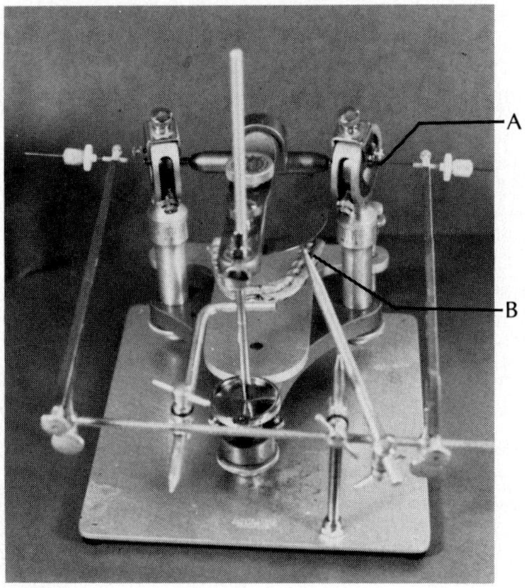

Fig. 6-32. Articulator on mounting stand. *A,* Hinge axis pins. *B,* Orbital indicator rod.

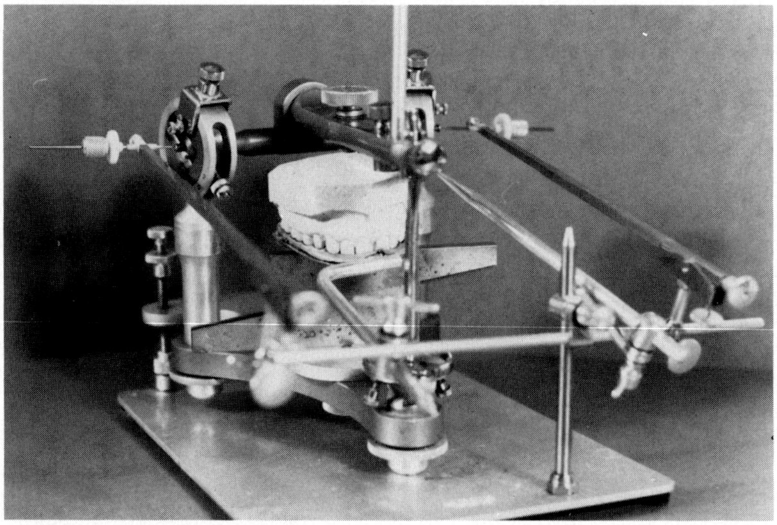

Fig. 6-33. Maxillary cast ready to be mounted.

the condyle locks are released, allowing the casts to occlude in centric occlusion, the incisal pin will again be close to zero (Fig. 6-34).

7. Open the upper arm of the articulator back so that the teeth of the mounted maxillary cast face upward. Fit the Coltoflax bites on the cast (step 14) (Fig. 6-35).
8. Fit the mandibular cast carefully atop the Coltoflax bites. Sticky wax a half dozen toothpicks to the front, sides, and back of the borders of the two models to secure them in position. Do not extend toothpicks beyond the base of the mandibular model (Fig. 6-36).

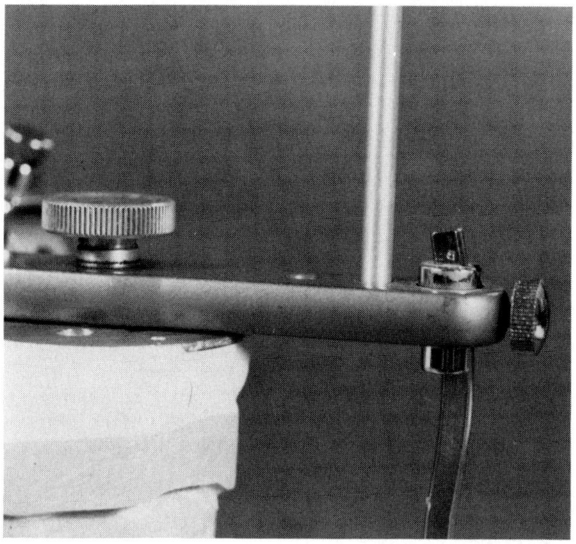

Fig. 6-34. Incisal pin is lengthened 3 mm.

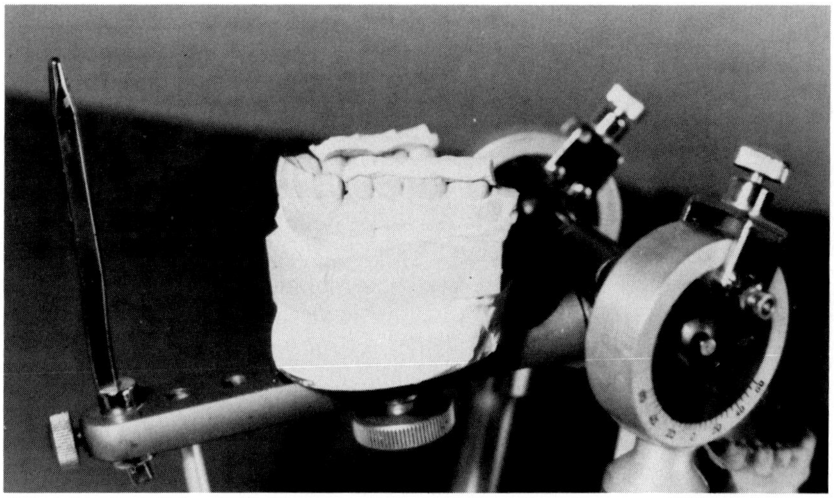

Fig. 6-35. Coltoflax bites on maxillary cast.

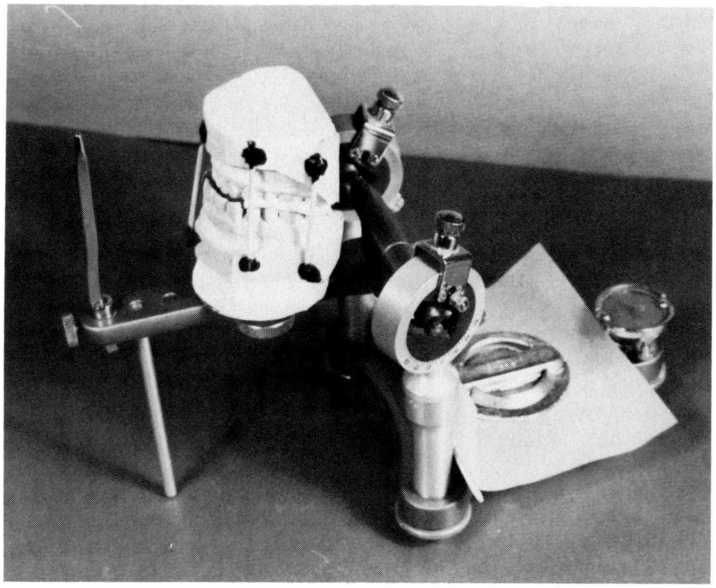

Fig. 6-36. Mandibular cast positioned in Coltoflax bites and secured with toothpicks.

9. Mix some fast-setting plaster, and place it on top of the mandibular cast and on the lower mounting ring. Close the articulator so that the two fresh mixes of plaster are united (Fig. 6-37).
10. When the plaster has set hard (40 minutes), remove the toothpicks and Coltoflax bites.
11. Release the incisal pin, and *carefully* allow the models to touch. They will touch on the first prematurity and in terminal hinge relation. Note the measurement on the incisal pin, but do not lock the pin (Fig. 6-38).

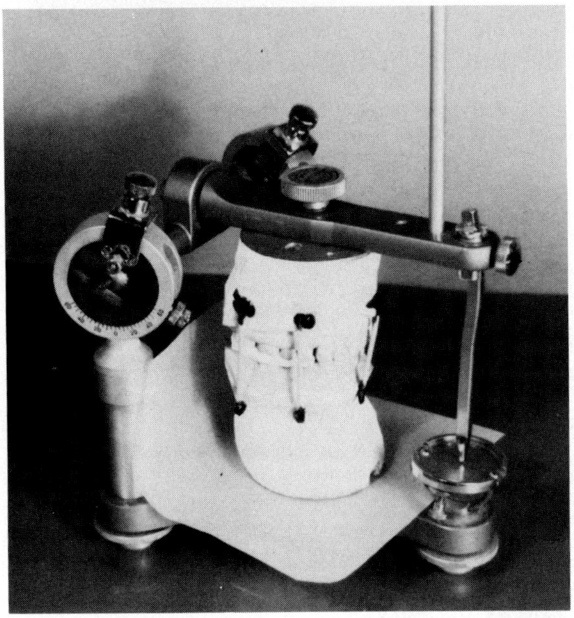

Fig. 6-37. Mandibular cast mounted.

12. Now unlock the condyles and the incisal pin, and the models will slide into centric occlusion. Note the new measurement on the pin. Also note the distance each condyle moves away from its stop. This is the amount of mesial slide (Fig. 6-39). NOTE: If the amount of movement on each side is equal, then the slide is completely mesial. If it is unequal, there is some lateral slide.

Articulator settings

1. Unlock the condylar inclination, and raise the pin off the incisal table. Place the protrusive bite between the casts, and close the mounted casts into the bite.
2. With one hand holding the maxillary cast securely into the protrusive bite, rotate the condylar inclination adjustment back and forth for the best settling of the cast into that bite. Lock that inclination setting (Fig. 6-40).
3. Repeat for the inclination setting on the other side.[20] NOTE: The technique for mounting the models of a patient with a pathological occlusion has been described. Because of interferences in the occlusion and stresses in the musculature, to continue with lateral bites and Bennett movement would be of doubtful accuracy and value. The models as they are now mounted show the casts in the same pathological relationship that the teeth exhibit in the mouth. This is the relationship which was a part of the cause of the temporomandibular joint dysfunction syndrome and discloses the occlusal problems that can now receive definitive study (Fig. 6-41).

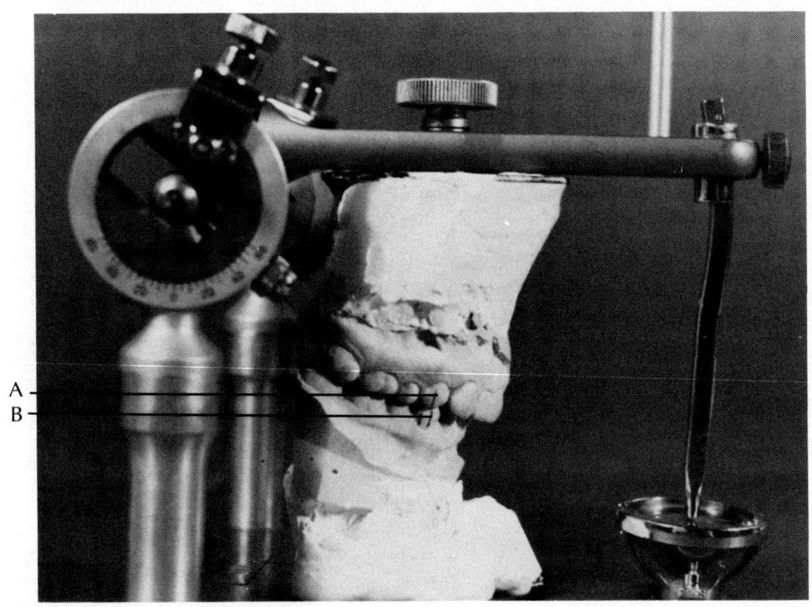

Fig. 6-38. Note orientation marks, *A* and *B*, in casts. Case is in centric relation position.

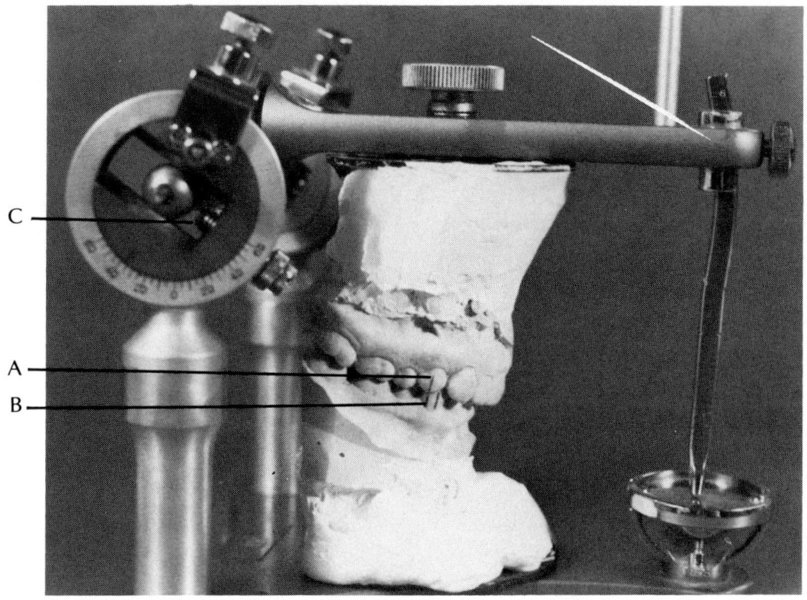

Fig. 6-39. Case is now in centric occlusion. Note change in orientation marks, *A* and *B*. Note new reading on incisal pin. Note distance between condyle and condyle stops, *C*.

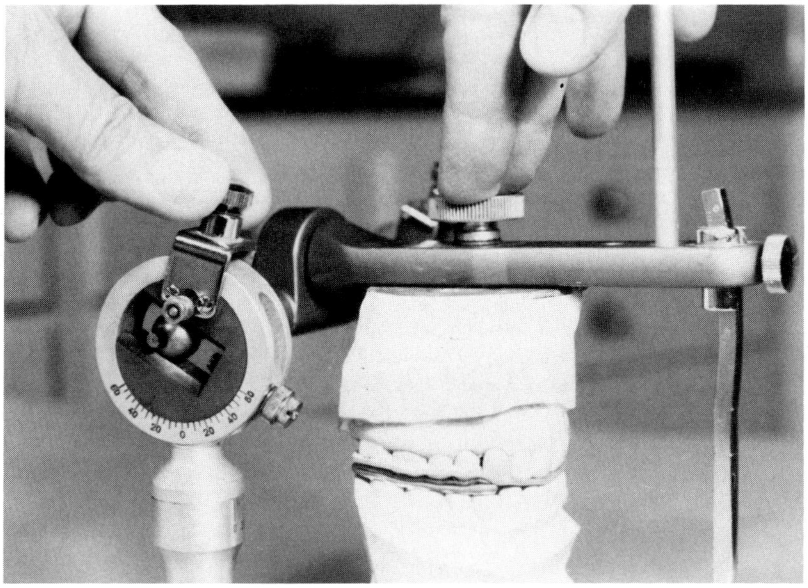

Fig. 6-40. Setting condylar inclination from protrusive bite.

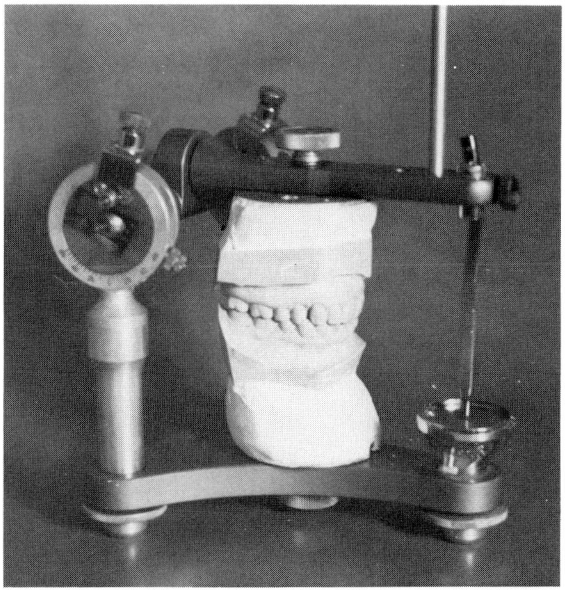

Fig. 6-41. Articulator adjusted. Case ready for study.

ACKNOWLEDGMENTS

I am grateful for the help of Aaron Cole, photography; Toni Snow, modeling; Dan Slotton, drawings; and Rex Ingraham, D.D.S., and Don Curnutte, D.D.S., Department of Occlusion, University of Southern California School of Dentistry, Los Angeles.

REFERENCES

1. Basehart, J.: Nonverbal communication in the dentist-patient relationship, J. Prosthet. Dent. **34**:4, 1975.
2. Bell, W.E.: Temporomandibular joint disease, 1960, The Egan Co.
3. Butler, J.H., Folke, L.E.A., and Bandt, C.L.: A descriptive survey of signs and symptoms associated with the myofascial pain dysfunction syndrome, J. Am. Dent. Assoc. **90**:636, 1975.
4. Crues, W.A.: "That's what you say . . .," J. Dent. Management **10**:29, 1970.
5. Dyer, E.: Personal communication, 1962.
6. Faeth, W.H.: Personal communication, 1969.
7. Kraus, H.: Physical methods. In Schwartz, L., and Chayes, C.M., editors: Facial pain and mandibular dysfunction, Philadelphia, 1969, W.B. Saunders Co.
8. Levy, P.H.: A form and function concept of occlusion and the temporomandibular relationships, J. Prosthet. Dent. **33**:149, 1975.
9. Miller, S.C.: Oral diagnosis and treatment planning, Philadelphia, 1936, Blakiston Co.
10. Morgan, D.H.: The great imposter, J. Calif. Dent. Assoc. **2**:52, 1974.
11. Noback, C.R.: The human nervous system, New York, 1967, McGraw-Hill Book Co.
12. Ramfjord, S.P., and Ash, M.M.: Occlusion, Philadelphia, 1968, W.B. Saunders Co.
13. Ricketts R.M.: Abnormal function of the temporomandibular joint, Am. J. Orthod. **41**:435, 1955.
14. Ricketts, R.M.: Roentgenography of the temporomandibular joint. In Sarnat, B.G., editor: The temporomandibular joint, ed. 2, Springfield, Ill., 1964, Charles C Thomas, Publisher.
15. Ricketts, R.M.: Personal communication, 1972.
16. Rieder, C.E.: Development of a simplified system for clinical evaluation of occlusal interrelationships. I. Acquisition of information, J. Prosthet. Dent. **33**: 264, 1975.
17. Sarnat, B.G.: The temporomandibular joint, ed. 2, Springfield, Ill., 1964, Charles C Thomas, Publisher.
18. Schwartz, M.S.: Functional analysis: case history, clinical and radiographic examination of the natural dentition and analysis made from hand held and mounted study models. In Ingraham, R., editor: Physiology of occulsion, Laboratory manual, Los Angeles, 1972, University of Southern California School of Dentistry.
19. Shore, N.A.: Head pain of temporomandibular joint origin, N.Y. State J. Med. **62**:3580, 1962.
20. Smith, B.J.: Adjustment of the lateral condylar guidances of dentatus AR series of articulators, J. Prosthet. Dent. **34**:208, 1975.

RECOMMENDED READINGS

Dikshit, J.V., and Mirza, F.D.: Muscle relaxant and rest position, J. Prosthet. Dent. **42**:5, 1979.

Farrar, W.B., and McCarty, W.L., Jr.: Inferior joint space arthrography and characteristics of condylar paths in internal derangements of the TMJ, J. Prosthet. Dent. **41**:5, 1979.

Garliner, D.: Myofunctional therapy, Philadelphia, 1976, W.B. Saunders Co.

George, J.P., and Boone, M.E.: A clinical study of rest position using the Kinesiograph and Myo-Monitor, J. Prosthet. Dent. **41**:4, 1979.

Greene, B.: Personal communication, 1980.

Guichet, N.F.: Biologic laws governing functions of muscles that move the mandibles, Part I, J. Prosthet. Dent. **37**:6, 1977.

Guichet, N.F.: Biologic laws governing functions of muscles that move the mandibles, Part II, J. Prosthet. Dent. **37**:7, 1977.

Johnstone, D.R., and Templeton, M.: The feasibility of palpating the lateral pterygoid muscle, J. Prosthet. Dent. **44**:3, 1980.

Lundeen, T.F.: Occlusal splint fabrication, J. Prosthet. Dent. **42**:5, 1979.

McNerney, W.J.: Help yourself to better health; blue print for health, vol. 28, no. 1, 1978, Blue Cross Association.

Nosedkin, J.N.: The evolution of occlusal dysfunctional therapy, J. Prosthet. Dent. **44**:1, 1980.

Scheer, W.L.: Personal communication, Oct. 1979.

Scott, A.J., III: Principles of the clinical examination, J. Prosthet. Dent. **37**:5, 1977.

Sheppard, I.M., and Sheppard, S.M.: Characteristics of temporomandibular joint problems, J. Prosthet. Dent. **38**:2, 1977.

Uthman, A.A., Mohl, N.D., and McCall, W.D., Jr.: Review of symptoms of muscle pain dysfunction, J. Prosthet. Dent. **41**:5, 1979.

Van Sickels, J.E., and Ivey, D.W.: Myofascial pain dysfunction: a manifestation of the short face syndrome, J. Prosthet. Dent. **42**:5, 1979.

7 The role of occlusion in diagnosis and treatment planning

DONALD C. CURNUTTE, D.D.S.

Occlusion has become a subject of major concern throughout the dental profession. In some dental schools today it is considered core subject matter. It is being taught as a conjoint program to undergraduate and graduate dental students, including the most modern concepts and philosophies in the science of occlusion as related to diagnosis and treatment planning and restorative dentistry. Many discerning practicing dentists are participating in continuing education occlusion programs on an international basis.

Since the majority of the disciplines of dentistry emphasize the significance of physiologically compatible jaw relations and interarch tooth contact to health and function of the gnathostomatic system, occlusion may well be the common meeting ground of most branches of dental science. Today a wide range of health professionals have begun to show a great deal of interest in occlusion or at least in the effects of occlusion on myofunctional and temporomandibular joint dysfunction and related myofascial pain and symptoms of the masticatory system. Some of these are the otolaryngologist, neurologist, myofunctional therapist, speech therapist, psychiatrist, psychologist, physiotherapist, and social worker. This is not surprising, considering the close anatomical proximity of the various components of the skull and head, as well as the complex physiological, neuromuscular, and biomechanical interplay between these anatomical components along with the psychic influences.

It is for these reasons that the role of occlusion should be considered an integral part of diagnosis and treatment planning for treatment of teeth, temporomandibular joint dysfunction, and myofascial pain, not only from the therapy standpoint but as preventive treatment as well.

GNATHOSTOMATIC SYSTEM

The gnathostomatic system (masticatory system) is composed of the teeth and their supporting tissues (including alveolar bone, periodontal ligament, and vascular supply), the temporomandibular joint, the neuromusculature and ligamentous arrangement, and the vascular supply of that system. It is considered biologically to be a stress system. Its tissues respond to excess stresses and forces the same ways as any other body tissues, by inflammation, infection, disease, trauma, and degenerative changes.

The gnathostomatic system must be viewed as a functioning unit. The physiology and function of all components of the system must be examined, as well as the influence one part has on another during function. The separate parts cannot be considered independently; it is impossible to study the occlusion of the teeth in function without noting the effect of mandibular function on that occlusion and vice versa.

The parameters of the science of occlusion are the anatomy, histology, physiology, pathology, growth, development, and biomechanics of the gnathostomatic system. To properly study or understand this system, it is necessary to go directly to the cell, or the biologics of the system. Tissues may respond to stress long before the patient is aware or dysfunction occurs in the system.

Occlusion is defined in the following ways:

1. Any contact between the incising or masticating surfaces of the upper and lower teeth
2. The relationship between the occlusal surfaces of the maxillary and mandibular teeth when they are in contact[1]
3. The contact relationships of the teeth resulting from neuromuscular control of the masticatory system[11]

Malocclusion is defined in the following ways:

1. Any deviation from a physiologically acceptable contact of opposing dentition
2. Any deviation from normal occlusion[1]
3. An interarch discrepancy of abnormal tooth position (morphological)

4. An occlusal form and/or intermaxillary relationship out of harmony with the individual pattern of jaw movement that results in occlusal interferences which may cause an occlusal dishormony

The concept of occlusion generally has been presented by the dentist as how the teeth contact during centric closure. It would appear that occlusion is a static phenomenon and that the teeth are in contact most of the time, which we know, of course, is not true. Occlusion is functional in nature. It is dynamic action in that teeth not only occlude or contact, but they also separate during mandibular movement. How they occlude and disclude has a great bearing on how the entire gnathostomatic system functions, and vice versa.

It must be remembered that teeth do not move. The upper teeth are firmly anchored to the maxillae, which are fixed anatomical components of the skull. The lower teeth are firmly anchored to the mandible, which itself moves freely. The lower teeth go along for the ride, so to speak, the mandible being their vehicle in flight. The occlusal contact and the disclusion of the teeth result from neuromuscular control of the masticatory system, which causes mandibular movement.

Functions of the teeth within the gnathostomatic system

Basically the teeth are passive instruments that perform their work only when mandibular movement occurs. Besides the important function of chewing, the teeth serve several other physiological and mechanical functions. They act as vertical stops for jaw closure, are sounding boards for phonetics, enhance esthetics, and provide anterior support for the mandible during protrusive and lateral excursive movement of the mandible as the anterior discluding factors of the teeth.

When the teeth are properly arranged within the dental arches, it is possible to have a mutually protected occlusion; that is, when the posterior teeth contact in mandibular closure, the anterior teeth do not contact, and vice versa. There should be no contact of posterior teeth during lateral or protrusive excursions of the mandible. For teeth to efficiently carry out their many functions within the system, it is important that they have cusps, ridges, grooves, and marginal ridges, whose morphological arrangements are geometrically compatible with jaw function.

When the occlusal surfaces of the teeth become worn, abraded, or fractured, or when teeth are missing, rotated, or tilted, they become less functional, and often excess horizontal forces are brought to bear on the teeth and components of the gnathostomatic system that may be destructive and may result in dysfunction of the system in part or in whole. Like any other system, it malfunctions at its own expense and may ultimately destroy itself.

It is therefore imperative that teeth are able to contact such that these destructive forces are absent or minimal and there is no damaging deflection of the mandible on full intercuspation of the teeth during centric-occlusion closure because of premature contact of some teeth in the arch.

It is also important that the posterior teeth do not collide with one another during disclusion, which would set up deflective and potentially destructive forces within the entire system. The cusps of teeth must be positioned to seat properly during closure, and they must not contact or rub each other during excursions of the jaw.

During chewing, the anatomical ridges on the occlusal surfaces of the teeth perform shearing functions, allowing food to be cut more easily. They work in conjunction with the stamp cusps (buccal cusps of lower teeth, lingual cusps of upper teeth) and the holding cusps (lingual cusps of lower teeth, buccal cusps of upper teeth). It is important that none of these components touch except during centric closure of the teeth. The grooves on the occlusal surfaces of the teeth, besides separating the cusps and ridges, serve as escape ways for the opposing cusps during mandibular excursions to prevent collision of opposing cusps and ridges.

If the cusps, ridges, and grooves are positioned in geometrical harmony with the pathways of movement of the condyles in their fossae, then collisions and deflective forces will not occur during closure or disclusion of the teeth.

Furthermore, it is physiologically desirable that the occlusal forces on the teeth during closure be directed vertically along the long axes of the teeth, thereby eliminating the horizontal or lateral forces, which are potentially destructive.

It is preferable that the stamp cusps of the teeth occlude within the confines of the perimeter of a fossa on the occlusal surface of the opposing teeth, not on marginal ridges nor into embrasures between the teeth. This ensures minimum sized point reciprocal contact areas of the teeth, which are confined to the intracoronal areas of any given tooth. This helps prevent tipping or rotating of teeth in the arch. It also helps direct the occlusal load along the long axes of the teeth, which lessens the amount of stress on the periodontium. Studies by Shaw, the anthropologist, indicated that the maximum amount of tooth contact over the entire arch should not exceed an area of 4 mm^2. There should be simultaneous positive centric contact on all posterior teeth, with each tooth sharing its part of the directed and distributed occlusal load so that no one tooth in the arch carries more or less than its share.

As soon as mandibular movement occurs when the teeth are in centric contact, there should be an immediate disclusion of the teeth without any further contact of the posterior teeth, with the condyles following the slopes of their eminences and the anterior teeth acting as the anterior guidance factors of the disclusion.

The foregoing is a brief description of the gnathological concept of a cusp-fossa functional occlusion. There are other concepts of occlusion in vogue in dental circles today. There are also those who disagree with the cusp-fossa concept. All concepts of treatment have a common goal, however—to reduce the stresses on all components of the gnathostomatic system by gaining neuromuscular balance, directing and distributing forces on the teeth and the periodontium, and lessening the destructive forces on the TMJ.

Experience and clinical results from treating occlusions and TMJ dysfunctions resulting from occlusal disharmonies have shown the gnathological concept of cusp-fossa occlusion to be highly successful in obtaining or maintaining neuromuscular balance within the system. It provides a logical means of directing and distributing the forces of occlusion, rendering them less damaging and destructive to all components of the system. It takes into account the anatomical form and geometrics of the fixed skull-fossa-condyle relations, as related to the teeth, and vice versa, without violating these fixed factors to obtain a physiological occlusion. It is also considered to be an efficient arrangement for the teeth to carry out their biomechanical functions with maximum efficiency and minimum stress.

MANDIBULAR MOVEMENT

The mandible has three types of functional movements: (1) masticatory, (2) nonmasticatory, and (3) reflex. The temporomandibular joints are the only joints in the body in which the articulating bone (mandible) can freely move out of its socket or fossa during function. To understand the science of occlusion and to clinically apply its principles of biomechanical function to diagnosis and treatment planning, the dynamics of occlusion must be considered from the standpoint of mandibular function and the interrelationship of that function to the contact relations of the teeth.

The mandible exhibits two types of geometrical movement—rotation and translation. The TMJ is often referred to as a *hinged-sliding joint*. Except for the hinged position of opening and closing (approximately the first 5 to 10 degrees of opening), which is usually rotational, the mandible usually presents a combination of timed, sequenced, simultaneous rotation and translation in three dimensions as the condyles move along the slopes of their respective eminences. Recent x-ray studies by Morgan[8] have shown that there is forward translation of the condyle when the bite is opened as little as 2 mm, or 2 to 3 degrees of opening. When the mandible is in its postural position, the condyle is positioned down and forward from the CR position.

The movement of the mandible is brought about by action of the various groups of muscles of the masticatory system operating through the afferent-efferent neural excitation process, as reflex, and through proprioception of the periodontal ligaments and the muscles themselves. Knowledge of the kinesiology of the jaw is a prerequisite to understanding occlusion in function, and it is a prerequisite particularly to understanding the three-dimensional geometrical patterns of the pathways of movement of the condyles along the anatomical slopes of the eminences and walls of their respective fossae. These pathways of movement are different but specific for every individual for given movements, depending on the peculiarities of the anatomical form and measurements of that individual.

The occlusion and disclusion of the teeth should be guided by these anatomical factors as condylar guidance. The translation and rotation of the condyles along the anatomical slopes of the eminences is what guides the directional movement of the mandible during all movement and thereby separates and occludes the teeth in the process.

The geometrical configurations of these anatomical slopes, the pathways the condyles follow along these slopes, the geometrical interplay from one fossa-eminence to the other during this movement (because the mandible is a single body), and the intercondylar width and general geometrical configuration and measurements of the mandible itself are often referred to as *the determinants of occlusion*.

It is these fixed anatomical and geometrical determinants which influence not only the degree and direction of jaw movement, but ultimately the degree, direction, and configurations of the morphological arrangement of the occlusal anatomy of the teeth, and consequently determine how the teeth occlude or separate during function.

Stallard and Stuart[12] and others worked out the geometrical principles of the determinants of occlusion years ago. Katz[6] has published an excellent text, *The Determinants of Human Occlusion,* which demonstrates in detail all the determinants (too numerous to completely list in this text).

Application of the determinants of occlusion leads to numerous rules, for example:

1. The steeper the angle of the eminences, the steeper the cusps and deeper the fossa of the teeth may be. Conversely, the flatter the angle of the eminences, the flatter the cusps and the shallower the fossa must be on the teeth.
2. The wider the intercondylar distance, the more distal the nonworking (or balancing) grooves must be on the lower teeth and the more mesial on the upper teeth. That is, the degree and directions, the degree of convexity or concavity

(curvatures), and the arcs of curvature of the ridges and grooves horizontally and vertically on the teeth are resultants of the size and directions of the arcs transcribed by the rotating condyle as the arc rotation center, the geometrical interplay of the anatomical slopes and condylar pathway angles between one joint and the other, and the radial distance of each given tooth from the arc rotation center.

TRANSFER OF SKULL-FOSSA-CONDYLE GEOMETRY TO AN ARTICULATOR

To properly study the geometrical interrelationship between the skull and the teeth, it is often necessary to use mechanical instrumentation that will allow the transfer of this geometry from the skull to a laboratory working instrument—an articulator. It is necessary to be able to accurately transfer the geometry, mount study casts of the patient's teeth, and maintain all spatial relationships intact statically and during function.

By establishing reproducible fixed anatomical landmarks and applying geometrical principles, it is possible to do this transfer accurately, as described in the following procedures.

Hinge axis and axis-orbital plane

When the condyles are in centric relation (their most retruded positions in their fossae), the horizontal (or transverse) axis is in its terminal position. This is also the position at which pure rotation occurs as a hinge movement of the mandible. This is referred to as the *terminal hinge position,* thus the term *hinge axis.*

The hinge axis is an imaginary line (horizontal axis) that passes horizontally through rotation centers of both condyles to the right and left when the condyles are in the centric relation position.

Fortunately the terminal hinge position is considered to be a physiological functioning position of the jaw, although most people do not always function from centric relation. This is a functioning position of the jaw in which there are no premature contacts of the teeth or other dysfunctions present in the system. It is a reproducible, fixed position. It can be relocated repeatedly and accurately by mechanical methods using a modified face-bow and styli that rotate when the jaw opens and closes. This apparatus is attached to the teeth by means of clutches. Therefore it can be used as a fixed anatomical skull landmark reference position, which can be permanently tattooed on the skin on each side of the face.

Once the hinge axis is located and marked, a third point is arbitrarily located and marked on the nose at approximately the level of the infraorbital foramen as a fixed anterior cranial reference point. The two posterior reference points (the hinge axis) and the anterior reference point geometrically establish an imaginary plane that passes horizontally through these three points. This cranial reference plane is referred to as the *axis-orbital plane.*

Establishment of this imaginary cranial reference plane gives the health care professional the means of accurately transferring the skull geometry to an articulator and makes it possible to use the articulator as a measuring device to obtain accurate geometrical measurements and skull-fossa relationships to that plane.

Axis-orbital face-bow transfer and mounting of diagnostic casts

By applying geometrical principles and the use of a mechanical device called a *face-bow,* it is possible to mechanically transfer the axis-orbital plane from the skull to an articulator. This procedure is referred to as an *axis-orbital face-bow transfer.*

Once adjusted to the face and the upper teeth, the face-bow is transferred and mounted intact to the articulator. Then diagnostic casts of the patient's upper teeth are mounted to the upper member of the articulator while supported by the bite fork portion of the face-bow. In this manner the teeth on the diagnostic casts maintain the same geometrical spatial relationships to the hinge axis and the axis-orbital plane as the teeth do in the skull. By making accurate interocclusal centric registrations, it is then possible to mount a lower diagnostic cast of the patient's teeth to the lower member of the articulator so that the true spatial relationships will be acquired, and an accurate tooth-to-tooth and arch-to-arch relationship will be acquired as well when the condyles are in the centric relation positions in their fossae. This is referred to as a *centric relation mounting* of diagnostic casts. Since they are related to the hinge axis, where only pure rotation occurs around the horizontal axis during closure, it is possible to determine which teeth make contact on centric closure in the centric relation tooth-contact position as the mandible (or articulator) arcs on the hinge axis. It is not unusual to discover that only two opposing posterior teeth touch on initial contact of the teeth during centric relation (CR) closure.

On full closure of the teeth to the centric occlusion (CO) tooth-contact position, or the fully intercuspated position, there may be a slide on the opposing surfaces of the teeth with a resultant deflection of the jaw to accommodate this position. There may be an anterior and/or lateral deviation of the mandible, which is observed by the different positions of the teeth from the CR to the CO tooth-contact positions.

The shift of the mandible and slide of the teeth are caused by guidance of the teeth moving along the inclined planes of the opposing teeth. The vertical dimension between the CR and the CO positions is at different heights, the CO being the more closed position. This shift between CR and CO tooth-contact positions is referred to as an *occlusal*, or a *centric, slide*. The result of this is that the condyles shift away from the centric relation positions in the fossae every time the patient brings the teeth together. This may set up forces on the neuromusculature and ligaments which can affect the function of the TMJ as well as bring lateral stresses to bear on the teeth, causing periodontal dysfunction mobility, wear, or fracture of the teeth. In some individuals this may be pathological to the gnathostomatic system, and because of host resistance and other compensating factors, some are not affected at all.

The posterior teeth should not guide the occlusion or the separation of the teeth. If they do, it is considered to be malocclusion, and it may be destructive.

Perhaps 90% of the population have an occlusal slide to varying degrees in their natural dentition. Most people live with it, and it may never become destructive. Others do well until they undergo psychic or physical stress, and some do not tolerate it well at all. Other stress factors may come into play at some time during the patient's lifetime that result in the pathological conditions of the gnathostomatic system. These are traumatic injury, systemic factors, the loss of strategically located teeth, or fractured teeth, which result in occlusal disharmony.

It is the diagnostician's duty to carefully observe these situations and arrive at educated decisions based on knowledge and experience as to the effects on the patient's oral health. They should not be ignored, because even though the patient is not always aware of changes and dysfunction within the system, the tissues are well aware of them, and they will respond accordingly.

CRITERIA FOR PHYSIOLOGICAL AND PATHOLOGICAL OCCLUSION

An essential aspect of occlusion is to establish accepted criteria for a physiological occlusion and for how the gnathostomatic system functions in health, as well as the necessary preparation for recognizing deviations from normal and pathological conditions that occur in various components of the system.

In the majority of patients there are few or no pathological conditions of the muscles operating the jaw. The practitioner is not always confronted with gross pathological conditions of the temporomandibular joint. However, there is a subtle pathological condition of function in nearly every mouth because of the malrelations between the opposing teeth themselves and between the interdigitation of the teeth and jaw motions.

The most common and most conspicuous pathological condition often is located in the teeth and the periodontium during the early and certainly the latter phases of dysfunction of the system. The best work of a dentist or physician is not in alleviating the well-established pathological conditions but in being able to discern by diagnostic skill those incipient and potential diseases which mark the patient as a victim of degenerative processes and disease. The diagnostician's work must be based on a thorough understanding of oral physiology. The concept of a physiological occlusion is presented as a yardstick to determine the need for treatment of the occlusion. In this approach the adult mouth that has demonstrated its ability to survive is recognized as normal.

Another definition of physiological occlusion is a state in which there is no pathological condition in any component of the gnathostomatic system that can be directly attributed to occlusal activity, no matter what the arrangement of the teeth.

Criteria for a pathological occlusion must be established as well to know where, when, how, and why to treat any given situation that results in a dysfunction of the occlusion or one that affects the occlusion. *Pathological occlusion* is defined as a state in which there is a pathological condition in any component of the gnathostomatic system that can be directly attributed to occlusal activity and that requires treatment.

Diagnosis

Diagnosis is based on (1) a thorough understanding of the tissue lesions, (2) an evaluation of the specific occlusal activity which is related to that lesion, and (3) appreciation of the systemic factors that modify the occlusal disharmonies and their pathological sequelae.

These three diagnostic considerations are profoundly interrelated, and they inspire speculation about the role of occlusion in the pathological situation that leads toward development of a concept of therapy which will be relevant to the needs of each individual patient.

The necessity for treatment is determined by taking a careful history and examining the tissues of the gnathostomatic system and by performing a functional analysis of the gnathostomatic system. Lesions associated with disturbances of the occlusion generally have multiple causes. The common causative elements generally found in varying degrees are occlusal interferences resulting in deflective jaw movement, heavy parafunctional activity such as bruxing and clenching, and at times, associated emotional disturbance. It should always be kept in mind that, as with any other disease process or injury, the effects of these etiological factors are modified by the adaptive capacity of the host.

For example, if the patient presents with facets of wear on the occlusal surfaces of the teeth caused by deflective occlusion or parafunctional activity but does not show any other pathological manifestations in other parts of the gnathostomatic system, such as TMJ dysfunction, pain, trauma, periodontal disturbances caused by primary or secondary traumatic occlusion, or impaired mandibular function caused by myofunctional discrepancy, then occlusal treatment is not necessarily indicated. The function and physiological condition of the gnathostomatic system in this case may be considered clinically normal for this individual.

In another individual who presents with gross occlusal wear without display of any further symptoms in the gnathostomatic system which may be related to that occlusal wear, except where the occlusal wear may result in a loss of vertical dimension, and possible pulpal exposure of some teeth because of heavy abrasion, obviously treatment is indicated. Perhaps treatment would consist of endodontic therapy followed by a full-mouth rehabilitation to reestablish vertical dimension and restore the occlusal surfaces of the teeth to physiological function by placing gold crowns and /or onlays on the teeth to restore the vertical dimension and geometrical harmony between the occlusal surfaces of the teeth and directional jaw geometry during movement of the mandible.

Of course this is an extreme example. At other times there may be symptoms manifested in the system because of a posterior bite collapse resulting from occlusal wear or missing or drifted teeth, with accompanying dysfunctions within the gnathostomatic system.

Other influencing factors in dysfunction are the following:

1. *Deep overbite* (vertical overlap) with the upper anterior teeth in linguoversion (Class II, division 2). Condyles are repositioned toward the rear of the fossa.
2. *Large overjet* (horizontal overlap) with the upper incisors forward of the lower incisors (Class II, division 1). There is no anterior disclusion of the teeth when the jaw moves forward, and the condyles are repositioned forward in the fossa.
3. *Posterior bite collapse:* No posterior stops for mandibular closure because of loss of teeth, tipped or tilted teeth, or grossly worn posterior teeth. This situation often causes trauma to anterior teeth with resultant pathological conditions, and the condyles are usually close to the eminence in the fossa. There is a loss of vertical dimension. This condition often produces a fulcrum, resulting in stress on the joint structures.
4. *Occlusal interferences* during the function of the mandible. This condition results in premature contacts of the teeth and occlusal slides that tend to deflect the jaw anteriorly and/or laterally. Changes in leverage can alter neuromuscular balance, producing muscle spasm, and may loosen, break, or wear teeth, stretch ligaments of the jaw, produce parafunctional habits, and cause dystrophic periodontal breakdown because of lateral forces on the teeth. Trauma must be sustained over a prolonged time to become damaging.

It requires a capable and well-informed diagnostician to determine the degree of health or disease of the system. Often consultations are required with other health professionals, and the diagnosis must be made with a combined approach. Often treatment is by combined therapy.

It has been estimated that occlusal dysfunction in varying degrees is the cause of 90% of TMJ problems as the primary factor or as a contributing factor. These situations must be diagnosed at an early stage, because it also has been determined that about 15% to 20% of the population suffers from TMJ dysfunction in varying degrees of severity, not to mention the great numbers of people who suffer varying degrees of periodontal disturbances caused by forces of occlusion as a contributing factor either as primary or secondary traumatic occlusion.

If heavy dental restorative procedures are to be undertaken in a mouth, occlusal treatment may be indicated before proceeding. For example, an occlusal adjustment may be made by selective grinding of the teeth to the CR position or orthodontic tooth repositioning as pretreatment before the restorative procedures.

In instances in which the patient exhibits symptoms of myofascial pain and/or TMJ dysfunction, occlusal adjustment and restorative procedures are often preceded by palliative treatment such as pharmacological, psychological, or physical therapy and interocclusal appliances for jaw repositioning and neuromuscular control. Before treating the teeth, treat the joints and muscles, being as conservative as possible. This is frequently necessary to position the condyles to the CR position before one can obtain proper geometrics of skull-fossa-condyle relations necessary to treat the teeth.

The need for treatment followed by a properly sequenced treatment plan can be determined only after a thorough diagnosis is made, which includes a functional occlusal analysis. A diagnosis must be predicated on what is right in the system as well as what is wrong. A good record system for gathering and synthesizing data should be incorporated into any diagnosis and treatment plan relevant to the patient problems, but it also can serve well in the legal sense, which is something to be aware of when undertaking this type of treatment.

Criteria and objectives of a functional anaysis

A functional analysis of the gnathostomatic system implies the taking of a careful history and the performance of an intraoral and extraoral examination of all the soft and hard tissues of the mouth. An occlusal analysis in the mouth should be an integral part of every oral examination with special regard to occlusal disharmonies and their possible sequelae in the form of functional disorders in any component of the system. It certainly should be a part of the examination of every patient who presents with myofascial pain and/or TMJ dysfunction.

The first question that must be answered is, "Does the patient present a physiological or a pathological occlusion?" That is, "Is there a pathological condition present in any of the components of the system that may be attributed to occlusal disharmonies?"

If no occlusion-related pathological condition is found, the tissues are functioning in a state of equilibrium; the forces generated by occlusal activity fall within the range of adaptability of the host. This situation cannot be improved on, and treatment is contraindicated. There is no need to proceed with the analysis.

If it is determined that there is an occlusion-related pathological condition in any of the tissues of the system, then an occlusal analysis must be performed on diagnostic casts of the patient's teeth that are accurately mounted on an articulator in the CR position. The procedures for mounting were described previously.

Diagnostic casts, whether hand held or mounted on an articulator, have limited value in determining the absence or presence of pathological conditions. Their value is in relating pathological conditions to existing disharmonies. The use of the articulator facilitates the accurate identification of the occlusal interferences. Although most interferences can be determined in the mouth, the mouth is a poor articulator. Everything is not visible. The articulator does not bend and torque like the jaw, the lingual aspect of the teeth is more visible, and it is easier to identify the interferences.

The occlusal analysis proceeds to locate and identify specific occlusal interferences during function. An attempt is made to relate the interferences to specific pathological conditions that may be present as a result of stressful forces generated by those interferences within the gnathostomatic system.

The examiner must attempt to answer the questions, (1) "What is (are) the cause(s)?" and (2) "What treatment is indicated?" A determination is made as to whether the interferences should be removed to treat the pathological condition, and the method by which this must be done is decided.

Only after these questions have been answered satisfactorily can a treatment plan be initiated that will be relevant to the needs of each individual patient.

An occlusal analysis is an adjunct to all other diagnostic aids and procedures. Besides taking a careful history and performing an oral examination, a radiographic survey also is required. This includes transcranial lateral oblique films, a full-mouth periapical survey, a bite-wing survey, and whenever possible a Panorex radiograph. If there is TMJ dysfunction, lateral head films and/or laminagraphic radiographs of the joints are most helpful. A functional occlusal analysis should be performed on diagnostic casts (1) when there is a pathological condition present in any of the tissues of the system as a result of occlusal activity, (2) when occlusal interferences are present, or (3) when there is to be a major reorientation of the occlusion by orthodontics, occlusal adjustment by selective grinding, restorative dentistry, surgical procedures (such as mandibular resection), or combinations of these methods.

It helps to arrive at a diagnosis and treatment plan whose results are predictable before performing certain irreversible procedures on the patient that may be wrong.

Conditions and symptoms to be observed and noted

Any of the following, either singly or in combination may occur as pathological conditions resulting from occlusal dysfunction. One or several components of the gnathostomatic system may be affected, and there may be an interrelationship of one part to another. The specific cause is not always readily apparent. The symptoms may vary as to the severity and degree. The patient may or may not be aware of some of the symptoms.

Pain in the region of the TMJ

Classic symptoms

1. Pain, headache, muscle spasm, particularly in the sternocleidomastoid, trapezius, masseter, and temporal muscles, as well as other muscles of mastication
2. Clicking, popping, snapping noises in TMJ
3. Dizziness and possible nausea
4. Earache, ringing in ears, a fullness or pressure backlog in the ear
5. Pain in tongue
6. Partial or complete inability to open or close the mouth; limited range of function of the jaw in one or more directions with or without pain
7. Radiographic studies showing condylar deviation:

malpositioned, remodeled condyle, worn condyle and/or eminence, and possibly compression and/or perforation of the articular disc

Occlusal considerations

1. Occlusal interferences during excursive jaw movements, particularly nonworking or balancing interferences during lateral movement, as well as working and protrusive interferences during excursive movements.
2. CO and CR positions of the teeth not coinciding during mandibular closure, resulting in an occlusal slide along the inclined planes of the occlusal surfaces of the teeth; possibly an anterior and/or lateral deviation of the mandible on closure of the teeth to the CO position
3. Improper horizontal overlap of anterior teeth (lack of anterior disclusion)
4. Excessive vertical overlap of anterior teeth (too much anterior disclusion); an anterior or posterior cross-bite
5. Facets of wear on occlusal surfaces of the teeth indicating that the patient may be a bruxer or have other parafunctional habits (often with large masseter muscles if a bruxer)
6. Mobility of the teeth because of primary or secondary traumatic occlusion, open contacts, diastemas, or gingival erosion
7. Fractured cusps (particularly stamp cusps) of teeth
8. Posterior bite collapse caused by missing, worn, tilted, or drifted posterior teeth with excessive contact of the upper and lower anterior teeth
9. Possible loss of vertical dimension with an increased freeway space
10. Nonfunctional restorations such as high gold crowns or bridges or improper ridge and groove directions of gold crown anatomy (iatrogenic)
11. Thickening of periodontal ligaments and possible dystrophic bone loss because of traumatic occlusion; possible gingival recession in some areas
12. Malposition of condyles in fossae (condyles not centered properly in fossae), as shown on TMJ radiographs
13. Possibly, pathological facets of wear in themselves
14. Deviate tongue patterns during swallowing, which may prevent teeth from touching because of lack of eruption, can result in open anterior bite and complete lack of anterior disclusion; tongue thrust, speech impediments; can accompany cleft palates and parafunctional discrepancies

Other considerations

1. Is the patient undergoing a psychological crisis of any kind because of stressful situations or emotional strain?
2. Was there traumatic injury to the TMJ, such as a fracture, or has the patient worn a Milwaukee brace for whiplash injury?
3. Are there congenital defects, such as the upper and lower jaws not matching in size, one side being retarded in growth, a macrogrowth, cleft palate, or cleft lip?
4. Are there congenitally missing teeth?
5. Has patient recently undergone oral surgery (particularly under general anesthesia), heavy-handed oral surgery, tearing of ligaments and stretching of muscles, or straining of TMJ?
6. Is the patient a mouth breather?

Treatment for pain of the TMJ may be as simple as getting the patient to discontinue certain parafunctional activity, or treatment may require physiotherapy or combined procedures from a multidisciplinary approach beginning with palliative treatment such as medication, occlusal repositioning splints, orthodontic and periodontic treatment, followed by occlusal adjustment by selective grinding, and finally a full-mouth rehabilitation to reorganize the pattern of the occlusion of the teeth to coincide with mandibular function (or the determinants of occlusion). Most cases lie somewhere in between. However, these situations do require that a thorough functional occlusal analysis be performed before treatment. The operator must be well informed and experienced in gnathological procedures and understand the skull-fossa-condyle geometry and the dynamics of the occlusal geography to these determinants. He or she must know what is normal, what is abnormal, which factors are fixed anatomically, and which factors are changeable. Treatment must be designed in such a manner that these principles are not violated, and this knowledge of the fixed anatomical factors must be used to establish harmony and physiological function between all components of the system—both the fixed and the changeable factors. The operator must know what can be changed while still maintaining geometrical and functional harmony in the system.

Occlusal adjustment

For a patient with a TMJ problem who presents with pain:

1. Complete examination, and compile data; take history.
2. Perform an occlusal analysis, including radiographic findings and other diagnostic aids.
3. Sometimes this is preceded by pharmacological therapy.
4. Interocclusal condylar repositioning splint may be used with point occlusal contact of posterior teeth and built-in anterior disclusion.

   a. This should be worn an average of 3 to 6 weeks with weekly observation and minor adjustments.
   b. It allows neuromusculature to regain equilibrium by reducing tissue stresses.
5. At this point of treatment by educating the patient to certain isometric and isotonic physiotherapy exercises and the discontinuance of a particular parafunctional activity, the TMJ problem sometimes may be considered to be under control.
   a. The patient may have to wear the splint only at night, only occasionally, or not at all; one of the considerations when wearing a splint too long is that the teeth may become intruded.
   b. This will maintain the equilibrium without further damage to the system; perhaps by ceasing bruxing at night, the patient's resistance will be sufficient to maintain this balance.
6. Sometimes the problem is solved only temporarily, and further treatment is required that involves a reorientation of the occlusion.
7. Occlusal reorientation may be performed by
   a. Selective grinding of the teeth
   b. Orthodontic tooth repositioning
   c. Restorative dentistry
   d. Combinations of the above
8. Assuming that orthodontic treatment is not necessary, an occlusal adjustment by selective grinding would be the next step in treatment.

Before adjusting the occlusion by selective grinding, two questions must be asked:

1. Is there any pathological condition in any component of the system resulting from the fact that CO and CR tooth-contact positions do not coincide (deflective occlusion)?
2. Is a major reorientation of the occlusion to be undertaken that will require using centric relation of the condyles as a reference position?

If the answer to either of these questions is yes, the occlusal adjustment must be performed at the CR position.

The occlusal adjustment first must be performed on mounted diagnostic casts following specific rules to obtain a mutually protected occlusion. The exact procedures for performing an occlusal adjustment are outlined in the manual *Physiology of Occlusion*,[4] following the rules of occlusal adjustment advocated by Stuart, Stallard, Thomas, and others. It entails following definite rules and sequences to obtain proper ridge groove directions on the teeth that are in harmony with jaw movement and maintain proper vertical dimension. The primary objectives of an occlusal adjustment are to promote healing and to maintain a neuromuscular balance within the system by distributing and directing the occlusal load over as many posterior teeth as possible while conserving tooth structure. After the adjustment is done on the diagnostic casts and charted, the patient's teeth may be adjusted by grinding in the mouth. Sometimes the goals of an occlusal adjustment are impossible to obtain because of positioning of teeth or arch discrepancy. It may be discovered that an occlusal adjustment in the mouth would be contraindicated. By performing first on the diagnostic casts, no irreversible damage has been done to the patient. It may be discovered that the patient requires orthodontic tooth repositioning before an occlusal adjustment to obtain a better tooth-to-tooth relationship.

In some instances an occlusal adjustment is only a step in the long process of restoring function to the patient's system. Often it becomes necessary to rebuild the occlusion of the teeth by restorative dentistry procedures. This may involve placement of gold crowns and/or onlays, fixed bridges, or removable partial dentures or combinations of these restorations. It may be preceded by orthodontic treatment and certainly by extensive periodontal treatment. All these procedures may be preceded by and accompanied by pharmacological treatment. At any rate these cases often require combined therapy performed by interdisciplinary means with consultation and cooperation of several professionals so that proper respect is given to the anatomical skull factors without violating any of the principles of occlusion. There must be a high degree of predictability to the completed case. The dentist who performs these procedures must be knowledgeable, experienced, and motivated, or the entire case may end up a greater failure than when treatment was started. The patient's needs should be supreme, and if the operator does not feel confident, the patient should be referred to someone who is knowledgeable in this field.

Rationale for pantographic recording. In most instances accurately mounting diagnostic casts in centric relation using a face-bow transfer and accurate interocclusal centric records is sufficient to perform an occlusal analysis and get a fairly good picture of the jaw and tooth relationships. It is often necessary to go further for a final diagnosis, especially if treatment is to be complicated.

It becomes necessary to transfer not only the static geometry of the skull-fossa relations to an articulator but also the dynamic three-dimensional anatomical and functional geometrical relationships.

The maximum amount of movement of the mandible in any given plane or direction is called its *border movement*. This movement is limited by the mandibular ligaments, capsular ligaments of the TMJ, muscles, and bone. Within the boundaries of the border movements there is a wide range of intraborder movement. Most movement occurs as intraborder movement.

Unlike intraborder movements, the border movements of the mandible are reproducible. Therefore they can be recorded and measured.

By applying geometrical principles and the use of mechanical apparatus and procedures it is possible to record and measure the degree and directions of the three-dimensional pathways of the border movements of the condyle in their respective fossae during function.

This mandibular movement recording is referred to as a pantographic recording. A pantograph is an instrument used to duplicate a map or drawing to the same or a different scale. The application here is to duplicate the condylar pathways of movement in the fossa-eminence or the topography of the fossa-eminence along given pathways during given jaw movements.

The recordings are scribed by styli on strategically located tracing plates, which are attached to mechanical side arms and anterior cross arms, which in turn are attached to the teeth by means of a cemented clutch. Thus when the jaw moves, the styli move also.

Fine lines are scribed on these plates which are actually segments of arcs transcribed by the rotating condyle and the geometrical interplay of the opposite condyle as they translate and rotate along the three-dimensional pathways of their fossae during movement. These lines are reproducible, since they are border movements of the jaw. They are always recorded at least twice for confirmation. Protrusion is not a border movement and is recorded only once. To be certain that the full border movement is recorded, especially the immediate side shift (or Bennett movement), it is necessary to induce this side shift by placing a light hand pressure on the nonworking side to the angle of the mandible, with the force directed toward the opposite, or rotating, condyle.

Essentially the pantograph separates the three-dimensional movement that occurs as simultaneous time-sequenced movement and breaks it down into its individual planes of movement on the tracing plates—the horizontal, vertical, and sagittal—for both condyles. It makes it possible to visually study the direction and degree of the time-sequenced movement in each single plane that occurs as three-dimensional movement in the skull.

The pantographic recording apparatus is related to the axis-orbital plane by use of a face-bow transfer, and then the entire apparatus is transferred from the patient and mounted to the articulator intact.

The articulator is designed to simulate jaw function. Its fossa controls can be made to operate in three dimensions. Mechanical adjustments of the fossa controls are accomplished to reproduce on the articulator the three-dimensional pathways of movement that were recorded from the jaw. Adjustments are made so that the styli follow the exact recorded lines on the tracing plates. The pantograph is a means of reproducing the curved pathways of movement within the fossae and obtaining the mechanical equivalents of the skull-fossa-condyle geometrical relations during function for any given individual. In other words, the pantograph transfers that patient's determinants of occlusion from the skull to an articulator and maintains with accuracy all the geometrical and spatial relationships between the skull geometry, the three axes of rotation, the hinge axis, and the axis-orbital plane.

After the articulator is adjusted, the pantograph is removed, and the diagnostic casts of the patient can be reattached, or a new mounting can be done from a new face-bow transfer and interocclusal centric registration.

Adjusting the articulator to a pantographic recording and mounting diagnostic casts make it possible to perform a definitive occlusal analysis in which an attempt is made to relate certain pathological conditions to occlusal interferences, to perform an occlusal adjustment on diagnostic casts to see if it is contraindicated in the mouth, or to do a diagnostic waxing up on a case that may need full occlusal reorientation by restorative dentistry procedures. It helps to arrive at a treatment plan in which the end result is predictable because all mistakes are made on the casts, not on the teeth when it might be contraindicated and would be irreversible.

It is also possible to mount casts of the patient's prepared teeth as master casts and to fabricate dental restorations that will be geometrically compatible with the patient's anatomical skull factors without violating any of the biomechanical, fixed anatomical, or physiological factors which exist for that patient. This can be accomplished when the determinants of occlussion for the given patient have been successfully transferred to a workable laboratory instrument in an accurate manner.

Now, if the angle of the eminence is 30 degrees, it is 30 degrees to the axis-orbital plane. A true rotation center distance (intercondylar distance) has been established. The degree and directions of the condylar pathways in their fossae have been recorded, measured, and transferred in relation to the axis-orbital plane, no matter what position the condyles assume during function. In a sense the anatomical and geometrical asymmetry of that patient has been transferred from the skull to the articulator, which is unique for that patient and serves as a prescription for any reorganization of the plane of occlusion or occlusal anatomy, without violating any of the fixed anatomical factors or the patient's determinants of occlusion.

Procedures for performing an occlusal analysis in the mouth

1. Instruct the patient to move the jaw in all directions. Note the range of movement. Is it painful to move? Is there any restricted movement? Record.
2. Measure the vertical dimension and freeway space.
   a. Make a small mark on the point of the chin and another mark on the lip just below the nose.
   b. Have the patient close the teeth to the CO position, and measure the distance between the two lines.
   c. Then have the patient lightly touch the lips with the teeth separated (say "Boston, Boston, Boston") and then maintain this position without moving.
   d. Measure again the distance between the two lines. The difference between the second measurement and the first is the measurement of freeway space. Record this measurement.
   e. Have the patient relax and swallow. Instruct the patient to leave the tongue in the position it seeks when swallowing. Separate the lips and note the position of the tongue. Is it between the teeth or in the upper anterior palatal regions?
3. Instruct the patient to open the mouth to its maximum opening, and measure the degree of this opening. The normal opening for adults is 45 to 60 mm, measured vertically between the anterior maxillary and mandibular teeth. Record this measurement.
4. Using the proper hand position, support the patient's mandible in an unstrained manner. With the patient's teeth slightly separated, program him or her into the terminal hinge (CR) position.
5. Instruct the patient to close the jaw, while hand supported, until the upper and lower teeth barely make first contact in the CR position. Observe the areas of initial contact and record. NOTE: Most likely all the posterior teeth will not be touching at this time.
6. From this initial CR contact position, instruct the patient to clench into the CO (fully intercuspated) position. Observe to see if there is any deviation of the mandibular teeth during this final closure such as anterior and/or lateral shift of the lower teeth. Record.
7. To measure the anterior deviation, have the patient first close to the CR position. Draw a vertical line on the buccal surfaces of the upper and lower first premolars on each side. Then have the patient close to the CO position, and draw a second vertical line on the buccal surface of the lower first premolar that is continuous with the vertical line on the upper premolar. (This line will be posterior to the first line.) Measure the distance between these two lines to obtain the measurement of the amount of anterior deviation or slide. Measure both sides and record.
8. To measure the amount of lateral deviation, place the teeth in the CR position, and draw a vertical line on the labial surfaces of the upper and lower central incisors. Have the patient close to the CO position, and draw a second vertical line on the labial surface of the lower central incisor that is continuous with the vertical line on the upper central incisor. Measure the distance between these two lines for the measurement of the amount of lateral deviation. Record. NOTE: It will be to the right or left of the original line, depending on the direction of the lateral shift.
9. To measure the amount of the overbite (vertical overlap) of the anterior teeth, instruct the patient to close the teeth to the CO position. With a sharp, soft marking pencil scribe a line horizontally along the labial surfaces of the lower anterior mandibular teeth, using the incisal edge of the upper maxillary incisors as a guide. Measure the distance between the scribed line and the incisal edges of the lower anterior mandibular teeth. This is the measurement of the amount of anterior vertical overlap in the CO position. Record.
10. To measure the amount of the anterior overjet (horizontal overlap), place a millimeter ruler at the edge of the upper incisors. Measure the distance from the incisal edges of the upper incisors to the labial surfaces of the lower anterior teeth. This is the measurement of the amount of anterior horizontal overlap in the CO position. Record. Repeat this procedure in the first molar area on each side to measure the amount of overjet of the posterior teeth. Record. Note if there is a posterior cross-bite.
11. Observe the occlusal surfaces of all the teeth in the upper and lower arch. Note the teeth that show facets of wear, both anteriors and posteriors. Record these on the chart.
12. Have the patient tap lightly in centric occlusion. Gently place the tip of the wet index finger against the buccal surface of each individual

tooth. In this way it is possible to record barely perceptible movement (vibration) of the teeth, or fremitus, during centric closure and lateral excursive movements. Record.

13. Observe for mobility of any of the teeth during centric closure or during lateral and protrusive excursions. Have the patient close teeth to the CO position and make protrusive and lateral excursions. Record teeth that have mobility and the degree of mobility.

Testing for interferences using Mylar tape

14. Place a strip of 0.0005-inch Mylar tape between the teeth, support the jaw, and have the patient close to the CR position. Instruct the patient to make a protrusive movement while attempting to pull the Mylar. If it grabs, there is protrusive interference. Repeat this procedure for all quadrants, and record the areas of interference.
15. Instruct the patient to make a lateral movement of the jaw from the CR position. Testing with the Mylar strip, note any nonworking and working interferences as the Mylar is progressively moved around the arch to test contact of each tooth. Repeat procedure with Mylar tape to test for working interferences. Record. NOTE: To be certain all the Bennett movement is introduced into these lateral movements, it is necessary to induce this side shift by producing a light pressure at the angle of the mandible on the nonworking side. The force is generated toward the working condyle on the opposite side.

Testing for interferences in the CR tooth contact position

16. Place the strip of 0.0005-inch Mylar tape between the teeth while supporting the jaw in the terminal hinge position. Have the patient open and close to the CR position, and progressively move the Mylar around the arch, testing contact of each tooth while attempting to pull the Mylar buccally from between the teeth without having the Mylar grab. Areas in which the Mylar tape grabs are areas of tooth contact in CR. Record.

Identifying interferences with marking ribbon

17. To mark the exact location of the occlusal interferences, it is necessary to use marking ribbon.
    a. *Protrusive interferences*. Place black marking ribbon between the teeth on both sides of the arch. Instruct the patient to move the jaw to an end-to-end position of the anterior teeth and then return it to the CO position. Support the jaw. If there are protrusive interferences, the markings will identify them as to number and position. Record. Note: Black marks on the mesial aspect of lower first premolars do not indicate protrusive interference but are part of the anterior disclusion as the mesial inclines of the premolars move against the distal inclines of the upper canines. Protrusive interferences appear on mesial inclines of the lower teeth and distal inclines of upper teeth.
    b. *Working and nonworking interferences*. Place green marking ribbon between the teeth on the right side and blue marking ribbon on the left side. Support the jaw, induce Bennett movement, and instruct the patient to make a right lateral movement. Working interferences will be identified by green markings on the teeth on the right side. Record. Nonworking interferences on the left are identified by blue markings. Record. Repeat this procedure for left lateral movement. Reverse the colored ribbon. Record.
        (1) Nonworking interferences generally occur on the mesial slopes, buccal inclines of the lingual cusps of upper teeth, and on the distal slopes, lingual inclines of the buccal cusps of lower teeth on the nonworking side.
        (2) Working interferences generally occur on the mesial slopes, lingual inclines of buccal cusps of upper teeth, and distal slopes, buccal inclines of lower teeth on the working side.
        (3) Occasionally working interferences appear on the distal slopes, buccal inclines of lingual cusps on lower teeth, and mesial slopes, lingual inclines of lingual cusps on the upper teeth on the working side of the arch. These are known as cross-tooth working interferences.
    c. *Centric interferences*. Place red marking ribbon between the teeth on both sides of the arch. Support the jaw, and instruct the patient first to close into the CR position, and mark. Then instruct the patient to close into the CO position, and mark. Record. The red will mark tooth contacts in the CR and CO positions. If there are interferences between CO and CR, there will be a long red mark along the mesial slopes, buccal inclines of the lingual cusps of the upper teeth, distal slopes, and lingual inclines of the buccal cusps of the lower teeth. These are the markings for an occlusal slide. Record.

18. Another method for checking the interferences is by the use of a loop of dental floss. For example, to check nonworking interferences, place the loop of floss posterior to the last teeth on the right side of the arch. Have the patient make a left lateral movement, and attempt to draw the loop of floss from between the teeth. If there is a nonworking interference, it will grab the floss and prevent its removal.
19. On the basis of the number and type of occlusal interferences, and in conjunction with the oral examination and radiographic findings, or because major restorative procedures are necessary in this case, at this time a decision is made to perform a definitive occlusal analysis on accurately mounted diagnostic casts before completing a diagnosis and making a treatment plan.

FUNCTIONAL OCCLUSAL ANALYSIS ON MOUNTED STUDY CASTS

To obtain a properly oriented centric-relation mounting of diagnostic casts on an articulator, it is ideal to establish a true hinge axis location and axis-orbital plane as a cranial reference before making a face-bow transfer and mounting the casts.

If the patient has a temporomandibular joint problem with associated pain or with inflammation and excess fluid in the joint, it may not be possible to program the jaw to the CR position until the TMJ is treated and becomes comfortable again. If the jaw cannot be programed to the CR position, the hinge axis location will be inaccurate.

To make a tentative diagnosis and perform an occlusal analysis on mounted diagnostic casts, it is often practical to do a quick-mount procedure. This involves establishing an arbitrary hinge axis location using one of several accepted procedures (a guess axis), thereby obtaining an arbitrary axis-orbital plane, taking a face-bow transfer in the usual manner, making interocclusal centric registrations, and mounting the diagnostic casts.

Most cases are first mounted as a quick mount, which is an accepted procedure. The casts can be mounted on any type of articulator that will accept a face-bow transfer, whether it is a fully adjustable arcon, a semiadjustable arcon, or even a nonarcon type. It is strongly suggested, whenever possible, to use at least the semiadjustable arcon type. Further adjustments can be made using wax checkbites to obtain angles of settings of the articulator to at least straight lines.

In most instances a quick mount of the casts is sufficient to allow the investigator to perform a tentative diagnosis and occlusal analysis. Casts mounted in this manner can be used to make an interocclusal repositioning splint, an antibruxing splint, or a night guard splint to treat the joints before any further treatment of the occlusion.

For a more definitive occlusal analysis, occlusal adjustment on mounted casts, diagnostic waxing up of the occlusion, and eventually a full-mouth rehabilitation, a true hinge axis location and accurate axis-orbital plane are necessary, and probably a pantographic recording would be required. This is one way to obtain accurate geometrics of jaw-skull relations on an articulator.

A true hinge axis and pantographic recordings should be established when:

1. There is a gross pathological condition in any component of the gnathostomatic system related to occlusal activity and requiring treatment of the occlusion to correct that condition.
2. There are gross facets of wear caused by occlusal interferences, and an occlusal adjustment is required.
3. There is to be a major reorientation of the occlusion by occlusal adjustment followed by major restorative dentistry procedures.

A quick mount of diagnostic casts should be sufficient in most instances to determine any further need for more sophisticated procedures. It can be used by anyone who understands the principles involved and has any kind of semiadjustable articulator.

The more sophisticated procedures require fully adjustable instrumentation to ensure accuracy of diagnosis, treatment planning, and treatment. It is up to the operator through knowledge and experience to make the decision to use more sophisticated procedures. All cases do not require it, perhaps only about 15% of all cases, but the operator must know which ones do and which do not. A full understanding of the principles of occlusion and instrumentation is a requirement to know which procedure to follow.

Procedures for performing an occlusal analysis on mounted study casts (centric relation mounting) on articulator

1. Loosen the incisal pin so it is not contacting the incisal table.
2. Close the articulator gently until the teeth on the casts make initial contact in the CR position. Note which teeth contact. Record.
3. At the CR position of contact drop the incisal pin until the incisal pin foot comes into contact with the incisal table. Observe the measurement indicated in this position on the vertical scale on the incisal pin. Record.
4. Close the articulator, and position the teeth in the CO position. Observe the measurement on the vertical scale of the incisal pin for this position. Record.

5. The difference between the two previous readings or measurements is the measurement of the vertical displacement of the lower teeth on closure from the CR position to the CO position. Record this measurement.
6. Using the proper hand positions to manipulate the articulator, move the lower member into protrusive and right and left lateral movements. Observe any working, nonworking, or protrusive interferences, and note presence or absence of cuspid rise and anterior disclusion.
7. Use 0.0005-inch Mylar strip to locate occlusal contacts in the CR position. Check each tooth in the arch. Record areas of contact.
8. To measure the amount of anterior shift or deviation of the mandible, place the teeth in the CR position. Draw a continuous vertical line on the buccal surfaces of the upper and lower first premolars on both sides of the arch. Then place the teeth in the CO position, and scribe a second line along the buccal surfaces of the lower premolars that is continuous with the vertical line on the upper premolars. Measure the distance between the two lines on the lower premolars on each side. This is the measurement of the amount of anterior slide of the teeth on each side during closure from CR to CO. Record these measurements.
9. To measure the amount of lateral shift or deviation of the mandible, place the teeth in the CR position. Draw a continuous vertical line on the labial surfaces of the upper and lower central incisors. Then place the teeth in the CO position, and scribe a second vertical line on the labial surface of the lower central incisor that is continuous with the vertical line on the upper incisor. This is the measurement of the amount of the lateral shift of the lower teeth on closure from CR to CO. Record. Note: This line will be either to the right or left of the first vertical line on the lower incisor, depending on the direction of the lateral shift.
10. To measure the amount of anterior overbite, close the articulator until the teeth are in the CO position. With a sharp lead pencil scribe a line horizontally along the labial surfaces of the lower anterior mandibular teeth, using the incisal edge of the upper maxillary teeth as a guide. Measure the distance between the scribed line and the incisal edges of the lower anterior teeth. This is the measurement of the amount of vertical overlap of the anterior teeth in the CO position. Record.
11. To measure the amount of the anterior overjet, place a millimeter ruler at the edge of the upper incisors. Measure the distance from the incisal edges of the upper incisors and the labial surfaces of the lower incisors. This is the measurement of the amount of horizontal overlap in the CO position. Record.

Locating interferences using Mylar tape

12. Place a strip of 0.0005-inch Mylar tape between the teeth. Move the lower member of the articulator into a right lateral movement. Check each tooth in the arch during lateral movements for working and nonworking interferences. Repeat for left lateral movement and protrusive movement. Record areas of contact.

Identifying interference with marking ribbon

13. Using different colored marking ribbons, mark and record the exact areas of occlusal contact and interferences for centric (CR) protrusive and lateral movements.
    a. *Centric interferences*. Place red marking ribbon between the teeth on both sides of the arch. Close the articulator until the teeth contact in the CR position. Observe the markings in the areas of contact and record. Then, keeping the red marking ribbon between the teeth, move the teeth into the CO position. Observe the markings in the areas of contact and record. NOTE: If there are interferences during the closure from CR to CO, elongated markings will be present along the respective inclines of the triangular ridges and stamp cusps. Record. This is the centric slide. The red centric markings distinguish these areas of contact from excursive contacts and indicate where the excursive contacts are part of centric contact.
    b. *Protrusive interferences*. Place black marking ribbon between the teeth on both sides of the arch. Move the teeth into the CO position, and observe an areas of protrusive contact or interferences. Identify and record.
    c. *Lateral movement interferences*. Place green marking ribbon between the teeth on the *right* side and blue marking ribbon on the *left* side. Move the lower member of the articulator into a right lateral movement and mark. Note and identify any interference markings in green for working interferences on the right side and record. Identify nonworking interference markings in blue on the left side. Record. Repeat for left lateral movement; identify and record.

This concludes the exercise for locating and identifying occlusal interferences for centric and eccentric movements. By this time a clear indication as to the degree of occlusal interferences should be evident.

The occlusal analysis on diagnostic casts should not stop here, however. The overall condition must be analyzed as to the actual tooth-to-tooth relationship, the jaw-to-jaw relationship, missing, fractured, drifted, tipped, tilted, or rotated teeth, contour of the gingiva, open contacts, and diastemas. In an attempt to make a complete study a thorough examination should be made of the radiographs to determine specific pathological conditions that may show up, such as thickened periodontal ligament spaces or bone loss. Furthermore, if there are pathological conditions of the TMJ or the neuromusculature, then an attempt must be made to relate specific occlusal activity to them. Radiographs of the TMJ are useful for this purpose in studying the different postures of the condyles in their fossae and in determining whether there are pathological conditions in the joint in the form of abraded or worn condyles and/or eminences or any other irregularities of the joint spaces or condyles.

SUMMARY

Not until all the factors of dysfunction have been thoroughly considered, including the emotional factors, and there has been a thorough occlusal and functional analysis of the gnathostomatic system, can a rational treatment plan be decided on.

It must be accepted that there are some cases in which treating the occlusion, even through combined therapy procedures, will not solve all the problems. Some problems, even though they may have been occlusally induced, are not correctable by ordinary occlusal treatment. Some cases are absolutely contraindicated for occlusal treatment, and they may require surgical intervention of one type or another. Sometimes if there is an ankylosed joint (either bony or fibrous), surgery may be the treatment of choice. Nevertheless, when any procedure is performed as treatment, the fixed anatomical factors must not be tampered with unless there is a follow-up occlusal analysis, and the occlusion should be placed back in harmony with the new anatomical geometric form resulting as a new anatomical fixed factor.

It must be kept in mind at all times that the biomechanics of jaw function and the function of the teeth operate as a working unit, that the system is biological, and that its tissues respond to stresses the same as any other biological mechanism. There is a definite relationship between all the components of the system—biologically, mechanically, and physiologically. It requires teamwork to properly diagnose and treat the many ills of the gnathostomatic system. The investigator must realize that occlusal disharmony is not the only cause of TMJ problems. There may be, and usually are, other factors to be investigated. An occlusal analysis is only a part of diagnosing what sometimes is a complicated series of causative factors of TMJ dysfunction and myofascial pain, but it is a part that cannot be ignored.

REFERENCES

1. The Academy of Denture Prosthetics: Glossary of prosthodontic terms, ed. 3, St. Louis, 1968, The C.V. Mosby Co.
2. Ferrein, M.: On movement of the lower jaw, translated by Joseph Simeon Landa, Paris, 1718, L'Imprimerie Royale.
3. Guichet N.F.: Principles of occlusion, Anaheim, Calif., 1970, Denar Corp.
4. Ingraham, R.: Physiology of occlusion, Los Angeles, 1972, University of Southern California School of Dentistry.
5. Ingraham, R., Curnutte, D., Walker P., Solnit, A., and Sockat, P.: A planned conjoint course in the undergraduate curriculum, Los Angeles, 1972, University of Southern California.
6. Katz, G.: The deteterminants of human occlusion, Los Angeles, 1964, Marina Press.
7. McCollum, B.B., and Stuart, C.E.: A research report, South Pasadena, Calif., 1955, Scientific Press.
8. Morgan, D.H.: Personal communication, 1977.
9. Pinto, O.: Physiology of mastication and mandibular function, Lecture to USC faculty, Sept. 27, 1975.
10. Posselt, U.: Physiology of occlusion and rehabilitation, ed. 2, Oxford, England, 1968, Blackwell Scientific Publications, Ltd.
11. Ramfjord, S.P., and Ash, M.M.: Occlusion, ed. 2, Philadelphia, 1971, W.B. Saunders Co.
12. Stallard, H., and Stuart, C.E.: Concepts of occlusion: What kind of occlusion should recusped teeth be given? Dent. Clin. North Am. **7**:591, 1963.
13. Stuart, C.E., and Stallard, H.: Conservation of natural and restored cusps in organized occlusion. Fortnightly Rev. Chicago Dent. Soc. **39**:11, June 15, 1960.
14. Stuart, C.E., and Stallard, H.: Principles involved in restoring occlusion to natural teeth, J. Prosthet. Dent. **10**:304, 1960.
15. Thomas, P.K.: Teaching and learning experiences in gnathology and restorative dentistry as member of Fresno Gnathological Research Group, Fresno, Calif., 1958-1976.

8 Radiographic procedures

LAWRENCE M. ROSEN, M.D., and DOUGLAS H. MORGAN, D.D.S.

This chapter describes the types of radiographic procedures used to study the temporomandibular joint area. Although the soft tissues and ligaments may play a role, the radiograph will show the bony abnormalities as well as the important dynamic changes that occur in the condyle, mandibular fossa, and articular eminence.

Seven different views of the temporomandibular joint are presented in one standard radiographic text,[20] and in another text there are five.[21] This is an indication of the difficulty in studying this particular structure and may be partly a manifestation of different workers in different medical or dental specialties with different areas of interest.

The temporomandibular joint lies close to the densest bone in the body, the petrous portion of the temporal bone. The problem is to get a clear view of this particular area free of the opposite side and to convey the functional dynamics of the joint in a reproducible manner, so that later studies can be made if necessary to make an objective assessment of the joint during the course of treatment.

TYPES OF TEMPOROMANDIBULAR RADIOGRAPHS

Cephalometric view

The cephalometric view is an arrangement in which a true lateral radiograph of the temporomandibular joint is shown in relation to the skull, the mandibular area, and the oral apparatus (Fig. 8-1). The bite and the temporomandibular joint are studied in the neutral position (Fig. 8-2).[27]

For this lateral head film the patient is put in a head positioner. The tube head is exactly 60 inches (152 cm) from midsagittal, the best position for a true x-ray view of the lateral head and for obtaining the film unmagnified. The 110-line SMIT-Roentgen grid is placed in front of the film to enhance the x-ray shot so it can be taken at a lower exposure (100 mA, 90 kV, $^{1}/_{5}$ second for 60 inches midsagittal).

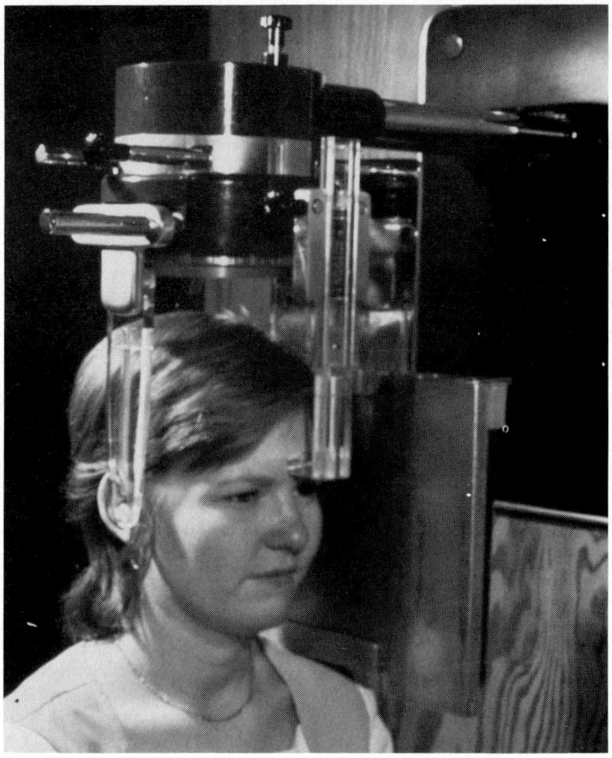

Fig. 8-1. Patient with head in cephalometric machine.

Intracanthus view

In the intracanthus projection the patient is studied in the open-mouth anteroposterior position (Fig. 8-3). The joint can be somewhat obscured by the overlying mastoid process, and slight changes in angulation and rotation are used to obtain another view of the lateral and medial poles of the condyle (Figs. 8-4 to 8-8). From these radiographs, changes in the condylar head can be detected by degenerative changes of the lateral pole of the condyle, erosion of the central portion of the condylar head, and variation in size of the right and left

Text continued on p. 137.

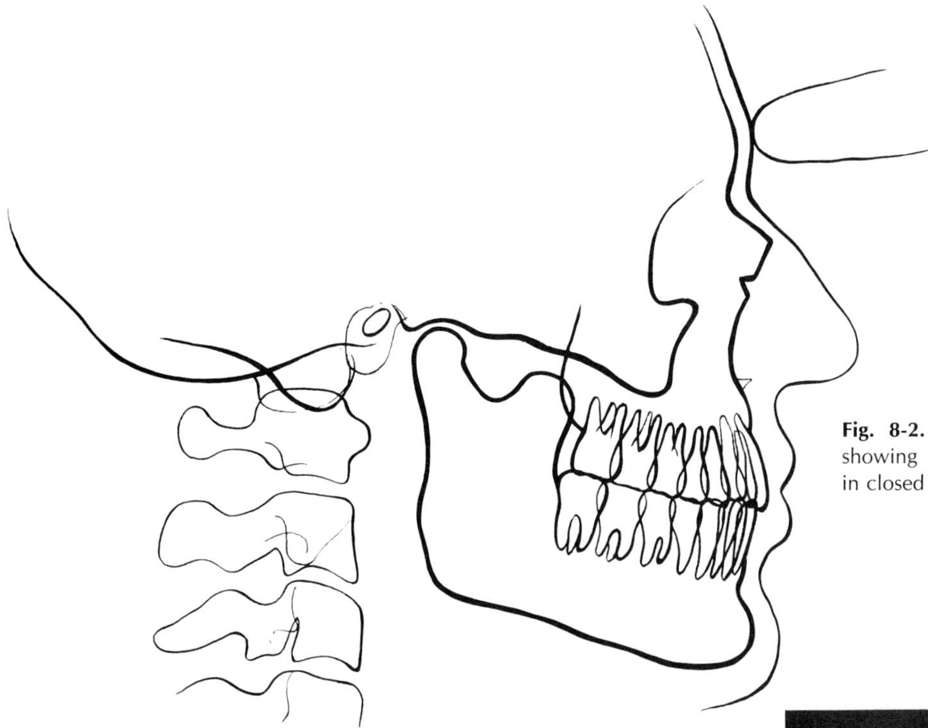

Fig. 8-2. Cephalometric profile view of head area showing relationship of maxilla and mandible to TMJ in closed position.

Fig. 8-3. Patient in open-mouth position for intracanthus projection.

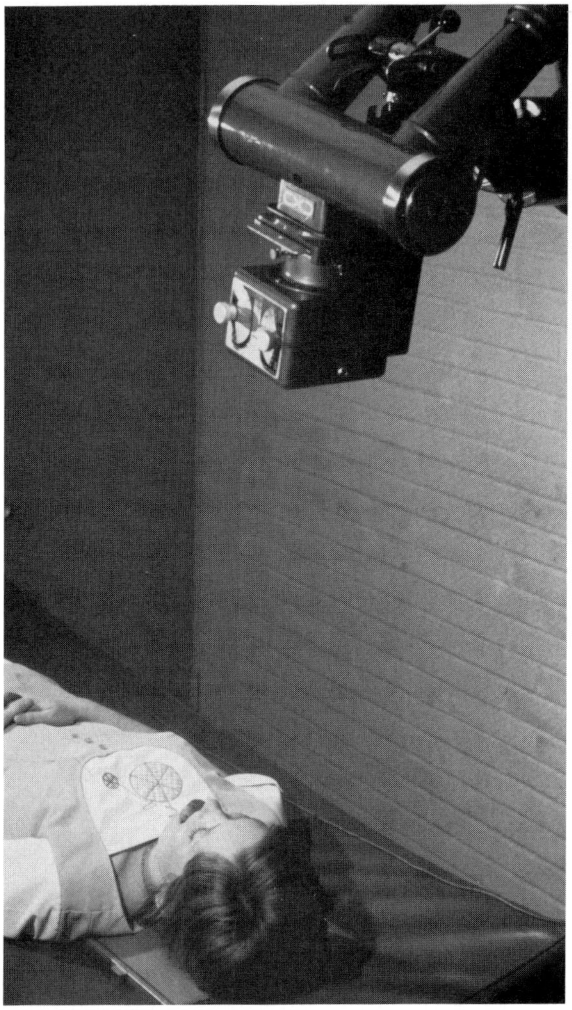

A 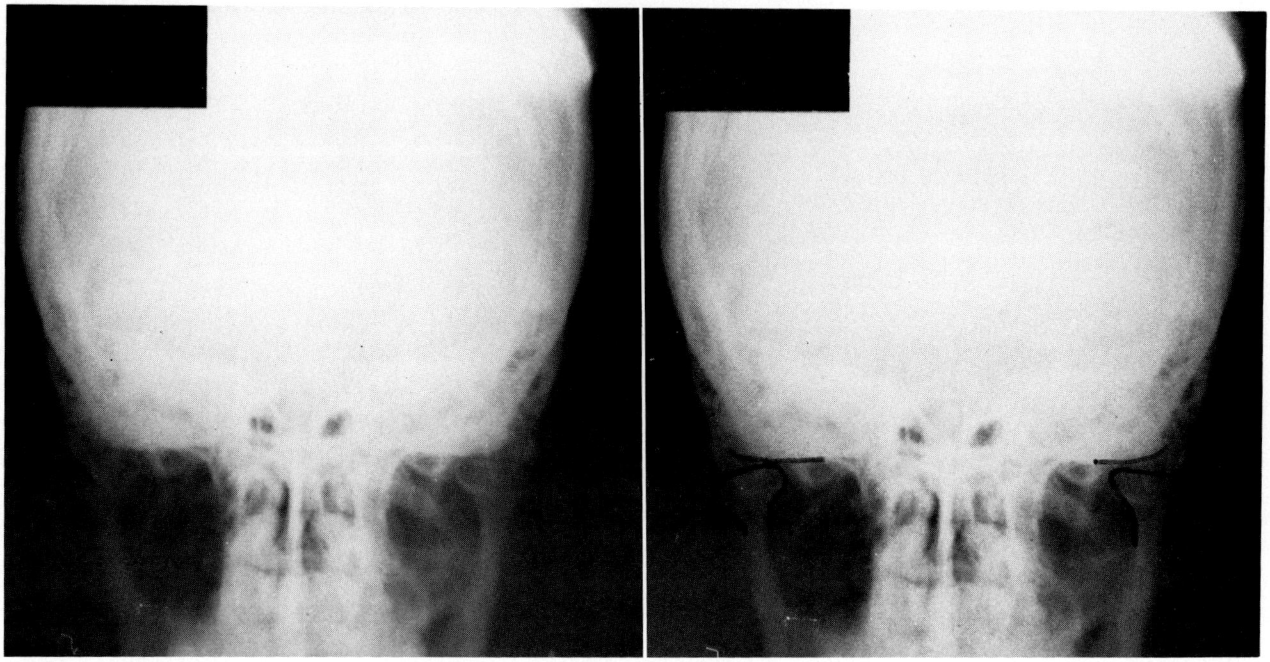 B

Fig. 8-4. A, Intracanthus view of patient showing mediolateral contour of condyles. This is a normal joint. **B,** Line drawing demonstrating shape of condylar head with normal contour.

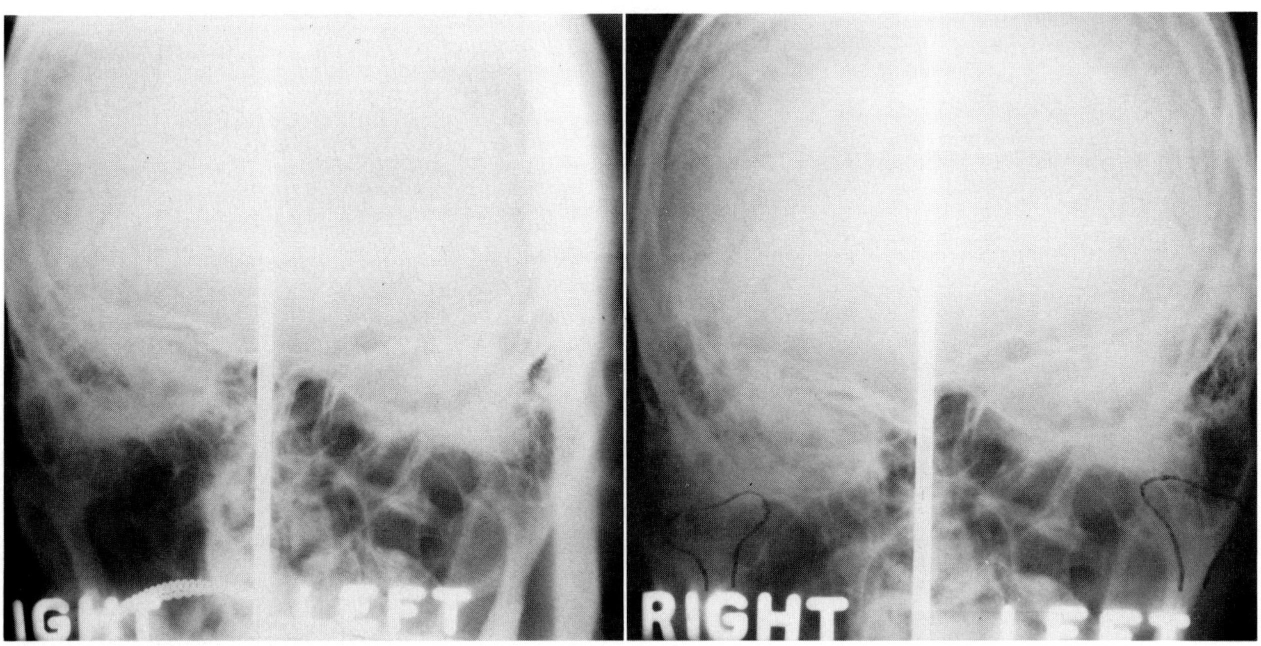

Fig. 8-5. A, Intracanthus view of patient (L.P.) having pain in left side of head. **B,** Intracanthus view of same patient showing flattening of lateral pole of left condyle; line drawing accentuating pathosis.

A 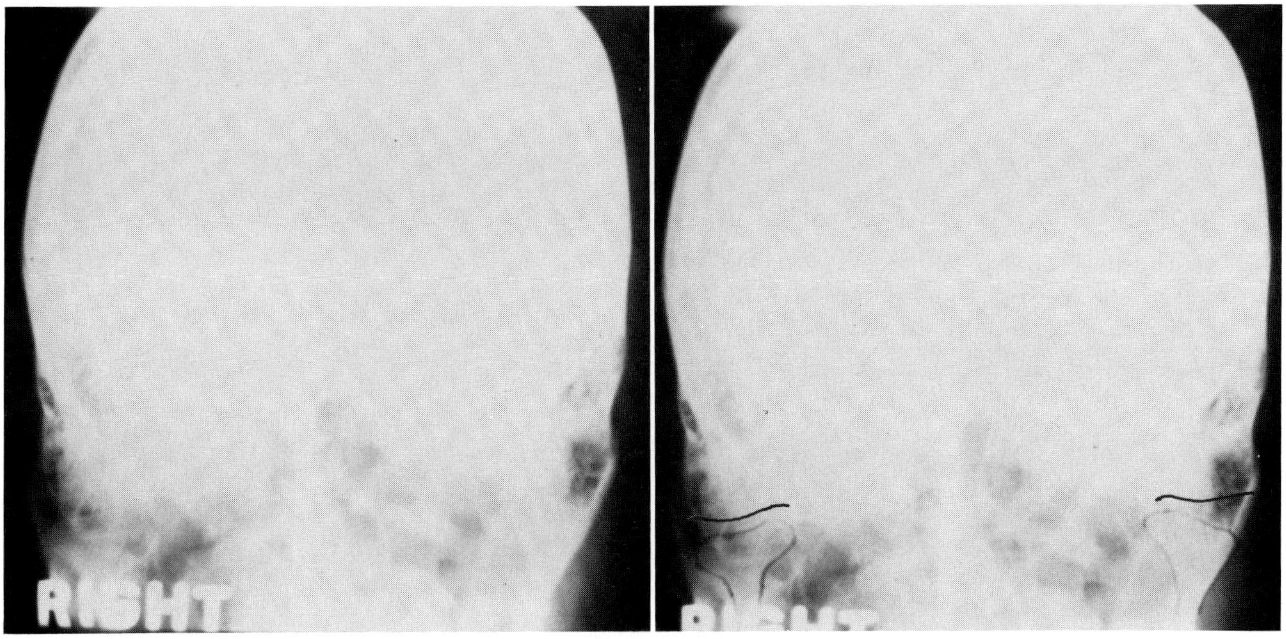 B

Fig. 8-6. A, Intracanthus view of patient (J.B.) with pain in right side of head and some symptoms in left side. **B,** Lines drawn on cephalometric view to accentuate condition reveal cupping out of center portion of condyle on right and flattening of lateral pole on left.

A 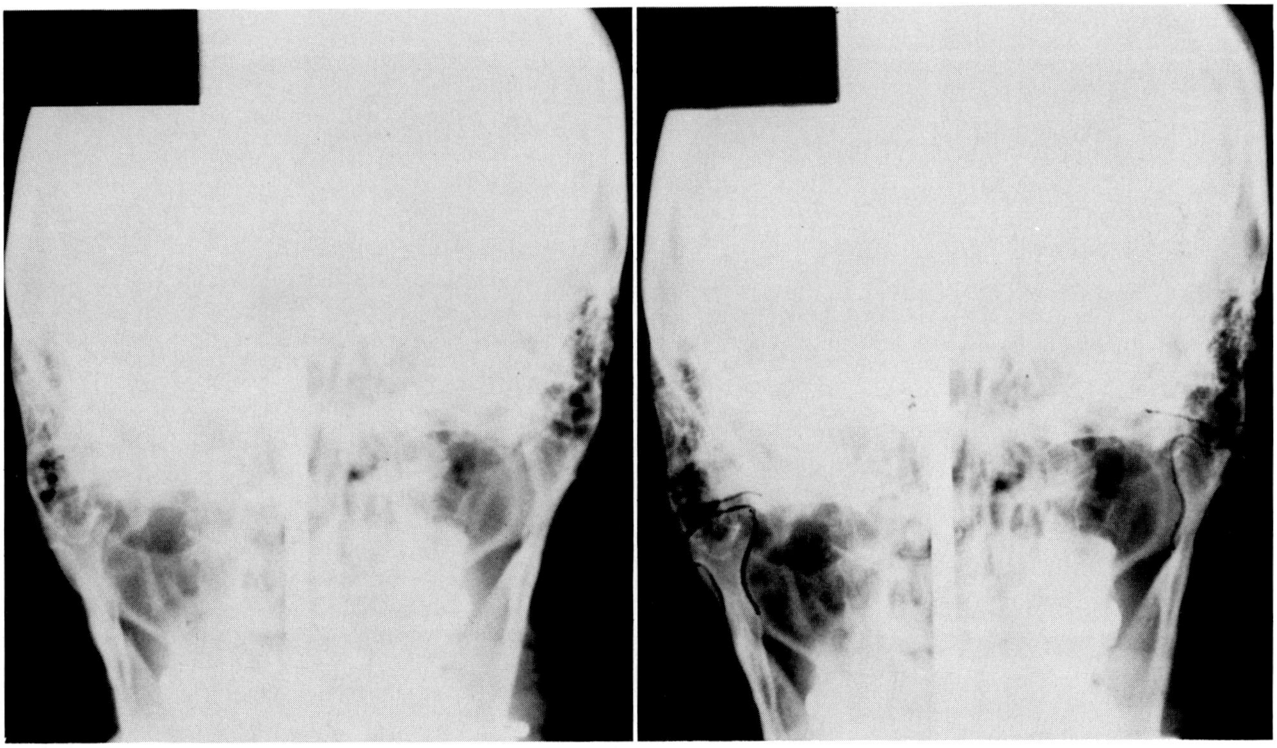 B

Fig. 8-7. A, Intracanthus view of patient having pain affecting both right and left joints. **B,** Lines drawn on cephalometric view to show cupping out of central portion of left condyle and flattening of lateral pole of right condylar head.

A

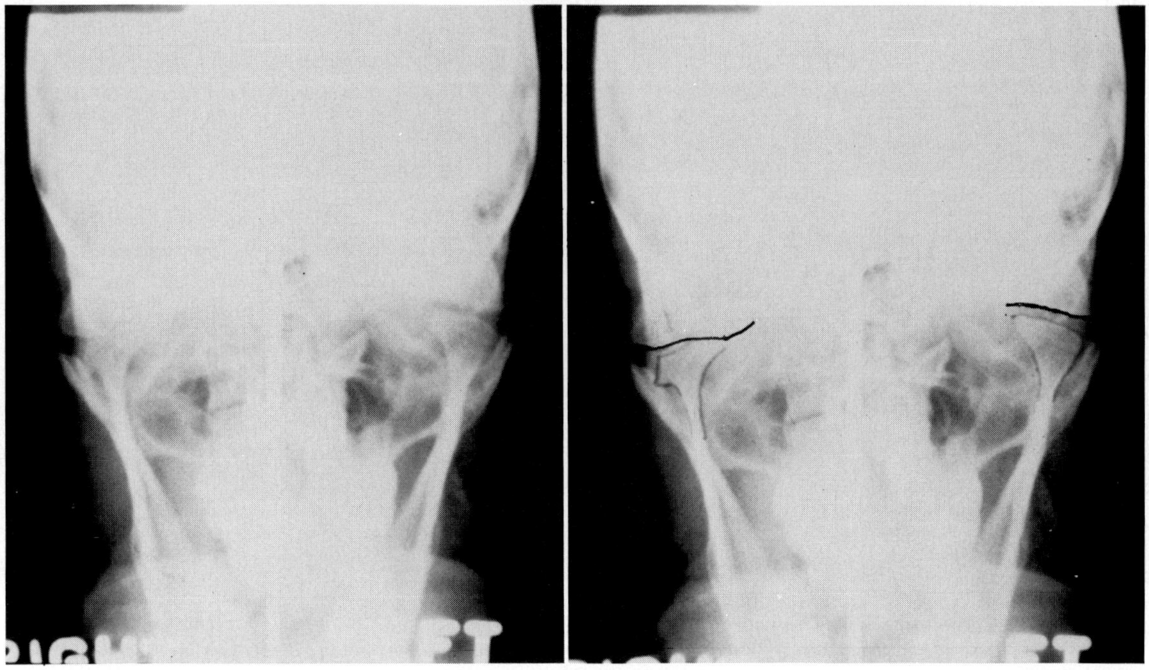

B

Fig. 8-8. A, Patient with severe pain in right head area, intracanthus view. **B,** Lines drawn on cephalometric view to show severe flattening of lateral pole of right condyle.

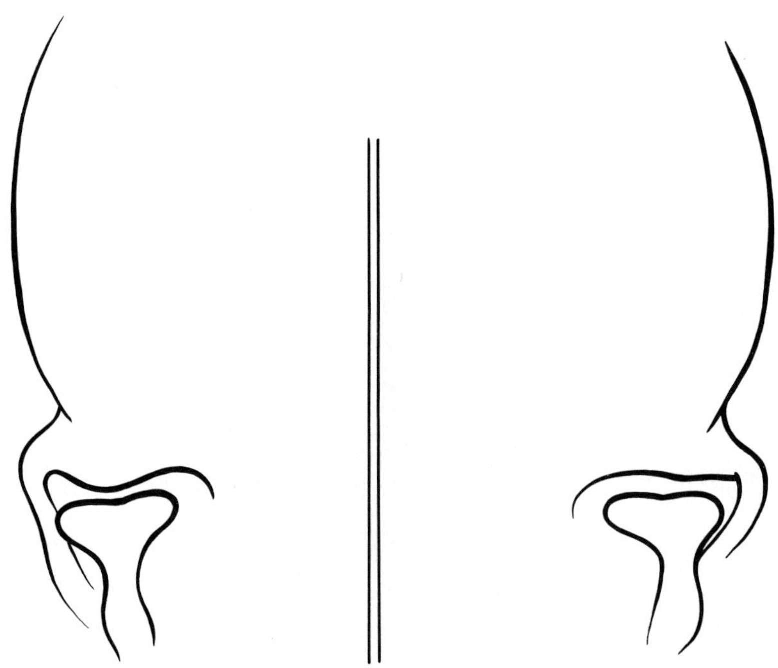

Fig. 8-9. Intracanthus view showing mediolateral condylar head, as well as mediolateral portion of articular eminence in some views.

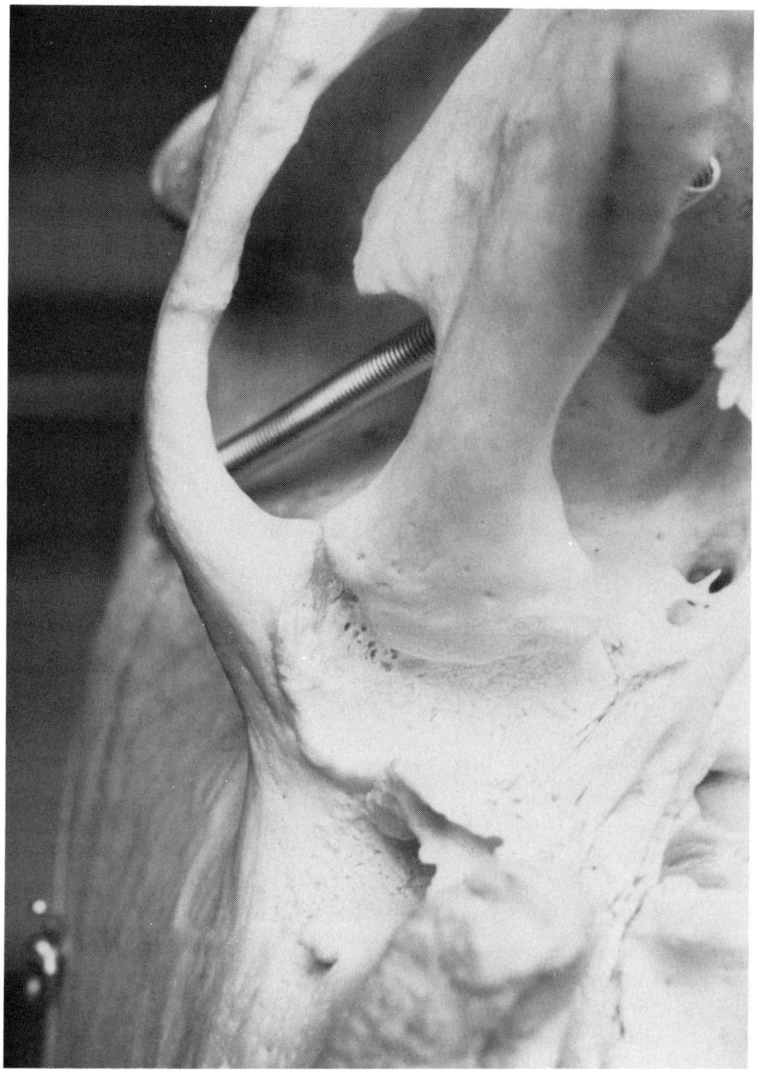

Fig. 8-10. Disarticulated skull showing erosion of lateral layer of cortical bone affecting eminences and erosion and flattening of lateral pole of condyle.

condyles (Fig. 8-9), as compared with the anatomical skull view shown in Fig. 8-10.

There are two ways to take this sort of x-ray film. Previously, patients lay down, and the picture was taken through the orbits. Now the better way is thought to be to position the patient in a head holder. The head positioner has ear posts that are emplaced, and the shot is aimed at the back of the head. The head is tipped down, and the patient opens the mouth for the picture. The open mouth drops the heads of the condyles out of the fossae to give an anteroposterior view of the condyles. The grid is used just as in the lateral cephalometric views, and the exposure settings are like those of the anteroposterior films.

Tomography, laminagraphy, or planograms

Tomography is a method by which the radiographs show parts of the bony anatomy at different levels from the table top. Essentially this is done either by having the patient move or by moving the tube around the patient. The fulcrum, or axis (center) of rotation, of the x-ray film and the x-ray tube is the only area that is not moved, and therefore it will be the only area in focus (Fig. 8-11). By altering the height of the fulcrum of this movement, all portions of the bony anatomy can be blurred out except that level of the fulcrum, and different portions of the bony anatomy can be clearly seen. The skull is an ideal anatomical structure for this process because of the complicated bony anatomy, which

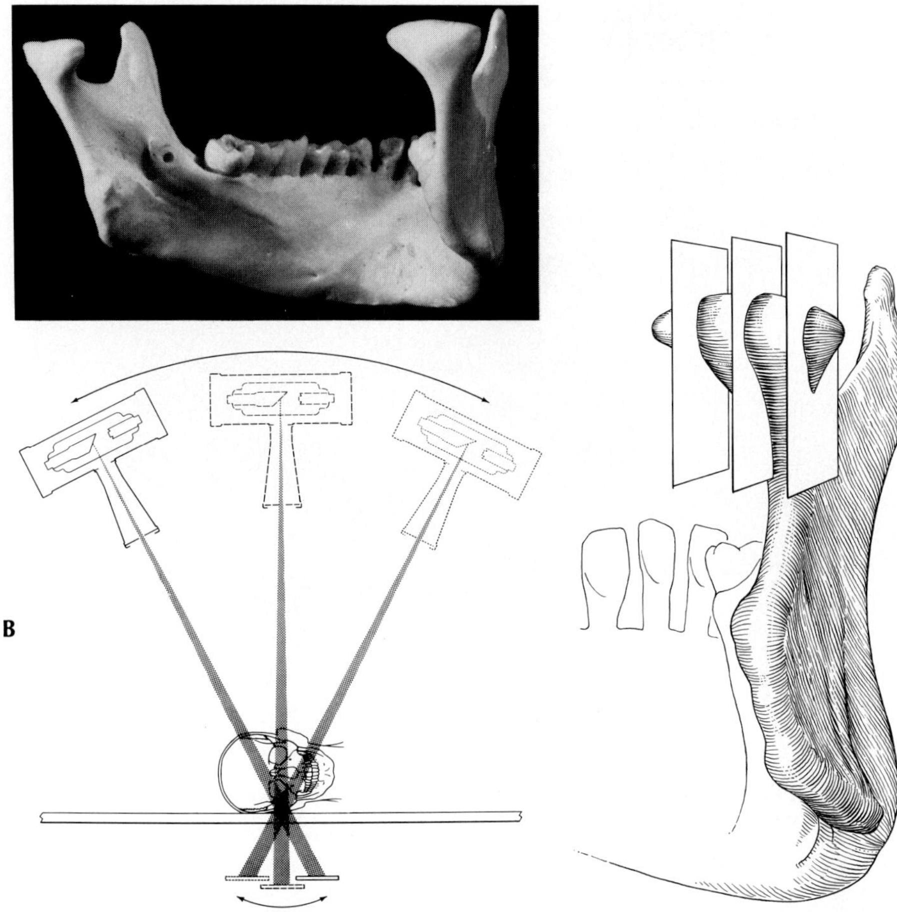

Fig. 8-11. Concept of sectioning of bone structure from tomogram techniques. **A,** Disarticulated dry skull mandible. **B,** Principle of tomography. **C,** Planes through head of condyle shown in this drawing of disarticulated mandible represent tomographic cuts in tomograms reproduced later. (From Coin, C.G.: Med. Radiogr. Photogr. **50:**26, 1974.)

has to be sorted out radiographically. Any portion of the skull in the lateral or anteroposterior position and, particularly, different portions of the mandible or condyle can be studied in this way.[11,29]

However, this technique does not reveal the dynamics of the joint. This particular method can be used to supplement the four-view transcranial lateral oblique method when additional backup information is needed. Nevertheless in certain cases such as tumor infiltration or congenital abnormalities tomography can be helpful. The amount of x-ray study done also can be limited by considerations of radiation. Therefore, this method is used less often, but it can be helpful for picking up bone changes that may indicate tumor infiltration or bony spur formation.[8,28,30]

For these films the technician focuses the unit on a particular part of the anatomy (the head of the condyle in this instance) and selects the appropriate distance so that only the one tiny area is in focus. Overall this method is somewhat comparable to the transcranial lateral oblique film, except that this one tiny area might be the only healthy area of the condyle, and with the rest of it missed, the examiner might not pick up a pathological condition in another area.

Panographic view

In the panographic study there is arc movement of the x-ray tube around the patient, and the view is used for better evaluation of the entire mandible. It gives a picture of the entire condyle laid out in one plane. However, the condylar anatomy is somewhat distorted (Fig. 8-12).

The mandible is a complex anatomical structure that varies among individuals, and this technique can be helpful in trauma cases in which the patient is unable to perform some of the motions that could be helpful

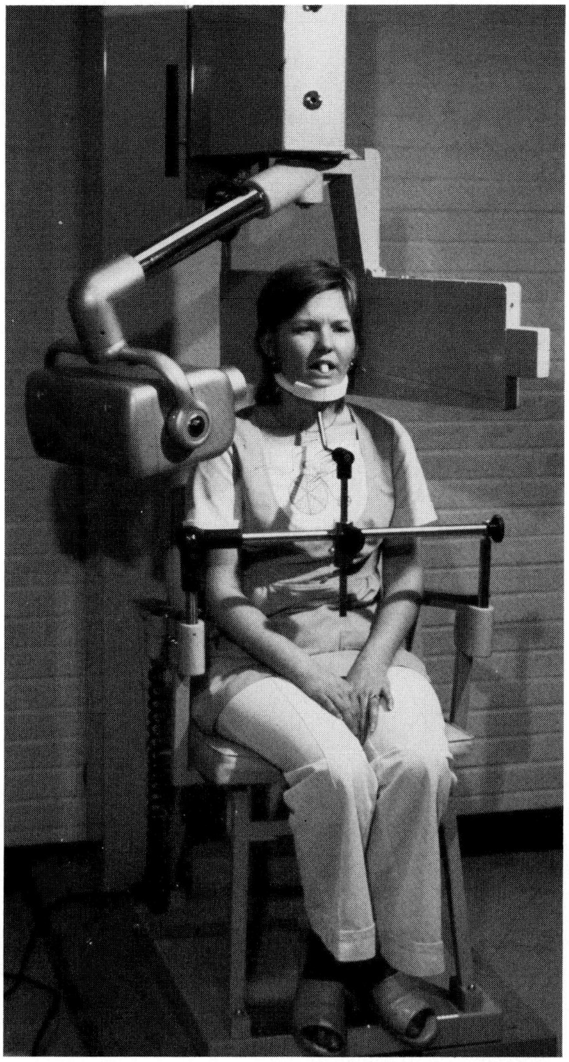

Fig. 8-12. Patient in position for panoramic radiograph of maxilla, mandible, and temporomandibular joints.

for a study of the dynamics. Still, the problems of fracture, distraction, and displacement can be evaluated.

Research has been done regarding the arthritic changes of the joint that occur in the lateral half of the condyle and articular eminence. In Sweden en bloc dissections of the temporomandibular joints of persons who had died of all causes were made. It was found that over 20% of these people had organic changes, usually in the lateral aspect of the condyle, the eminence in the upper portion of the joint, the disc in between, or a combination of these abnormalities.[10]

Several machines for obtaining Panorex views are available: the SS White Panorex Unit, the GE Panelipse, and the Siemens Orthopantomograph. In the SS White Panorex Unit the patient is placed in a center position head and chin rest, The cassette film is positioned according to height and the exposure determined according to the patient's size. The film and tube head are rotated around the patient's head. The chair shifts so that the tube head bypasses the spinal column, which results in a white area in the middle of the film. There is some magnification but not a great deal.

The GE Panelipse film is on a cylindrical drum. There is no break in the center of the film, but it slows as it goes around the spinal column, and it does take an x-ray film of the column also. Both the Panorex and Panelipse units are comparable as far as information and slight magnification.

The Orthopantomograph has more magnification. The patient stands, and the film cassette is curved. It can be positioned for special views of the TMJ, but although it is good for picking up fractures, it is not particularly good for seeing subtle changes in the relationship between the head of the condyle and the fossa.

Transcranial lateral oblique views*

The McCormack temporomandibular joint board† has a 25-degree angulation (Fig. 8-13), a modification of Updegrave's apparatus.[31] The angulation is used so that the structure of each temporomandibular joint can be thrown into relief and away from its mate, resulting in less distortion. The external auditory canals are used for points of fixation to stabilize the head. The patient's individual anatomy is used, rather than arbitrary points that could vary between patients, since asymmetry is a rule in every skull.

The x-ray tube is placed at a true vertical angle and 22 inches (56 cm) from target to film, with no variation from this. The patient positions the ear on the ear rod, and the head is then rotated until the temple rests on the board. The other ear rod is then placed in the ear, and the angle is noted and recorded so the x-ray view can be accurately reproduced later (Fig. 8-14).

The submentovertex view is taken to determine the amount of rotation of each condyle (Fig. 8-15). To take the submentovertex view, the ears must be marked. A ¼-inch ball bearing glued to the end of a cotton roll and then placed in the ear is ideal. A tracing is then done to find the correct angle. A line is drawn from the center of one ball bearing to the other. Another line is drawn through the long axis of each condyle. A measurement is taken where the two lines intersect. This gives the correct angle to place the patient's head for the x-ray exposure. After many submentovertex views have been taken to determine the amount of rotation of the condyles, a relationship between the shape of the patient's head and the amount of rotation of the condyles is found. This extra film can be eliminated in most cases.

The standard series in the transcranial lateral oblique radiographs consists of eight views. First, on the upper left the teeth are closed lightly on 2 mm of bite wax. This wax-bite opening is taken to simulate a

*Information and technical advice for the use of the McCormack temporomandibular joint board was supplied by Jo Register, D.L.X.T., Glendale Oral X-Ray Laboratory, 633 N. Central Ave., Glendale, Calif. 91203.

†McCormack temporomandibular joint board available through Ron McCormack, McCormack Enterprises, 2182 El Camino Real, Oceanside, Calif. 92054.

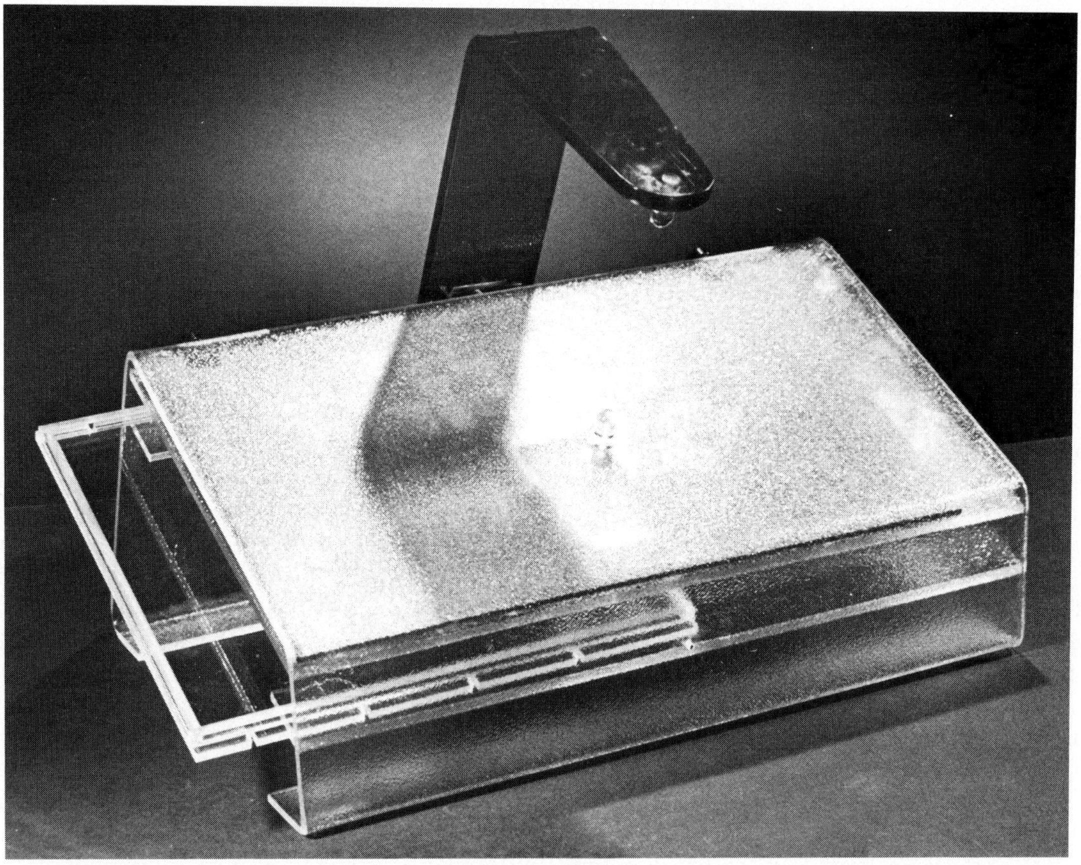

Fig. 8-13. McCormack temporomandibular joint board with ear posts to position patient's head accurately on board.

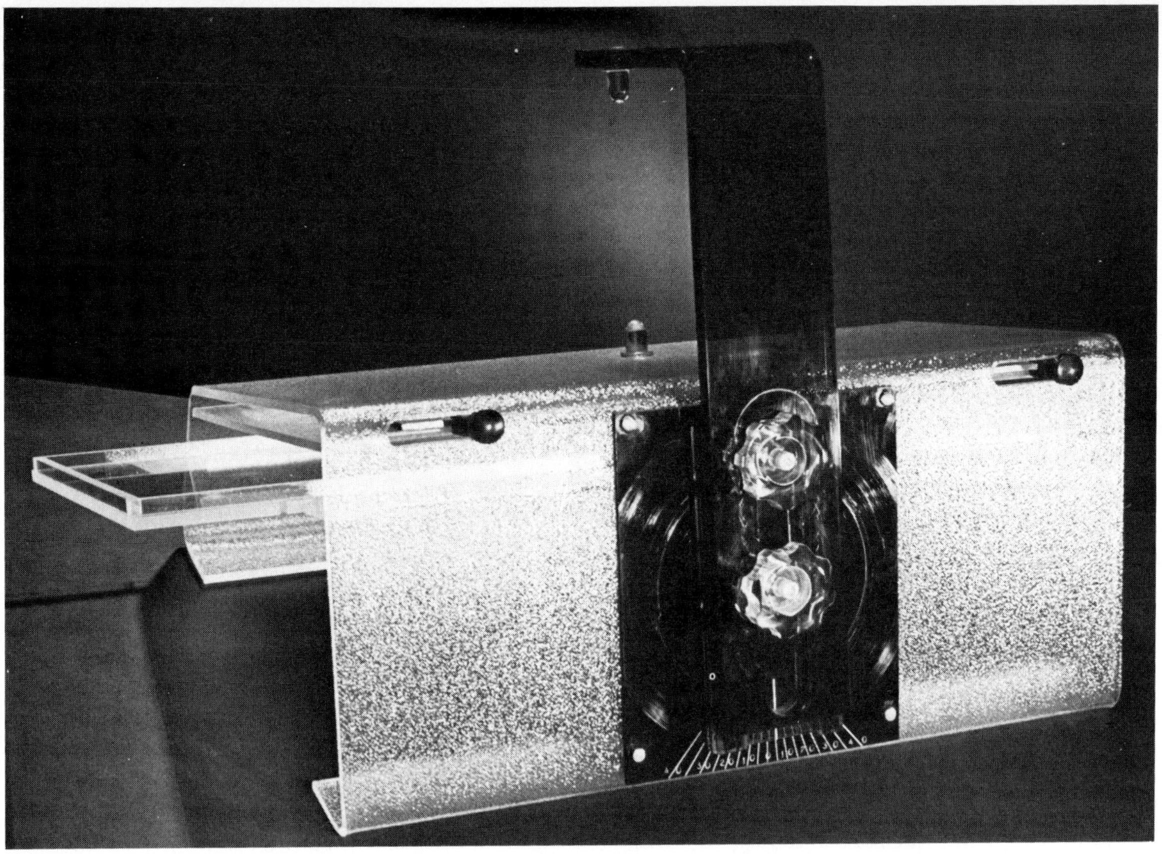

Fig. 8-14. McCormack temporomandibular joint board showing angulation measurements for angulating ear posts to position patient's head properly on head board.

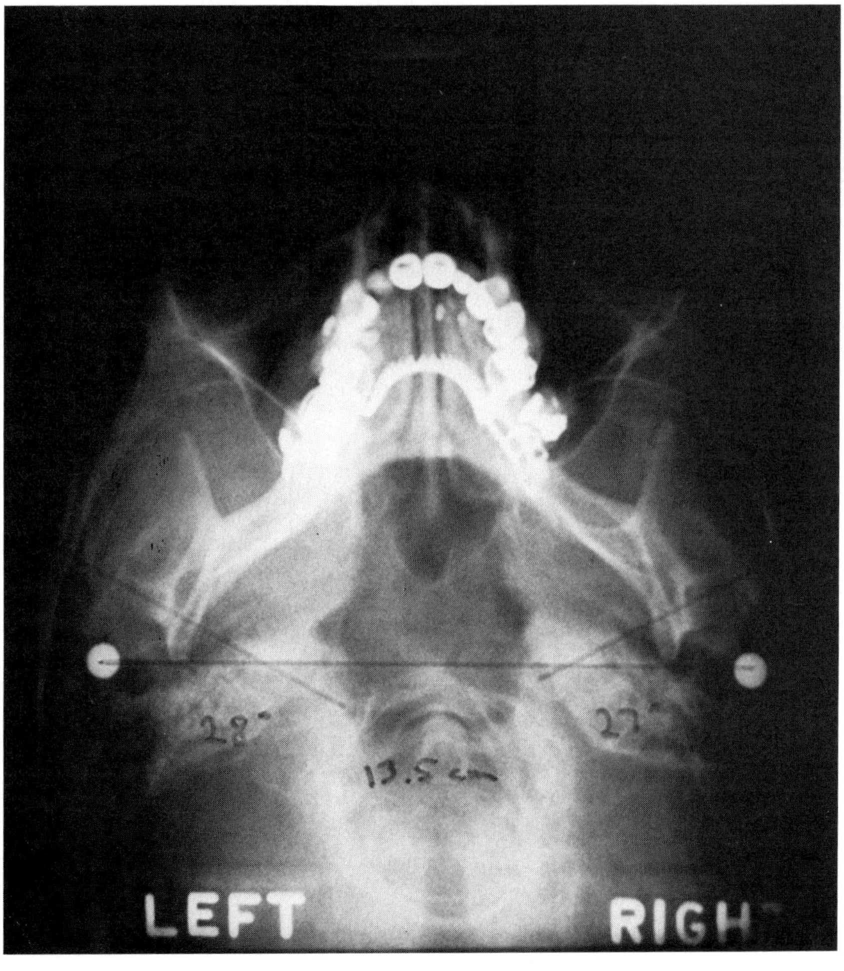

Fig. 8-15. Submentovertex view showing measurement of angle of condyles to line drawn between auditory meatus.

splint bite, since the usual splint is approximately 2 mm thick. This gives an idea of the condylar position if a splint is to be used. In the second view the teeth are closed in occlusion. In the third view the teeth are open 12 mm interincisally. In the fourth view the mouth is wide open 31 mm interincisally unless the patient has a limited opening, in which case that width is measured and recorded. The same procedure is then done on the right side. With this apparatus the TMJ is clearly seen in the vast majority of patients.

Normally the condyle lies within the joint space 1.5 mm anteriorly, 2.5 mm superiorly, and 7.5 mm posteriorly. This last measurement is made from the center of the auditory canal. Experience has shown that a measurement of 2.5 to 3 mm from the posterior head of the condyle to the postglenoid area is within normal limits. There is normal linear sclerotic outline to the mandibular fossa, articular eminence, and condyle.

By standardizing the amount of mouth opening (which is then reproducible), judgments can be made as to the orientation of the joint space with respect to the condyle and articular eminence and as to the amount of movement of the condyle with wax-bite opening, half opening, and wide opening. Such changes in the joint's condylar function in the half-open (12 mm) and wide-open (31 mm) views and a narrowing of the disc space in the closed view should be noted. The disc spaces should maintain themselves similarly as the condyle translates over the slopes of the articular eminences. Bony changes, such as the flattening of the anterior head of the condyle and of the descending or ascending slopes of the eminences or any type of erosion, can be detected. The most common areas of erosion are at the anterior aspect of the condyle and the descending slope of the articular eminence, with variations. There can be erosion on the posterior portions of the condyle and fossa as well.

The transcranial lateral oblique view technique is valuable, since results can be reproduced. The patient's head position, as well as the angles of radiation, are carefully determined, and the source of radiation is measured so that the patient may have the same type of radiograph taken at a later date for a comparison of any bony and/or functional changes that may have occurred in the joint during that time.

Fig. 8-16 shows a transcranial lateral oblique radiograph with three views, and Fig. 8-17 presents the same view as a line drawing. Fig. 8-18 shows the standardized eight views (four positions for each side) of this technique. This angulation focuses most clearly on the anterior aspect of the condyle and the descending and ascending slopes of the eminences. A fifth view of the

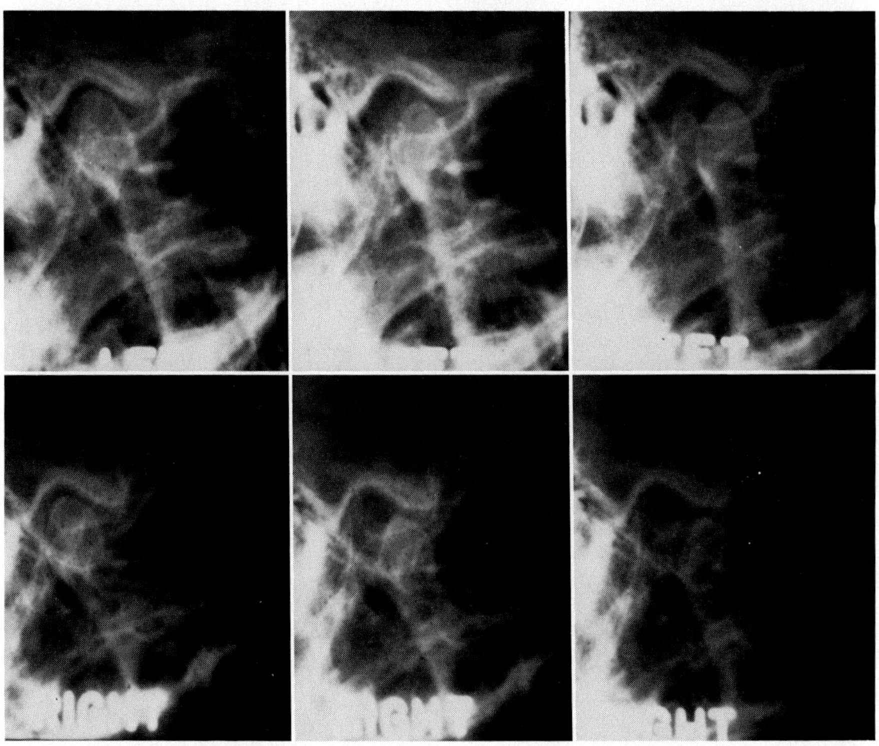

Fig. 8-16. Transcranial lateral oblique radiographs with three views of patient with different mouth openings.

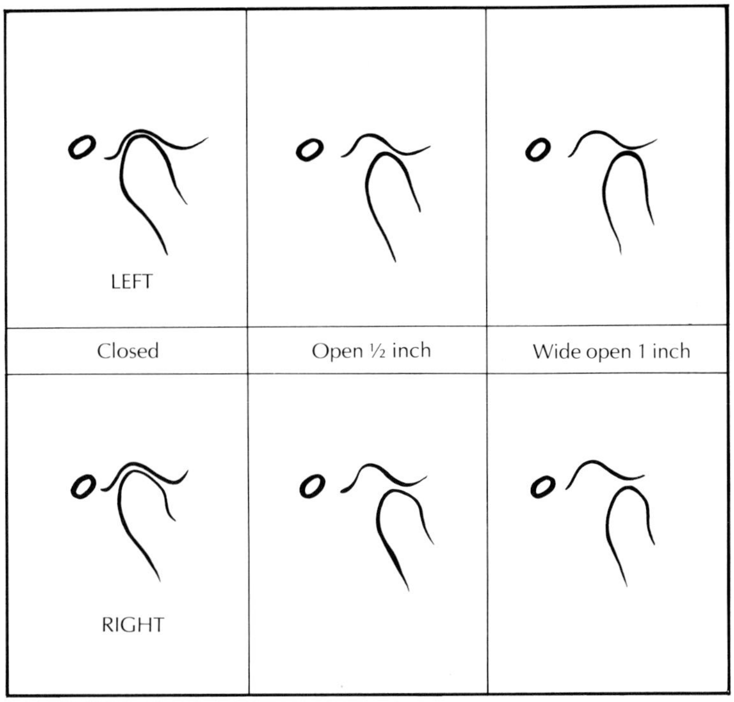

Fig. 8-17. Line drawings of radiographs in Fig. 8-16 showing mouth open ½ to 1 inch.

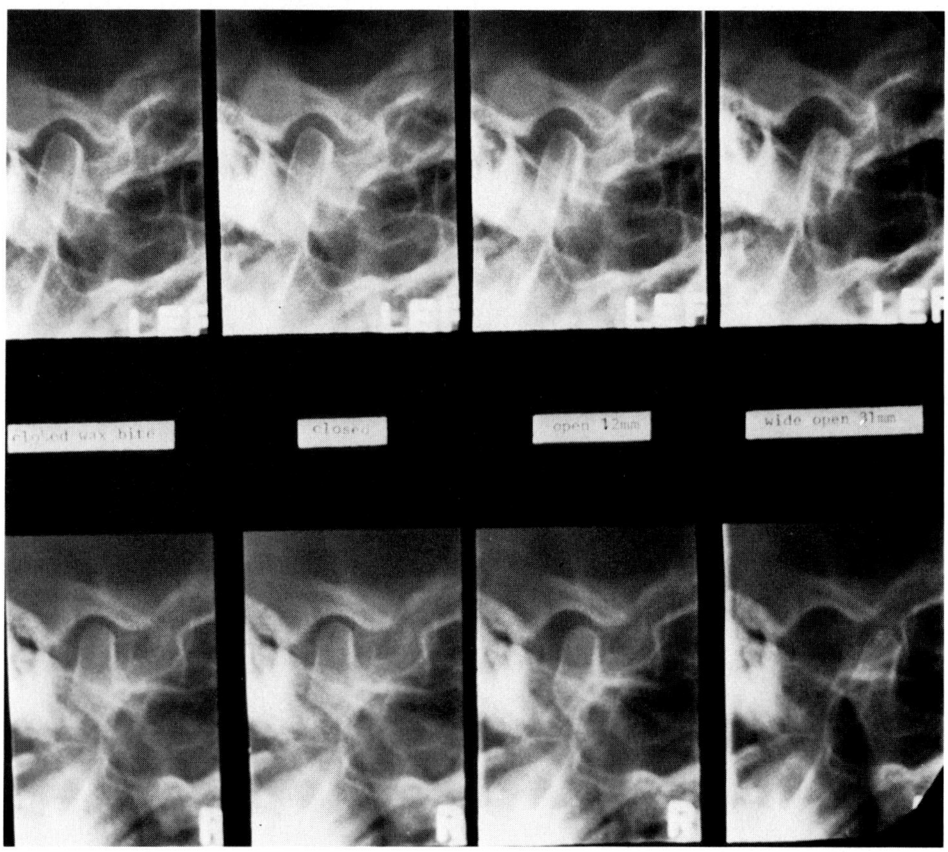

Fig. 8-18. TMJ x-ray views showing standardized eight views. In closed position, film shows clear cortical outline in posterior fossa area of both joints.

same patient in the closed position, taken with this same board but with the angulation slightly changed, focuses more on the posterior fossa area (Fig. 8-19). In the right joint x-ray film note particularly the posterior fossa area, which shows a slight change in shape and a fuzziness of the cortical layer of bone, indicating some osteogenic activity that did not appear in the other x-ray views. This view also shows changes in the posterior head of the condyle.

New transcranial lateral oblique systems. Recently two commercial head-holding systems, which can take TMJ x-ray films using standard dental x-ray machines, have been developed. The system developed by the Rinn Corporation (Elgin, Ill.) involves a head-holding device that uses the office x-ray machine to take transcranial lateral oblique views with a special film cassette. This technique requires that a new small film be placed in for each functional view of the TMJ (Figs. 8-20 to 8-22). The system of the Denar Corporation (Anaheim, Calif.)

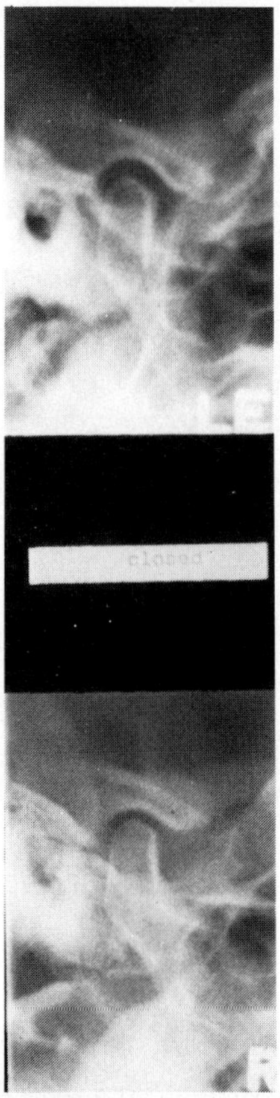

Fig. 8-19. With modified view in closed position right posterior fossa area shows some erosion.

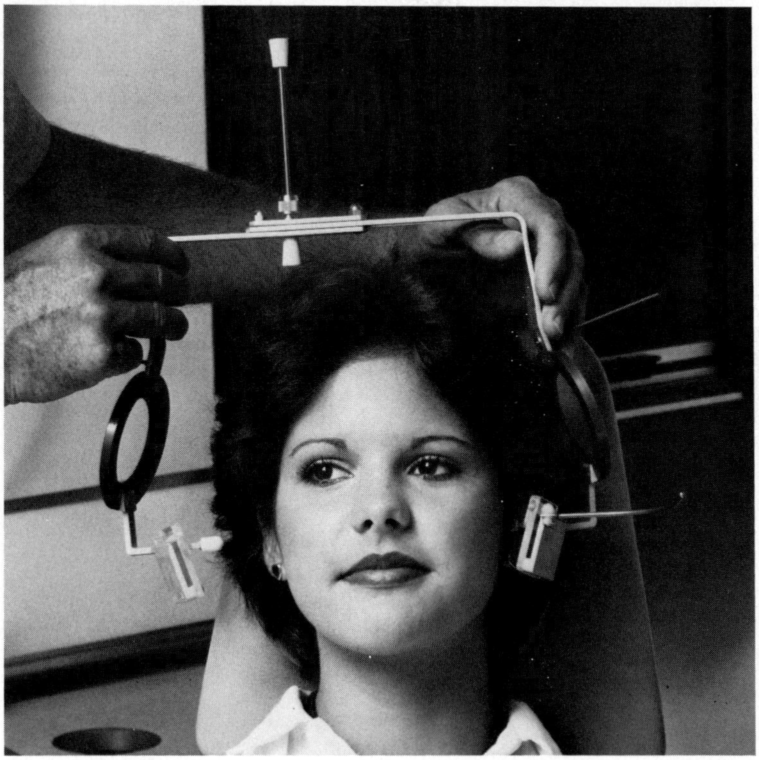

Fig. 8-20. Preliminary positioning of the Condy-Ray instrument. (Courtesy Rinn Corp., Elgin, Ill.)

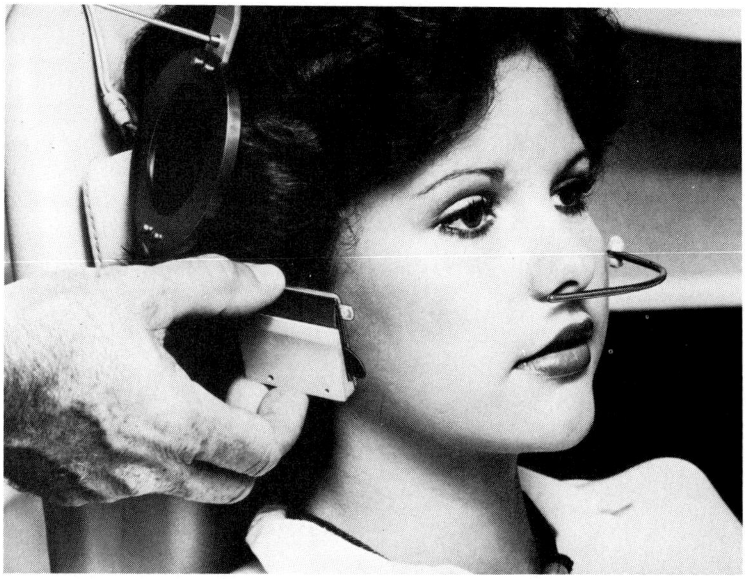

Fig. 8-21. Film cassette placed on side to be x-rayed. Film numbering device can now be adjusted to number the exposure. (Courtesy Rinn Corp., Elgin, Ill.)

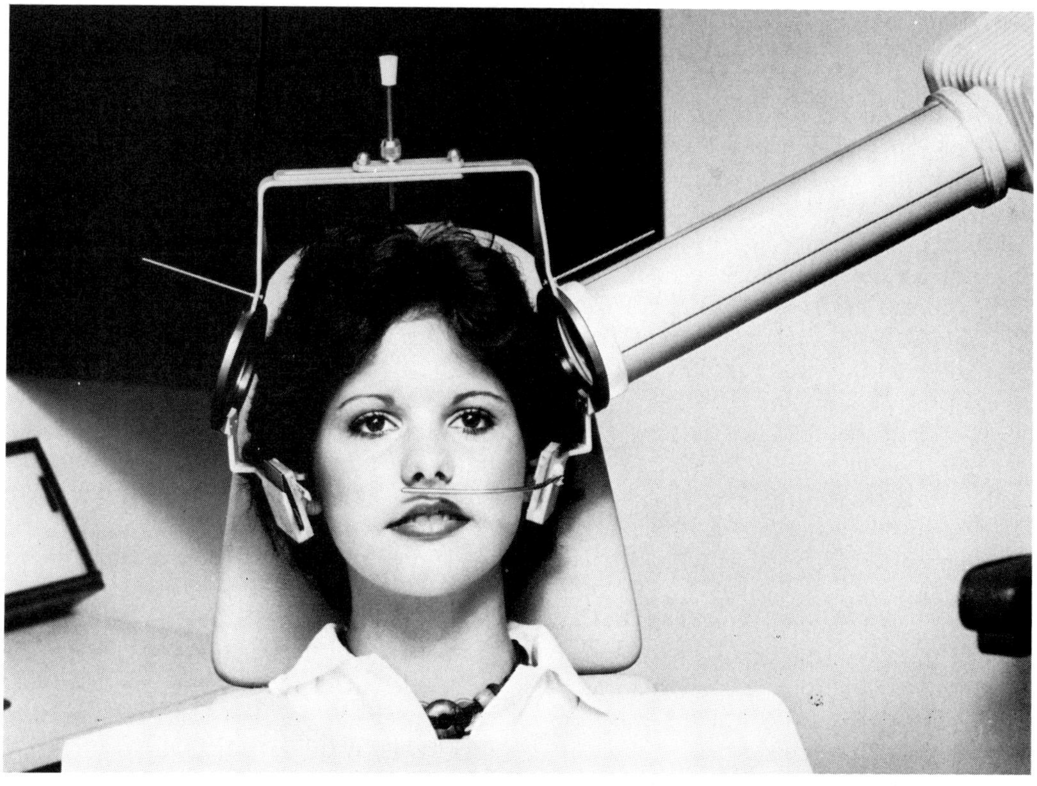

Fig. 8-22. Final exposure being made with long cone. (Courtesy Rinn Corp., Elgin, Ill.)

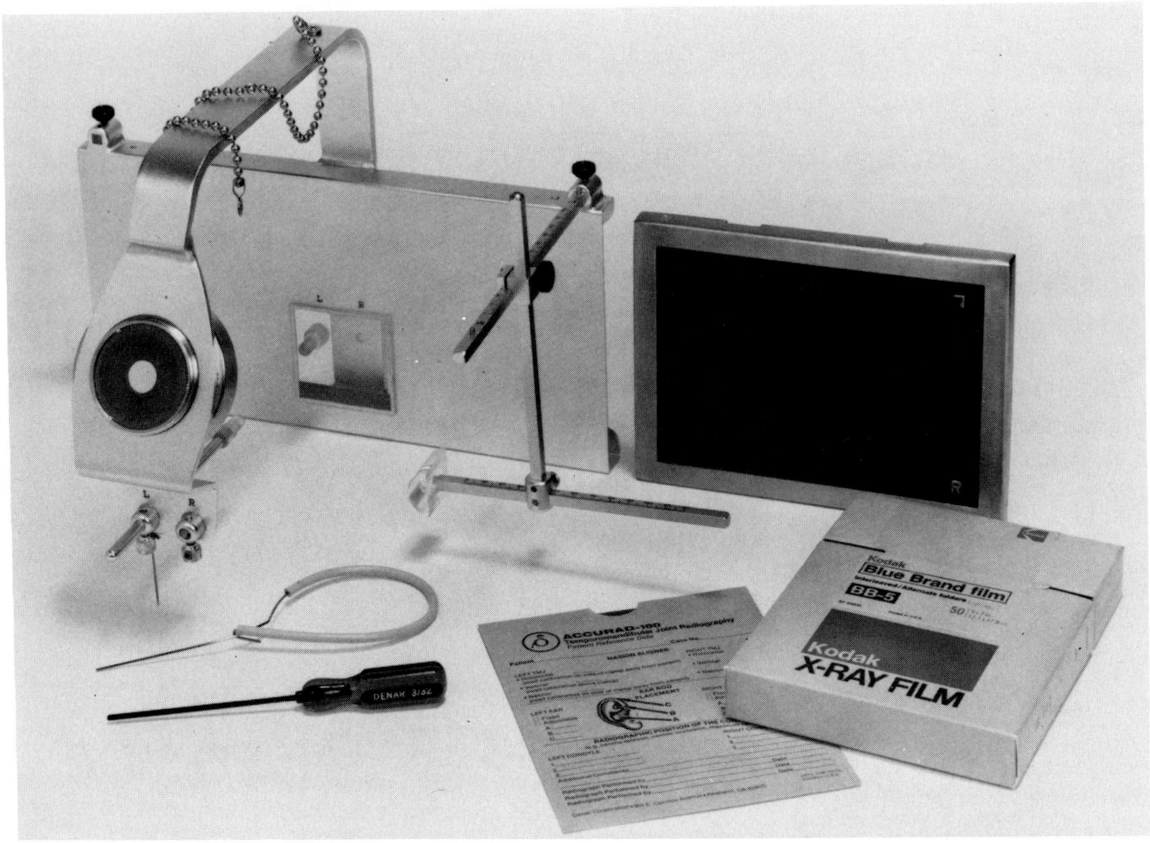

Fig. 8-23. Accurad-100 unit of Denar Corp. with film cassette. (Courtesy Denar Corp., Anaheim, Calif.)

uses a larger film and three pictures each of the right and left condyles to show its functional views (Figs. 8-23 to 8-25).

Both systems offer an excellent way to obtain an initial diagnostic film in the dental office with a minimum of equipment and expense and are recommended as a helpful means of having a record of the TMJ to discover any dysfunction or disease of the joint. An x-ray view of the TMJ should be taken as part of a complete examination of the patient, and these systems offer a relatively convenient way of doing so.

Cephalometric tomography

The x-ray Sectograph* can be used for radiographing other cephalometric structures, but it is uniquely suited for radiographing the temporomandibular joint. It eliminates many of the distortions involved in angulating a patient's head on a slant board. It also minimizes distortions from magnification used in other techniques. The x-ray beam comes in a straight line from approximately a 5-foot focal distance.

*Quint X-Ray Co., Inc., Los Angeles, Calif.

The patient is seated and lined up prinicipally by head supports on either side of the head. On the inner surface of these supports dowels project out, to be inserted into the ear's external canals to align the patient so that the midsagittal plane is parallel to the film. Then the entire head is rotated 20 degrees oblique to the film. By being able to duplicate the head alignment in this fashion, radiographs can be taken at a later date with the patient in the same position, so that any changes can be ascertained as being caused by intervening treatment or structural changes rather than possibly having been caused by positional differences. This reproducibility of position is also a major asset of this technique.

Adjusting the cut in or out can be done if the first set of pictures are slightly fuzzy or out of focus. The initial cut usually lies between 3.25 and 3.75 mm, although some formulations may give slightly different distances. The temporomandibular joint laminagraphs are done with the closed, at-rest, and wide-open mouth positions. A full-articulation (six picture) series of laminagraphs is made for suspected temporomandibular joint problems.

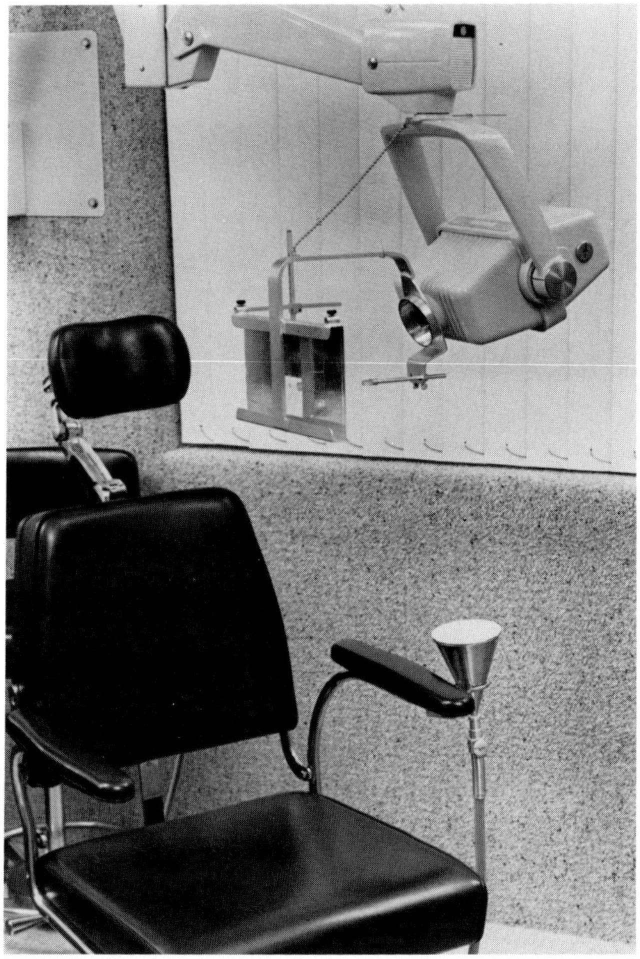

Fig. 8-24. Accurad-100 unit attached to dentist's x-ray unit. (Courtesy Denar Corp., Anaheim, Calif.)

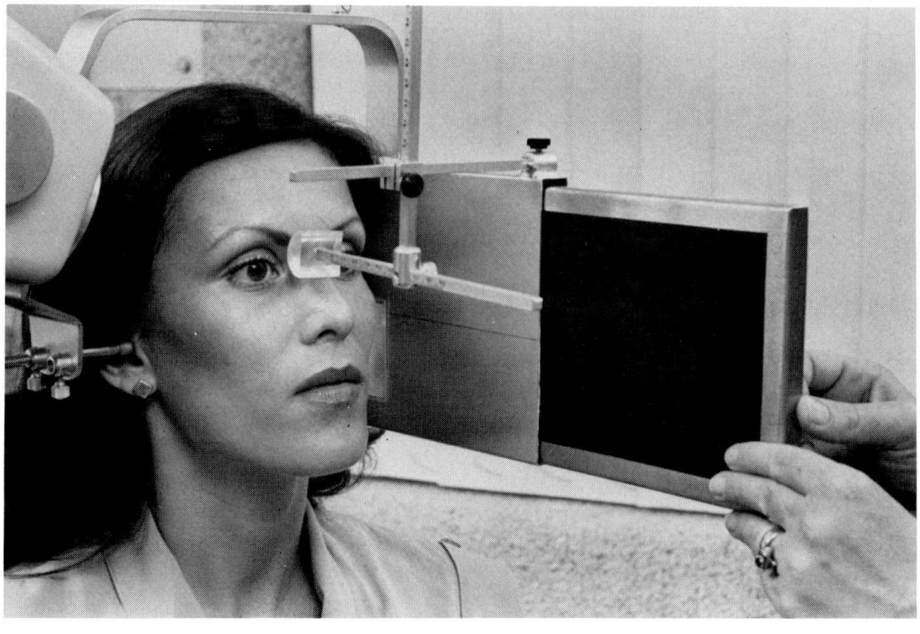

Fig. 8-25. Patient in position, about to have transcranial lateral oblique x-ray views taken. (Courtesy Denar Corp., Anaheim, Calif.)

Xeroradiography

The xeroradiographic method uses a selenium-coated plate and a charged plastic powder or toner, producing variations in shades of blue (Figs. 8-26 and 8-27). The bone will appear blue or white, and the soft tissues also will be seen more clearly than on the usual radiograph. This has been used successfully in evaluation of tissues of the breast. Small malignancies that are not palpable can be detected.

This technique is just beginning to be used for the evaluation of the soft tissues of the face and may be of value when used for the temporomandibular joint as well. It is one area worthy of further investigation to produce a method by which soft tissues can be studied and abnormalities in them picked up radiographically.[4] Of note, however, is that although the picture itself is impressive, the radiation factor is much more than that of standard x-ray exposures, and they are more expensive.

Recently, with the assistance of the White Memorial Hospital Radiology Department (Los Angeles) physician Merlyn Woesner, his chief technician Oseas Barnedo, and Jo Register (owner and chief technician of the Glendale Oral X-Ray Laboratory), we were able to take a series of transcranial lateral oblique films using xeroradiography techniques. To more clearly compare, one set was taken with standard x-ray exposure and technique and another with the xeroradiography technique. It was hoped that the disc tissue could be seen in this approach, but in this set of films it was not apparent. A clear outline of the bony structures of the joint can be seen, and it can be noted in the upper left joint that the opening movements are reversed. The upper left joint film (Fig. 8-28) shows the mouth open 31 mm.

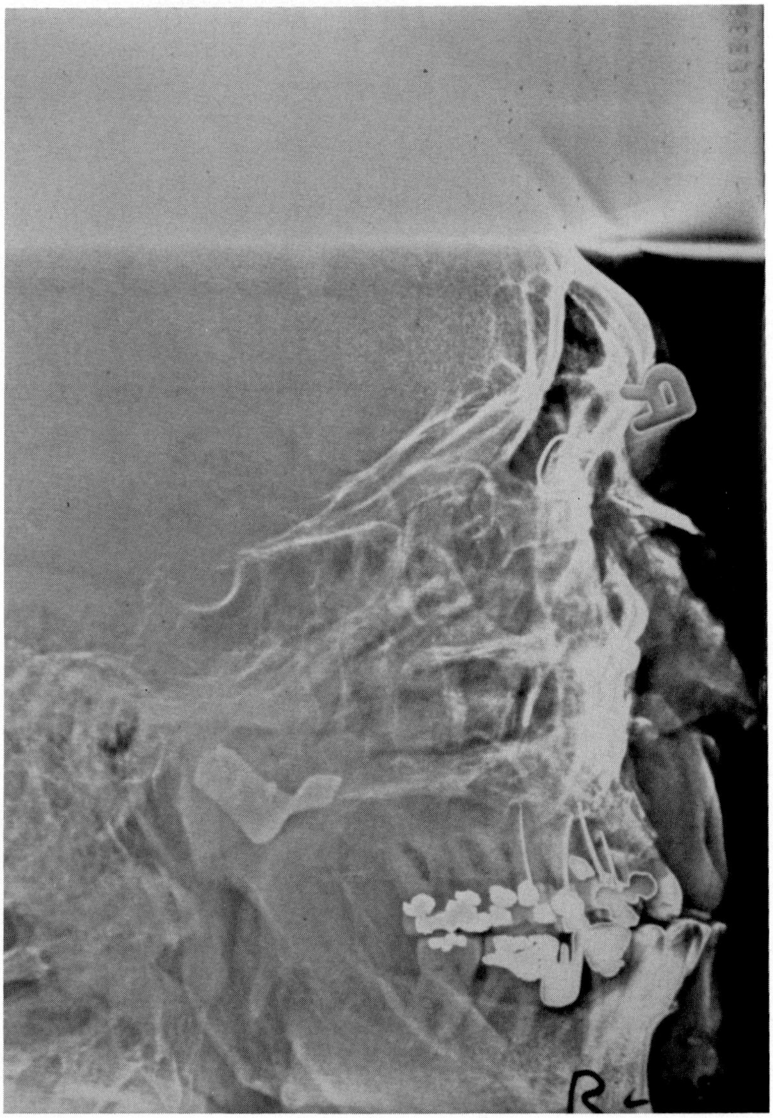

Fig. 8-26. Xeroradiograph of patient (J.P.) with mouth closed who had bony ankylosis after severe facial trauma.

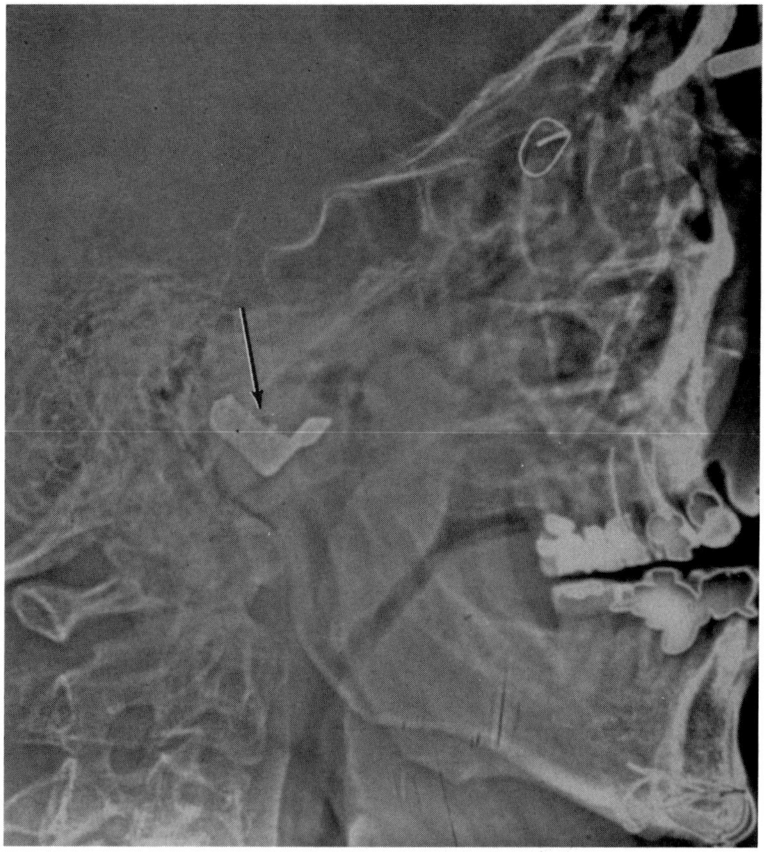

Fig. 8-27. Xeroradiograph showing patient (J.P.) with mouth partially open after osteoarthrotomy of joints and placement of right-angle prosthesis.

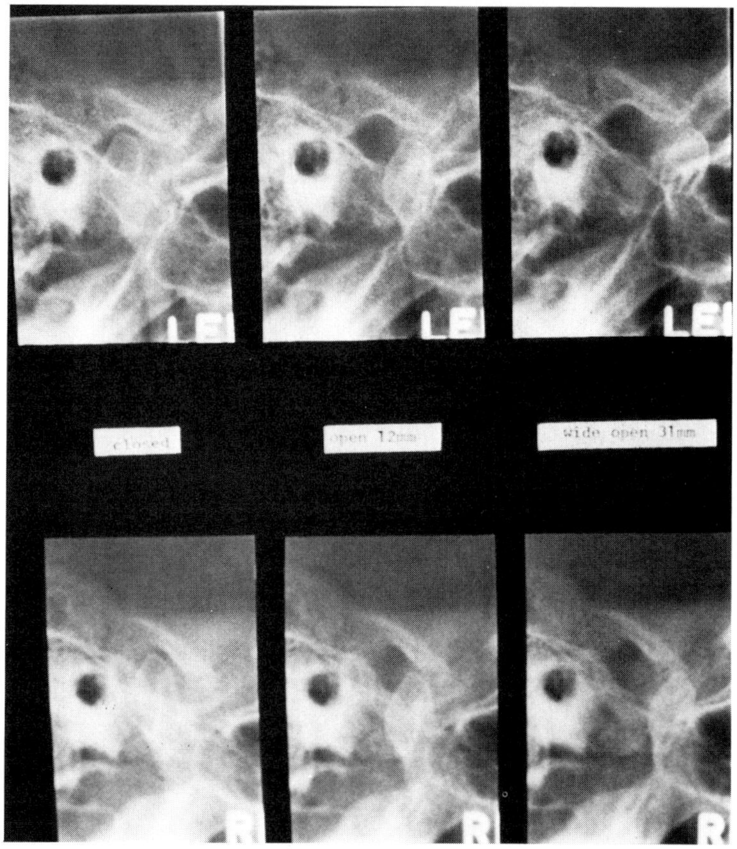

Fig. 8-28. Specialized TMJ films showing flattening of left eminence and flattening of anterior aspect of left condyle.

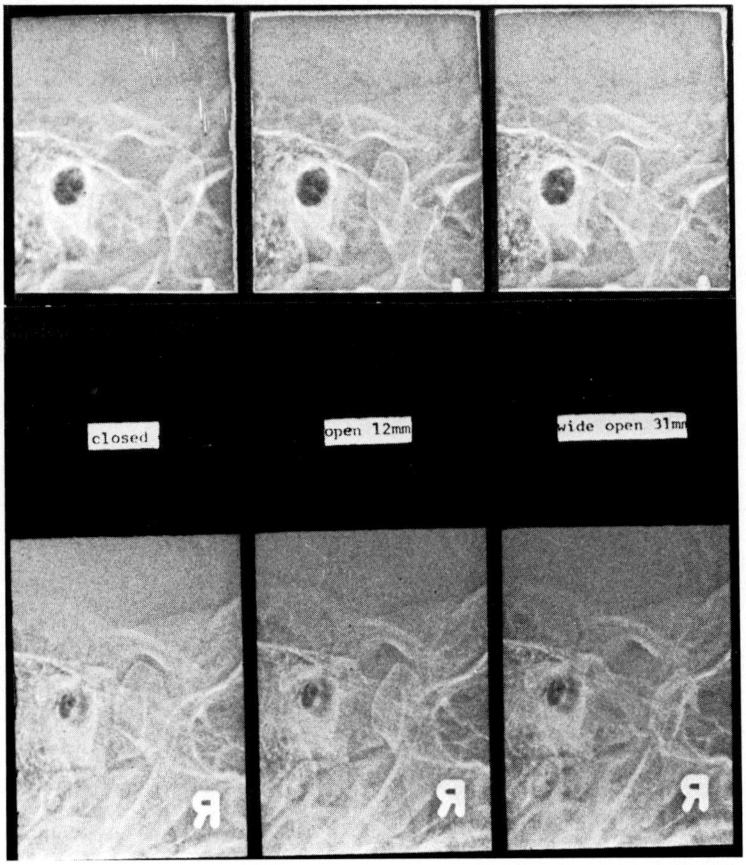

Fig. 8-29. Xeroradiography films showing erosion of right posterior fossa area, flattening of anterior head of right condyle, and erosion of articular eminence. It is of interest to compare standardized transcranial lateral oblique views and xeroradiography views of same patient.

The upper right film (Fig. 8-29) shows the mouth in the closed position.

Magnification radiography

One system that is reported by Murphy and others[22] as providing superior TMJ images at acceptable levels of exposure is the RSI microfocus magnification system fitted with a special positioning unit for lateral radiography of the TMJ.

Direct radiographic magnification, contrasted to conventional contact radiography, recently has gained increased acceptance because of technological advances in x-ray tube design, the development of rare-earth screens, and renewed interest in the detailed and early radiological diagnosis of arthritic and metabolic disorders. Direct microfocus magnification results in an image with improved resolution, decreased noise, enhanced visual appreciation and perception of detail, and greater diagnostic value.

For the TMJ positioning unit the basic design of the Updegrave unit is modified so that the Plexiglas positioning apparatus is affixed to a metal frame, which is shorter than the standard object tray and has angled-forward corners to allow room for the patient's shoulder (Fig. 8-30). Unlike the Updegrave with its standard 15-degree angle, this magnification head support surface is hinged along the front to allow incremental 5–degree angle changes along the coronal plane of the skull to enable correction of TMJ profiles not accommodated by the other fixed standard. Thus the TMJ object tray can be moved on its metal frame toward and away from the machine chassis to adjust for skull size from pediatric to large adult patient (Figs. 8-31 and 8-32). TMJ magnification from 1.5 to 2.7 times is possible.

The issue of increased radiation exposure to the patient, an inherent part of geometrical magnification radiograhy, cannot be ignored. However, rare-earth screen and very fast film combinations are now available that are much more efficient than the older calcium tungstate systems. At two images (open and closed) per TMJ, the total entrance dose is approximately 2000 mrem for magnification versus 600 mrem

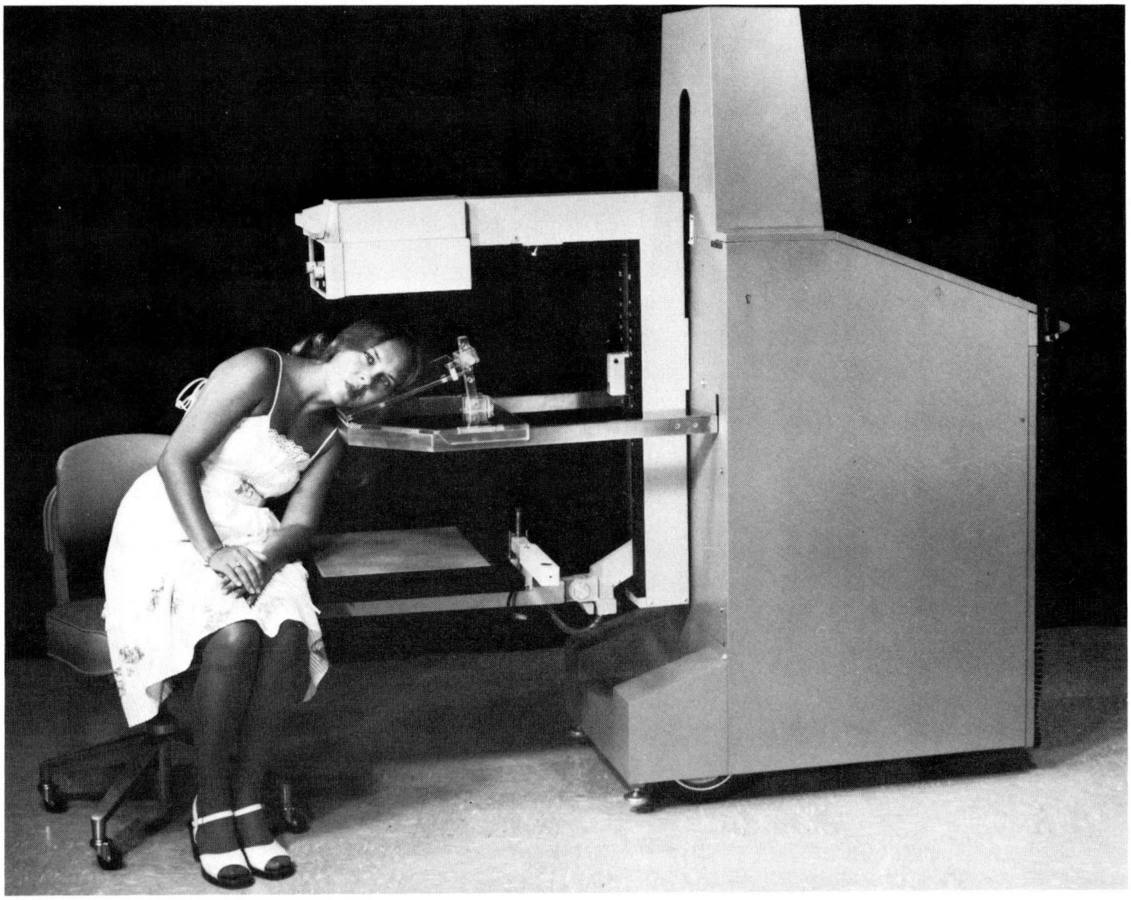

Fig. 8-30. RSI microfocus magnification system adapted for transcranial lateral oblique radiography of TMJ, demonstrating ease of access and positioning because of shortened object tray and angled-forward corners. (From Murphy, W.A., et al.: Radiology **133:**524, 1979.)

for contact radiography. The improved image and increased diagnostic information are felt to be worth the increased exposure, which is still within an acceptable range. Moreover, with the advent of TMJ magnification radiography, tomography is seldom necessary.

The combination of microfocus magnification and a lateral positioning device solves the need for both minute radiological detail and dependable positioning of a small anatomical part. Figs. 8-33 to 8-38 show both normal and abnormal conditions of the TMJ with this image system.

Arthrography

The first clinical use of TMJ arthrography to be reported was by Norgaard[23] in the 1940s. More recently TMJ arthrography has been used by Wilkes,[33] Farrar and McCarty,[17] Dolwick and others,[12] and Blaschke, Solberg, and Sanders.[5] This procedure basically involved the injection of a water-soluble, iodine-containing contrast medium (dye) into the joint space. The procedure is effective and safe but rather technically difficult to do.

The technique of Blaschke, Solberg, and Sanders[5] involves placing dye in both the superior and inferior joint spaces. Fig. 8-39 shows the placement of an angiocatheter into the lower joint space; Fig 8-40 shows the same for the superior joint space. Fig. 8-41 demonstrates the injection of a small amount (usually 0.3 to 0.5 mm) of water-soluble radiographic contrast medium into the lower joint space. Figs. 8-42 and 8-43 are the arthrograms and diagrams of a normal TMJ, moving from closed to open. It should be noted that fluoroscopy is used to see the correct position of the angiocatheter in relation to the upper and lower joint spaces during insertion. Also, tomography is used after the dye has been placed. Consequently the Blaschke group's

Text continued on p. 156.

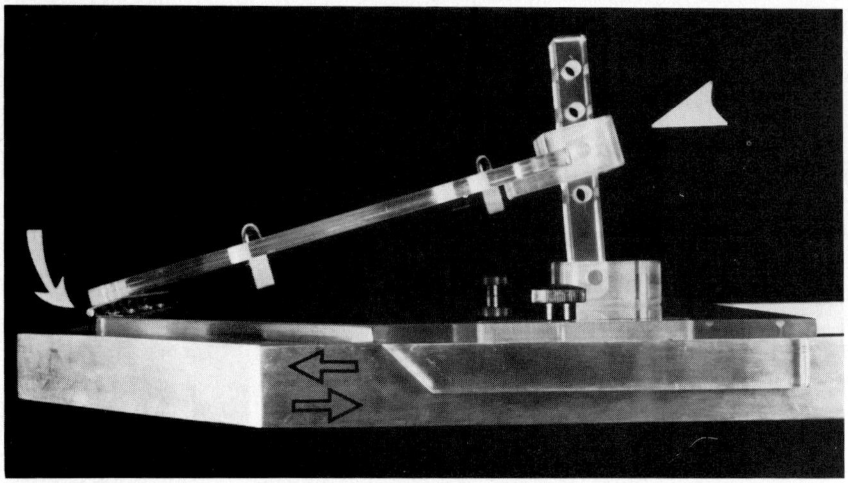

Fig. 8-31. TMJ magnification positioning device, lateral view. Hinged head support surface *(curved arrow)* permits 5-degree changes measured by moving sliding peg-in-hole *(arrowhead)*. Plexiglas unit can slide along arms of its metal frame *(open arrows)*. (From Murphy, W.A., et al.: Radiology **133:**524, 1979.)

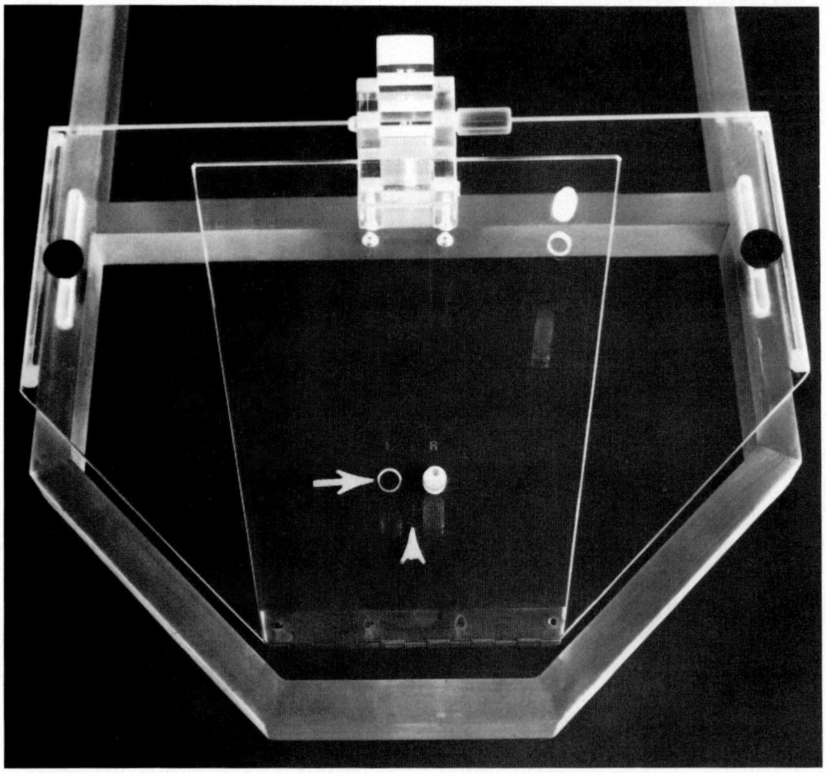

Fig. 8-32. TMJ magnification positioning device, surface view. Crosshatch *(arrowhead)* localizes central beam to TMJ. Threaded left and right ear plug holes *(arrow)* accept interchangeable pediatric and adult-size ear plugs. (From Murphy W.A., et al.: Radiology **133:**524, 1979.)

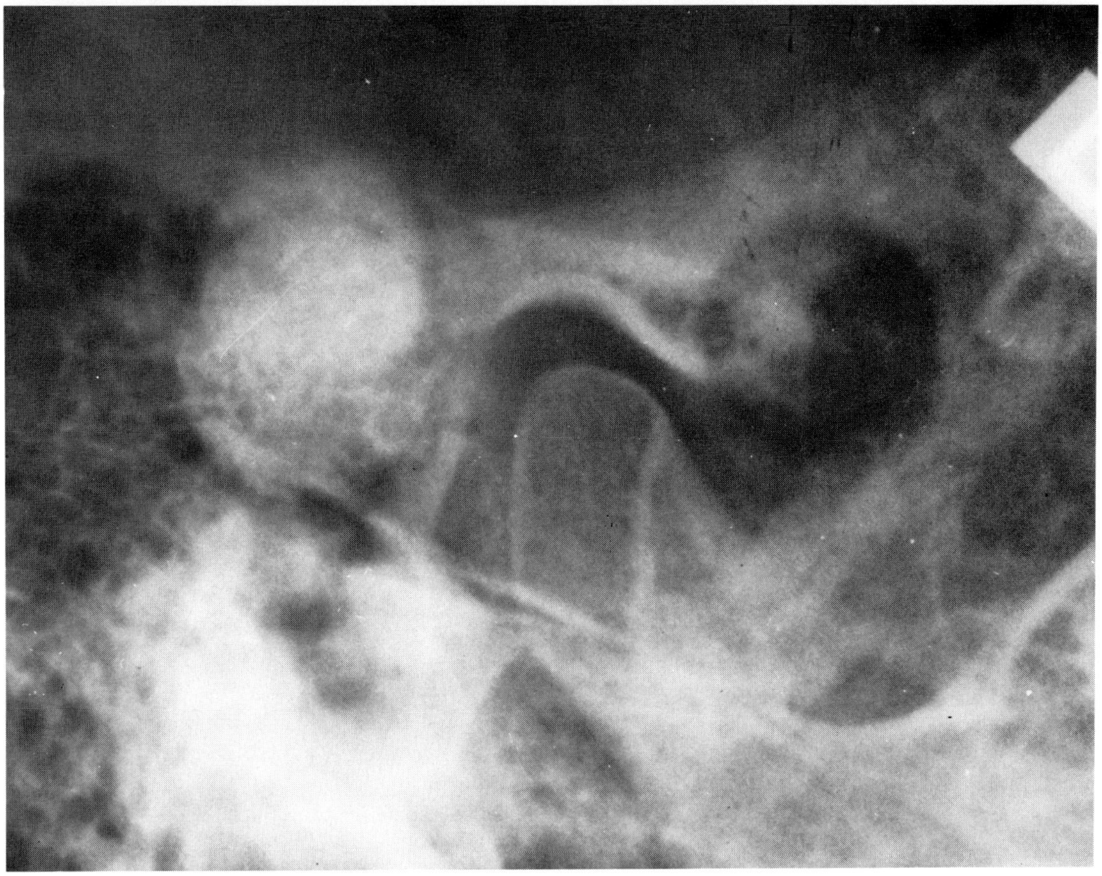

Fig. 8-33. Magnification radiograph showing TMJ in closed position with some demineralization over ascending slope of eminence and posterior fossa area. (Courtesy Dr. W.A. Murphy.)

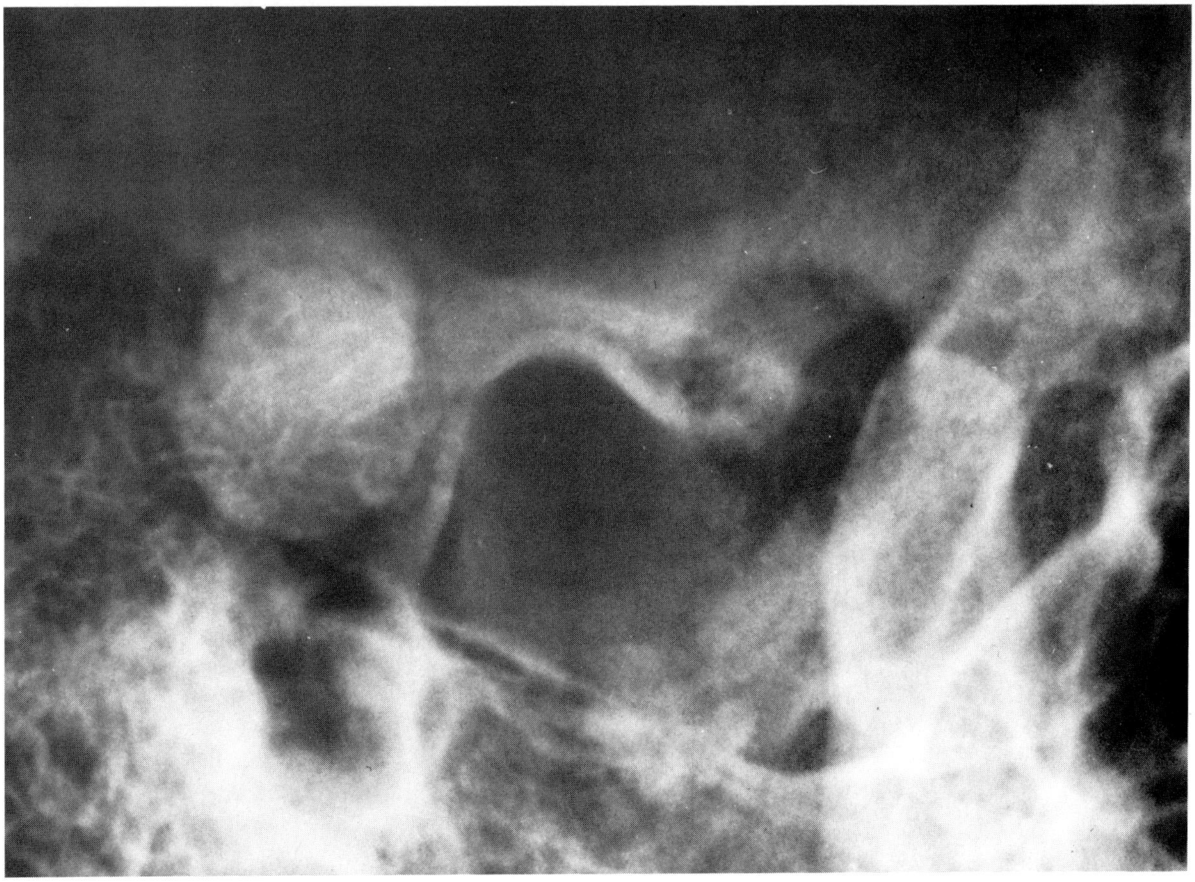

Fig. 8-34. TMJ in open position showing excessive forward translational movement. (Courtesy Dr. W.A. Murphy.)

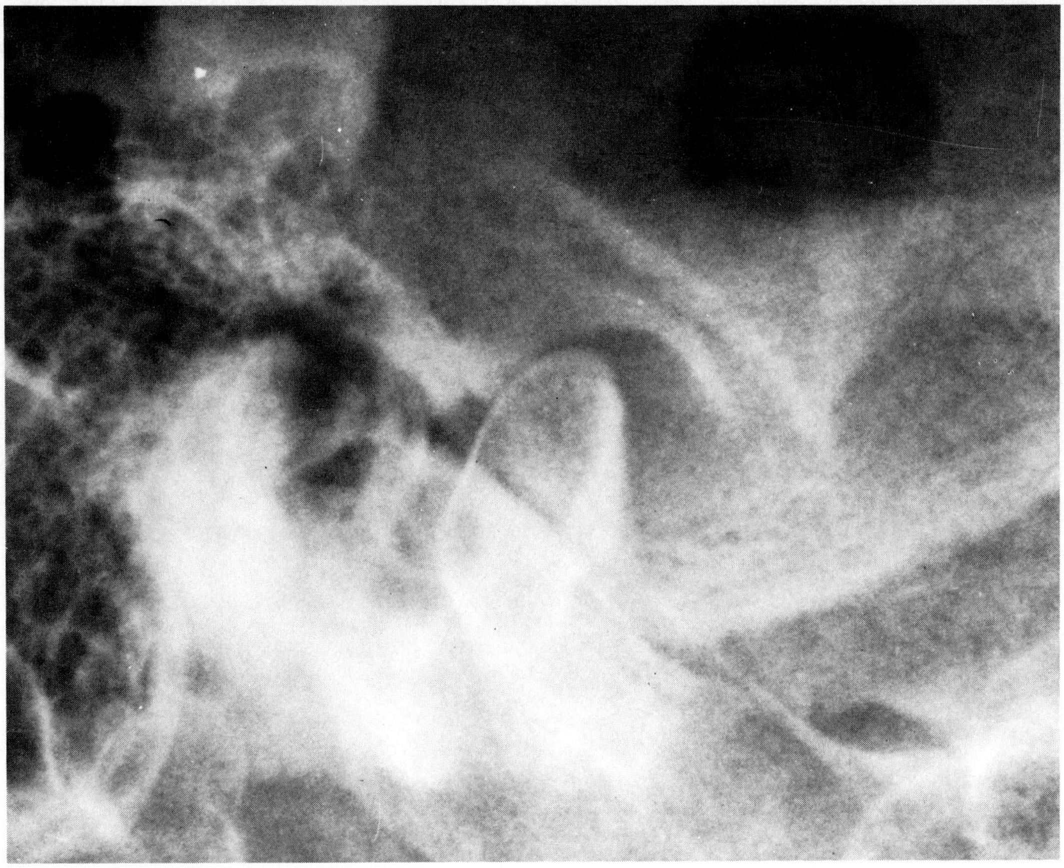

Fig. 8-35. Magnification radiograph showing retroposition of condylar head because of dislocated meniscus. (Courtesy Dr. W.A. Murphy.)

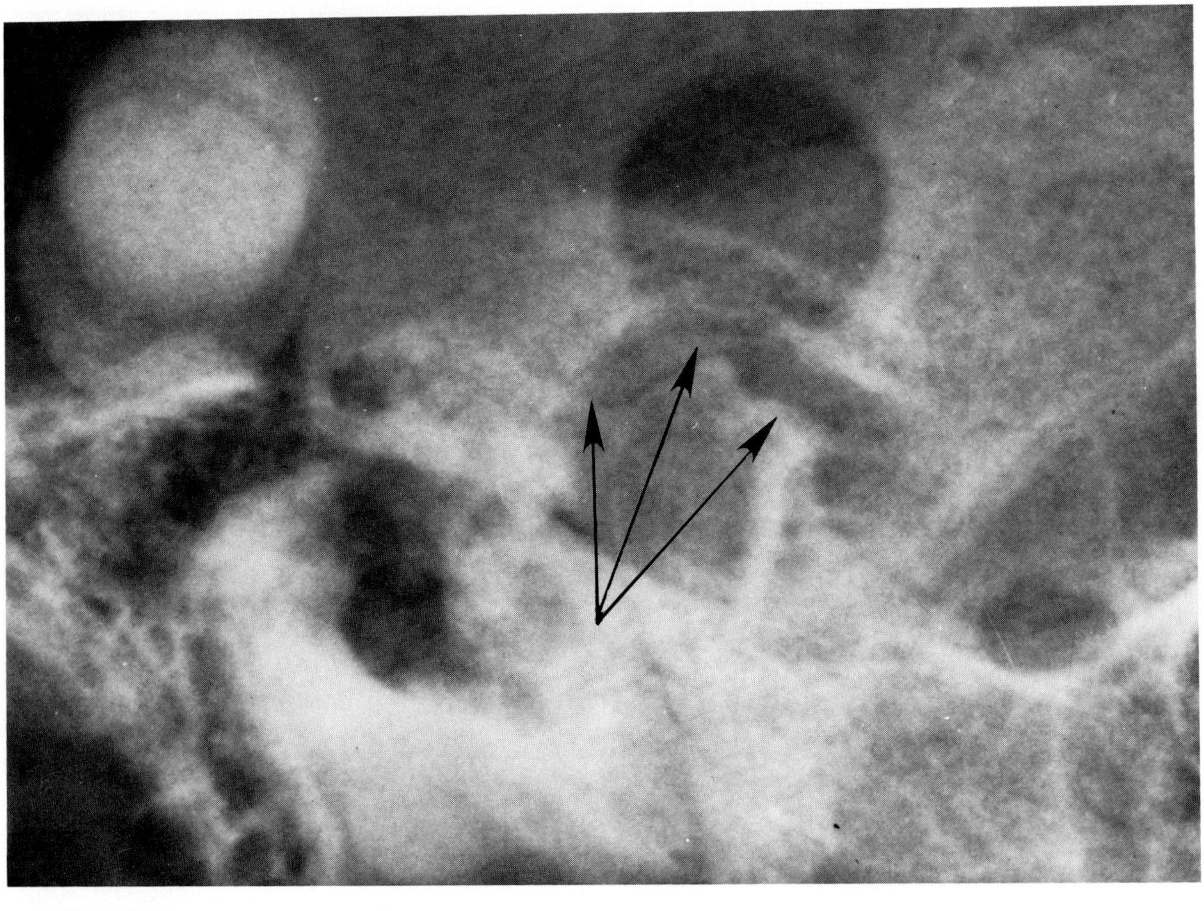

Fig. 8-36. Magnification radiograph showing erosive or inflammatory arthritis of TMJ. Note irregularity of cartilage (joint) space and erosions of condylar head and mandibular fossa. (Courtesy Dr. W.A. Murphy.)

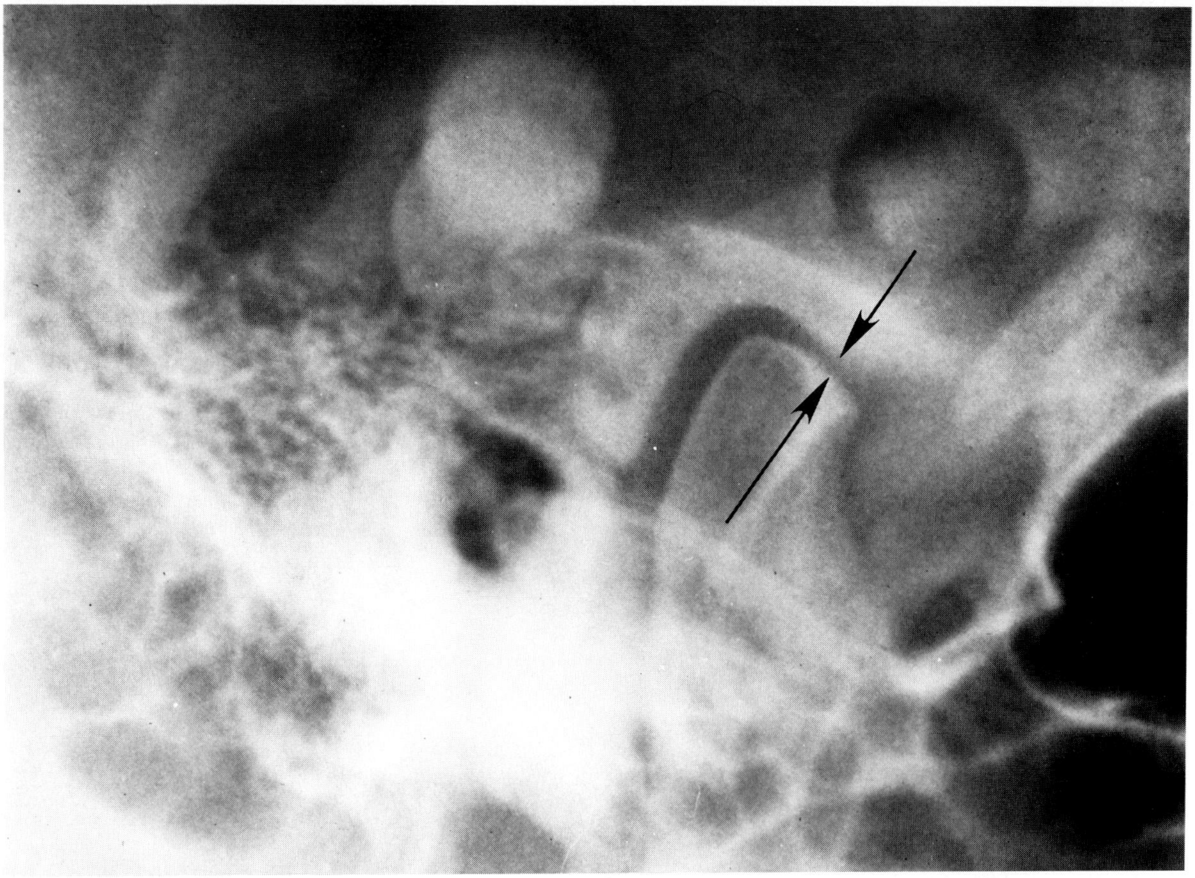

Fig. 8-37. Magnification radiograph showing early osteoarthritis of TMJ. Note cortical thickening of anterior condylar head and erosion of opposing surface of temporal eminence. (Courtesy Dr. W.A. Murphy.)

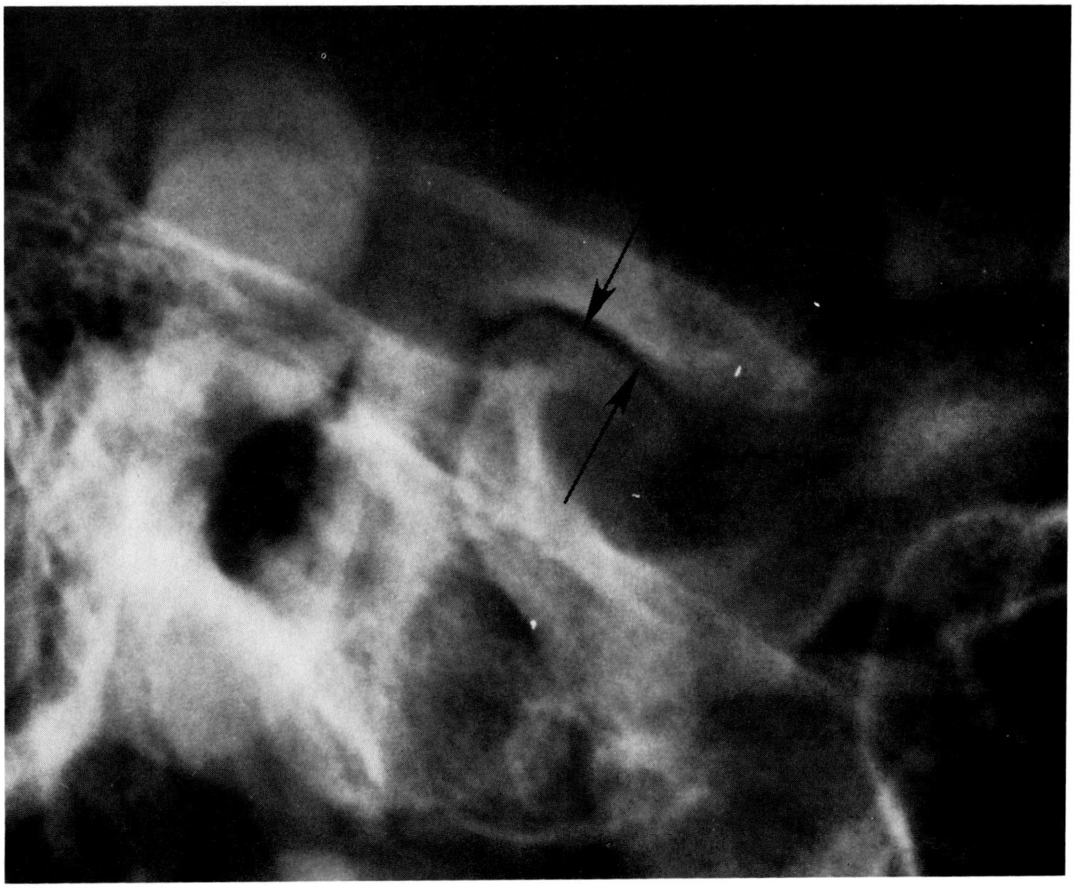

Fig. 8-38. Magnification radiograph showing osteoarthritis (degenerative joint disease) of TMJ. Note very narrow cartilage (joint) space with considerable spur formation on condylar head. (Courtesy Dr. W.A. Murphy.)

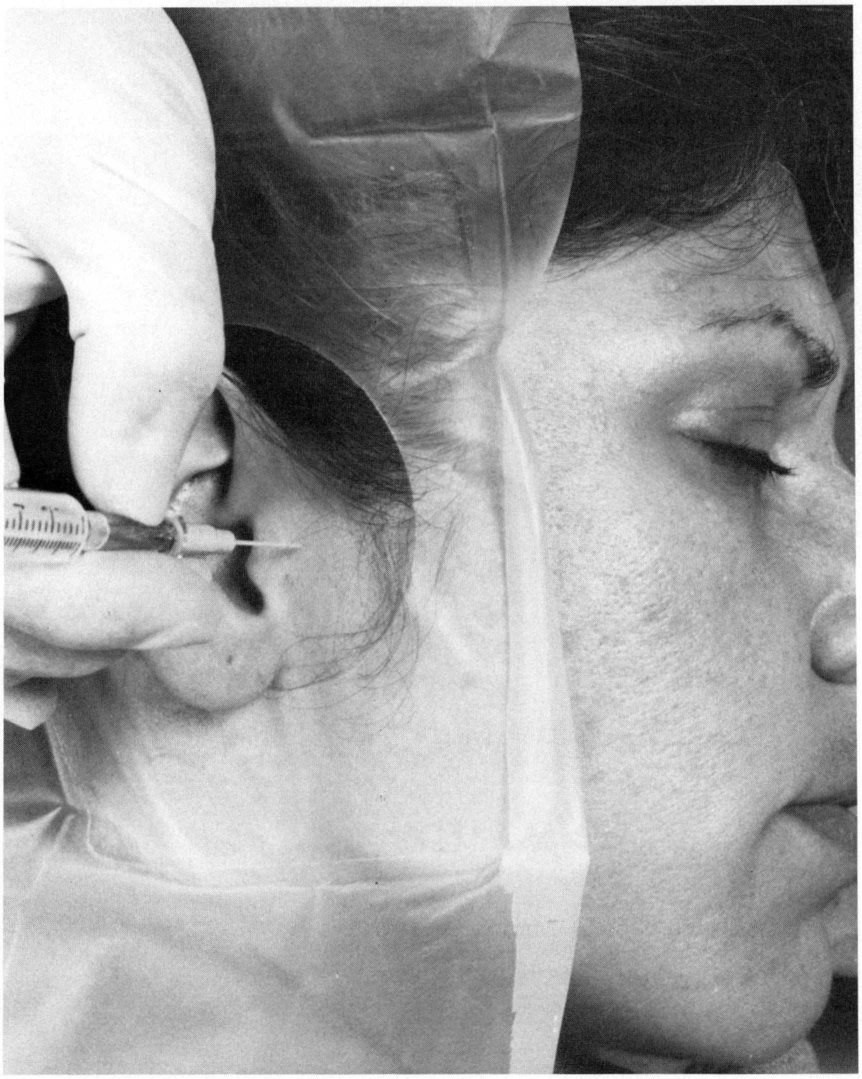

Fig. 8-39. Placement of angiocatheter into lower joint space.

technique would require the use of a radiology department for the necessary equipment. Figs. 8-44 and 8-45 show the arthrogram and drawing of disc anterior displacement with reduction.

The use of arthrography does not eliminate the need for taking accurate transcranial lateral oblique views or laminagraphy. These x-ray examinations also should be taken, since the radiopaque material obscures osseous structures that will show up in other views.

Arthrography is helpful in confirming early disc derangements before bony changes have occurred. This technique also helps in analyzing treatment modalities for internal derangement of the disc, including surgical repair of a damaged disc.

Transcutaneous arthroscopy

Transcutaneous arthroscopic examination of the TMJ recently has been described by Johnson.[18a] His listed indications for this procedure are unexplained TMJ pain, subluxation of the TMJ, degenerative arthritis, torn temporomandibular meniscus, tumor, and intraarticular hemangioma. The joint is distended with saline by a no. 21 needle. The patient is positioned supine and given general anesthesia, and the passive opening and closing of the mandible provides orientation for the arthroscopist. The jaw should be passively opened to widen the space at the point of entry of the needle and allowed to come into a closed position after capsular penetration. The needle's point of entry is an-

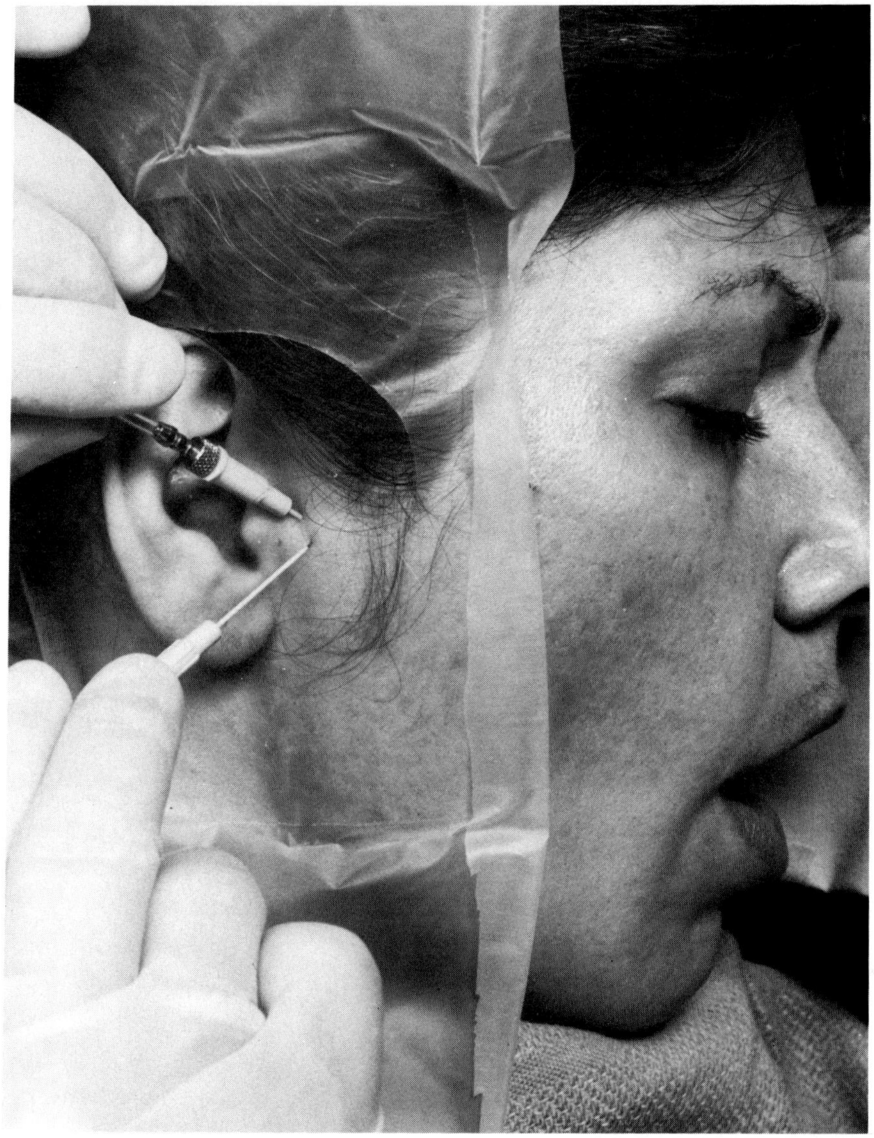

Fig. 8-40. Placement of angiocatheter into superior joint space.

terior and slightly lateral to the TMJ on the surface of the cheek. The direction from that point is posterior and angled 15 degrees toward the joint.

The needle is then removed, and the cannula system follows the same course. Confirmation of entry can be made by x-ray examination but is best established by palpation. Even with x-ray control or image intensification techniques there is still great demand for palpation skills because it is very easy to slide deep to the joint and into the area of the oral cavity. An x-ray film taken at the time of the needle passage can determine the exact entry site into the anterior portion of the TMJ. It is a common surgical procedure to approach the TMJ from the posterior direction, but the anterior approach enables a wider capsular target by opening the mouth for the transcutaneous arthroscopy.

Care should be taken to make only a minimal puncture in the skin with the no. 11 blade, since a deep puncture into the subcutaneous tissue might lacerate portions of the facial nerve. The angle of penetration should be superficial enough to avoid penetrating deep into the TMJ. There may be considerable swelling and extravasation of saline around the joint after the procedure, but it should resolve within a day.

Johnson's findings[18a] in the normal TMJ is that there is a fine vascularity throughout its entire synovium. The meniscal surface, whether superior or inferior, is smooth with little vascularity. The articular

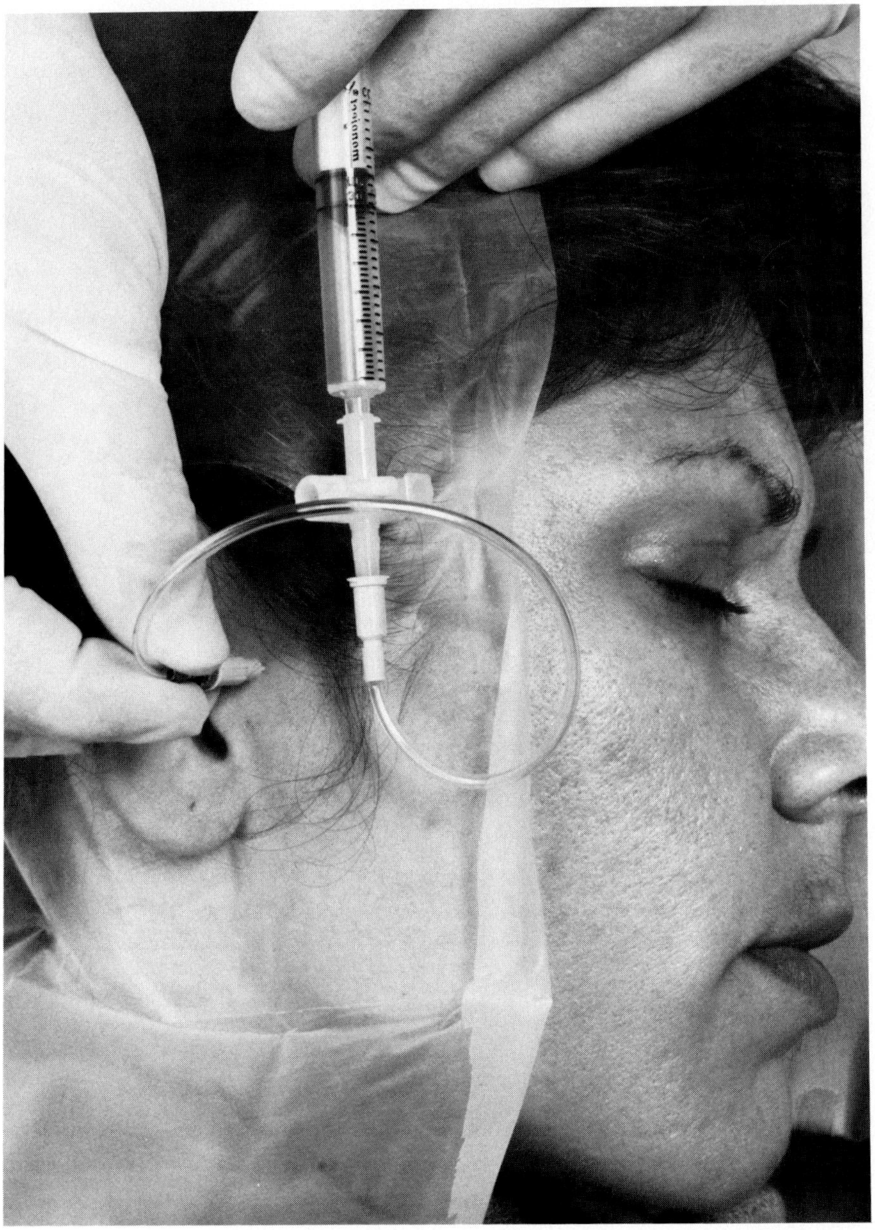

Fig. 8-41. Injection of small amount of water-soluble radiographic contrast medium into lower joint space.

surface of the temporal bone is rather small and poorly defined and flows right into the synovium. The condyle of the mandible is more easily defined as articular cartilage. The synovial space goes down 1 cm around the neck of the mandible, inferior to the condyle. A puncture in the inferior portion of that joint can actually show bone of the neck of the mandible, and by moving the scope up, the reflection of the articular surface can be seen.

The pathological findings noted by Johnson[18a] in four patients given arthroscopic inspection showed that patients with subluxation have abrasions of the meniscal surface as well as fibrous bands across the joint. A fibrinoid type of exudate was seen in two of these patients. The youngest, a 5-year-old boy, was inspected 6 weeks after resection of a hemangioma that went down to the level of the joint. Since the ENT surgeon did not want to unnecessarily resect the joint, arthroscopy was able to confirm that there was no hemangioma in the joint and therefore no need for further resection.

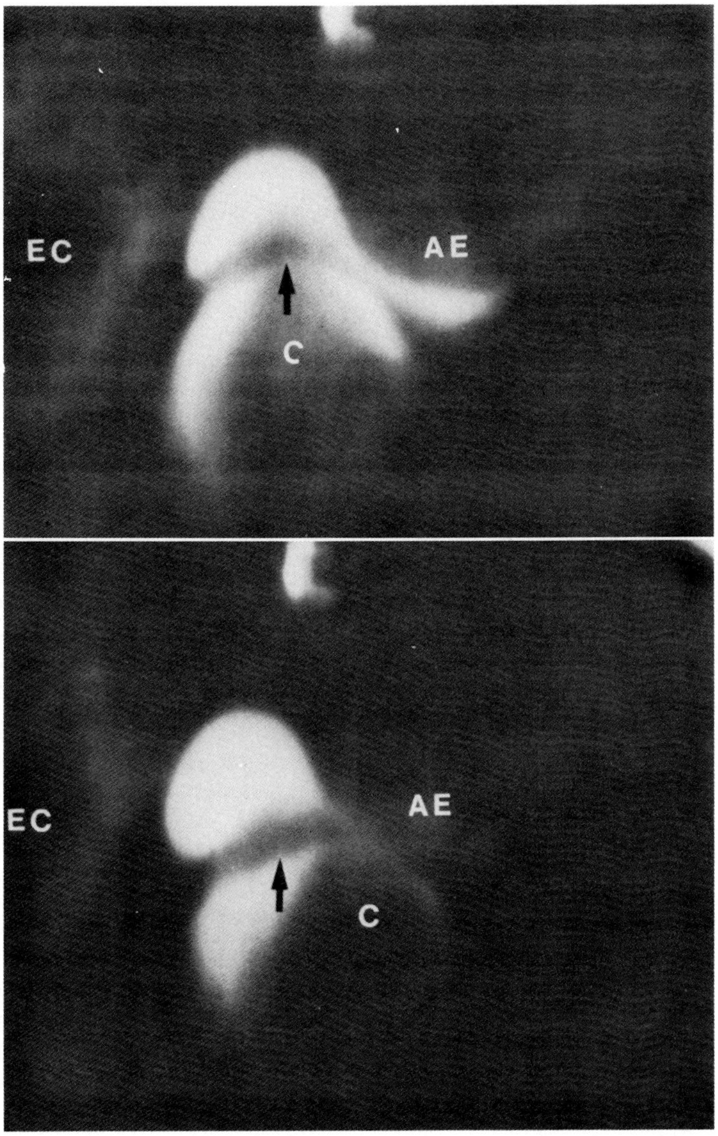

Fig. 8-42. Normal TMJ arthrogram. *Top,* Both upper and lower joint spaces are moderately opacified; jaws are opened approximately one finger breadth of interincisal distance. Portion of contrast medium is seen in anterior recesses. Posterior band *(arrow)* of disc is positioned directly above condyle. *Bottom,* Jaws are opened further, and condyle is anteriorly translated to greater extent, obliterating contrast in both anterior recesses. Posterior band of disc *(arrow)* trails behind condyle. *C,* Condyle; *AE,* articular eminence; *EC,* external ear canal. (From Blaschke, D.D., et al.: J. Am. Dent. Assoc. **100:**388, 1980. Copyright by the American Dental Association. Reprinted by permission.)

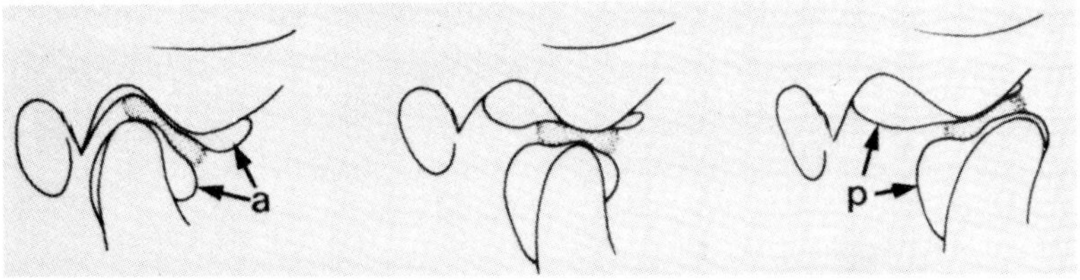

Fig. 8-43. Normal TMJ arthrogram sequence. Note bulging of anterior recesses *(a).* Posterior recesses *(p)* have assumed characteristic shapes. (From Blaschke, D.D., et al.: J. Am. Dent Assoc. **100:**388, 1980. Copyright by the American Dental Association. Reprinted by permission.)

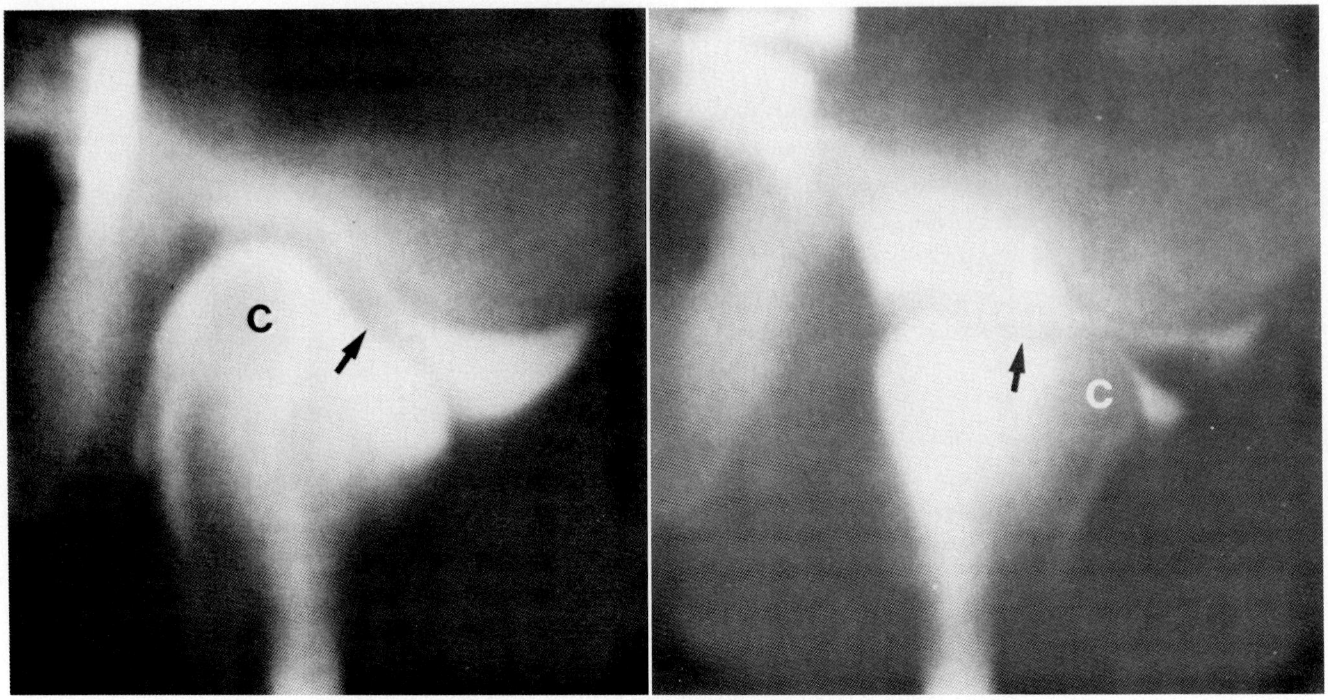

Fig. 8-44. Arthrogram of disc anterior displacement with reduction. (From Blaschke, D.D., et al.: J. Am. Dent. Assoc. **100:**388, 1980. Copyright by the American Dental Association. Reprinted by permission.)

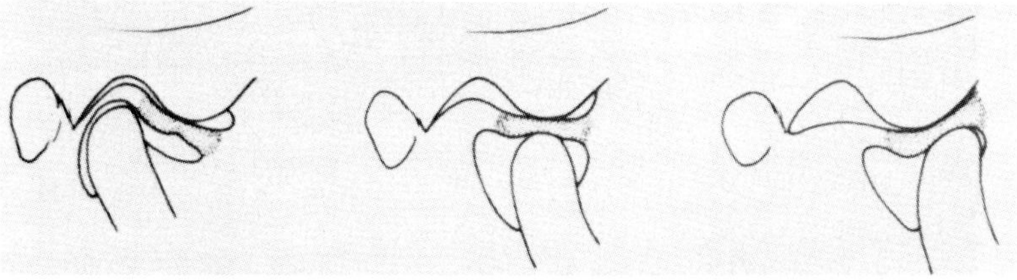

Fig. 8-45. Drawing of disc anterior displacement with reduction. (From Blaschke, D.D., et al.: J. Am. Dent. Assoc. **100:**388, 1980. Copyright by the American Dental Association. Reprinted by permission.)

COMPARISONS

Discussing their findings on a comparison between conventional oblique transcranial radiographs, tomograms, and histologic sections, Eckerdal and Lundberg have stated*:

The probability of making a correct radiographic diagnosis from the conventional system is low if a pathological change is located exclusively centrally or medially. In 33 cases in the present investigation, different pathomorphological changes, including sclerosis, erosions, deviation of form and osteophytes, occurred exclusively in the medial and central parts. These medial and central pathological changes were not observed in the conventional radiographs, with the exception of one case in which an anterior osteophyte was seen as a "gross" structural detail. It should be added that a lateral location of a pathologic trait does not guarantee that it will be perceived in conventional radiographs (4 cases). However, in most instances, diagnosis of the joints, based on conventional radiographs, is correct when the depicted lateral part has structural and relational characteristics which are representative of the whole joint.[19,32]

In tomography the central two-thirds of the joint are well defined with sharp image contours, whereas the structures of the lateral parts are blurred; the blurring is greatest in the peripheral sections. This was graphically demonstrated by

*From Eckerdal, O., and Lundberg, M.: Dentomaxillofac. Radiol. 8:47-48, 1979.

Eckerdal[13] for the different projection and morphologic combinations. In the literature there are indications that the essential joint diseases mostly have their primary location in the lateral part of the joints.[9] Oberg et al[24] reported 18 lesions, 13 lateral and 5 central. None were found medially. Bauer,[3] on the other hand, examined osteoarthritic patients and found the highest frequency of osteophytes in the central part of the joints. The differing results could be explained by the differences between the two materials and the structural changes being studied. The results of Bauer are supported by clinical tomographic observations and also by the results of the present investigation. According to Oberg, 72% of lesions are located laterally and thus demonstrable in conventional radiographs. In our study, the figures of 78% and 81% were reported.

Earlier investigations have concluded that the tomographic technique offers more diagnostic reliability than the conventional methods when applied to the temporomandibular joints.[14,25,32] The present investigation strongly supports this conclusion. The probability of false negative findings in conventional radiographs was calculated. An interesting question is how this knowledge might interfere with the clinical considerations. Is there enough support now for individualized examination procedures? It cannot be denied that the conventional is favored because of its simplicity. The superiority of tomography in the reproduction of small and gross structural changes in the central two-thirds of the temporomandibular joints strongly supports the use of this method in the diagnosis of suspected arthritic changes. While such an examination will give a concomitant and reliable image of the relationship between the joint components,[16] a logical consideration is to omit some or all of the conventional images. A development such as this has occurred in diagnosis of the larynx and the vertebral column.[18,26]

RECENT DEVELOPMENTS: RADIONUCLIDE BONE SCANNING*

Radionuclide bone scanning is a safe, simple, sensitive technique that measures the extent, the aggressiveness, and even the existence of skeletal abnormalities. The introduction of bone scanning first came about when radiologists realized that a more sensitive diagnostic tool was needed for the detection of bone pathology. Borak[7] reported that there is a need to lose about 50% of the calcium salts (demineralization) from bone before a lesion will be visible on a radiograph. Thus entire medullary cavities could be filled with tumor, and such a pathologic condition would not be seen on routine radiography until there was spread to or erosion of the cortical bone. The need for a superior diagnostic tool for the detection, localization, and even definition of the extent of involvement of bony abnormalities becomes immediately evident.

Bone scanning is based on pathophysiological changes that occur in bone. Tumors, cysts, and degenerative changes from trauma, infection, etc. will erode or destroy existing bone and concurrently stimulate the formation of new reactive bone. It is in this new reactive bone that radionuclide pharmaceuticals concentrate to the greatest degree. This concentration, that is, the increased uptake of radiopharmaceuticals, forms the basis of bone scanning (Figs. 8-46 and 8-47). In addition to seeking areas of increased osteoblastic activity, the radiopharmaceuticals concentrate in areas where there is increased blood supply. This is a very important point in diagnosing vascular lesions and inflammatory disease and for differentiating malignant from benign lesions. Since the malignant lesions are characteristically extremely vascular and hyperemic, they will concentrate the radioisotope much more rapidly than the benign lesion.

Historically, several radiopharmaceuticals have been used in the study of bone pathology. With the introduction of various phosphate compounds of technetium in 1971, bone scanning has become a very viable, sensitive diagnostic tool. Technetium 99m has many advantages, the most important being that it is widely available, is safe, has a satisfactory half-life, and provides excellent resolution for scintigraphy. Technetium diphosphonate is the most sensitive agent in detecting bone pathology and currently is being used in most radiology departments. Gallium is another bone-seeking radioisotope; however, it is also very selective for inflammatory lesions. Gallium is picked up by the neutrophil and thus will readily identify inflammatory changes. It is also picked up by some specific soft tissue tumors like lymphoma and accordingly can be used to stage Hodgkin's disease.

For years radiologists and orthopedic surgeons have used radionuclide bone scanning as a diagnostic modality in their treatment of synovitis, osteoarthritis, and degenerative joint diseases of the extremities. We advocate a similar approach for the detection of bone pathology of the temporomandibular joint. Bloom[6] showed that the correlation is extremely accurate between positive, or "hot," bone scans of the TMJ and degenerative changes in the condylar head or anterior glenoid fossa as evidenced by postsurgical histopathological study (Figs. 8-48 to 8-51). Coincidental to Bloom's findings that bone scanning showed greater sensitivity than radiography in recognizing degenerative changes in the TMJ was the discovery that the anterior portion of the glenoid fossa undergoes the initial osseous degenerative changes, which then proceed to the condylar head.

Many disease processes involving the TMJ can readily be studied by radionuclide bone scanning. Specifi-

*Section contributed by Charles D. Hasse, D.D.S., Past Chief Resident, Oral Surgery, Veterans Hospital, Long Beach, and University of California Irvine Medical Center.

A

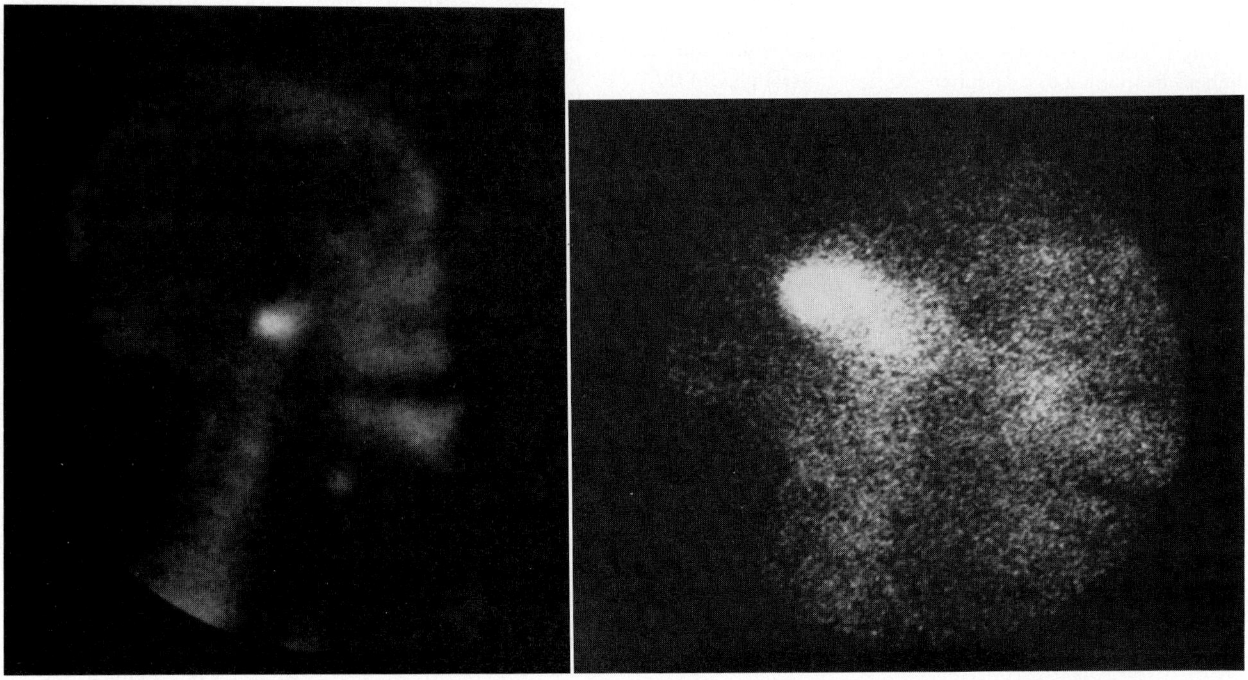

B

Fig. 8-46. Right lateral views of technetium 99m bone scans for patient with hyperplastic condyle. Note "hot spots" in area of TMJ.

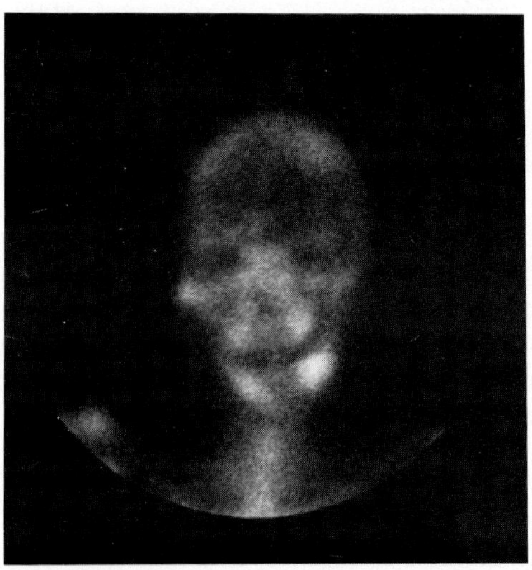

Fig. 8-47. Frontal view of patient with left mandibular body fracture and right subcondylar fracture. Positive scan is indicative of combined osteogenic and osteoblastic activity. (Courtesy Charles D. Hasse, D.D.S.)

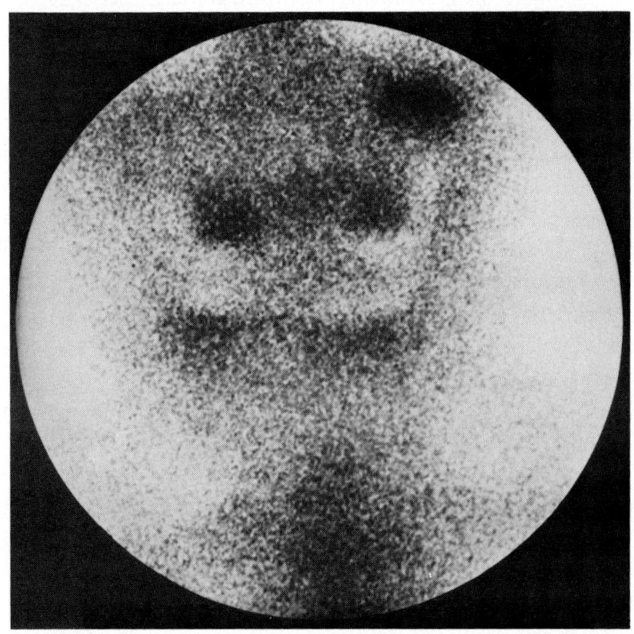

Fig. 8-48. Anterior skull projection showing greatly increased activity of left temporomandibular joint compared with right temporomandibular joint. Cause of "hot spot" was condylar hyperplasia. Refer to Fig. 8-50. (Courtesy Charles D. Hasse, D.D.S.)

cally, scanning is beneficial in the diagnosis of neoplasia, trauma, inflammatory disease, and metabolic disease. From an interpretation standpoint it can be difficult to differentiate between an abnormality in the head or neck of the condyle versus the articular tubercle or mandibular fossa of the temporal bone owing to their close anatomical proximity. Recently Alexander[1] and Alexander, Fratkin, and Hall[2] introduced a TMJ marking technique which eliminates this problem, since it provides more accurate delineation of the temporomandibular joint and the associated structures.

The patient with TMJ pain remains a diagnostic challenge to the clinician who deals with the management of this problem. Frequently this challenge can lead to frustration on the part of the dentist or physician if no radiographic or clinical cause for the patient's symptoms can be pinpointed. These patients often are directed to seek unwarranted psychiatric counseling for their psychogenic pain syndrome. With the routine use of radionuclide bone scanning as part of our TMJ workup, early detection of disease is possible, and the initiation of appropriate therapeutic measures can begin before irreversible temporomandibular osseous changes take place.

A

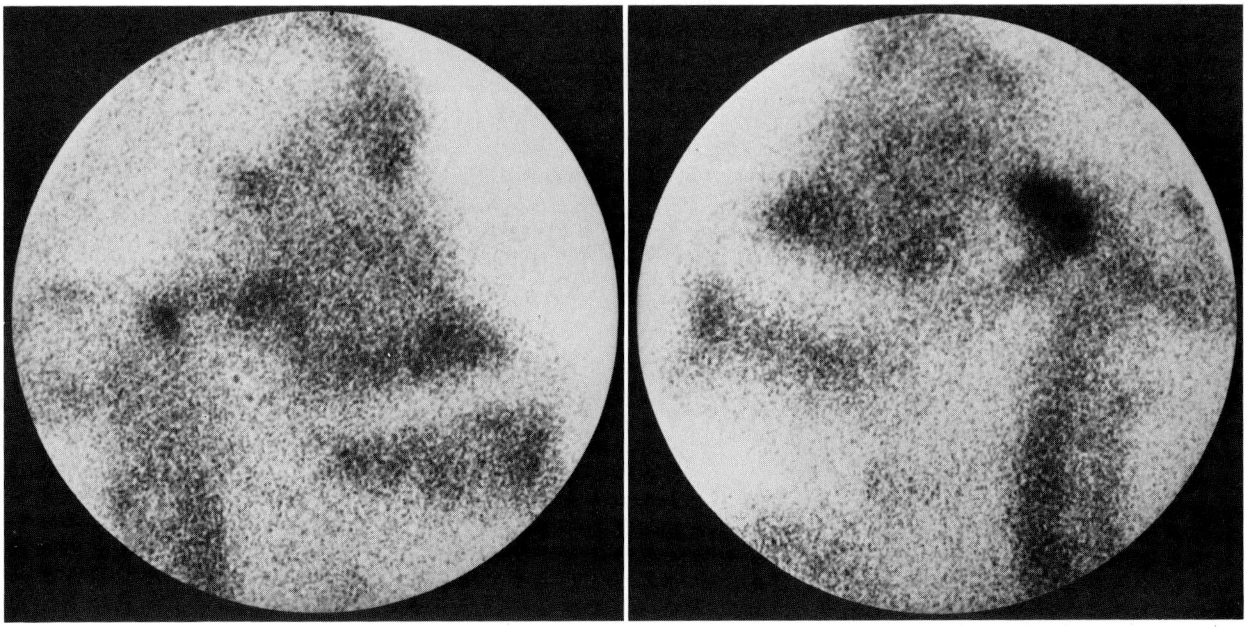

B

Fig. 8-49. A, Right lateral technetium 99m bone scan showing normal right condyle. **B,** Left lateral scan showing abnormal left condyle. (Courtesy Charles D. Hasse, D.D.S.)

A

B

C

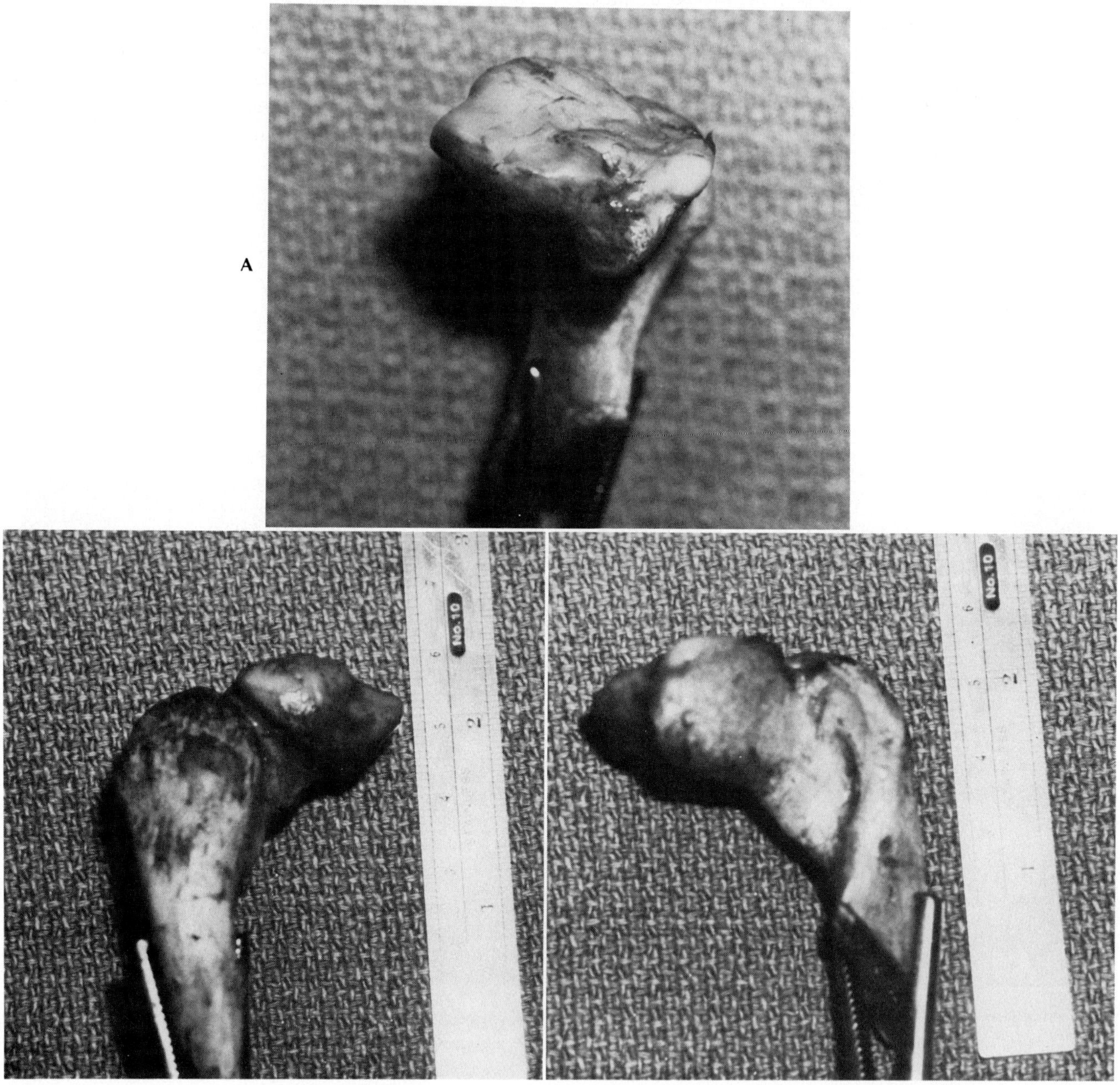

Fig. 8-50. Posterior **(A),** right **(B),** and left **(C)** lateral views of condylar head with aberrant bony growth. Extensive osteogenic activity secondary to trauma resulted in gnarled, lobulated growth on condylar head. Technetium 99m bone scans for this patient were extremely "hot." (Courtesy Charles D. Hasse, D.D.S.)

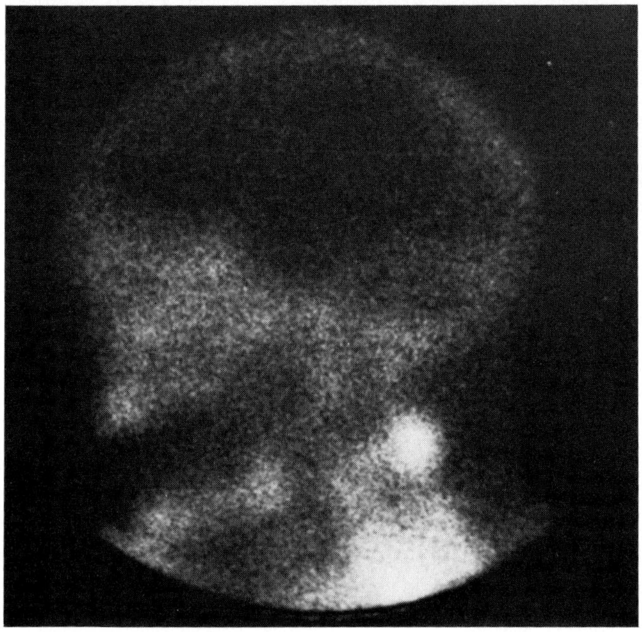

Fig. 8-51. Left lateral bone scan showing extreme osteogenic activity in cervical spine area. Patient was referred for evaluation for head and neck pain. Early degenerative changes in cervical spine were responsible for symptoms. (Courtesy Charles D. Hasse, D.D.S.)

REFERENCES

1. Alexander, J.M.: Radionuclide bone scanning in the diagnosis of lesions of the maxillofacial region, J. Oral Surg. **34**:249, 1976.
2. Alexander, J.M., Fratkin, M.J., and Hall, D.L.: Temporomandibular joint marking for radionuclide bone scintigraphy, J. Oral Surg. **37**:753, 1979.
3. Bauer, W.H.: Osteoarthritis deformans of the temporomandibular joint, Am. J. Pathol. **17**:129, 1941.
4. Binnie, W.H., Stacey, A.J., Davis, R., and Cawson, R.A.: Applications of xeroradiography to dentistry, J. Dent. **3**:99, 1975.
5. Blaschke, D.D., Solberg, W.K., and Sanders, B.: Arthrography of the temporomandibular joint: review of current status, J. Am. Dent. Assoc. **100**:388, 1980.
6. Bloom, C.Y.: The application of bone scintigraphy in the diagnosis of TMJ disorders, Transactions of the American Association of Oral and Maxillofacial Surgeons, 61st meeting, New Orleans, Sept. 1979.
7. Borak, J.: Relationship between clinical and roentgenological findings in bone metastases, Surg. Gynecol. Obstet. **75**:599, 1942.
8. Brader, A.C.: Application of the principles of cephalometric laminagraphy to studies of the frontal planes of the human head, Am. J. Orthod. **35**:249, 1949.
9. Carlsson, G.E., Lundberg, M., Oberg, T., and Welander, V.: The temporomandibular joint: a comparative anatomic and radiologic study, Odont Rev. **19**:171, 1968.
10. Carlsson, G.E., Oberg, T., Bergman, F., and Fajers, C.M.: Morphological changes in the mandibular joint disc in temporomandibular joint pain dysfunction syndrome, Acta Odontol. Scand. **25**:163, 1967.
11. Coin, C.G.: Tomography of the temporomandibular joint, Med. Radiogr. Photogr. **50**:26, 1974.
12. Dolwick, M.F., et al.: Arthrotomographic evaluation of the TMJ, J. Oral Surg. **37**:793, 1979.
13. Eckerdal, O.: Tomography of the temporomandibular joint, Medicamundi **16**:144, 1971.
14. Eckerdal, O.: Tomography of the temporomandibular joint: correlation between tomographic image and histologic sections in a three-dimensional system, Acta Radiol. (Suppl.) **329**:1, 1973.
15. Eckerdal, O., and Lundberg, M.: The structural situation in temporomandibular joints, Dentomaxillofac. Radiol. **8**:42, 1979.
16. Eckerdal, O., and Lundberg, M.: Temporomandibular joint relations revealed by conventional roentgenologic techniques: a comparison with tomography and the morphologic background, Dentomaxillofac. Radiol. (In press.)
17. Farrar, W.B., and McCarty, W.L.: Inferior joint space arthrography and characteristics of condylar paths in internal derangements of the TMJ, J. Prosthet. Dent. **41**:548, 1979.
18. Hemmingsson, A.: Roentgenologic methods in examination of the larynx: comparative phantom investigations in the frontal projections, Acta Radiol. Diagn. **12**:673, 1972.

18a. Johnson, L.: Diagnostic and surgical arthroscopy, ed. 2, St. Louis, 1981, The C.V. Mosby Co.

19. Lewis, G.R.: Temporomandibular joint radiographic technics: comparison and evaluation of results, Dent. Radiogr. Photogr. **37**:8, 1964.
20. Merrill, V.: Atlas of roentgenographic positions and standard radiologic procedures, ed. 4, St. Louis, 1975, The C.V. Mosby Co.
21. Meschan, I.: Radiographic positioning and related anatomy, Philadelphia, 1968, W.B. Saunders Co.
22. Murphy, W.A., Adams, R.J., Gilula, L.A., and Barbier, J.Y.: Magnification radiography of the temporomandibular joint: technical considerations, Radiology **133**:524, 1979.
23. Norgaard, F.: Arthrography of the mandibular joint, Acta Radiol. **25**:679, 1944.
24. Oberg, T., Carlsson, G.E., and Fajers, G.M.: The temporomandibular joint: a morphologic study on a human autopsy material, Acta Odont. Scand. **29**:349, 1971.
25. Omnell, K.A., and Petersson, A.: Radiography of the temporomandibular joint utilizing oblique lateral transcranial projections: comparison of information obtained with standardized technique and individualized technique, Odont. Rev. **27**:77, 1976.
26. Reichmann, S.: Tomography of the lumbar intervertebral joint, Acta Radiol. Diagn. **12**:641, 1972.
27. Ricketts, R.M.: Variations of the temporomandibular joint as revealed by cephalometric laminagraphy, Am. J. Orthod. **36**:877, 1950.
28. Ricketts, R.M.: Laminagraphy in the diagnosis of temporomandibular joint disorders, J. Am. Dent. Assoc. **46**:620, 1953.
29. Ricketts, R.M.: Present status of laminagraphy as related to dentistry, J. Am. Dent. Assoc. **65**:56, 1962.
30. Ricketts, R.M.: Roentgenography of the temporomandibular joint. In Sarnat, B.G., editor: The temporomandibular joint, ed. 2, Springfield, Ill., 1964, Charles C Thomas, Publisher.
31. Updegrave, W.J.: Temporomandibular articulation, x-ray examination, Dent. Radiogr. Photogr. **26**:41, 1953.
32. Weinberg, L.A.: What we really see in a TMJ radiograph, J. Prosthet. Dent. **30**:898, 1973.
33. Wilkes, C.H.: Arthrography of the temporomandibular joint in patients with the TMJ pain-dysfunction syndrome, Minn. Med. **61**:645, 1978.

9 Interpretation of radiographs

DOUGLAS H. MORGAN, D.D.S.

A major cause of temporomandibular joint disease is skeletal malrelationships as well as dental malrelationships. The relationship of the condyle to the articular eminence–mandibular fossa can be displaced from its normal position. If the condyle shows displacement from its normal position in either an anterior, superior, or posterior direction (and there is no history of trauma), a bite and/or a skeletal problem might be suggested.

CASE 1: D.B.

The diagnosis made in the case of D.B. was cervical arteritis. He had been seen by numerous physicians and had taken many medications. Eventually he was referred to us by his neurosurgeon, who recognized the temporomandibular joint as a possible source for the patient's complaints.

The radiographs in Fig. 9-1 shows the new fourth view, the closed wax-bite view. In this projection the patient lightly touches the teeth on two thicknesses of dental wax (2 mm). This will reproduce what would happen to the relationship of the condyle within the fossa if that individual had a splint of 2 mm thickness. One of the effects of a splint is to open the bite, making the external pterygoid muscle pull the condyle forward. In the teeth-closed view the posterior disc space can be seen to be narrower than the anterior disc space. The posterior space is narrow in both the left and the right sides. As the patient touched on the wax, the condyle moved forward slightly. Interestingly, all that was done to help this patient's neck pain was to put him on a resilient dental splint. The final result shows in the fifth view. He is occluding lightly on the splint. The condyle is now in a more normal position within the articular eminence–mandibular fossa complex.

A

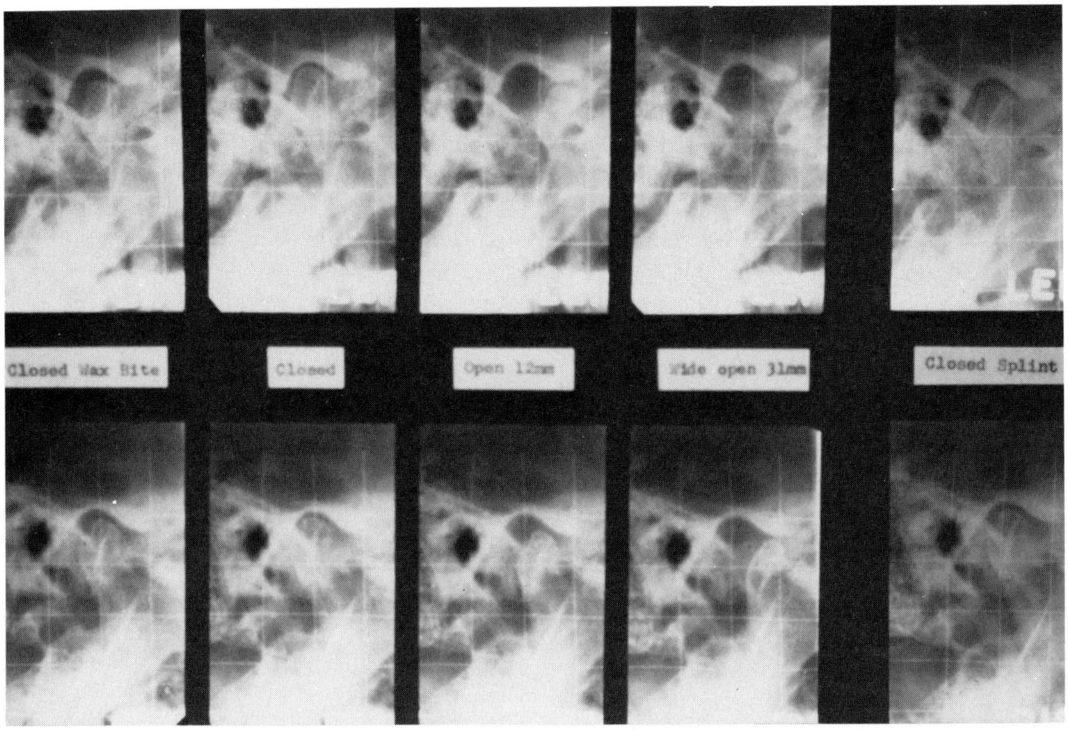

B

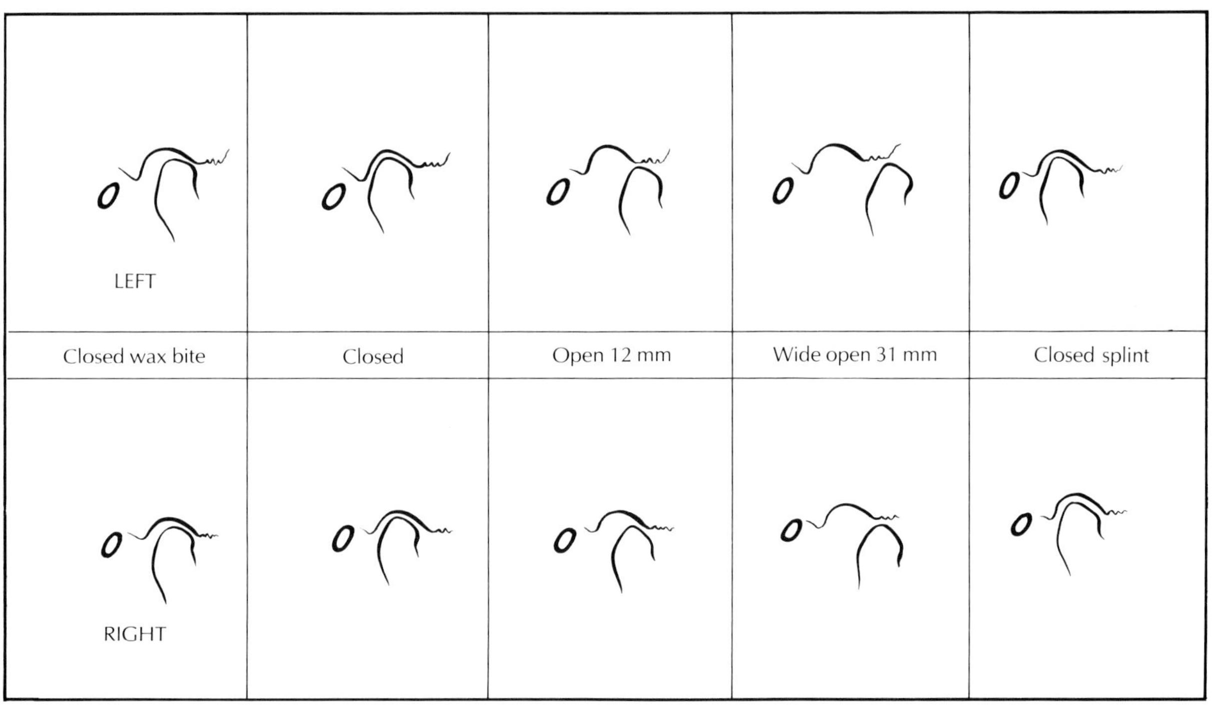

Fig. 9-1. A, Transcranial lateral oblique films of patient (D.B.) with tentative diagnosis of cervical arteritis showing added view, closed wax-bite view with 2-mm opening (first view), and fifth view, with patient's teeth touching on resilient dental splint. **B,** It can be seen in closed view that condyle is slightly posteriorly displaced in fossa. Closed splint view of approximately 1.5 mm opening shows condyle moving slightly anteriorly, increasing posterior disc space. There is also some erosion of cortical bone in both eminences.

CASE 2: A.R.

A.R. had severe pain on the left side of her head that had been diagnosed variously as migraine, tic douloureux, and atypical facial pain. It was not suspected that the pain could be referred from the temporomandibular joints (Fig. 9-2).

On the right side can be seen the normal anterior, superior, and posterior joint space. The normal condylar motion occurs in the ½-inch opening, wide-open view. In the left joint a narrowing in the joint space can be seen all along its perimeter; this is a bone-on-bone relationship. When this occurs, it indicates degeneration and/or perforation of the meniscus. The anterior and lateral half of the joint usually is where the damage occurs. In the half-open view there is no disc space seen between the articulating bone surfaces. This lack of space is maintained throughout the entire movement. It can be imagined what is occurring in that joint. There is also significant erosion of the postglenoid fossa area.

On the left temporomandibular joint, bone-on-bone contact can be seen; on the right there is normal joint space. The fibrocartilage disc between is degenerated and/or perforated. The disc or meniscus is not separating the articular surfaces properly, resulting in the bone-on-bone contact.

Figs. 9-3 to 9-8 give three views each of the right and left sides enlarged. Although the patient has no pain on the right side, there is some demineralization of normal sclerotic outline on the postglenoid area of the fossa, on the anterior aspect of the condyle, and on the ascending slope of the eminence. This is because of remodeling and hyperemia and is seen in joints in other parts of the body. The unique aspect this joint is that there is translational movement inside the joint, and therefore a dynamic study is important.

Text continued on p. 173.

A

B

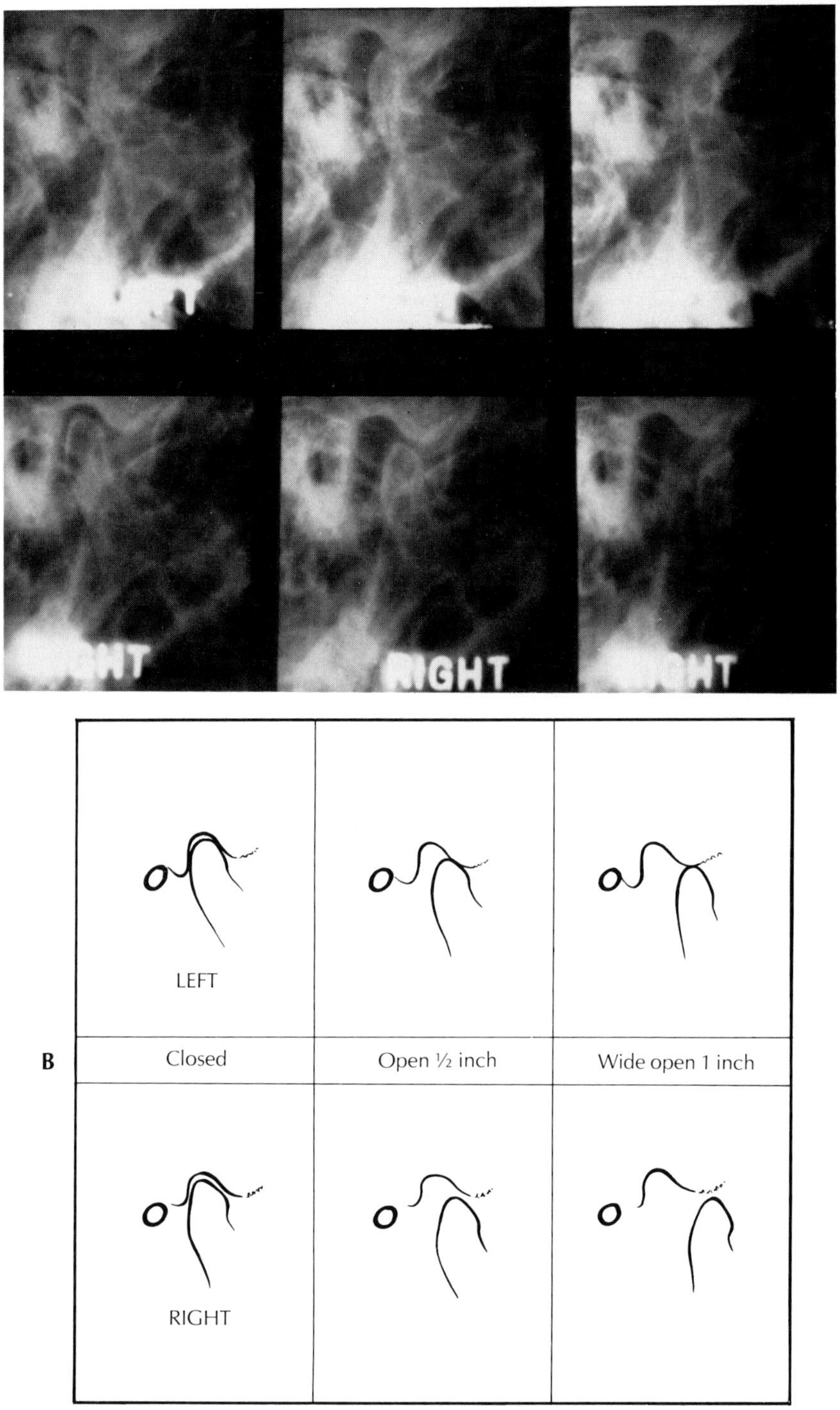

Fig. 9-2. A, Transcranial lateral oblique films showing three views (old type), revealing pathosis primarily in left joint and some flattening of right condyle (A.R.). **B,** Bone-to-bone contact of anterior head of condyle to descending slope of eminence shown in left joint. Some erosion of cortical bone over ascending slope of eminence and some flattening of anterior surface of right condyle can be seen.

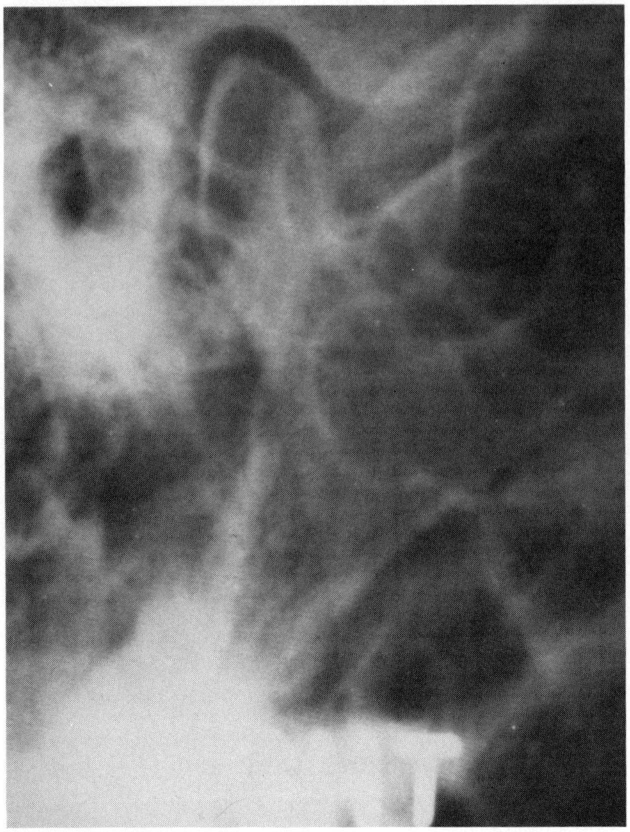

Fig. 9-3. Right side of patient (A.R.) with teeth lightly in occlusion.

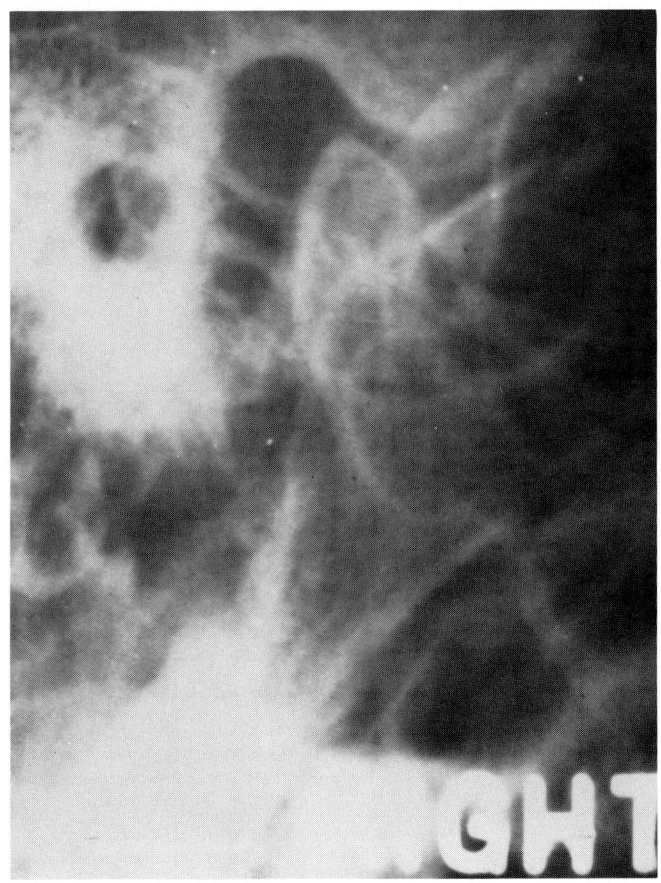

Fig. 9-4. Right side with mouth interincisal opening $^{1}/_{2}$ inch.

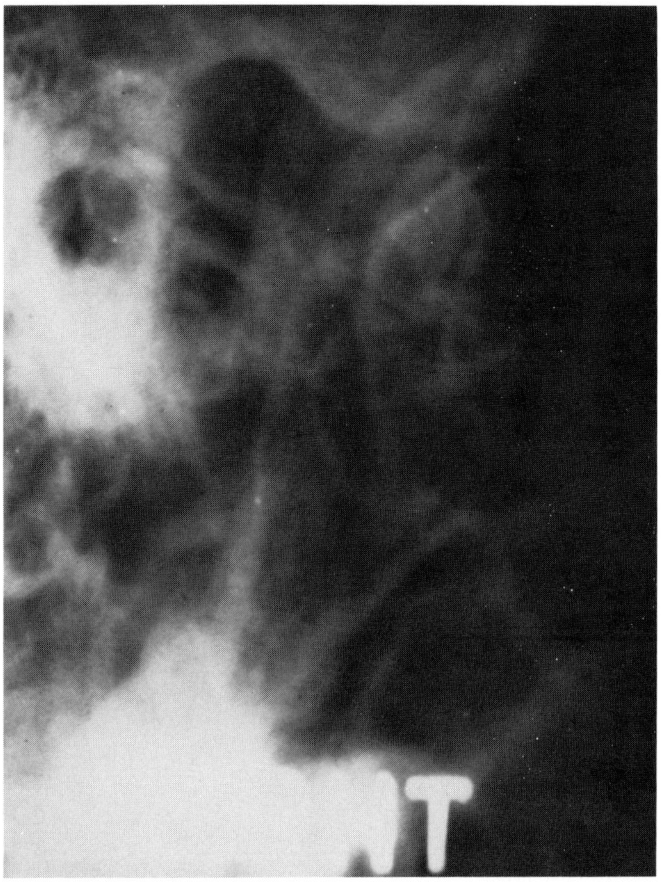

Fig. 9-5. Right side with mouth interincisal opening 1½ inches.

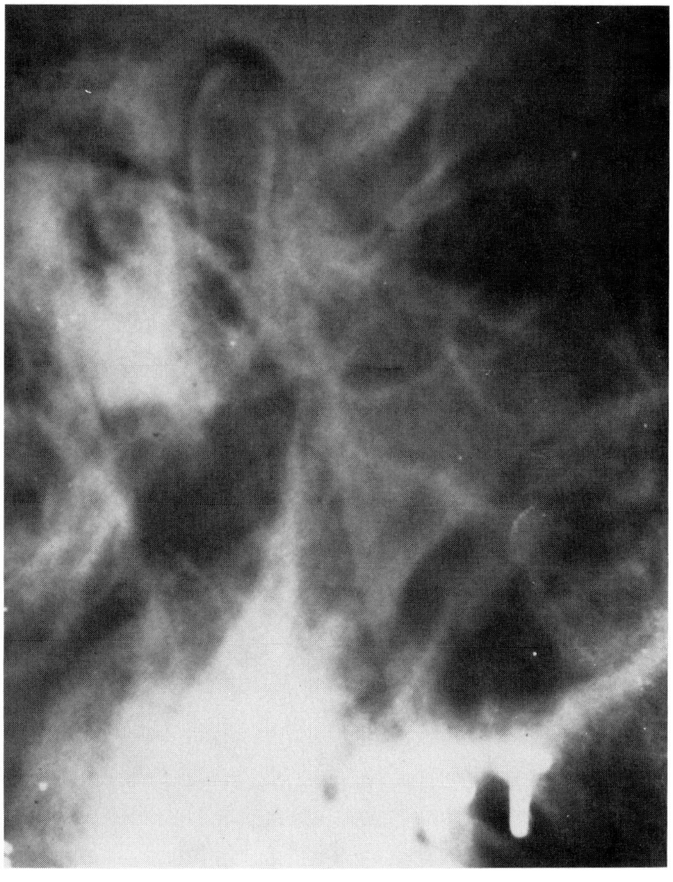

Fig. 9-6. Left side of same patient (A.R.) with teeth lightly in occlusion.

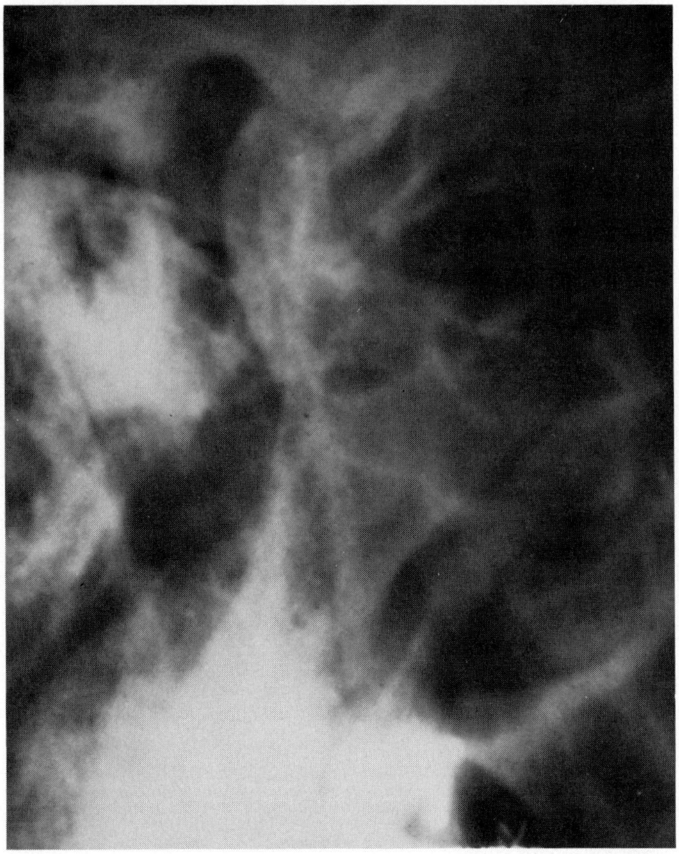

Fig. 9-7. Left side with mouth interincisal opening 1/2 inch.

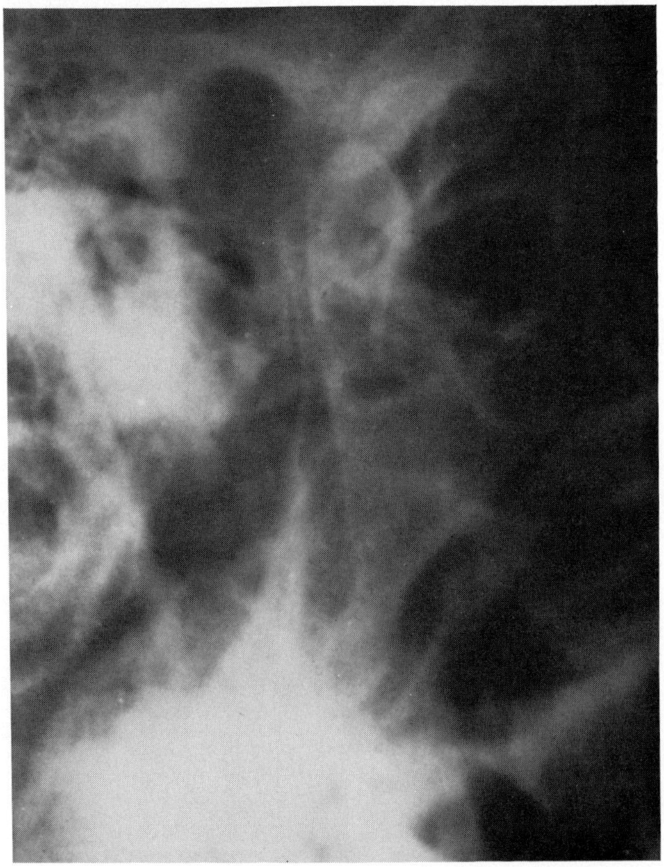

Fig. 9-8. Left side with mouth interincisal opening 1 1/2 inches.

CASE 3: A.G.

Fig. 9-9 is a cephalometric radiograph depicting a closed bite. The central incisors come down some distance over the lower incisor teeth. These radiographs are used routinely by the orthodontist as well as by dentists and physicians involved in this work.

Fig. 9-10 is the cephalometric tomogram of the patient using functional views similar to the transcranial lateral oblique views. This shows the joint space with the patient at rest, nearly a bone-on-bone relationship, which is maintained with a wide-open view. There is a discrepancy in the size of the condyle, which appears smaller than normal on the right. This could be a congenital abnormality, or it could be associated with the arthritic process. The joint space is decreased on both sides, and the area of the articular eminence and the mandibular fossa can be seen. These films give a functional view not ordinarily seen with tomograms. They have been done by a special dental laboratory using a technique that was developed by Ricketts.[2]

Fig. 9-11 is the regular transcranial lateral oblique film. The anterior condylar motion is shown on both sides with the closed wax-bite view. On the right side the narrowing of the anterior joint space and a flattening of the condyle can be seen. On the left side the anterior joint space is maintained. There is a slight anterior movement of the left condyle in the wax-bite view. This places the condyle in a more central position in the fossa. Opening the bite 2 mm on this side would be helpful. On the right side, opening the bite 2 mm would advance the condyle too far forward and not be helpful. These are some of the more common findings and are fairly easy to evaluate with the four-view transcranial lateral oblique study.

In comparing the cephalometric tomograms and the transcranial lateral oblique views it can be noted that a much clearer picture is obtained of the lateral joint surface with the latter. In the tomograms the picture is more difficult to interpret, and the viewer is dependent on one cut or section, which may miss the area in which the disease process exhibits itself. Consequently, if there is a choice between the use of the transcranial lateral oblique views or the cephalometric tomograms, we would elect to use the former. The tomograms could be used as backup pictures if the disease process is not exhibited in the lateral half of the joint surface and it is necessary to take a series of cuts of the medial aspect of the joint.

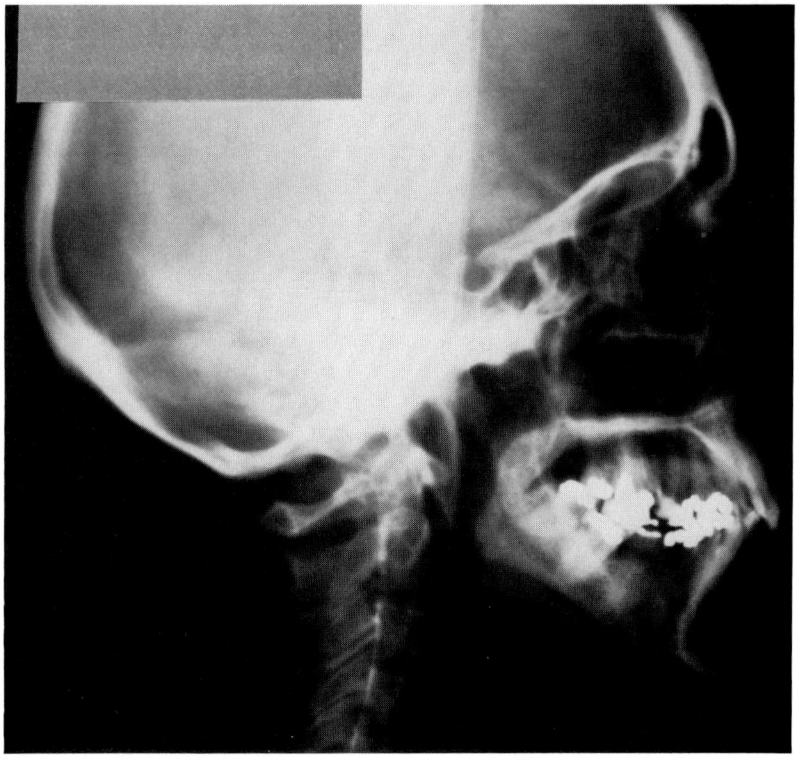

Fig. 9-9. Cephalometric radiograph depicting closed bite. (A.G.).

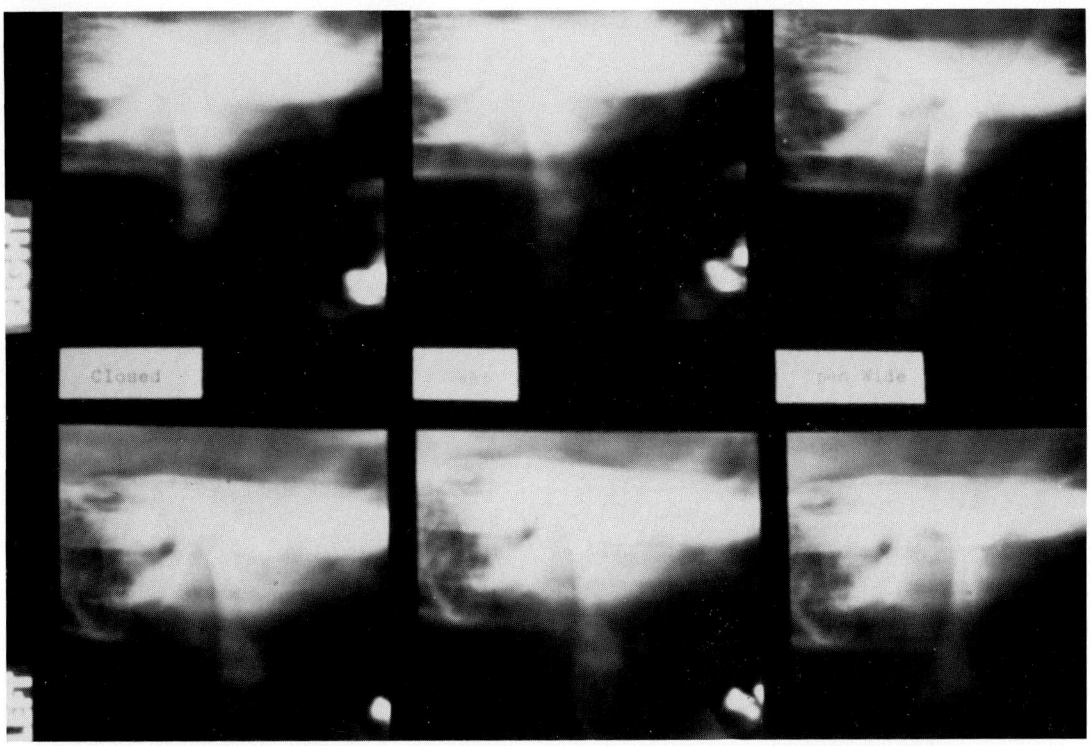

Fig. 9-10. Cephalometric tomogram showing condyles in three positions: teeth closed, rest position, and wide-open position. It is difficult to read these x-ray films because of the exposure.

A

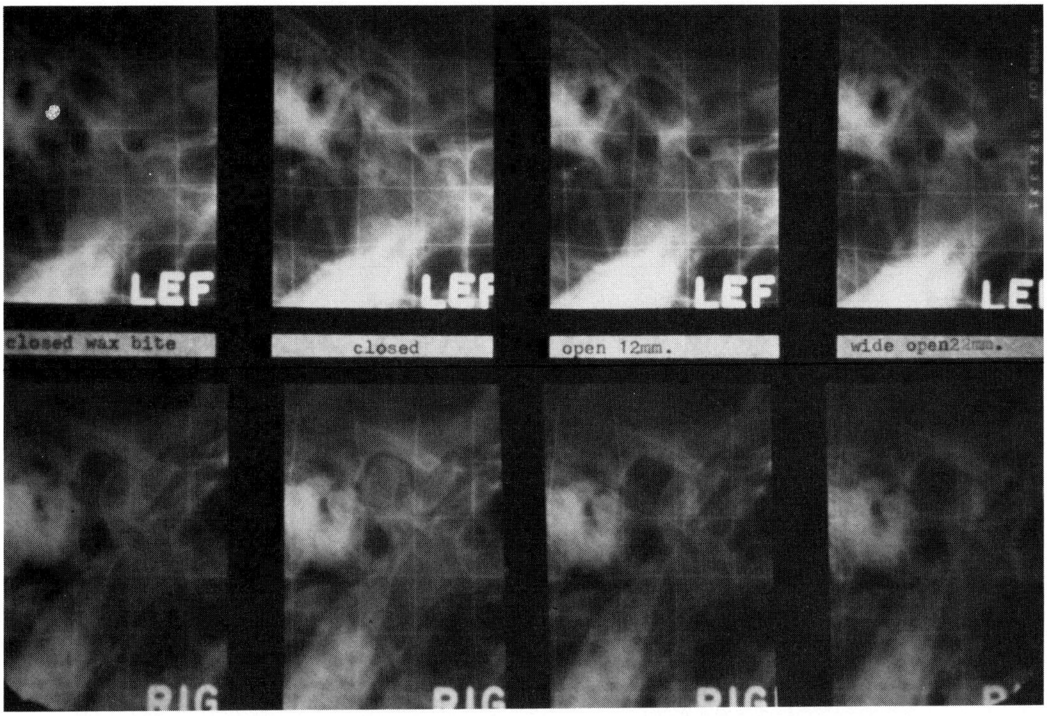

B

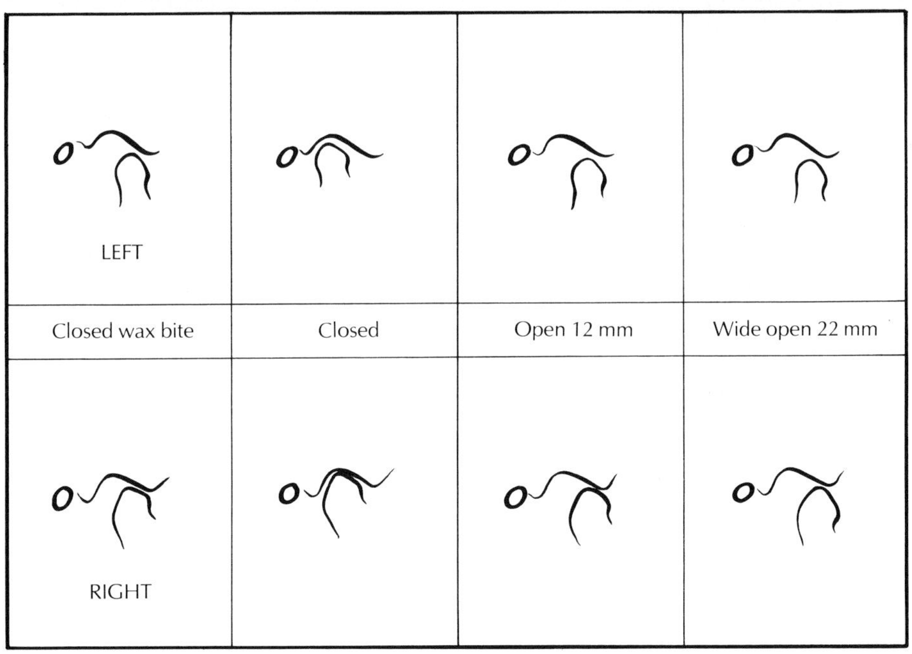

Fig. 9-11. A, Transcranial lateral oblique films of same patient (A.G.) with cephalometric tomograms showing fourth (wax-bite) view. **B,** Flattening of anterior head of condyle shown in left joint. In closed view of right joint, flattened anterior head of condyle and minimum disc space can be seen in translational views.

CASE 4: J.M.

J.M. had had symptoms for 37 years. He had dropped out of high school and could not attend college because of the pain, which would become most acute after dinner. He tried to obtain help from numerous sources. He had worn a dental splint, but in his case the splints caused more symptoms.

Fig. 9-12 shows the cephalometric radiographs. Observing the jaw, it is seen that the patient has an end-to-end bite, which almost looks like a prognathic mandible (a Dick Tracy jaw). In analyzing the radiographs it is seen that it is not a true prognathic mandible. For some reason, possibly spasms of the external pterygoid muscle, he had moved his jaw forward, creating an end-to-end bite.

On the transcranial lateral oblique films (Fig. 9-13) the following observations can be made. In the closed view it can be seen that the condyle has moved forward both in the right and left sides. In the closed wax-bite view, simulating a dental splint, the condyle would move forward even more. This made the use of splints counterproductive because in this instance their use only accentuated the existing problem. With this patient, treatment is being planned to adjust the occlusion, perhaps with some device that could retrude the condyle into the fossa. Once the condyle is back into its normal skeletal relationship, he could be evaluated for other treatment.

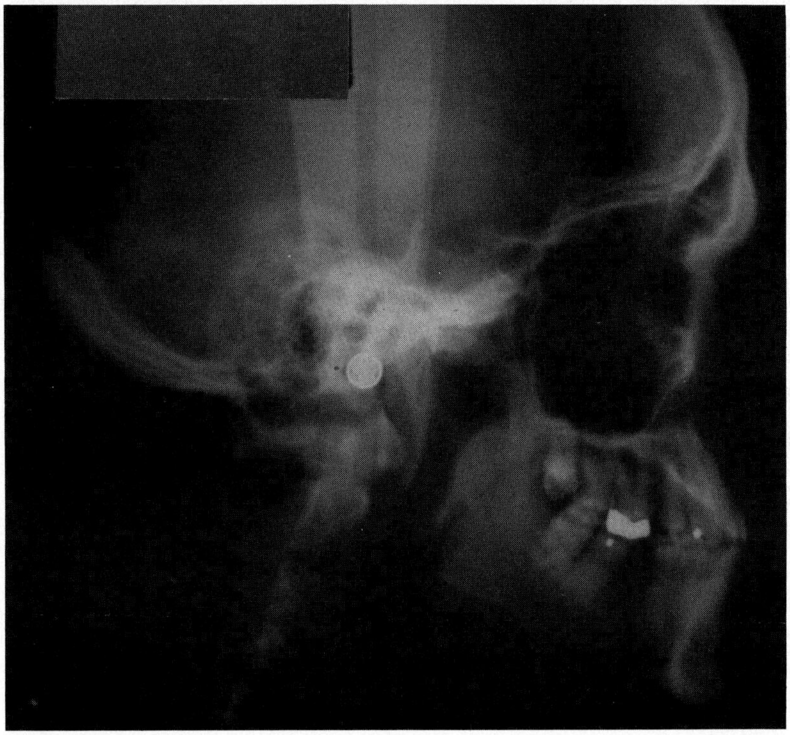

Fig. 9-12. Cephalometric radiograph (J.M.) showing what appears to be a prognathic mandible.

A

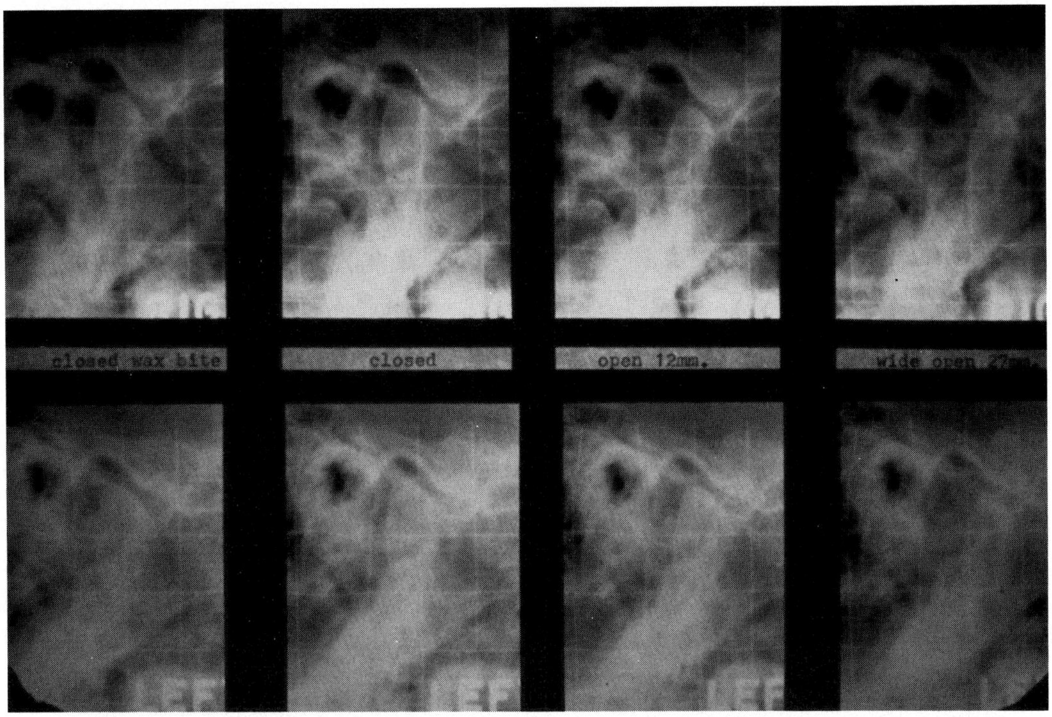

B

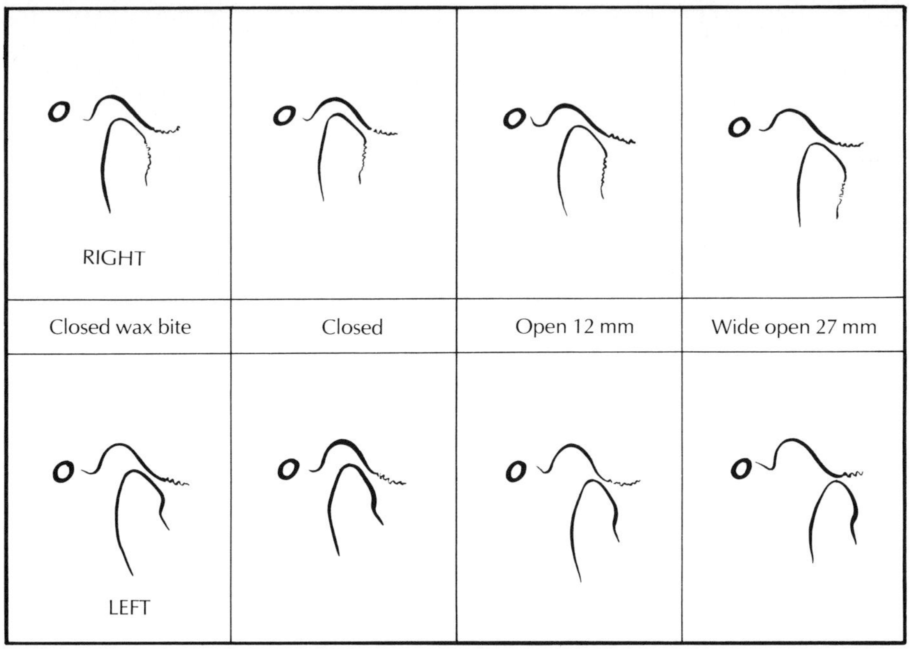

Fig. 9-13. A, Transcranial lateral oblique films (J.M.) showing abnormal anterior position of condyle with relationship to fossa in closed position. **B,** Closed wax-bite view (approximately 2 mm) shows abnormal forward translation of condyle. Flattening of anterior surface of both condyles and erosion of ascending slope of eminence also can be seen.

CASE 5: U.P.

Fig. 9-14 is a unique Panorex film of an individual with congenitally missing condyles. Yet what is most interesting is that this person has fairly normal occlusion. This is a rarity because when both condyles are resorbed or removed surgically, the result is usually an open bite and a retruded mandible.

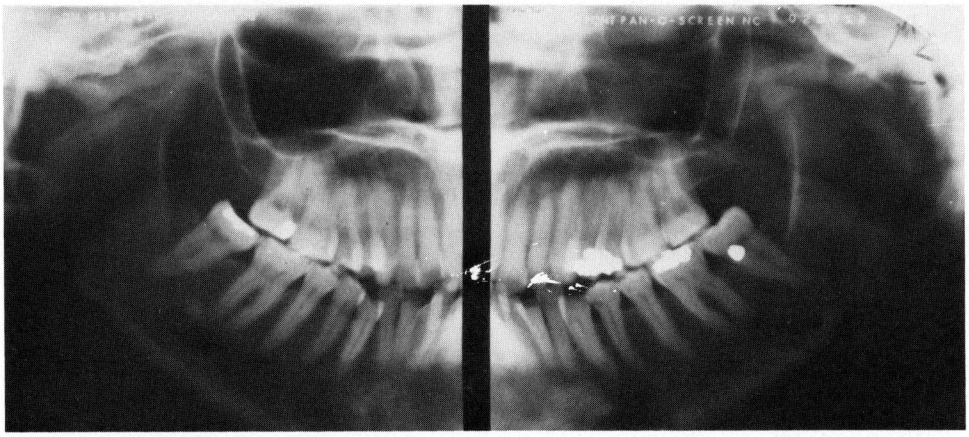

Fig. 9-14. Panorex of individual (U.P.) with congenitally missing condyles.

CASE 6: J.D.

This young man was afflicted with a Class III mandible, or prognathism. His lower jaw was jutting out. However, this is not readily apparent, since his mustache has disguised some of the outline's imperfections. His concern was not the prognathic jaw but the severe ear pains he suffered.

His TMJ questionnaire presented an interesting history. As well as the pain in the ear, for which he had been to numerous ear specialists, there was also pain in the neck, a grating sound in the left joint, and soreness of the facial muscles for the previous 6 years. He had been to an orthodontist. It was his ENT specialist who suspected that his temporomandibular joints might have something to do with his ear problems.

Fig. 9-15, a cephalometric radiograph, makes it easier to observe the prognathic protrusion of the mandible. Orthodontic analysis shows that the latter is a Class III (prognathic) mandible. Orthodontists are helpful in analyzing jaw relationships, particularly when skeletal malrelationships are not readily apparent.

This cephalometric tomogram uses Ricketts' technique.[3] The posterior joint space can be seen, although there is difficulty in seeing the anterior joint space (Fig. 9-16).

Further information is derived from the transcranial lateral oblique film (Fig. 9-17). The narrowing of the joint or disc space can be seen. There is extreme flattening of the eminences. There is some flattening of the condyle and, again, some narrowing on the joint space in the open-mouth view.

The joint space should be maintained evenly in anterior translation. If at any point there is significant narrowing, bone-on-bone contact, or significant widening, this is important. It indicates that pathosis is present.

This case is interesting because the patient had a grating sound, or crepitus, in the left joint. Yet it appears that the eminence is almost flat on one side and nonexistent on the other. In any event, statements have been made that Class III individuals, having prognathic jaws, do not have temporomandibular joint problems, since the condyles do not translate over the eminences in a normal way. This is not always true. This patient's eminences were flat, not from being worn down by

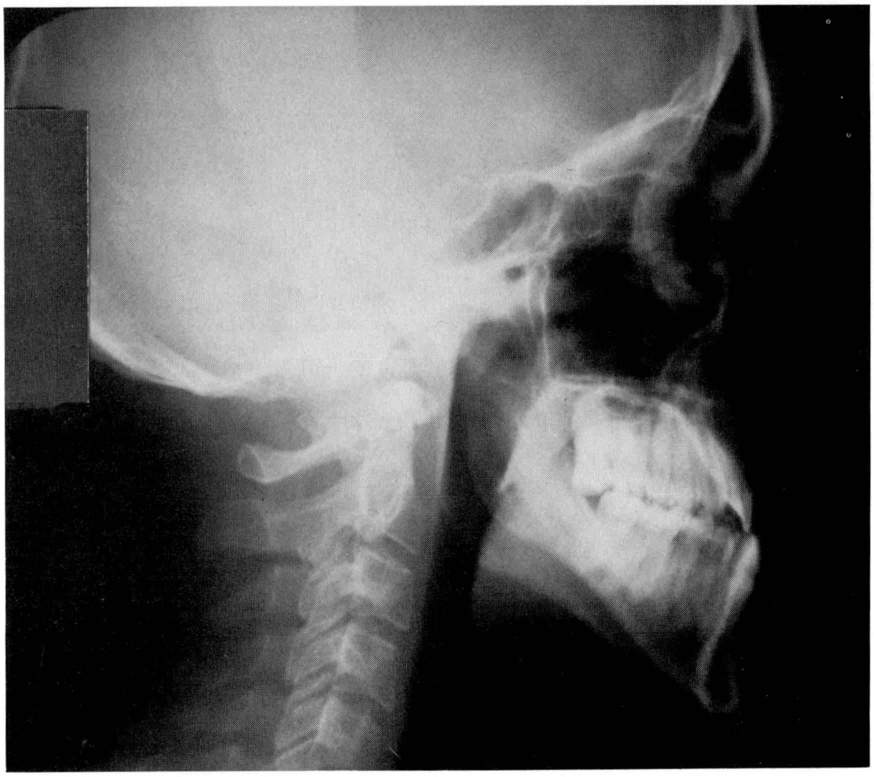

Fig. 9-15. Cephalometric radiograph of patient (J.D.) showing true prognathic condition of mandible in relation to maxilla.

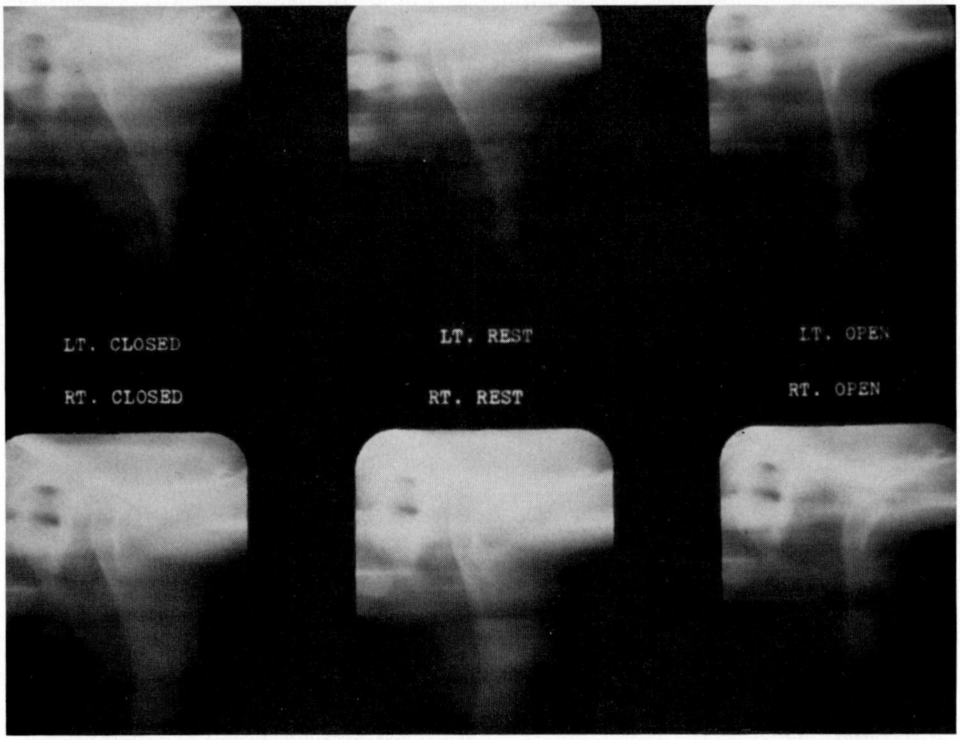

Fig. 9-16. Cephalometric tomogram of same patient (J.D.) showing three functional views. Note how difficult it is to see anterior joint space.

A

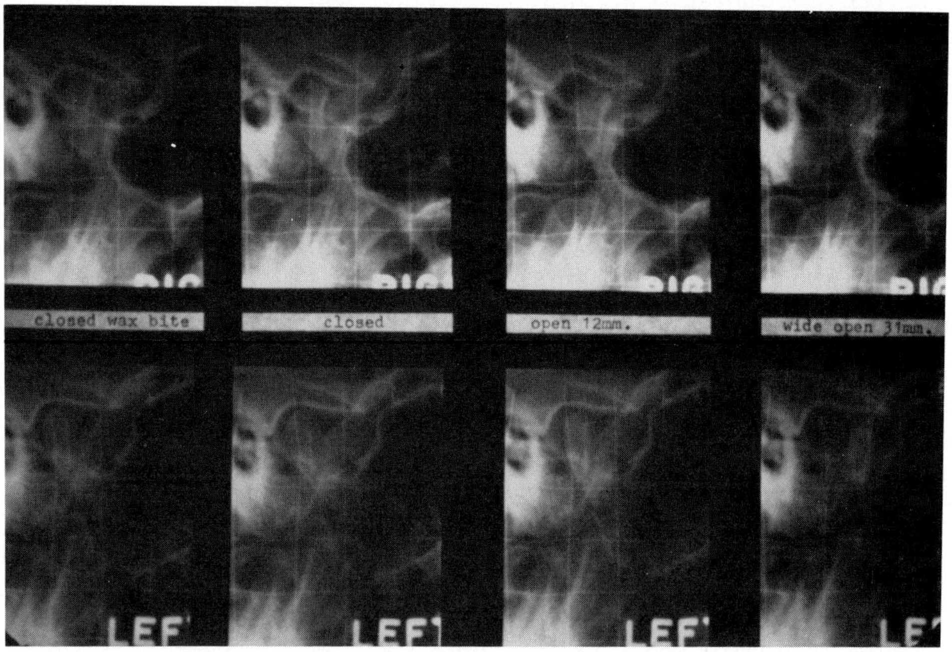

B

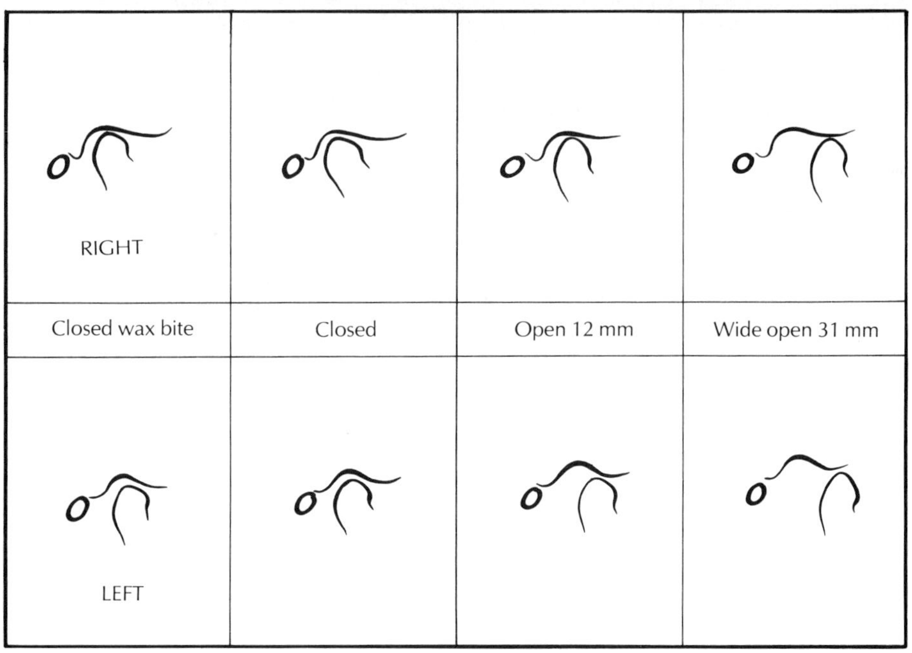

Fig. 9-17. A, Transcranial lateral oblique radiographs of individual (J.D.) with Class III occlusion, showing flattening of both eminences, particularly left. **B,** Asymmetrical condylar functioning can be seen in 12-mm view. Bone-on-bone contact of condyle to eminence can be seen in wide-open (31-mm) view in right joint.

overuse but from never having been developed. The condyles translating over the eminences stimulate their growth and development.

This young man had a restoration of the eminences on both sides and has been helped (Fig. 9-18). Orthognathic surgery also may be done to restore the mandible to a more normal position. In one prior case of a prognathic jaw operated on with insertion of a TMJ prosthesis, correction of the prognathism was not necessary after the arthritic problem was helped.

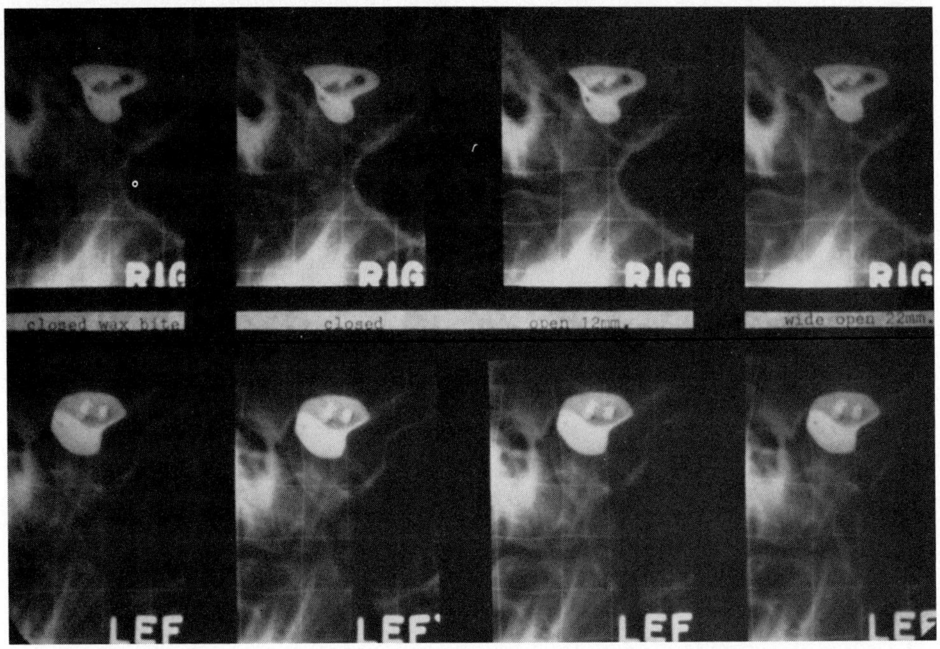

Fig. 9-18. Postoperative transcranial lateral oblique films with articular eminence prosthesis restoring shape of eminence, with functional views.

CASE 7: A.F.

A.F., a young woman, had a bone tumor of the temporomandibular joint. It can be seen that the regular films taken in the hospital are not too helpful diagnostically (Figs. 9-19 and 9-20). The tumor was on the right side. In the anteroposterior view it is difficult to see the temporomandibular joint (Fig. 9-21). An anteroposterior view using xeroradiography of this joint showed the tumor clearly on the right side (Fig. 9-22).

In this case acupuncture anesthesia was used. She could not open her mouth and had generalized rheumatoid arthritis. It would have been impossible to orally or nasally intubate her; otherwise a tracheotomy would have to have been performed. During the operation with A.F. under the acupuncture anesthesia no premedication and no local anesthesia were used. Some electrical stimulation of the needles was applied. The patient was able to talk to the surgeons throughout the entire procedure and open her mouth and afterward needed no pain medication. The pathosis was a benign tumor (an osteoma). It had distorted the anatomy of the condyle and the areas of the zygoma. Multiple views of the tomograms and xeroradiographs were taken to sort it out to obtain more information (Fig. 9-23).

Fig. 9-24 shows the normal side, in which the condyle can be seen again, as well as the area of the articular eminence–mandibular fossa. The utility of the four-view method with xeroradiography is being explored to determine whether additional information can be obtained.

Fig. 9-25 is a radiograph of the same patient using the specialized TMJ films. It shows the left joint well. However, the right joint, where the tumor is located, is not seen as clearly as with the xeroradiography. Different techniques must be used for different problems.

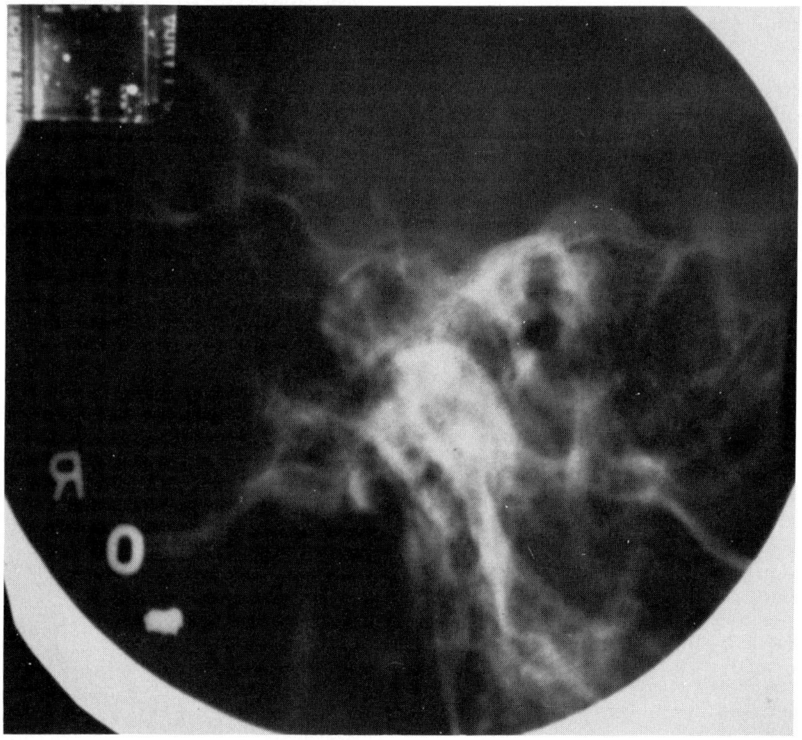

Fig. 9-19. Lateral view of right temporomandibular joint of patient (A.F.), using standard radiographic hospital techniques.

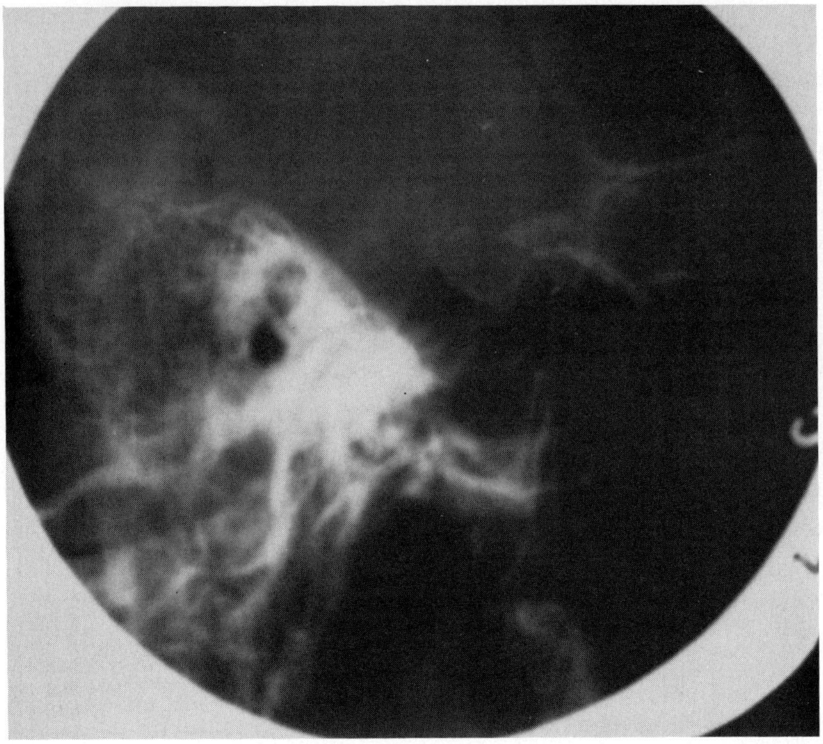

Fig. 9-20. Lateral view of left temporomandibular joint of same patient (A.F.), using standard radiographic hospital techniques.

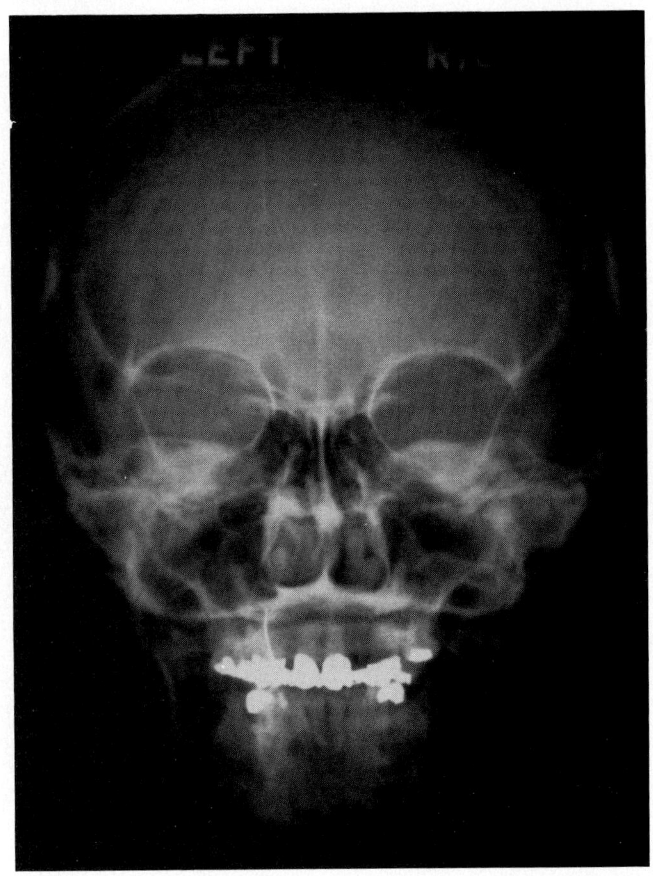

Fig. 9-21. Anteroposterior view of patient (A.F.).

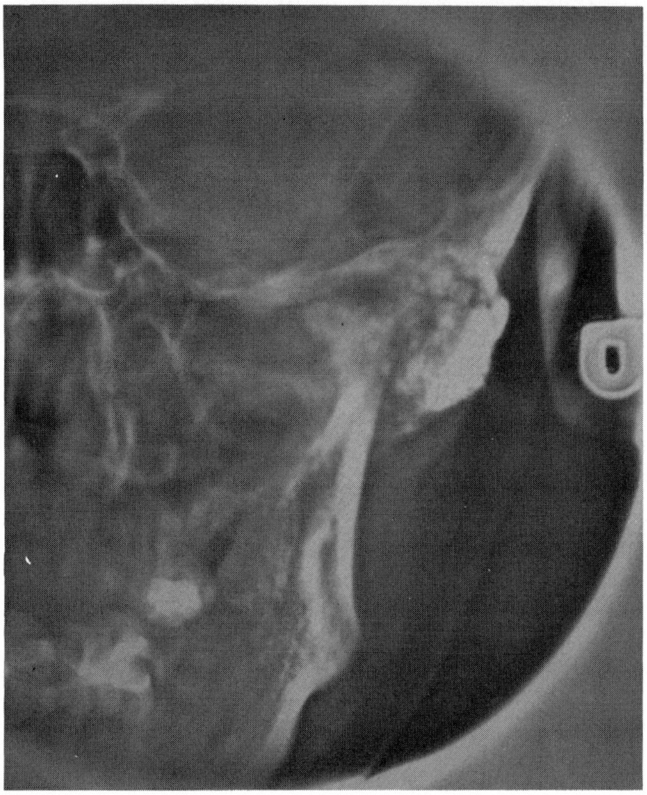

Fig. 9-22. Anteroposterior view employing xeroradiography technique. Condyle and bony tumor can be clearly seen.

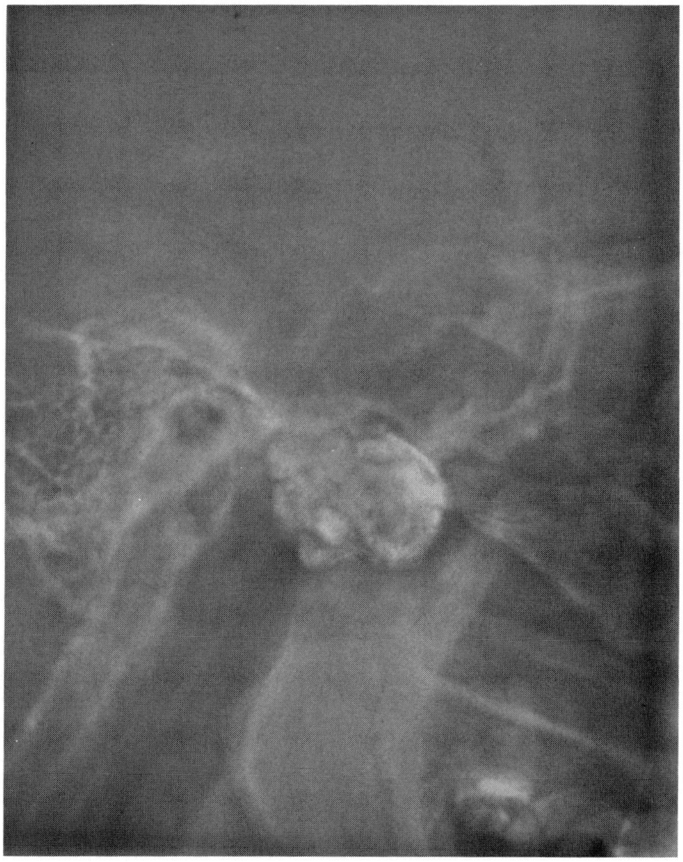

Fig. 9-23. Xeroradiography of tomographic section of right temporomandibular joint showing extent of tumor.

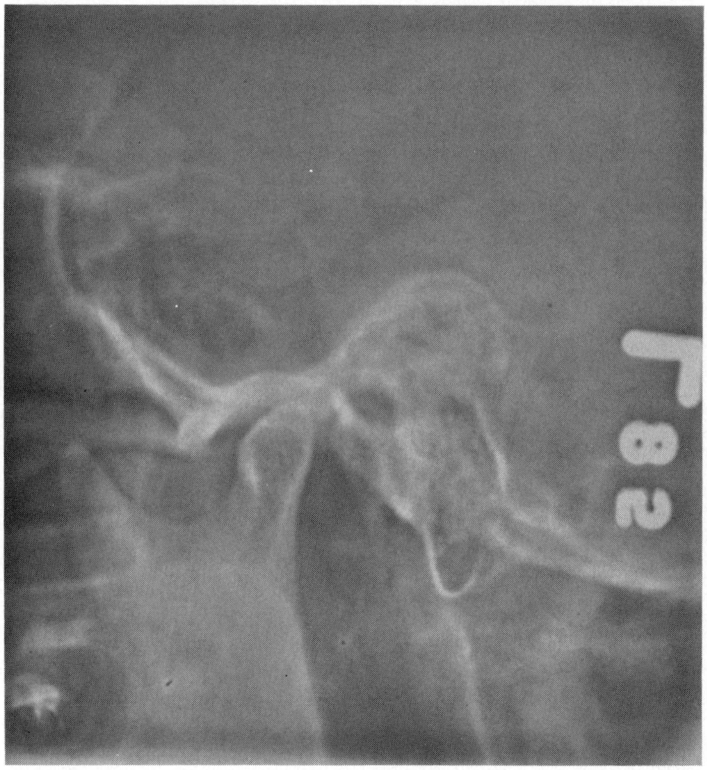

Fig. 9-24. Tomogram of left temporomandibular joint (normal side), using xeroradiography technique.

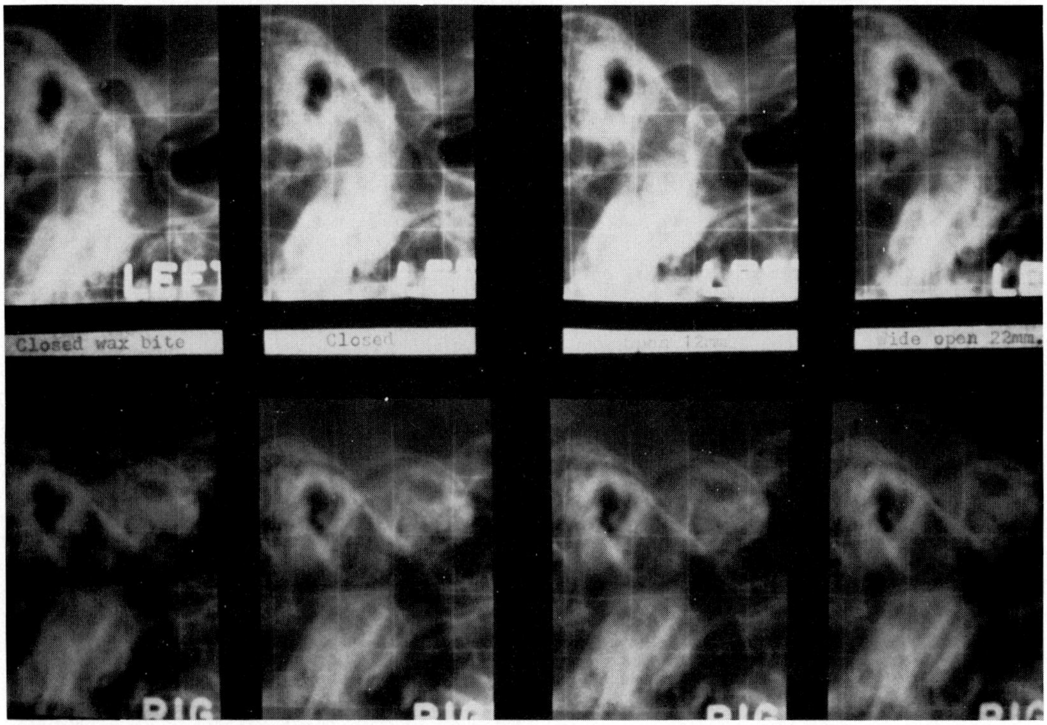

Fig. 9-25. Transcranial lateral oblique films with four views of patient (A.F.).

CASE 8: S.B.

S.B., a young woman, was unable to open her mouth. Standard hospital radiographic techniques were employed in these radiographs (Figs. 9-26 and 9-27). It is hard to discern the temporomandibular joint in the center of the picture, which demonstrates the difficulty in evaluating this type of radiograph. This is a good case for illustrating the importance of diagnostic TMJ radiographs. In this view of the temporomandibular joint the landmarks cannot be seen readily. The radiographic interpretation would be difficult, and equivocation would have to be used. From these films it would be difficult to know whether the patient had a bony or fibrous ankylosis or whether the right, left, or both joints were involved. Specialized TMJ films were taken with her mouth forced open 1/4 inch (Fig. 9-28). It was noted from the films that both eminences were almost flat and the disc spaces diminished (Fig. 9-29).

The right condyle did translate, so it was decided to operate only on the left condyle. The anesthetist attempted to blind-nasally intubate her for nearly an hour. It was necessary to do a tracheotomy. Five days after surgery she was able to open over 1 1/2 inches (Fig. 9-30). It is interesting to note that succinylcholine (Anectine) did not break the spasm of her jaw. In some individuals it may be that the muscle group of the jaws is the last striated muscle to be affected by the drug.

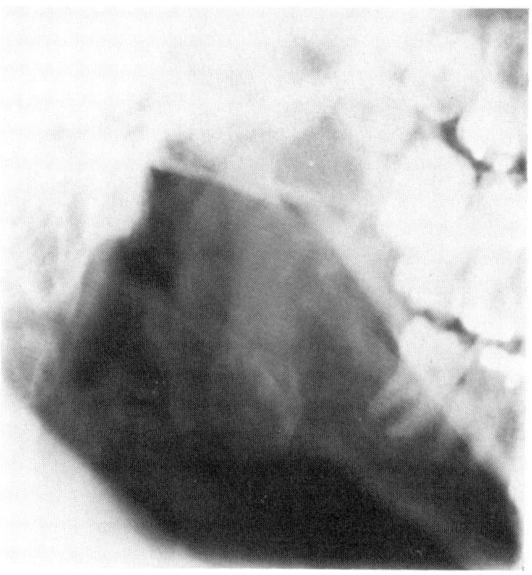

Fig. 9-26. Closed view of right temporomandibular joint of S.B., using standard radiographic hospital techniques.

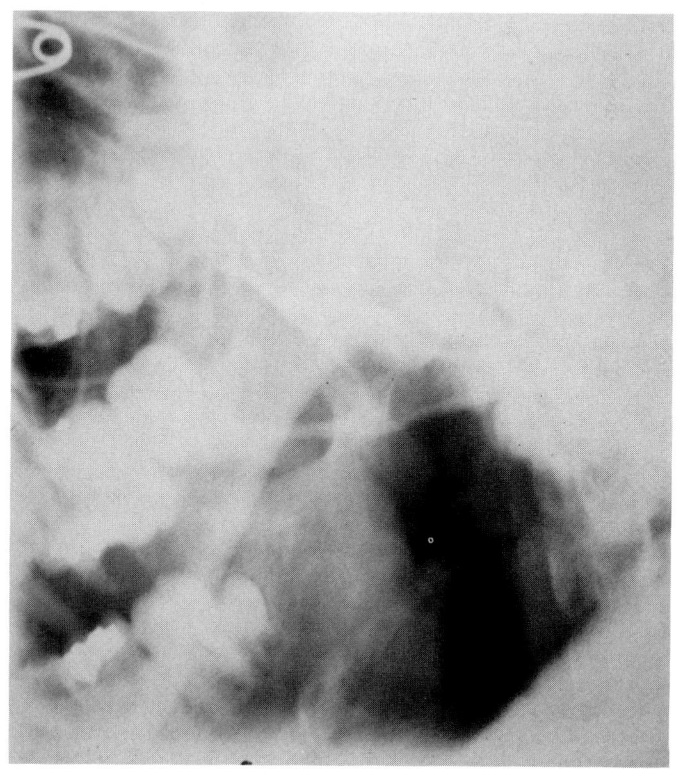

Fig. 9-27. Closed view of left temporomandibular joint, using standard radiographic hospital techniques.

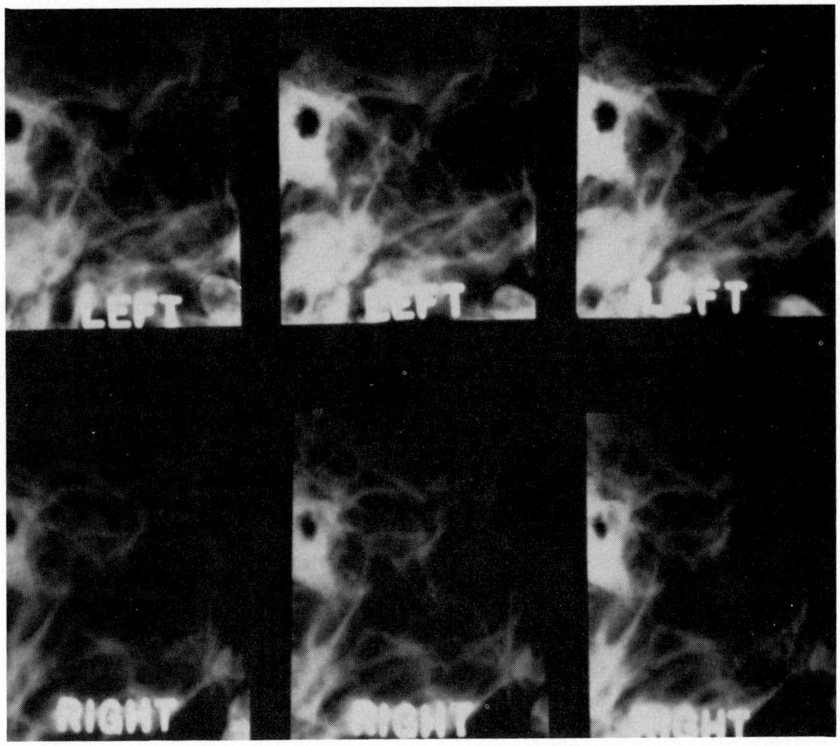

Fig. 9-28. Transcranial lateral oblique films of patient forcing mouth open approximately $^{1}/_{4}$ inch.

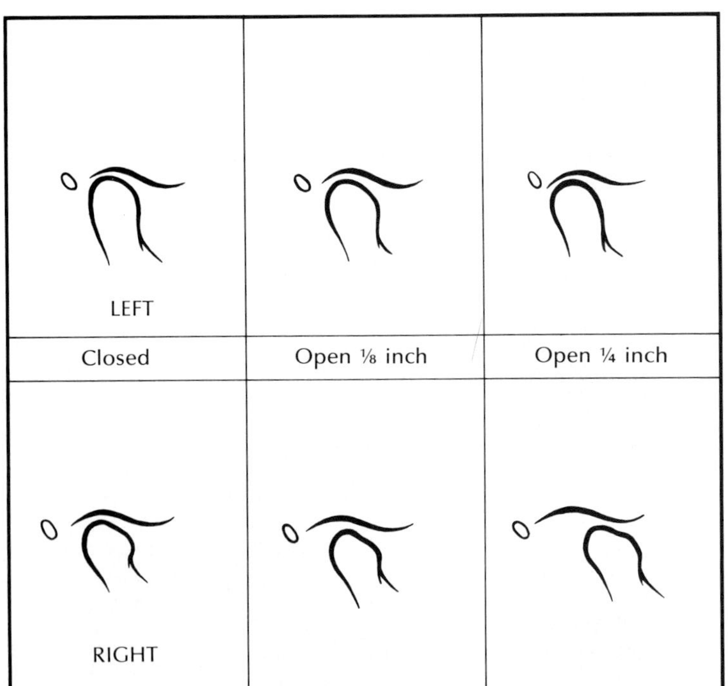

Fig. 9-29. Line drawings of transcranial lateral oblique films showing flattening of eminences, some disc space, and some movement of right condyle.

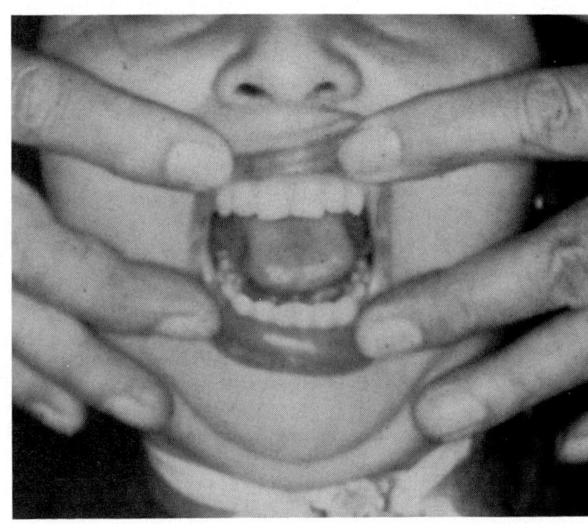

Fig. 9-30. Patient (S.B.) 5 days after surgery, able to open mouth interincisally over $1^{1}/_{2}$ inches.

CASE 9: G.S.

The report to the referring physician on a temporomandibular joint x-ray examination of this patient stated the following:

Examination: Temporomandibular joints: neutral, open-mouth, and closed-mouth positions, Towne views.
Radiological consultation: The temporomandibular joints are well visualized on the various views. The articular margins and articular heads of the condyles are well visualized and appear well preserved. No evidence of sclerotic change or erosion of the margins can be identified. There is limitation of excursion.
Summary: No evidence of osseous abnormality. Limitation of excursion noted in the open-mouth views.

The radiographs that the radiologist used were excellent. In the closed and open views they showed that there was diminishing of the disc space on the right side. However, the radiologist probably attributed this lack of disc space to a change in angulation of the patient's head in relation to the cassette (Fig. 9-31).

As the report then stated, this lady had severe headaches on the right side, but "The joints are visualized in the various views" (Fig. 9-32). "The articular margin and articular head of the condyle are visualized and appear well preserved. No evidence of bony change or erosive margins could be identified." After receiving this letter of negative pathosis, the patient went to a psychiatrist, thinking that her problems must be emotional.

With the transcranial lateral oblique films of the same woman (Fig. 9-33, *A*) it can be seen that the joint space is reduced. There is almost a bone-on-bone configuration on the right side where there is some condylar motion. The apparent decrease in condylar motion, which was thought to be possibly within normal limits for this patient, is misleading. Condylar motion has occurred, but the joint space is narrow, so that there is a different problem here. It is not a condylar motion problem, suggesting ankylosis or a muscle spasm. However, there is some alteration of the joint. If the patient is in pain, he or she will open only as much as can be done comfortably. Sometimes the patient will be able to open to a minimum amount, and this will be recorded.

Fig. 9-33, *B*, is a line drawing describing the same process. The irregularity shown here is probably more of a demineralization of the joint. Condylar motion is occurring. Again, the joint space narrowing indicates the pathosis.

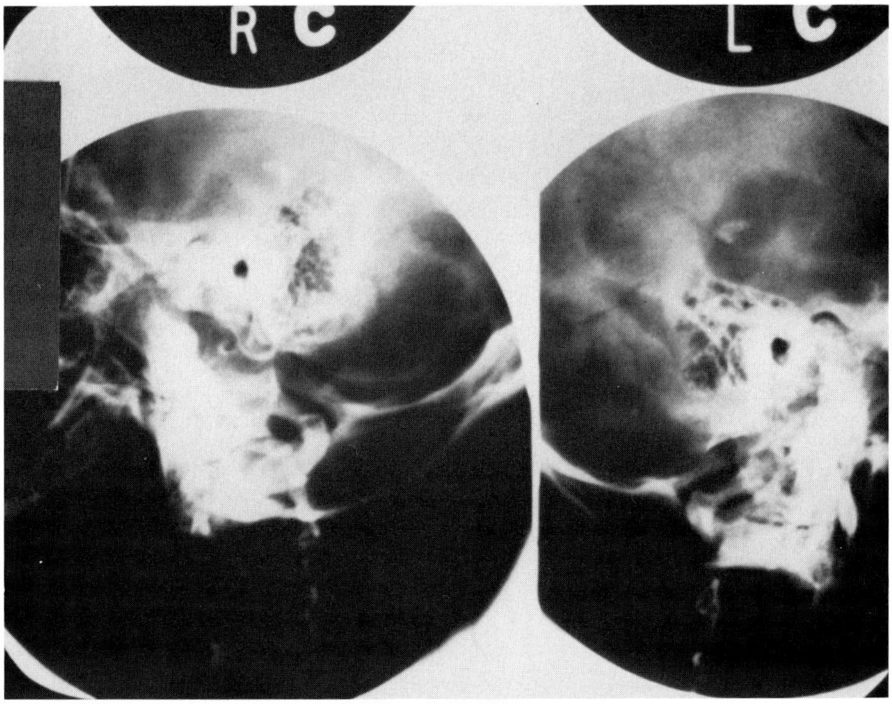

Fig. 9-31. Right and left temporomandibular joints shown in closed view, using standard hospital radiographic technique.

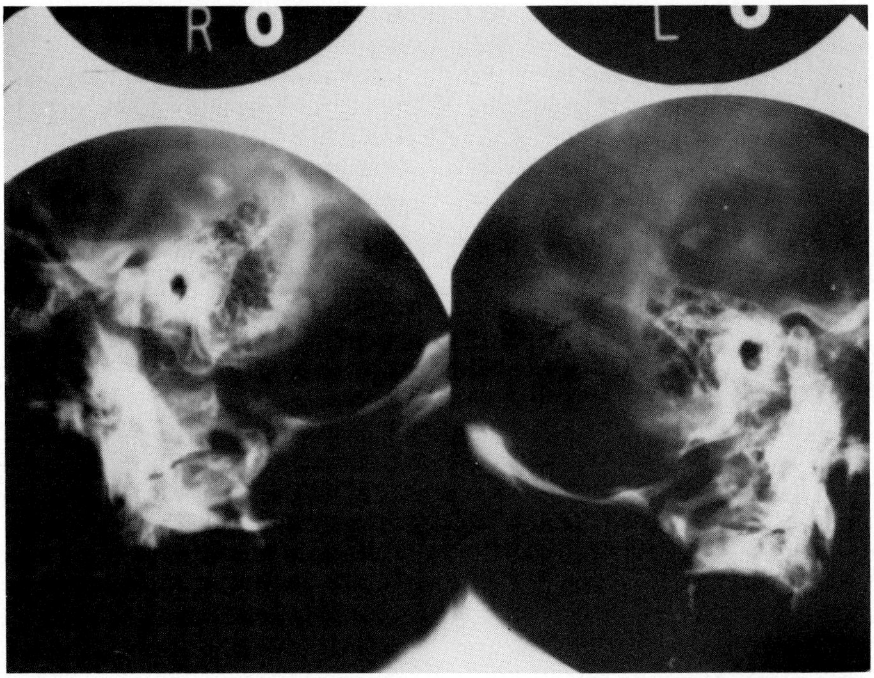

Fig. 9-32. Right and left temporomandibular joints shown in open view, using standard hospital radiographic technique.

A

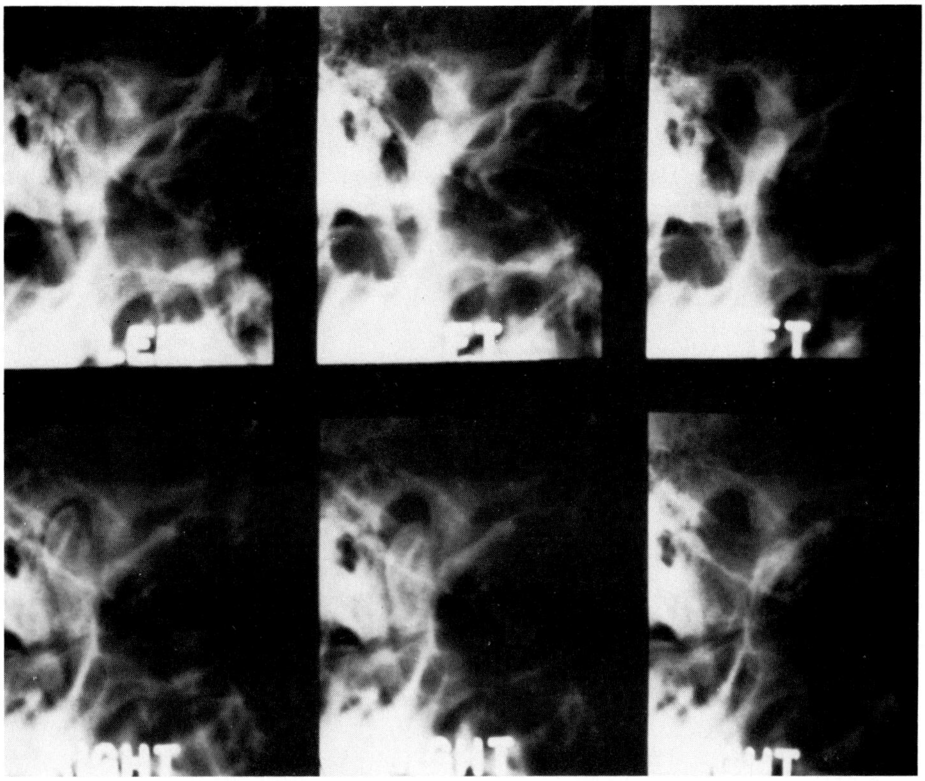

B

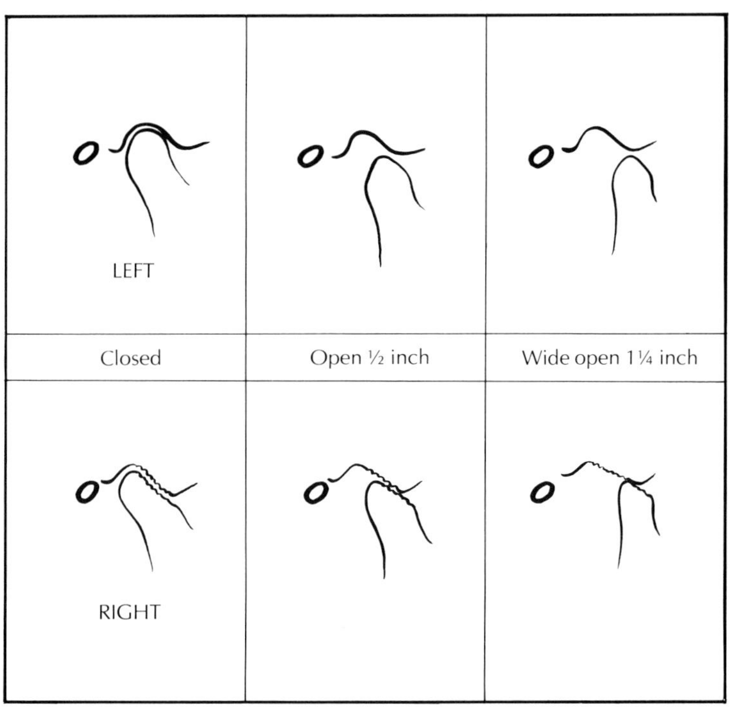

Fig. 9-33. A, Transcranial lateral oblique films of patient (G.S.) showing diminished disc space in right joint and flattening and erosion of right eminence (with some flattening and erosion of left eminence also). **B,** Line drawings of transcranial lateral oblique films accentuating what is seen in x-ray technique. There appears to be bone-on-bone contact in right joint.

CASE 10: C.S.

C.S. was referred by an oral surgeon. Radon seeds can be seen in the upper right TMJ area. The young woman had had a mixed-cell tumor of the left parotid gland removed surgically some years previously. When she developed pain in the right side and swelling, the surgeons thought it was the same problem as on the opposite side. They removed the parotid gland and introduced radon seeds to prevent a recurrence. This was accomplished, but there was no change in the patient's signs and symptoms.

The problem can be seen in these radiographs (Fig. 9-34, *A*). The narrowing of the joint space has occurred on this side, and the narrowing is maintained through the excursion of the condyle. There is decreased condylar motion as well. It also can be noted that the right articular eminence is flattened. This young woman's symptoms mimicked a parotid tumor because the synovial pressure within the capsular ligament caused swelling. After TMJ surgery and placement of a prosthesis her symptoms subsided. This is an example of why disease of the temporomandibular joint is designated "the great imposter."

A

B

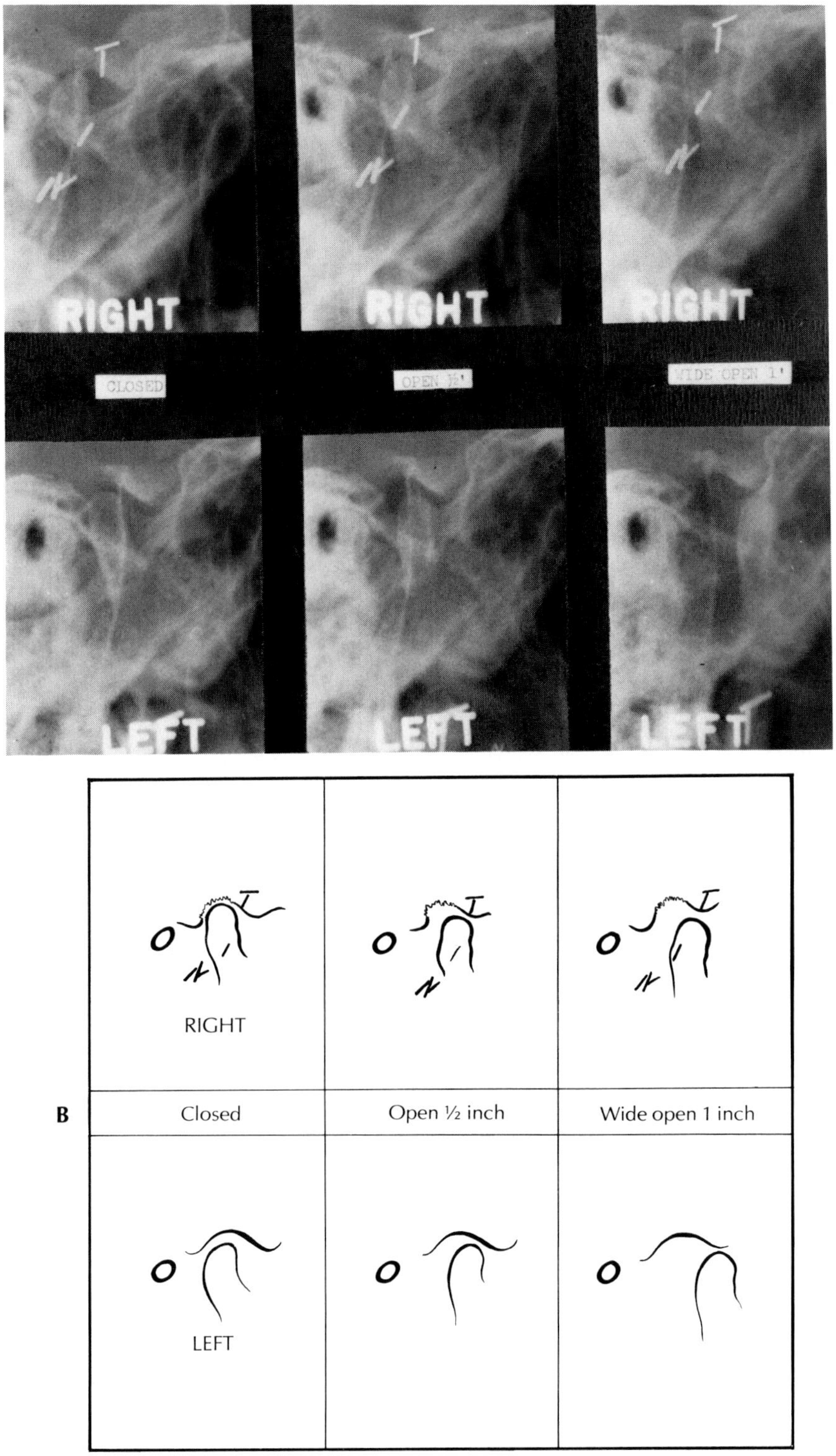

Fig. 9-34. A, Transcranial lateral oblique films of patient (C.S.) showing radon seeds after parotidectomy and diminished disc space, erosion of cortical bone over right eminence, and flattening of eminence. **B,** Line drawings show in closed view condyle tightly placed in fossa. There is erosion of cortical bone in upper aspect of fossa as well as flattening of articular eminence. In left joint can be seen diminished disc space in all views but minimum damage to cortical layer of bone over joint surface.

CASE 11: C.A.

C.A. had been seen by a large otological medical group, which had done a complete diagnostic workup (Fig. 9-35, *A*). The patient's primary symptoms were dizziness and some ringing in his left ear, but no pain. Had it not been for the medical group's awareness of the various symptoms of temporomandibular joint pathology, the man might still be without help.

In this study there is a narrowing of the joint space, and in the wide-open mouth view there is almost a bone-on-bone relationship. The condylar motion on both sides is somewhat decreased (more on the right side compared with the left). The decrease in the joint space indicates a soft-tissue change. The narrowing of the joint space is always significant (Fig. 9-35, *B*). Another change that can occur is the deformity of the bony anatomy—the articular eminence, mandibular fossa, or condyle. Irregularity or demineralization in the narrowing of the joint space can be seen. This points out the importance of good radiographs. Without these radiographs there would have been little clinical evidence that this man's dizziness, or vertigo, had anything to do with the temporomandibular joint. His dizziness was eliminated by placement of an articular eminence prosthesis on the left side. He still has slight tinnitus in one ear.

A

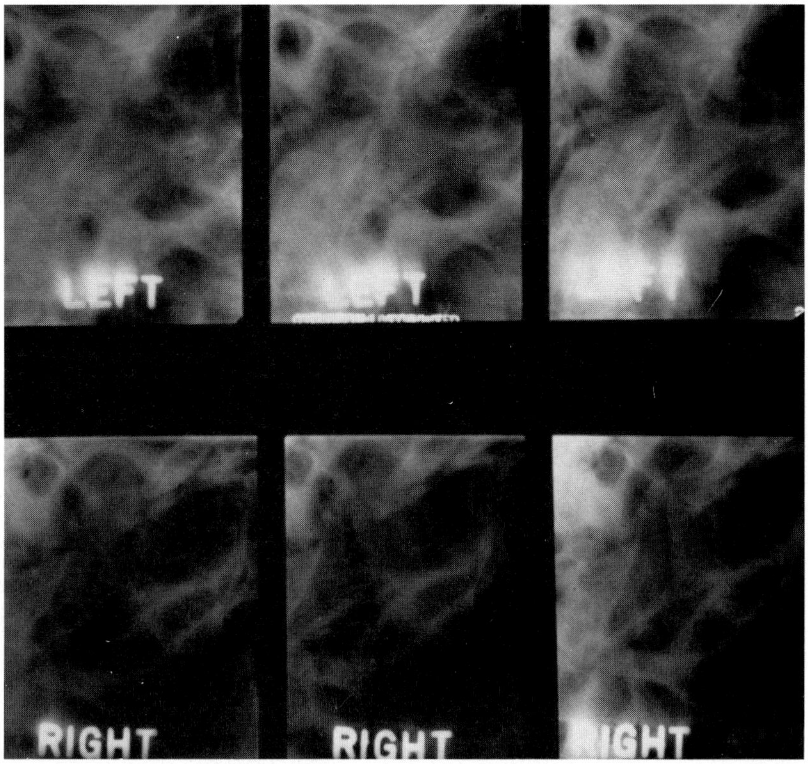

B

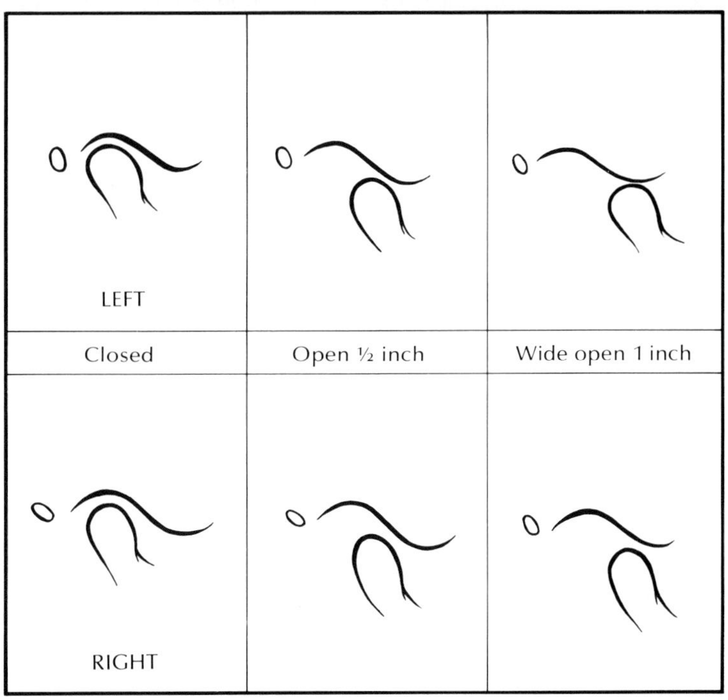

Fig. 9-35. A, Transcranial lateral oblique films of patient (C.A.) showing erosion of left eminence. **B,** Line drawings of patient (C.A.) showing flattening of anterior condylar head, diminished disc space, and bone-on-bone contact of left condyle to eminence in wide-open view.

CASE 12: M.C.R.

Fig. 9-36, *A*, presents views of a woman who had severe tongue pains on the left side. She was chronically subluxated on the left side. On this side in the closed-mouth position it is seen that the condyle is subluxated, and only slight motion has occurred on opening her mouth. On the right side the condyle's location is somewhat more normal, but there is still abnormality. Movement of the condyle is slight. This again illustrates the importance of the dynamic as-

A

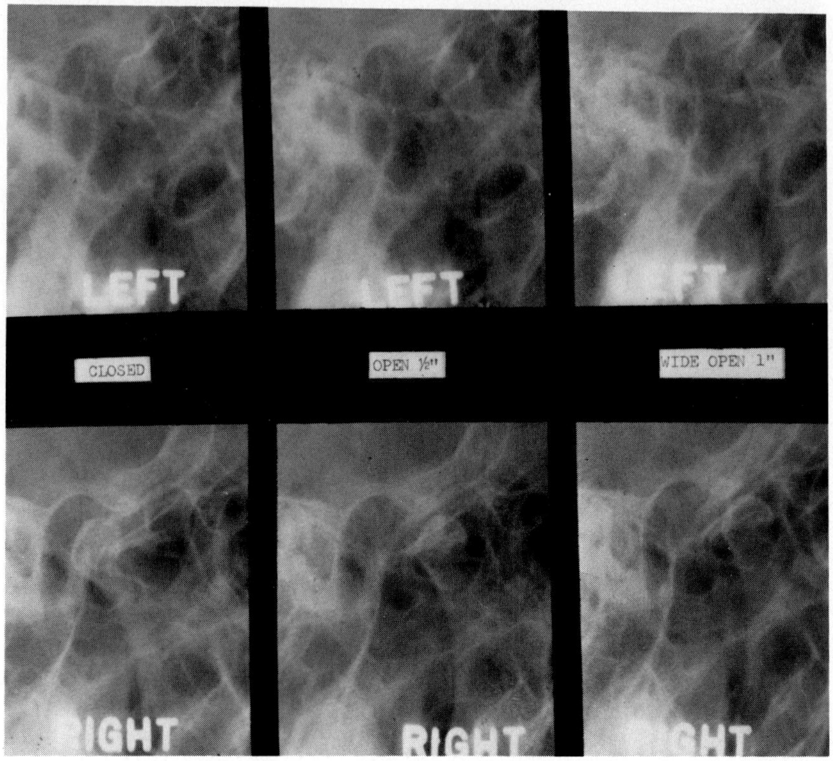

B

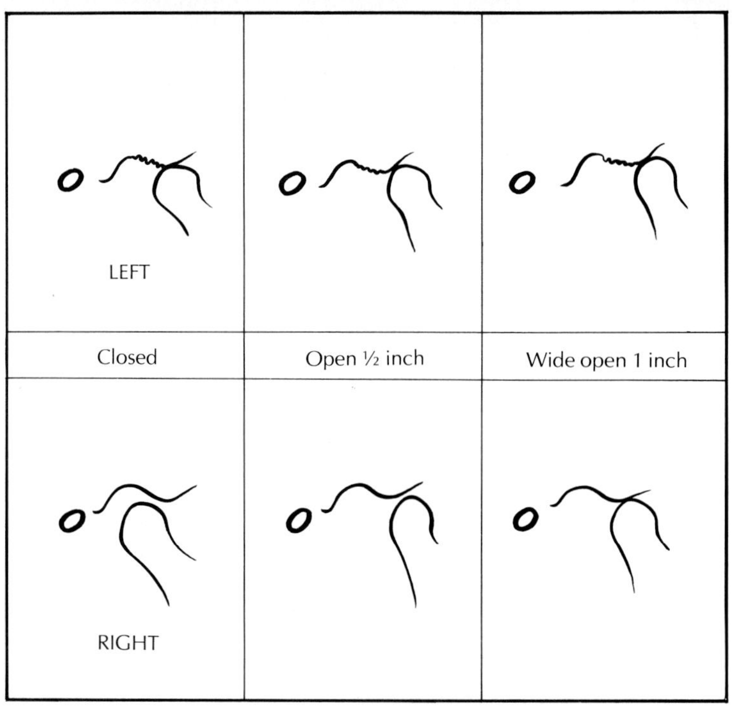

Fig. 9-36. A, TMJ films showing severe chronic subluxation of left condyle and, to lesser degree, right condyle. **B,** Line drawings showing bone-on-bone contact to eminence and abnormal functioning of both right and left joints.

pects of this particular radiography (Fig. 9-36, *B*).

In the radiographs taken after restoration of the joint with a prosthesis the condyle is back in its normal position. One interesting aspect of this case is that the woman had a bad occlusion initially, but it did not seem too abnormal at the time (Fig. 9-37). Apparently she had adapted and was chewing satisfactorily in her opinion. The left condyle is seen in a normal position with more normal movement within the articular eminence–glenoid fossa.

A

B

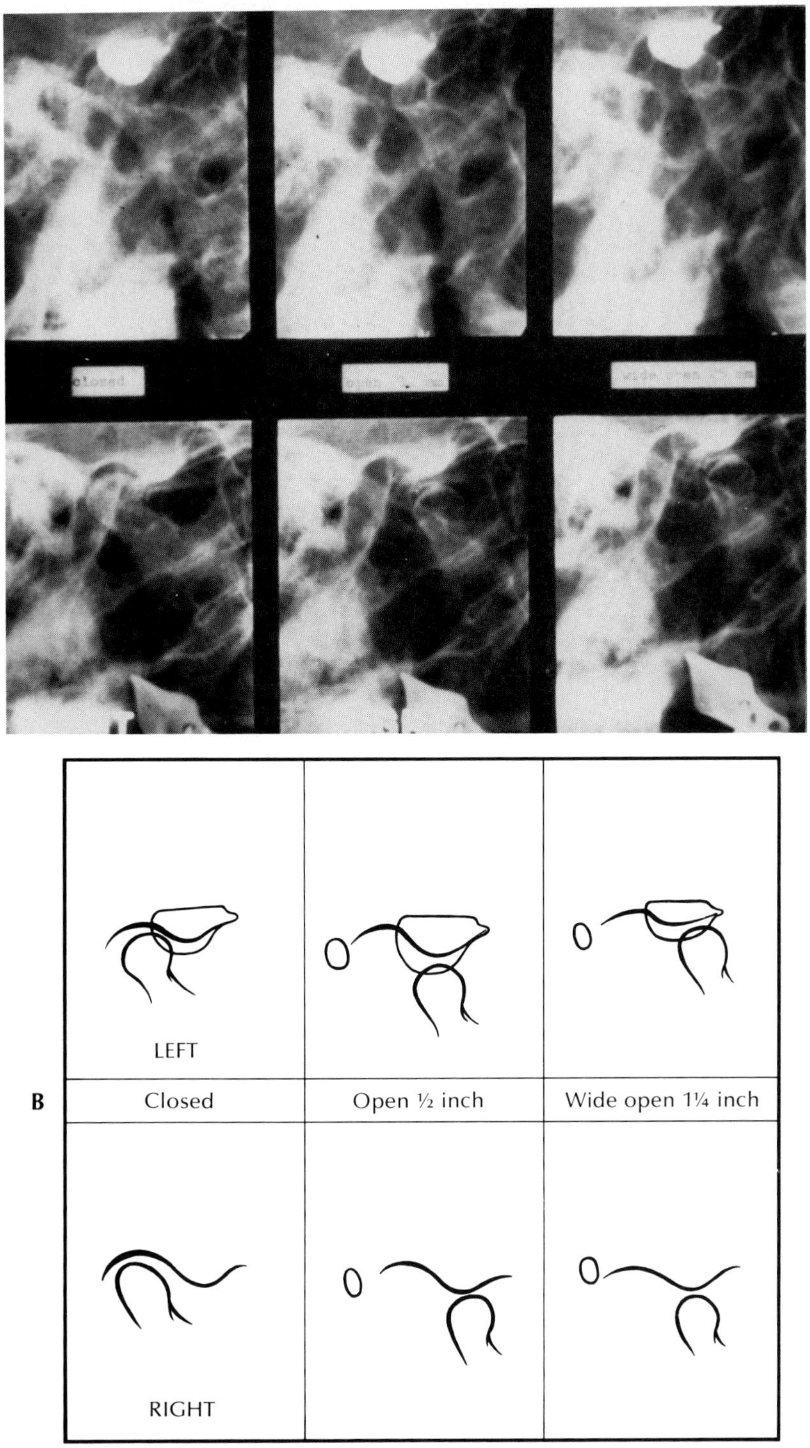

Fig. 9-37. A, Transcranial lateral oblique films of patient (M.C.R.) showing both condyles in normal position, functioning normally. **B,** Line drawings depicting normal functional movement after restoration of left articular eminence with implant.

CASE 13: E.K.

The specialized TMJ radiographs in Fig. 9-38 depict an ex-Navy nurse who is a registered narcotics addict. The radiopaque material obscuring some of the views was used in myelography, an x-ray procedure of the spine, since she had severe pain of her head and neck. The reason for her pain could not be determined, and she became addicted to narcotics.

The radiographs reveal severe compression of the disc in the right joint. Most of the pain was on the right side, with some pain on the left. On both sides the condyle is in an anterior position in the closed-mouth view. This is because of the pull of the external pterygoid muscles. There is also a flattening of the eminence in the left joint. The woman refused treatment; she had adjusted to her addiction.

A

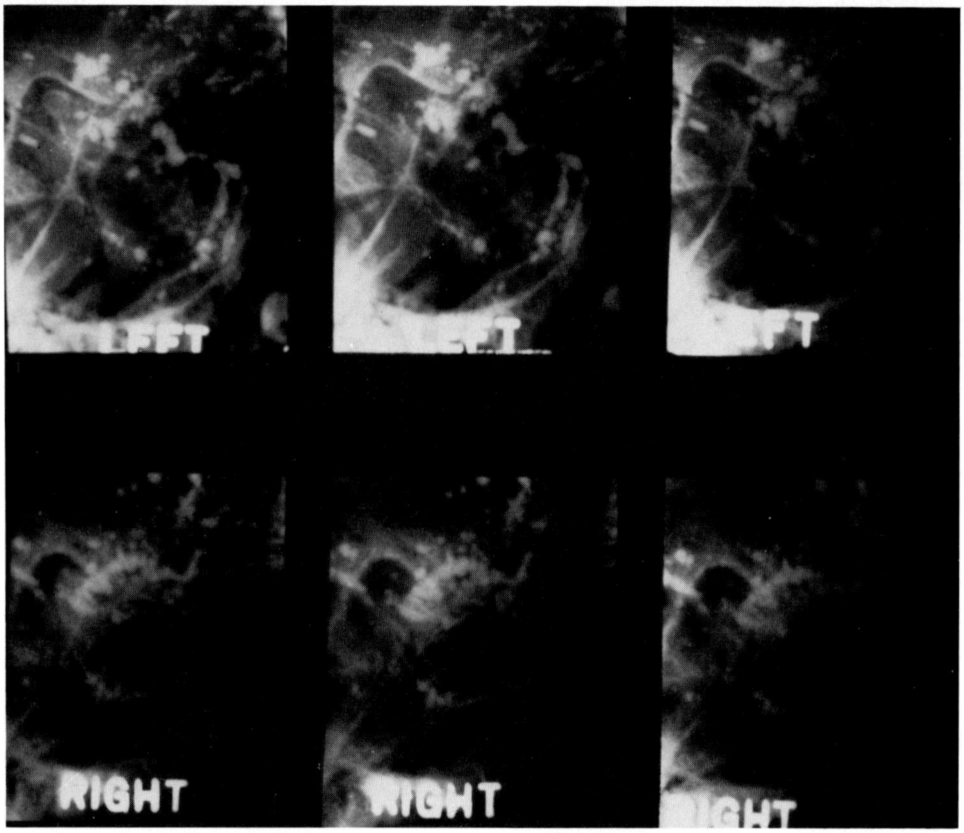

B

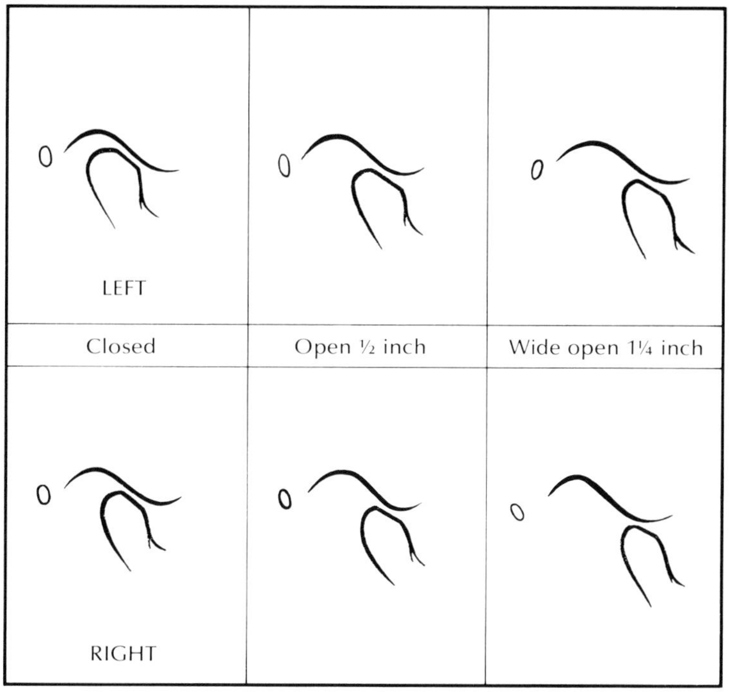

Fig. 9-38. A, Transcranial lateral oblique films of patient (E.K.) showing in closed view abnormal anterior position of both right and left condyles. Condyles are obscured by opaque medium. **B,** Line drawings of radiographs showing flattening of both eminences and diminished disc space, particularly on right side, and flattening of anterior aspect of both condyles.

CASE 14: J.A.

This young man had a history of recurrent Bell's palsy affecting the left side of his face. In his first attack he was completely paralyzed for $1^1/_2$ months. Gradually the muscle function returned, with some weakness. However, he had attacks several times a year. He had been complaining of an earache in the left ear since the first attack of Bell's palsy. The radiograph revealed a diminished disc space in the left joint compared with the right (Fig. 9-39).

The condylar movement was asymmetrical. There was also a flattening of the left articular eminence and erosion of the cortical layer of bone over the descending and ascending slopes of the eminence. Surgery was performed with insertion of an articular eminence prosthesis, primarily to help with the ear pain. The ear pain subsided. Interestingly, there were no further attacks of Bell's palsy, and the weakness of the facial muscles was eliminated.

It is interesting to note that some of the anatomical research states there are branches of the facial nerve that go to the capsule of the temporomandibular joint.[4] It is possible that some types of Bell's palsy are caused by a temporomandibular dysfunction. The patient's sister had a similar problem with ear pain and Bell's palsy. A similar procedure was performed, and she was relieved of her symptoms also. Their younger brother also was affected but was helped by nonsurgical treatment.

A

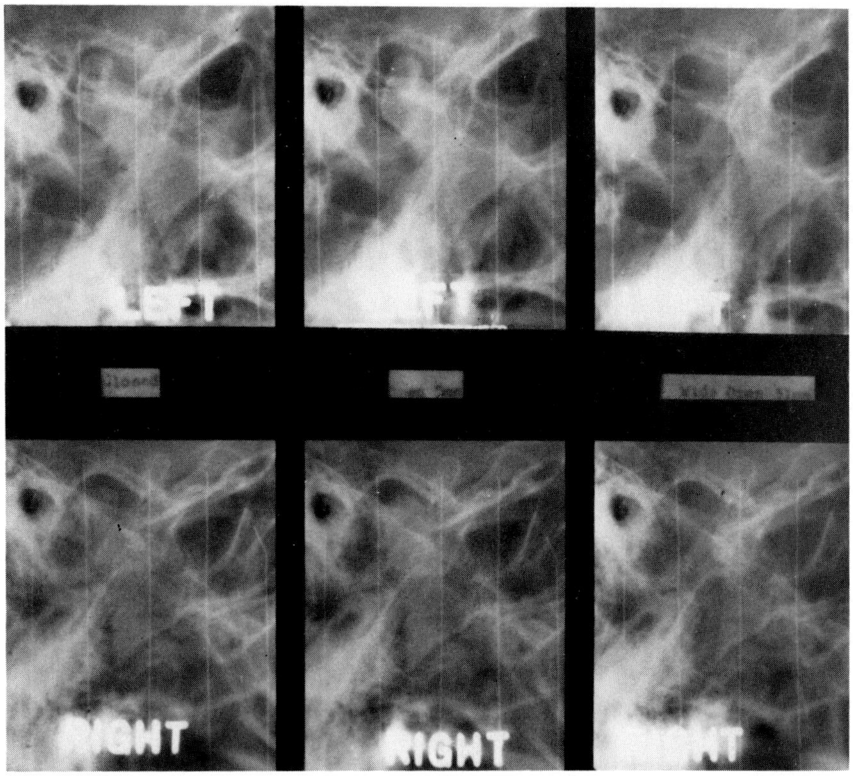

B

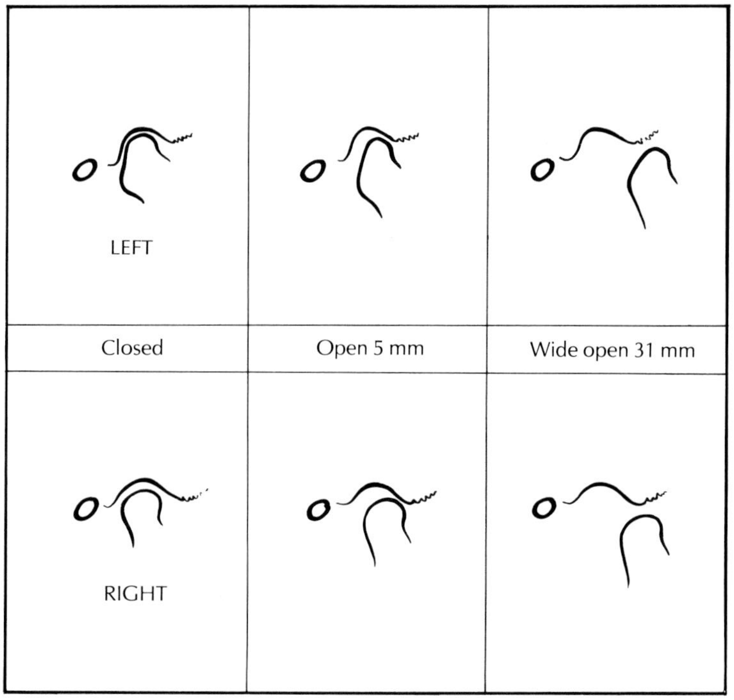

Fig. 9-39. A, Transcranial lateral oblique films of patient (J.A.) showing diminished disc space in left joint and flattening of condylar hear. **B,** Line drawings showing in both right and left joints erosion of cortical layer of bone over ascending slope of eminence.

CASE 15: B.N.

A 12-year-old girl was referred by an oral surgeon who had seen her for several months. Her main symptom was chronic subluxation, which was so severe that it occurred several times a week. Her teeth had been wired together, but the wires were broken by the subluxation. She had been to at least 15 specialists in the previous year, had dropped out of school, and was undergoing psychiatric treatment.

Specialized TMJ radiographs showed a flattening of both articular eminences (Fig. 9-40). There was significantly more flattening in the right joint, with osteogenic activity affecting the periphery of the eminence, a slight lagging in functional movement of the right condyle in comparison with the left, and a clicking sound in both joints on movement.

She had a history of bruxism and tooth clenching during the prior 6 years. It appeared that these habits had worn down the eminences. Therefore it was easy for the external pterygoid muscles to go into spasm and pull the condyles out of position. Surgery was performed on only the right joint. A prosthesis was inserted, and it restored the contour of the eminence. Since the surgery, the patient has been free from functional problems, and her pain has subsided.

A

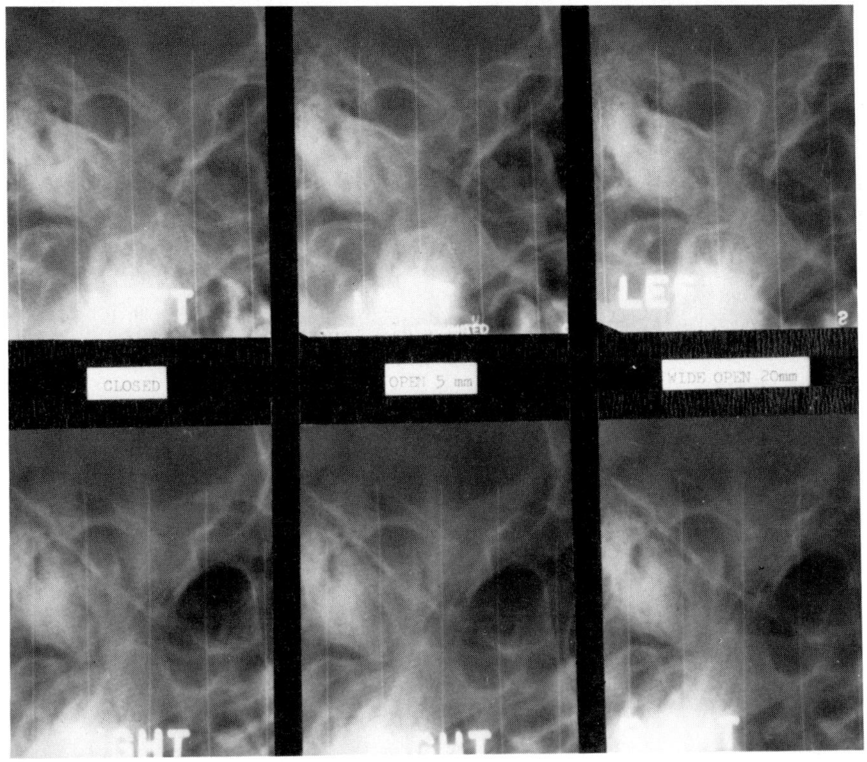

B

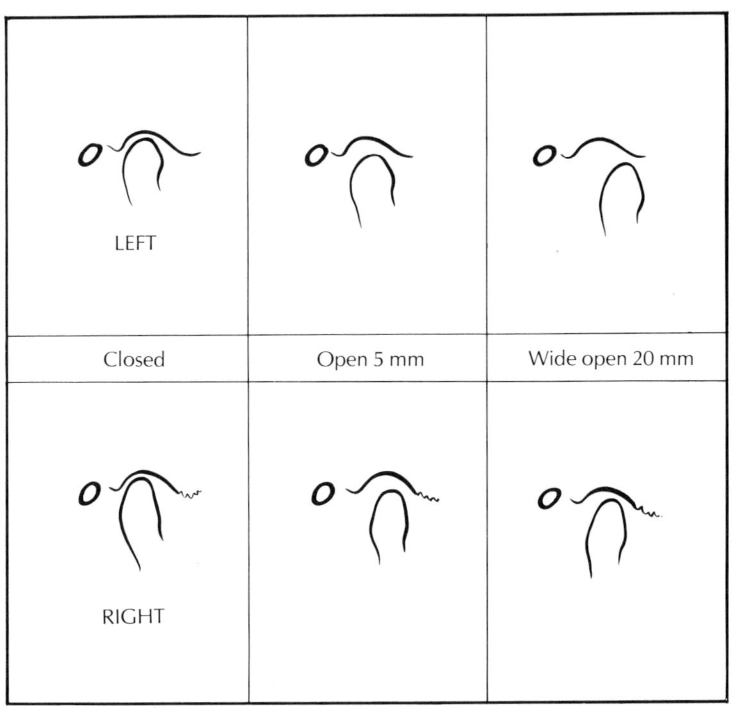

Fig. 9-40. A, Transcranial lateral oblique films of patient (B.N.) showing flattening of both eminences, more significantly on right, and erosion of cortical bone affecting right eminence. **B,** Line drawings depicting in left joint some flattening of anterior head of condyle. In wide-open (20-mm) view right condyle can be seen rotating, not translating. There is asymmetry in shape between right and left condyles.

CASE 16: C.R.

After an auto accident this 31-year-old woman had a 2-year history of severe pain in both joints, with particular trouble on the left side of the head, eye, and ear with pressure blockage and ringing. She was able to open 35 mm, with a 2-mm deviation to the left. The specialized x-ray films show that in both joints there is a flattening and erosion of the cortical bone over the eminences (Fig. 9-41). Note in the closed view in the right joint that the condylar head is anteriorly displaced. It is also interesting to note that when the patient occludes lightly in the 2 mm thickness wax-bite view, the right condylar head moves back to a more normal position in the fossa. In the 31-mm view the left condylar head translates further over the eminence than does the right one. In both joints there is bone-on-bone contact as the condylar head translates over the eminence. She did not respond to nonsurgical treatment. At the time of surgery it was observed that there was osteoarthritis of both joints with severe tearing and compression of the meniscus that could not be repaired. Bilateral arthroplasties and meniscectomies with insertion of articular eminence prostheses were performed. She had relief of her symptoms after this procedure.

A

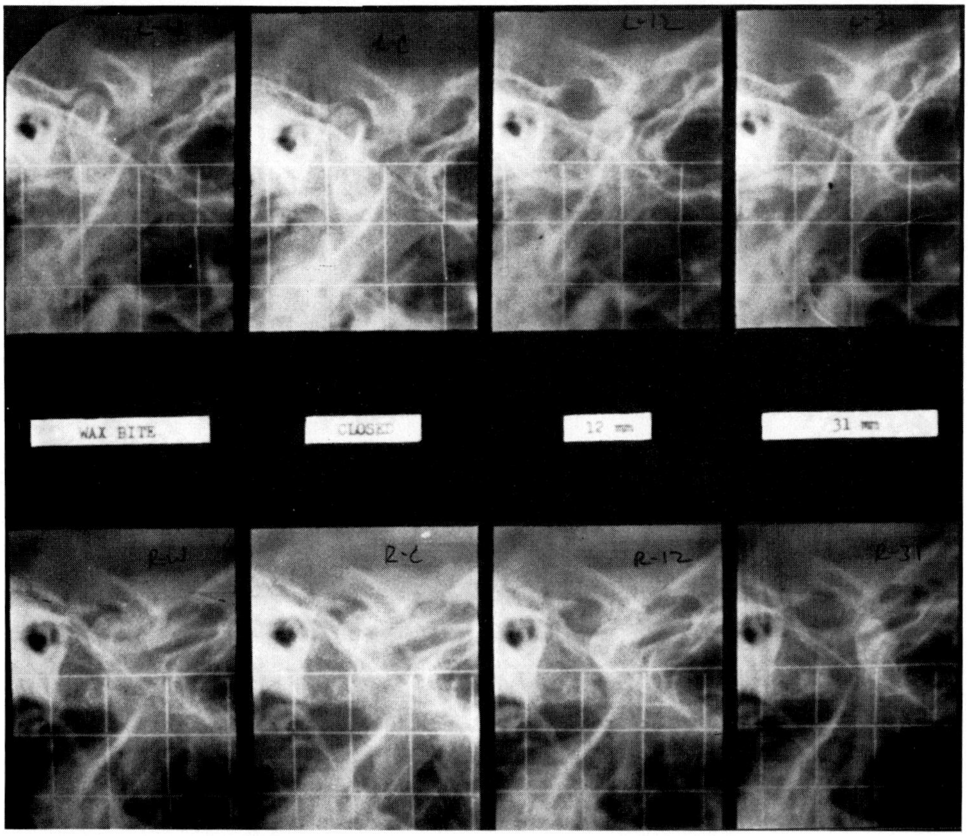

B

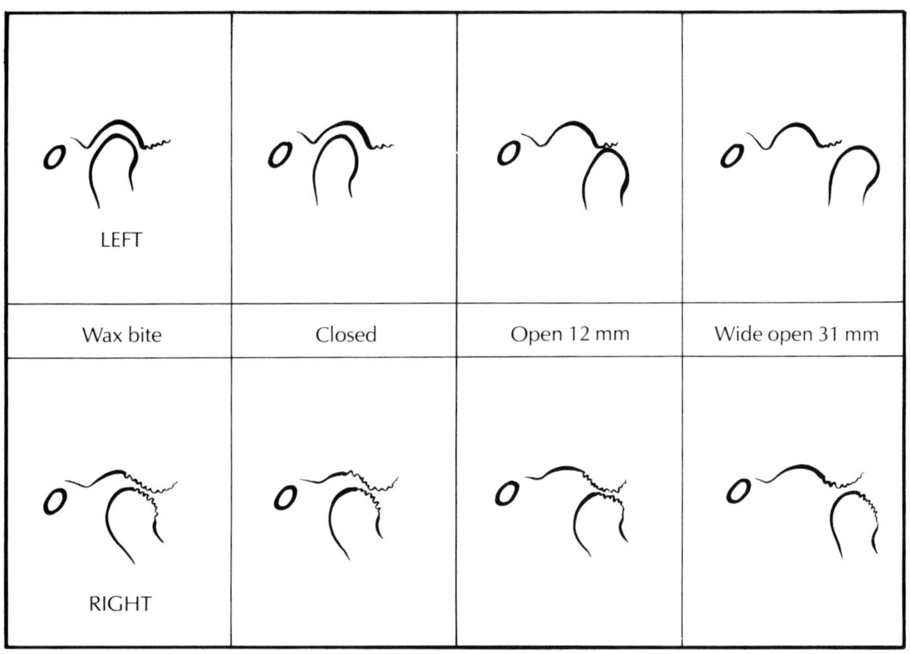

Fig. 9-41. A, Specialized TMJ film shows in left joint, closed view, condylar head slightly posteriorly displaced; 12-mm view reveals bone-on-bone contact of condyle to eminence; in 31-mm view can be seen overextended position of condyle in relation to eminence. Right TMJ closed view shows anterior displacement of condyle in relation to articular eminence. There is bone-on-bone contact of anterior portion of condyles to slopes of eminences. **B,** Line drawings show in right joint a right angle flattening of eminence. There is erosion of cortical layer of bone over eminence. In right side there is flattening of eminence, flattening of anterior condylar head, and erosion of cortical layer of bone over both eminences and anterior condylar heads. Erosion of posterior wall of fossa can also be noted in right joint. In 31-mm view the asymmetrical position of left and right condyles can be seen.

CASE 17: C.C.

This woman had a 15-year history of headaches, neck pain, and dizziness, with ringing in the ears. Her mouth opened 31 mm with a 1-mm deviation to the left. Specialized TMJ x-ray films in the closed view of the left joint reveal that there is even disc space anteriorly, superiorly, and posteriorly (Fig. 9-42). In the closed wax-bite view there is a slight translation of the condyle over the eminence and increased disc space posteriorly. As the condyle translates, the disc space slightly increases in thickness, as noted in the 31-mm view. This may be because of a slight increase of synovial fluid within the joint capsule or some hypertrophy of the disc. There were no joint sounds. In the closed view of the right TMJ it can be noted that the anterior head of the condyle is nearly contacting the descending slope of the eminence. In the closed wax-bite view (2-mm opening) the right condylar head translates forward more than the left joint. In the 12-mm view there can be seen slight asymmetry of opening between the right and left sides. In the 31-mm view the disc space has widened. There is also some erosion noticed on the ascending slope of the right eminence. If nonsurgical procedures do not give relief, some type of surgical repair of the joint may be necessary.

A

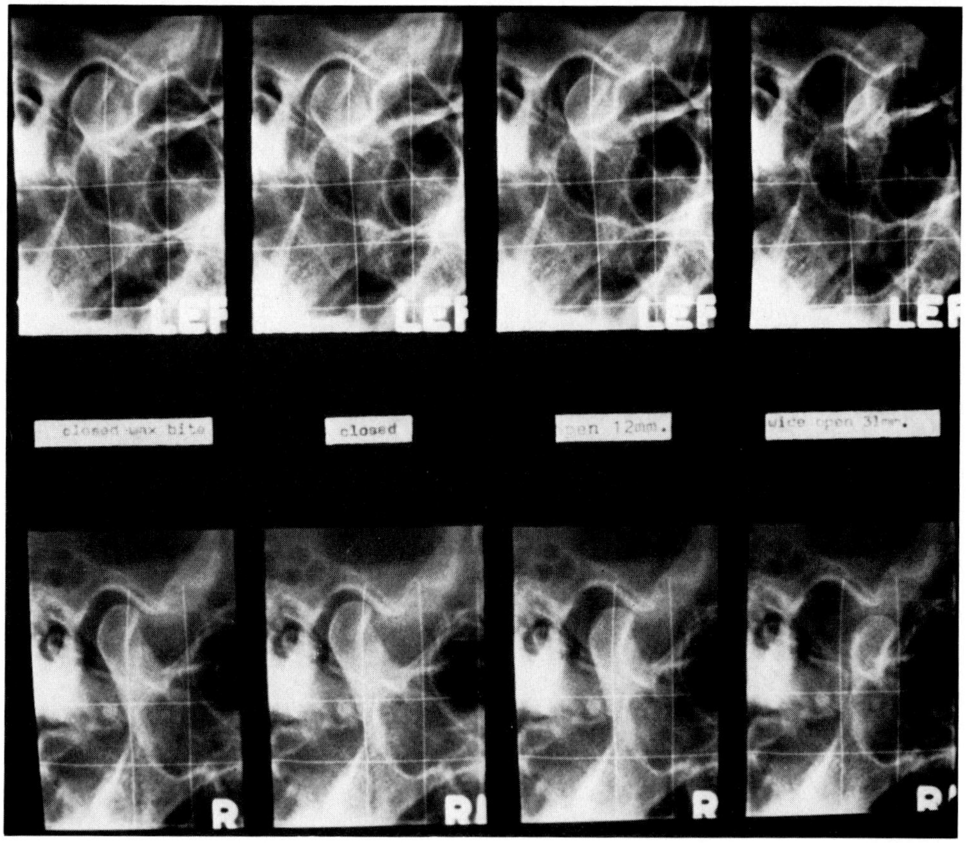

B

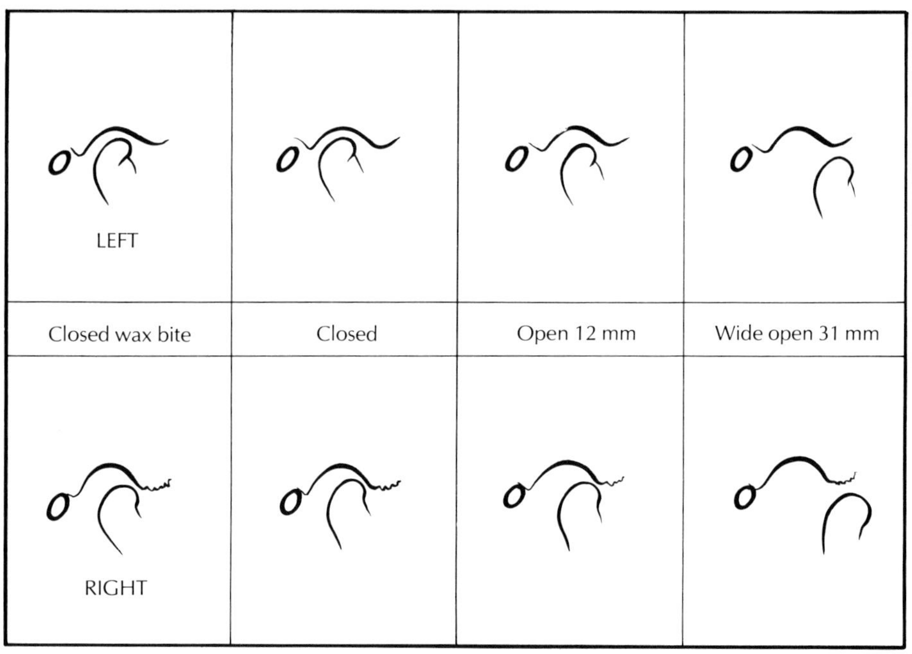

Fig. 9-42. A, Transcranial lateral oblique x-ray films showing in left TMJ, closed view, slight posterior position of condyle to fossa-eminence. Closed wax-bite (2-mm) view shows condyle translated minimally forward (a better condylar position). In open (12-mm) view, condyle is seen translating over eminence, and in wide-open (31-mm) view, condyle is translating to height of eminence. Note that disc space anteriorly is always of same thickness. In right TMJ closed view, condyle is translated slightly forward with minimum disc space anteriorly. In closed wax-bite view, condyle is translated forward excessively. In open view, condyle is translated forward with minimum disc space. In wide-open view it is translated forward with normal disc space. **B,** In line drawings of left joint, closed wax-bite view shows best condylar position. Cortical outline of bone of fossa and articular eminence are within normal limits. Right side depicts minimum disc space between anterior condylar head and descending slope of eminence in first three views. There is erosion of cortical layer of bone over ascending slope of eminence. Right condyle in 31-mm view is rotating abnormally.

CASE 18: R.M.

This woman was not particularly troubled by pain, but she had been bothered by a popping sound in the left joint for as long as she could remember. Six months previously she found it was becoming very difficult to chew or to open her mouth widely. She was able to open 29 mm with a 2-mm deviation to the left. Her specialized TMJ x-ray films show a flattening of the anterior head of the condyle on the right side (Fig. 9-43). On her opening 2 mm in the closed wax-bite view the condylar head appeared not to translate forward. In the wide-open view (29 mm) the condylar head only rotated and was retruded within the fossa. Compare the condylar position to that in the 12-mm view. There are a number of factors that can cause this condition. It may be that the external pterygoid muscle will not contract further, in an effort to prevent more damage and flattening of the anterior condylar head. There is a possibility of some disc derangement in the right joint, although there were no clinical signs such as popping or grating. Arthrograms could be helpful in determining if there were such disc dysfunction in the right joint. In the left joint a more normal shape is seen on the condylar head. Again, it can be noted in the 29-mm wide-open view that the condyle does not translate forward but rotates. This may be a result of disc derangement, since there was a popping in this joint. If nonsurgical treatment is not helpful, surgical repair of the joint, with a possible repositioning of the meniscus, will be recommended.

A

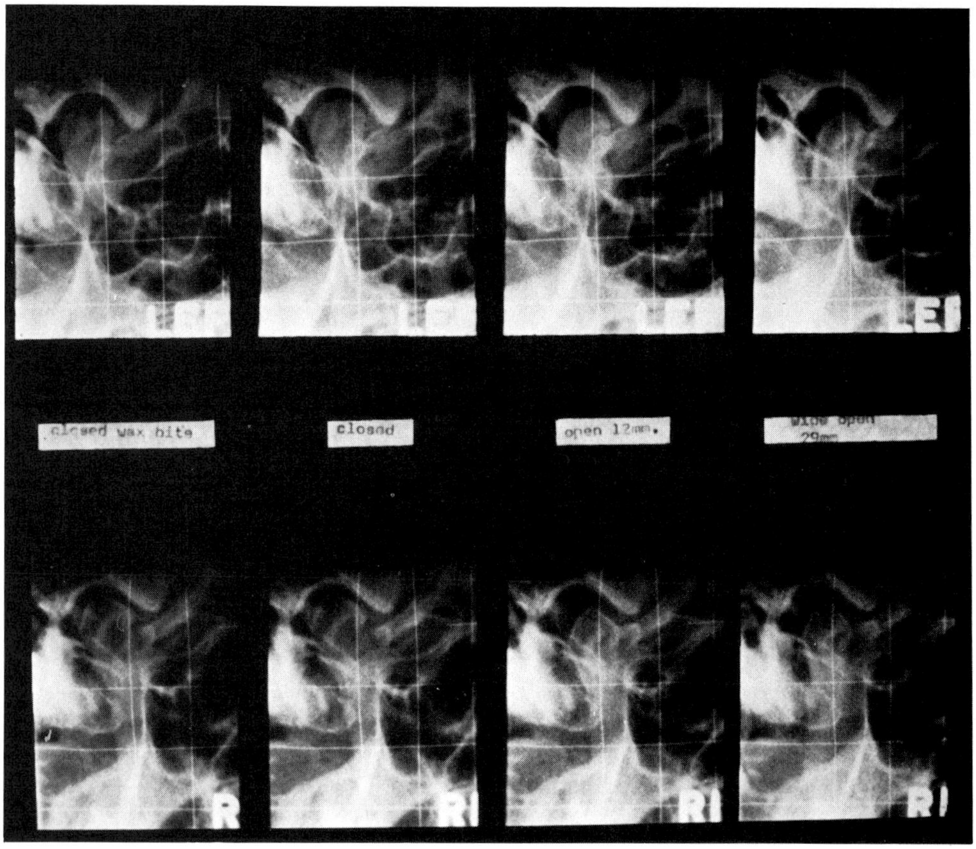

B

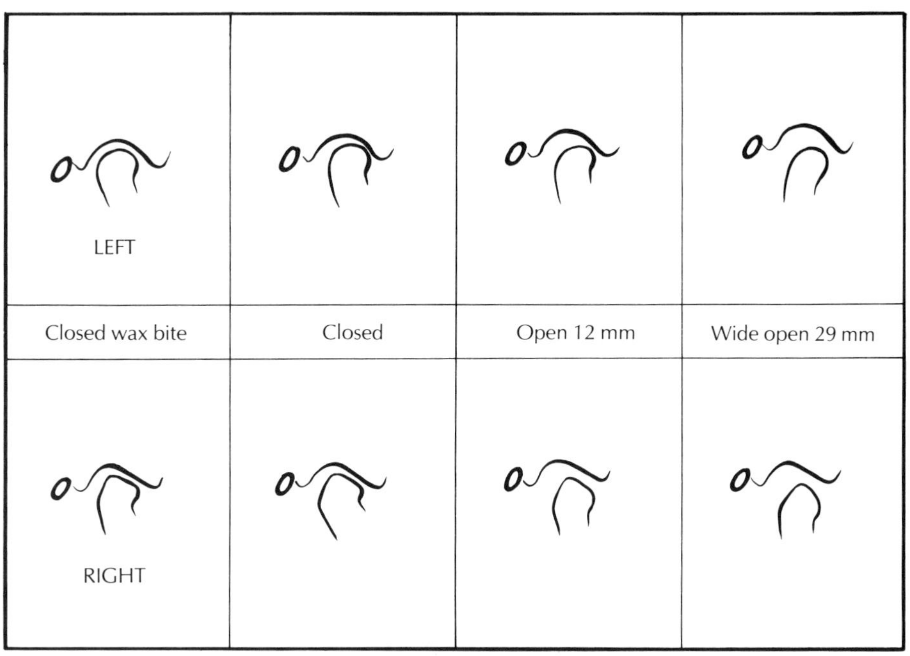

Fig. 9-43. A, Transcranial lateral oblique x-ray films showing in left view, closed position, diminished disc space between anterior condylar head and descending slope of eminence. Wax-bite (2-mm) view shows better position of condyle in relation to fossa-eminence. Wide-open (29-mm) view shows condyle rotating, not translating, and widened disc space. In right joint, closed view, is seen flattening of anterior condylar head and also flattening of posterior condylar head. Wide-open view also shows condyle rotating, not translating, and slight retrusion. **B,** Line drawings confirm significant difference of shape between left and right condyles. Wider than normal disc space in both joints can be seen in wide-open views, indicating abnormal functioning of joints.

REFERENCES

1. Morgan, D.H.: Surgical correction of temporomandibular joint arthritis, J. Oral Surg. **33**:766, 1975.
2. Ricketts, R.M.: Variations of the temporomandibular joint as revealed by cephalometric laminagraphy, Am. J. Orthod. **36**:877, 1950.
3. Ricketts, R.M.: Present status of laminagraphy as related to dentistry, J. Am. Dent. Assoc. **65**:56, 1962.
4. Schmid, F.: On the nerve distribution of the temporomandibular joint capsule, Oral Surg. **28**:63, 1969.

10 Differential diagnosis of TMJ disease

S. JAMES VAMVAS, D.D.S., F.A.C.D.

LISTENING TO THE PATIENT

Differential diagnosis of the temporomandibular disorders has been and is still one of the most perplexing and challenging problems facing medicine and dentistry. Much has been written on this subject, with varied opinions as to its causes, creating disagreement and controversy on the subject. The many complex symptoms presented in each individual case require the use of every avenue of examination at the dentist or physician's disposal in making an accurate diagnosis. Nerves, muscles, and bone changes all are involved individually and collectively.

Before one can adequately determine the course of procedure in the treatment for the pain or dysfunction of the temporomandibular joint syndrome, an intelligent analysis of the individual's complaint must be reviewed. No better start can be made than by allowing the patient sufficient time to tell the story about his or her discomfort. The principal reason that a patient seeks advice is for the relief of pain or other distressing symptoms. Pain and discomfort are subjective symptoms and must be given serious consideration in evaluating the problem.

Listening is an art in itself and can be most rewarding. Many clues can be found in the patient's statements, and these will prevent the practitioner from making too hasty a diagnosis. The patient's story in most cases can lead to an accurate diagnosis or reason for the pain and dysfunction. Regardless of whether the discomfort is considered to be real or imagined, it must be taken incontrovertibly for granted that for the individual seeking help, the discomfort and pain are real.

One cannot afford to make a hasty decision if one is to be honest with one's self and honest with the patient in making a diagnosis of the cause of temporomandibular joint pain or disturbance. Patience in listening to the individual's story can give a true lead that will conclude in an accurate diagnosis.

ANATOMY AND PHYSIOLOGY OF THE TMJ

Muscular involvement

In myofascial pain dysfunction 85% of the temporomandibular joint pain or discomfort can be traced to involvement of the musculature directly and indirectly used in the movements of the jaw. According to Kawamura,[10] "Muscle pain may create a vicious circle. Muscle pain induces a sustained reflex contraction of the jaw muscle, which in turn increases muscle pain, which further contributes to sustained reflex contraction with pain gradually radiating into adjacent areas. . . . If jaw muscle inactivity is unbalanced, the teeth may occlude defectively, and *uncommon* parts of the stomatognathic structure may be stimulated."

Findings by Greene[7] were that research during the past 15 to 20 years has indicated that most so-called temporomandibular joint problems are caused by fatigue and spasm in the masticatory muscles and do not involve the joint itself.

The muscles that may be involved in myofascial pain are the masseter, internal pterygoid, external pterygoid, temporal, suprahyoid, infrahyoid, sternocleidomastoid, scaleni, and rhomboid.[10] Most of the jaw muscles are short, flat, thick muscles that can induce strong force by their contraction. The oxygen consumption of the masseter muscle greatly exceeds that of the limb muscles, indicating some differences in their energetic functional processes.

The mandibular elevators are the masseter and internal pterygoid muscles (for protrusion) and the temporal (for retrusion). The mandibular depressors are the external pterygoid (for protrusion) and the digastric (for retrusion). The temporal and external pterygoid muscles are involved in lateral deviation.

The temporal muscle suspends the mandible against gravity in a sling. In opposition to this, the masseter and the internal pterygoid muscles, which are attached to the angle of the mandible, induce the strong, biting force in forceful chewing.

The superficial belly of the masseter muscle arises from the lower border of the anterior two thirds of the zygomatic arch of the maxilla and attaches to the lateral surface of the lower part of the mandibular ramus, as far down as the angle of the mandible. The deep belly of the masseter arises from the inner surface of the zygomatic arch and attaches to the lateral surface of the coronoid process of the mandible and upper part of the mandibular ramus.

The major muscle responsible for moving the mandible away from the pressure areas between the teeth is the external pterygoid muscle.[1] If the upper and lower teeth do not mesh together precisely, the external pterygoid muscles will contract to move the mandible forward or laterally away from these prematurely contacting teeth. This constant contraction results in the muscle contracting around its own blood supply, with eventual muscle fatigue. Bruxism and clenching of the teeth are subconscious efforts on the part of the patient to erase prematurely contacting tooth surfaces.

The external pterygoid, especially its inferior head, is the main trigger muscle used in opening the mouth. Although it is possible for any of the jaw muscles to go into a spasm as a result of bite disharmony, the muscle most frequently involved in the temporomandibular joint syndrome is the external pterygoid.

Jaw opening is assisted by the suprahyoid muscles. Within this coordinated muscle group, the digastric muscle is dominant, and it functions in the forced opening of the mandible when the hyoid bone is fixed by the infrahyoid muscle group. The lower jaw is protruded primarily by the simultaneous bilateral contraction of the external pterygoid muscles. The masseter and the internal pterygoid muscles also help draw the jaw slightly forward.

Retrusive movement of the mandible is accomplished by contraction of the posterior belly of the temporal muscle, in which the muscle fibers run almost horizontally. The posterior fibers of the temporal muscle draw the condyle backward during retrusion. The digastric and other suprahyoid muscles also are involved in retrusion.

Lateral movement of the mandible is essential for grinding food and is achieved by the action of the external and internal pterygoid muscles on one side and the contralateral temporal muscle. When the mandible moves to the left side, the right external pterygoid muscle, acting together with the right internal pterygoid muscle, moves the chin across the midline toward the left side.

Capsular ligaments

Synovitis also may be present within the capsular ligament, with no injury to the disc or the articular surfaces of the joint. This condition is reversible.[9]

The surface of the deep part of the glenoid fossa lacks fibrous cartilage. However, the surfaces of the posterior slope of the articular tubercle and the articular surface of the condylar head are covered by fibrous cartilage, which suggests that these parts of the joint are able to provide resistance force.

The articular disc is an oval plate and, with the exception of the posterior part, is made of a dense, fibrous collagenous tissue. The posterior edge of the disc attaches to the capsule by means of a thick, loose, connective tissue that permits forward movement of the disc with contraction of the external pterygoid muscle. Thus the disc and the condylar head are always drawn forward by the external pterygoid muscle. The disc is divided into two parts in back. The upper part of the disc attaches to the temporal bone, and the lower part attaches to the posterior surface of the condylar neck.

The ligaments of the temporomandibular joint are the articular capsule (capsular ligaments) and the temporomandibular, sphenomandibular, and stylomandibular ligaments. The articular capsule is a fibrous membrane that extends from the condylar neck at some distance from the articular surface to the outer periphery of the glenoid fossa. The capsule is considerably thinner and looser in front than in back.

Movements of the joint

The normal temporomandibular joint moves freely, without strenuous effort and without pain. The basic character of joint movement is a hingelike rotation. The posterior fibers of the temporal muscle help draw the condyle backward into the glenoid fossa and particularly help remove pressure from the head of the condyle when the teeth are strongly clenched. At maximum opening of the mouth the condylar head is usually just against the peak of the articular tubercle.

In disorders of the temporomandibular joint the mobility of the joint itself is more or less disturbed, as well as the spatial relation of the disc and the condylar head. In the normal movement of the mandible the upper and lower heads of the external pterygoid muscle act in harmony, and the articular disc moves forward together with the condylar head; thus the condylar head always holds a constant relationship to the central part of the disc. However, once this harmonious function of the two heads of the external pterygoid muscle is disturbed, the condylar head may collide with the edge of the disc at the beginning or end of the mandibular opening and closing. In such disturbances of the external pterygoid muscle a clicking sound in the joint is produced.

The physiological rest position of the mandible is the position in which all gnathostomatic structures are in balanced condition. We also may assume the presence of some muscular dysfunction if the patient is unable to guide the jaw easily from rest position to centric occlusion.

DIFFERENTIAL DIAGNOSIS

Malocclusion

Malocclusion may be an important factor in pain. Examination of the dentition should be made, noting missing teeth and open or closed bite. One of the most frequently encountered conditions resulting in pain in the temporomandibular joint is lack of posterior teeth.[9] Mastication is then accomplished by thrusting the mandible forward, using the available anterior teeth for chewing. This action, in turn, pulls the head of the condyle forward, stretching the ligament and muscle attachments. This abnormal action of the muscles of mastication and nerve endings can create pain in the area of the temporomandibular joint. Individuals who have worn dentures for a long time because of overclosure of the bite may have this same resultant pull, creating the same effect on the temporomandibular joint.

Occlusal interferences are not necessarily abnormal. If the patient has adapted to the occlusion, and if there is no sign of associated mandibular dysfunction, there is no indication for the elimination of the interferences.

It is also important to note that whenever occlusion is altered, there will be some change in the proprioceptive impulses arising from receptors in the periodontal membranes. These changes also can bring about a risk of spasm.

Trauma

Blows to the mandible may injure the joint and result in temporomandibular joint pain.[9] The injury may be transitory, or it may produce permanent damage to the meniscus, which may initiate long-term joint symptoms. Surgical procedures in the mouth and throat, intubation for general anesthesia, bronchoscopy procedures, and protracted dental procedures may produce undue tension on the joint and initiate joint pain.

Whiplash

There is adequate proof that whiplash injuries are responsible for many TMJ pain dysfunctions. Intermittent or constant pain many times will accompany such injuries.

There is a similarity between some symptoms of whiplash and of TMJ dysfunction. Two signs remote from the TMJ and from hysterical manipulation can be noted. In many patients the internal pterygoid muscle and submandibular salivary gland are swollen or painful on palpation. When TMJ dysfunction is unilateral and unmistakable, these signs often will be found on the same side, suggesting therefore that such occurrence is not unrelated. The relationship of TMJ dysfunction and whiplash can be explained as deceleration effects on the mandible and thus on the TMJ either through direct injury or through neurological involvement.[16]

In the treatment of whiplash, cervical traction also may produce TMJ arthropathy. When cervical traction is used in the treatment of neck injuries, a primary TMJ arthropathy may be aggravated, or a secondary arthropathy may result. Traction may be used if provisions are made to protect the temporomandibular joint from trauma through the use of bite plates or soft splints.[6]

Muscle stretching

The myofascial trigger areas are thought to be small, hypersensitive areas located in the fascia between muscle bundles. It is theorized that irritation of these hypersensitive areas may be caused by many factors, such as excessive stretching of the muscle, injury from injection, extremes in temperature, fatigue, nervous tension, and complications of menopause.[18] Some authorities believe that pain arising from these trigger areas may bombard the central nervous system and produce referred pain. This pain may also stimulate the muscle from which it arises into spasm.

Forceful or sustained contraction

Various emotional tensions may increase muscle tonicity and lead to pain and dysfunction. This is evidenced by the twitching or bulging of the masseter muscle under known stress. Prolonged periods of tension may be a factor in joint pain-dysfunction syndrome. Soldiers faced with combat and persons with pressing domestic or financial problems frequently manifest TMJ pain, lower back pain, and the like.

To explore the role of psychological factors in mandibular pain-dysfunction syndrome (MPDS), a group of 27 female patients with manifest MPDS was compared with a group of 27 healthy women in a battery of personality inventories.[13] The MPDS patients had significantly higher scores in the Neuroticism, Somatic anxiety, Psychic anxiety, and Muscular tension variables. They also had significantly higher scores in one of the two aggressive variables, Hostility. No group differences were found in the extraversion variables.

A striking difference was found in the High superego strength scale, in which the healthy patients obtained significantly higher scores, indicating a tendency to be more conscientious, responsible, orderly, and serious. A similar indication is implied by their significantly higher ratings for unpleasantness in thrill situations.

The symptoms, usually unilateral, are muscle tenderness and a dull aching pain in the preauricular area, often radiating to the ear, face, head, neck, and shoulders. There are also often clickings, irregularities, or limitation of movement in the temporomandibular joint. It was concluded that the high anxiety and muscle tension demonstrated in the patients were probably of great importance in the development of MPDS, even if it may be assumed that MPDS symptoms have further accentuated these characteristics.

Myositis

Myositis, or fibrositis of masticatory muscles, is most frequently seen in young or middle-aged persons.[9] It is characterized by a dull ache in the affected part and limitation of movement. Pressure on the involved muscle elicits pain. The cause of the inflammation is unknown, and symptoms usually subside gradually with application of heat, gentle massage, and administration of salicylates.

Subluxation or chronic dislocation

Dislocation of the mandibular condyle is nearly always associated with pain. In fact dislocation is frequently caused by pain resulting from an abnormal excursion, stimulating the muscles into severe contracture or spasm and thus trapping the condyle head anterior to the eminence.[18]

Bruxism

Bruxism is abnormal clenching, grinding, and gnashing of teeth thought to be caused by a combination of emotional stress and local disharmony in the masticatory apparatus. Of the two factors, the unconscious reaction to mental stress or emotion may be predominant. Hypertonicity of the masticatory muscles appears to be a constant finding.[18] Once the pattern is established, it appears to be self-perpetuating and manifests signs of extensive occlusal wear, possible periodontal involvement, and increased muscle tonicity.

Pressure

Tension or pressure on the articular disc and connective tissue of the capsule in the posterior region may cause TMJ damage. The anterior periphery of the disc receives pressure when the condylar head moves forward to the posterior slope and tip of the eminence. This portion of the disc is subject to wear, fraying, and cracking.

It has been demonstrated that nerve fibers are found in the periphery of the disc. It is assumed that pressure on this portion of the disc is the principal reason for pain occurring in the joint.

Vertigo

Vertigo may be caused by differences in the impulses conveyed to the vestibular center of the brain by one ear as compared with the other.[9] The conduction system of the ears that conveys these impulses is situated in close relationship to the temporomandibular joint. Dental occlusal and TMJ abnormalities, which usually occur unilaterally, may irritate and injure the adjacent conduction system of one ear more than the other. This results in a difference or imbalance of vestibular impulses, which causes vertigo.

The dental-TMJ causes of vertigo are overclosed, traumatic dental occlusion and traumatic malrelationships of the temporomandibular joint with the adjacent structures of the ear. These dental causes are activated by trauma, fatigue, intrapsychic strain, emotional stress, fingernail biting, cigar and pipe smoking, and organic diseases that lower the vestibular threshold.

Osteoarthritis

Osteoarthritis (also known as *hypertrophic arthritis* or *degenerative arthritis*) is a chronic arthropathy, usually occurring in elderly people with degenerative and hypertrophic changes in the bone and cartilage. In some instances there is considerable thickening of the synovial membrane. It is essentially a degenerative process, differing in this respect from those inflammatory forms of arthritis, for which some bacterial agent is responsible.

The term *arthrosis* of the TMJ has been defined as a primarily noninflammatory degenerative disturbance of the normal function of the joint. It should be remembered, however, that the disturbance may derive not only from the joint itself but also from other functional parts of the gnathostomatic system. It is the disturbed normal function of the joint that is first revealed by clinical examination, and after treatment it is the rehabilitation of this function that is the most easily recognized result of the therapy.[12]

The following dysfunction symptoms may occur: (1) crepitation, crackling, or clicking in one or both joints, (2) pain or tenderness in one or both joints on opening or chewing and on palpation, (3) pain or tenderness in one or both joints, (4) luxation and subluxation, (5) difficulty in opening mouth, (6) locking in one or both joints at certain positions, (7) pain in one or both joints on biting on hard or tough objects, (8) symptoms from the ears, (9) impaired hearing, (10) tooth grinding or pressing, (11) headache, (12) dizziness, (13) strain, stiffness, or tiredness in neck or back of the head, (14) strain or tiredness in one or both joints, (15) burning tongue, or (16) a deviation of the mandible on biting occlusion or opening.

The most important predisposing factor is old age, since the wearing quality of the joint is diminished. Arthrosis is found in 80% to 90% of the population over 60 years of age. Most cases of pain and muscle dysfunction are found in younger people. Trauma history should be checked in these cases, since it is questionable whether their discomfort originated in the joint.

First, a careful examination also should be undertaken by an ear specialist so as to eliminate, where possible, all causes other than purely dental ones. There still will remain a limited number of cases, but in these dental treatment can reasonably be expected to yield a favorable result. This therapy consists to a large extent of the restoration, by one means or another, of the lost physiological vertical dimension.[12]

There may be perforation of the disc without bone changes, resulting in a crepitus of the joint. There also may be erosion of the cortical layer of the joint in the form of condylar erosion (anterior, superior, or posterior), articular eminence erosion (descending or ascending slope), or mandibular fossa erosion (superoposterior wall). Changes in the shape of the condylar head, spurs, and lipping may be seen radiographically. The general practitioners of both dentistry and otolaryngology usually have been disappointed with radiographic evaluations of patients suspected of having pathological conditons of the TMJ.[4] On occasion, however, the condyle seems to have almost disappeared. Narrowing of the joint space is often seen. Xerography and laminagraphy can provide added information. Specialized TMJ radiographs are described in Chapter 9.

In some instances there is considerable thickening of the synovial membrane, resulting in chronic synovitis. There also may be functional discrepancies, such as malocclusion, limited mandibular motion, or deviation on opening. Except for trauma, the cause is unknown. It is postulated that the effects of age and wear caused by skeletal malrelationships of the jaw, microtrauma, and bruxism may cause some of the pathological conditions. Excess weight may have some effect on the weight-bearing joints. It is not a true inflammation but, essentially, a degenerative process.

The joint cartilage is gradually destroyed, and the joint surfaces are replaced by sclerosed bone. As the condition progresses, bone spurs may develop, or demineralization of the cortical bone may occur. Ankylosis is not encountered. Symptoms may be mild or absent, or there may be pain and tenderness, which appear and disappear at intervals. Bony changes can occur in the late stages of chronic infectious arthritis, just as chronic osteoarthritis can become secondarily infected.

Rheumatoid arthritis

Rheumatoid arthritis (also known as chronic infectious arthritis, atrophic arthritis, or arthritis deformans) is a chronic disease of the joints characterized by inflammatory changes in the synovial membrane and periarticular structures and by atrophy and rarefaction of the bones.[2] The temporomandibular joint is involved more frequently in rheumatoid arthritis than in any other form of joint disease.

The disease manifests itself in the earlier stages as a migratory swelling and stiffness of the joints, in the later stages by more or less deformity and ankylosis. Rarely is only the temporomandibular joint affected; in the majority of cases the disease is polyarticular.

Rheumatoid arthritis accounts for 30% to 40% of all rheumatic disorders. It is essentially a disease of middle age, usually affecting those between 25 and 50 years old, with the average age of onset being 35. Women are affected more than men by three to one. The cause is unknown. It is believed that the disease results from an atypical antibody reaction to bacterial infection affecting the colloidal interfibrillar substance of the connective tissue.[2] There may be several predisposing causes:

1. Severe physical or emotional shock preceding the onset
2. Fatigue (mental or physical)
3. Trauma, which lowers the local resistance of the joint (and the infection becomes localized in the area of injury)
4. Infections such as acute coryza, tonsillitis, sinus infection, influenza, pneumonia, or typhoid fever
5. Exposure to dampness, rain, or cold
6. Constitutional infirmity
7. Heredity (the disease is said to run in families)
8. Climate (the disease is rarely encountered in the tropics)

The major clinical features are severe local and systemic symptoms, which begin slowly. One or more joints become swollen and painful, accompanied by fatigue, muscle stiffness, and loss of weight. There also may be a slight elevation of temperature (37.2° to 37.8°C [99° to 100°F]), with rapid pulse, slight elevation of sedimentation rate, atrophic skin, and generalized lymph adenopathy.[2]

Rheumatic fever

Rheumatoid arthritis must be differentiated from subacute rheumatic fever, a distinction that is not always easy to make. In both conditions the patient may give a history of tonsillitis followed by an acute arthritis with fever and swelling of the joints. In rheumatic fever, however, the temperature is higher, the sweating is more profuse, and cardiac complications are frequent. The therapeutic test is valuable. Treatment with sodium salicylate or aspirin usually gives instant and permanent relief from rheumatic fever. In rheumatoid arthritis, however, these drugs produce only a temporary improvement.

There may be no radiographic evidence of the disease in the early stages. As it progresses, however, there is evidence of marginal resorption. There will be punched-out areas of cortical bone, a narrowing of the joint space, and possible progression to ankylosis.

	Rheumatoid arthritis	*Osteoarthritis*
Average age of onset	Young adults	Condition of aging
Weight	Normal or underweight	Usually overweight
Focuses of infection	Usually present	Usually absent
Condition of bones	Rarefaction	Condensation of articular margins
Joints involved	Any joint in body	Chiefly knees, spine, fingers
Type	Migratory	Localized
Appearance of joints	Periarticular swelling	No swelling
Course	Usually progressive	Stationary
Termination	Ankylosis and deformity	No ankylosis; usually no deformity

Infectious arthritis

Infectious arthritis is the least common of the arthritic conditions affecting the temporomandibular joint. The infectious process may result from direct extension or hematogenous spread.[9] Organisms that may be responsible are staphylococci, streptococci, *Neisseria meningitidis, Neisseria gonorrhoeae,* diplococci, mycobacteria, and spirochetes. Generalized disease such as gonorrhea, syphilis, tuberculosis, rheumatic fever, scarlet fever, and measles may be complicated occasionally by joint involvement, or joint disease may result from local extension of infections from the middle ear, mastoid, or parotid gland.

Juvenile rheumatoid arthritis

When rheumatoid arthritis occurs in children,[2] certain features differ from the picture usually seen in adults. The constitutional symptoms, particularly fever, are likely to be more severe and indeed may precede the development of arthritis at times by several weeks or months. A variety of nonspecific skin rashes, usually of the erythema multiforme type, may be seen. Nodules are rare. Uveitis is frequent and may lead to blindness. Evidence of cardiac involvement with pericarditis or valvular lesions is more common, as is enlargement of the lymph nodes, liver, and spleen. The eponym *Still's disease* has been applied to juvenile rheumatoid arthritis in which such visceral involvement is prominent; there is general agreement that the range of manifestations in rheumatoid arthritis in children is just as varied as in the disease in adults and that separation of this combination as a disease entity is not justified. Monoarticular involvement at the onset of the disease is more frequent in children than in adults.

Certain skeletal abnormalities occur in children primarily because of interference with the normal rate of growth in secondary bone centers. The rheumatoid inflammation in proximity to these centers may temporarily accelerate their rate of growth and then may cause premature closure of the epiphysis. This may result in failure of certain bones, such as the mandible, to develop fully. Also particularly striking in juvenile rheumatoid arthritis is the predilection for involvement of the cervical spine, leading to ankylosis of the cervical vertebrae; other portions of the spine are spared. Tests for rheumatoid factor are positive in a lower percentage of children with rheumatoid arthritis than in adults.

Ankylosis of the TMJ

Ankylosis of the TMJ is infrequent but serious. If it occurs in children during the formative years, crippling deformity of the mandible can result. It is disabling at any age because of the inability to open the mouth and masticate food properly.[9] There are two types of ankylosis—fibrous and bony. Fibrous ankylosis is caused by the restriction of mandibular movement because of fibrous attachment between the head of the condyle, glenoid fossa, and possibly the articular eminence. The disc may be absent. Some hinge motion is present, but excursive motion of the condyle is impossible. Fibrous ankylosis may precede bony ankylosis, and a combination of fibrous and bony attachment between the condyle and glenoid fossa is at times present.

Bony ankylosis is a fusion of the condylar head and the articulating portion of the temporal bone by an osseous bridge. Occasionally ankylosis is manifested by only a slight overgrowth of the condylar head as it fuses to the glenoid fossa. In other cases the head may be grossly enlarged, with complete absence of normal contour. The neck also may be greatly expanded and lacking in normal contour.

Possible causes of ankylosis are (1) rheumatoid arthritis, primarily, (2) rheumatic fever, (3) pyogenic infection, (4) fractures of the condyle, or (5) prolonged immobilization of the badly comminuted condylar head.[9]

Fractures

High on the list of complaints is that of TMJ pain or dysfunction caused by injuries from a direct blow to the area, including resultant fractures in the region of the condyle. In the majority of cases in which the fractured condyles are permitted to heal in their fractured relationship (where the central occlusion is maintained in centric relation), the neuromuscular system has great capacity to adapt itself to new anatomical restrictions.

In the absence of a fracture a blow will cause edema, swelling, and contraction of the musculature.

Acute gouty arthritis

Hyperuricemia caused by reduced urate secretion in patients not overproducing uric acid is frequently encountered among Filipinos, Chinese, and Japanese. TMJ pain appearing in this susceptible population, particularly after thiazide therapy as well as surgery and the other usual precipitating events, should suggest an episode of acute gouty arthritis. This is a common and remediable cause of TMJ pain dysfunction syndrome occurring among populations with these ethnic backgrounds.[3]

Tumors

Osteomas are most common, developing on the condylar head and causing limitation of movement. Because of the insidious onset and the slow progress of the symptoms as well as the difficulties of diagnosis, neoplasms of this type are usually large before they are discovered. The use of passive stretch here is useful. If the limitation of movement is caused by a bony obstruction, it is possible to feel the sudden dead stop caused by the obstruction. There is no rebound when finger pressure is released. When muscle spasm is responsible for the limitation, evidence of elasticity can be felt, and there is a pressure rebound of the mandible when finger pressure is released.[18]

TRIGEMINAL AND ATYPICAL FACIAL NEURALGIAS

The recent independent studies of Roberts and Person[15] and Ratner, Person, and Kleinman[14] present observations and data supporting the possibility that preexisting dental and oral pathological conditions may be major contributing factors in the onset of both idiopathic and atypical facial neuralgias. Their studies provide the first evidence to support earlier contentions of neurologists such as Harris[8] and Kinnier-Wilson and Bruce[11] that dental and oral disease might be important contributing factors in the onset of trigeminal neuralgia and also of atypical facial neuralgia.

In Roberts and Person's study[15] of 16 patients with idiopathic trigeminal neuralgia and 21 patients with atypical facial neuralgia it was found in nearly all instances that the painful phenomena associated with both disorders were closely related to the presence of maxillary or mandibular bone cavities at previous tooth-extraction sites. Roberts and Person note that although standard dental diagnostic x-ray examinations are usually negative in both idiopathic trigeminal and atypical facial neuralgias, roentgenographic changes *can* be detected in jaw bones that ordinarily might be considered to be within the range of normal variations, but which in these patients with histories of facial pain reflect the existence of the pain-related bone cavities. In some cases frank radiolucencies may be visible at bone-cavity sites, which under other circumstances might be dismissed as unrelated to the pain experienced by the patient. But when these cavities have been detected by radiography, palpating them nearly always elicits the same pain pattern of which the patient has complained. Figs. 10-1 to 10-12 illustrate such roentgenograms in their use at detecting changes in the jaw bone that, without pain symptoms, might be considered within the range of normal variations.

These areas, once detected, can then be exposed, usually under local anesthesia using an intraoral surgical approach. Roberts and Person[15] report that in each in-

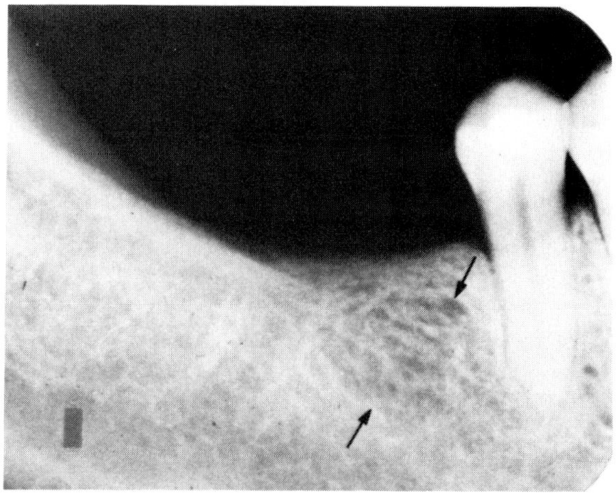

Fig. 10-1. Trigeminal neuralgia in left mandible, premolar and molar regions. Circumscribed radiolucent area *(arrows)* is distal to second premolar.

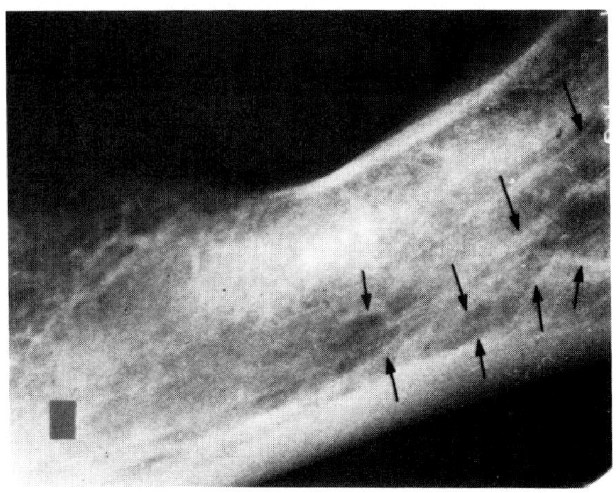

Fig. 10-2. Trigeminal neuralgia in right mandible, premolar and molar regions. Irregularly shaped radiolucent areas *(arrows)* extend from molar to premolar areas.

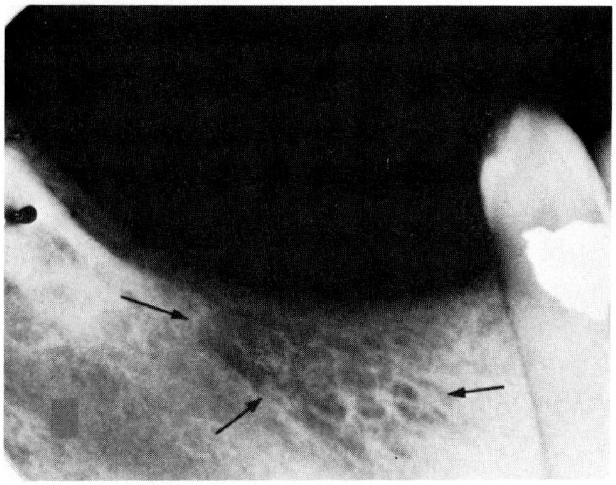

Fig. 10-3. Atypical facial neuralgia in left mandible, premolar region. There is irregularly shaped radiolucency *(arrows)* distal to second premolar.

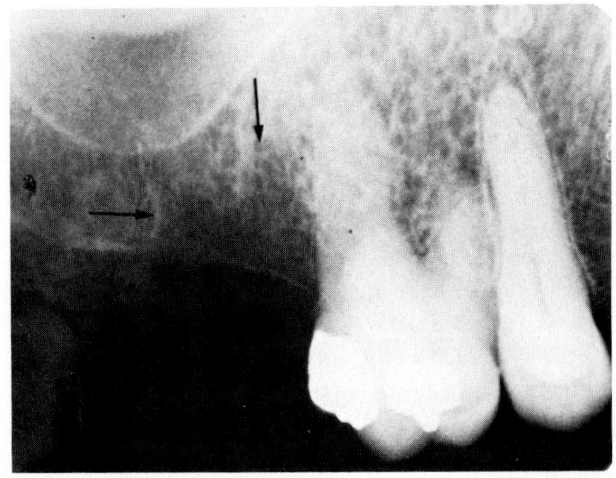

Fig. 10-4. Atypical facial neuralgia in left maxilla, molar region. Arrows point to irregular triangular radiolucency, distal to first molar.

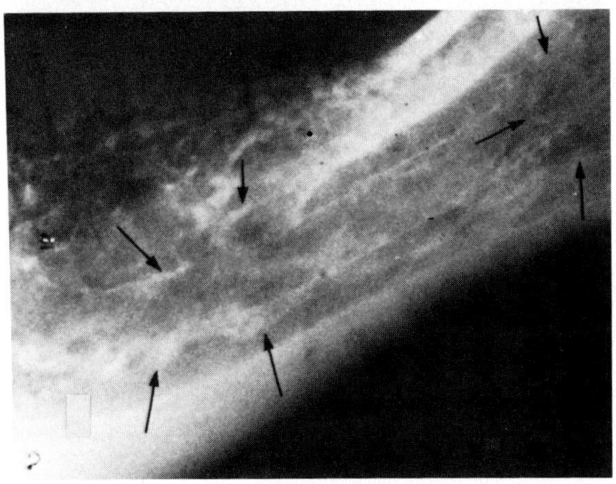

Fig. 10-5. Trigeminal neuralgia in right mandible; two cavities are present. In canine and premolar region irregular radiolucency is seen, with sparse, thickened, and disorganized trabeculae. Posteriorly in molar region a cavity was found in area shown by three arrows.

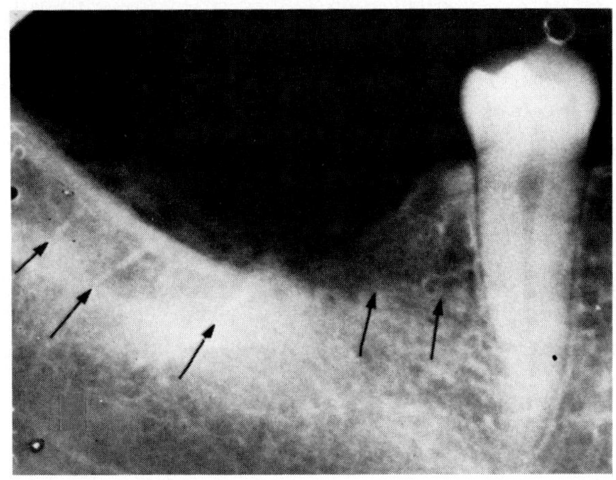

Fig. 10-6. Atypical facial neuralgia in left mandible. Distal to second premolar is triangular radiolucency. More posteriorly in molar region a second cavity was found where vestiges of lamina dura are seen.

A

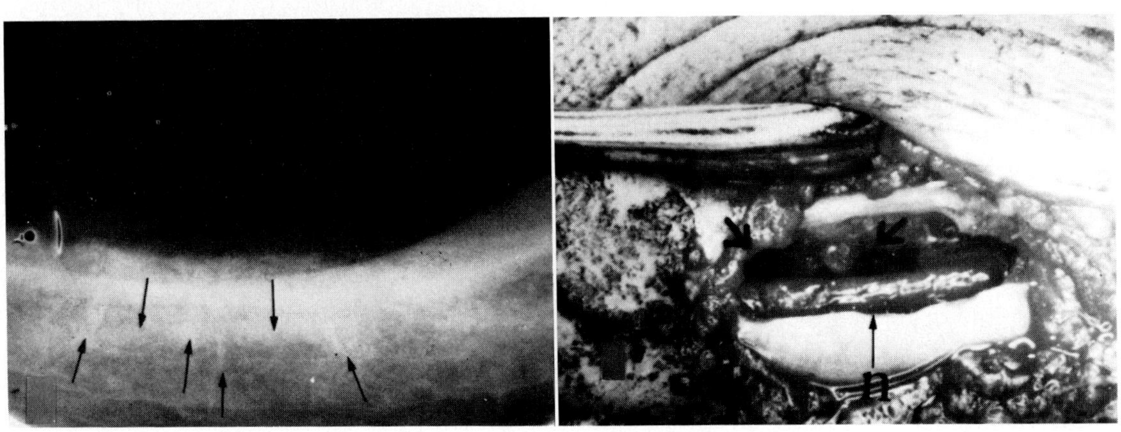

B

Fig. 10-7. Atypical facial neuralgia. **A,** Right mandible, molar region. Vestiges of lamina dura *(up arrows)* are seen, below which is diffuse radiolucency *(down arrows)*. **B,** Photograph of these areas. On exposure of area indicated by arrows in **A,** two cavities *(arrows)* were seen, which were sockets of extracted molar teeth. Superiorly, they opened onto surface of mandible. Inferiorly, they entered mandibular canal, whose wall was almost entirely destroyed by disease process. Much necrotic bone was curetted, leaving mandibular nerve *(n)* coursing freely through body of mandible, as shown.

A 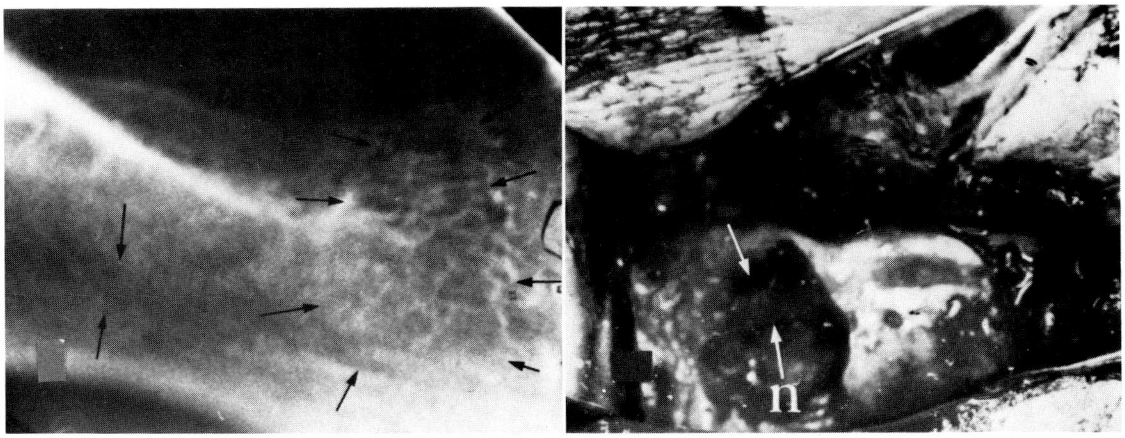 B

Fig. 10-8. Trigeminal neuralgia. **A,** Left mandible, premolar and molar regions. Two cavities are shown by arrows. Anterior most (premolar) region is almost circular, whereas posteriorly a diffuse, horizontal shadow extends to border of anterior cavity. **B,** Corresponding photograph of region of mandible made during surgical treatment of bone cavity. Arrow points to base of cavity that is remnant of socket of extracted tooth. Also, in Fig. 10-7, *B,* socket communicated directly with space surrounding mandibular nerve *(n),* whose wall was almost entirely destroyed by disease process.

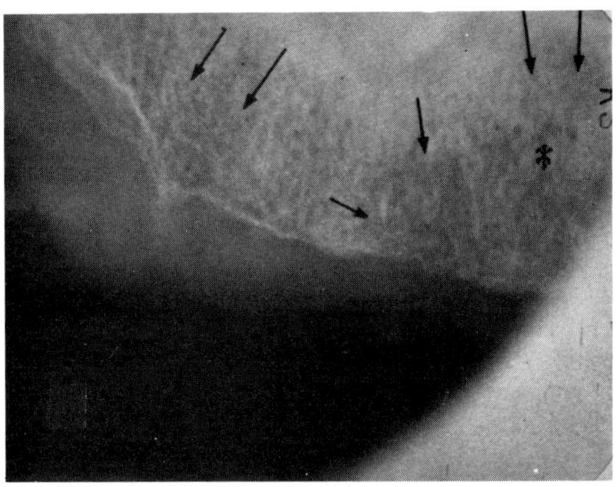

Fig. 10-9. Trigeminal neuralgia, upper left premolar and molar regions. Two confluent cavities exist *(arrows).* There is also a group of random, small radiolucent spots in premolar area *(asterisk).*

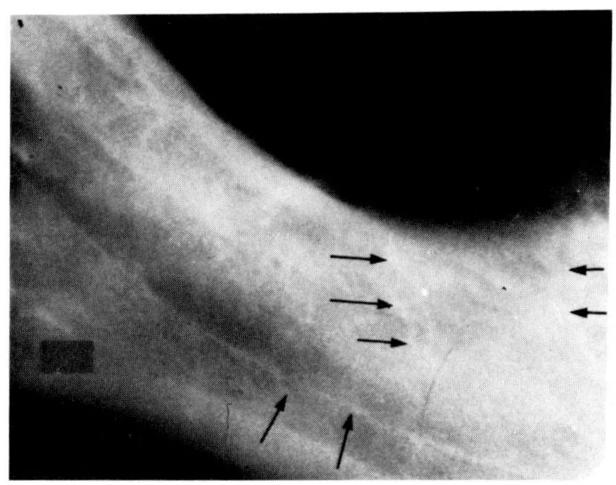

Fig. 10-10. Trigeminal neuralgia in left mandibular region. Bone trabeculae form two vertical lines from alveolar crest toward mandibular canal and demarcate site of nonhealed molar socket. Bottoms of sockets were continuous with mandibular canal.

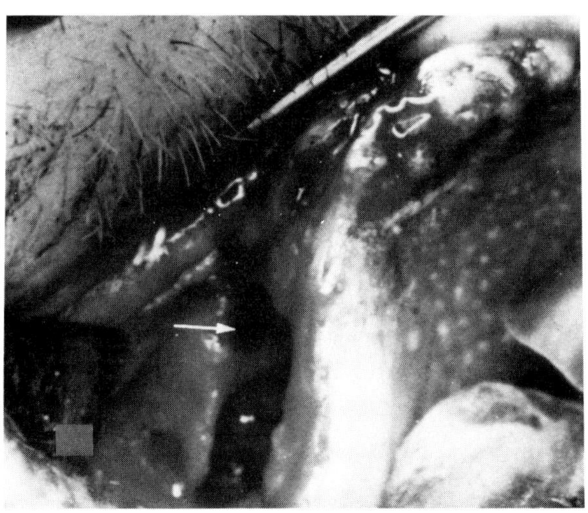

Fig. 10-11. Trigeminal neuralgia. Photograph of left maxillary premolar and molar areas corresponding to radiolucent areas in Fig. 10-9. Anterior circular radiolucent area of Fig. 10-9 is represented here by arrow, and its distal extensions to tuberosity region are evident. Anterior-most cavity *(arrow)* existed as such when area was first exposed. Its distal extension consisted of soft, necrotic-like, very vascular bone, which disintegrated during curettage, resulting in cavity extensions seen in photograph.

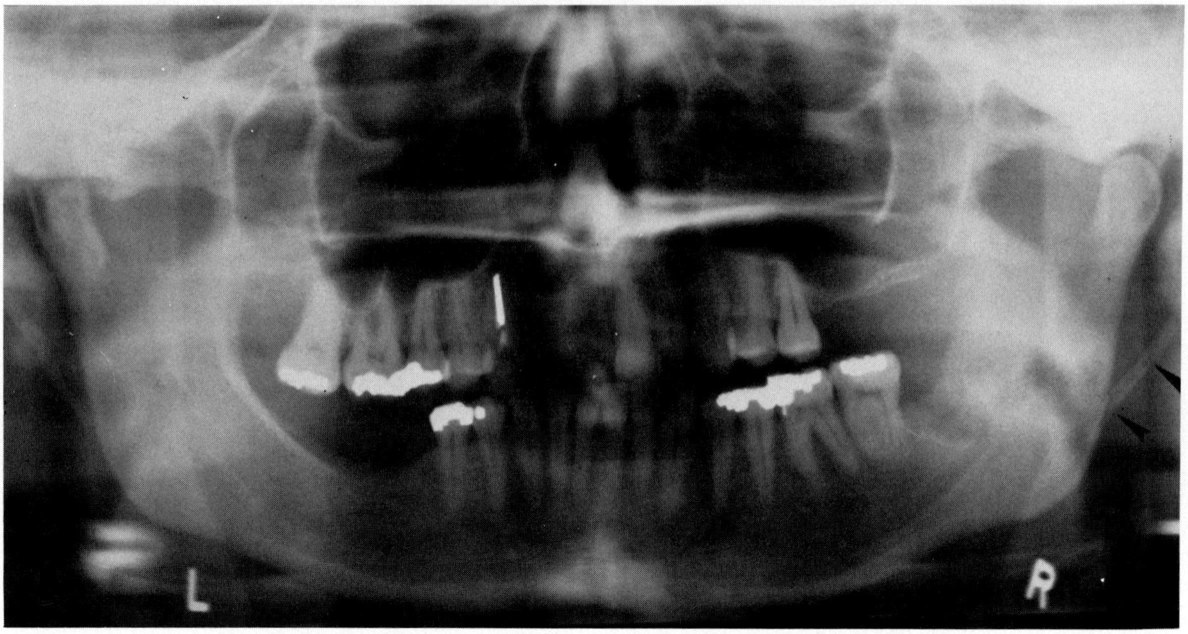

Fig. 10-12. Preoperative radiograph of symptomatic elongated right styloid process.

stance the areas were found to consist of bone cavities at the sites of previous tooth extractions, with dimensions of up to 2 cm or more and with narrow fistulous extensions or tracts from the cavity channel leading in irregular fashion through adjacent bone for distances up to another 2 cm. In the lower jaw these narrow tracts always opened into the mandibular canal. In the upper jaw the tracts often ended in a second bone cavity, which might be larger than the first; at times the fistulous tract would even continue into a third cavity, possibly communicating with the nasal cavity. Nerve fibers often are exposed in the walls of the cavities as a result of the bone destruction.

The treatment used was standard oral surgical procedures for curettage of the cavities and administration of antibiotics. All tracts and cavities were carefully curetted until bone of normal consistency was reached, and then the curetted voids were first thoroughly irrigated with sterile distilled water and packed with a solution of chloramphenicol (Chloromycetin) and absorbable gelatin sponge (Gelfoam). The overlying gingiva was repositioned and sutured.

Complete pain remissions for periods varying from 2 months (for the most recently treated cases) to 9 years were reported in Roberts and Person's patient sample.[15] For those in whom pain returned in the same pattern, the original lesion or lesions were reexposed, recuretted, and treated. But if a new pain pattern emerged, it usually was found to be related to a different bone cavity, perhaps not initially detected. Such a cavity also was exposed and treated. Disappearance or decrease of pain occurred immediately or within 1 week following surgery in most cases. The observations and results of this study suggest that dental and oral pathosis may play a role in the genesis of trigeminal and atypical facial neuralgias.

EAGLE'S SYNDROME

Eagle's syndrome, or symptomatic elongated styloid process, may present a wide variety of symptoms, including difficulty in swallowing, sore throat, glossodynia, headache, and severe hemifacial pain.[5] The most consistent symptom reported has been pharyngeal pain. TMJ dysfunction, impactions, oral infections, and oral neoplastic disease also can be associated with these symptoms.

The normal styloid process is no more than 30 mm in length, and many individuals have no styloid process at all. Most are no longer than 10 mm. Often the stylohyoid ligament is ossified, and the process is elongated. If this process angles either laterally or medially, it can encroach on the external or internal carotid artery, and vascular pain will occur as pressure is brought to bear on the artery. Manipulation of the process will elicit typical symptoms. Diagnosis of Eagle's syndrome is made by palpating the tonsillar fossa.[17] A hard protuberance in this area indicates an abnormal styloid process. The normal styloid process cannot be palpated in the pharynx. Panographic radiographs can substantiate the presence of elongated styloid processes as well as give their accurate measurement and position (Figs. 10-11 to 10-15).

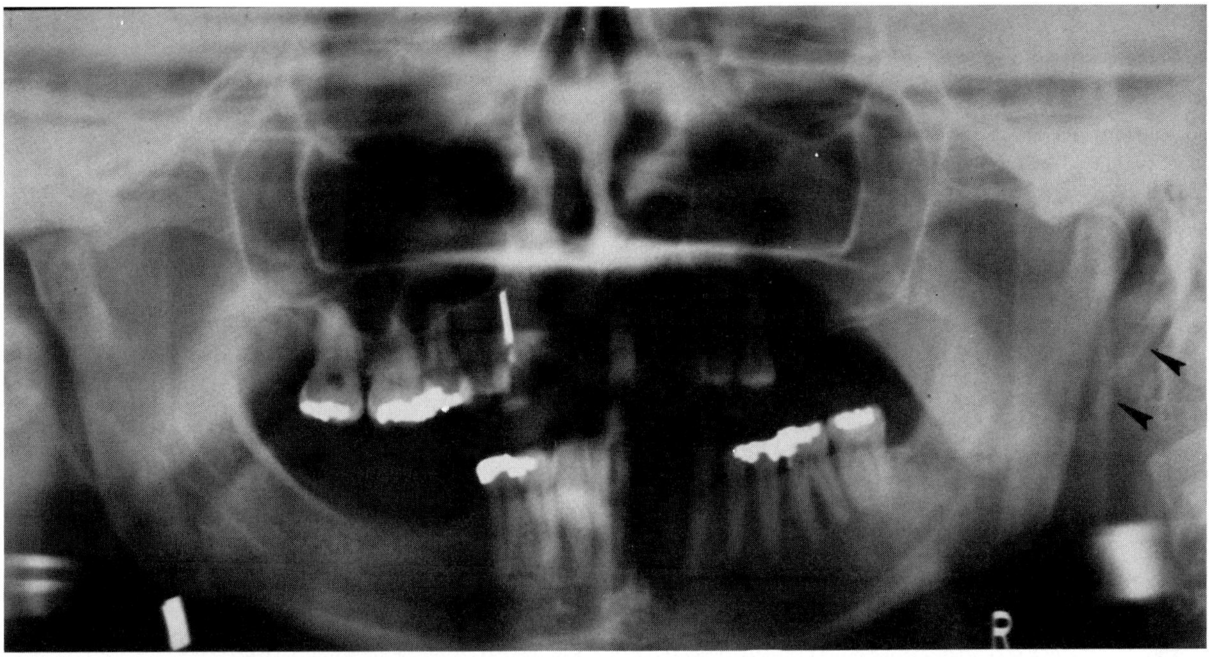

Fig. 10-13. Postoperative radiograph of surgical stump of styloid process following resection.

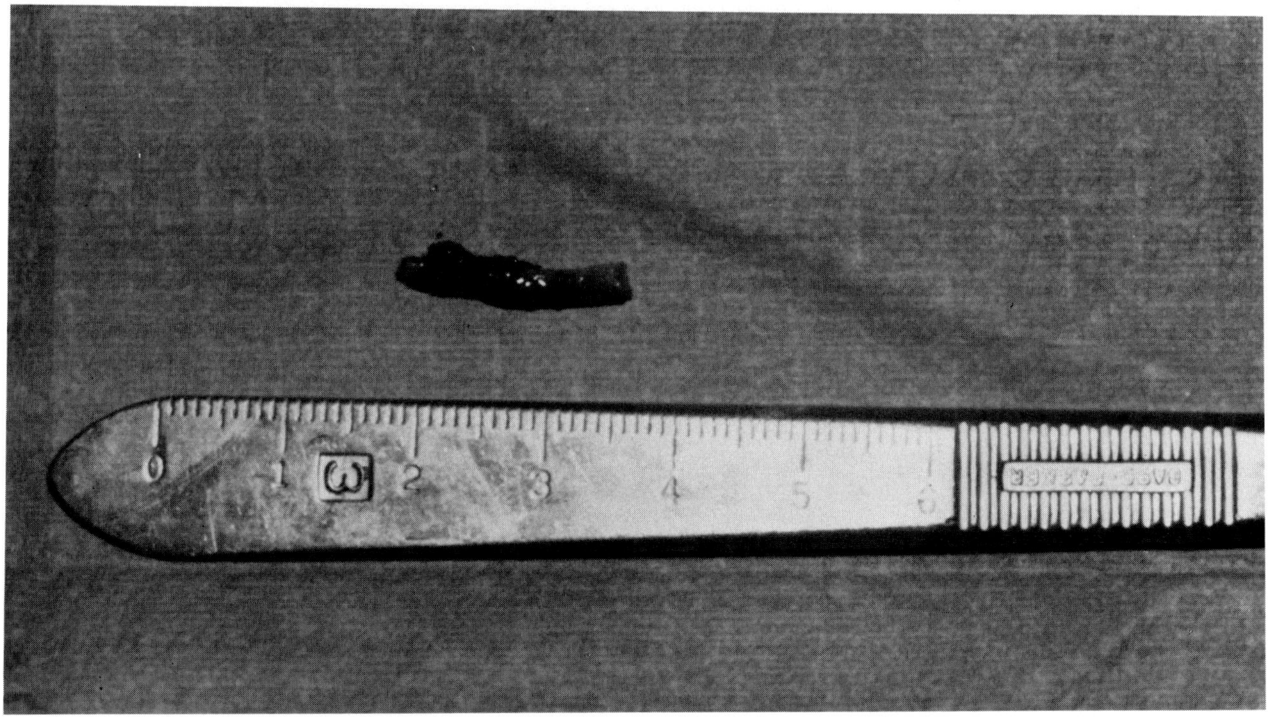

Fig. 10-14. Surgical specimen of styloid process removed via transoral approach at tonsillar fossa. (Case courtesy Charles D. Hasse, D.D.S.)

A

B

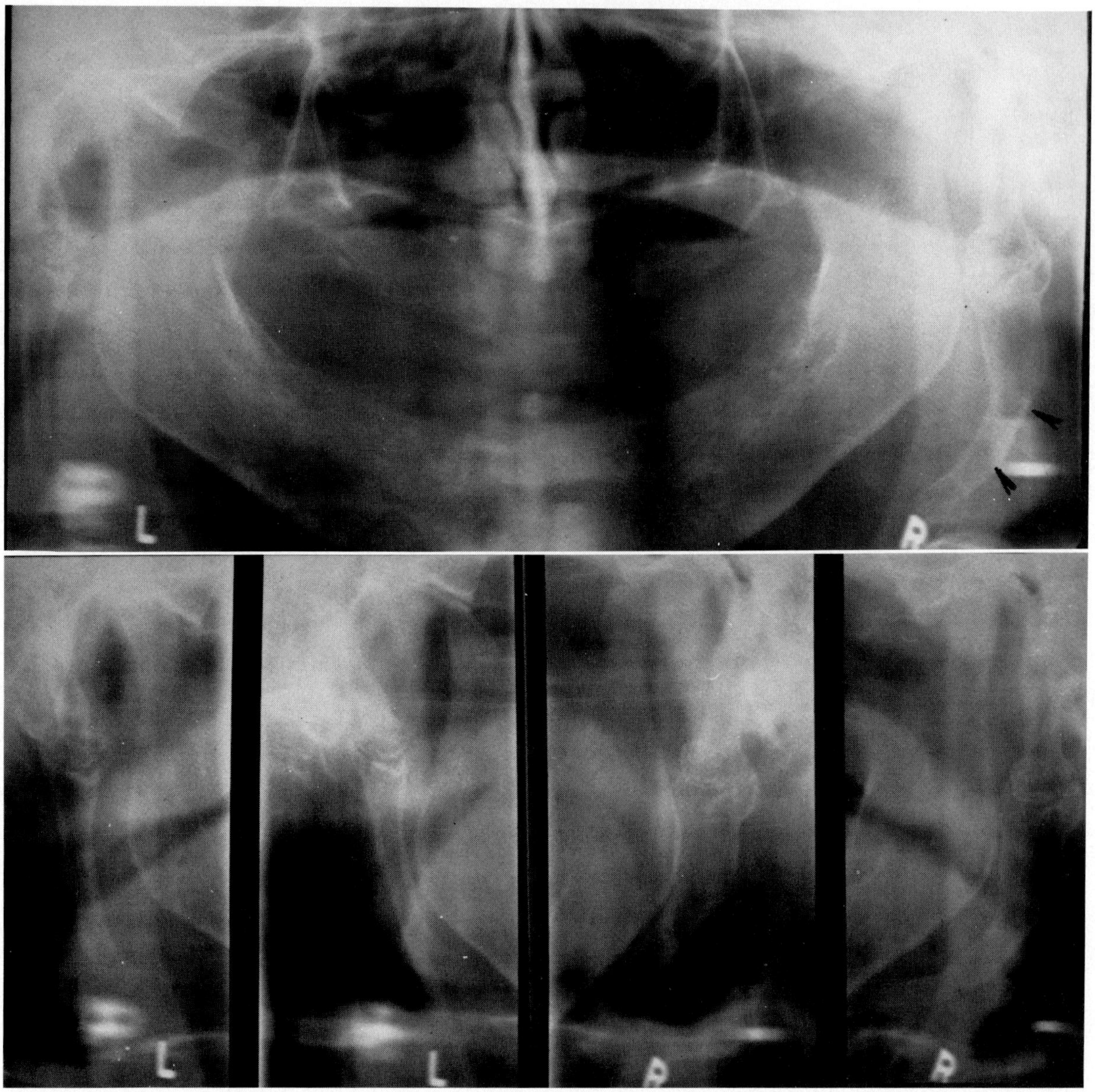

Fig. 10-15. A, Second case in which panographic views show massive elongation of styloid-stylohyoid complex. Remarkably, patient was asymptomatic, and surgery was not indicated. (Case courtesy Charles D. Hasse, D.D.S.)

REFERENCES

1. Alpert, R.L.: The temporomandibular joint pain dysfunction syndrome, J. So. Carolina Med. Assoc. **68**:379, 1972.
2. Beeson, P., and McDermott, W., editors: Cecil-Loeb textbook of medicine, ed. 13, Philadelphia, 1971, W.B. Saunders Co.
3. Chun, H.: Temporomandibular joint gout (letter to the editor), J.A.M.A. **226**:3, 1973.
4. Compere, W.E.: The radiologic examination of the temporomandibular joint, Trans. Pac. Coast Otoophthalmol. Soc. **53**:99, 1972.
5. Eagle, W.W.: Elongated styloid process: symptoms and treatment, Arch. Otolaryngol. **67**:127, 1958.
6. Frankel, V.H., Shore, N.A., and Hoppenfeld, S.: Stress distribution in cervical traction: prevention of TMJ pain syndrome, Clin. Orthop. **32**: 114, 1964.
7. Greene, C.S.: The temporomandibular joint syndrome, J.A.M.A. **224**:622, 1973.
8. Harris, W.: Neuritis and neuralgia, London, 1926, Oxford University Press.
9. Irby, W.B., and Baldwin, K.H.: Emergencies and urgent complications in dentistry, St. Louis, 1965, The C.V. Mosby Co.
10. Kawamura, Y.: Mandibular movement: normal anatomy and physiology and clinical dysfunction. In Schwartz, L., and Chayes, C., editors: Facial pain and mandibular dysfunction, Philadelphia, 1968, W.B. Saunders Co.
11. Kinnier-Wilson, S.A., and Bruce, A.N.: Neurology, vol. 1, Baltimore, 1955, Williams & Wilkins Co.
12. Lindblom, G.: A longitudinal research of dysfunctional disturbances (arthrosis) in the temporomandibular joint—their diagnosis and treatment results up to 1969, Sven. Tandlak. Tidskr. **64**:559, 1971.
13. Molin, C., Shalling, D., and Edman, G.: Psychological studies of patients with mandibular pain dysfunction syndrome, Sven. Tandlak. Tidskr. **66**:11, 1973.
14. Ratner, E.J., Person, P., and Kleinman, D.J.: Oral pathology and trigeminal neuralgia. I. Clinical experiences, J. Dent. Res. **55B**:299, 1976.
15. Roberts, A.M., and Person, P.: Etiology and treatment of idiopathic trigeminal and atypical facial neuralgias, In press.
16. Roydhouse, R.: Whiplash and temporomandibular joint dysfunction, Lancet **1**:1394, 1973.
17. Russell, T.E.: Eagle's syndrome: diagnostic considerations and report of case, J. Am. Dent. Assoc. **94**:548, 1977.
18. Schwartz, L.: Disorders of the temporomandibular joint, Philadelphia, 1959, W.B. Saunders Co.
19. Tylman, S.D., et al., editors: Year book of dentistry, Chicago, 1965, Year Book Medical Publishers, Inc.

11 The ear, nose, and throat

LELAND R. HOUSE, M.D., and **WILLIAM P. HALL, M.D.**

It has been clearly shown[3,8,11] that the majority of patients with temporomandibular joint disease present with symptoms that they think originate in structures of the ear, nose, or throat. It is therefore important for anyone dealing with TMJ patients to have a thorough understanding of the anatomical relationship between the ear and the TMJ, to be familiar with the meaning and causes of the more obscure symptoms of tinnitus and vertigo, and to be aware of the elements and techniques of a good ear, nose, and throat (ENT) examination. The purpose of this chapter is to acquaint the reader with a review of pertinent anatomy and symptoms and to outline the steps involved in the ENT examination in hopes of stimulating the practitioner interested in the TMJ to acquire the skills needed to perform an ear, nose, and throat examination and therefore provide better patient care.

RELATIONSHIP OF TMJ AND ENT STRUCTURES

Many intimate anatomical relationships involving bones, fasciae, ligaments, muscles, vessels, and nerves give a reasonable explanation for the reflex reactions that account for symptoms referable to the ear from pathological conditions or dysfunction in the TMJ, or vice versa.

Anatomy

The temporal bone has four parts: the squamous, the mastoid, the petrous, and the tympanic portions. From the lower part of the squamous bone projects the zygomatic process. Below the root of the zygomatic process is the mandibular fossa. The TMJ is located between the mandibular (or glenoid) fossa in the temporal bone (which also houses the middle and inner ear) and the condylar process of the mandibular bone. The condyle of the mandible rests in the fossa of the temporal bone against the temporomandibular joint and its fibrocartilaginous disc, or meniscus (the TMJ disc), which bears the force or friction of the movements of the condyle in the joint. The TMJ is thus in close proximity to the external ear, the ear canal, the tympanic membrane (eardrum), and the tympanic cavity. Behind the external ear and the TMJ is the mastoid portion of the temporal bone, and projecting inward is the petrous portion.

Fig. 11-1 is a schematic drawing of the ear showing relationships of the external ear, the cartilage of the external ear, and the skin lining with its hair follicles and glands. The bony canal begins where the cartilage is attached. Across the deep end of the canal is the tympanic membrane. The ossicles and space form the middle ear, which through the eustachian tube opens to the pharynx. Deep to the middle ear is the inner ear with the cochlea, the semicircular canals, and the nerve leading to the brain.

Anatomically and functionally, the ear is divided into three parts: external, middle, and internal. The external ear consists of the pinna, or ear cartilage, which is covered by perichondrium and periosteum, and the fascia, which includes the various glands and components of the skin. The middle ear begins with the tympanic membrane, to which is attached a chain of three ossicles supported by ligaments and joints. They are suspended in the middle ear in such a way that sound vibrations picked up by the tympanic membrane are conveyed through the middle ear space and transmitted to the inner ear. The inner ear is composed of the cochlea (shaped like a snail's shell) and the vestibular labyrinth with the three semicircular canals. These bony structures of the inner ear are filled with a fluid, *perilymph*. Suspended in this fluid is a delicate membranous labyrinth that takes, more or less, the shape of the bony labyrinth. Inside this membranous labyrinth is another fluid, *endolymph*. The fragile nerve structures that receive sound, motion, and positional stimuli are supported in the endolymph-filled structures.

The oval window is the separation between the middle ear and the inner ear. Sound vibrations are trans-

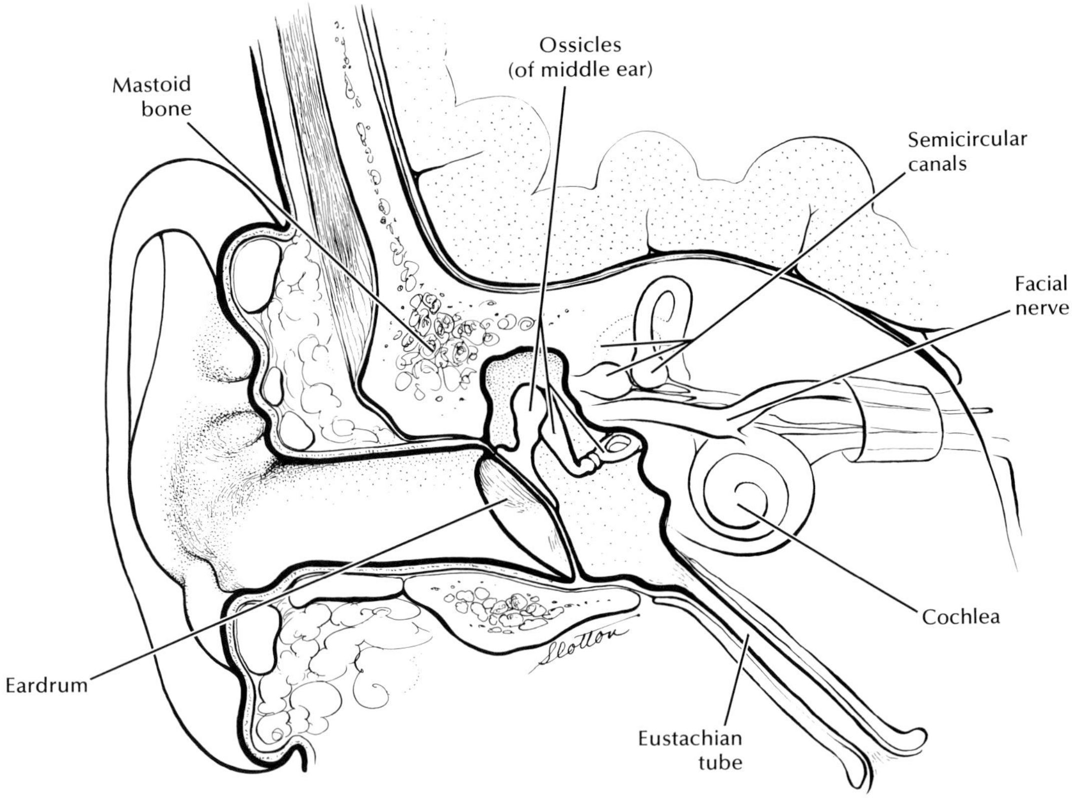

Fig. 11-1. Schematic of ear.

ferred by movements of the stapes in the window. The eustachian tube has muscle structures around it that are related to the muscles of the palate, the styloid process, and the muscles of the pharynx. The mucous membrane of the eustachian tube, like the mucous membranes in the nose and pharynx, is subject to swelling and functional changes, which may account for sensations of fullness and obstruction from fluid collecting in the middle ear. All these factors may be influenced one way or another by TMJ dysfunction and muscle tensions.

The facial nerve also passes through the temporal bone. The chorda tympani nerve stretches across the middle ear in close proximity to the ossicles. The mandibular-malleolar ligament has a relationship with the capsule and ligament of the TMJ and is a possible explanation for some of the ear sensations experienced in biting or chewing[12] (Fig. 11-2). Temporomandibular joint abnormalities may contribute to pain or discomfort by way of this relationship.

There are various intimate nerve relationships and reflex connections with the autonomic nervous system and the ear. The tympanic plexus makes connections from the glossopharyngeal nerve, the autonomic plexus around the carotid artery, and the petrosal nerves. The chorda tympani crosses through the middle ear. The stapedius muscle is supplied by a branch from the facial nerve, and the tensor tympani muscle is supplied by the mandibular nerve by way of the otic ganglion. The external ear is supplied by the great auricular and the auriculotemporal nerves. Disturbed body physiology, stress, and tension may be responsible for symptoms around the ear from adverse effects on these nerves.

SYMPTOMS

Symptoms of TMJ disorders that are common also to ear, nose, and throat problems are tinnitus, vertigo, impaired hearing, fullness in the ear, and pain. It is important to point out that these are symptoms, not pathological entities, and as such are subjective rather than objective. These symptoms occur in a variety of conditions: central nervous system disorders, pathological conditions of the external, middle, and inner ear, head and neck tumor problems, sinus disease, dental problems, metabolic aberrations, allergies, and emotional problems. With the exception of impaired hearing, which can be evaluated by audiometry, these symptoms cannot be directly measured or tested objectively, and one must rely on a careful history, physical examination, and, when indicated, special tests, x-ray examinations, and procedures to make a diagnosis.

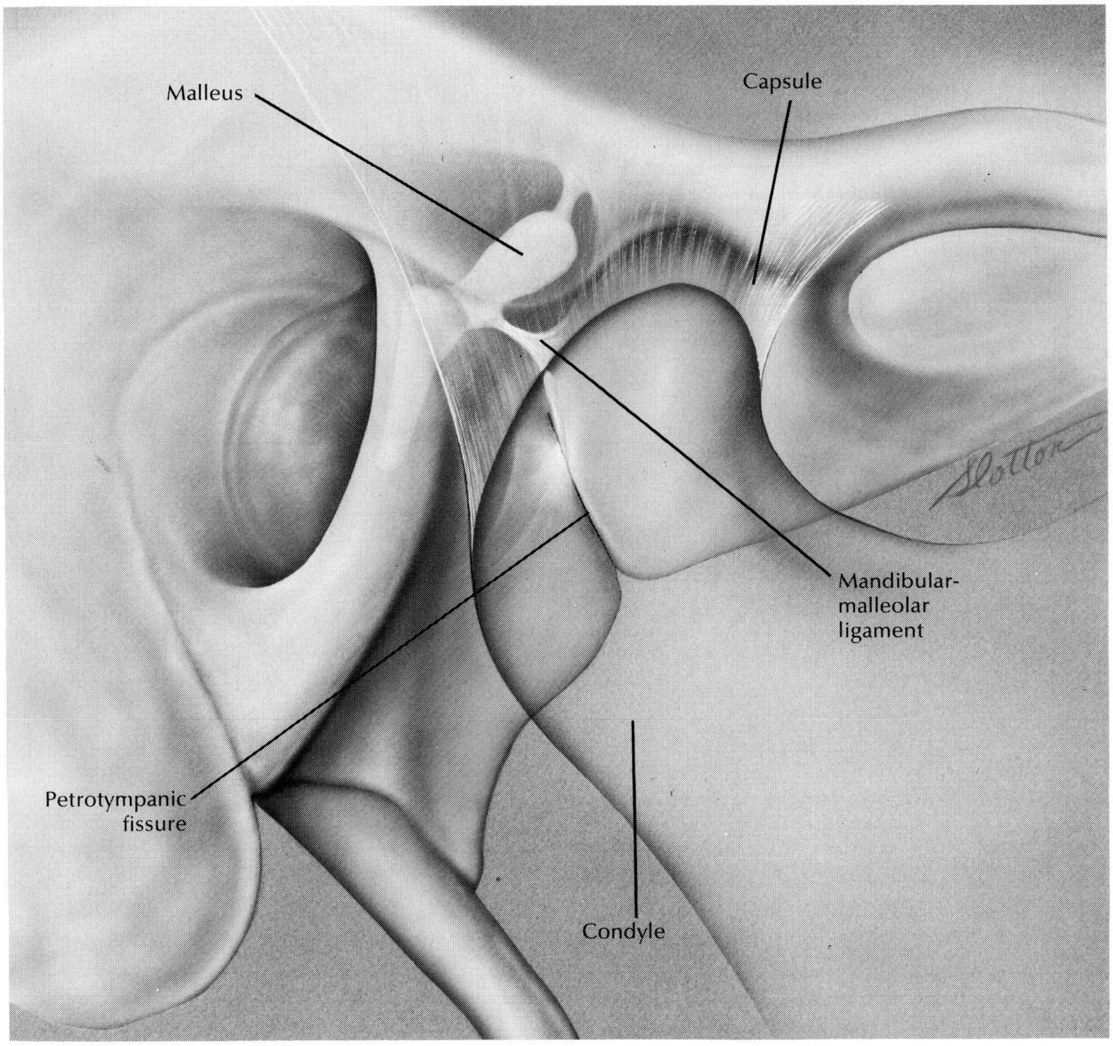

Fig. 11-2. Fibrous connection between mandibular-malleolar ligament and joint capsule.

Tinnitus

Tinnitus is defined by *Black's Medical Dictionary* as a noise heard in the ear without any objective cause. It may be described by the patient as ringing, buzzing, hissing, pounding, or a variety of other sounds. It is important to elicit a description of the character of the noise heard by the patient. Pulsating tinnitus synchronous with the pulse is characteristic of inflammatory disease of the middle ear or with vascular lesions of the middle ear or carotid artery system. A bruit may be heard on auscultation over the common carotid artery in the neck and confirms the presence of a vascular lesion producing this type of tinnitus. A hissing sound, often likened to the sound of steam escaping, indicates arteriosclerotic changes in the blood vessels supplying the inner ear and is usually associated with the high-pitched sensorineural hearing loss of presbycusis. Buzzing or roaring is most often used to describe the sound heard in Meniere's disease but is by no means diagnostic. Ringing is the term most frequently used by patients to describe their tinnitus and is almost invariably the type of sound heard by patients with TMJ syndrome. The tinnitus, or ringing sound, in TMJ disease may be constant or intermittent and may be related to the patient's pain or described as completely separate and unrelated.

The details of what takes place within the inner ear and central nervous system when tinnitus is perceived are poorly understood. Stimuli arising from a multitude of locations follow different pathways to the cerebrum, where interpretation as a noise takes place. Tinnitus is the most variable of otological symptoms and the least predictable symptom to respond to medical or surgical otological treatment. It also has been found to be the symptom least responsive to TMJ surgery.

There is a type of sound, separate and distinct from tinnitus, that can be objectively detected by the examiner with a stethoscope, that is, the crepitus, popping, or clicking heard when the jaws open and close as the condylar head advances over a damaged disc and returns to the mandibular fossa. This sound is properly correlated with TMJ dysfunction rather than with ear disease.

Vertigo

Vertigo is defined by *Black's Medical Dictionary* as a condition in which the affected person has a false sensation of his or her own movements or of those of surrounding objects; in other words, this is a subjective illusion of body motion involving either the person or the environment.[10] The patient, however, does not complain of vertigo but uses the term *dizziness* to describe this symptom as well as other symptoms such as syncope and ataxia. Light-headedness and many other forms of dizziness do not represent true vertigo and must be excluded by careful history taking. The patient with TMJ syndrome frequently experiences true vertigo, and it is not uncommon for vertigo rather than pain to be the chief complaint.

The differential diagnosis of vertigo is beyond the scope of this chapter, but Spector[15] includes the TMJ in his comprehensive review. On the other hand, Facer and Maragas[5] categorize the causes under systemic, neurological, ophthalmological, otolaryngological, and psychogenic headings without mentioning the TMJ. Could TMJ vertigo be therefore psychogenic? Indeed, it is so impossible to separate the anxiety and tension prominent in the TMJ patient from the vertigo experienced as a symptom that this may be the cause of the vertigo. However, the anatomical connection of the TMJ to the malleus through the anterior malleolar ligament makes one speculate on whether a more direct association is present, and hypotheses based on these anatomical relationships have been offered.[2-4,6,9]

Although vertigo is purely subjective and cannot be verified by testing, it is often accompanied by nystagmus, the only objective sign of vertigo.[11] Nystagmus, a slow movement of the eyes toward one side and a rapid return to the midline, can be observed, induced, recorded, and measured. The slow phase occurs as a result of labyrinthine impulses to the ocular muscle nuclei in the brain stem, and the return, fast phase is initiated by the central nervous sytem. At this time the best method to clinically evaluate nystagmus is electronystagmography.[13] Study of the pathological conditions of the TMJ has failed to reveal any electronystagmographic abnormalities, and therefore this test and other available vestibular tests are used in the patient with TMJ disease to verify or exclude other entities producing vertigo.

Impaired hearing

Hearing loss may be measured objectively by audiometry performed in a soundproof booth. Measurable hearing loss attributable to TMJ problems has not been demonstrated, but subjective improvement in hearing, although not verified audiometrically, is not an uncommon occurrence after successful TMJ surfery or treatment. This may be caused by a feeling of well-being after relief of pain, relaxation of muscles of mastication and the palate affecting the eustachian tube, relief of annoying tinnitus, or a combination of all these factors.

The main function of audiometry in the patient with TMJ syndrome therefore is to diagnose or rule out coexisting otological pathosis. Radiographs of the mastoid bone and, on occasion, tomograms of the temporal bone may be ordered to distinguish symptoms arising from chronic ear infections or vestibulocochlear nerve tumors from conditions in the TMJ.

Fullness in the ear

Patients often complain of a feeling of fullness in one or both ears, with or without a subjective hearing loss. This symptom may indicate eustachian tube dysfunction, middle or inner ear disease, as well as nonotological causes, and proper otological work-up, including audiometric testing, is indicated.

Pain

The pain of TMJ disease may be perceived in a variety of locations of the head and neck and has been tabulated in Chapter 22 as well as discussed in other chapters of this book. Although a complete differential diagnosis of pain is beyond the scope of this chapter, a few pertinent points are worthy of consideration. Earache is frequently a symptom of TMJ disease as well as many otological and nonotological entities. The external and middle ear are innervated by cranial nerves V, VII, IX, and X and the cervical plexus. Since there are no pain fibers innervating the inner ear, pain cannot be a symptom of inner ear disease. Referred pain to the ear, however, may originate from any structure or area supplied by these nerves. Unilateral headache, if associated with nausea, is suggestive of migraine or other vascular causes. True trigeminal neuralgia as well as atypical facial neuralgia is a diagnosis of exclusion, and a thorough search must be made for underlying pathosis. "Sinus" headache is a frequent complaint of patients but is not usually associated with sinus disease. When nasal structures are the source of pain, the nasal mucosa has been found to exhibit a much higher sensitivity than that of the sinus mucosa.[7] In addition to the location, the character of the pain is an important diagnostic consideration, as well as the duration.

ENT EXAMINATION

A good ear, nose, and throat examination is an essential part of the evaluation of the patient with suspected TMJ disease. Although the technique of the examination is essentially the same in each patient, there are three distinct situations in which the examination is indicated: (1) in the evaluation of a patient with symptoms related to the head and neck area but with as yet undiagnosed pathological conditions, (2) in a patient with symptoms that change, or when new symptoms appear in a patient with known TMJ disease, and (3) for preoperative evaluation when surgery of the TMJ is considered. It is important therefore to have an otolaryngologist or someone else skilled in the techniques of examining the ear, nose, and throat as part of the team treating the patient with TMJ disease. Any able-bodied physician or dentist certainly possesses the dexterity to perform an ear, nose, and throat examination and with supervision, practice, and persistence would have no trouble mastering the technique.

The equipment involved is simple and inexpensive. A good light source is mandatory, and nothing matches the quality, economy, or versatility of a simple head mirror and 100-watt incandescent light bulb placed to the side and behind the patient's head. A simple tray of instruments is needed, including ear speculum, 512-cps tuning fork, wire applicator with cotton, ear curette, nasal speculum, nasal decongestant spray or drops, tongue depressor, 2 × 2-inch gauze, and nasopharyngeal and laryngeal mirrors (Fig. 11-3). Details of the technique of each step of the routine ENT examination are available in any standard ENT textbook, but particularly recommended is the one by Boies, Hilger, and Priest.[1] In the TMJ patient particular emphasis is given to searching for pathological conditions producing pain or vertigo, and this is emphasized here.

It should be pointed out that before, during, and after the actual ear, nose, and throat examination the astute clinician performs an overall assessment of the patient, including general appearance, physical health, mental status, and nutrition, and is on the lookout for clues indicating systemic disease.

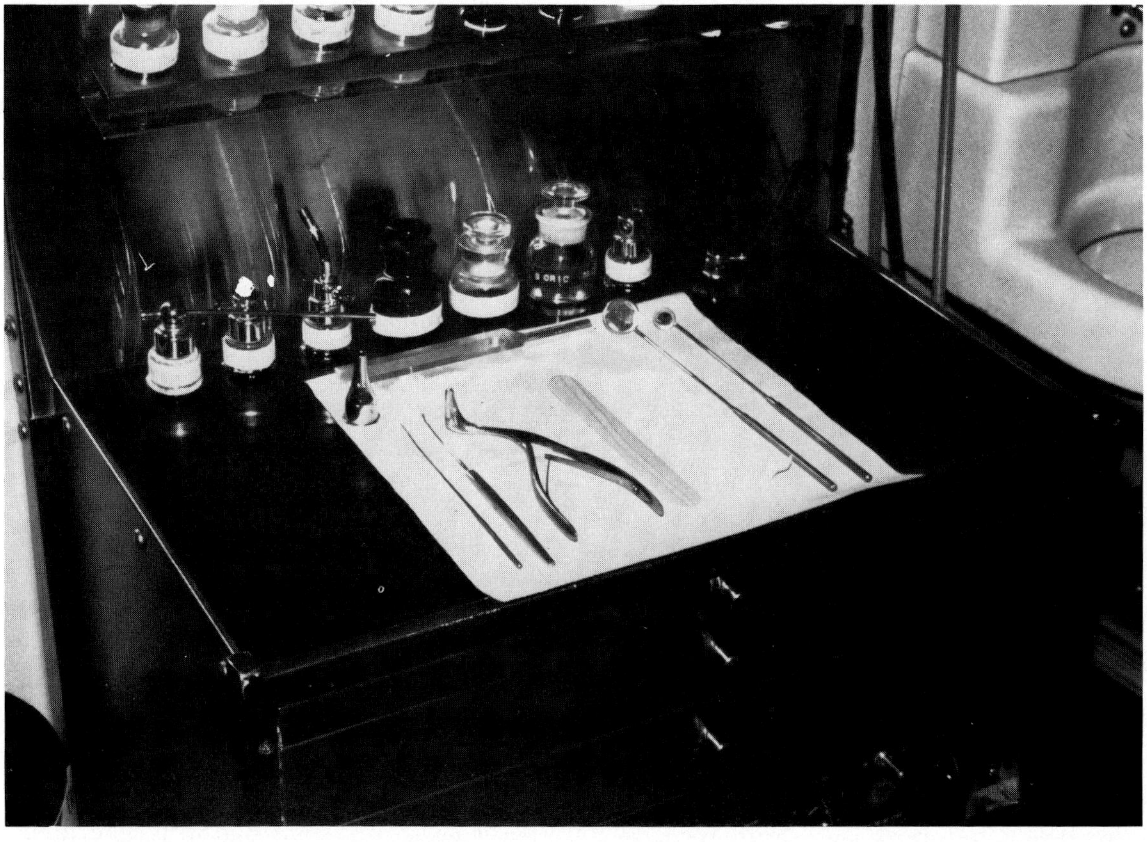

Fig. 11-3. Instruments necessary for complete ENT examination in TMJ patient.

The ear, nose, and throat examination generally begins with otoscopy (Fig. 11-4). Impacted cerumen, foreign bodies, or inflammation of the ear canal can all produce earache. The tympanic membranes are carefully observed as to their color (normally pearly gray) with a good light reflex. Inflammation, perforation, bulging, or retraction should be readily apparent. It is extremely rare for active mastoid or middle ear disease to be present with a normal eardrum. Fluid may collect in the middle ear and may at times be detected by visualizing the bubbles or a fluid level, although it more commonly presents as amber, blue, or pink discoloration associated with decreased mobility of the tympanic membrane.

The tip of the mastoid bone is palpated and tuning fork tests performed, comparing bone conduction with air conduction in each ear (Rinne's test), testing for lateralization with the tuning fork placed against the skull or incisor teeth in the midline (Weber's test), and evaluating the difference of intensity of sound heard in the two ears. Palpation of the temporomandibular joints and involved muscles is performed, the extent of the examination depending on the situation. Details of the TMJ examination appear in Chapter 6.

Intranasal examination (Fig. 11-5) is performed using the nasal speculum, with particular emphasis placed on looking for spurs or deviations of the nasal septum that impinge on the turbinates, producing pain. In many cases it is necessary to use a topical decongestant spray such as phenylephrine (Neo-Synephrine) to properly examine the nose. The external nose must not be neglected as a source of facial pain. The so-called tension nose is caused by an overdeveloped nasal septum externally tenting up the skin over the nasal pyramid, which produces tension on the skin and soft tissues, stimulating the cutaneous nerve endngs (Fig. 11-6). A tension nose is diagnosed by a positive "ooh" sign, that is, the tip of the nose moving downward when the patient says "ooh."

Intraoral inspection is performed with the assistance of a tongue depressor, with the structures of the mouth, teeth, pharynx, tonsil, and tongue all being carefully visualized (Fig. 11-7). Particular emphasis is placed on searching for neoplasms and on detecting pathological dental conditions. Palpation of the base of the tongue is particularly revealing, since a malignancy in this area may produce earache without throat symptoms and may be easily palpated even when not detectable by inspection. Palpation of the tonsillar fossa should be performed when an elongated styloid process is suspected as a cause of pain. The nasopharynx and larynx are inspected using appropriate mirrors (Figs. 11-8 and 11-9). Considerable practice and experience are required to master this technique and properly visualize all structures in this area. Emphasis is on detection of a possible

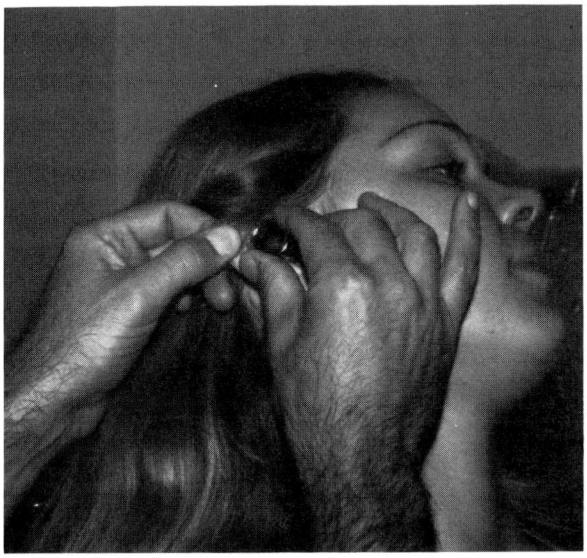

Fig. 11-4. Otoscopy using head mirror and speculum. Advantage of using head mirror as light source is that both hands are free for instrumentation.

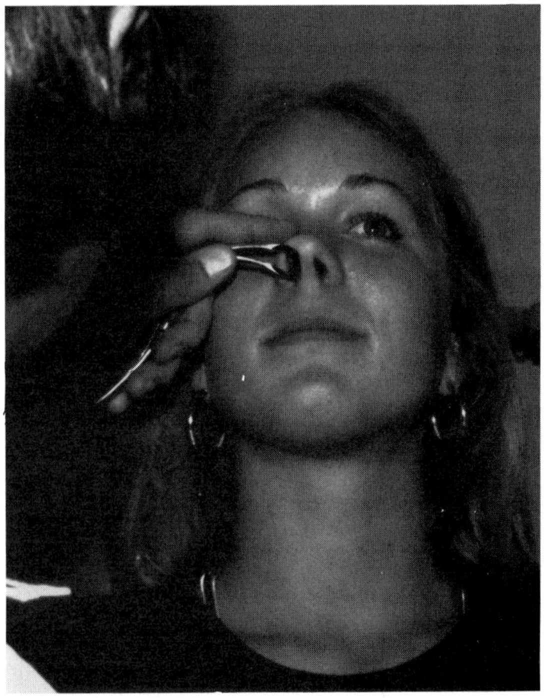

Fig. 11-5. Anterior rhinoscopy using curved nasal speculum and head mirror. Left hand is used to hold speculum, and right hand is free for instrumentation or for introduction of decongestant spray or other intranasal medications.

A 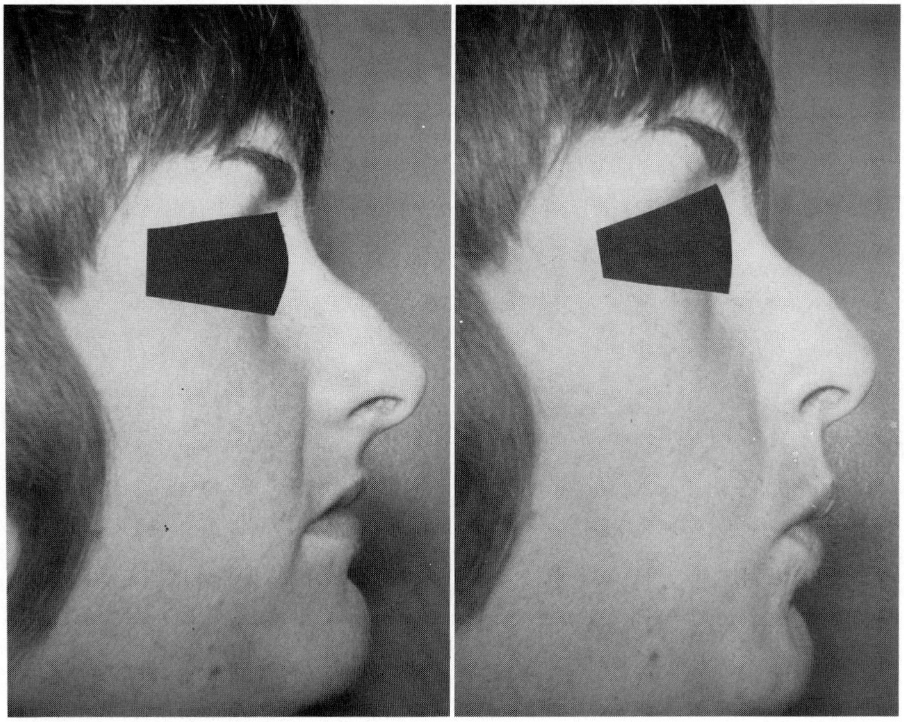 B

Fig. 11-6. *Tension nose* is demonstrated here. **A,** Normal position of nose with lips at rest. **B,** When patient says "ooh," tip of nose drops down.

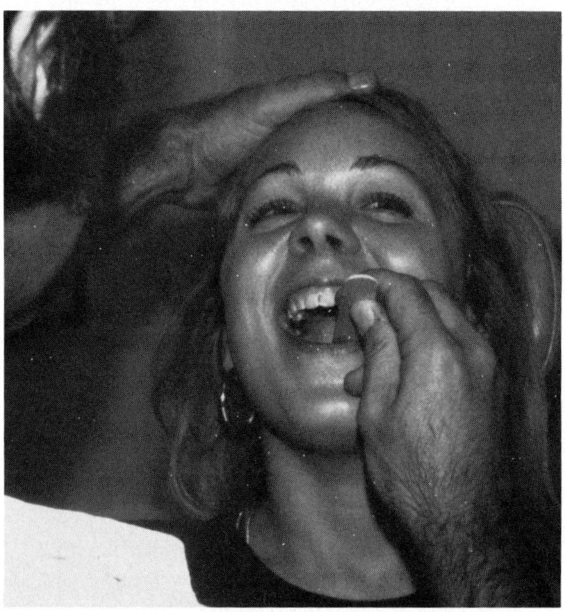

Fig. 11-7. Tongue depressor is used to facilitate oral examination.

tumor as well as on determination of the condition and function of the vocal cords.

Palpation of the anterior and posterior neck completes the ear, nose, and throat examination. The anterior neck is carefully examined for enlarged lymph glands, thyroid enlargement or masses, salivary gland masses, or other lesions. The posterior neck is examined particularly in regard to the posterior cervical musculature, since the spine, cervical arthritis, myositis, or fibrositis all may produce symptoms confused with TMJ disease, which may coesist with disorders of the TMJ.

Although there are typical patterns of pain distribution with the pathological entities mentioned, sufficient variation exists to make the clinical examination vitally important in making the diagnosis. Just as one cannot exclude the TMJ as a source of symptoms mimicking many diseases of the head and neck, so also a good ear, nose, and throat examination must be done to exclude a variety of diagnosable and treatable conditions that may be confused wtih TMJ disease.

SUMMARY

It is important to be aware of the relationship of the TMJ to certain areas of the ear, nose, and throat where similar symptoms can be produced or to which they can

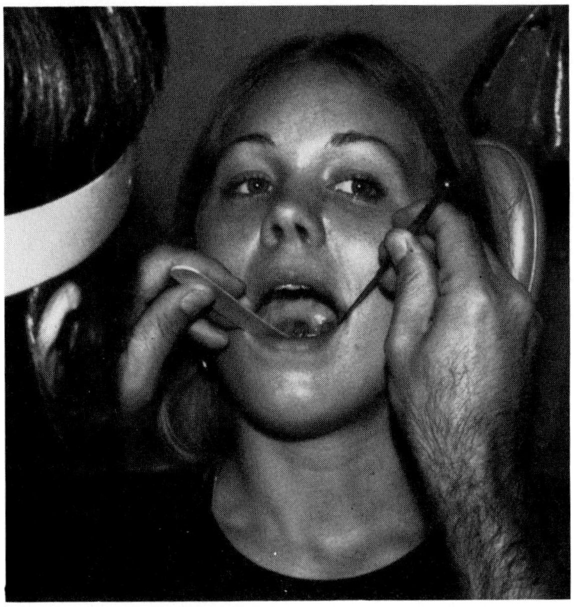

Fig. 11-8. Indirect nasopharyngoscopy illustrating use of tongue depressor with left hand and nasopharyngeal mirror introduced beneath palate.

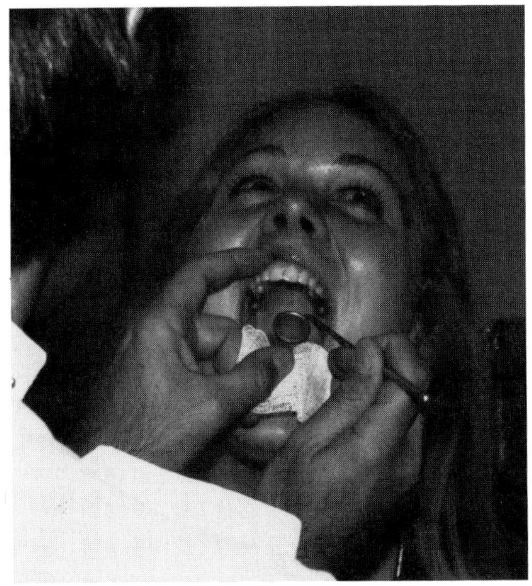

Fig. 11-9. Indirect laryngoscopy illustrating gentle grasping of tongue with 2 × 2-inch dry gauze strip and insertion of laryngeal mirror.

be referred. There is still a great deal to be learned in the treatment of TMJ disease, but is a logical conclusion that improved patient care is an extension of correct diagnosis.

REFERENCES

1. Boies, L.R., Hilger, J.A., and Priest, R.E.: Fundamentals of otolaryngology, Philadelphia, 1964, W.B. Saunders Co.
2. Cawthorne, T.: Modern trends in disease of the ear, nose, and throat, London, 1954, Butterworth & Co., Ltd.
3. Costen, J.: Neuralgias and ear symptoms associated with disturbed function of the temporomandibular joint, J.A.M.A. **107**:252, 1936.
4. Costen, J.B., Clare, M.H., and Bishop, G.H.: Transmission of pain impulses via the chorda tympanic nerve, Ann. Otol. Rhin. Laryng. **60**:591, 1951.
5. Facer, G.W., and Maragas, N.T.: The dizzy patient, Postgrad. Med. **57**:73, 1975.
6. Goodfriend, D.J.: Role of dental factors in cause and treatment of ear symptoms and diseases, J. Am. Dent. Assoc. **21**:204, 1934.
7. McAuliffe, G.W., Goodell, H., and Woolf, H.G.: Experimental studies on headache pain from the nasal and paranasal structures, Assoc. Res. Nerv. Dis. Proc. **23**:185, 1943.
8. Morgan, D.H.: Temporomandibular joint surgery: correction of pain, tinnitus and vertigo, Dent. Radiogr. Photogr. **46**:27, 1973.
9. Myrhaus, H.: Locale of perife syptomu ved kievelleddsarthro, Finsk, Tanal. Forhandl., vol. 98, 1955.
10. Nelson, J.R.: A comprehensive approach to the treatment of dizziness, Hawaii, 1975, American Medical Assocation Clinical Convention.
11. Norris, C.W., and Eakins, K.: Head and neck pain: TMJ syndrome, Laryngoscope, vol. 84, 1966.
12. Pinto, O.: A new structure related to the temporomandibular joint and the middle ear, J. Prosthet. Dent. **12**:95, 1962.
13. Pulec, J.: Clinical electronystagmography, Laryngoscope **78**:2032, 1968.
14. Rubin, W.: Otolaryngol., Med. Clin. North Am., vol. 6, 1973.
15. Spector, M.: Dizziness and vertigo, New York 1967, Grune & Stratton, Inc.

12 The orthopedic influence

VICTOR W. MINTZ, D.D.S.

The paucity in reporting of the temporomandibular joint syndrome in the medical and dental literature is proof that the condition is grossly overlooked. It has been called a "no-man's land," situated as it is between otolaryngologists, who often pass it by, and dental professionals, who mostly lend it lip service. Morgan[4] calls it "the great imposter," which indeed it seems to be in its ability to mimic many other syndromes with a variety of signs and symptoms. One such disguise is the drug-resistant headache, which causes the patient, treated but unrelieved, to suffer long periods of chronic craniofacial pain. This may eventually advance or precipitate neurotic behavior, for which the patient is labeled a neurotic by another group of our professional colleagues and advised to learn to live with the problem. Before simply categorizing some of these ill-fated patients, it would behoove us to examine the problem more deeply and carefully and admit our lack of sophistication in this area rather than condemn these patients as incurable neurotics.

Temporomandibular joint syndrome may be defined as a pain-dysfunction phenomenon characterized by severe to excruciating pain in the temporomandibular joint and cranial-facial-cervical areas. It is associated with clicking and popping, tinnitus, vertigo, and some episodes of syncope. Also affected may be various areas of referred pain, such as the preauricular and postauricular areas, the zygomatic arch, the mandibular, temporal, and frontal areas, behind the eyes, the vertex of the head, occipital areas, the back of the neck and shoulders, the sternocleidomastoid muscle, and the trapezius muscle. There may even be a tingling in the fingers.

The symptoms may seem bizarre, but an examination of the musculoskeletal and neurological symptoms will produce the explanation that the temporomandibular joint syndrome can and does camouflage trigeminal neuralgia, glossopharyngeal neuralgia, and occipital neuralgia. Because of the complex nature of temporomandibular joint syndrome and the multiplicity of its symptoms, a multidisciplinary approach is necessary in the treatment of such a patient. Fragmentation of interest must be avoided in the diagnosis and treatment of this syndrome.

Although the dental profession has been closest to the problem, it has been pursued only by a small percentage of those professionals. It is mentioned and taught to some degree in the dental schools, but it has not been emphasized sufficiently to impress the practitioners with its importance. Indeed, even certain dental techniques can cause potential harm to the temporomandibular apparatus. The making of interocclusal records, which is done by introducing material between the teeth of the opposing jaws, can cause dislodgment of the condyles in the glenoid fossae. Other techniques (such as pantographic tracings or Gothic arch tracings) that involve a centric bearing screw on which the patient must exert pressure also alter the condylar relationship. The employment of materials for so-called bite relationships, when used unilaterally, causes a torquing of the mandible. Thus in spite of some knowledge of the mechanics of the masticatory system, the dentist may still disregard the importance of the temporomandibular relationship in everyday treatment. Our medical colleagues, on the other hand, aware of the problem known to them mainly as Costen's syndrome, place little importance on it and, generally, if they encounter it, will make a referral usually to a dental practitioner. However, the dentist may be provincially tooth oriented and thus accept the temporomandibular joint syndrome as being directly caused by prematurities or interfering cusps and other existing problems with the occlusion of the maxillary and mandibular teeth. The dental profession must alter its concept of jaw relations as having an influence only on the immediate structures such as the maxilla, the mandible, and the teeth. It is a fact that improper jaw relationships will directly affect these parts in the causation of a painful syndrome involving these and other outlying structures. The treatment of these abnormal relationships is truly an orthopedic procedure, since the greater percentage of cases deal primarily with muscle rather than with the joint per se. It behooves us to acquaint ourselves with the anatomy, physiology, and kinesiology of all the related structures, so that we may pursue all the ramifications as to the possible causes and effects of the temporomandibular joint syndrome.

The causes of temporomandibular joint syndrome may be listed in four main categories: (1) dental origin—traumatic occlusion and its trauma-producing effect directly on the joint; (2) orthopedic origin—muscle involvement causing mandibular malposture as well as cranial-cervical malposture; (3) traumatic origin—physical injury or trauma to the patient affecting the shoulders, neck, head, and jaw (for example, whiplash); and (4) pathological origin—degenerative diseases such as arthritis, congenital defects, and fractures of the condyle or other related structures. Suffice it to say that the first three categories may all interrelate and that the initial cause may trigger off and contribute to the others. However, to treat the patient successfully, the overall picture must be considered and understood. Even the pathologically caused problems will ultimately tie the dental and orthopedic factors together.

The problems of dental origin are discussed only as they contribute to the ultimate breakdown of the orthopedic problem regarding the muscles of the head and neck as well as of the shoulders. However, this chapter dwells mainly on the muscular mechanism of the orthopedic involvement. Premature contacts of the teeth in final closure of the jaws cause a chronic irritation of the heads of the external pterygoid muscles. This will cause some spasms, and therefore the meniscus (or disc) will not move harmoniously with the head of the condyle, resulting in a clicking and popping and ultimately causing further inflammation and spasm in the function of the muscle. The mandibular malposture thus produced, in turn, results in malocclusion and interference with the teeth as they intercuspate. Repetition of the cycle continues, and a chronic interference with proper muscular action and function perpetuates the problem, which results in unequal destructive distribution of forces on the chewing mechanism. Aside from disturbing the process of chewing, it also develops noxious stimuli to the central nervous system. This continued stimulation produces a constant neurological pattern of activity that does not permit a period of rest. This endless inflow of impulses results in the production of undesired effects such as spasm or pain. This becomes a vicious cycle, and the continuation of activity may result in what has been described as *occlusal neurosis*.[5] Mandibular movement is dictated by the muscles of mastication until the final phase of jaw closure. Then the inclined planes of the teeth determine the final position of the mandible in its relation to the maxilla. If there is any discrepancy between the muscular jaw closure position and the position established by the inclined planes of the teeth, the muscle fiber length is altered, and function is affected. The result is a pain-spasm-pain cycle. This is particularly true in cases of bruxism in patients who are teeth grinders and clenchers.

The physiology of the masticatory system is involved with four functions: (1) mastication, (2) swallowing, (3) speech, and (4) respiration. However, since most people are preoccupied with the parafunctional habit of bruxism, we must consider this action as a physiological function of the masticatory system. The system consists of the central nervous system, the bones, the temporomandibular joints, the muscles and ligaments, the periodontium, and the teeth; all these are involved in function. In the act of mastication and deglutition not only are the teeth and jaws involved but also all the muscles of the head and the neck, which include the cheeks, lips, hard and soft palate, tongue, and hyoid bone, to which the mandible and tongue are attached. Deglutition, respiration, and speech also involve the musculature of the throat, the larynx, and muscles of the face. Anatomically, the head is balanced on the spine by virtue of the atloidooccipital joint, and all these structures are involved in the functions of the masticatory system. Cinefluorographs have been made in the past demonstrating the action of the jaws, the head and the neck, and even the hand and arm in the act of incision and mastication. These pictures also indicate the movement of the mandible, the hyoid mechanism, and the esophagus. In one group of pictures the portrayal of the hand holding an apple grasped between the teeth shows that the teeth are embedded in the apple until the hand pulls away from the head, and the head pulls away in an opposite direction to literally tear the fragment of food that the individual is holding and eating. The amount of closure into the food depends on the texture, and the amount of pull or jerking motion of the head also depends on the texture of the food. This clearly demonstrates that the teeth rarely, if ever, come together while chewing or incising and that in the action of chewing, the head and neck, as well as the structures just mentioned, are all involved. Therefore any syndromes that interfere with the function of the masticatory system may involve pain radiation of the head and neck as well as of the mouth, tongue, throat, and ears. As remote as these symptoms may appear, it is readily seen that they are directly related. When left undiagnosed and untreated, they even cause psychosomatic disturbances. A tongue thruster, a deviate swallower, a patient with malocclusion, or a patient with a mandibular malposture may well be a candidate for such syndromes, particularly if these noxious stimuli are continuously overstimulating the central nervous system. This will result in hyperactivity of muscle, which in turn will create pain and spasm.

This complexity is further explored by Kraus[2] when he states, "In this painful spasm, pain of muscular contraction reduces further muscle contraction over the short reflex arc and this contraction, in turn, increases pain and furthers more contraction, producing a vicious circle." Once the pain-spasm-pain cycle begins, the mandibular malposture causes an upset and imbalance in all the muscles of mastication, that is, the temporal, the masseters, the internal pterygoids (the elevator muscles of the mandible), and the external pterygoids (the depressors of the mandible). This, in turn, alters the function and activity of the suprahyoid muscles and, alternately, the infrahyoid muscles. With the interference of the hyoid groups, alteration of the position of the hyoid bone will lead to a mandibular malposture or stress in the functions of the tongue, which also could lead to dysfunction in the acts of swallowing and speech. At the same time that all these msucles are affected, the resultant alteration of the center of gravity of the skull (or alteration in the position of the cranium) places greater action or function on the slack muscles of the neck and the cervical spine. These prolonged chronic contractions in the cervical slack muscles cause tension and, again, result in the pain-spasm-pain syndrome. Concomitantly this process also affects the scaleni muscles, the sternocleidomastoid muscles, and then the trapezius muscles, which affect the shoulders and the upper back. Reference areas of pain can extend down into the arm and even into the fingers.

Frost[1] states, "As muscle pain increases the muscle becomes weaker, eventually to the point of pseudo-paralysis." He also states that the disuse caused by the prolonged bone pain also causes local muscle atrophy, which often can be seen and palpated. He then continues, "Prolonged muscle pain leads to atrophy of the affected muscle and often also of its anatomically and functionally contiguous synergists. It is accompanied by the development of an osteoporosis of the bones to which the muscle is attached or which it actuates." Frost further states, "A muscle whose tendon contains a painful lesion acts as though the muscle itself contained the lesion. Where it is anatomically feasible the joints actuated by the painful tendon, or muscle, are held by other muscles and by adjusting body attitude in space, so as to relieve tension on the affected muscle.

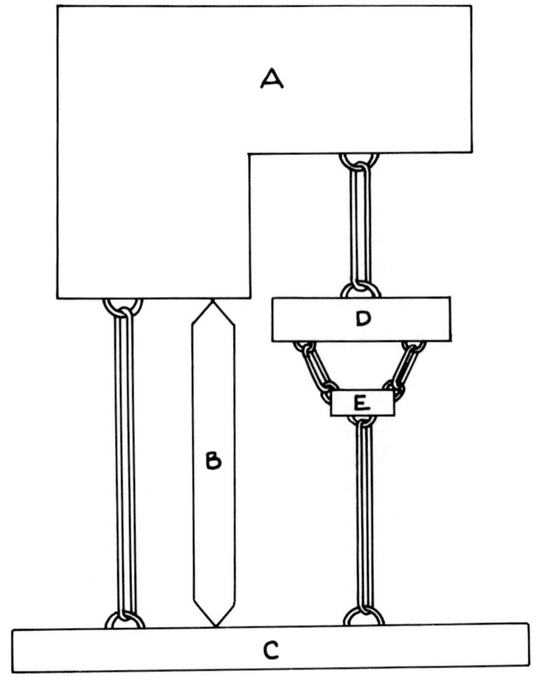

Fig. 12-1. Diagrammatic representation of muscular balance of head and neck region. *A,* Head (minus upper face); *B,* vertical column; *C,* shoulder girdle; *D,* mandible; *E,* hyoid bone. (From Current advances in dentistry, Telephone Extension Program, University of Illinois College of Dentistry, 1949.)

Prolonged tendon pain will lead to atrophy of the attached muscle, and often also to come osteoporosis in the region of its bony attachment."

Fig. 12-1 illustrates diagrammatically how muscular balance is necessary to maintain good muscle function and must be maintained by good body mechanics. This entire apparatus must be in complete balance, otherwise overstimulation of the essential muscles will result in contraction and spasm. "If a muscle has been in spasm for some time or if a muscle has been tense and shortened for a period of time it will lose its physical elasticity. It will not be able to yield to passive stretch after giving up tension but will remain contracted."[2]

Travell[6] states, "When musculoskeletal structures function under stress they give rise to pain that is referred to a distance remote from its source and, hence, local treatment is likely to be ineffective because it is applied to the region where pain is felt rather than to the place where it originates."

An examination of the anatomy of the musculoskeletal system will bear out the logic and explanation of the foregoing description. Further evaluation of the mechanics will help one understand that the TMJ syndrome can be caused by factors that may even begin at the postural level. A shortened leg or severe back injury or chronic lower back problems may cause scoliosis of the spine. This can alter the position of the cervical vertebrae and the position of the cranium and finally result in a mandibular malposture, which can affect the muscles of mastication, cause spasm and chronic irritation, and trigger the pain-spasm-pain cycle. It therefore should be understood that interfering cusps can trigger this complete chain reaction throughout the musculoskeletal system. But this reaction can also originate in the back or shoulders and progress in reverse to the mandibular malposture, which again can result in improper intercuspation of the teeth.

By this mechanism, it may be understood that a TMJ problem also can be caused by trauma, particularly in cases of whiplash, any severe blow to the head, or any fall involving a skull injury. Or it can be caused by a repetitive maintenance of an unorthodox position in a job or exercise that may tend to overstimualte any of the muscles in the previously described chain reaction. In short, the TMJ syndrome can develop from an orthopedic postural problem that affects the muscles which are necessary to maintain good posture and good health.

"When a part of the body, such as the mandible, assumes an abnormal position in relation to the rest of the body, it upsets the correct postural maintenence of the body against gravity. To maintain equilibrium and balance, it calls on one set of muscles to function at the expense of others. It puts a strain on these muscles and creates in them a state of increased tension (hypertension) and in the antagonistic muscles a state of decreased tension (hypotension). By upsetting structural relationships and neuromuscular balance, it may cause various symptoms. As a matter of fact, the occurrence of muscle spasm, distant referred pain and direct injury secondary to disturbed posture are every-day experiences to workers."[5]

Referring to Fig. 12-1 again, muscular balance is of utmost importance because if this system is upset in any manner, the result will be muscle spasm and pain. Myalgia caused by myositis can be treated with quick relief if an early diagnosis is made. If not, the patient may suffer for a long time, with the chronic irritation of the muscles finally resulting in severe muscle spasm, affecting the patient's emotional behavior as well. Many of these patients describe the pain as headache, and point to various areas of the head and neck as the areas of pain. Unfortunately for the patient these areas of pain are the pain reference areas and may be treated by the practitioner locally rather than at the point of origin. Travell[6] defines mechanical headaches as a "repetitive mechanical derangement of the musculoskeletal system." That is, faulty body mechanics are an essential cause of head pain. She further states that "under recurrent mechanical stress, two neck muscles (the trapezius and the sternocleidomastoid) and one of the masticatory muscles (the temporalis) account for most headaches of this kind." To this list should be added the external pterygoid muscle.

"A person with a headache often finds himself a medical orphan. He is fortunate, indeed, if the headache is transient. Otherwise, he may find himself on an excursion to an ophthalmologist, otolaryngologist, dentist, psychiatrist, osteopath and chiropractor. Thereupon, he is x-rayed, massaged, analyzed, fitted with glasses, relieved of his turbinates and his teeth and too often emerges with his headache intact."[3]

This is sad but true. Travell and Rinzler[7] show a pain reference in and around the maxillary teeth that is caused by spasm in the temporal muscle. Case histories have shown patients, after exhaustive dental treatment, including endodontic therapy, apical surgery, and eventually the removal of maxillary teeth, to be left with their pain intact. An injection of 2% lidocaine (Xylocaine) with no vasoconstrictor into the anterior fibers of the temporal can give relief. Similarly, patients with pain reference areas around the zygomatic arch and preauricular areas have had their turbinates removed, only to remain in pain. Correction of the temporomandibular joint syndrome gives these patients relief and renders them free of pain. Patients suffering from whiplash may wear a cervical collar for long periods because the pain persists around the occipitocervical area. Proper TMJ syndrome treatment and correction of the mandibular malposture in some of these patients render them greater comfort and also freedom from pain.

Recently, through the efforts and interest of a few persons in the dental and medical professions involved in headache research and treatment clinics, the temporomandibular syndrome has gained a more prominent role in diagnosis and treatment. The medical orphan is, at last, becoming legitimized.

REFERENCES

1. Frost, H.M.: Musculoskeletal pain. In Alling, C.C., III, editor: Facial pain, Philadelphia, 1968, Lea & Febiger.
2. Kraus, H.: Muscle function of the temporomandibular joint, Dent. Clin. North Am., p. 553, Nov., 1966.
3. Moench, L.G.: Headache, ed. 2, Chicago, 1951, Year Book Medical Publishers, Inc.
4. Morgan, D.H.: The great imposter: diseases of the temporomandibular joint, J.A.M.A. **235**:2395, 1976.
5. Stoll, V.: The importance of correct jaw relations in cervico-oral-facial orthopedia, Dent. Concepts **8**:3, 1965.
6. Travell, J.: Mechanical headache, Headache **7**:23, 1967.
7. Travell, J., and Rinzler, S.H.: The myofacial genesis of pain, Postgrad. Med. **2**:425, 1952.

13 Psychogenic factors contributing to the etiology and symptoms of temporomandibular joint pain-dysfunction syndrome

ROGER A. MARUM, Ph.D.

This chapter is based on the clinical findings of a 2½-year study involving 84 patients diagnosed as having temporomandibular joint pain-dysfunction syndrome. The overall purpose of the study was to understand the multifaceted somatic and psychological conflicts that these patients experience.

CLINICAL OBSERVATIONS

Temporomandibular joint pain-dysfunction patients have been examined, instructed, advised, at times reprimanded, supported, and comforted by a myriad of different professionals in the medical and dental fields. Their autobiographies reflect the frustration of lost travelers, moving in the dark, stumbling blindly down a foreign path. Much like Bunyan's pilgrim, they try to fend for themselves, often becoming resigned to the station of a lonely wayfarer whose whole life is a long, transforming pilgrimage plagued with endless questions but few answers and solutions.

These patients frequently become skeptical of their physicians, wary of new treatment procedures, and cynical about life. They develop a hopeless attitude toward life as their attempts to find relief and assistance are met with further frustration. Lengthy assessment procedures, diagnostic evaluations, endless questions, and numberless palpating, probing fingers become part of the regimen that is their day-to-day life. More often than not, each new medical, dental, or therapeutic intervention elicits new questions and treatment modalities but offers few substantive results, let alone a cure.

It is imperative to realize that the patient's pain may be part of a defensive maneuver to avoid other less acceptable thoughts or impulses. For the patient's full and comprehensive diagnosis and treatment one must examine the possibility that the role of "victim" may be part of a more intricate and ensconced defensive maneuver. Accepting the patient's perception of reality would reinforce that defensive stance and militate against the chances for accurate diagnosis and effective treatment.

After successive frustrating and sometimes fruitless attempts to obtain relief, these people begin to question their own credibility. They begin to harbor feelings of self-doubt. On occasion, when others doubt the legitimacy of their pain, they may question their own capacity to decipher that which is real from that which is not. Many times they will withdraw, expressing inordinate wariness of professionals, family, and friends, all of whom are seemingly helpless to assist them. Friends and family become adversaries rather than allies. The odyssey in search of a cure becomes a lonely one.

As the patient continues this lonely search for relief and a cure, the professional becomes increasingly more impotent in the patient's eyes. The patient's (victim) outlook in fact may be a reversal of what actually occurs. The professional becomes the victim, rendered ineffectual by the patient's ubiquitous somatic problems. It is feasible that this reversal then becomes symbolic of the patient's unconscious strategy.

These patients often are mystified by their disease or dysfunction and welcome the entrance into their lives of someone who seemingly knows what the trouble is and who willingly takes charge. The attending clinician's interventions and care are consciously sought while being thwarted at a deeper, unconscious, and conflicting level.

The conflicting needs reflected in this kind of behavior confirm the oral dependency needs demonstrated by Ross, Bentley, and Greene[3] in their work with a veteran. Typically, these patients have unsatisfied dependency needs that become displaced to the oral region but that also are acted out in other day-to-day facets of their life.

The patients are often and justifiably concerned about the expenses incurred. However, in a majority of cases there is an insurance carrier that covers a significant portion of the total account, again placing the patient in the position of being dependent on some external source for care. Financially, the insurance makes sense and is often fortunate for the patient, enabling medical treatment that otherwise might not be affordable. From a clinical point of view the patient-carrier relationship can become the target onto which more primitive needs and impulses are displaced.

The patients exude helplessness as well as obvious expectations. There is an ever-present hope that this time the results will be different or more enduring. They have placed their well-being in the hands of the professional and in spite of past disappointments expect effective, positive results. Often the clinician is bigger than life to them. The patients appear to have little or no control over whatever it is that has been causing them discomfort. The professional who undertakes their treatment therefore must be invested with considerable power. The treating clinician becomes to some the personification of the idealized parent. Because of the nature of the temporomandibular joint pain-dysfunction syndrome, alleviation and/or cure often is not forthcoming. Once again the relationship between clinician and patient (parent and child) "fails." This may be unwittingly designed to enhance the unconsciously produced treatment failure that will or might come.

The patient's attitude of helplessness also may be a defensive maneuver, a denial of some of the more primitive oral sadistic impulses. Binger[1] discusses the mouth as it relates to human instincts and passions, one of which is the desire to injure or kill. The immobilizing of the patient's mouth may be in fact a reaction formation.

When the patient enters the office, there is an implied change in the chain of responsibility. Whereas once the continuum was *me, my body,* and *my doctor,* the *me* part is no longer a participant but rather an observer.

Sometimes the patients, while describing their medical journey, will identify with the pain. Rather than saying, "I *have* intractable pain," they will quite frequently state, "I *am* intractable pain." It is as though their whole being were the soma (that is, there is a regression to body ego).

During the initial moments of the clinical meeting it becomes evident that patients are often mystified and confused by their problems. There is the explicit wish to have their problems solved, which frequently means "solve me." Implicit in this is the unconscious oral sadistic wish to destroy the expert or authority (that is, the parent). Every[2] considers the primitive, oral aggressive instinct fundamental to the etiology of dysfunctions of the mouth.

The patients sometimes hide their fears, doubts, and vulnerability behind a bravado. Erudite questions with regard to medical procedure and physician credentials are commonplace. A frequent question is, "How many like us have you seen?" The patients each perceive themselves as having unique pain; after all, many have sought to resolve their problems but have failed. Yet they also want to know that they are not different, strange, or anomalies (that is, they wish to be reassured in their attempted defense, that is, regression to body ego).

Patients usually want to trust the clinician but initially are wary, suspicious, and sometimes fearful that "dark" secrets will be uncovered. Perhaps this reflects the fear that their oral sadism will be uncovered. Jones, in Chapter 25, discusses the patient's use of an oral character defense. The patients examined in this current study also appeared to suggest an oral character defense of the biting, aggressive type. Seeing a physician for psychological reasons may mean to them that their problems are "all in their heads," which implies that their pain is not real. The psychologist or psychiatrist is their last chance, and this suggests that they are "hopeless cases" (enhancing the victim role).

During sessions with the clinician the patients are intrigued by the questions and information requested. Although much of the medical history has been repeated often, the request for autobiographical information is usually new and stimulates their curiosity. Some wonder what value this new information can have, since the emphasis moves from the somatic to a more personal knowledge of self. Many, although their curiosity is piqued, resist the task and express annoyance and anger. The inanimate, impersonal forms (paper and pencil tests for assessment) appear to be readily accessible targets for suppressed anger. Although the patients are compliant and at times enthusiastic, despite reservations, when the paper and pencil tasks begin, a noticeable resignation and resistance starts to surface.

The frustrations and confusion of the patient seem to come forth during this portion of the assessment more than during the clinical interview. Frequently the patient will verbally negate the importance of the forms and questions, assuming a cavalier attitude toward the task.

A majority of these patients have experienced personal or family problems that warrant some therapeutic intervention. It is the contention of the examiner that emphasis on physical problems provides a defense against openly examining the deeper, internalized conflicts and struggles. The questions and statements to which the patients respond seem to penetrate those somatic defenses, at least to the extent that the resistance and avoidance become more overt. There is a unilateral reluctance to divulge too much. This may be said for almost any clinical population. These patients, however, appear to be significantly more reluctant to explore personal issues. The physical pain they have experienced provides an acceptable issue on which to focus their concern.

Although these patients all consciously want assistance and alleviation of the symptoms that have plagued them, there appears to be a common fear that they will reveal too much of themselves in the process. Perhaps this fear is most evident among those patients whose speech is barely intelligible or whose mouths are almost locked in a closed position. The somatic expression of keeping one's mouth shut has added significance for these patients. The body responds and carries out the unexpressed wish of the psyche.

Over a period of time and after many varied forms of examination and treatment these patients believe that no one trusts their assessment of the pain and discomfort they experience. They become suspicious and doubt that their complaints are given credibility. They look on the clinician with the preexisting idea that the legitimacy of their complaints is being questioned. The fact that this clinician emphasizes the psyche and not the body further reinforces this belief.

It is imperative for the examiner/clinician to be supportive (that is, to listen and attend closely) and to create an atmosphere in which these fears and doubts can be expressed and examined. The patient's potential for establishing a working rapport with the clinician cannot be determined in one session, nor will it occur within a period of weeks. The patient's evident distrust and wariness can only be noted and explored in a very limited and cautious manner. Although they have many defenses, these patients frequently demonstrate a fragility and vulnerability, at times giving the impression that their somatic defenses are holding together a fragmented and splintered ego.

They perceive the clinician as possessing some capacity to see through them. This appears to indicate that they have some idea, however unacceptable, that there is more to the problem than physical trauma. It also may be a veiled wish to be penetrated and understood. The patients appear to invest the clinician with the powers that they deny themselves.

Temporomandibular joint pain-dysfunction patients are noticeably uneasy in face-to-face confrontations. Not only do they frequently experience the process as a questioning of their credibility, but also the pain etched on their faces often gives their physiognomies a grotesque, distorted look that is embarrassing to them. To sit face to face wearing the evidence of their pain and suffering is traumatic and frightening for them. Eye contact is difficult, and there is a tendency among the patients to avoid the clinician completely.

On many occasions the patients may break down in tears as limited catharsis begins. The mere fact that someone would listen in an empathic manner elicits more than the patients intend to divulge. The surprise and relief commensurate with the expression of emotion are universal. There is a moment of relaxation of defenses as the patients let go of the girding bonds that have held them together through chronic pain and lengthy travail. There is a sense that a deeper, unconscious pain is surfacing, and the relief is evident even though the process is reluctantly undertaken. Even those patients who are able to open and close their mouth at will appear to demonstrate an underlying wish to open up and be heard.

Even with this modicum of relief the firmly entrenched defenses limit insight and understanding. Constant emphasis on the physical problems and body pain is the rule more than the exception. If the patient perceives that the clinician questions the legitimacy of the physical complaints, detailed medical reports are produced as evidence.

It is not uncommon for the problems and inconveniences presented by temporomandibular joint pain-dysfunction to reflect the pain, turmoil, and chaos of the patient's personal life. In several cases if the patient had not had temporomandibular joint problems, it is likely that he or she would have had some other abiding affliction, reflecting inner turmoil. The patient's life circumstances may have been in disarray for some time prior to the onset of the joint problems. The physical problem and/or trauma is evident and well documented; it is the underlying, contributing etiological factors that are not as evident.

The patients have reason to be unhappy, cantankerous, and angry. They have experienced considerable trauma and abuse and often have received symptom relief only to have the pain return later. There are, however, indications of underlying feelings of anger and rage that may relate to deeper and more long-standing grudges, abuses, and trauma. Unfulfilled dependency needs, early childhood rejection, and ubiquitous feelings of unworthiness and inadequacy seem to be inordinately represented in this select population.

The pain and discomfort in their mouth and jaw may reflect the unending search for the consistent, nurturing parent they never had as a child. It may also be a defense against oral sadistic wishes. The pain and travail they endure is almost like a punishment. Many of the patients express the thought, "Why me?" They puzzle over what they may have done to be singled out to experience this disease and affliction. This perception suggests an unconscious wish or impulse for which patients feel they should be punished. There accompanies this process a reluctance to give up the somatic pain. The pain and body problem is less threatening and endangering than the underlying impulse to which it may be tied.

There is no question that these patients experience tremendous discomfort and physical pain brought on by deteriorated physiological systems and processes. Their bodies are no longer temples, but hair shirts, and serve as constant reminders of their vulnerability.

It is also apparent that the problem involves a multitude of factors. Psychological stress, ever-present tension, etc., contribute to the somatic problems confronted by these patients. Their seemingly endless quest for symptom relief and elusive cure takes them through the gamut of medical, dental, and mental health providers. The diverse etiological factors present necessitate multidisciplinary intervention.

CASE HISTORIES

People who experience the multifaceted problems that accompany temporomandibular joint disease also experience tumult and chaos in their personal lives. This disruption, if not precipitated by the disease, is certainly exacerbated by internal conflict, emotional distress, and/or interpersonal conflicts.

The following case studies serve to illustrate the myriad ways in which temporomandibular joint syndrome, a physical problem involving organic pathogenesis, must certainly embody psychological factors. These factors may be causative or may be functional developments that occur commensurate with the onset or prolongation of the organic problems.

Case 1

Mrs. A. is a 38-year-old married woman who has one child by a previous marriage. Mrs. A. left her parents at an early age to attend college. Following 2 years of study she left college to marry and has held various jobs ever since. For a period during the 1960s she was involved in counterculture and antiwar (Vietnam) activities.

Mrs. A. reports that she has no recollection of any serious medical problems during childhood and adolescence, although she does recall experiencing the trauma of enuresis until age 7. She reports that her parents were quite strict, that her father was not very affectionate or attentive, and that her mother was very critical and emotionally demanding. She has one sibling, a sister, with whom she is very close and who she considers her best friend.

Mrs. A. states that she was rebellious and defiant during her childhood and adolescence, and that even as a young adult she struggled with authority. On occasion she has contemplated suicide and perceives herself to be inordinately criticized and scrutinized by others. She describes herself as very tense, prone to periods of intense rumination and withdrawal from others, and at times unwilling to relate to others, preferring to be an introvert and to "shut the world out."

Mrs. A. states that her temporomandibular joint problems began 6 years ago. Since then she has been experiencing severe head and neck pain. The initial diagnosis involved dental problems correctable by effecting change in her dentition. At that time work was also done to alleviate muscle tension and muscle abuse resulting from excessive jaw clenching and the grinding of her teeth. Shortly thereafter she underwent surgery to repair bone damage. The surgery was only marginally effective in correcting the condition.

Mrs. A. reports that she has a hopeless feeling about her life. She seems to think that it is her destiny to always have something different or peculiar about her. Her experience in the underground became a life-style commensurate with these perceptions. Her temporomandibular joint problems began shortly after she and her husband "surfaced" and left the counterculture movement. She did not see herself as fitting into the straight world and became wary of people around her.

The intense pain and physical trauma that she experienced during the last 6 years have etched themselves on her face, giving her a contorted, Quasimodo-like expression. Her physiognomy has become a reflection of her perception of herself. Whereas once she inaccurately perceived people as viewing her as strange and different, they now do so, giving credence to her long-held, although irrational, belief in her strangeness.

The organic problems associated with temporomandibular joint syndrome in this instance have allied themselves with preexisting unconscious struggles and fears, offering formidable opponents to treatment. The patient's visage has literally become an ever-present symbol of the repressed internal struggle of her unconsciousness.

Case 2

Mr. B., a married man in his 60s with several children, reports that he and his wife have enjoyed a good life together. He has been a successful businessman for 40 years and has held numerous important positions in community groups. Mr. B. states that he started with very little and through hard work and good fortune has established a successful, ongoing business that has made "the good life" possible.

As a member of a large family, Mr. B. did not have very much during his childhood and adolescence and reports that he learned early about the value of money. He has been quite benevolent with his own children, only to see them squander their monies through poor investments and frivolous living. Mr. B. questions his success as a father, believing that he failed to pass on his own values and standards to his children, thereby leaving them ill equipped to deal with the often harsh realities of the world. He has cut off all relationships with two of his children because of their profligate ways.

Mr. B. has a long history of medical problems involving treatment for weight loss, cardiovascular problems, and prostate surgery. Approximately 20 years ago he began experiencing some difficulty with his teeth. Within the last 10 years he has experienced severe oral and facial pain as well as orofacial dyskinesia. Along with the dyskinesia were symptoms indicative of some temporomandibular joint problems. His tongue thrusting appeared to be related to the temporomandibular problems as well as being a method of exacerbating the problems in weakened muscle and cartilaginous tissue. Although he has been treated by physicians, dentists, psychotherapists, and various other specialists, he has received little assistance in halting the embarrassing and frustrating tongue thrusting. The various treatments have provided some temporary relief but have caused considerable pain and frequently have left him feeling even more discomfort after the immediate relief dissipated. He reports that his body has experienced a great deal of pain and trauma, leading him to a sense of hopelessness when confronted with the thought that he may never be "whole" again.

Mr. B. has been a well-known and much sought-after extemporaneous speaker in the large midwestern city in which he lives. He also has enjoyed the accolades and plaudits that come to one who frequently holds important civic positions demanding public presentations and speeches. It was at such an occasion that the tongue thrusting first appeared and began to severely limit his ability to speak and communicate. While sitting on the dais awaiting his turn to speak, he began to lose control of his tongue and some of his orofacial muscles. Although he had never been nervous before, his initial reaction was to attribute the problem to "a case of nerves." Over a period of time the tongue thrusting became more intense, at times lasting for several minutes before ceasing and permitting normal mouth and tongue movements to resume. The periods when normal speech and facial control were possible became fewer and of shorter duration, whereas the periods when he experienced the dyskinesia increased and were of longer duration.

The tongue thrusting perhaps represents a deeper, unconscious wish to dismiss or do away with others. The gesture in itself is a condescending, denigrating one usually reserved for those in disfavor.

The tongue thrusting radically changed Mr. B.'s life. No longer able to participate in civic and social functions, which had brought him much pleasure, he began to withdraw, experience periods of depression, and become more dependent on his wife. She acted as his interpreter and eventually was at his side virtually all the time. Mr. B. began to feel like a dependent child, unable to feed or care for himself. This could be a defensive maneuver designed to immobilize and defend himself against aggressive and unacceptable oral sadistic wishes.

On one occasion, while discussing the problems confronted by him as he became more dependent, he asked to speak with the examiner privately. After the departure of his wife he leaned over, addressed the examiner, and in a clear, succinct voice said, "Sometimes she makes me so mad I could scream!" His next few sentences were spoken with clarity and precision. Mr. B. spoke openly about his wife's driving ("terrifies me") and her incessant worrying about money matters. When it was pointed out to him that his speech was clear, showing no sign of dyskinesia, he appeared nonplussed and became quiet. The next time he spoke his speech was once again garbled by the tongue thrusting.

The cause of the tongue thrusting is unclear. There is medical evidence indicating a pathological condition. It also appears probable that there are some functional aspects of Mr. B.'s problem which have their basis in the manner in which he defends against the expression of unacceptable thoughts and impulses. For years Mr. B. entertained people with his wit and humor, rarely if ever saying an unkind word or apparently harboring an unkind thought. This may very well have been a reaction formation designed to deal with unconscious anger. Unacceptable thoughts were repressed and unconscious restraint exercised over threatening impulses. Something began to change within the last few years, and it would appear that the somatic problems entailed in orofacial dyskinesia became the means of defense against the surfacing and experiencing of that which was repressed.

Case 3

Mr. C. is a 33-year-old computer programmer. He is the married father of two who states that he has deeply held religious beliefs and is involved in church activities for both personal and professional reasons.

Mr. C.'s wife and two sons have had extensive medical problems that have required frequent medical attention as well as frequent geographical relocations. Mr. C.'s medical problems date back to his childhood.

Mr. C.'s childhood was marked by deprivation, poverty, and a detached relationship with his parents. He describes his father as an ineffectual man who was incapable of making decisions and appeared to be controlled by events and circumstances rather than vice versa. His mother is described by him as worthless and of dubious moral repute. Neither parent appeared able and/or willing to give much to their son. He grew up deeply resenting his background and harboring an intense dislike for both parents.

Mr. C.'s medical problems began early and include various orofacial and musculoskeletal surgeries as well as chronic pain and several localized paralyses. He has experienced the gamut of treatment interventions to alleviate the chronic pain and correct what he believes to be congenital defects.

By his own report, Mr. C. has become an expert in every professional area in which he has been involved. He states that he has been responsible for writing, editing, and publishing academic and professional texts in various fields and is currently well known for his expertise in the area of computer science that is his specialty. Although often inhibited by his physical and medical problems, he reports that he has always overcome obstacles on the way to success and that he doesn't believe that anything is impossible for him.

Mr. C. is prone to grandiose statements and appears to have an inflated and somewhat narcissistic view of himself. It would appear that the physical trauma which he has experienced has been related to some extent to internal struggles and conflict. His emphasis on a continuing series of somatic problems and his imminent victories over them provide the stage for his acting out an unrealistic and at times inappropriate view of himself and his world. Emphasis is placed on the body and somatic problems in an apparent defense against the deeper, more ensconced conflict and pain related to a deprived childhood that was marked by abuse and psychological trauma. A propensity to overcompensate for deeper fears of inadequacy and worthlessness is evidenced in the ongoing need to overcome with superhuman effort obstacles presented by his medical problems.

Mr. C.'s temporomandibular joint problems appear to have distinct psychological and organic components. Although the pain and discomfort endured by Mr. C. have been great, their presence appears to be more acceptable than looking into and dealing with underlying, unconscious areas of psychological conflict. Mr. C. had limited insight into the internal struggles being defended against by his ever-present physical problems.

Repression and denial function as defenses to thwart the rise to consciousness of unacceptable thoughts and impulses related to the experiences of early childhood and adolescence as well as issues of current prominence. Emphasis on his temporomandibular joint problem and other previous orofacial problems appears to obfuscate some deeper and more primitive oral aggressive impulses.

When physical pain and disease are combined with evident psychological disturbances, treatment is difficult and frequently impossible. Body pain and trauma become part of the vast network of defense mechanisms used to repress unacceptable thoughts and impulses. In this case Mr. C., an angry man, denies his rage and covers his fears of inadequacy and self-doubt by portraying himself as a Herculean figure capable of all things.

Case 4

Mrs. D. is an attractive married woman in her mid-20s. She and her husband of 6 years were separated shortly before she began treatment for temporomandibular joint syndrome. Mrs. D. is a college graduate who has a responsible middle-management position with a large international company. She appears to be a conscientious and diligent worker.

Mrs. D. is the older of two children. Until recently her brother lived at home with her parents. She states that her family has always maintained close ties and that family members expect and demand much of each other. Both her parents work and have done so since she was a young adolescent. When she was between the ages of 5 and 10, her father was frequently out of town for business purposes. On occasion the family would move on a moment's notice to accommodate her father's occupational demands. Mrs. D. recalls that those moves and the often transient life-style they fostered were upsetting to her and her brother and seemed to disrupt her parents' relationship. On several occasions Mrs. D.'s mother would send her to plead with her father not to leave. This would be to no avail, with her father explaining that it was necessary and that he would return as soon as possible. There were several instances when Mrs. D. would function as the intermediary for her parents when the changes in their life-style would create severe arguments and fights. She stated that many times she felt responsible for holding the family together and experienced her father's absence as a personal rejection.

There were also periods when the patient's father was unable to find employment. During these periods he would escape the castigating remarks of his wife by seeking out his daughter and treating her as his ally and confidante as well as his source of support and understanding. An alliance formed out of this relationship. The resultant oedipal strivings and conflict caused considerable internal struggle for Mrs. D. as she grew into adulthood.

While working her way through college, she married her childhood sweetheart. She was the sole source of income during the first years of their marriage. It became increasingly apparent that Mrs. D.'s husband was immature and somewhat childlike in his view of the world and his place in it. Mrs. D. became the one who took care of the couple's affairs (such as business and social matters), and her husband became more dependent and childlike. Because her husband came from a deprived single-parent home, she felt sorry for him and deeply responsible for providing for him. She hoped that in time he would "grow up" and that their life together would be as she had originally hoped.

During the years she was married, Mrs. D.'s father frequently requested her presence at family functions, at times stating that he would not attend unless his daughter went with him. Mrs. D. felt responsible for her father's happiness and complied, frequently choosing her father and family's company to that of her husband.

Mrs. D. reported that she had always been in sound physical health and was surprised one morning when she awakened and discovered that she was unable to open her mouth. Although aware that she clenched her jaws and ground her teeth at night, she had never before experienced any orofacial pain or discomfort. In time she was able to move her jaw and was capable of speech and eating, but she also began to experience painful headaches, causing nausea, vomiting, and some general body discomfort.

The physical problems occurred at approximately the same time that she and her husband were considering moving to another city. This move, to accommodate Mrs. D.'s husband's continuing education, would have necessitated moving away from her parents. Her father, with a history of medical problems was hypertensive, overweight, and prone to high blood pressure. She worried about his condition and felt that she should be near him until his condition improved, despite the fact that he refused to seek medical assistance. Mrs. D. decided that it was time to separate. The decision to remain while her husband left, although painful, appeared to be best. Shortly therafter she sought treatment for temporomandibular joint syndrome.

Mrs. D.'s physical condition was brought on by both physical and psychological factors. The excessive grinding and clenching appeared to have taken some toll on the meniscus in both jaw joints. The reasons for the pathological condition and the sudden onset of the symptoms appear to have their basis in the preexisting internal struggles of the patient.

During the first session of Mrs. D.'s psychological evaluation she reluctantly talked about the dissolution of her marriage and the concomitant pain involved. She also expressed hopelessness and anger toward her husband and perceived herself to be a failure for not succeeding in the marriage. After that session she had a telephone conversation with her estranged husband, and to her surprise and later delight, she voiced her rage toward him and slammed the receiver back on its hook. Within several hours her mouth began to open, and the stiffness and discomfort began to dissipate. That experience precipitated her work in therapy.

Mrs. D., a woman of considerable ego resources, was able to weather a traumatic childhood, and then during her early adult years, in the midst of external chaos, worked to unravel the dynamics of the internal conflicts that were in part responsible for her temporomandibular joint problems.

For years she figuratively kept her mouth shut while married to a man whose behavior and attitude toward life closely resembled the passive childlike manner in which her father faced life and family responsibilities. Her inordinate sense of responsibility for her father's well-being and happiness was transferred to the relationship with her husband, compelling her to stay in a relationship that offered her little, if any, return. As the relationship with her husband changed and broke apart, she was able to examine the deeper ties to her father, their mutual seductiveness, and the resultant emptiness and rage that stemmed from that relationship. As her work in therapy progressed, there was less and less resistance to uncovering her unconscious wishes and fears, and the symptoms that had preoccupied her began to dissipate.

On the surface Mrs. D. became more willing and able to express theretofore unacceptable emotion. Of greater importance and significance for her was that she had the ego strength to look beyond the somatic struggle and invest herself in the arduous and often bittersweet struggle of unraveling her unconscious.

REFERENCES

1. Binger, C.: Personality and oral disease, Ann. Dent. **4**:175, 1946.
2. Every, R.G.: The significance of extreme mandibular movements, Lancet **2**:37, 1960.
3. Ross, G.L., Bentley, H.M., and Greene, G.W.: The psychosomatic concept in dentistry, Psychosom. Med. **15**:168, 1953.

PART THREE

TREATMENT

14 Gnathological treatment

WILLIAM S. SEIBLY, D.D.S., Ph.D. and ROBERT A. JAMES, D.D.S., M.S.

The gnathological methods of TMJ therapy consist of all restorative procedures designed to enhance the harmony of the occlusion. Both equilibration and reconstruction of the dentition are implemented, since malocclusion is a consistent finding in TMJ disorders. Treatment is designed to decrease the trauma directly resulting from occlusal disharmony and to eliminate habits that perpetuate continued hyperfunction of the system.

Chronic overfunction in itself may be sufficient to initiate TMJ symptoms. Certainly, hyperfunction is a significant contributory problem. Patients suffering from TMJ problems usually exhibit bruxism, teeth clenching, or constant toying with specific cusps, especially if malocclusion exists. Restoration to occlusal harmony reduces function to manageable levels, reduces symptoms, and prevents acute exacerbations from occurring.

TMJ disease is a multifactorial problem. Likewise, gnathological techniques are one of several methods of treatment, used singularly or more frequently in conjunction with other approaches. The practitioner must choose the appropriate procedure, know the limits of that procedure, make a reasonable prediction of the results, and know how to correctly implement these techniques. Attempting gnathological treatment without a proper understanding of such parameters frequently results in additional symptoms.

This chapter explains the basics of gnathological techniques: (1) the geometry of mandibular movement and the resultant occlusal patterns and methods for recording these patterns, (2) concepts and variations of occlusion, (3) principles and methods of equilibration, (4) principles and methods of occlusal reconstruction, and finally and most important (5) the limitations of gnathological treatment of TMJ problems. The reader is referred to several excellent manuals on the minutiae of the various topics.

GEOMETRY OF MANDIBULAR MOVEMENT

A knowledge of the factors influencing the shape of the envelope of mandibular movement must be mastered, especially those which relate specifically to occlusal contact. These factors include three-dimensional spacial concepts, with changes in time.

Several factors influence the path followed by any specific cusp in relation to the opposing tooth. Clinically, these factors exert their influence simultaneously, but understanding can be facilitated if each of these factors is considered individually, using familiar gnathological terminology.

Hinge axis

The hinge axis is the center of rotation for the mandible during the first phase of opening. It is visualized as a straight line passing through both condyles. This hinge axis moves with the mandible. Thus when the patient is opening in a protrusive relationship, the hinge axis moves more anterior in relation to the maxilla (Fig. 14-1). The hinge axis exists, can be located, and is consistent through decades of adult life, although slight changes are seen in severe TMJ disease.

Eminence

Movable bony joints are covered and protected by cartilaginous articular surfaces. The path of articular movement is dependent on muscles, ligaments, the shape of the bony parts, and the thickness and uniformity of the cartilage. In the TMJ the sigmoid curvature of the cranial portion of the joint dictates the vertical displacement of the condyle during anterior (protrusive or lateral) movements. The curvature of the eminence is similar but slightly different for each individual.

Rotational centers

Lateral movements of the mandible are produced by a forward movement of one condyle with a minimum

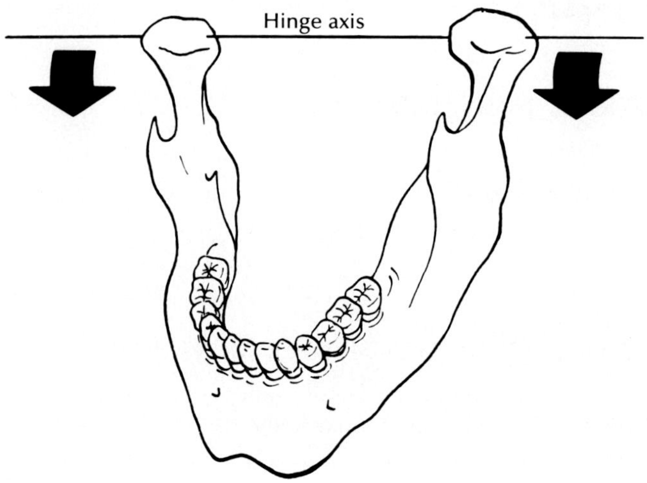

Fig. 14-1. Hinge axis is visualized as straight line passing through both condyles and is center of rotation for mandible during first phase of opening.

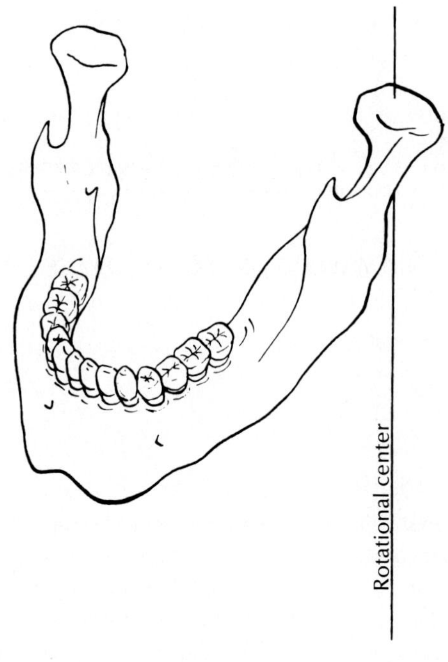

Fig. 14-2. Lateral movements of mandible are produced by forward movement of one condyle and minimum movement of other condyle. Moving condyle *orbits* around rotational center.

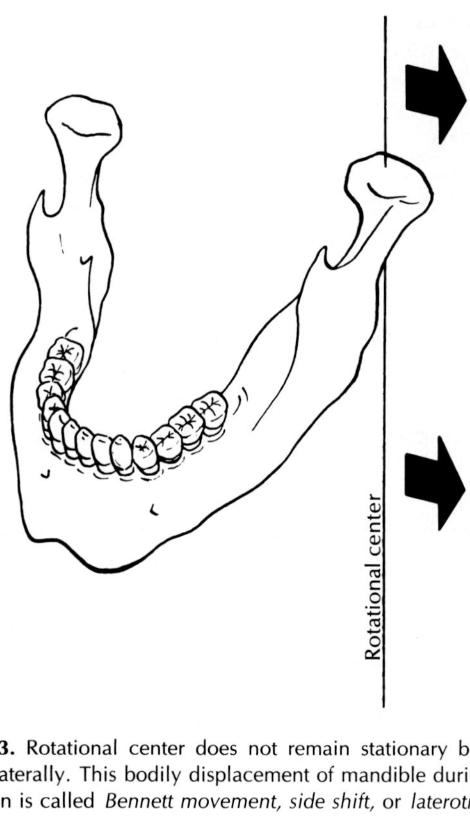

Fig. 14-3. Rotational center does not remain stationary but is displaced laterally. This bodily displacement of mandible during lateral excursion is called *Bennett movement, side shift,* or *laterotrusion.*

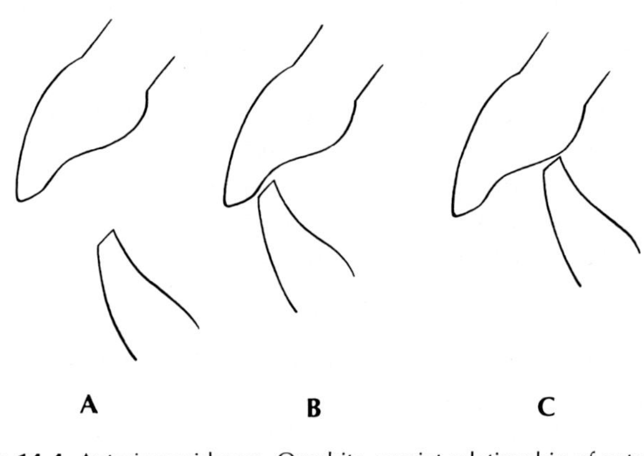

Fig. 14-4. Anterior guidance. Overbite-overjet relationship of anterior teeth influences direction of mandibular movement during protrusive and lateral excursive movements of mandible. **A,** Open bite with no anterior guidance to influence direction of mandible. **B,** Normal relationship. **C,** Influence of lingual concavity of maxillary incisors in instances of increased overbite.

movement of the other condyle. Visualized from above, the moving condyle can be described as orbiting about the fixed, or pivoting, condyle. This pivot around a vertical axis is called a *rotational center* (Fig. 14-2). The rotational center is a concept, a good approximation, and an excellent learning tool, although the center is not fixed, nor necessarily coincident with the hinge axis, nor even measurable.

The *pivoting* side refers to the somewhat stationary condyle or to that side of the mandible. This is frequently called the *working* side, occasionally the *lateral* side. *Orbiting* refers to the forward-moving condyle or to that side of the mandible and is synonymous with the terms *idling, balancing,* or *contralateral* side.

Bennett movement

In lateral excursion of the mandible if the pivoting condyle is accurately pivoted, any point on the mandible (such as cusp tips) would trace a segment of an arc around that pivot point. Precise recordings of human mandibular movements consistently reveal lines with segments more nearly straight than true arc segments and not infrequently display a concavity rather than the expected convexity. This rotational center, or pivoting point, usually does not remain stationary in lateral excursions but is displaced laterally. Therefore, in addition to the forward excursion of the orbiting side, the mandible moves bodily in the direction of the pivoting side (Fig. 14-3).This bodily displacement of the mandible during lateral excursions is called *Bennett movement, side shift,* or *laterotrusion*.

Frequently Bennett movement is most pronounced at the inception of the lateral excursion, developing what is called an *immediate side shift,* and is disproportionate to the anterior and inferior condylar changes. The orbiting condyle in such cases, when viewed from above, traces a curve initially forward and medial, which then turns more forward as anterior translation of the orbiting condyle continues.

Anterior guidance

In protrusive movement two factors dictate the path followed by the mandibular teeth: *anterior guidance* and the *eminence angle*. Anterior guidance is determined by the horizontal and vertical overlap of the anterior teeth and curvature of the lingual concavity of maxillary incisors.

Fig. 14-4, *A*, illustrates an anterior open bite where there is no anterior guidance. Fig. 14-4, *B*, illustrates the more normal anterior relationship. As the incisal edges of the lower anterior teeth move forward, vertical displacement occurs, with resulting separation of the posterior teeth. Fig. 14-4, *C*, illustrates the influence of the lingual concavity of maxillary incisors in instances of increased overbite. As the incisal edges of the lower anteriors move forward over the cingula of the upper anteriors, there is little initial separation; as protrusion continues, the amount of posterior separation accelerates until an edge-to-edge relationship is reached. Further protrusion results in closure as the edge-to-edge position is passed. Anterior guidance is thus entirely dependent on the arrangement and morphology of the anterior teeth.

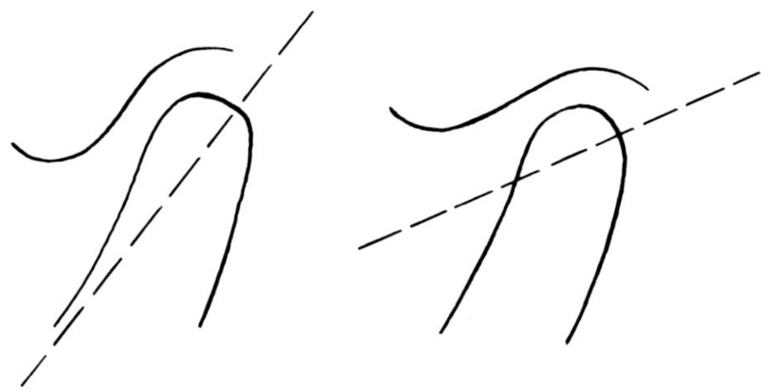

Fig. 14-5. Eminence angle is idealization of general sigmoid slope of eminence and is generally considered in relation to horizontal plane. It is dependent on cranial anatomy rather than on dentition. The steeper the eminence angle, the greater the vertical separation of posterior teeth as condyle translates across eminence.

Eminence angle

The eminence angle is an idealization of the general sigmoid slope of the eminence. Generally, it is considered in relation to a horizontal plane and is dependent on cranial anatomy rather than on dentition. The steeper the eminence angle, the greater the vertical separation of the posterior teeth as the mandible translates in protrusion (Fig. 14-5).

A basic principle is that the closer a tooth is to a determinant of occlusion, the greater will be the influence of that determinant. For any individual tooth the anteroposterior position in the dental arch becomes significant. From Fig. 14-6 it will be noted that the second and third molar teeth are never as near the eminence angle as the premolars are to the anterior guidance. Therefore anterior guidance is the most important factor influencing the relative cusp height.

Increased anterior guidance and increased eminence angles will allow taller cusps, and a decrease in these factors will demand shorter cusps. As stated earlier, the eminence angle is generally referenced to a horizontal plane; however, it takes on greater significance as it is referenced to the occlusal plane. Fig. 14-7 illustrates how this angle influences the protrusive path followed by mandibular teeth. A greater angle will allow greater posterior separation of the dental arches

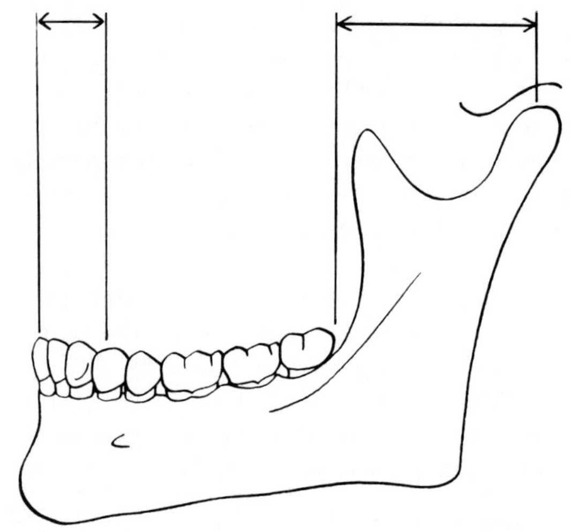

Fig. 14-6. The closer the tooth is to determinant of occlusion, the greater the influence of that determinant. Second and third molar teeth are never as near eminence angle as premolars are to anterior guidance. Therefore anterior guidance is the most important factor influencing relative cusp height.

A

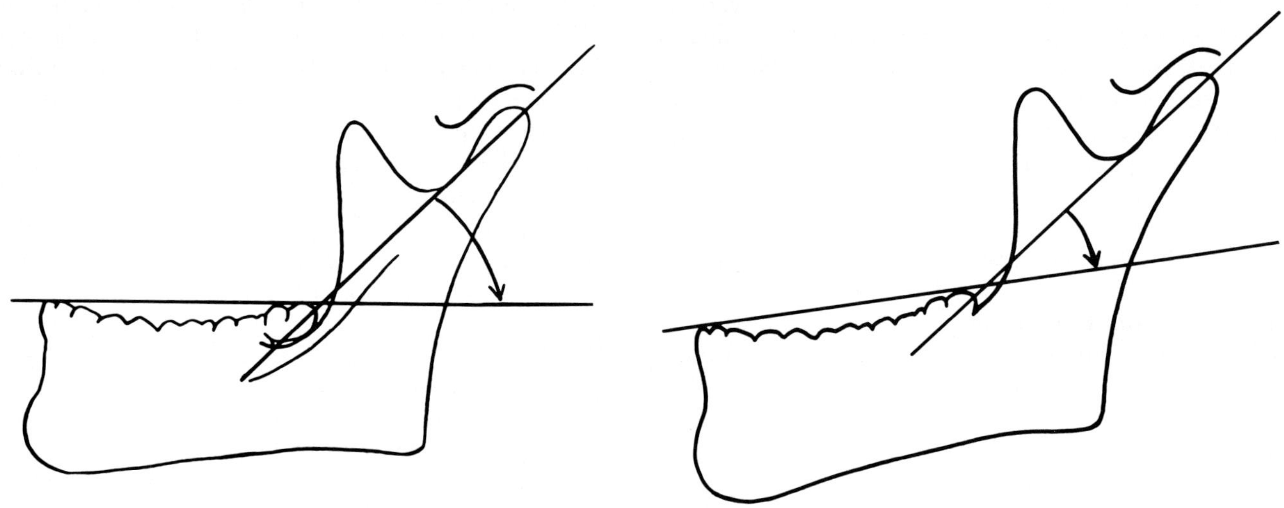

B

Fig. 14-7. Eminence angle and occlusal plane. **A,** Greater angle would allow steeper cusps. **B,** Shallower angle would demand shorter cusps.

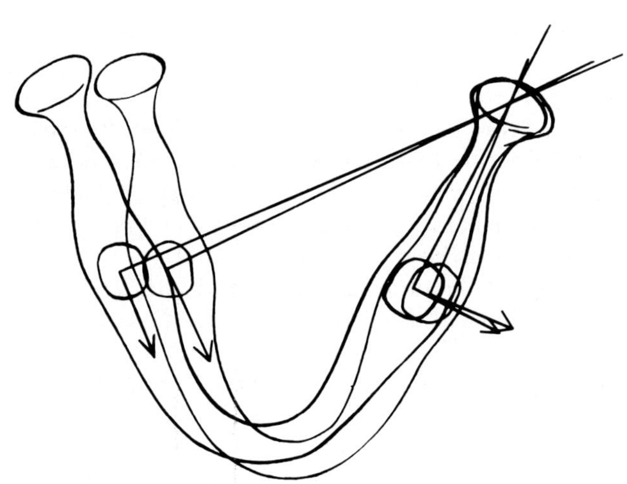

Fig. 14-8. Intercondylar distance influences both working and idling excursions. This is probably least significant of all factors, and arch width is usually more significant.

and thus allow for taller cusps, and conversely, a lesser angle will provide less separation and will demand shorter cusps.

In lateral excursions only one condyle is translating, and all factors just mentioned apply, along with two additional determinants: *intercondylar distance* and *Bennett movement*.

Intercondylar distance

Fig. 14-8 illustrates the effect that intercondylar distance has on the pathway followed by the teeth in both the oribiting and pivoting arch segments. With increased distance, the mandibular cusps of both the orbiting and pivoting sides move in a more anterior direction in relation to the maxillary teeth, and therefore both the working and idling grooves of the maxillary teeth are directed more mesially.

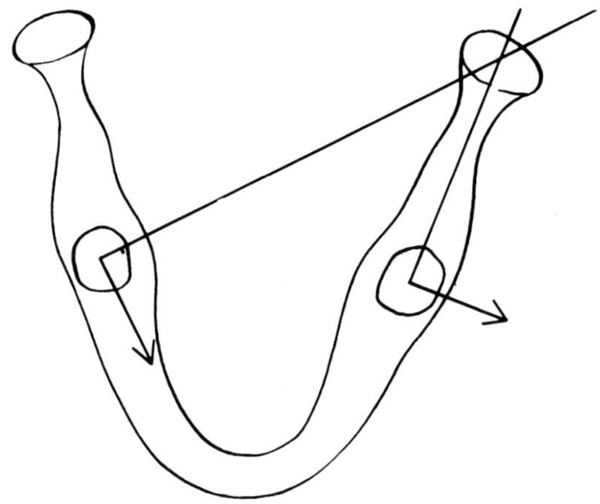

Fig. 14-9. Orbiting condyle exerts its greatest influence on idling side. Direction of idling teeth approximate that of orbiting condyle, and magnitude of movement is greater on idling side.

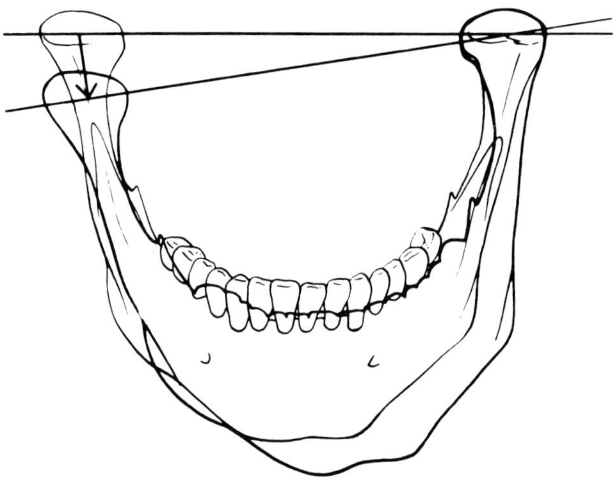

Fig. 14-10. Vertical separation takes place as condyle slides forward and downward, resulting in greater vertical separation of posterior teeth on idling side.

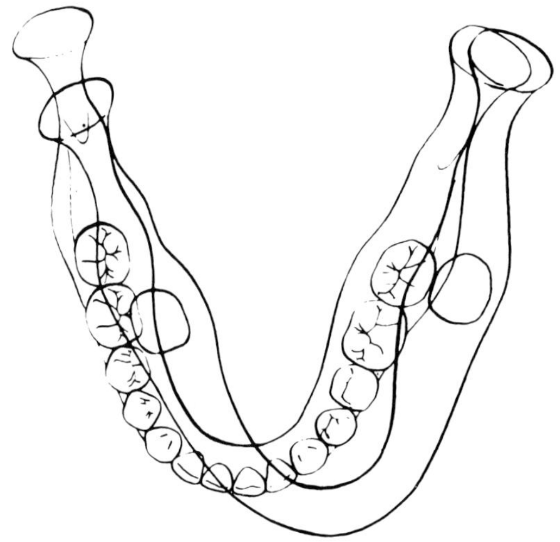

Fig. 14-11. Lateral displacement (Bennett movement) of mandible during lateral (pivoting) movements. See Fig. 14-3.

The change in direction is relatively small and probably less significant than other factors. Moreover, changes in arch width will affect changes in occlusal patterns. These changes are based on the same principles as those affecting intercondylar distance.

The closer a tooth is to a determinant of occlusion, the greater will be the influence of that determinant; therefore cusps in the arch segment nearest the orbiting condyle are more greatly influenced by its path than are teeth on the working side (Fig. 14-9). Of perhaps greater significance, however, is the vertical component (Fig. 14-10). As the orbiting condyle travels forward down the eminence angle, a significant vertical occlusal separation occurs on the idling side, whereas on the working side the predominant vector is lateral, with little vertical separation. This early separation on the idling side is significant in preventing idling occlusal interferences.

Just as the hinge axis moves with the mandible (Fig. 14-1), so the rotational center moves laterally (Fig. 14-11). This laterotrusion will complement the already predominant lateral vector on the working side and results in less vertical occlusal separation (necessitating shorter cusps) and in more distally directed working and idling grooves on the maxillary teeth.

Compound movement of pivoting condyle

Finally, laterotrusion seldom occurs in a purely horizontal direction. In addition to the lateral displacement, the working condyle may vary upward, down-

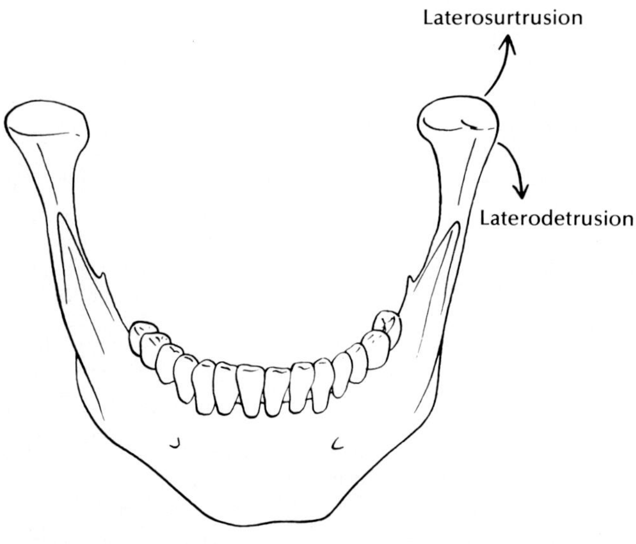

Fig. 14-12. Mandible combines laterotrusion with upward, downward, forward, or backward variations. Laterosurtrusion demands flatter occlusal morphology; laterodetrusion allows taller cusps.

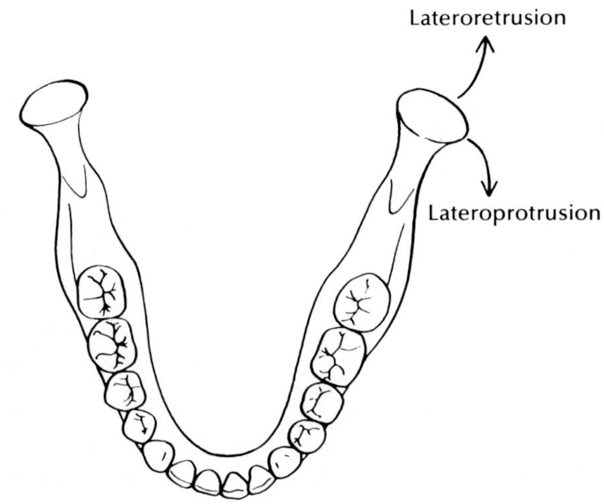

Fig. 14-13. Lateroretrusion and lateroprotrusion influence direction of cuspal excursions.

ward, forward, or backward. These variations are called, respectively, *laterosurtrusion, laterodetrusion, lateroprotrusion,* and *lateroretrusion* (Figs. 14-12 and 14-13).

These variations occur primarily on the working side and can have a significant effect on the working occlusal morphology. Laterosurtrusion is antagonistic to vertical separation provided by either the eminence angle or anterior guidance and, if severe, can completely negate their effect and thus demand relatively flat occlusal morphology. Conversely, laterodetrusion will complement these same determinants and allow for taller cusps. Similarly, lateroprotrusion and lateroretrusion will affect groove direction.

Summary

The TMJ is a ginglymoarthrodial joint. This not only allows the mandible to pivot around the hinge axis during the initial opening movement but also permits a sliding motion of the condyles with continued opening or with protrusive movements. This protrusive path of the condyles mimics the sigmoid shape of the eminence. The condyles also may be brought forward individually, and since the mandible is a fairly rigid structure, one condyle tends to pivot, while the other orbits around the pivoting condyle. This produces lateral excursions. The mandible does not necessarily pivot at a fixed rotational center but usually shifts toward the pivoting side. This side shift (Bennett movement) is often more pronounced at the beginning of lateral excursions (immediate side shift). It rarely follows a straight line and can significantly modify cuspal pathways.

The pivotoing condyle does not necessarily move parallel with the hinge axis during Bennett movement but typically follows a divergent path, which may be slightly upward (laterosurtrusion), downward (laterodetrusion), forward (lateroprotrusion), or backward (lateroretrusion). These variations originate from the pivoting condyle, and although the movement of the entire mandible is changed slightly, their occlusal effect is seen on the working side. These variations are camlike movements, and a simplistic upward, downward, forward, and backward definition for this component of movement fails to convey the concept of actual direction and timing. The curvilinear anatomy of the TMJ is consistent with such observations, and these movements are almost predictable.

HINGE-AXIS RECORDING

Several articulating instruments are capable of simulating mandibular movements, but the degree of accuracy depends on the precise manipulation of each phase, such as locating the hinge axis and mounting the maxillary cast in relation to the axis.

The methods of hinge-axis location are classified into two broad groups: arbitrary and rotational techniques.

Arbitrary techniques

Arbitrary methods can approximate the hinge axis within a radius of about 1 cm and are superior to mounting casts in an articulator without any attempt at a hinge-axis relation. Such methods may be categorized as follows:

1. Arbitrary measurements can be made from other locatable structures, such as 13 mm anterior to the external auditory meatus on a line extending from the outer canthus of the eye to the top of the tragus of the ear.[1]
2. Mechanical devices: References are made mechanically to anatomical landmarks and are transferred directly to an articulator. A well-known example is the Quick Mount face-bow,* designed to transfer this relationship from patient to articulator with a minimum of time and effort. With this device, reference is made to the external auditory meatus and the nasion (the deepest portion of the saddle of the nose).
3. Radiographic extrapolation: If cephalometric films are used to locate the distance and direction of the center of the condylar head from the external auditory meatus, errors will occur. The assumptions are that the radiographic center of the condyle coincides with the center of rotation and that the ear bar on the apparatus can be related to the soft tissue later. The added complexity of this method of estimation is not usually justified.
4. Palpation: This technique is based on a similar assumption that the lateral tip of the condylar head approximates the hinge axis. Each condylar head is located by palpation, and the overlying skin is marked preparatory to face-bow transfer to an articulator.

Rotational techniques

Rotational techniques all are based on the concept that the center of rotation (hinge axis) can be best detected by condylar rotation. Three methods employ rotational techniques:

1. Pointer-reference methods[6]: Flat references with grid markings are rigidly fixed to the cranium (or maxillary teeth) and positioned on the sides of the head in the TMJ area. Pointers, placed perpendicular to the references, are attached to the mandible. When the mandible is arced in its terminal hinge-axis position and the tip of each pointer is at the exact hinge axis, they will appear to remain stationary in relation to the grid markings. Occasionally grid paper is applied to the face itself.[4] Although it is easier, this introduces an additional error from soft tissue movement.
2. X-ray grid[2]: By replacing the paper grid with an x-ray film packet and the pointer with a metal plate perforated in a gridlike configuration, the arc pattern produced by a single opening is easily demonstrated. This research method has displayed great accuracy.
3. Electronic transducer[8]: With the output of positional and rotational transducers monitored by a digital computer, a precise determination of the hinge axis is possible. Although currently too involved for routine clinical use, such research-oriented methods may eventually replace manual techniques.

The mandible can be arced only about 10 degrees in the terminal hinge-axis position before translation of the condyles occurs. Also, the pointer scribes arcs of shorter lengths when approaching the hinge axis, and these arcs are difficult to determine near the hinge axis. Positioned only 1 mm from the axis, the pointer's arc length is less than 0.3 mm (0.012 inch). Finally, many patients show great difficulty hinging smooothly through this arc. Some patients' movements are almost impossible to record, and ironically these usually are the ones in the greatest need of this measurement.

Vertical reference

The positioning of a maxillary cast on an articulator can be repeated only when the hinge-axis transfer is accompanied by a vertical reference; otherwise the cast could be rotated about the axis anywhere within the limits of the articulator. Variables such as the eminence angle have meaning only if the maxillary cast is relocatable in reference to a vertical line or a point. Conceptually, the hinge axis forms one side of a plane that is fixed in space by another point. The other point must be any fixed and relocatable point; the corner of the eye, the inferior border of the orbit, the nasion, a tattooed point on the nose, and even the teeth themselves all have advantages and drawbacks. Obviously one must be consistent in any particular case and use the *same* vertical reference.

Techniques that exclude the vertical reference demand a resetting of the articulator variables with each mounting. This may be entirely adequate when additional mountings are not anticipated and only lateral checkbites are used.

The complexity of the case must be considered when determining the articulating technique to be used.

1. If no change in vertical relationship is to occur and no reference to lateral movements is to be made, a hinge axis is unnecessary. Many single-tooth castings are mounted in a crude hinge that relates casts only in centric.
2. If maxillary and mandibular casts are exceptionally accurate and marked facets of wear exist, the movements of the teeth can be approximated by hand, and a hinge axis and even the articulator

*Whip-Mix Corp., Louisville, Ky.

could be omitted for single-tooth castings. The technique of hand-held casts is not considered valid by those who thoroughly understand occlusion. Interestingly, those who know refuse to guess.

3. To duplicate the functional paths of mandibular movement, a correct hinge axis is necessary. Various chew-in methods offer a compromise in which excursions are recorded in the counterdie and are used to define the occlusion for single castings in which a cusp-fossa relationship is ignored.
4. A highly accurate hinge-axis mounting is required for a change in vertical dimension (opening or closing the bite), for extensive occlusal reconfiguration, or for any full-arch prosthesis.

In summary, when casts are mounted on an articulator, the hinge axis transfer is the most important step. Without this, all other adjustments become guesses.

RECORDING OF MANDIBULAR EXCURSIONS

All methods of recording mandibular movements require a firm mechanical attachment of a recording device to the maxilla (or the cranium) and to the mandible, usually by anchoring it to the teeth. The movement of the mandibular portion of the instrument in relation to the cranial reference is recorded. The border movements, which are the most lateral displacement of the mandible throughout the lateral excursion sequence, are captured, together with some protrusive reference. From these records a suitable articulator can be adapted to duplicate with great accuracy the mandibular movements of that particular individual. But there are great variations in the methods used for obtaining the records and individualizing the articulator. The following methods are typical of these approaches and represent general concepts rather than descriptions of all manufactured devices.

1. The Stuart[7] technique is the most widely known. The recording device scribes lines on six small black plates—lateral to each TMJ, two on the hinge axis line, and two anterior to the face. A layer of chalk is deposited on each plate, and a perpendicularly placed stylus marks the resulting pathway. After the recorder is removed from the head and attached to the articulator, the articulator is adjusted to precisely follow the scribed lines. The articulator has mechanical fossalike compartments on the upper member, which may be tilted or rotated to simulate a particular functional pathway, and certain replaceable plastic and metal portions are individually ground. Once adjusted, the articulator settings are noted. When the cast is completed, the record of these settings and the individually ground parts are retained as part of the patient's record.
2. The TMJ instrument* records the mandibular movements in autopolymerizing plastic. An inverted cup of soft plastic is placed lateral to the head on the hinge-axis line, and a sphere mounted to the mandibular portion of the articular molds the pathway into the plastic by repeated mandibular excursions until the plastic has hardened. After the recorder is transferred to the articulator, the molded plastic guides are used as a template to mold an additional plastic replica in the area of the TMJ. This has the advantage over the Stuart instrument of eliminating any mechanical adjustment; however, there are problems of plastic rebound and shrinkage.
3. The Dentonamics instrument† used special burs in air turbine hand-piece heads to record the mandibular movements in clear plastic blocks. These blocks, one on each side of the hinge-axis line and one in the anterior midline, provide the reference by which plastic eminence blocks are machined. Thus the manual setting of the articulator is eliminated. The ability to replace eminence blocks without any other adjustments is a great advantage, especially when using a single articulator for several cases. One disadvantage is in the mechanical rigidity required to minimize the vibration of the bur in the plastic block, and the grooves never appear as precise as with the lines generated by the Stuart instrument.
4. A number of electronic methods are being developed that will allow the acquistion of mandibular movement data.[8] The methods currently are involved, expensive, and not as consistent as mechanical devices. Eventually an electronic sensor system should replace the other methods and be accurate, easy to use, and of reasonable cost so as to make the system available in many more circumstances.

CONCEPTS AND VARIATIONS OF OCCLUSION

Experimental observations develop statistical averages, but the average occlusion is not necessarily ideal. Unfortunately, descriptions of "ideal" occlusion usually reflect philosophical attitudes rather than objective observations. However, several types of occlusal generalizations can be identified.

*TMJ Corp., Thousand Oaks, Calif.
†Dentonamics Corp., Inglewood, Calif.

Mutually protected occlusion

In the mutually protected occlusion[1,2,4] all the teeth occlude in centric relation, the majority of the occlusal stress being exerted on the posterior teeth and touching but lightly in the anterior segment. In other (eccentric) positions the anterior teeth provide a cam or ramplike effect, which opens (discludes) the posterior teeth. Therefore the centric force is directed to the posterior teeth and the eccentric forces to anterior teeth. It appears that the anterior teeth are more sensitive to force applied perpendicularly to the long axis of the tooth than are posterior teeth.[3] Mutually protected occlusion allows for the design of sharply cusped teeth, which have greater masticatory efficiency than flatter teeth.

Flat occlusion

Flat occlusion is not a natural occlusion but is the result of extensive wear or dental intervention. No human is born with flat occlusal surfaces on teeth. Many clinicians advocate this flat-cusp occlusion with every cusp in contact with opposing teeth through every mandibular excursion.

Conditions of severe alveolar bone loss, advanced periodontium destruction, and greatly reduced periodontal attachment may severely threaten any successful anterior disclusion, as in the mutually protected occlusion. The efficiency of cusp-fossa occlusion is lost, however, and hyperfunction causes lateral masticatory forces to be amplified, especially in the molar regions.

Open-bite cases

Occasionally the anterior teeth do not touch in any excursion. Tongue-thrusting habits are often implicated, and this etiological factor must be recognized and the cause removed. Orthodontic treatment in the younger patient can be successful. Older patients with open-bite occlusion are some of the most difficult to properly treat. Teeth are not easily moved, habits are not easily changed, and results are often, at best, a compromise.

Occlusion modified by tooth loss or tooth movement

Causes of modified occlusion include full and partial dentures, migration of the remining teeth, extensive dental treatment, and orthodontically reorganized occlusion. The modification may be beneficial, but nevertheless it produces alterations in the natural occlusion and usually results in some degree of malocclusion.

Long centric occlusion

Cusped teeth, although more efficient in cutting through a bolus of food, produce greater lateral displacement and instability in full dentures. Dental clinicians recognized early that a flatter occlusal table increased the stability of full dentures but reduced the masticatory efficiency. Efficiency was enhanced by adding grooves to flat teeth and reducing the total occlusal width. One effective solution has been the introduction of a sharp-edged tooth on one arch opposed to a flat surface on the other. In posterior restorations in natural dentition this principle has been applied to individual cusps, where sharp cusp tips articulate in a shallow, flat fossa. This arrangement is described as a long centric occlusion because posterior tooth contact is not merely a point contact, as in the mutually protected occlusion, or a broad contact into all eccentric positions, as with the flat dentition, but a small sliding contact in and around centric relation.[5]

Comments

Frustration occurs when it is recognized that each of these conflicting techniques can produce successful results in selected cases. A statistical evaluation of successes and failures using a sufficient number of cases has not been published, and one can only refer to clinical experience. In our opinion the mutually protected occlusion offers the finest results. As with all techniques, proper case selection and technical excellence are indispensable for achieving gratifying results. However, TMJ problems are multifunctional, as is treatment. It must be noted that although the healthy individual can accommodate a wide range of variation with reasonable success, the TMJ problem case demands that much greater attention be paid to occlusal harmony. The mutually protected occlusion capitalizes on the unique role of the anterior teeth for the following reasons:

1. Anterior teeth act as an anterior ramp, similar to the eminence angle, to remove occlusal contact from the posterior teeth.
2. The uniquely sensitive proprioceptive mechanism of the anterior teeth monitors and inhibits excessive stress in eccentric movements.
3. The position of these teeth, far ahead of the masticatory muscle insertion, reduces the effective force in that area. Conversely, molars are directly in line with the muscular tension. Therefore lateral forces in the posterior area can be much more severe yet less keenly perceived.

Mutually protected occlusion or even long centric occlusion is not possible to implement completely without functional anterior occlusion.

PRINCIPLES AND METHODS OF EQUILIBRATION

The method of equilibration described here aims at establishing a centric occlusion that is congruent with centric relation.

Centric occlusion, also called *habitual, acquired,* or

customary centric, has been defined as the position of the mandible when the teeth are in maximum intercuspation. This position is dictated by the teeth, not the temporomandibular joint, and provides the vertical stop for mandibular movement. Without teeth for guides, no precise habitual centric occlusion can be located. Excessive wear of the occlusal surfaces of teeth produces a diffuse area of centric occlusion. Malocclusions with severe symptoms are occasionally seen in which more than one centric occlusion can be located.

The muscles of mastication are heavily regulated by muscle spindle and other proprioceptive feedback mechanisms and are able to adapt to tooth-dictated occlusion with surprising accuracy and repeatability.

Centric relation is dictated by the temporomandibular joint and associated ligaments and has been defined as the interarch relationship in the rearmost, midmost, and uppermost position of the mandible. This position coincides with the terminal hinge axis, which is the most posterior unstrained hinge-axis position. In most individuals centric occlusion differs from centric relation, and the mandible must move forward from hinge-axis closure to achieve centric occlusion. In such cases the external pterygoid muscles usually contract slightly to avoid the initial contact of terminal hinge-axis closure. When centric relation and centric occlusion coincide, the hinge-axis closure ends in a distinct contacting of all teeth simultaneously. Under these circumstances a favorable environment develops that minimizes the antagonism of proprioceptive information originating from the teeth (periodontal ligament), the TMJ, and the muscles and ligaments involved in mandibular movement.

One important feature of centric relation is its reproducibility. Situated at a precise corner of the envelope of mandibular movement, it can be located at a slightly opened position and be defined within reasonable changes in vertical limits. It usually remains stable throughout life, as does the hinge axis.

Temporomandibular joint harmony

Many people during their lifetime tolerate a centric occlusion that differs from centric relation, with seemingly little or no ill effects. However, a few individuals are unable to harmonize the discrepancy between joint, muscle, ligament, and tooth proprioception. Muscular tension and compulsive cuspal grinding are believed to result from this mismatch.

Occlusal problems

Tooth-grinding habits, bruxism, and chronic clenching can increase the wear rate drastically. As enamel is worn away, the dentin is exposed, and the wear is further accelerated. Contrary to popular opinion, eating usually is not the greatest source of wear; normal eating requires only about 5% of a person's total time. Occlusal wear can only be reduced by diminishing these destructive tooth-grinding habits. Unfortunately these destructive habits are most difficult to modify. The clinical observation is quite valid: "Teeth don't wear in, they wear out."

Periodontal complications

Opinions vary among periodontists as to the role excessive occlusal loading plays in initiating damage to supporting tissue. However, nearly all agree that it is a significant factor in existing periodontal disease. Severe occlusal hyperfunction will result in a pathological condition of the weakest link, regardless of whether it is the temporomandibular joint, the teeth, or the periodontium.

Rationale for accepting an acquired centric occlusion

1. Avoid unnecessary changes in the absence of adverse symptoms. If no problems of the TMJ, occlusal wear, or marked periodontal disease exists, and if the mouth is relatively quiet, equilibration is not indicated.
2. Multiple tooth restorations with cuspal involvement may require modification of the entire occlusion. Minor restorations in themselves do not justify lengthy equilibration procedures.
3. Consider the age, medical condition, and above all the mental attitude of the patient. Superficial correction may only aggravate a potentially dangerous problem. Many temporomandibular joint syndrome patients relate their first symptoms to dental treatment.
4. A careful evaluation must include the amount of occlusal change and other dental work required, the limits of treatment, and a realistic appraisal of the patient's ability to tolerate both the occlusal changes and the other dental procedures needed to implement the treatment plan. If it appears that the patient would be unable to endure the required treatment, it may be better to employ an alternative treatment plan that is compatible with the acquired centric.

All equilibration techniques involve irreversible procedures, and careful evaluation must be made before instituting these procedures. Articulated diagnostic casts are invaluable in making this evaluation.

Articulated diagnostic casts

Several advantages can be gained from a hinge-axis mounting of study casts on an articulator that has been set by lateral checkbites to approximate the eminence and side shift angles:

1. Mandibular movements are easier to manipulate with articulated casts compared with the mouth, especially when complicated by the muscular hyperfunction present with TMJ problems.
2. All areas of occlusion are more easily visualized, compared with the mouth. The lingual view of occluding teeth can be seen only on casts.
3. The articulator provides an aid in the location of premature contacts.
4. Deflective malocclusion from prematurities displaces the mandible somewhat during closure. Although this is nearly impossible to estimate in the mouth, the condyle and fossa portion of the articulator readily shows the amount of condylar displacement.
5. Preliminary equilibration on mounted casts indicates the amount of tooth structure to be removed from each location and the proper equilibration sequence and provides an estimate of final results.
6. Splints or recording clutches may be fabricated with slight changes in vertical opening without additional bite registrations.

The following armamentarium is useful for equilibration procedures:

1. Adjusted articulator with mounted casts
2. Marking (and detecting) media
    a. Articulating paper (various types)
        (1) Plastic
        (2) Typewriter ribbon
    b. Occlusal indicating wax
    c. 0.0005-inch plastic shim stock*
3. Mirror
4. Holder for marking medium
5. Light source
6. Loupes (optional)
7. Rotary cutting instruments
    a. Diamonds
        (1) Wheel
        (2) Finger stone
    b. Burs
    c. Polishing
        (1) Finishing burs
        (2) Abrasive (rubber) wheels
        (3) Abrasive compounds

Centric equilibration

The patient should be placed in a semireclining position, which allows comfort for both the clinician and the patient. If equilibrating directly into a centric relation, the operator may employ the following techniques. With the mandible relaxed and the chin gently grasped between the thumb and medial surface of the first finger, the mandible is manipulated in an up-and-down arcing motion. Care must be exercised to avoid forced posterior displacement of the mandible. At first the arcs should not allow dental contact. Such contact can best be avoided by placing the index finger of the opposite hand between the patient's incisor teeth. The TMJ patient has learned to associate pain with occlusal contact and will find it extremely difficult to relax and allow the operator to manipulate the mandible in a seemingly threatening manner. With the operator's finger preventing occlusal contact, the patient feels reassured and protected. Once it has been verified that the mandible is indeed relaxed and arcing freely, the finger can be gradually withdrawn to allow the arcing mandible to close until the first posterior contact is made.

This manipulation must be achieved in an extremely gentle manner, or the patient will be unable to release control of the mandible. The operator ascertains when this first contact is made by both sound and feel. With the patient's chin held gently between the thumb and forefinger as described, the operator will be able to perceive contact through them. Some place the thumb lightly on the necks of the lower incisors to facilitate contact detection. Coupled with this tactile sensation, the operator should listen carefully for a dull, often muffled sound, which is typical of premature contacts.

It is often helpful to solicit the patient's assistance by asking if the contact that is being demonstrated by the repetitious arcing manipulation is on the right or left side of the arch. The side contacting first is so obvious to the patient that he or she will assume the operator also knows. Often buccal or lingual contacts may be interpreted as "left" or "right." Further helpful information may be gained by asking, "Is it touching toward the front or back of your mouth?" "Can you put your finger on the tooth that is being touched?"

Having determined the general area, the operator places a marking medium interdentally and repeats the procedure until the first contact is recorded.

Places to reduce. With rare exceptions, premature posterior occlusal contacts result in a shift or slide of the mandible, with at least one component in an anterior direction. By demonstration of this component in two dimensions (Fig. 14-14) it can be readily visualized that only prematurities on mesial slopes of maxillary teeth and distal slopes of mandibular teeth can result in an anterior shift of the mandible. In a similar manner, premature contacts of the right arch that result in a left-slide component can only be caused by prematurities on palatal slopes of maxillary teeth and buccal slopes of mandibular teeth (Fig. 14-15), whereas premature contact on the left side that results in a left-slide component can only be caused by buccal slopes of maxillary

*Artus Corp., Englewood, N.J.

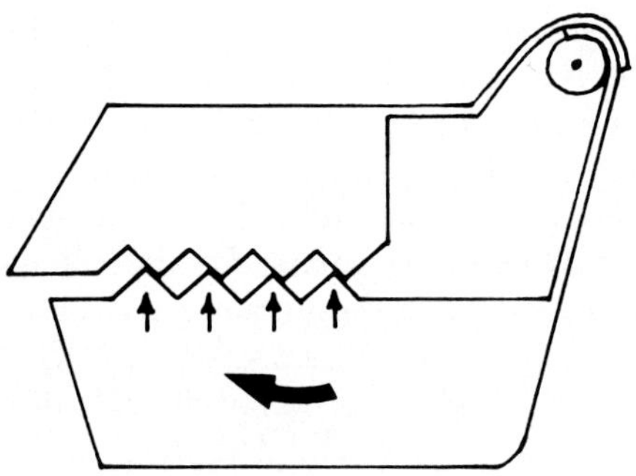

Fig. 14-14. Premature contacts *(small arrows)* on mesial slopes of upper cusps and on distal slopes of lower cusps will result in anterior displacement of mandible.

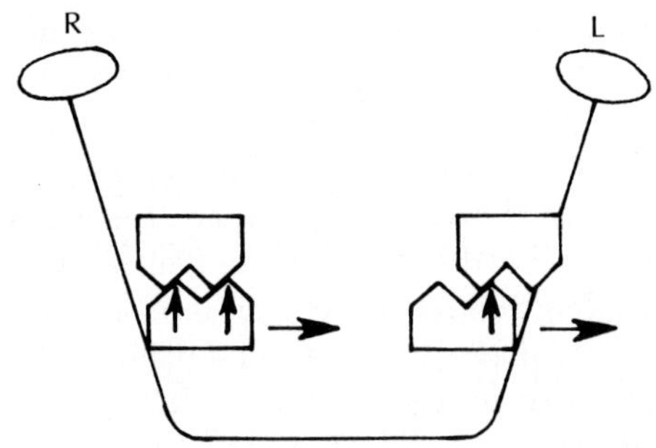

Fig. 14-15. Cusp slopes causing lateral interferences are determined both by direction of slide and by arch segment containing interference.

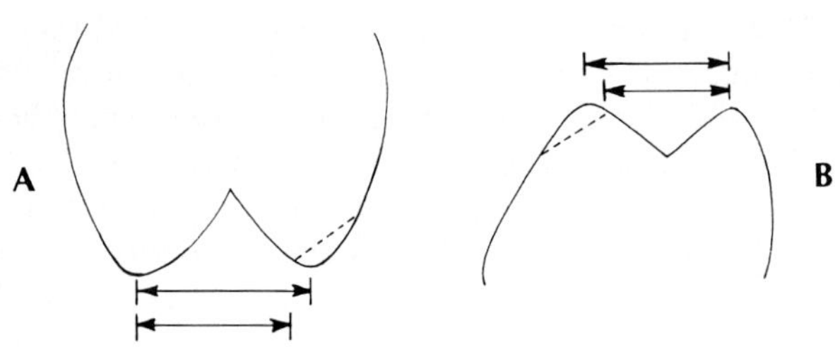

Fig. 14-16. Occlusal table can be narrowed by reducing palatal slopes of palatal cusps in upper arch, **A,** and buccal slopes of buccal cusps in lower arch, **B.**

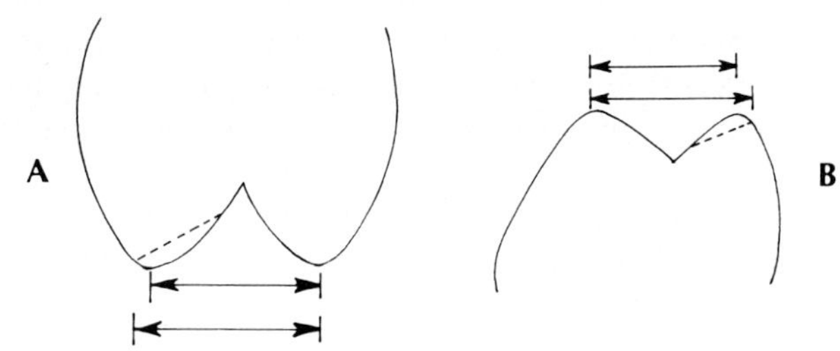

Fig. 14-17. Conversely, reducing palatal slope of buccal cusps of upper teeth will result in widening of occlusal table, **A,** as will reduction of buccal slopes of lingual cusps of lower teeth, **B.**

teeth and lingual slopes of mandibular teeth.

A slide with a right component will elicit premature contacts on the opposite slopes, as just described. Since the slope causing lateral shift is dependent on both arch and direction, confusion can easily result.

A simple rule can be followed that will result in the removal of the proper area of the cusp. If the operator thinks in terms of narrowing the occlusal table, the rules previously outlined will be followed. The occlusal table is narrowed by reducing the palatal slope of the palatal cusp of maxillary teeth and by reducing the buccal slopes of the buccal cusp of mandibular teeth (Fig. 14-16). Reducing the palatal slopes of buccal cusps of maxillary teeth will widen the occlusal table (Fig. 14-17, *A*) as will reduction of the buccal slopes of lingual cusps of mandibular teeth (Fig. 14-17, *B*). Contacts in the *B* area do not affect the width of the occlusal table and thus are equally reduced on both maxillary and mandibular teeth. This "narrowing of the occlusal table" rule also can be followed in cases of cross-bite.

The most frequently encountered interference is between the mesial slope of the lingual cusp of the maxillary first premolars and the distal slope of the mandibular canines. Since the closing arc of the mandible tends to separate these slopes, what at first appears to be a major interference often proves to be easily corrected (Fig. 14-18). This fact emphasizes the importance of properly mounted study casts in a hinge-axis relation, since no other method exists that can predetermine which interferences are readily amenable to simple equilibration techniques.

Principles of equilibration. To eliminate a slide, it is generally necessary to continue reduction of posterior contacts until anterior contact is made. Clinically, the operator will notice a distinct change in both the quality and volume of the sound generated by tapping the teeth together in the manner described. This difference is sound is obvious even to the inexperienced operator and results from the additional contact of the anterior teeth.

In severe maxillary anterior protrusion it may not be feasible to gain centric relation contact of all anterior teeth without closing the vertical dimension. If the maxillary anterior protrusion is not too severe, centric-relation contact can usually be gained on the distolingual slopes of the maxillary canines, and such contact frequently will be adequate to provide a somewhat stable occlusion and eliminate the anterior slide.

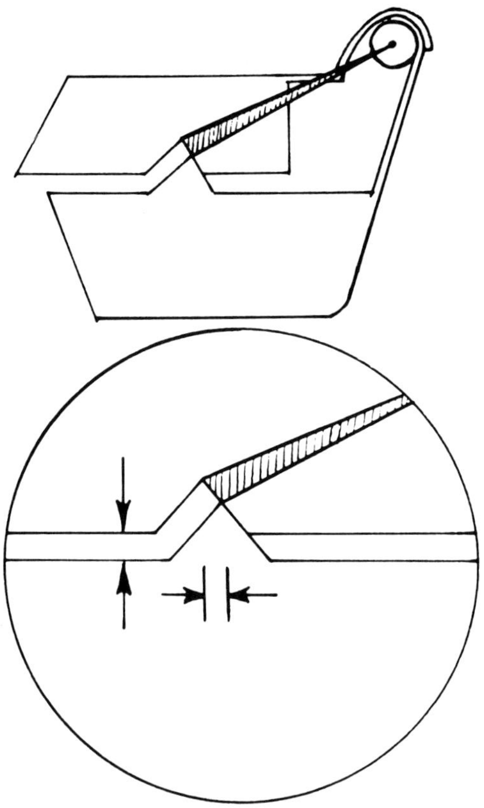

Fig. 14-18. Closing arc of mandible has both vertical and horizontal components. Therefore interference resulting in mesial slide may frequently require minimum reduction, since horizontal component of closing arc complements closure obtained from reducing mesial slope of upper arch and distal slope of lower arch.

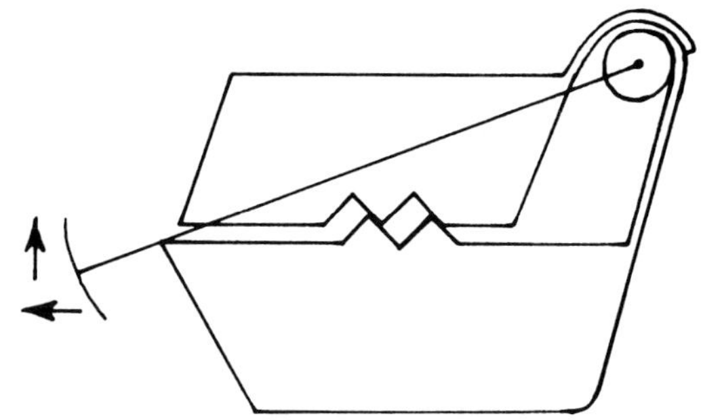

Fig. 14-19. In cases of anterior cross-bite, although anterior component of closing arc complements equilibration procedures, it will aggravate anterior cross-bite as bite is closed from first contact.

Anterior cross-bite. With an anterior cross-bite the anterior teeth are frequently the primary cause of an anterior slide and therefore must be reduced before or during posterior equilibration. In such cases it is necessary to determine whether it is feasible to change the anterior teeth from a cross-bite relation or an end-to-end or even normal occlusal relation by equilibration techniques alone. In some cases anterior full-coverage restorations are preferable.

A normal anterior occlusal relation usually can be achieved only in cases in which the incisal relation is edge to edge and where there is very little overbite. Seldom are posterior interferences found with an end-to-end bite. It must be recognized that the closing arc of the mandibular incisors has not only a vertical component but also a nearly equal forward component, which tends to compound any anterior cross-bite problem (Fig. 14-19). Therefore the amount of closure beyond first contact must be carefully evaluated. Mounted study casts will best aid in this determination.

Diminishing the vertical dimension (closing the bite). Proper equilibration should result in only slight closure of the centric vertical dimension. If elimination of a slide by subtractive techniques will result in excessive vertical closure, then such treatment is contraindicated, and one of the additive techniques should be employed.

Anterior teeth. Subtractive techniques should be avoided in anterior teeth. If it is deemed necessary to remove anterior tooth structure in a normal anterior relationship, then it is obvious that the lingual aspect of maxillary incisors must be removed, and the labioincisal area of lower anteriors must be removed.

A serious error frequently made is to apply the rules for posterior teeth to the maxillary canines.

Generally, equilibration is carried out until the canines contact in centric relation. If it is determined to equilibrate beyond that point, then unless group function is the desired goal, the mesial slope of the maxillary canine must be kept inviolate, since removal in this area will result in loss of this tooth's contribution to disclusion. If the operator follows a technique in which lateral interferences are eliminated first, working toward a centric relation, this principle must be carefully followed. If a balanced occlusion is the goal, the anterior teeth will be equilibrated concurrently with the posterior teeth; this can probably best be accomplished by allowing the patient to translate the condyle with teeth contacting on interimposed marking media.

Flat and worn dentition. Subtractive equilibration techniques are contraindicated in most patients with already flat dentition. Overclosure should be strongly suspected as a contributing cause of TMJ symptoms. It is virtually impossible to eliminate slides without further closure in such cases.

Broad areas demonstrated by occlusal indicator media. The general rules of equilibration are to remove from mesial slopes of maxillary posterior teeth and distal

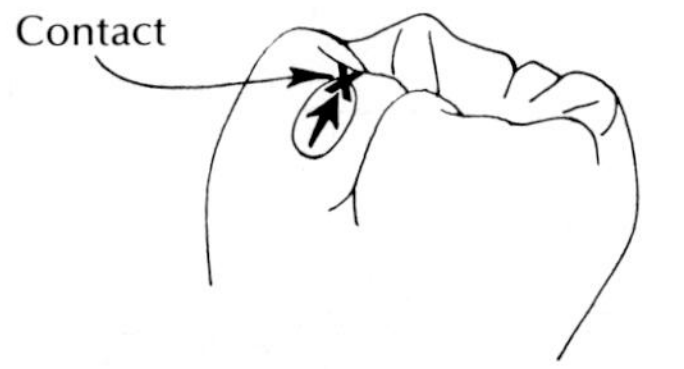

Fig. 14-20. Broad centric relation premature contacts. When broad contact areas *(large circle)* occur as result of manipulating mandible in centric-relation position, enamel should be removed starting at apical extension and progressing occlusally in direction of arrow, leaving final contact at X. This results in narrowing of occlusal table without loss of cusp height.

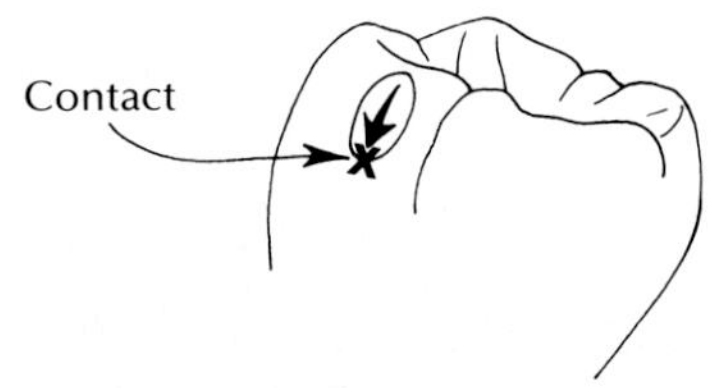

Fig. 14-21. When broad contact area *(large circle)* results from excursive movement, cusp height must be reduced. This is accomplished by removing tooth structure from occlusal portion and working in direction of arrow, preserving contact area as marked by X.

slopes of mandibular posterior teeth and to narrow the occlusal table. These general rules can be followed in a straightforward manner when prematurities result in point contacts. However, when closure or excursions result in broad-area contacts, the rules differ with the method being employed.

Broad centric relation premature contacts. When broad contact areas are demonstrated while manipulating the mandible in centric-relation closure, the basic rules apply, that is, narrow occlusal table. Tooth structure should be removed starting at the apical portion of the contact, leaving the coronal extension undisturbed (Fig. 14-20).

Broad contact resulting from excursive movement. However, when broad contact areas result from excursive movements of the mandible, the cusps must be shortened and the A contact maintained. Thus the coronal portion of the contact area is to be removed, leaving the more apical extension undisturbed (Fig. 14-21). Narrowing the occlusal table tends to sharpen and maintain cusp height, whereas elimination of lateral interferences tends to flatten or shorten cusp height.

Gnathological equilibration

Equilibration techniques are all designed to distribute the occlusal forces more equitably and reduce overloading on individual teeth. These methods are subtractive, removing but not replacing enamel, and the thickness of enamel imposes a severe limit on the permissible range of modification. The indications for occlusal equilibration are to correct restorative errors, to reduce lateral forces on selected teeth, to establish a more ideal occlusion before extensive restorative procedures, and to eliminate slight discrepancies in the occlusion. Gnathological equilibration differs from other equilibration techniques by employing articulated casts, by preserving and implementing cusp-fossa occlusion, and by adjusting centric last.

Accurately mounted casts provide the finest method of detecting occlusal discrepancies. By equilibrating these discrepancies on the articulator first, errors in the reduction of occlusal surfaces are detected in the casts, not in enamel. In addition, stone casts show contours more easily than the teeth, which, because of their color and translucency, make it difficult to see occlusal detail.

Many equilibration techniques destroy occlusal detail. The aim with gnathological equilibration is to preserve and enhance such detail and to progress toward a cusp-fossa occlusion rather than to simply flatten the teeth. This is accomplished by selectively reducing slopes of cusps and ridges. The effective cusp tip position may be shifted as much as 1 mm, and then by proper manipulation of the slopes and ridges surrounding the opposing fossa, the occlusal relationship can be greatly improved. Deepening grooves to develop the convexity of cusps and ridges is truly time consuming but is essential to avoid the flat surfaces, which frequently invite hyperfunction.

When adjusting centric first, extreme care must be exercised in adhering to the principles set forth earlier, or final modifications of lateral and protrusive excursions will destroy centric contact. If the aim is to produce a decidedly flat occlusion, the loss of an occasional centric contact on teeth in most cases will be compensated for by natural tooth movement. Gnathological equilibration approaches the task with a different philosophy. When all anterior modifications and eccentric interferences are eliminated, none of the subsequent centric changes can introduce additional eccentric interferences. Therefore interferences in protrusive excursion are removed first, followed by each of the lateral excursions, and the slight centric adjustments are made last. A precise centric contact may be developed for each tooth.

Eqilibration sequence

1. Test *protrusive* excursion for interference. Begin with the most extended (end-to-end) relationship, and as interferences are removed, progress toward centric

a. Adjust the distal slopes on maxillary posterior teeth.
b. Adjust the mesial slopes on mandibular posterior teeth.

2. Test lateral excursion for interference. Begin with a position equivalent to a cusp-to-cusp relationship of the canine teeth on the working side, and proceed toward centric relation.
   a. Idling, or orbiting, side interference
      (1) Adjust the mesial slopes on the maxillary teeth. Attempt to develop deeper grooves on the lingual cusps of maxillary teeth to allow lower cusps to pass freely by this mesial slope reduction.
      (2) Adjust the distal slopes on the mandibular teeth. Develop deeper grooves on the lingual slopes of the buccal cusps to permit the upper cusps to pass freely by distal slope reduction.
   b. For the working, or pivoting, side interference adjust the buccal cusps of the maxillary teeth so as to perfect the interdigitation of the lingual cusps. Slight recontouring of the lingual grooves on the upper cusps might be necessary.
3. Repeat for the *opposite lateral* excursion.
4. Repeat steps 1 through 3 until a smooth intermeshing of the cusps occurs in all excursions.
5. Test *centric* relation.
   a. Gross defects are usually a result of centric occlusion being slightly protrusive to centric relation.
      (1) Adjust the mesial slopes of maxillary teeth. This corresponds to removing tooth structure from the portion distal to the fossae, which become deepened slightly and moved distally.
      (2) Adjust the distal slopes of mandibular teeth. This corresponds to removing tooth structure from the portion mesial to the fossae, which again are deepened but moved mesially.
   b. Final centric contact is developed only by deepening the fossae to produce a cusp-fossa relationship with tripodized contacts. The centric contact should be slightly closed compared with the original centric relation to provide the rearmost, uppermost, and midmost unstrained position of the mandible when in maximum intercuspation.

Finishing. The final result must have equal contact pressure on both sides and between anterior and posterior areas. Notations are made at each step of the equilibration procedure on the mounted casts, and these together with the mounted casts are used at the dental chair as guides for the actual intraoral equilibration. Thin articulating paper and 0.0005-inch plastic shim stock are helpful in the final phases of the procedure on both the casts and the actual teeth.

On extensive equilibration projects repetition of the mounted cast evaluation may suggest minute improvement in the equilibrated occlusion. Alternatively, leaving the enamel slightly unpolished and examining after 2 weeks often reveal areas of excursive wear and heavier contact. Only minimum removal of tooth structure is required at this stage, typically to merely take the polish from the heavy contact areas. Diamond stones are efficient for initial gross reduction but leave an intolerably rough surface, which necessitates a substantial additional loss of tooth structure when repolished. Mounted white Arkansas stones and flame-shaped finishing burs leave a finer finish and an almost polished result. The finishing bur is invaluable to perfect the developmental and supplemental grooves and to produce a convex contour of the ridges.

Although at first glance a prolonged and complex technique, experience has shown that gnathological equilibration produces a precise occlusion. The tendency of many equilibrated cases to require almost unending touch-up adjustments is greatly reduced with this method. The total time might actually be significantly less using gnathological equilibration.

Advantages. Equilibration has several advantages compared with the alternatives. Compared with reconstruction involving cast restorations, equilibration requires considerably less irreversible tooth removal and, in properly selected cases, can offer immediate improvement or elimination of symptoms. Furthermore, if excessive tooth structure removal is necessary in selected areas, cast restorations can be subsequently used.

Compared with removable splints, equilibration offers the obvious advantage that correction can be made without opening the bite and, again, can be accomplished without intervening laboratory procedures.

The main disadvantage is that equilibration involves purely subtractive measures with the accompanying potential for loss of vertical dimension.

PRINCIPLES AND METHODS OF OCCLUSAL RECONSTRUCTION

Gnathological reconstruction in cases of TMJ dysfunction presents certain complicating problems and requires more extensive and meticulous treatment planning. The following checklist shows the steps and sequences required in such a treatment plan. This outline must be modified to fit the specific requirements of each individual case.

Treatment checklist

Study casts. Mounted casts are used to provide a preliminary analysis of the occlusal problem and for the construction of appliances if needed.

Preliminary amelioration of the TMJ problem. Complete gnathological reconstruction in the acute phase of TMJ disease is not recommended. Rather, preliminary techniques (splints or equilibration) should be implemented to relieve the acute phase. Besides quieting the symptoms to allow recording, one can determine the changes in vertical dimension that would be acceptable and the toleration of a particular patient for any type of treatment.

Recording of the mandibular movements. Until the mandibular movements are recorded, few definitive data are available to evaluate true occlusal patterns. In addition, patients with TMJ problems often show an erratic pattern of mandibular movement. In any particular case, or even for a particular condyle, a successful recording must be repeatable. In TMJ problem cases displaying nonreproducible tracings, the recording can be used only as a preliminary measurement to be followed by an additional recording at a later stage in the reconstructive process.

Study casts mounted on a fully adjusted articulator. Based on the information gained from accurately mounted study casts on a fully adjusted articulator, two important preliminary decisions must be made. First, should one proceed or terminate treatment? Are the problems occlusally oriented, or are there other overriding etiological factors? Second, will occlusal splints and equilibration suffice, or will reconstruction be required? If reconstruction is contemplated, the exact approach is postponed until after the diagnostic waxing up is completed.

Diagnostic waxing up. Briefly, the teeth on the sets of articulated casts are prepared as they would be in the mouth. Two sets of casts are prepared identically; one is a restorative guide, and on the other all teeth are restored in wax in proper arch-to-arch, cusp-fossa relationship. This essential step will indicate whether a certain approach is practical or even possible. Many occlusal problems are not solved by gnathological techniques alone. These include many cross-bite situations, severe arch size discrepancies, or certain esthetic problems. The diagnostic waxing up establishes the correct amount of tooth reduction for the restorations. If greater tooth reduction is required, both sets of prepared casts are trimmed. The set of casts without wax serves as a guide during tooth preparation to optimize the balance between adequate tooth reduction and preservation of tooth structure. The diagnostic waxing up enables the operator to predict answers to questions of occlusion, esthetics, and tooth preparation. Adequate preparation reduces chair time and frustrations. It is wise to take more time for planning than for doing.

Final decision concerning the treatment plan. At this point the dentist should know (1) how many teeth are involved, (2) what procedure is to be used on each tooth, (3) how much tooth structure, if any, is to be removed, (4) the sequence in which each of these procedures is to be done, (5) the general design of the whole treatment, and (6) various options, such as type of materials, location of connectors, teeth to splint, and tooth reinforcement. A detailed treatment plan should be entered as part of the patient's record. NOTE: Up to this time no irreversible procedures have been initiated except that of minor equilibration. The decision is now made to proceed or to limit further treatment to minor equilibration. It is far better to agree that further treatment would be a poor choice before irreversible treatment begins. Never begin a case if it can't be conceivably improved.

Initial emergency procedures. This includes any surgical intervention, the removal of teeth, endodontic treatment, periodontal therapy and management, and treatments of other dental conditions that have not been completed previously. The maintenance of hopelessly involved teeth until this time is unnecessary. Patients showing inadequate oral hygiene are always poor candidates for reconstruction, and ample time must be provided for them to demonstrate their aptitude and motivation.

Preparation and impression. The treatment plan is now implemented. The anterior teeth establish anterior guidance and the rate of opening (disclusion) and, together with the functional pathways of the mandibular joint, determine the pattern of disclusion of all the posterior teeth. Therefore, if the guiding planes of the anterior teeth are to be restored, that should be done first. The number of teeth to be prepared at each appointment is based on several factors. The temporary coverage for prepared teeth provides little protection for the TMJ patient; therefore the time from the beginning of preparation to the placement of all the provisional castings should be as short as possible. The comfort and endurance of both patient and operator also must be considered. Occlusion is developed on opposing teeth simultaneously; therefore it is necessary to complete opposing arches or segments together. Single quadrants should not be attempted individually. Regardless of the number of teeth prepared, full-arch impressions and full-arch bite registrations are required to develope an occlusal pattern that will function harmoniously.

Placement of provisional castings. The interval from the beginning of tooth preparation until the placement of provisional castings should not exceed a week. A relapse into the acute phase of a TMJ problem thus can usually be avoided. These castings, although constructed as well as possible, will not receive the marginal finish or the permanent cementation of the final castings. If facings are required during this phase, plastic generally is preferred to porcelain, since it is quicker and easier to fabricate. To facilitate the removal of the provisional castings, small hemispheres the size of a no. 6 round bur are left protruding from the axial surfaces. An easily removed temporary cementing medium must be employed.

Remounting provisional castings. The accumulated errors of impressions, mountings, and the casting technique result in an imprecise occlusal relationship. After being fitted in the mouth, the occlusal surfaces of the crowns are keyed with the use of an occlusal remount jig, which holds all the crowns in their proper relationship while an impression is taken (Fig. 14-22). With a previously taken bite registration and hinge-axis relation these crowns are mounted again on the articulator in precisely the same relationship as in the mouth. This technique will allow for laboratory equilibration and can bring about precise occlusion in a cusp-fossa relationship. This often over looked step is necessary for gnathological reconstructions, and it is especially essential for patients who suffer from TMJ problems. Indeed, this procedure is frequently repeated within several months to ensure a complete harmony of occlusion. The TMJ case usually requires a longer period of maintenance with the provisional castings than does a patient who is not suffering from these problems. It is during this provisional casting period that the occlusal and TMJ problems must be minimized. If required, an additional recording should be completed after the TMJ symptoms have subsided. Progress should be delayed until occlusal harmony and regression of symptoms are definitely apparent.

Constructing final restorations. With cast restorations in place as provisional coverage, the time required to fabricate the final crown does not become a serious problem. Such restorations can be meticulously idealized. On these castings all the detail that is required of final gnathological restorations may be leisurely implemented. Porcelain is used for facings rather than the plastic that was chosen for the provisional restorations. Since equilibration is subtractive only, many prefer to construct the final restorations with a fraction of a millimeter opening in the anterior segment, which provides slight additional material to be equilibrated after the remount procedure.

Remounting final restorations. Although similar to the remounting of the provisional castings, these permanent crowns are refined later in the laboratory after the patient has been dismissed, protected by the replaced provisional castings. The final castings may be remounted several times to achieve the finesse of occlusion that is always required. By this unhurried approach opportunity is given for a more critical examination of the marginal integrity of every crown, the position and contour of each casting, and the shade of each facing. The laboratory equilibration procedure results in a much finer attention to detail and finesse, which is sought in gnathological reconstruction.

Temporary cementation of final castings. With TMJ

A

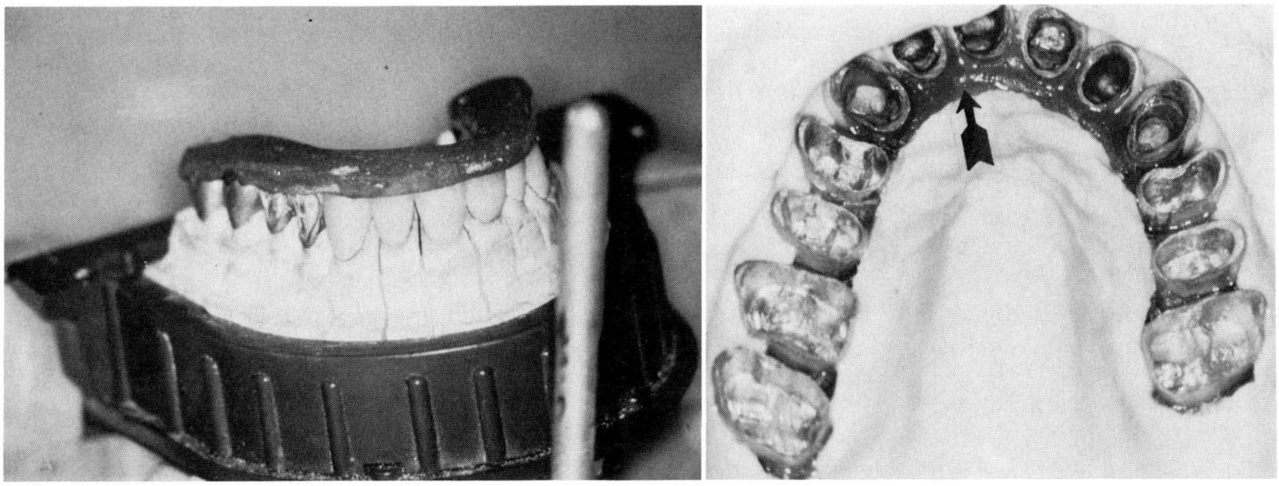

B

Fig. 14-22. Remount jig. **A,** Acrylic remount jig is fashioned on articulator before taking it to mouth. After crowns have been completely seated on their respective teeth, wash is taken inside jig, which will key crowns according to their position in mouth. **B,** Impression is then taken with jig in position. Jig is withdrawn with impression, and crowns are reassembled on jig as shown. Arrow indicates keyed side of jig. Model is then poured and mounted from bite registration and hinge axis.

problem patients it is wise to delay final cementation of the permanent castings. No permanent cementation should ever occur until the patient is entirely asymptomatic because further remounts might be necessary and are impossible after final cementation. Equilibration and repolishing of the castings in the mouth are done with difficulty and frequently tend to destroy rather than enhance the occlusion.

Final cementation. Before cementation the small round knobs on the sides of the crowns, which were to facilitate removal, are carefully polished away. Cementation may be implemented on a segmental scheme, usually the same as was the preparation of the teeth, that is, anteriors first. No more than two crowns are seated simultaneously to allow time for adequate seating and marginal finishing. Cementing many crowns in the mouth at one time invariably results in inadequate seating and margins that are not properly finished, which negates much of the effort expended to achieve the finesse of occlusion.

Recall. Patients are recalled for the following three reasons:

1. To periodically determine if the standard oral hygiene has been maintained in theory and application. This includes a prophylaxis and an examination for caries. Good oral hygiene will minimize the secondary caries incidence; however, the necessity of intervention in even incipient lesions must be emphasized to the patient.
2. To detect any recurring TMJ symptoms early.
3. To ascertain the degree of wear that has occurred since the last visit. All things mechanical will show wear proportional to the amount of force, the amount of time this force was applied, and the distance traveled. Ideal occlusion tends to minimize habitual grinding and resultant wear. In addition, masticatory overloading is reduced by the increased efficiency of precise cusps, ridges, and grooves that are seen in the cusp-fossa technique.

Tripodization (three-point contact of cusps in opposing fossae)

In developing an occlusal pattern having a cusp-fossa relationship, an attempt is made to provide each working cusp with an antagonist fossa into which it can center when the arches are in centric relation. This cusp-fossa occlusion avoids placing cusp tips in an end-to-end relationship or on marginal ridges where their wedging effect might force food between contacts.

Tripodization refers to a three-point contact within each cusp-fossa system. It is not desirable for a cusp to engage a fossa with broad surface area contact. Such a relation tends to mash rather than cut and increases the

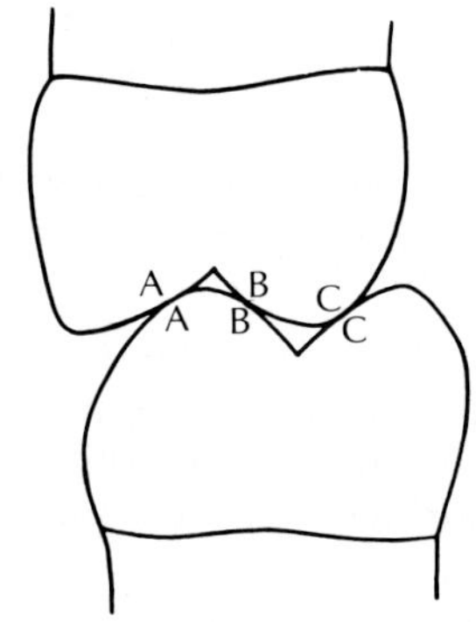

Fig. 14-23. Classic location of *A, B,* and *C* contact areas. *A* and *C* contacts complement one another and are antagonistic to outnumbered *B* contact.

load on the support system. Tripodization allows the teeth to masticate more efficiently. A single-cusp contact on an inclined surface lacks stability, since teeth move when subjected to slight but sustained forces. Conversely, three contacts surrounding the cusp tip will result in a lateral and vertical stabilization not possible with a single-point contact.

With two or more such cusp-fossa systems on a tooth, each with three-point contact, it is possible to develop a stable occlusion that introduces no lateral forces on the teeth when thy are in centric closure. Most premolars have this double tripodization, and molars may have four or five such cusp-fossa systems.

If all the posterior teeth occlude simultaneously in tripodized cusp-fossa relationships, and if the anterior teeth provide a smooth disclusion path that lifts the posterior teeth apart rather than sliding, then the only lateral stress momentarily placed on the posterior teeth occurs when a bolus of food directs chewing cycle forces onto the teeth. These brief instants of stress in the infrequent exercise of mastication are well within the acceptable range of function and health.

A close inspection of this tripodization reveals a tendency for these contact points to be disproportionately aligned. Viewed from the proximal aspect, posterior teeth show the following contacts: *A*, the lingual slope of the upper buccal cusps occludes with the buccal slope of the lower buccal cusps; *B*, the buccal slope of the upper lingual cusps occludes with the lingual slope of the lower buccal cusps; and *C*, the lingual slope of the upper lingual cusps occludes with the buccal slope of the lower lingual cusps.

These contacts frequently are referred to as *A*, *B*, and *C* (Fig. 14-23). The *A* and *C* contacts are on nearby parallel inclined planes, and the reciprocating *B* contact is outnumbered. Thus the importance of the *B* contact to occlusal stabilty should not be overlooked. Additionally, the occlusal view reveals that *B* contacts

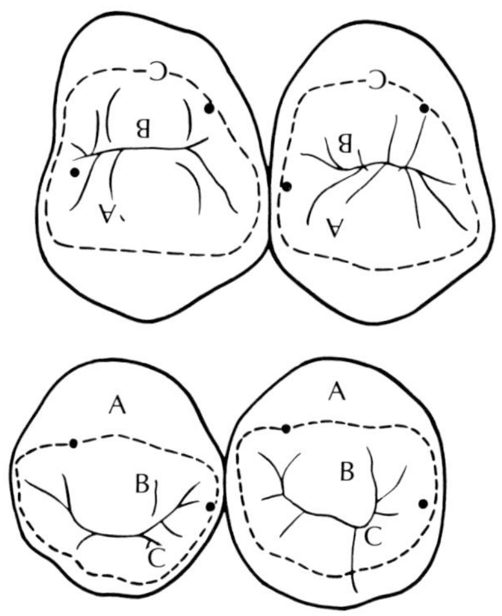

Fig. 14-24. Importance of *B* contact is further emphasized in case of premolars where tripodization allows five contacts for each premolar, only one of which is *B* contact.

overlap. Thus on the premolar the two cusp-fossa systems have only five (not six) contacts, only one of which is the *B* contact (Fig. 14-24). For these reasons this *B* contact integrity is stressed, and failure to maintain *B* contacts produces malocclusion.

LIMITATIONS OF GNATHOLOGICAL TREATMENT

The degree of success in any particular TMJ case involves many factors, and not everything is understood concerning the reasons for TMJ problems or exact results to be gained from any specific treatment. It would be helpful to be able to recognize cases for which no great benefit can be anticipated or cases in which treatment will have severe limitations. However, such absolute prognostic guidelines seldom exist in the healing arts.

Likewise, the correction of occlusal disharmony, in itself does not guarantee the alleviation of all TMJ problems. This is expected, since occlusal problems usually are contributory together with other etiological factors. The reduction or removal of any single factor should, and usually does, lessen the severity of symptoms, often to such a degree as to be proclaimed a clinical cure. Indeed, many cases are resolved only to this level. Additionally, the destructive nature of TMJ inflammation, as with any bony joint disease, frequently can result in permanent changes, frustrating a total return to former function.

Failures to cure TMJ cases by correcting the occlusion, by either equilibration or reconstruction, usually stem from either an inadequate technical precision, an inability to modify other factors (often more significant than occlusion), or an inability to recognize the limits of a particular treatment for a specific case.

Minimal occlusal deviation

Minimal occlusal deviations are perhaps the most easily treated. Equilibration is usually the treatment of choice, perferably with the use of splints through the diagnostic phase. Restorations, where indicated, should be incorporated into the treatment plan. One quickly learns to consider simple cases with a degree of suspicion. Hinge-axis mounting of casts in at least a straight-line articulator in centric relation is much more dependable diagnostically than merely a clinical evaluation. By using casts, the amount of deviation from ideal can be determined, the test equilibration can be completed, and a reasonable assessment of final results can be made before oral instrumentation. Occasionally cases of apparently slight occlusal deviation are encountered clinically, but after the quiescence of acute symptoms and analysis with an articulator, the deviations prove to be much more complex. Minimal occlusal deviations, when properly diagnosed, respond well to careful equilibration and minimal replacement of restorations.

Two pitfalls must be avoided: (1) equilibration of contraindicated cases, and (2) poor implementation of (or failure to complete) potentially successful cases. Either situation can precipitate an acute exacerbation of symptoms rather than their amelioration.

More involved occlusal discrepancy

Although reconstruction of dental occlusal anatomy is decidedly indicated in more involved occlusal cases, one must never ignore the influence of other etiological factors; otherwise reconstruction can be an insufficient treatment to the detriment of patient, practitioner, and profession. Typically, the use of diagnostic splints, myofunctional therapy, orthodontics, oral surgery, and preliminary equilibration is included as needed before actual tooth preparation.

Reconstruction has the advantage of a much greater range in the ability to idealize the occlusion compared with equilibration. Restorations may be additive, not merely subtractive. The vertical dimension may be varied (the bite may be opened or closed). Minor alignment problems may be effectively corrected with crowns. Problems of occlusal disharmony beyond the limits of equilibration are best treated in this way. There are, however, limits to the use of restorative dentisty to harmonize the occlusion. In cases of TMJ dysfunction consider the following limitations:

1. Psychological factors may limit one's ability to reconstruct or even equilibrate the occlusion. It is our opinion that no irreversible procedures should be attempted until the psychological factors present a favorable climite for success. Some patients would never present a favorable prog-

nosis. However, in patients exhibiting protracted pain with repeated failure of treatment, frustration and despair can produce emotional havoc in otherwise stable individuals. The emotional state is better assessed after first reducing the TMJ symptoms.

2. There are physical limits to both equilibration and restorative dentistry. Surgery, orthodontics, or both are frequently required to produce an environment suitable for gnathological procedures. An example of this is the marked discrepancy of the dental arches, such as in many severe Class II malocclusion cases in which there is no practical way to occlude the anterior teeth in centric relation. Cross-bites and all teeth tilted out of their proper vertical axis are best corrected orthodontically before restorative procedures are undertaken. Never start a case that cannot be finished successfully.
3. The acute phase of TMJ inflammation is best treated by other reversible methods first. In this state mandibular movements cannot be recorded well, occlusal relations are distorted, and the prolonged opening of the mouth required for restorations only complicates the problem. In such cases splints and occasionally minimal equilibration of interfering cusps are the only occlusal treatment suggested.
4. Expense, time, or both may limit the treatment. Although the cost of reconstructing the occlusal surfaces on at least all the posterior teeth is a limitation for patients, the time factor may be a problem that is overlooked. Often, many months are a minimum time. The tendency to abbreviate the treatment time can erroneously eliminate the important remount phase. Thus the essential time necessary for finesse is sacrificed.
5. Factors limiting the success of any restorative procedure are often a greater liability in gnathological treatment. A proper diagnostic sequence is essential. Consider the implications of overlooking *systemic diseases,* such as leukemia, cancer of the mouth, diabetes, or circulatory disorders. Nothing can modify the prognosis of an otherwise superb result as much as the severe *periodontal involvement* of even one essential abutment tooth. Evidence of insufficient oral hygiene or of generalized or localized bone loss certainly will modify or even cancel a favorable prognosis. Reconstruction is not indicated where oral hygiene lags. A *high caries susceptibility* does not change with ideal restorative dentisty, and in many cases the caries rate is modified only slightly by improved oral hygiene. In cases with a history of rampant caries, the longevity of results may be decidedly limited, and frequent recall examinations are required.

In summary, although extremely demanding, gnathological procedures provide an important remedial approach, which, when coordinated with other diagnostic and treatment methods, offers great potential for the amelioration of symptoms caused by myofacial pain dysfunction.

REFERENCES

1. Boucher, C.O., editor: Swenson's complete dentures, ed. 6, St. Louis, 1970, The C.V. Mosby Co.
2. Gregory, G., Shyrock, E.F., and Baum, L.: Hinge axis analysis: new procedure for location, J. South, Calif. State Dent. Assoc. **37**:59, Feb., 1969.
3. Kawamura, Y., Nishiyama, T., and Funakoshi, M.: A study on topognosis of human tooth, J. Osaka Univ. Dent. School **7**:1, 1967.
4. Lau, V.M.S., Aufdemberg, T.W., and Baum, L.: Simplified technique for hinge axis location and face bow transfer. In Kilpatrick, H.C.: Work simplification in dental practice, ed. 3, Philadelphia, 1974, W.B. Saunders Co.
5. Ramfjord, S.P., and Ash, M.M.: Occlusion, ed. 2, Philadelphia, 1971, W.B. Saunders Co.
6. Sharry, J.J.: Complete denture prosthodontics, New York, 1968, McGraw-Hill Book Co.
7. Stuart, C.E.: Accuracy in measuring functional dimensions and relations in oral prosthesis, J. Prosthet. Dent. **9**:220, 1959.
8. Tajan, Y.: Measurements and registration in odontostomatology: electronic apparatus review of odontostomat, Midi France **30**:42, 1972.

15 Splints

EUGENE P. WAGNER, D.D.S., F.A.C.D.,
S. KENDRICK CRANDALL, D.D.S.,
and RICHARD B. OLIVER, D.D.S.

In years past, dentistry has had as its domain the oral cavity proper, and its concern was limited to the tissues found therein. The teeth were given paramount importance, and all structures were thought of as static elements. Further observations have shown us the interrelationship of all the individual elements that make up the gnathostomatic mechanism, and the spotlight today is on the total system as a dynamic functional entity. The teeth are no longer thought of alone but as one corner of a triangle, with the temporomandibular joints as the other corners. This triangle moves in three-dimensional patterns by way of muscle action, which is dictated by afferent sensory inputs from the teeth and by external psychological factors. Pathological activity of this system has been shown to cause a multitude of symptoms and syndromes, which have been bunched into the general category of myofascial pain.

DIAGNOSIS

Our awareness of myofascial pain problems is in its infancy, and knowledge regarding the relationship of the myriad symptoms to their causative factors is still in a primitive stage. It has long been a tenet in medicine that the most important part of treatment is diagnosis. This is doubly true in situations in which the treatment can involve irreversible tissue alterations. Treatment after improper diagnosis will be ineffective at best and destructive at worst.

Many cases lend themselves to easy diagnosis and are amenable to mechanical treatment, that is, occlusal alteration. Other cases appear to be easily diagnosed but fail to respond to all attempts at correction. It is apparent in these cases that a key causative factor has been overlooked and that the practitioner is proceeding with a faulty understanding of the problem. This can lead to disastrous results for the patient and possible legal consequences for the dentist.

IDEAL RELATIONSHIP

The ideal relationship of the jaws when the teeth are occluded is reached when, with the mandibular muscles in equilibrium at their resting length, subsequent isotonic contraction of the muscles causes the mandible to close without interference to the height of the interocclusal space.

In a physiologically ideal occlusion no contact is encountered until closure terminates with solid simultaneous contact of all the opposing teeth. This is known as the myocentric position. Because closure to this position begins with the musculature in a state of relaxation (balanced tonus) and continues with free muscle contraction, uninfluenced by proprioception, the resultant myocentric position is most compatible with maintaining a state of relaxation of the musculature. The most physiologically advantageous occlusion is one that requires the least amount of accommodative avoidance by the musculature.

The first step in registering the most physiologically benign position of occlusion is to establish equilibrium of the mandibular muscles at their resting length. When this rest position of the mandible is attained, it then becomes the null, or neutral, launch position from which an isotonic contraction of the mandibular musculature will carry the mandible through the interocclusal space to the ideal position of occlusion. Establishment of a stable launch pad (rest position) is an essential prerequisite to registration of a repetitive myocentric position.

The questions then arise of how to find a physiologically benign occlusion and whether centric relation, centric occlusion, or some other predetermined position should be used.

Centric relation

Definitions of centric relation range from an unstrained position, to the most retruded position of the mandible from which lateral movement can be made, to the rearmost, uppermost, and midmost position. By and large, regardless of variations in the definitions, the basic concept calls for positioning the mandible at its posterior border stop. Centric relation usually is defined in terms of condylar position with the provision that the occlusion should be coordinated along the borders in harmony with the gliding movements of the condyles against their articular surfaces.

Up until recently, because of a lack of precise instrumentation, the hypothesis that functional occlusion should be arranged with the mandible in its most retruded border position had not been adequately tested by measurement. With the development of the Mandibular Kinesiograph, this instrumentation problem has been overcome. Studies have been done on 160 subjects. *None chewed, swallowed, or carried on parafunction in the centric-relation position*.

The question arises: if the occlusion is built to centric relation, will it continue to function there? So far, an adequate sampling of cases built to the centric-relation position has not been done, but of the few cases that have been recorded from 5 weeks to 2 1/2 years after adjustment of reconstruction, all were functioning from 1 to 1.5 mm anterior to centric relation.

The Mandibular Kinesiograph recordings done so far indicate that centric-relation occlusion constitutes an iatrogenic malpositioning of the mandible that is not tolerated by the musculature. The recordings also show that the more the mandible is forced posterior, the more it is misdirected away from the functional target. Damage to the musculature and to the stability of the occlusion appears to be a quite common side effect of centric-relation positioning of the mandible. Damaging side effects should be a matter of concern and investigation.

Centric occlusion

The closure of the mandible to an existing centric occlusion may or may not represent a favorably oriented muscular position. The existing centric occlusion may constitute a deviated position of the mandible, tolerated because of the accommodative avoidance conditioning of the musculature. Because of proprioceptive input, a centric occlusion that represents a deflection from myocentric position will be accommodated, within limits, by the musculature, even though the musculature pays a price for that accommodation.

Centric occlusion and myocentric occlusion ideally should, and often do, coincide. On the other hand, a lack of coincidence between centric and myocentric occlusion may be quite marked, or the discrepancy may be expressed as fractions of a millimeter. *Lack of coincidence may be in vertical and lateral dimensions as well as in an anteroposterior dimension*. If centric and myocentric occlusion do not coincide and the occlusion is then altered or established at the myocentric position, then the myocentric position becomes the new centric occlusion or proprioceptive position, with a consequent relaxation of the musculature.

SPLINT PURPOSE

To facilitate diagnosis and prevent needless, irreversible tissue alterations, several types of splints and bite planes have been designed. These appliances share all or some of the following effects:

1. Provide the ideal relationship of the jaws when the teeth are occluded
2. Create a physiological environment where the muscles can be in a relaxed state
3. Remove any interferences or proprioceptive disharmonies
4. Provide a freeway space compatible with normal oral functions
5. Place the condyle in a better physiological position with respect to the articular eminence–mandibular fossa and the disc
6. Diagnose the extent of occlusally caused symptoms
7. Relieve symptoms caused by mandibular dysfunction.

The short-term result is the elimination of muscle spasm and pain caused by the hyperactivity of certain muscle groups. This is an invaluable diagnostic sign that the case is indeed treatable by an alteration in occlusion and indicates what that change should be. The longer term result is to allow the inflammation of the temporomandibular joints to subside and the condyles to return to their proper position in their fossae. This is a prerequisite if definitive treatment is to be successful.

Several appliances are described here, ranging from a very simple emergency-type appliance requiring minimum knowledge and equipment for fabrication to those requiring more advanced understanding and sophisticated equipment.

Lucia jig

Also referred to as a deprogrammer, the Lucia jig is the simplest of all the occlusion-altering appliances but is capable of providing dramatic results in acute cases of trismus of the mandible. It consists of a smooth acrylic ramp placed on the lingual aspect of the upper incisors.

It is made by bringing acrylic resin, hardened to the doughy stage, to the mouth on either a tongue blade or a plaster spatula that has been coated with petroleum jelly to prevent the material from sticking. The acrylic is placed against the teeth and part of the palate. With

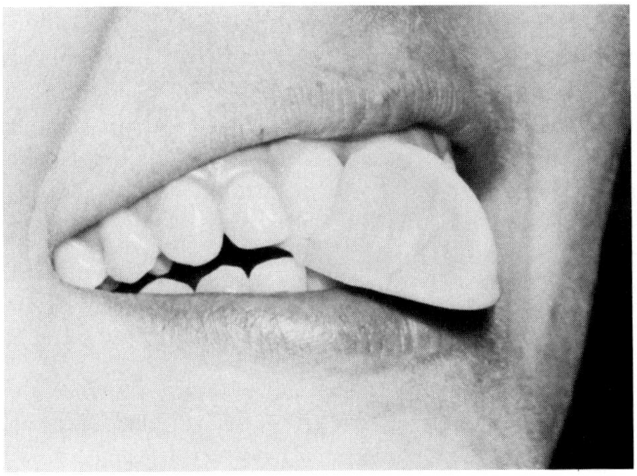

Fig. 15-1. Lucia jig (deprogrammer) in place.

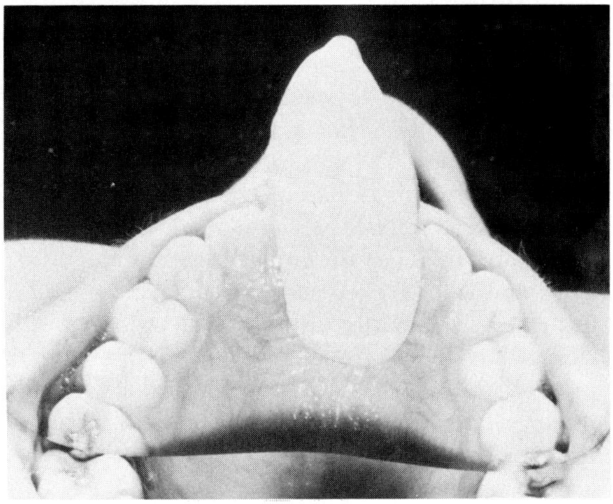

Fig. 15-2. Lucia jig, occlusal view, showing smooth ramp.

the fingers of the free hand, mold some of the acrylic up over the incisal edges of the central incisors to act as a stabilizer. Keep the acrylic from drooping over the sides of the plaster knife. Before the acrylic reaches its final set, a trial removal will ensure that no undercuts are involved. When finished, the appliance, which is held in place with denture adhesive, should be just thick enough to provide complete posterior disclusion, wide enough to allow contact of all four lower incisors with the ramp, and smooth enough for comfortable sliding of the teeth (Figs. 15-1 and 15-2). As the patient slides the jaw forward and back, the new proprioceptive pattern will replace the accustomed one, muscle relaxation will begin, and in a short time the patient will be able to open wider. If sufficient relaxation can be attained, and if time permits, one can go further with treatment. If not, then the patient can take the appliance home to use if needed until an appointment can be scheduled.

On occasion a patient will present with trismus so severe that insufficient freeway space exists to allow fabrication of this appliance. In such cases a tongue blade, cotton roll, or anything possible is placed between the teeth to sufficiently alter the proprioceptive inputs to allow some relaxation. Often, alternating the application of ethyl chloride refrigerant spray with massage to the masseter and temporal areas will provide the necessary initial relaxation.

Anterior bite plate

Often called the frontoplateau splint, the anterior bite plate has the same basic function as the Lucia jig but is of more sophicated design. It is similar in design to a Hawley-type retainer with the addition of sufficient acrylic lingual to the upper incisors to provide a ledge and ramp against which the lower incisors will function. The lingual table of acrylic is made thick enough so that in centric closure all the posterior teeth are kept lightly out of contact. The acrylic is continued up the lingual inclines to form a ramp from canine to canine sufficient to provide disclusion of the posterior segments in all eccentric excursions. Bringing the acrylic just over the incisal edges of the anterior teeth will increase stability and retention, lessen the chances of moving the anterior teeth labially, and protect the lingual gingiva from pressure trauma. No acrylic is placed over the occlusal aspects of the posterior teeth. Clearance should not be excessive, and the lingual ramp should be as smooth as possible to minimize proprioception and the tendency to brux on the appliance. All splints should be minimum in bulk, well contoured, and polished to minimize awareness of tongue, lips, and cheeks.

This appliance has the advantage of ease of fabrication and adjustment because of no posterior tooth contact. This aspect is also its greatest drawback, since it can allow eruption of the posterior teeth. Its use therefore must be limited to a short duration of 1 or 2 weeks if worn continuously, slightly longer if worn only at nights. This should be ample time to accomplish its purpose of allowing muscle relaxation by altering the occlusal sense.

Soft or resilient splint or night guard

The soft or resilient splint or night guard is a bruxism guard made of soft resin. It may be fashioned for either upper or lower teeth and is designed for even centric contact of all the teeth. The philosphy behind the appliance is that a soft occlusal surface will lessen the proprioceptive input and subsequent bruxing activity. The fact that the material is soft leads many dentists to the incorrect assumption that the occlusion need not be perfected, since the material is forgiving. If one is going to the trouble of fabricating the appliance to reduce pressure sensation, then one must adjust the occlusion meticulously to maximize this goal. Another positive effect of the splint is that it opens the bite approximately 2 mm. This can cause the condyle to translate slightly forward. If the condylar head is posteriorly placed when the teeth are closed, this forward movement centers the condyle in a better position. Also, if a hard splint is to be used later, it will give the clinician an idea of how much to open the bite with the other device.

A new approach to the resilient splint is the hydrostatic appliance. This appliance consists of fluid-filled cells interposed and worn between the teeth. Using Pascal's law, which states that an enclosed fluid distributes force equally and simultaneously in all directions, the hydrostatic cells have the ability to equally distribute occlusal forces to all the teeth. Since the fluid medium is totally flexible, the appliance is continuously self-adjusting to changes in muscle and joint requirements as resolution takes place. This appliance is still in the research phase and not available for general use. The soundness of the principle involved lends it strong promise for the future.

Posterior pivot

In the past the posterior pivot appliance called for bilateral single-point contacts on the most distally placed teeth and was made either as a removable appliance out of acrylic or as a more permanent one cast in metal. The theory behind this appliance was that the posterior contacts would act as fulcrums, and that muscle pressure on closing would cause the condylar heads to drop down out of the fossae and relieve pressure there. This idea is contrary to what anatomy dictates. In fact, the force vectors of the principal closing muscles (masseter and temporal) act in just the opposite manner and tend to seat the condyles into the fossae. This approach therefore had no basis in fact. Any positive results that it might bring are probably the short-term results that the patient enjoys when any change is made that allows the originally fatigued muscles to relax. This success, however, is short lived, since the new proprioception leads to a different bracing pattern and a new pain profile. In addition, this concentration of force on two units in the power zone and none on the others will lead to intrusion and extrusion of teeth and a worsening of the original occlusal situation. A more rational approach is the use of the Shore appliance.

Shore appliance

The Shore appliance covers all the occlusal surfaces in either the maxillary or mandibular arch. This appliance provides the operator with great flexibility. By gripping all the teeth in one arch, it acts as a true splint, preventing tooth movement and maximizing the number of posterior teeth occluding. In its usual form all teeth will have uniform centric contact, and anterior guidance will provide posterior disclusion in all eccentric movements. However, it is a simple matter to place any combination of teeth in group function on the working side or complete disclusion of any particular tooth or teeth because of mobility or sensitivity. Opening of the bite can be accomplished without fear of extrusion of posterior teeth.

The appliance is begun on a full-arch model by fabricating an acrylic palate having wrought stainless steel wire clasps in the molar region and ball clasps distal to the canines. The acrylic is carried to the height of contour of the posterior teeth and is left just shy of the anterior teeth except for a 5-mm wide strip that is extended over the incisal edge of the central incisors (Fig. 15-3). This programmer acts as the Lucia jig did and allows the mandible to relax and slide freely in all excursions. The patient is rehearsed in these movements until they can be made smoothly.

The appliance is tried in the mouth for fit (Fig. 15-4), all teeth are coated with petroleum jelly, and a roll of doughy acrylic is adapted to the occlusal surfaces of the upper teeth, overlapping the border of the splint. The patient is closed into centric relation and instructed to move in all eccentric excurions (Fig. 15-5). With the programmer as a guide one can quickly provide a functionally generated path of occlusion for the appliance. After hardening, all excess acrylic is removed, and the posterior segments are trimmed to allow contact in centric relation only (Figs. 15-6 and 15-7).

To make a lower appliance, mount opposing models in centric relation with a slight open-bite relationship.

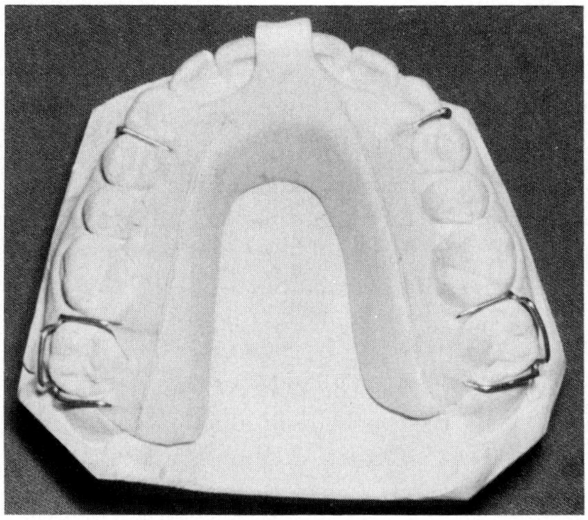

Fig. 15-3. Shore appliance as it appears after laboratory phase.

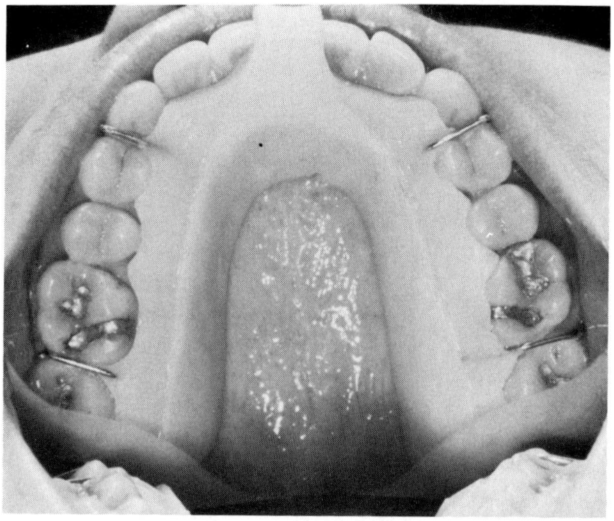

Fig. 15-4. Shore appliance in position before addition of occlusal portion.

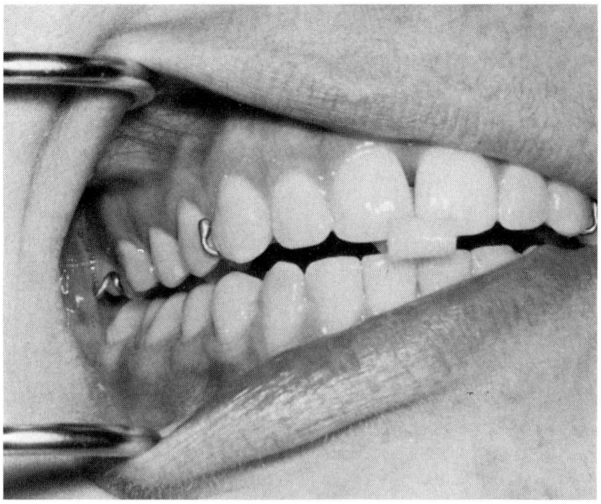

Fig. 15-5. Shore appliance in place showing programmer.

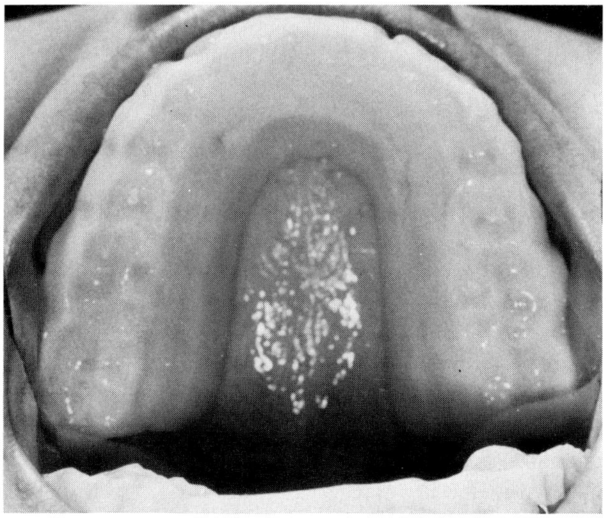

Fig. 15-6. Shore appliance completed, occlusal view.

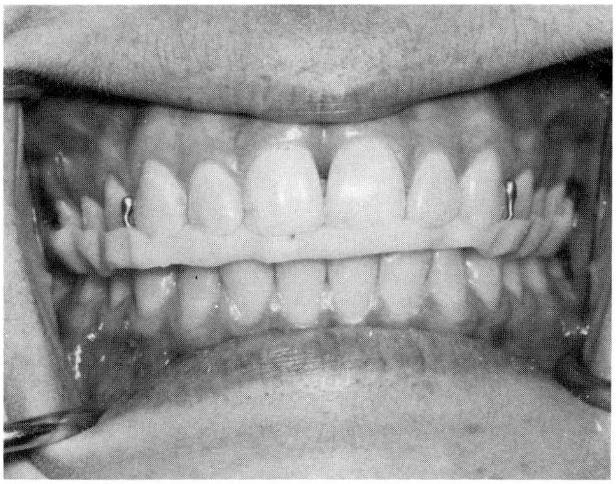

Fig. 15-7. Shore appliance completed, centric relation.

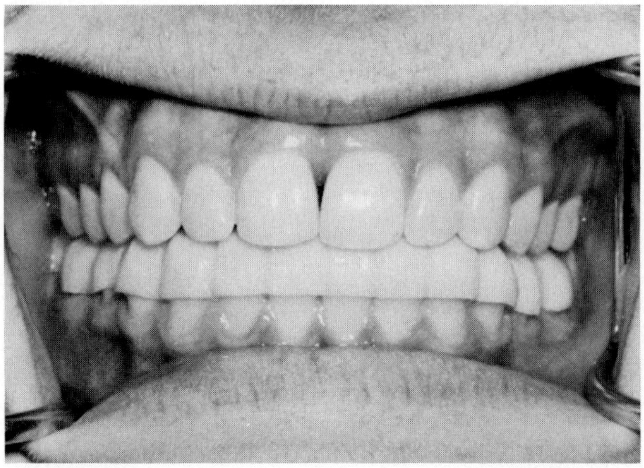

Fig. 15-8. Lower full-coverage splint in centric relation.

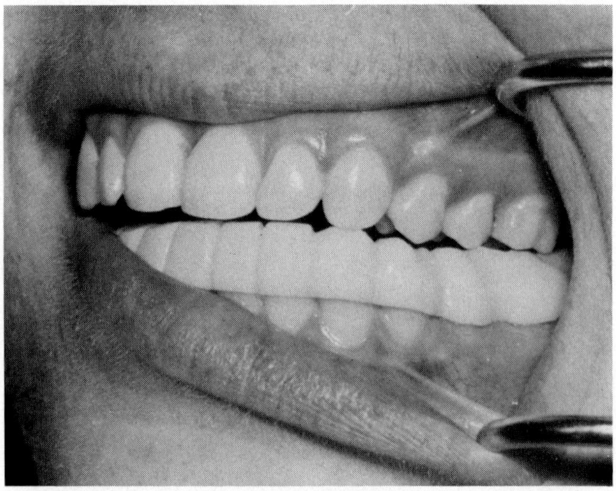

Fig. 15-9. Left lateral excursion illustrating cuspid lift characteristic.

Any articulating instrument with a positive vertical stop is adequate. A roll of doughy acrylic then is applied to the lower model, and the upper model is closed into it to the predetermined vertical dimension. The excess material is adapted to buccal and lingual surfaces. After hardening, the appliance must be sculptured so that it overlays the teeth yet is as cosmetic as possible. The posterior teeth are altered to eliminate all contact in lateral excursions while retaining all centric contacts (Figs. 15-8 to 15-10).

The appliance is worn continuously for a week, and then the patieent is questioned regarding any changes in symptoms. A thorough pretreatment examination and complete records regarding signs and symptoms are invaluable at this time. All too often the patient is quick to forget how severe the symptoms were once he or she begins to obtain relief. Also, many signs, such as muscle pain or palpation, joint sounds, tooth sensitivity, and mobility, are not reportable by the patient and must be checked again by the clinician. As treatment progresses and symptoms subside, the occlusion will need to be adjusted. This can be done either by selective grinding or by replacing the entire occlusial portion of the splint. With experience, the latter often becomes the more expedient approach.

Jankelson Splint

Before a splint is prescribed, a Myo-Monitor is used to establish equilibrium of the mandibular muscles at their resting length and determine an ideal occlusal position.

The Myo-Monitor. The Myo-Monitor* is an electronic instrument designed to generate an electrical current corresponging to the natural nerve stimulus that produces muscle contracton in the body. It produces controlled current pulses adjustable to between 0 and 30 mA. Pulses 2 msec long are provided at intervals of 1.5 seconds. The instrument is powered by four 1.5-V flashlight batteries. The interval between pulses allows the muscles sufficient resting time between contractions so that they can respond indefinitely without fatigue.

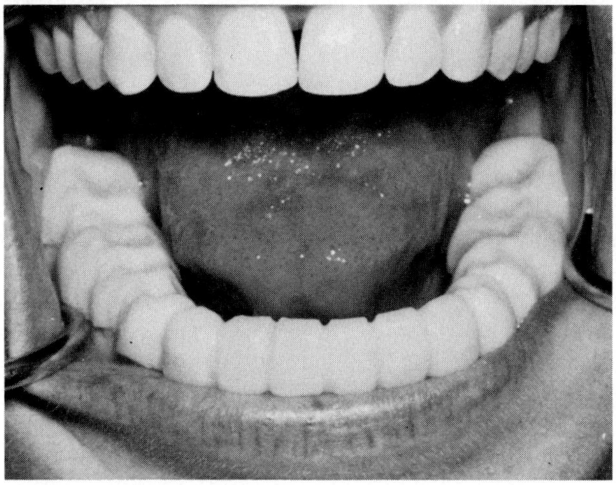

Fig. 15-10. Occlusal view. Note scooped-out occlusal form necessary to eliminate lateral interferences.

Contact with the patient is established with two electrodes placed symmetrically on the skin of the face just in front of the tragus of the ears, with a third opponent electrode placed at the nape of the neck. Through these electrodes the instrument provides simultaneous stimulation to the facial nerve and the

*For more detailed information on the uses of the Myo-Monitor and Kinesiograph in the treatment of TMJ dysfunction, refer to Chapter 32 or contact Myo-Tronics Research, Seattle, Wash.

trunk of the fifth nerve over the opening of the mandibular notch after it has emerged from the skull through the foramen ovale. When properly adjusted, the pulse current produces repetitive contraction of all the muscles involved in mandibular movement and guides mandibular closure to the correct occlusal position dictated by the musculature alone. It is important to understand that the muscles do not contract singly but all act simultaneously. Jaw closure is the result of contraction of a group of muscles.

Automatic involuntary closure of the mandible is an important objective in clinical dentistry. The Jankelson Myo-Monitor has been developed to meet this need.

Making the splint. Once it has been determined that a splint is needed, the following procedure is used:

1. Make a set of casts of the patient's dentition.
2. A pencil is used to mark on the lower cast the border to which the splint will be extended. It is clearly seen that the pencil marking follows the gingival margins of the posterior teeth then goes up to the tips of the incisors from canine to canine. It then goes down and again follows the gingival margins of the posterior teeth on the other side. This line indicates the border of the splint on the lingual side.
3. Once the pencil markings have been completed, lubricate the lower cast with separating medium. Alcoat may be used here.
4. Templates* are used to construct the wafer to mold over the lower cast. Lay the template with the shape of the lower arch cut out in it on the counter.
5. Make a thin wafer (about 1.5 to 3 mm thick) of acrylic in the shape of the lower arch.
6. Lay the acrylic over the lower cast, conforming it to the shape of the cast with your fingers.
7. After molding the acrylic over the lower cast, you can see the pencil marking, to which the acrylic is trimmed with a hot no. 25 Bard-Parker blade by following these pencil markings.
8. Once the acrylic has hardened over the lower cast, you should be able to lift it off without any problem.
9. Fig. 15-11, *A*, shows the completed wafer. Take the wafer off the lower cast, and with a hand piece and bur, trim off the flash and smooth all the sharp edges of the wafer.
10. Fig. 15-11, *B*, shows that meanwhile the patient has been pulsing for 30 to 45 minutes and is now prepared to have the splint pulsed in.
11. Note the freeway space between pulses of the Myo-Monitor, and either measure with calipers tape strips attached to the nose and chin (Fig. 15-11, *C*) or measure the space between upper and lower incisors.
12. Now put the wafer into the patient's mouth, and wipe the surface of the wafer dry with tissue paper.
13. Mix more orthodontic resin and pour it into a no. 412 Monoject syringe. When the acrylic reaches the putty state, inject it over the wafer (Fig. 15-11, *D*) and build it up to at least the thickness desired.
14. If the acrylic is too soft, it has a tendency to slump over the sides of the wafer. Put lubricant on your fingers and build up the acrylic to at least the desired height.
15. Once the acrylic is in the mouth, instruct the patient to let the jaw relax. Now put the calipers that already have been registered to the relaxed rest position back on the nose and chin tape. You will see that it usually falls short of the rest position. The patient has been pulsing all this time. Now instruct the patient to just let the jaw relax up a little at a time until it reaches the same rest position registered in step 11.
16. Once you have brought the patient's jaw to the same rest position, increase the pulse of the Myo-Monitor so the jaw rises from the rest position through a freeway space of 1 to 1.5 mm. This will automatically register the occlusion into the splint to the correct vertical position. You can easily determine the amount of interocclusal space given the patient by watching the rise of the calipers each time the mandible rises under the influence of the Myo-Monitor stimulus.
17. Once the acrylic gets to the rubbery state in the mouth, take out the splint.
18. The coronoplasty technique of adjusting the splint so it has a cusp-to-fossa relationship is now used. Fig. 15-11, *E*, shows equilibration of the splint. It is easy to see the formation of the buccal cusp on the splint. This is the area that fit into the fossae of the natural dentition of the patient. With a pencil, mark the tips of the buccal cusps.
19. Mark the depth of the fossae with a pencil. This is where the lingual cusp tips of the upper teeth fit into the splint.
20. With an acrylic bur, remove the excess buccal surface to the cusp tips. Do not touch the buccal cusp tips.
21. The buccal cusp tips now fit into the fossae of the upper teeth. All the excess acrylic that once overlapped the buccal surface of the upper teeth has been ground away.

*Available at Myo-Tronics Research, Seattle, Wash.

22. Grind away the bulk of the acrylic on the lingual side of the splint by rounding the lingual cusp tips to about the height of the buccal cusp tips. Grind the acrylic back away from the fossae, allowing free entry into the fossae by the lingual cusp tips of the upper teeth.
23. Take the no. 9 bur from Lefrom Laboratory and break up the inner proximal areas of the splint by grinding grooves in these areas.
24. After defining the interproximal areas by using the coronoplasty technique of occlusal adjustment, first groove, second spheroid, and third point the cusp tips. Put in the details of the anatomy of the teeth by grooving and leaving point contacts on the buccal cusp tips without eliminating them completely. Then spheroid from groove to groove, putting a spheroidal shape to the cusps. Next, point the cusp tips; do not grind away the buccal cusp tip contacts or the depth of the fossae. These are the vertical stops.
25. Do final adjustments in the mouth, removing any interference in and out of the new centric occlusion (Fig. 15-11, *F*).
26. The splint is hardly noticeable. The patient should be instructed to wear the splint 24 hours a day, even while eating, and to keep the splint clean. Occasionally it is helpful for the clinician

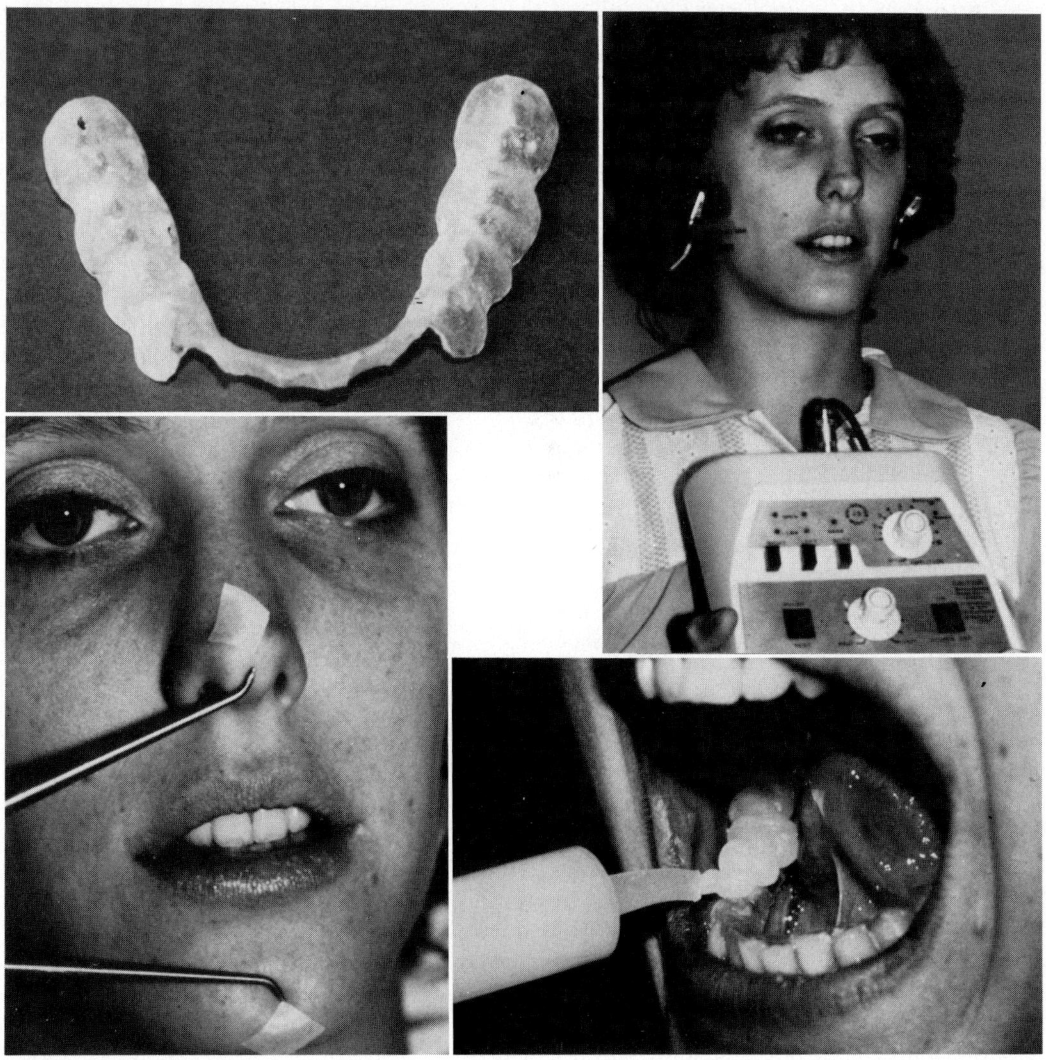

A

B

C

D

Fig. 15-11. A, Splint base before construction of occlusion. **B,** Patient pulsing with Myo-Monitor. **C,** Measuring freeway space. **D,** Injecting soft acrylic onto splint base.

to put fluoride gel into the splint and let the patient wear that for a few minutes before cleaning it.

27. Fig. 15-11, *G* and *H*, shows radiographs of the condylar position with the splint out and the splint in.
28. Adjust the splint every week or so as needeed. After a few weeks it may be desirable to grind off the occlusal portion of the splint and pulse into a new occlusion as the musculature adapts to the myocentric position.
29. Final treatment may entail equilibration, orthodontics or reconstructive dentistry.

The Weiss neuromuscular removable mandibular repositioner*

The temporary mandibular repositioner accommodates physiological occlusion, carving into the appliance's occlusal surface the means by which free entry into maximum intercuspation of the dentition can be accomplished. The temporary splint obtains and holds the neuromuscular position of the mandible, aiding the patient in deglutition. Parameters thus are established on which to base the design of a permanent appliance.

*This section was contributed by Michael H. Weiss, D.D.S., F.I.C.C.O., private practice, Phoenix, Ariz.

E F G H

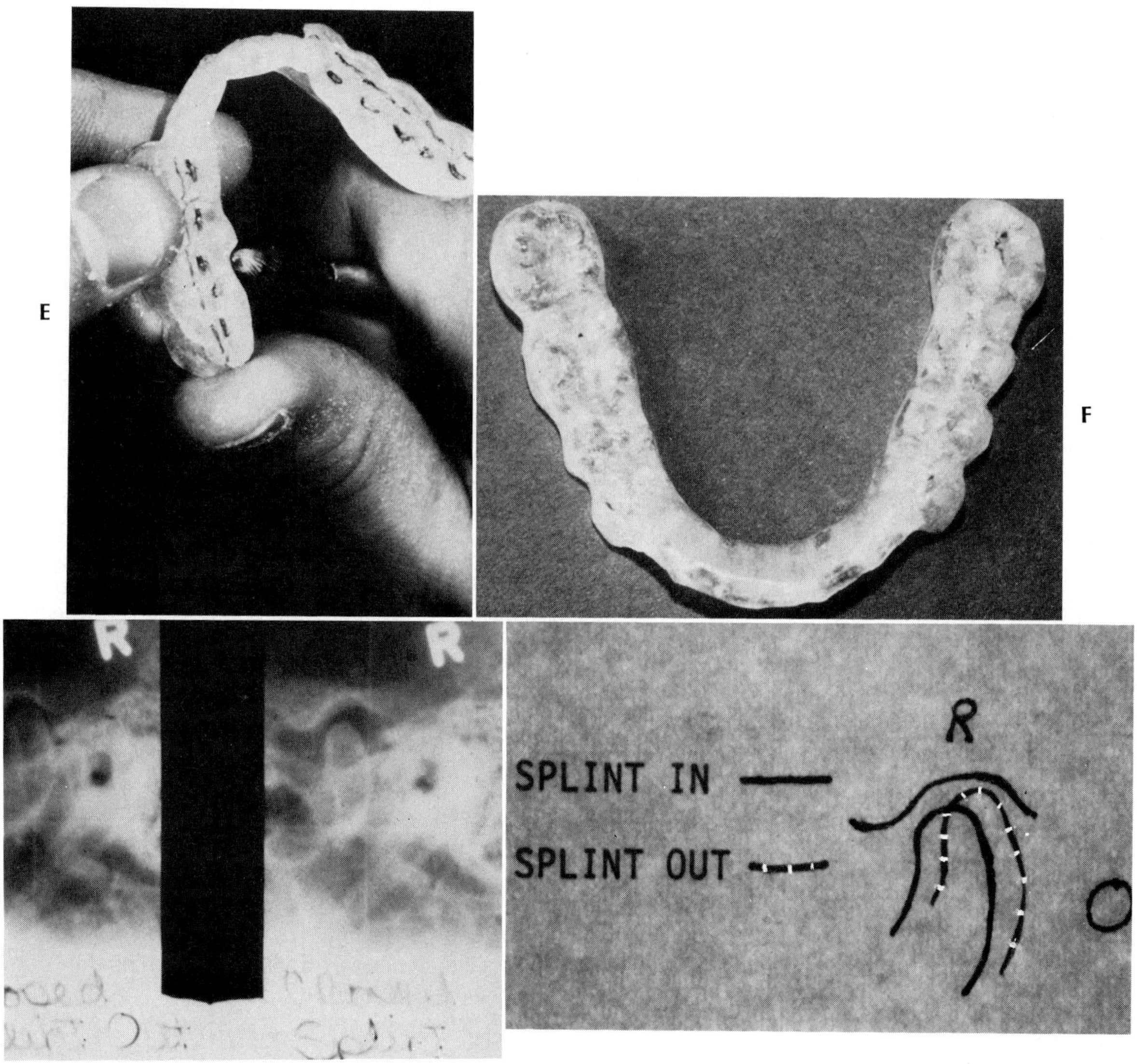

Fig. 15-11, cont'd. E, Equilibrating splint. **F,** Completed splint. **G,** Radiograph of condyle with splint out and splint in. **H,** Radiographic tracing with splint out and splint in.

Because it is a diagnostic tool, the temporary splint becomes unstable after a short period of use. If, while the patient is wearing it, the objective and subjective symptoms have been relieved, the dentisi must consider a more permanent alternative. Treatment options include altering the occlusal surface of the temporary splint to allow the natural eruption of the posterior teeth, orthodontic procedures, fixed coronal restorations, or the removable, neuromuscular mandibular repositioner.

Design, fabrication, and application of the removable, permanent neuromuscular repositioner allow the patient to achieve a solid platform and relief from MFPD-TMJ symptoms without the trauma and cost of full-mouth restorations.

The repositioner takes time and in-depth design planning. The close cooperation of the dental laboratory is essential. The dentist must emphasize to the technician that each procedure during its fabrication must be rigidly followed to achieve positive results.

The repositioner designed by Michael Weiss, D.D.S., consists of a chrome and steel substructure that is entirely tooth-borne to ensure maximum rigidity and a base for the superstructure.

The superstructure is fabricated of a new material consisting of very fine particles of silicon dioxide—so fine that it could be classified as a colloid—combined with Bower's plastic formula. This combination is extremely solid but can be occlusally altered even though retaining a high polish after occlusal adjustment.

The posterior teeth of the MFPD-TMJ patient are usually inclined lingually as a result of the tongue being interposed occlusally during deglutition. This presents a problem when fabricating the removable repositioner. Since the appliance must be both stable and rigid, the metal overlays supporting the superstructure should cover as much tooth surface as possible without extending into undercuts. In most cases the lingual portion of the lower posterior appliance should be recontoured to lower the height of tooth contour, since no lingual clasps are used on this appliance.

Laboratory and clinical procedures for fabrication of this appliance are interdependant and therefore presented alternately.

1. Clinical
   a. Lower study model survey is made (Fig. 15-12).
   b. Coronoplasty is used to accommodate metal onlays and clasps.
   c. Elastomeric upper and lower dental impressions are made.
2. Laboratory
   a. Epoxy resin models are made for accuracy and abrasive resistance (Fig. 15-13).
   b. Lower epoxy model survey is made; undercut wax slightly over survey line and interproximal portion of anterior and posterior teeth.
   c. Refractory model is returned to dentist.
3. Clinical
   a. Place framework outline on refractory model.
   b. Obtain relaxed rest position with Myo-Monitor (Fig. 15-14).
   c. Register neuromuscular occlusal deglutition position (Fig. 15-15).
   d. Transfer registration to models and secure with sticky wax.
4. Laboratory
   a. Articulate models on rigid, hinged, nonadjustable articulator with anterior and posterior vertical pin stops (Fig. 15-16).

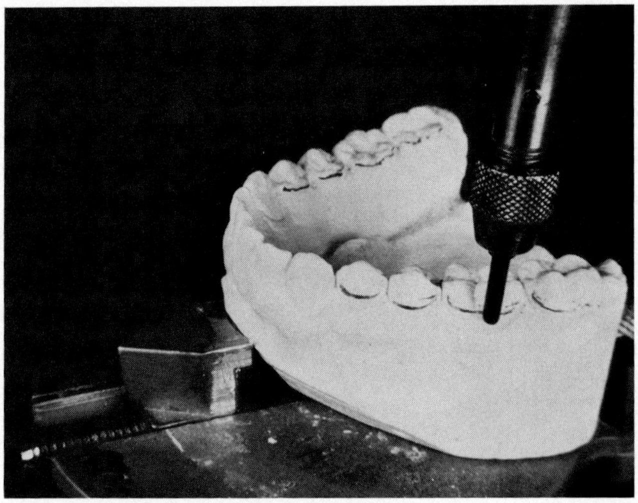

Fig. 15-12. Survey lines on precoronoplasty lower study model.

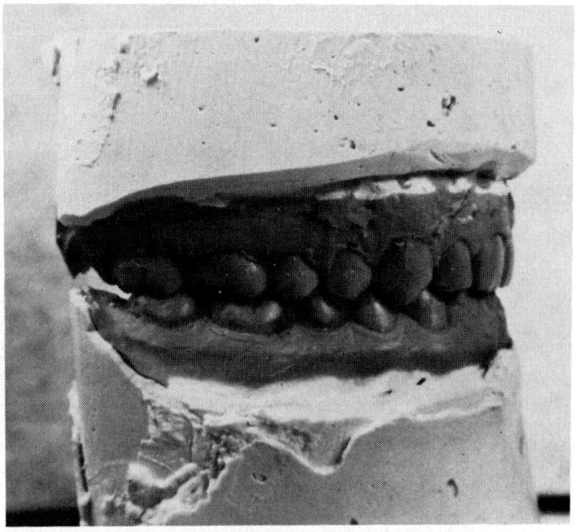

Fig. 15-13. Preneuromuscular registration position; epoxy resin models occluded.

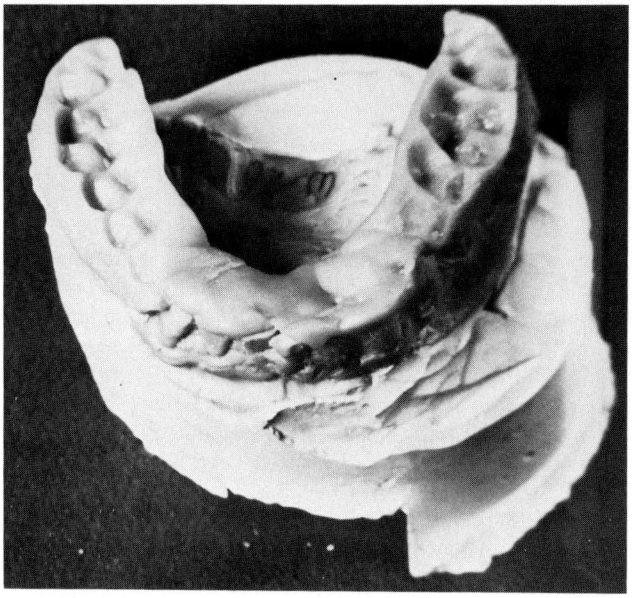

Fig. 15-14. Myo-Monitor pulsed acrylic bite registration.

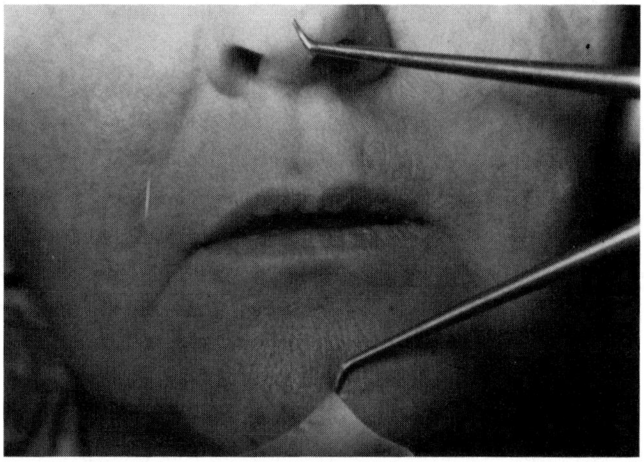

Fig. 15-15. Registering neuromuscular relaxed rest position.

b. Wax prelubricated epoxy lower cast to accommodate cusp-fossa relationship and interocclusal clearance for superstructure.
   (1) Transfer wax overlay to refractory cast.
   (2) Complete tooth-supported waxing up.
   (3) Add rentenive clasps and retentive beads for posterior onlays.

c. Complete the cast metal framework (Fig. 15-17).

5. Clinical: Check framework on patient's dentition for fit and stability.
6. Laboratory
   a. Fabricate superstructure of neuromuscular mandibular repositioner (Fig. 15-18).

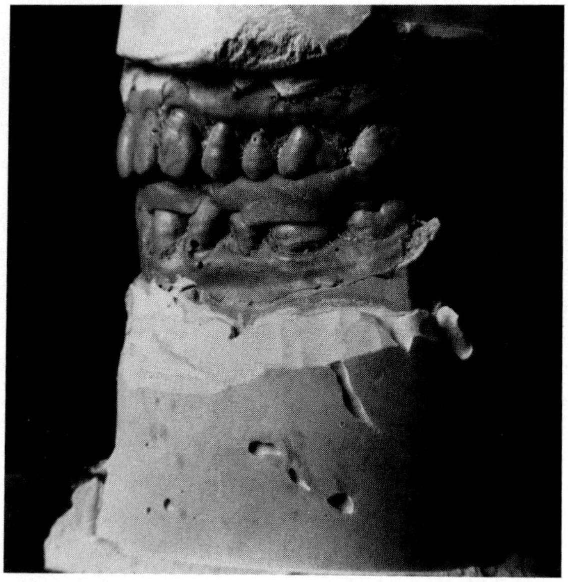

Fig. 15-16. Mounted articulated models.

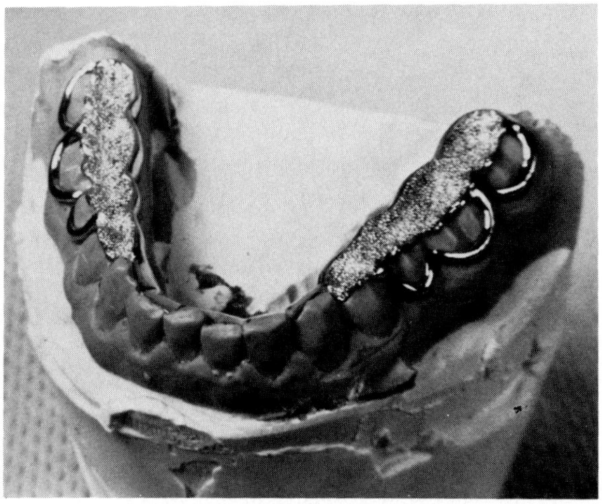

Fig. 15-17. Cast metal framework with finish line and retentive beads.

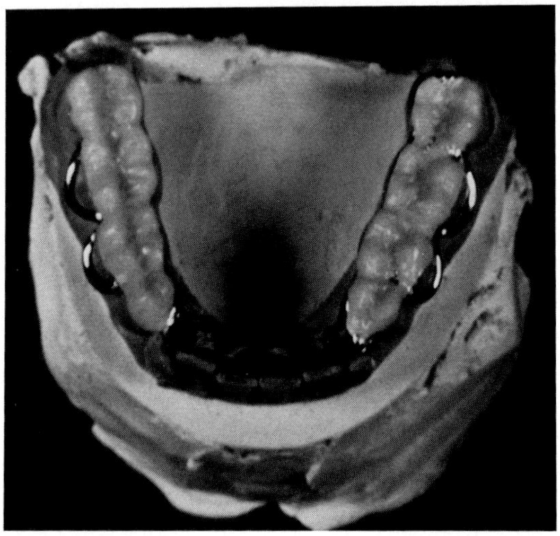

Fig. 15-18. Weiss appliance fabricated.

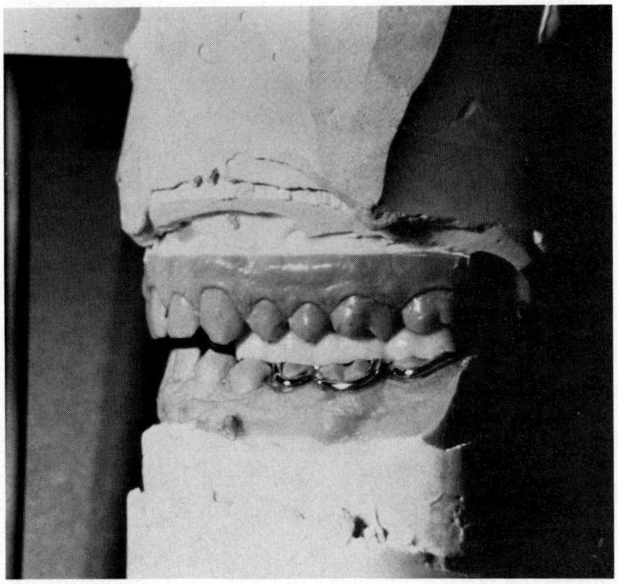

Fig. 15-19. Completed Weiss neuromuscular removable mandibular repositioner.

   b. Stabilize metal framework on prefabricated lower epoxy model with corrective clear orthodontic acrylic wash (Fig. 15-19).
7. Clinical
   a. Check neuromuscular mandibular repositioner for proper mandible-skull alignment and correct cusp-fossa relationship using Myo-Monitor and Mandibular Kinesiograph analysis.
   b. Schedule periodic patient recalls to check objective and subjective responses to neuromuscular appliance.

Conclusions. The neuromuscular removable mandibular repositioner benefits the MFPD-TMJ sufferer in the following ways:

1. It accommodates the patient's muscular need to function normally during deglutition.
2. It helps the patient without the cost and trauma of coronal tooth preparation.
3. It alleviates the time and cost of orthodontic treatment.
4. Finally, the appliance is removable. If the patient decides at a later date to move into another area of treatment, the appliance can be removed without damaging the oral cavity.

CASE HISTORIES

Case 1

A 30-year-old woman presented herself at the emergency hospital at 11 PM with intense pain in the general area of the upper left molar and the left temporomandibular joint. There were no caries or previous restorations. The occlusion was apparently normal in all aspects. The external pterygoids were tender to palpation. On the assumption that muscle spasm was the immediate cause of her pain, impressions for making a plastic upper flipper overlay were taken. Meanwhile temporary relief from pain was given by medication and moist heat to the afflicted area. The patient returned the next day for the appliance, and a few days later it was apparent that her acquired centric relation was considerably different from her true centric relation. In discussing her past symptoms, the patient indicated that there had been no pain; however, she had been aware of some clicking and popping and thought her jaw was "double jointed." The acute pain on this occasion probably was caused by additional emotional stress that exceeded her ability to adapt.

Case 2

A 63-year-old woman presented with left temporomandibular joint pain. This pain on occasion was so intense that she had lost 2 or more days of work a month over a period of 7 or more years. Occlusion was poor. She was missing several posterior teeth and had a pronounced overclosed bite. The immediate modality of treatment was the use of the Shore appliance to gradually restore vertical dimension an centric relation. Progress was gradual. The patient was seen approximately every 2 weeks for adjustments to the appliance, sometimes repeating the entire Shore process. The vertical dimension was varied until the patient and dentist thought the optimum position had been realized. With comfort achieved and no adjustment required for several weeks, a cast overlay lower partial was constructed to maintain this comfortable position.

SUMMARY

This chapter presents several tools to be used in the diagnosis and treatment of myofascial pain and temporomandibular joint pain. The multifactorial nature of these problems is such that a change in occlusion will not always bring success. We do no favor to our patients, ourselves, or dentistry as a whole by recommending large occlusal reconstructions that are unsuccessful. One is merely asking for trouble by treating definitively before determining whether the case is amenable to occlusal treatment. The appliances mentioned are convenient, reversible mechanisms to aid a rational treatment program.

RECOMMENDED READINGS

Guichet, N.: Occlusion—a teaching manual, Anaheim, Calif., 1967, Denar Corp.

Lerman, M.D.: The hydrostatic appliance: a new approach to treatment of the TMJ pain-dysfunction syndrome, J. Am. Dent. Assoc. **89:**1343, 1974.

McHorris, W.H.: TMJ dysfunction—resolution before reconstruction, delivered at Sixth International Gnathological Conference, Mexico City, Nov., 1973.

Ramfjord, S., and Ash, M.: Occlusion, ed. 2, Philadelphia, 1971, W.B. Saunders Co.

Schwartz, L.: Disorders of the temporomandibular joint, Philadelphia, 1959, W.B. Saunders Co.

Schwartz, L., and Chayes, C.: Facial pain and mandibular dysfunction, Philadelphia, 1969, W.B. Saunders Co.

Shore, N.A.: Temporomandibular joint dysfunction and occlusal equilibration, ed. 2, Philadelphia, 1976, J.B. Lippincott Co.

16 Considerations in the treatment of muscle spasm

ERIC PAUL SHABER, D.D.S.

In assuming the responsibility of treating patients who present with pain syndromes about the head, face, and neck, it is incumbent on one to be intimately aware of the complexities of the anatomical, myophysiological, and neurophysiological mechanisms that are brought to bear in providing a rational approach to therapy. It is well established that a myriad of disorders can predispose a patient to facial pain. These include muscle spasm, emotional stress, dental malocclusion, facial neuralgias, the arthritides, trauma, infection, neoplasm, ear and sinus disorders, salivary gland disease, congenital deformities, vascular disorders, and postural discrepancies.

It is recognized that the symptoms of these various factors are delicately intertwined. However, with the use of a consistently thorough history and physical examination, coupled with the knowledge of muscular pain referral patterns, the more esoteric causes can be eliminated. It is the purpose of this chapter therefore to present a method of providing definitive therapy for the single most prevalent common denominator of facial pain (myofascial pain-dysfunction syndrome): muscle spasm.*

THE HISTORY

The history deals with the patient's chief complaint and onset and duration of symptoms. Information such as location of pain, character of pain, and precipitating factors should be elicited. Previous treatment attempts and their sequelae are to be noted.

Careful observation of the patient may raise one's index of suspicion with regard to a primary myofascial syndrome. What is the *postural cant* of the head on the shoulders? Is there a shoulder level discrepancy? Can a history of lower back and/or foot pain be elicited? Do the hips appear to be discrepant?

It must be emphasized that during this time an evaluation of the patient's psychological status may provide insight in accumulating pertinent diagnostic data. This portion of the evaluation should be accomplished in an atmosphere free of anxiety-provoking factors. The importance of psychogenic overtone cannot be overemphasized in the genesis of myofascial pain.[16]

Excellent detailed outlines such as those of Burket and associates[5] and Schwartz[17] will provide the reader with a means of compiling a complete history. Sir William Osler's often quoted, "Listen to the patient; he is giving you the diagnosis," is particularly applicable when diagnosing facial pain. With the knowledge of a thorough history, the examiner may now perform a systematic physical evaluation, focusing attention on key symptoms brought out in the history. *A methodical, well-organized physical examination is most important, in that many patients suffering from facial pain have been treated by many specialists; and for the sake of sparing the patient undue redundancy, the examiner may tend to be cursory in approach. Professionalism, thoroughness, and an attitude of confidence must be conveyed.*

PHYSICAL EXAMINATION

The physical examination actually begins in the consultation room; it is here that the experienced clinician may gain some insight into the patient's physical disorder. It is important to understand that the human body functions as one beautifully compliant machine, and obviously deficiencies in one part of this machine affect all other parts. Specific systems of the body cannot be isolated from others.

Once in the operatory, the following observations should be noted and questions asked:

1. Postural evaluation (Figs. 16-1 and 16-2). The single most common perpetuator of muscle spasm throughout the body is the mechanical

*References 1, 10, 14, 17, and 18.

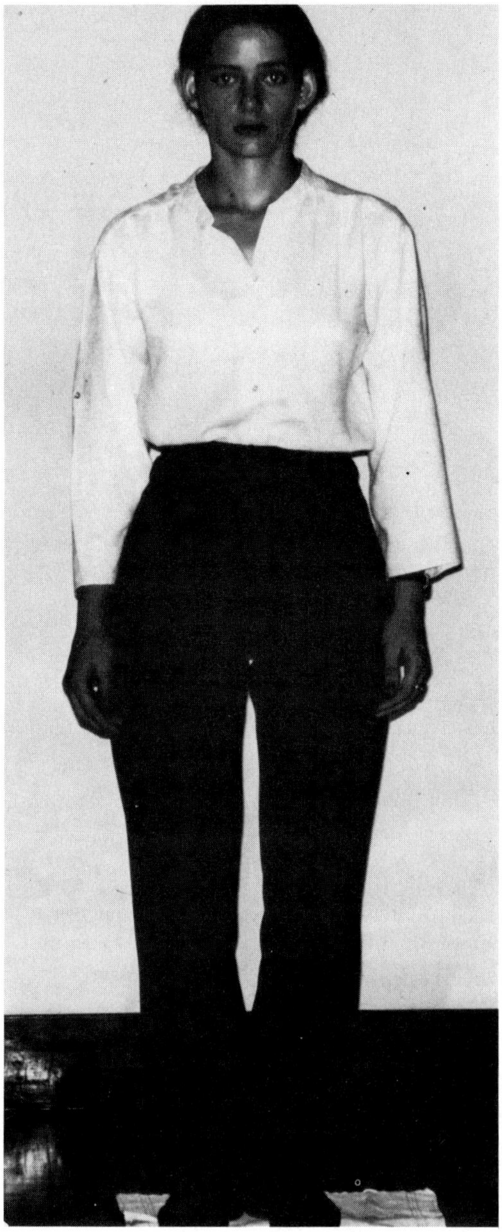

Fig. 16-1. Posture of patient with complaint of head and neck pain.

disorder caused by limb-length discrepancy. Conscious efforts to determine lower limb length are tremendously valuable in obtaining long-term curative results.

a. Hip height based on the levels of the iliac crests and position of the anterosuperior iliac spines must be ascertained. What is the level of the scapulae bilaterally? Does the head show an aberrant cant (tilt), denoting peculiar muscle vectors at the atlantooccipital articulation? Is one leg longer than the other?
b. Feet should be examined by a competent clinician to determine if any inherent disorders are present.
c. Muscles of primary interest include the long peroneal, iliopsoas, quadratus lumborum, semispinal musculature, levator scapulae, rhomboids, and, of course, muscles of the neck (trapezius and sternocleidomastoid), which rapidly spread muscular irregularity to the gnathostomatic system.
d. Radiographic examination of the posture may begin with a scanogram of the lower limbs to determine leg length discrepancy. This scanogram should include the iliac crests and the ankles bilaterally. This survey must be taken while patient is weight-bearing.

2. Inspection of head, face, and neck (Fig. 16-3). Are there notable asymmetries, suggesting abnormal facial growth, trauma, infection, or muscular hypertrophies?
3. Mandibular excursions
   a. Opening. Is the opening movement smooth, painless, and free from deviation? If pain is present, what is its character and location? A measurement of the maximum interincisal opening (MIO) within pain limits should be noted. A range of approximately 40 to 55 mm for MIO can be considered normal.[22]
   b. Closing. Is the patient able to bring the jaws together without manipulation of the mandible? Are teeth tender when maximum intercuspation is obtained?
   c. Lateral movements. Is the range of motion similar bilaterally? (Lateral and protrusive movements should be observed with patient's teeth in slight contact.)
   d. Protrusive movements. Can the patient perform a protrusive motion without deviation?
4. Temporomandibular joint examination (Fig. 16-4)
   a. Direct palpation
      (1) Pretragus area
      (2) Directly over the condylar head
      (3) Through the external auditory meatus. Do the condyles glide smoothly, or is a snapping motion palpable? Can translation be ascertained? Is there pain? Does the overlying tissue show signs of inflammation (Fig. 16-4, *A*)?
   b. Indirect auscultation. With the bell of a stethoscope placed over the temporomandibular joints, auscultation may reveal clicking sounds or crepitation, which may be indicative of some osteodegenerative process (Fig. 16-4, *B*).[10,17]

A 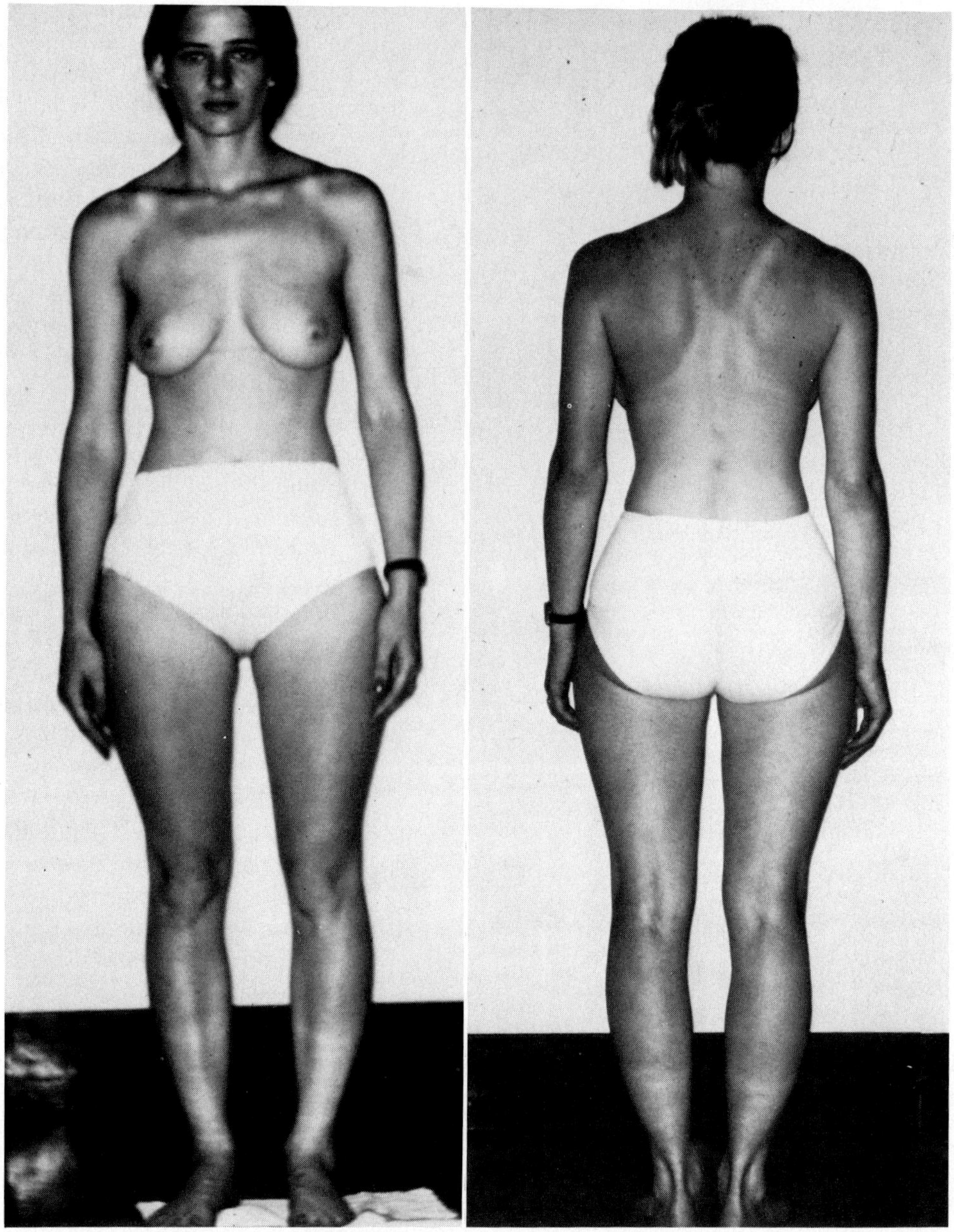 B

Fig. 16-2. Front **(A)** and back **(B)** views reveal profound skeletal and/or muscular irregularities that often are seen in chronic myofascial pain-dysfunction patients.

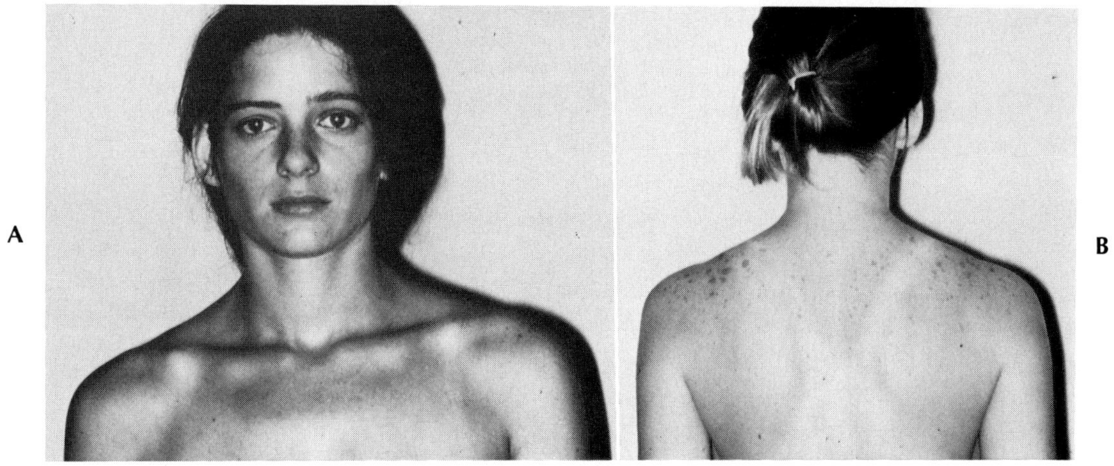

Fig. 16-3. A, Close-up frontal examination of head, face, and neck. Note discrepant levels of superciliary ridges, distinctive head cant, and relative position of clavicles. **B,** Note difference in shoulder heights and levels of scapulae.

5. Digital muscular examination. Attempts should be made to define trigger zones (spastic areas) and the associated pain referral patterns. Pain referral patterns follow predictable anatomical pathways for most muscles and manifest symptoms at some distance from their trigger zones.
   a. Temporal muscle (Fig. 16-5). The temporal muscle acts primarily as an elevator (closer) of the jaw, although its function as a mandibular retruder cannot be overlooked. The temporal muscle originates in the temporal fossa and inserts on the coronoid process of the mandible. It is important to note that this muscle is capable of referring pain to the *entire* maxillary dentition (depending, of course, on which fibers are affected) and is the prime muscle responsible for the common temporal headache.
   b. Sternocleidomastoid muscle (Fig. 16-6). This muscle acts primarily to rotate and stabilize the head as a result of its effect on the atlantooccipital articulation. The sternocleidomastoid consists of a sternal division and a clavicular division. Pain referral patterns are diffuse, but correlation to chin, ear, and preauricular pain is notable. It is this muscle which is often involved with vertigo symptoms.
   c. Trapezius muscle (Fig. 16-7). This muscle has its attachments superiorly at the occipital region and inferiorly at the scapula. Its action is that of raising the shoulders. It is considered by many as the seat of the classic tension headache. Note that pain to the angle of the mandible can be referred.
   d. Masseter muscle (Fig. 16-8). The masseter muscle has two distinct portions: a superficial and a deep layer. The masseter muscle has its origin at the zygomatic crestal border with some fibers originating slightly posterior to the zygomaticotemporal suture. Insertion of this muscle is at the angle of the inferior border of the mandible, where it forms an elevating (closing) sling with the internal pterygoid muscle. Observation of the pain referral patterns of this muscle is interesting. The superficial portion tends to refer pain to the posterior dentition of both the maxilla and the mandible. This is the second masticatory muscle yet mentioned with an odontogenic referral pattern. The deep layer of this muscle refers pain to the region of the ear, and it is one of two muscles (the first being the sternocleidomastoid) capable of simulating ear pain.
   e. Internal pterygoid muscle. The internal pterygoid muscle has its origin on the medial surface of the lateral pterygoid plate and its insertion at the inferior border of the mandible, where its fascia is contiguous with that of the masseter muscle. Its action is primarily elevation, but assistance in lateral movements is noted. Pain referral patterns for this muscle are rather vague with most reference to the external pterygoid, floor of the nose, throat, condylar area, and ear.
   f. External pterygoid muscle (Fig. 16-9). The external pterygoid muscle is anatomically and kinesiologically misunderstood. The external pterygoid has two divisions, a superior and an inferior. The superior division has its origin

A

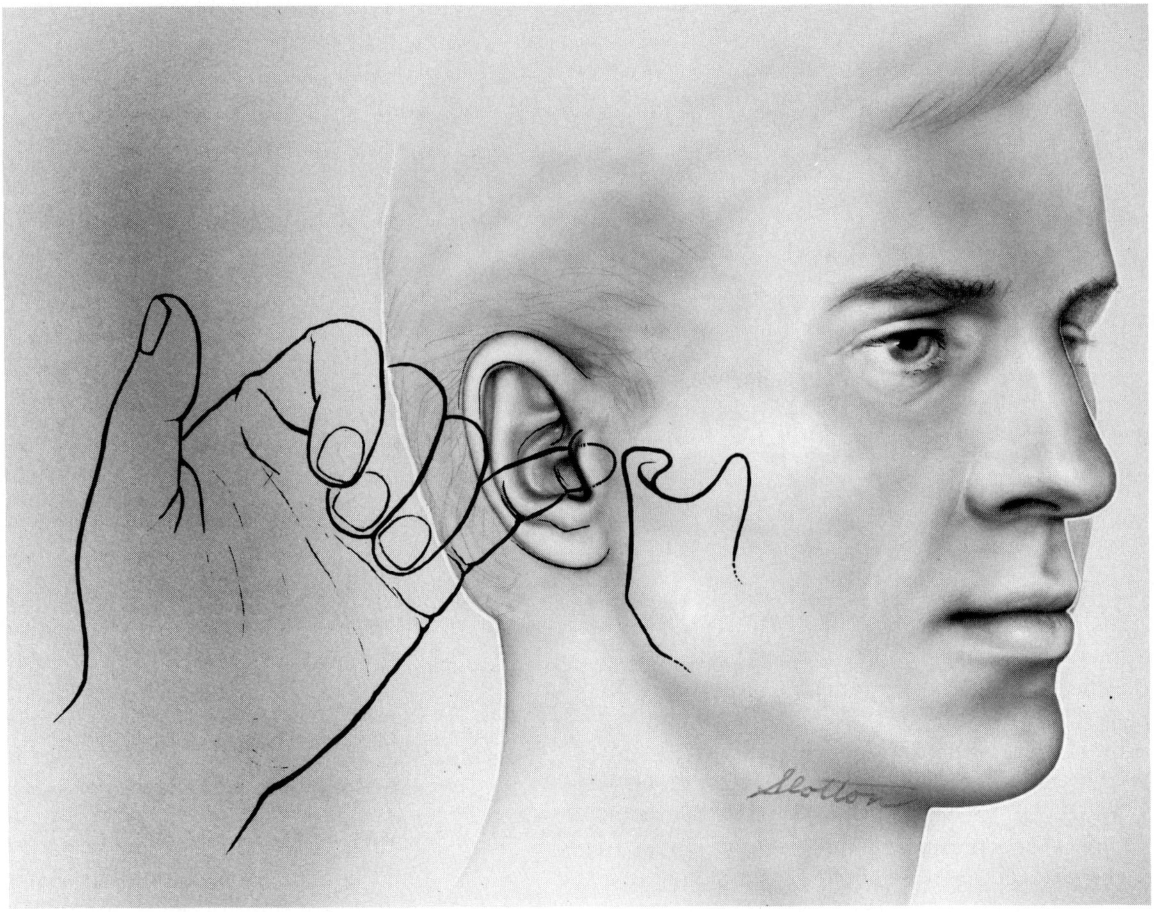

Fig. 16-4. Examination of temporomandibular joint. **A,** Manual palpation through external auditory meatus to evaluate intracapsular disease and orthopedic disorders.

at the infratemporal crest and its insertion at the articular disc (meniscus). The inferior head of this muscle originates at the lateral surface of the lateral pterygoid plate and inserts at the condylar head. It is an incoordination of these two distinct muscular heads that can cause clicking, subluxation, and dislocation of the condyle. Absolute knowledgeability of the prime pain referral pattern of this muscle is a clinical necessity. The external pterygoid muscle refers pain to the area of the temporomandibular joint. It is the primary muscle of the head, face, and neck to do so. Unilateral spasm of this muscle will cause a mandibular deflection to the contralateral side; bilateral spasm initiates a protrusive movement or a premature translatory excursion. Chronic spasm of this muscle can cause the symptom of tinnitus.

6. Oral examination. Is the occlusion "normal" for this patient? Have there been any recent dental restorative procedures? Do the teeth show signs of bruxing or grinding? Is there dental infection (caries, periodontitis, pericoronitis)? Are there signs of parafunction (cheek biting, tongue indentation, accelerated attrition)?
7. Otolarngological examination. Visualization of the tympanic membranes of the ear to rule out infection, foreign bodies, or excess cerumen is indicated. It should be noted if the pharynx and tonsils are inflamed or purulent.
8. Radiographic examination. A series of polytomographic radiographs are taken of each joint at prescribed mandibular positions. These TMJ tomograms are available with reproducibility. From these radiographs one can determine condylar integrity at any cranial depth, and it is possible to detect trauma, ankylosis, neoplasms, and degenerative bone changes. Attention should be focused on the joint space surrounding the con-

B

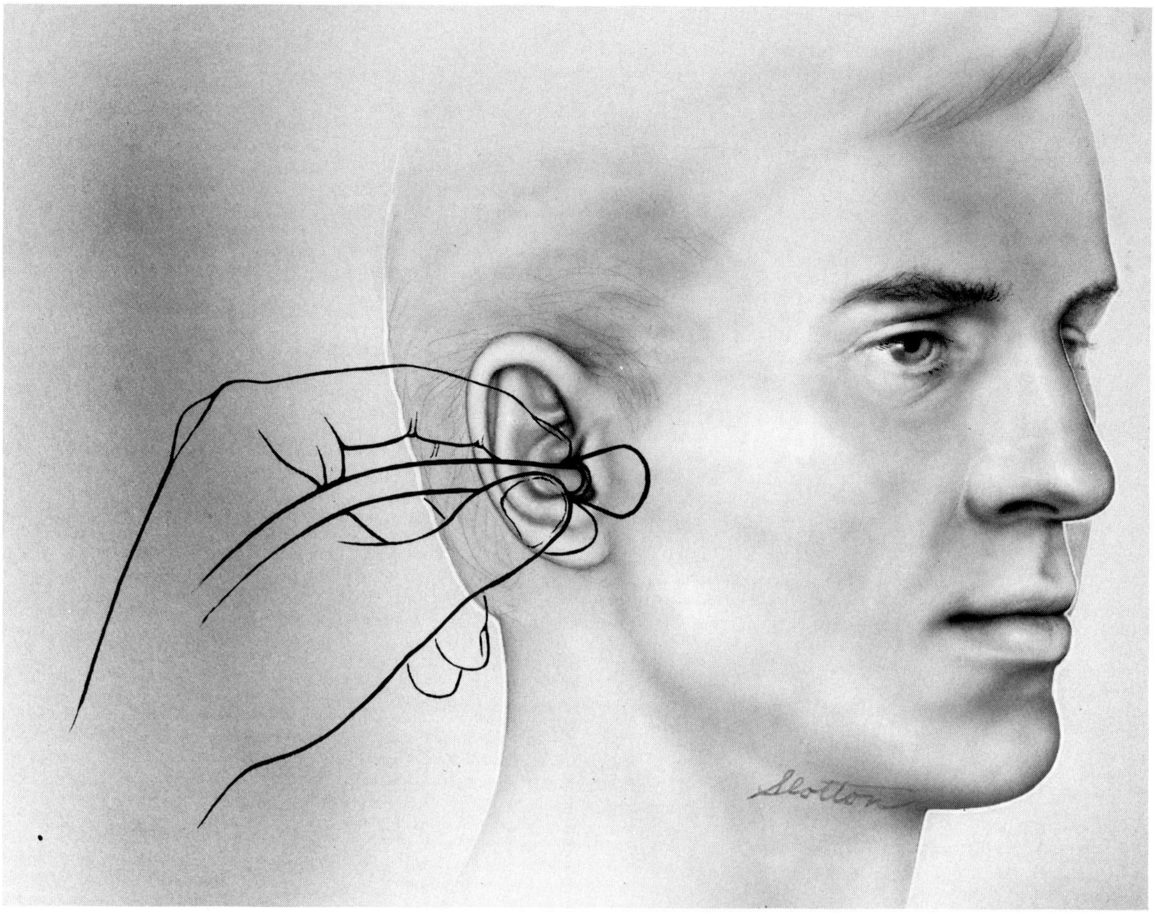

Fig. 16-4, cont'd. B, Auscultation with bell of stethoscope placed adjacent to glenoid fossa to detect clicking (muscular, orthopedic, or discal) and crepitation indicative of osteodegenerative bone changes.

dyle. One must not forget that the condyle articulates with the anterior slope of the glenoid fossa. In other words, the condylar head (capitulum) is in articulation with the posterior portion of the eminence (tuberculum). The space posterior to the condyle must be open to house comfortably the retrodiscal tissue within the glenoid fossa. Posterior and superior deflection of the condylar head in the fossa should alert the clinician that the mandibular position is faulty.

9. Laboratory studies
   a. Latex fixation. It is known that symptomatic temporomandibular joints can be attributable to rheumatoid arthritis.[10] It is not infrequent that the temporomandibular joints are initially involved.[1]
   b. Sedimentation rate. Elevated sedimentation rate may cause one to suspect an osteodegenerative process. If this test is positive, an inflammatory process may be occurring in the temporomandibular joints, and a serum electrophoresis may be indicated.
   c. Antinuclear factor (ANF) with titer. An elevation in this test may denote the possibility of an active autoimmune process.
   d. Serum calcium level. Calcium is essential in maintaining the integrity of the cell; hypocalcemia must be corrected.
   e. Minnesota Multiphasic Personality Inventory (MMPI). This gives an indication of whether the patient will be refractory to physical therapy without prior or concurrent psychological counseling; it is an integral diagnostic tool.
   f. Arthritis radiographic series. A competent survey of hands, hips, and lateral lumbar spine will usually reveal generalized osteodegenerative changes when present.
   g. Vitamin level. Hypovitaminosis of vitamins B_1, B_6, C, and folic acid all have been associated with malfunction of muscle systems.

Text continued on p. 296.

A

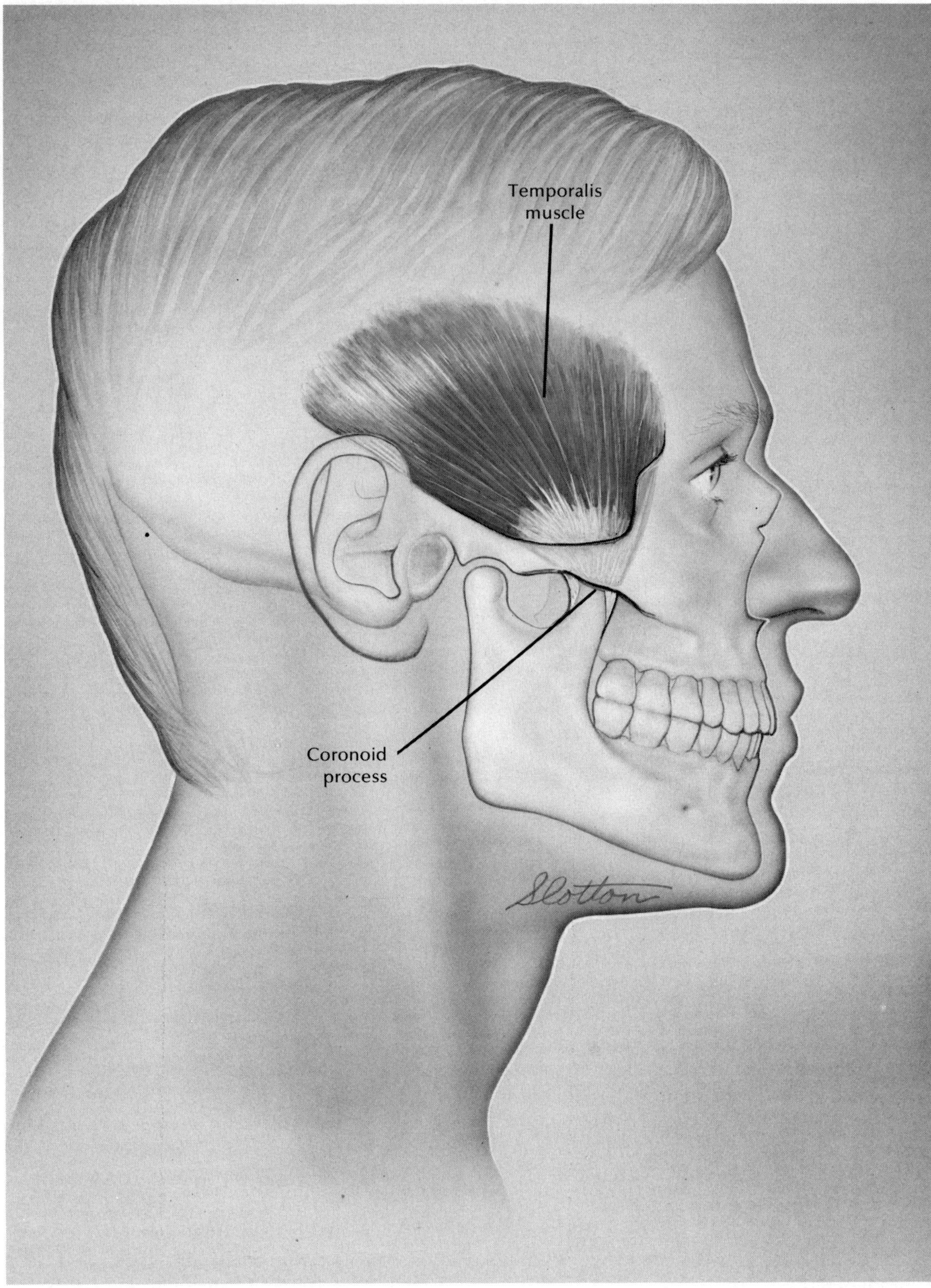

Fig. 16-5. Anatomical depiction of temporal muscle. **A,** Temporal muscle with origin in temporal fossa and insertion on coronoid process of mandible.

B

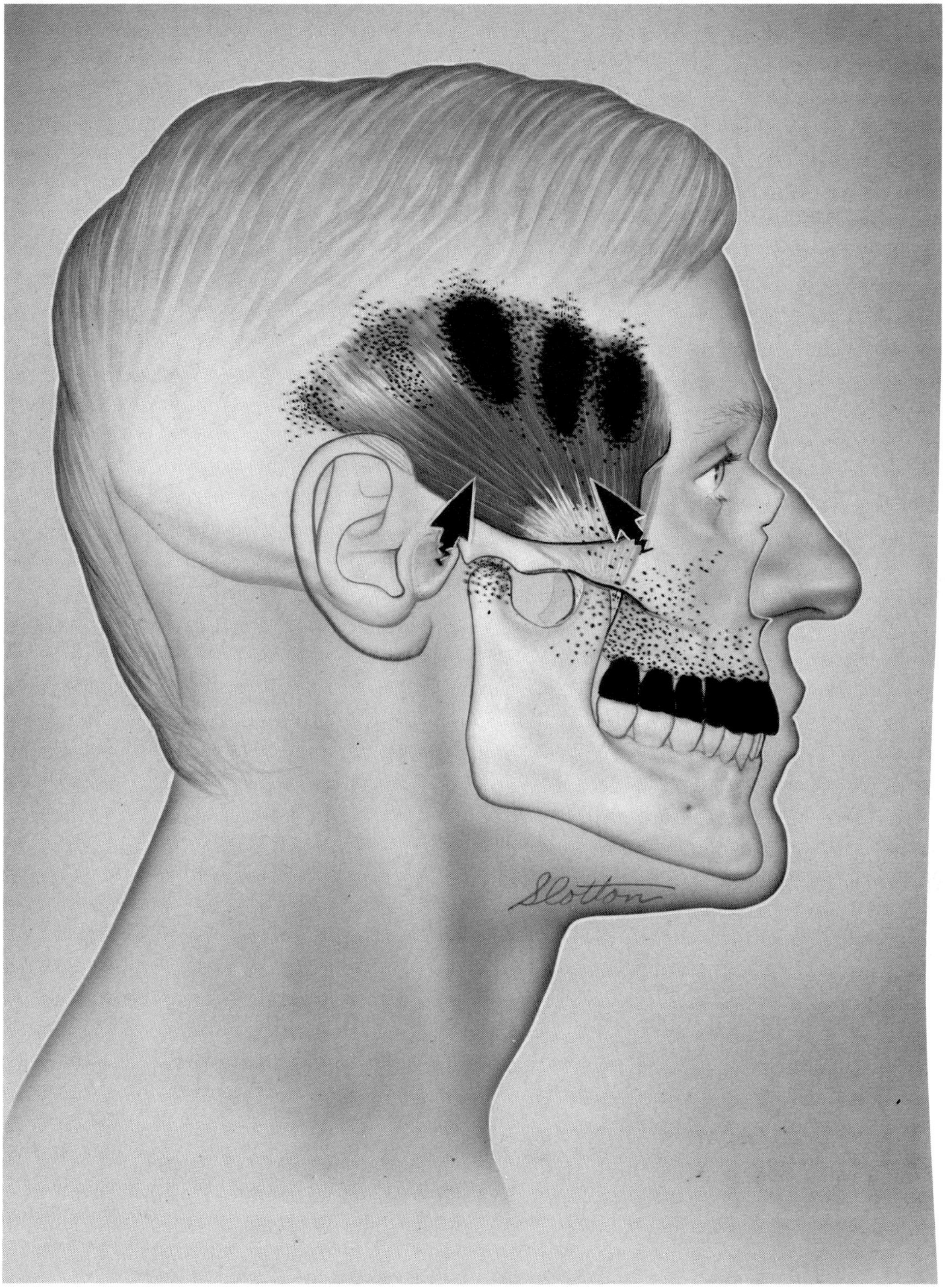

Fig. 16-5, cont'd. B, Arrows depict trigger zones; stippled areas delineate pain referral patterns. Other than area of temple, most commonly involved structure is maxillary dentition.

A

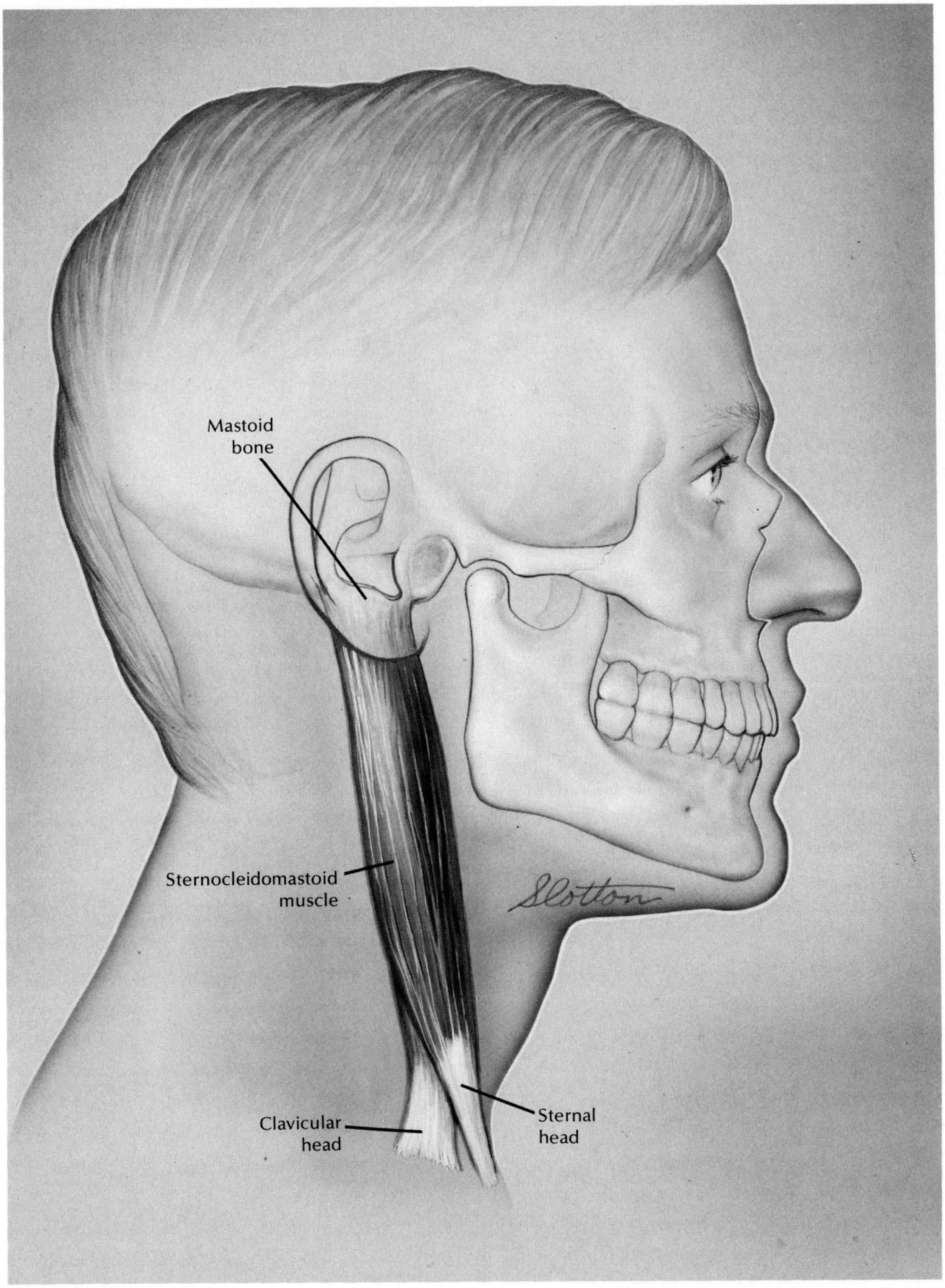

Fig. 16-6. Anatomical depiction of sternocleidomastoid muscle. **A,** Sternocleidomastoid muscle with origin at mastoid and two divisions: sternal and clavicular.

B

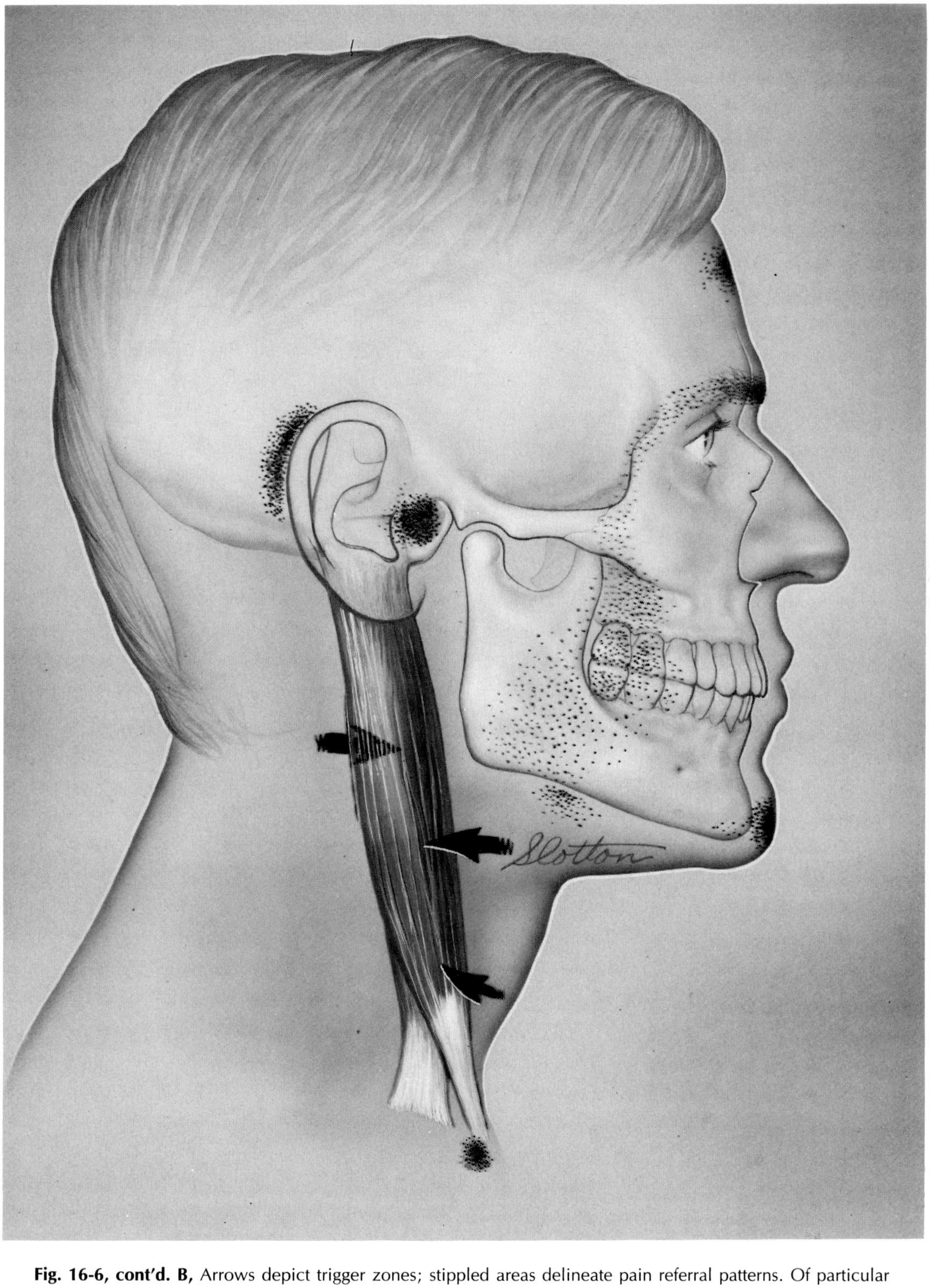

Fig. 16-6, cont'd. B, Arrows depict trigger zones; stippled areas delineate pain referral patterns. Of particular significance is localization of pain to chin and preauricular regions. Sternocleidomastoid muscle may often precipitate otalgia, which is easily confused with organic disorders of ear. When this muscle is in chronic spasm, vertigo may occur.

A

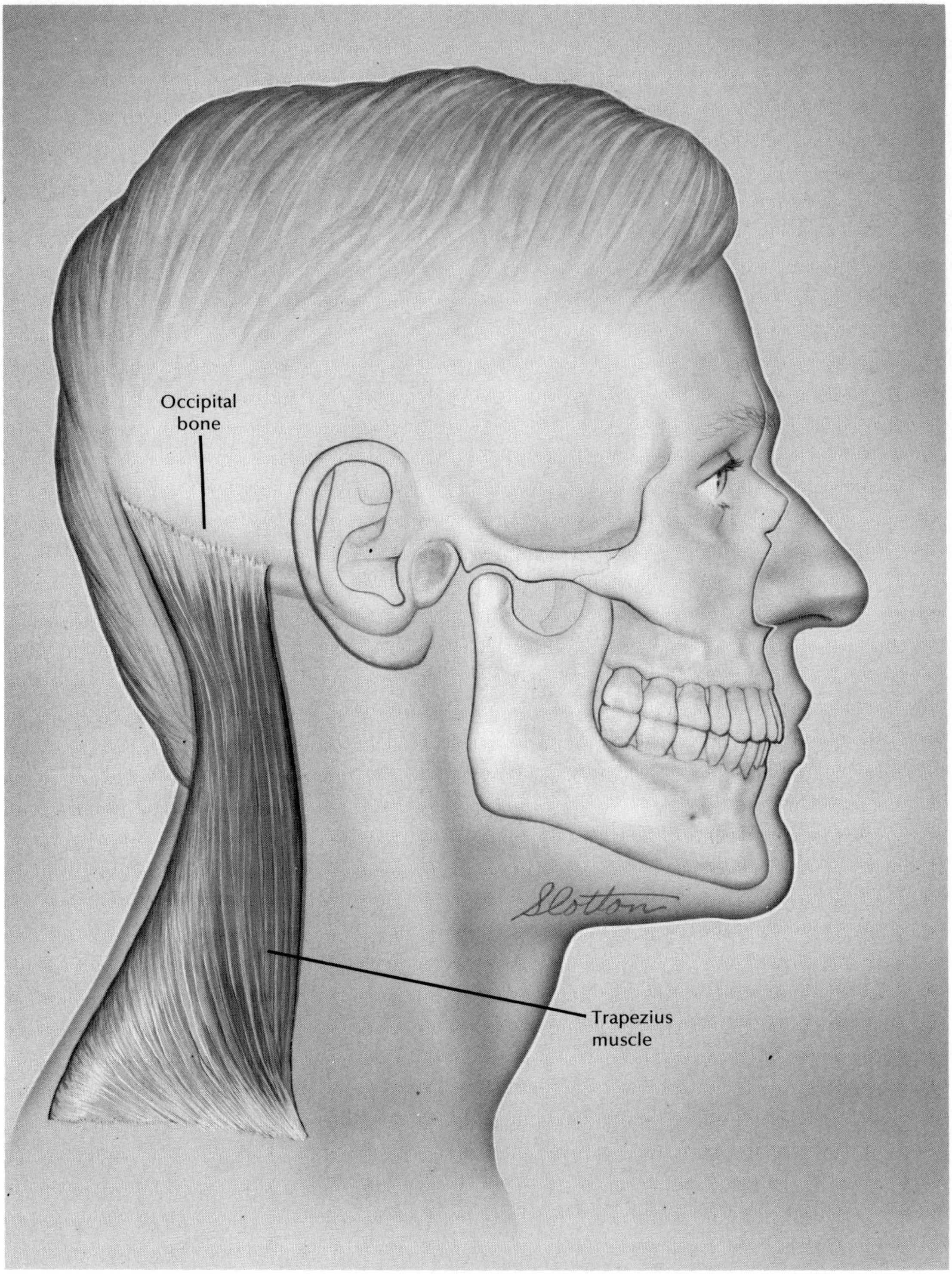

Fig. 16-7. Anatomical depiction of trapezius muscle. **A,** Trapezius muscle originates on occipital bone and finds its insertion at scapula. It is a diffuse muscle covering much of posterior neck.

B

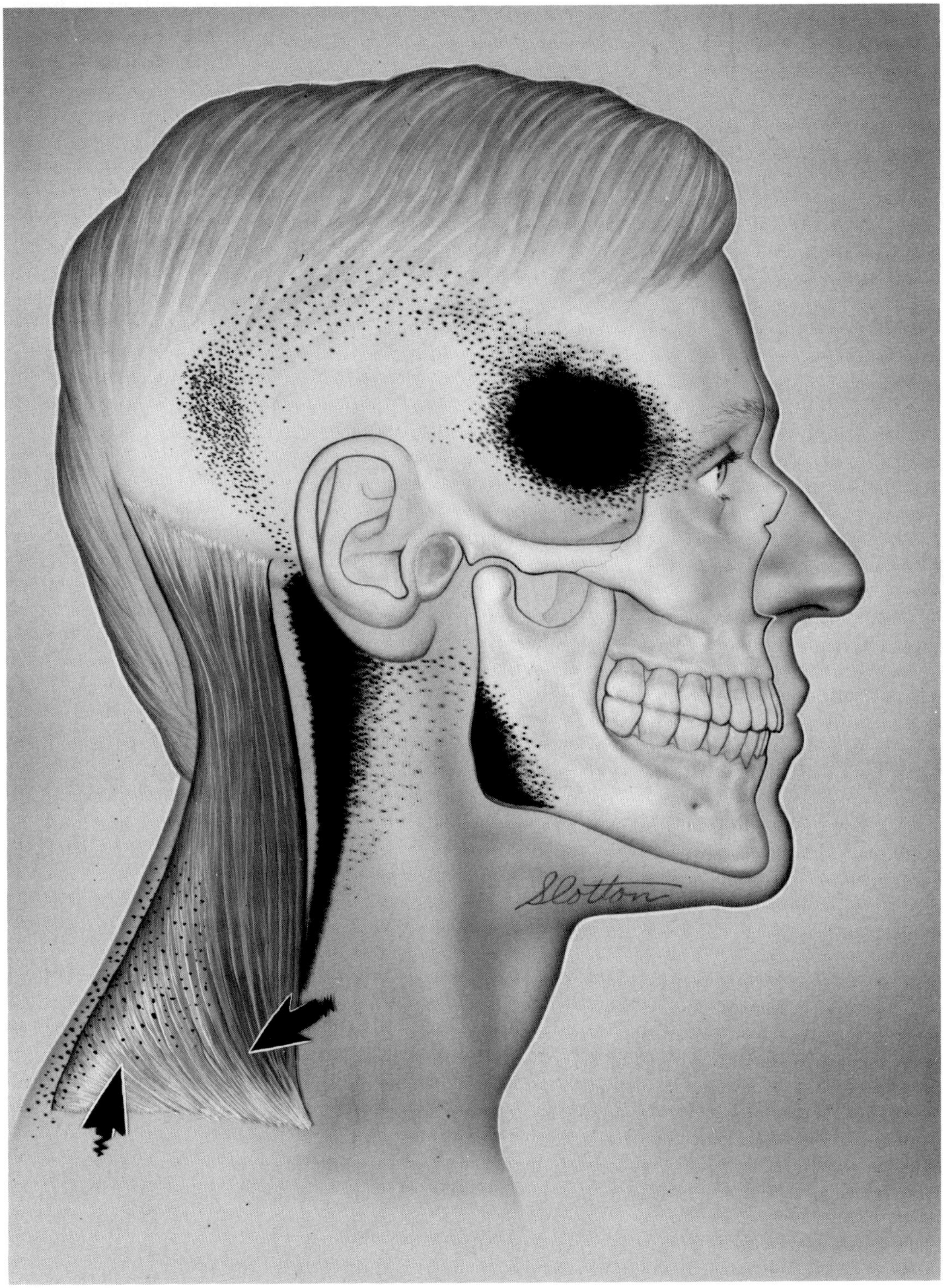

Fig. 16-7, cont'd. B, Arrows depict trigger zones; stippled areas delineate pain referral patterns. Lateral orbital pain and localized vague pain at angle of mandible are often diagnostic.

A

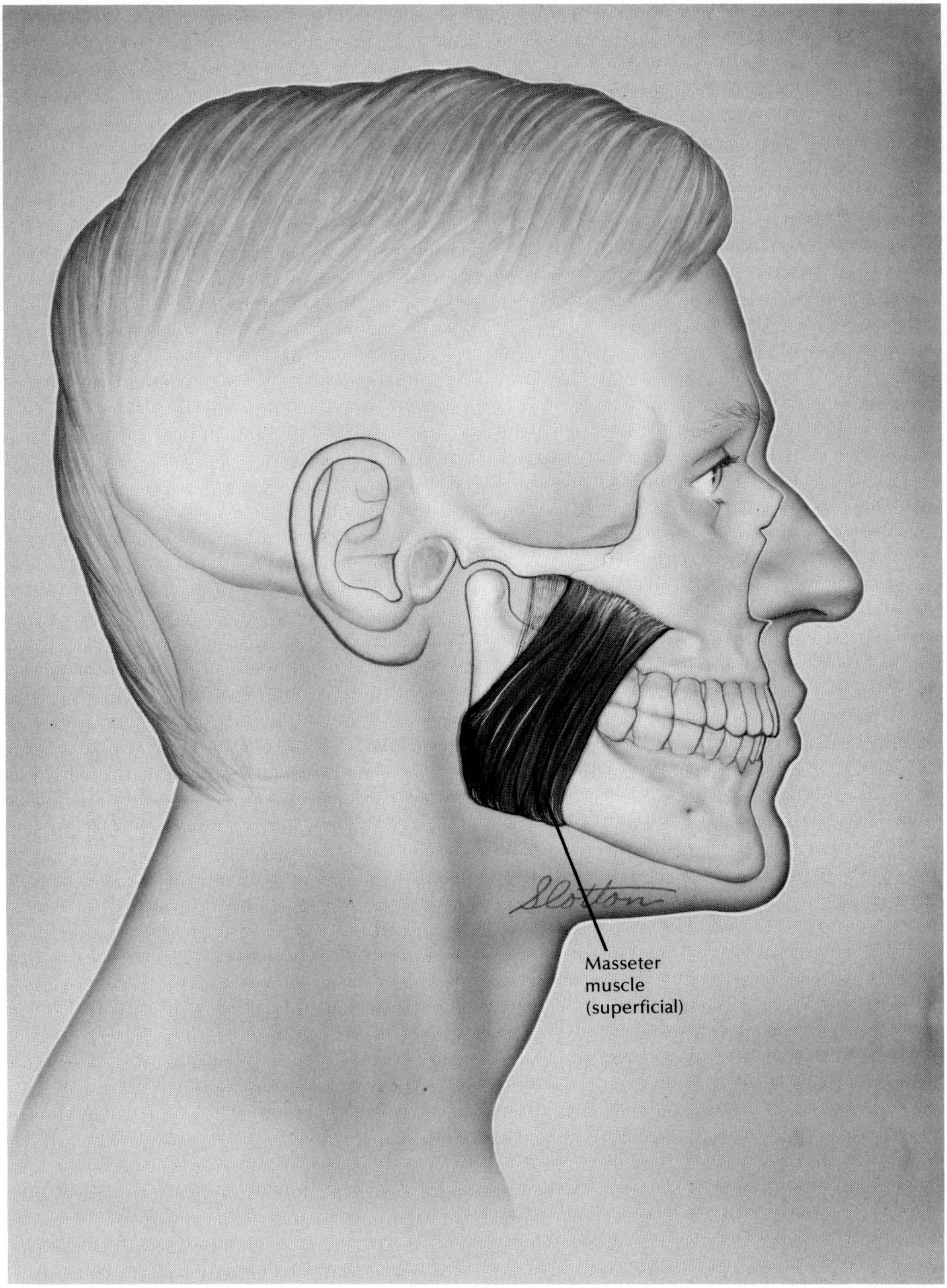

Fig. 16-8. Anatomical depiction of masseter muscle. **A,** Superficial layer of masseter muscle originates at zygomatic buttress with insertion at angle of inferior border of mandible.

B

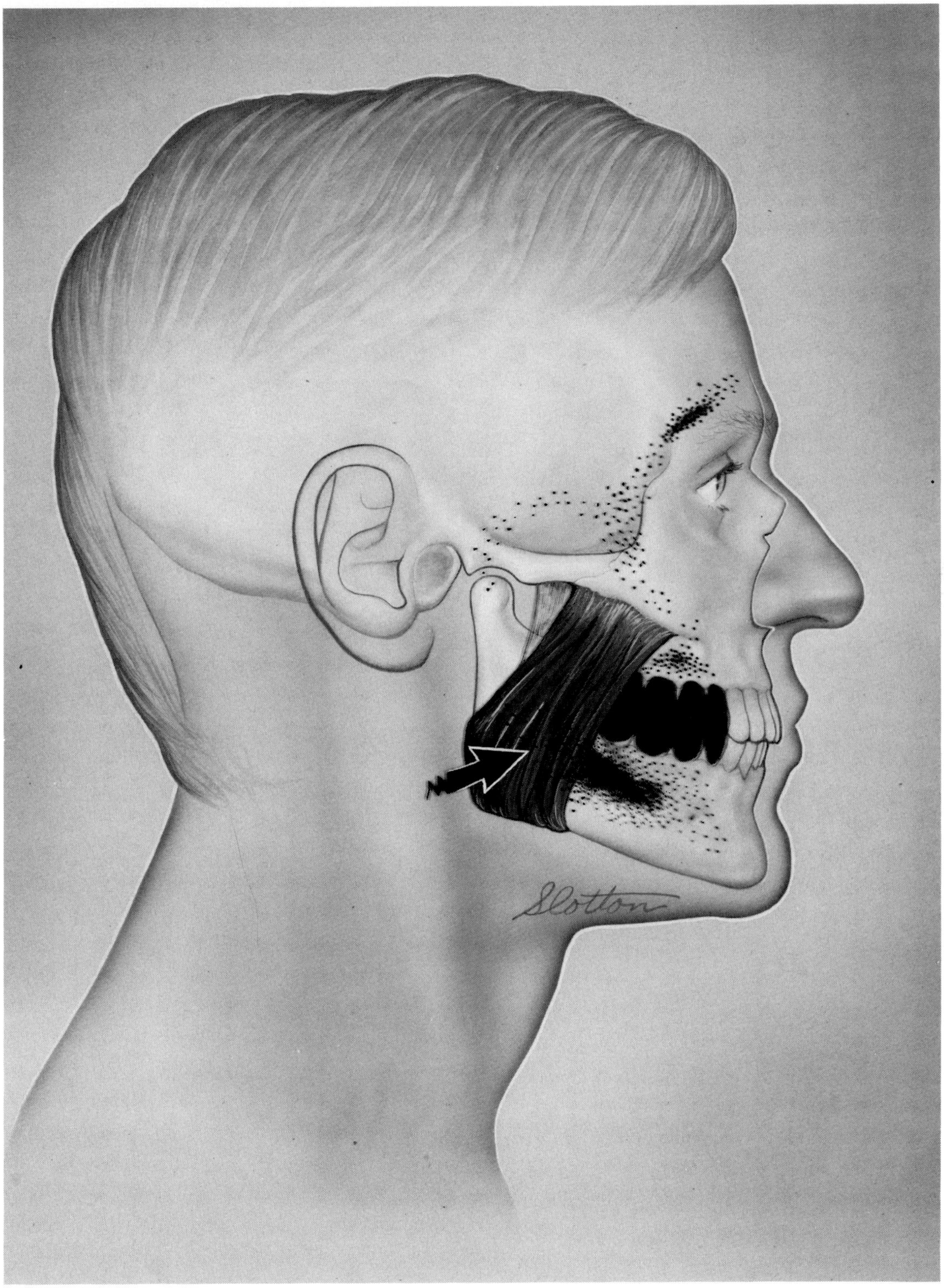

Fig. 16-8, cont'd. B, Arrow depicts trigger zones; stippled areas delineate pain referral patterns. Referral regions are particularly concentrated in both maxillary and mandibular posterior dentitions. *Continued.*

C

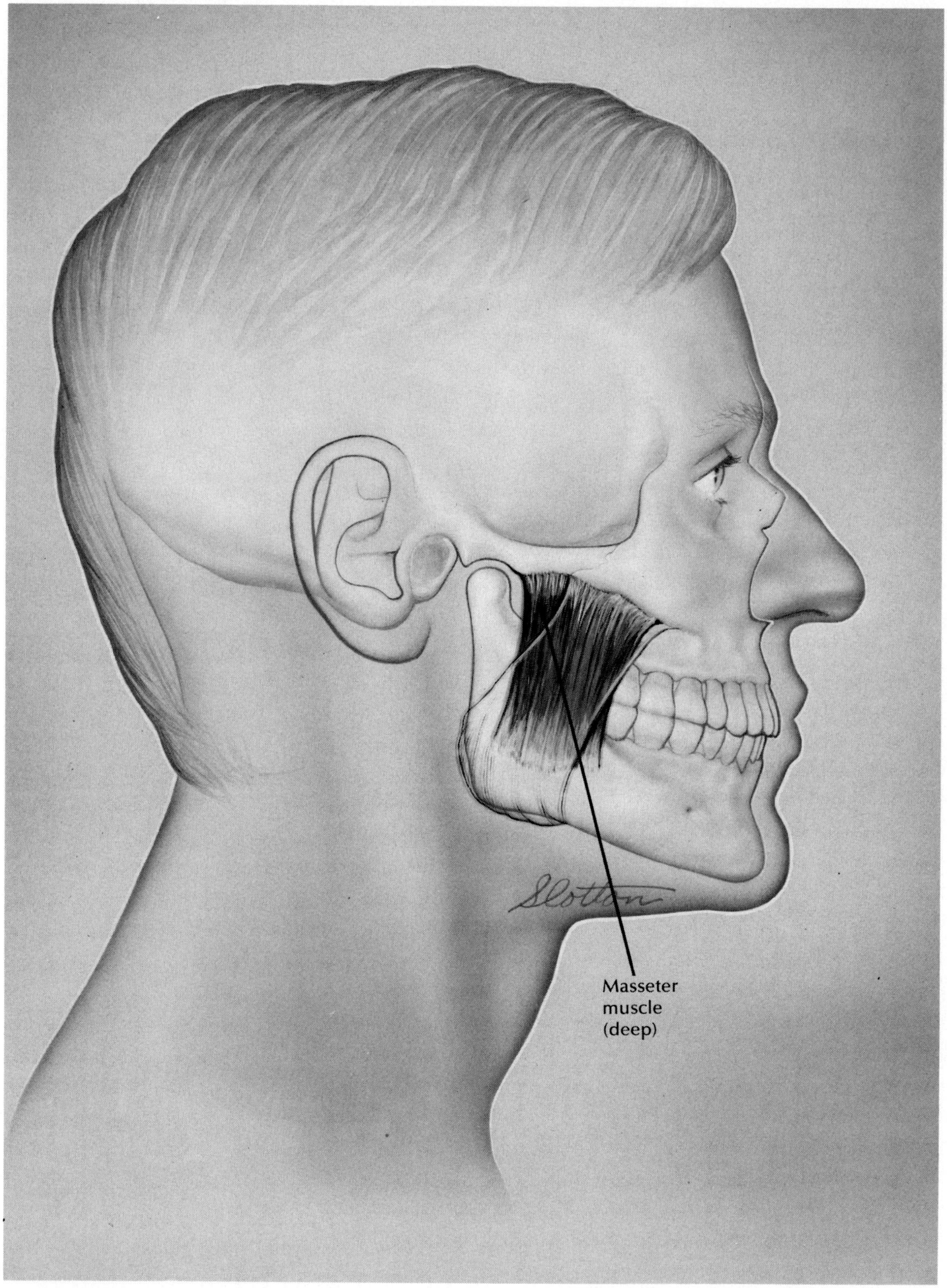

Fig. 16-8, cont'd. C, Deep layer of masseter muscle. This muscle has its origin on zygomatic buttress with its terminal fibers extending just posterior to zygomaticotemporal suture. Insertion is just deep to its superficial component.

D

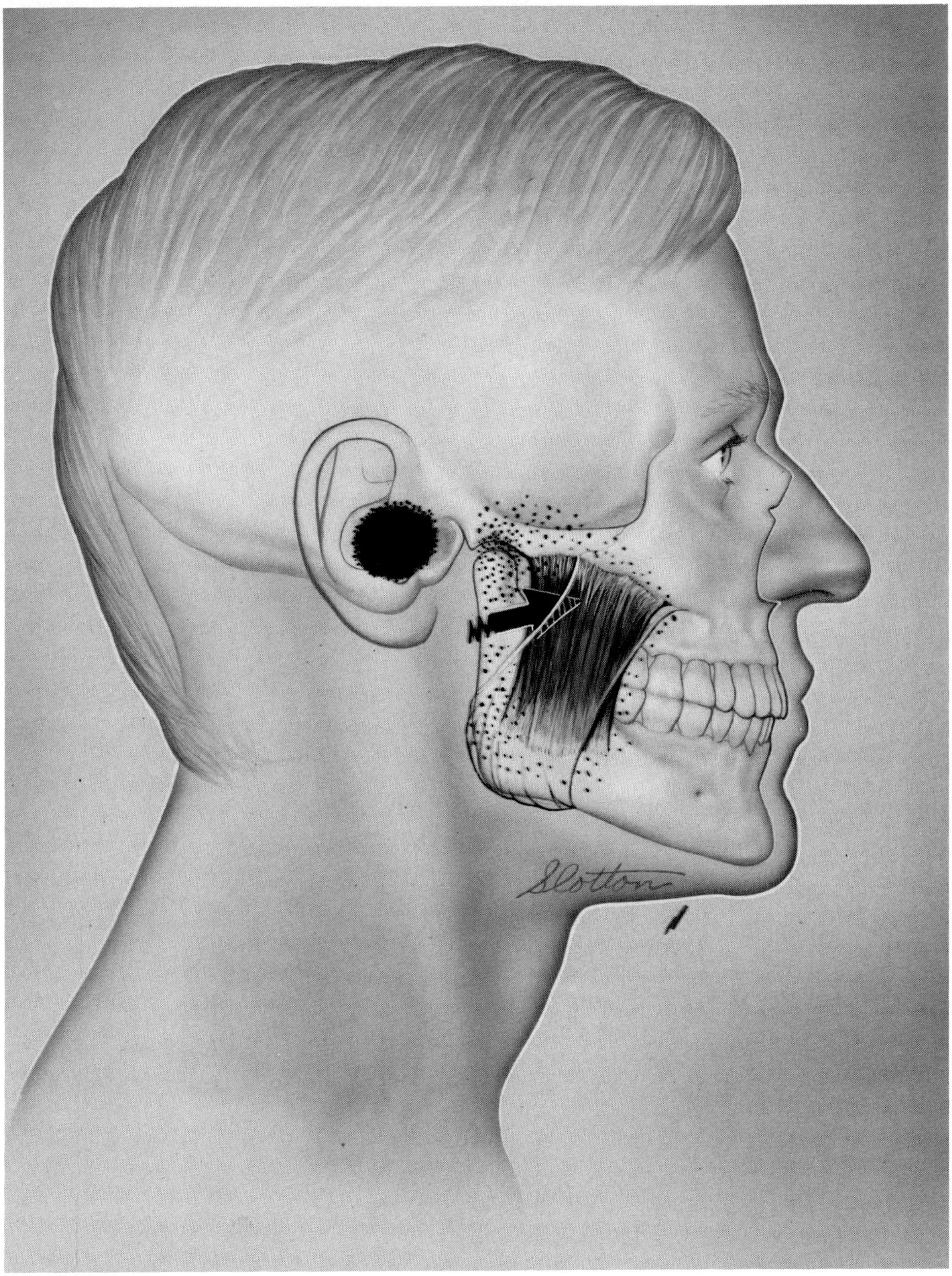

Fig. 16-8, cont'd. D, Arrows depict trigger zones; stippled areas delineate pain referral patterns. Intense pain localized about ear is symptomatically classic in this muscle.

A

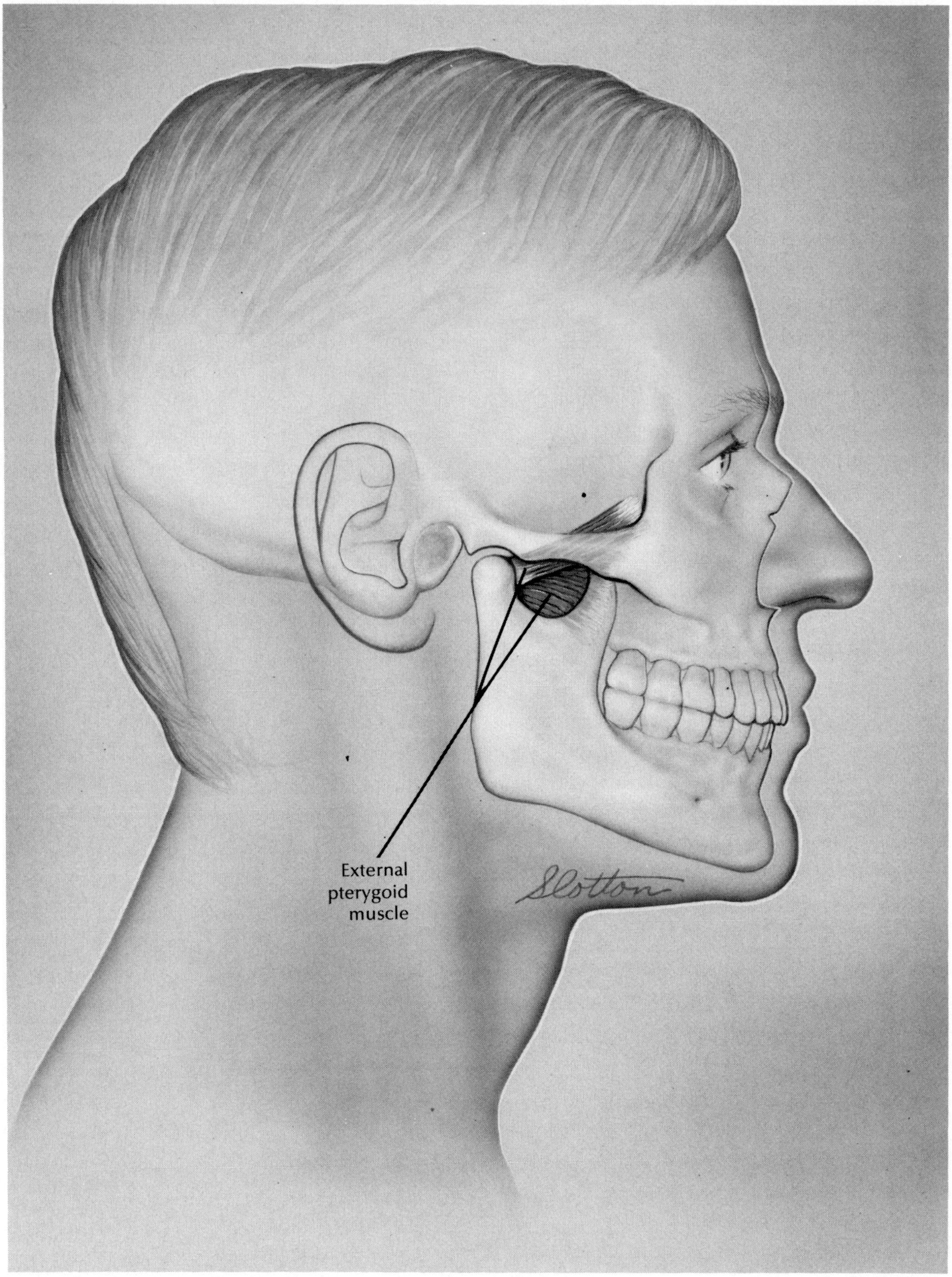

Fig. 16-9. Anatomical depiction of external pterygoid muscle. **A,** This muscle is composed of two separate heads: the superior head, which finds its origin at infratemporal crest and its insertion on articular disc (meniscus), and an inferior, larger head, with its origin on lateral surface of lateral pterygoid plate and insertion on condylar head.

B

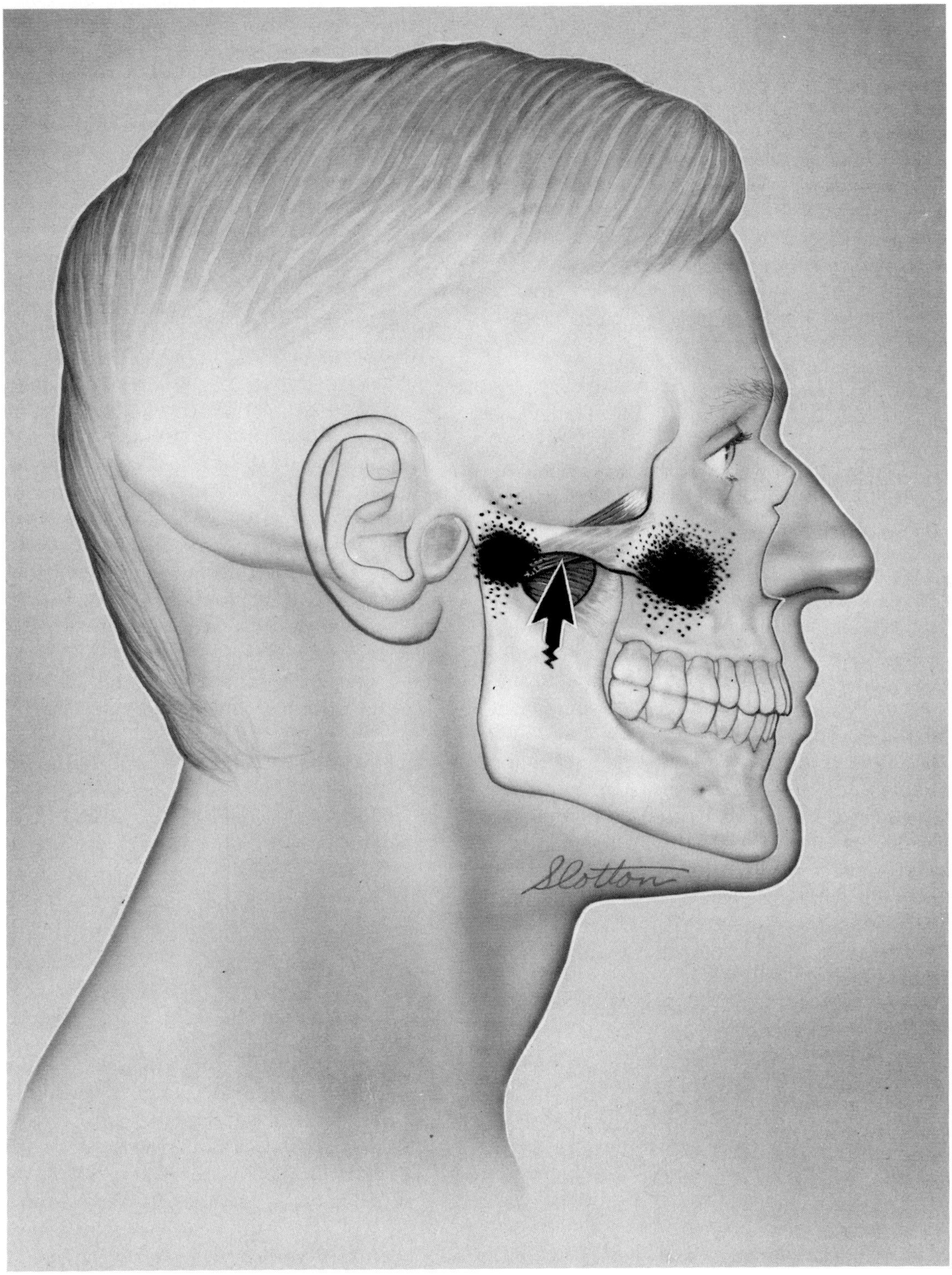

Fig. 16-9, cont'd. B, Arrows depict trigger zones; stippled areas delineate pain referral patterns. Pain about temporomandibular joint is frequently diagnostic. Complaints of fullness in area of zygomatic buttress are not uncommon.

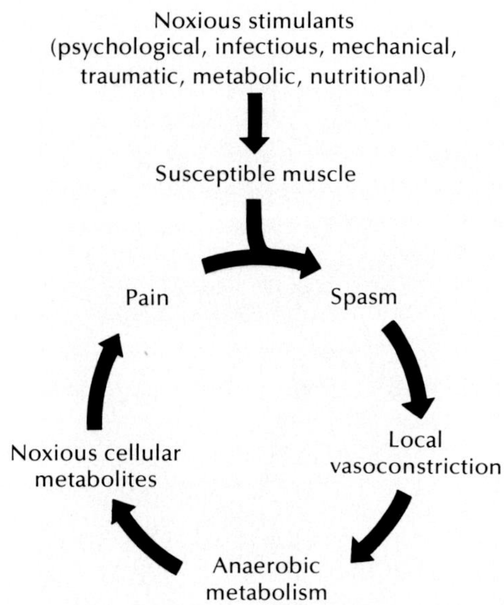

Fig. 16-10. Pain-spasm-pain cycle is a vicious deteriorative biochemical cycle resulting in muscular spasm and subsequent pain referral patterns.

h. Uric acid level. Hyperuricemia may often trigger myospasm.
i. Thyroid activity level. Abnormally high levels of T_3, T_4, and TSH denoting hyperthyroidism can predispose many patients to muscular spasmodic episodes.

With the history and physical examination completed, the clinician must take definitive steps to *interrupt* the disease cycle (Fig. 16-10). Prompt problem solving, consultation, and referral to the proper practitioners is tantamount to quality treatment. The success of treatment in many cases appears to be related to the period when treatment is initiated. Many observers believe that the earlier in the disorder treatment is started, the greater the likelihood of success. This apparently is independent of the treatment modality instituted.[6]

We actively begin to treat this disease with the knowledge that there exists between the temporomandibular joint and its musculature an elaborate feedback mechanism. It is through this feedback mechanism that this sensitive sensory system continually attempts to right itself in the face of induced shifts in condylar position. *This is a protective physiological process*. However, if this process were deranged and allowed to continue indefinitely, it could (and often does) cause marked limitation of motion with spread of spasm to other muscles and may eventually involve the entire gnathostomatic and body postural apparatus. Guarding, or overprotection from painful trigger zones, by the patient may indeed limit suffering from myospasm, but it may also cause gradual, permanent contracture and ultimate limitation of mandibular movements (hypokinetic disease).[9] Immobilization, either by external appliance or by conscious and subconscious inhibition of voluntary movement, is a major factor in the rapid progression of painful muscle spasm to painless permanent contraction.

TREATMENT OF MYOSPASM

Psychophysiological treatment

As previously mentioned, a first consideration for those treating facial pain secondary to muscle spasm is the establishment of a propitious therapeutic atmosphere. Patient and practitioner develop attitudes from the moment they meet, and it is for this reason that the conveyance of honesty and concern be immediately accomplished. As has been suggested, complete separation of myospasm from concomitant psychogenic factors is improbable. It is therefore imperative for one to consider the strong possibility of a biphasic disorder.

Levine[10] proposed five procedures likely to aid the patient who is predisposed psychologically to somatic disorders such as ulcers, colitis, migraine headache, dermatitis, TMJ syndrome, or lower back pain.[10,12]

1. *Reeducate* the patient as to the mechanisms involved and factors causing or aggravating the patient's disorder. Patients do not readily believe, nor do they understand, vague statements about the connection between anxiety and pain. An explanation of the mechanisms involved will be more convincing and reassuring if it is couched in language appropriate to the patient's education and intelligence. This understanding will better prepare the stressed patient to fight the temptation of searching for magic cures.
2. *Reassure* the patient as to the benign character of myospasm The patient should be reassured that no permanent facial deformities or dysfunctions will arise. The clinician must convey confidence and competence, being certain not to placate the patient merely to gain approval.
3. *Ventilation* of the patient's fears may have a cathartic effect in certain cases. Even when a patient is fully aware that the fears are irrational, verbalization can be therapeutic.[17]
4. *Suggestion* may act as a powerful therapeutic tool. The calm assurance with which the practitioner works suggests to the patient that improvement is bound to occur. Let suggestion act in a natural, quiet fashion rather than trying to use it in some spectacular way, such as the use of various placebo techniques.
5. *Interpretation* as to the degree of psychophysiological overtone should be cautiously ascertained

by the nonpsychiatrically trained person. Although the dentist or physician is in no position to suggest to the patient the answer to life's problems, the fact that the practitioner has helped the patient focus attention on a possible cause is invaluable. The therapist who expresses an opinion about the psychophysiological component of a disorder will spare the patient much confusion and pointless consultations.

Myophysiotherapy

Proper management of myospasm and myalgia depends on accurate localization of the affected muscles (physical examination). Therapeutic exercises in the treatment of myospasm aim to restore painless and adequate mandibular movements by improving the properties required for function of the masticatory muscles and represent the cornerstone of conservative therapy.[8]

By having the patient use rhythmic, coordinated mandibular movements, muscle spasm can be physiologically diminished or eliminated. It is initially important to carefully instruct the patient as to the *exact* methodology you choose for him or her to use. An excellent initial exercise entails having the patient place the tongue as posteriorly as possible in contact with the palate while keeping the mandible in a retruded position. By assuming this position, the patient's articular movements are mainly rotary and limited by the constraints of the internal pterygoid muscle. The patient is told to open the mouth slowly, rhythmically, within pain limits, 10 times in succession. Next the patient is told to repeat such exercises with the addition of one critical modification—voluntary resistance.

The use of voluntary resistance to the opening movement is based on the physiological principle of *reciprocal muscle inhibition* (reflex inhibition).[7,17] On depressing the mandible, for example, the contracton of the depressor (suprahyoid) muscle group causes an inhibition of th elevator muscles. It is by this principle of prime muscle movers inhibiting their antagonists that joint movements are made possible. It follows, then, that if a muscle is subjected to a greater degree of inhibition, its relative relaxation will increase proportionately. This muscular relaxation will increase circulation to the antagonist system, and it is during this period of active reflex inhibition that the noxious stimuli (biogenic amines) present in and about the trigger zone can be eliminated by now-dilated intramuscular blood vessels. As more muscle fibers are relaxed and fewer remain in spasm, the patient will notice that mandibular movements gradually become rhythmic and painless. The interested reader is referred to Schwartz' text[17] for detailed exercises aimed at treating specific spastic muscles.

I use a *series* of therapeutic exercises consisting of 10 unassisted movements followed by 10 voluntarily resisted movements. The patient is instructed to perform during the day and to do three series of exercises at bedtime.

The amount of resistance that a patient is instructed to use should be of great enough intensity to allow for increased circulation to spastic musculature, thus ensuring ATP synthesis and facilitating muscular relaxation (Chapter 3). Conversely, the resistance must not be of such magnitude as to make smooth gliding movements impossible. "Muscle fiber is delicate, sensitive, and responsive. It can be coaxed but not driven."[15]

Physical agents

For treatment of myospasm the use of moist heat seems to be most advantageous. Heat should be applied directly adjacent to trigger zones, not referred pain areas. It has been speculated that temperature changes can alter the amount of vasodilator substances held within tissue spaces.[13] It is known that heat applied directly to the face can only be significantly therapeutic for the more superficial muscles, that is, the temporal, masseter, and cervical muscles. For the effective treatment of myospasm of the deeper muscles (the pterygoids) the use of ultrasound diathermy may be indicated.[2,3]

The use of heat to the trigger zones seems best used as a conditioner for other treatment modalities, for example, myophysiotherapy. The patient is instructed to place the heat over a particular area for no less than 10 minutes preceding therapeutic exercies. This 10-minute period allows the physical agent adequate time to be of therapeutic value but simultaneously affords time for the patient to relax and psychologically prepare for exercise.

Intramuscular injection and dry needling

Intramuscular injection of local anesthetic agents into painful trigger zones has become therapeutically efficacious. Travell[21,22] demonstrated that accurate infiltration was often effective in permanently terminating the pain-spasm-pain cycle. Physiologically, the mechanism by which intramuscular injection can eliminate painful myospasm is undoubtedly complex, but two main phenomena may be suggested. Initially, the local anesthetic agent pharmacologically breaks the cycle by clocking nerve impulse conduction and removing the pain from the area. The elimination of pain, although only transient, may allow the patient sufficient time to regain normal function. Second, and of equal importance is the fact that local anesthetic agents, such as procaine and lidocaine (Xylocaine), act as vasodilators and muscle relaxers. A local anesthetic agent must be used *without* its vasoconstrictor components, since these chemicals would only create further tissue ischemia and increased ATP deficit with an intensified accumulation of biogenic amines.

The technique of dry needling at one time was considered useful for its placebo effect, but it is now known to be therapeutically sound from a physiological basis. By piercing spastic muscle fibers with a needle, a shift in the concentration of intracellular potassium results, with an alteration of the membrane conduction potential, and nerve conduction is blocked temporarily, thereby interrupting the pain-spasm-pain cycle.[22] Many techniques of intramuscular injection and dry needling have been described.[1,17,22]

A short period of reflex inhibition exercises should precede anesthetic injection. It is important to first isolate the trigger zone and then gently probe with a needle in search of the most hypersensitive tissue. Once defined, a slow infiltration of anesthetic solution is deposited. The trigger zone is gingerly peppered with the needle alternately with the infiltration of anesthetic solution. This technique of probing for pain, aspiration, filtration, and dry needling should be continued until all pain from the trigger zone is eliminated. When the pain referral pattern is obliterated, the patient then is instructed to begin a series of exercies. With the cycle interrupted, the patient will be able to increase MIO, and dysfunction will be minimized. After the most acute trigger zone has been treated, the patient may state that pain referred from other zones also has been minimized or eliminated. Systematic intramuscular injections are continued on other trigger areas until the patient is able to more physiologically and anatomically duplicate painless mandibular excursions. This technique is the most aggressive and efficacious therapy for acute spastic episodes.

Vapocoolant spray

The use of vapocoolants (such as ethyl chloride or Fluori-Methane) is considered therapy with a physical agent to effect counterirritation.[19,22] Fluori-Methane spray seems to be preferable because of its ability to penetrate tissue more deeply and thereby perpetuate dissociative stimuli and allow painless muscle movements.[4] This neurophysiological property of counterirritation acts to eliminate painful stimuli from trigger zones because of a massive afferent barrage sent from the area cooled. Since pain and temperature sensation travel by the same spinal pathways (the spinothalamic tract), it is theorized that response to pain impulses originating from the trigger zone is competitively inhibited, thereby interrupting the pain-spasm-pain cycle.

The technique calls for the patient to be placed in a comfortable position with the eyes and nose shielded. The vapocoolant is applied in a stream at a distance of about 45 cm (18 inches). The spray is applied with slow, sweeping movements from the trigger zone to the region of referred pain. During this time the patient is instructed to prepare for active stretching exercises. When the movements become painless, the spraying is stopped. The procedure may be repeated with careful observation to avoid skin frosting. The use of vapocoolant spray is uncomplicated and offers good physiological and clinical responses.

Pharmacotherapy

There are many agents now available that are purported to be of assistance when treating myofascial syndromes. It is beyond the scope of this chapter to cover all these compounds. Because of its lack of extrapyramidal effects and its usefulness in the symptomatic relief of tension and anxiety, at this time diazepam (Valium) appears to be a most useful pharmacological agent. In addition, it is a useful adjunct for the relief of skeletal muscle spasm caused by reflex spasm to local pathological conditions (such as mechanical, infectious, nutritional, or psychogenic). This agent may best be used in therapeutic dosages during the patient's most stressful periods. It has been our experience that the use of chemicals is indeed limited, with the exception of diazepam and therapeutic vitamin and mineral supplementation.

Biofeedback

A relatively new and apparently useful modality in treating myofascial pain-dysfunction syndromes is biofeedback. This is a method whereby the patient may observe his or her physiological muscular responses on some form of visual or auditory display. Practitioners of this treatment form believe that the patients do not merely guess the level of their response to therapy but actually have correct information displayed for them.

The concept of muscle potential is explained to the patient as being the possible relationship between muscle tension and perceived pain. Electrodes are placed in the usual fashion in constantly duplicable positions on similar muscles with the use of a template. Next, a muscle potential is recorded on a digital millivoltmeter so that the patient can observe the actual amount of muscle tension at any given moment. Thus, as the patient tenses the muscle, he or she will observe a numerical increase on the millivoltmeter. While the patient is relaxing the muscles, the figure approaches zero. With an awareness of actual levels of muscle potential, the patient can ascertain what activities result in the lowering of muscle potential and can become fully aware of the muscle sensations associated with each level of tension.[6] The use of masticatory muscles,

muscles of facial expression, or torso muscles seems to provide effective relaxation training results.

Nutrition

If muscular tissue is to respond in a therapeutic fashion, proper nutrition is a most integral part in assisting this response. It has been said the muscle is an energy machine. When this machine is well oiled and bathed in the proper fuel, its strength, resiliency, and integrity (that is, functional adaptative capabilities) will be enhanced.

By using current concepts of muscular metabolism and cellular biology, a rational, scientifically based nutritional regimen for the treatment of the myofascial pain-dysfunction syndrome can and should be an instituted.

SUMMARY

A method for the diagnosis and treatment of muscle spasm has been described. *Recognition of trigger zones and pain referral patterns is essential for accurate diagnosis and therapy.* Attempts should be made to correlate clinical symptomatology with known physiological, biochemical, and molecular responses. Therapy is directed toward interrupting the pain-spasm-pain cycle and reestablishing normal muscle function.

The muscles of the body work as an intricately linked web. When a group of muscles as significant as the gnathostomatic group are kinesiologically disturbed, subsequent and often profound postural changes can occur. Observation of these changes and prompt multidisciplinary appraisal are recommended.

ACKNOWLEDGMENT

I would like to acknowledge Carol Satriani for her gift of enlightenment.

REFERENCES

1. Archer, W.H.: Oral surgery, ed. 4, Philadelphia, 1961, W.B. Saunders Co.
2. Bell, W.H., and Ware, W.H.: Management of temporomandibular joint pain dysfunction syndrome, Dent. Clin. North Am. **15**:487, 1971.
3. Bierman, W., and Licht, S.: Physical medicine in general practice, ed. 3, New York, 1951, Paul B. Hoeber.
4. Broken, N., and Bierman, W.: Temperature changes produced by spraying with ethyl chloride, Arch. Phys. Med. **36**:288, 1955.
5. Burket, L.W., et al.: Oral medicine: diagnosis and treatment, ed. 6, Philadelphia, 1971, J.B. Lippincott Co.
6. Guyton, A.C.: Textbook of medical physiology, ed. 4, Philadelphia, 1971, W.B. Saunders Co.
7. Kraus, H.: Principles and practice of therapeutic exercises, Springfield, Ill., 1950, Charles C Thomas, Publisher.
8. Kraus, H., Prudden, B., and Hirschhorn, K.: Role of inactivity in production of disease—hypokinetic disease, J. Am. Geriatr. Soc. **4**:463, 1956.
9. Laskin, D.M.: Etiology of pain-dysfunction syndrome, J. Am. Dent. Assoc. **79**:147, 1969.
10. Levine, M.: Psychotherapy in medical practice, New York, 1942, The Macmillan Co.
11. Lewis, T.: Blood vessels of the human skin and their responses, London, 1927, Shaw & Sons, Ltd.
12. Lupton, D.E.: A preliminary investigation of the personality of female temporomandibular joint dysfunction patients, Psychother. Psychosom. **14**:199, 1966.
13. Lupton, D.E.: Psychological aspects of TMJ dysfunction, J. Am. Dent. Assoc. **79**:131, 1969.
14. MacKenzie, W.C.: The action of muscles, London, 1918, H.K. Lewis & Co.
15. Morgan, D.H.: Dysfunction, pain, tinnitus, vertigo corrected by mandibular joint surgery, J. South. Calif. Dent. Assoc. **29**:505, 1971.
16. Physicians' desk reference, Oradell, N.J., 1977, Medical Economics Co.
17. Schwartz, L.: Ethyl chloride treatment of limited, painful mandible movement, J. Am. Dent. Assoc. **48**:497, 1954.
18. Schwartz, L.: Disorders of the temporomandibular joint, Philadelphia, 1966, W.B. Saunders Co.
19. Selye, H.: The physiology and pathology of exposure of stress, Montreal, Canada, 1950, Acta, Inc.
20. Travell, J.: Pain mechanisms in connective tissues. In Ragan, C., editor: Connective tissues: transactions of the second conference, New York, 1952, Josiah Macy, Jr., Foundation.
21. Travell, J.: Temporomandibular joint pain referred from the muscles of the head and neck, J. Prosthet. Dent. **10**:745, 1960.
22. Travell, J., and Rinzler, S.H.: The myofascial genesis of pain, Postgrad. Med. **11**:425, 1952.

17 Treatment of muscle spasm

YALE S. PALCHICK, D.D.S., F.A.G.D.

It is becoming more apparent that pain in the muscles of the head, neck, and shoulders comprises a large proportion of the complaints of pain and/or discomfort presented by patients to the practitioner. Many times examination of patients with these complaints reveals no organic disease of the teeth or gums, no disease of the circulatory system, and no disease of the peripheral or central nervous system. There may be no evidence of pathological conditions of the mandibular articulation. As a result, the symptoms exhibited by the patient often are classified as psychosomatic, and diseases of the skeletal muscles are not even considered as a potential source of pain, whereas the resultant muscle spasm may well be the primary source of pain.[6]

According to Bonica,[1] pain is the net effect of incredibly complex interactions of ascending and descending neural systems, biochemical, physiological, and psychological mechanisms, as well as neocortical processes that involve dynamic activities in most parts of the nervous system that occur simultaneously. By the time the pain is perceived, it has been submitted to the actions of many of these neural systems. Consequently it cannot be artificially dichotomized into sensory pain and pain associated with emotional components. Bonica states further, "There is a recent trend to believe that most, if not all, patients with persistent pain develop 'chronic pain behavior' exclusively as a result of environmental reinforcers. This does an injustice to patients with arthritis, cancer, chronic visceral disease, orofacial pain, causalgia, and a host of other chronic pain syndromes in which the persistent complaint of pain is not due to learning, but rather due to persistent dysfunction of the nociceptive system." Thus muscle spasms can be understood as an etiological entity and not purely a neurotic behavior pattern.

The treatment of muscle spasms, as any treatment, is dependent on the results obtained from the taking of both a medical history and an examination. The many inputs to muscle disease, among which are the teeth, the temporomandibular joint, and other associated oral structures as well as the patient's posture, occupation, and emotional responses, must be evaluated. A nutritional evaluation is also necessary for a complete diagnosis. Certain organic diseases and infections must be ruled out. Drug intake and other environmental factors must be weighed. Trauma to the head and neck must be evaluated as far back as the patient can remember. As stated by Travell,[9] "Effects of trauma can be cumulative."

Once the diagnosis has been determined, the outline of treatment is made, and with the help of the patient, treatment is set into motion. In considering the type of treatments it must be kept in mind that skeletal muscles may be in spasm because of stress disorders that may be either organic or environmental. Muscles are subject to noxious stimulation of various sorts—mechanical, emotional, infectious, metabolic, nutritional, or more likely a combination of several of these stresses—and react by shortening and developing spasms. Muscles in spasm exhibit an overactive stretch reflex or resistance to passive lengthening. When any part of a muscle is shortened beyond its physiological limit, the pain may be very intense. Usually pain associated with skeletal muscle spasm is referred and appears as a target area far from the source. Referred pain originates in a small zone of hypersensitivity, known as a trigger area (myglosen), which is located within a muscle or fascia.[5]

Trigger areas are caused by trauma or chronic stress that has resulted in a shortening of muscle fibers (ranging from a few to a great many), leading to limited motion and/or pain and discomfort. It is important to understand that shortening of muscles under stress is the result of homeostatic protection (splinting) against injury. This protective splinting tends to gain momentum so that increasing numbers of related muscle groups develop spasms and facilitate the pathway of the spasm-pain-spasm cycle. Inhibition of normal fight or flight responses mandated by our civilization results in residual muscle tension. This muscle tension is frequently localized as trigger areas.

The referred pain pattern in one person is the same as in another. The trigger area and the target area of pain can follow the same pattern, whether the noxious stimulus is applied directly to the muscle or whether it reaches the muscle indirectly from the viscera or brain via the central nervous system.[9]

Painful spasms and the results of these spasms usually outlast the precipitating event. Selye states, "Injury initiates the deteriorative biochemical cycle." The passage of time in itself does not bring about recovery.

A clear understanding of these basic principles is needed both to facilitate treatment and so as not to end treatment too soon. The practitioner must be sure that the signs, of which the patient is not aware but which can be elicited by the examining practitioner, as well as the symptoms presented by the patient are eliminated. Should the signs go unattended for a long period, the tissue may degenerate, and motion may be limited. Thickening of the skin (fibrositis) may become a problem, and thus the prognosis would be poor. If the practitioner were to depend on clinical symptoms alone, the treatment would be aborted. As a consequence, the pain would return and the treatment deemed ineffective and discontinued.

The accompanying questionnaire has been developed based partially on the preceding philosophy.

HISTORY AND EXAMINATION FORMS

This section discusses the medical history and examination forms and demonstrates how the forms are used in the first step of planning treatment.

Sir William Osler pointed out that the patient will give many leads toward diagnosis. Careful analysis of the conditions and symptoms noted on the medical history and examination forms will eliminate those which should be treated by another medical entity.

In addition to recognizing the symptoms that the patient presents, the practitioner must also be aware of signs. Long before clinical discomfort of pain is in evidence, the signs will reveal existing problems and will enable the practitioner to predict future symptoms that the patient may present. The dental practitioner should be very careful to distinguish signs of discomfort or pain that are not within the realm of dental practice. There are many organic causes, in addition to the environmental stresses, that lead to pains around the head and neck that do lie within the confines of the dental practitioner's treatment.

Care should be taken that any signs or symptoms which exhibit causes and/or mechanisms that are beyond the understanding or evaluative capacities of the examining practitioner do not lead to conclusions that symptoms are of a psychological rather than an organic etiology. It is very important that prejudgment is not made about the patient, even on a limited basis. Each patient is complex, and each comes to the examining room as a composite of the influences and traumas experienced. Elfenbaum stated that, "The patient with a disease also is at dis-ease."

As mentioned previously, the history and examination forms are used to start the outline of treatment. Many of the questions asked are self-explanatory; however, some of these questions are discussed here in terms of their relative significance in making the diagnosis and/or determining the prognosis.

Business information

The first part of the history consists of questions relating to information needed for office records. Obtaining the social security number, the name of the patient's insurance company, and the type of insurance, as well as information regarding financial accountability, will save much in the way of time and energy when it comes to filling out insurance forms, billing, etc.

The practitioner may find that the name of the spouse or parent, business address, and business and residence telephone numbers are a convenience should it be necessary to reschedule an appointment or discuss the patient's progress with a family member during working hours.

A complete list of the patient's physicians and dentists is convenient for extending professional courtesy to one's colleagues in keeping their records current.

The marital status, number of children, and occupation of the patient are invaluable in giving insight to the patient's responsibilities and in determining work habits that may lead to stress and influence pain around the head and neck.

Patient history

The history is best taken by the practitioner. It is especially important for the practitioner to gain total insight to the patient's problems. Sometimes the most significant insight is gained from a casual remark made by the patient during an examination and/or history taking which may or may not be considered important if the history is taken by someone other than the practitioner. It is of particular assistance to tape-record the taking of the history. A recording will permit the practitioner to review the comments made by the patient, which otherwise would be difficult to notate in the rapid-fire discussion by many patients of their problems. Of course, the patient's permission should be received to tape-record the history, and the patient should be further advised that the information is being recorded to aid in the consolidation of information and in the accumulation of data in a more thorough manner so that the patient's needs may be more thoroughly met and as a possible aid to other patients who may have the same problems.

As the history of the patient is taken, it is best for the practitioner to sit facing the patient, on an eye-to-eye level. In many cases the hand-to-arm position (the hand of the practitioner on the arm of the patient) increases the patient's confidence in the practitioner and elicits more patient response. If at all possible, with the permission of the patient, the spouse, a very close friend if the patient is unmarried, or a parent if the patient is a minor should be asked to be present. This provides a rapport between the patient and the advisor or consultant, since the patient now has someone who has been exposed to the problems from which the patient suffers. The advisor or consultant in turn becomes more deeply aware of the many small things that lead to the discomfort of the patient.

It should be noted that the accompanying questionnaire is designed to gain information about the patient's true condition by asking questions that examine the same aspect of the condition in several different ways and at different places within the questionnaire. The comments made here regarding the patient's responses are organized according to topic and include the pertinent questions at the various points in the questionnaire (identified by the corresponding letter and number).

It is difficult to ascertain and understand the amount of pain suffered by any patient and its effects on that patient. By asking the patient to describe the reason for the visit, the practitioner takes the first step in gaining insight to the patient and the patient's problems and in determining whether the patient would benefit from treatment.

Asking the patient for a personal opinion regarding reaction to stress (L37) is another aspect of understanding the patient and projecting the prognosis. Furthermore, should the patient be accepted for treatment, the answer to this question may assist the therapist or practitioner in detecting stressful conditions while the patient is undergoing treatment. The cause and effects of the stress can then be explored to a greater degree to avoid overlooking other causes.

Should the patient affirm that pain increases when opening the mouth (J11, 12), the dental practitioner can be assured that the muscles of the head and neck which are contributing to the discomfort of the patient are within the parameters of dental practice. However, should the patient indicate difficulty in swallowing (J11, 12, L17, 18), the practitioner should be aware that the patient may be exhibiting symptoms of anxiety, (after other functional and organic problems are eliminated by referral to a physician and/or by palpating the anterior neck muscles), and this may be a consideration in whether the patient would profit from treatment. Another indication of anxiety is a positive response to the question pertaining to difficulty in breathing (L13). Follow-up questions include a comparison to tight bands around the chest or difficulty in taking a full breath. Negative responses would rule out the anxious patient and/or respiratory or organic complications.

Some degree of self-preservation is involved in being selective and in accepting only those patients who will best benefit from the investment of time and energy by the practitioner and therapist. Carefully eliminating those patients whose conditions indicate that they are not within the realm of the dental practitioner is vital.

A very straightforward question such as, "With a bad headache, do you do your dishes before going to bed?" (L32) can help establish a true pain picture. If the pain is of great intensity around the head or neck, a patient normally would leave everything in the way of household chores and would attempt to treat or escape the pain. Should the patient state that all duties are finished before retiring, the practitioner can surmise that the pain may not be as intense as described, that the patient may be a victim of a compulsive neurosis, or even more simply that the patient feels that the alternative of leaving the duties undone would create more tension.

The answers to more specific questions, such as "Do you have frequent headaches?" (B), assist in giving the proper weight to the response. Determining the frequency, duration, and area of the head involved provides information that is used in evaluating the vascular components involved and the degree to which these components lie within the jurisdiction of the dental practitioner.

The rule of thumb in determining whether a patient suffers from a vascular headache is to ask whether the patient feels better being up or lying down (L33). If a vascular headache or migraine component is indicated, a determination must be made as to whether it is caused by vasoconstriction or vasodilatation. The patient would be better referred to a physician for an evaluation of the cause of the pain.

Certain vascular components that come into play in the early morning hours prompt inclusion of questions regarding the time of day, night, morning, or afternoon (J6, L31) when the pain is most severe. Another reason for including these questions is to assess cause and effect. For instance, should the patient sleep with covers over the head (L25), this may indicate insufficient oxygen intake, which may be a primary reason for pain on awakening. If this question were omitted, the practitioner might be left with an entirely false impression regarding the cause of pain.

Frequent nausea or vomiting (L26) in the nonpregnant patient also would indicate that a vascular component or other organic cause is present in addition to, or in conjunction with, muscular discomfort.

Selye stated that "Injury initiates a cycle of pain-spasm-pain." The precipitating event, however, may be long forgotten by the patient; therefore answers to the question regarding blows to the head (C) are significant in determining the trauma experienced by the patient in the past that may be a contributing factor to the discomfort in the present. Later in the history form the question of trauma is addressed in another manner by asking about patient involvement in accidents (L2, 3). This is just another way of exploring the multiple factors that affect the muscles around the head and neck, which actually may have begun many years previously and may have caused muscle splinting, limited motion, and pain. The length of time involved between onset and treatment may give the practitioner some idea of the length of treatment that will be necessary to alleviate the symptoms.

Investigating other trauma or contributing factors is handled by a request for the listing of all doctors, medicines and hospital stays (F, G, H, L38-40) with which the patient was involved for the last 3 years. Additional follow-up questions at this point can expand the history prior to the 3-year span. In this way the practitioner can begin to understand how long the patient has suffered and how much the patient has accomplished in the way of treatment. This information is valuable in making a diagnosis and in determining the type of treatment to be prescribed, as well as determining the type of consultants to be contacted. Patient records can be requested and evaluated.

A patient who has suffered from a kidney or bladder infection or who has been subjected to a catheterization (L27) may exhibit problems in the head or neck as a result of a rise in blood pressure caused by the presence of bacteria. This patient should be referred to a urologist.

The difference between isometric contraction where the muscle contracts with no movement (clenching) and isotonic contraction where the muscle contracts with movement (grinding) is the reason for including questions regarding clenching and grinding the teeth (K1-3). It is frequently overlooked that the clenching patient generates more problems than the grinding patient, since more than 5 to 7 seconds of isometric contraction will result in the physiological responses of trauma to the muscle fibers and all the consequences that follow.

Isometric contraction and referred pain patterns to the head, neck, and dentition caused by sleep patterns (L16) are investigated by determining if the patient maintains pressure on the side of the head and neck for extended periods. Jackson[4] maintains that the cervical spine is not supported in any position during sleep without a supplemental device. Therefore normal sleep positions, in and of themselves, are stressful, and the use of a Cervi-Pillow may be considered for the patient.

Other postural problems might be engendered by occupational positions or telephone habits (L14, 15). Isometric contractions that lead to patient discomfort may be the result of occupational and/or recreational tasks. For instance, if the patient must maintain a constant position, uses a clutch to shift, sits in bucket seats, or carries a comb or a wallet in a hip pocket while driving (L23), these could be factors contributing to problems with the neck and head.

Some of the long nerve fibers that give rise to leg cramps (L11) may be affected by body positon and/or the nutritional state of the patient. Therefore a nutritional evaluation is indicated.[2] Limb length disparity (L24), common in at least 77% of the total population, also may result in cramping and/or tenderness in the shorter limb. Limb length disparity and/or muscle imbalance (with negative neurological findings) may be the cause for bumping into walls or into a door jamb when passing through an exit (L30).

Personal habits such as smoking (L21) and excessive coffee intake (L22) may contribute to vascular problems and hypoglycemia. If the heavy coffee drinker were to eliminate the intake of coffee, vasodilation usually would occur, removing the vasoconstricting influence of caffeine with its subsequent discomfort and pain as a result of this added vascular component.

Even a small, although distasteful, habit such as picking the nose (L29) can have major consequences. There are certain trigger areas in the turbinates of the nose that refer pain back into the antrum, which could be mistaken as pain from the masseter muscle rather than referred pain.[9] This referred pain also could arise from a sinus condition.

Referred pain also can be confusing and difficult to diagnose in the case of tearing or dry eyes (K6). Provided that the patient history or consultation with an ophthalmologist, has ruled out any pathological conditions as the cause for these symptoms, the practitioner may consider the autonomic concomitant in the referred pain patterns from the sternocleidomastoid muscle as the cause of these symptoms.[9]

Another autonomic concomitant of the trigger area of the sternocleidomastoid muscle is an injected eye where the bleeding appears only in the temporal canthus of the eye and on the same side as the sternoclei-

HISTORY FORM

Date ______________ Social security no. ______________

Name ______________ Marital status ______________

Address ______________ Telephone ______________
Street City State Zip code

Occupation ______________ Date of birth ______________

Spouse's name and address ______________

Parent's name and address ______________

Business address ______________ Telephone ______________

Spouse's business ______________ Telephone ______________

Are you covered by major medical insurance? ______ Name of company ______________

Person responsible for account ______________

Your physician ______________ Telephone ______________

Address ______________

Your dentist ______________ Telephone ______________

Address ______________

Referred by ______________

Reason for this visit ______________

Answer every question, please

Please answer as many questions as possible with *yes* or *no;* for more detailed answers to any questions, use the accompanying blank sheet of paper.

A. Have you had Arthritis ______ Sinus infection ______ Ear infection ______ Blood vessel disease ______

Hepatitis ______ Other ______________

B. Do you have frequent headaches? ______ Area of head ______________

Duration ______________

C. Have you ever had a severe blow to the head? ______ What part? ______ When? ______

D. Are you allergic to any medication(s)? ______ Which? ______________

E. Are you now taking any medication(s)? ______ Which? ______________

F. Have you consulted a neurologist? ______ Who? ______________

G. Have you consulted a psychiatrist? ______ Who? ______________

H. Have you ever had temporomandibular joint treatment? ______ Give details and results ______________

I. Is there any family history of similar conditions? ______________

J. *Pain symptoms*

1. Where does the pain start? ______________
2. Is there pain in the joint in front of right ear? ______________ Left ear? ______________

3. Describe pain: Sharp ______ Dull ______ Aching ______ Deep ______ Superficial ______
   Other ______
4. How often do you have pain? ______
5. Is pain constant? ______ Intermittent? ______
6. What time of day or night is pain most severe? ______
7. Is pain unchanged? ______ Increased? ______ Decreased? ______
8. Does pain start abruptly? ______ Gradually? ______
9. Does pain disappear abruptly? ______ Gradually? ______
10. What relieves the pain? ______
11. What increases pain? Yawning ______ Eating ______ Speaking ______ Shouting ______
    Singing ______ Other ______
12. Does opening of mouth cause pain? ______ Does swallowing? ______
13. Do your teeth hurt? Upper teeth ______ Lower teeth ______
14. Have you ever had a feeling of pressure or tenderness about the right eye? ______ Left eye? ______

K. *Other symptoms*

1. Are your jaws clenched on awakening? ______
2. Clenching or grinding teeth during sleep? ______ During waking hours? ______
3. Any feeling of tiredness in jaw muscles? ______
4. Have you noticed any change in saliva? None ______ Increased ______ Decreased ______
5. Salty taste in mouth? ______ Coppery taste? ______
6. Any excessive tearing from eyes? ______ Dry eyes? ______ Which? ______
7. Do you ever get dizzy? ______ How often? ______ Does the room move, or do you? ______
8. Ringing noises in right ear? ______ Left ear? ______
9. On opening or closing of your mouth, popping or whooshing noises in the right ear? ______ Left ear? ______
10. Stuffiness in right ear? ______ Left ear? ______
11. Changes in hearing in right ear? ______ Left ear? ______

L. *General*

1. Do you see spots in front of your eyes? ______
2. Have you ever had an accident? ______
3. Have you ever been hit in the face? ______ When? ______
4. Does your scalp itch? ______
5. Do you have trouble combing your hair? ______
6. Do you get bloodshot eyes? ______

Continued.

7. Do you get a stiff neck? ______ Which side? ______

8. Do you get blurred vision? ______ Tunnel vision? ______

9. Do your jaws feel rusty in the morning? ______ Evening? ______

10. Do you get earaches? ______ Which side? ______

11. Do you get leg cramps? ______ How often? ______

12. Are your teeth sensitive to cold? ______ Hot? ______ Sweets? ______

13. Do you have trouble breathing? ______

14. Do you work in the same position for long periods of time? ______

15. Do you talk on the telephone for long periods of time? ______

16. Do you sleep on your side? ______ Right? ______ Left? ______ Position of knees ______
    Position of hands ______

17. Does food or water stick in your throat? ______

18. Do you have trouble swallowing? ______ What? ______

19. Have you ever had a feeling of numbness in your fingers? ______

20. Do you have backaches? ______ Where? ______ How often? ______

21. Do you smoke? ______ How many cigarettes a day? ______

22. Do you drink coffee? ______ How many cups a day? ______

23. Do you do a lot of driving? ______

24. Do you know if one leg is shorter than the other? ______

25. Do you sleep with covers over your head at night? ______

26. Do you get nauseated or vomit? ______ How often? ______

27. Have you ever had a kidney or bladder infection? ______ When? ______
    Were you catheterized? ______

28. What was done? ______

29. Do you pick your nose? ______

30. Do you often bump into walls or doors? ______ Which side most frequently? ______

31. Is your pain worse in the morning or afternoon? ______

32. With a bad headache, do you do your dishes before going to bed? ______

33. Do you feel better being up or lying down? ______

34. Do you often burp? ______ Get flatulent? ______

35. Do your eyes get tired? ______

36. Do you use eye drops for any conditions regularly? ______ Occasionally? ______

37. How do you react to stress? ______

38. List all doctors seen in the last 3 years and their findings on accompanying sheet.

39. List all medicines taken in the last 3 years on accompanying sheet.

40. List the time spent in the hospital in the last 3 years.

41. Is there anything that I have not asked that I should know? Explain ______

domastoid muscle spasm. Other reasons for bloodshot eyes (L6) must be carefully eliminated.

If the patient sees spots in front of the eyes (L1), determining the type of spots is important. Black floaters are quite normal and are part of the aging process. However, colored flashes of bright orange or red and movement of zigzag lines indicate that a referral to an ophthalmologist is in order to rule out any other pathosis before treatment is undertaken. Blurred or tunnel vision (L8) indicates a vascular component and needs attention from a consulting physician.

Dizziness (K7), especially if the sensation is described as that of the patient moving as opposed to the room moving, is another example of a symptom that needs a thorough examination by an outside consultant, in this case a neurologist.

Should the patient indicate numbness in the fingers (L19), the practitioner must again consider the neurological aspects, since the patient may have a problem in the brachial plexus or a space lesion that should be investigated, preferably by a neurologist. With a negative neurological report, investigate the impact of sleep or work patterns.

Questions regarding hair care, including shampooing, drying, and back-combing, are used in the patient/practitioner discussion to augment the question about combing the hair (L5) to detect if there have been long-term contractions of the temporal or trapezius muscle, since this condition frequently manifests itself as sensitivity to the movement of the superficial layer of the scalp.

Stiff necks (L7) or torticollis shed light on possible reasons for limited motion and discomfort. The posterolateral neck and the sternocleidomastoid muscles should be given attention.

Teeth that are sensitive to cold (L12) are the indirect result of a passive hyperemia caused by trauma to the dentition over some time. Once the trauma is relieved, the sensitivity dissipates.

The answers to the question about anything else that could be important (L41) may have both medical and legal implications. First, it is important that the patient be aware of a shared responsibility in regard to treatment. Second, the question gives carte blanche for patient input and may be the place where a bit of vital information is imparted that the other questions, for one reason or another, did not cover. Third, this question is included as a preventive measure against legal repercussions should the patient become disillusioned with the treatment or results and attempt to assign blame by claiming that some symptoms were overlooked. Should the patient not care to share such information, the practitioner usually cannot be held legally responsible.

EXAMINATION

After the medical history has been taken, pertinent information gleaned from the history (such as the point of origin of the pain, time of pain onset, and duration and progression of pain) is transferred to the examination form using the diagrams for reference points (Fig. 17-1). Explore with the patient items of merit that arose during the history taking and note them on side one of the form.

The examination actually begins by observing the patient as he or she walks into the office, noting the gait, balance, position of head and neck, and size of facial and neck muscles. The features will also reveal the state of "dis-ease."

The patient then is asked to perform several tasks. With shoes and coat removed, standing with feet and toes together, the patient is observed by the practitioner from a distance of 4 or 5 feet to determine if either shoulder is higher than the other (Fig. 17-2). After noting this, the practitioner then locates both the right and left iliac crests with an index finger while the therapist or assistant observes, again at a distance of 4 or 5 feet, to determine if there appears to be any variance in height (Fig. 17-3). Occasionally anteroposterior x-ray views of the pelvic girdle may be required to determine the relative height of the iliac crests. If so, the technician should be instructed to take the x-ray views with the patient standing with feet together. Even the looser structures can directly affect craniomandibular problems; 77% of the population of the United States have lower limb disparity, with resultant abnormal head and neck positions and peripheral entrapment neuropathy (soft tissue entrapment of nerves between muscles). If a shoe lift is indicated, it should be made of hard leather and should not exceed 6.3 mm (1/4 inch) in thickness. The shoe lift normally is prescribed for the heel; however, on occasion it is necessary to prescribe a lift for the whole foot.

Still standing with feet together, facing the practitioner, with hands on either side, the patient is simply asked to close the eyes. By standing directly in front of the patient, the practitioner can determine if there is any imbalance on either side or front to back (Fig. 17-4). It is important that absolute silence be maintained to negate the use of any sound reference points to maintain balance. As an additional check for imbalance, the patient is then asked to take three steps forward and three steps backward with the eyes still closed. Should there appear to be some imbalance, a mouth prop is inserted to open the patient's mouth between 6 and 20 mm if possible, and the patient is asked to repeat the tasks just mentioned, with the practitioner noting if the postural imbalance is corrected by changing the proprioceptive afferent messages. This test

Yale S. Palchick, D.D.S.
3455 Granger Road
Akron, Ohio 44313
(216) 666-0035

EXAMINATION SUMMARY AND
DISTRIBUTION OF PAIN AREAS

Name______________________________

Date_______________________________

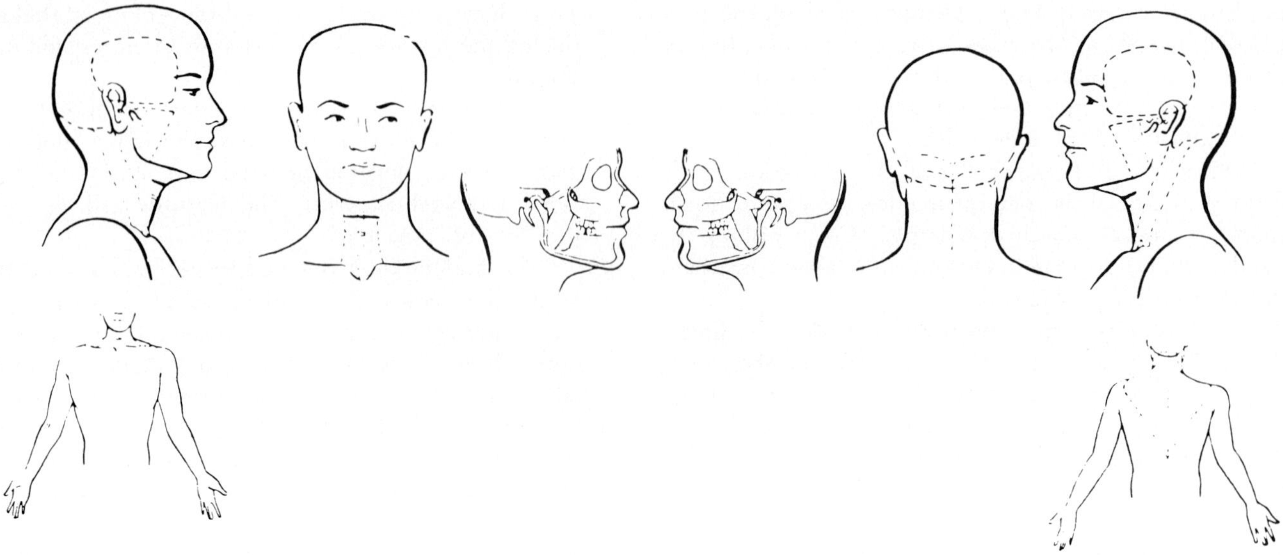

Should you desire a free copy of the forms we use, send your request with a self addressed, stamped 9 x 12" envelope to Dr. Yale S. Palchick at the address above.

A

Fig. 17-1. Examination form. **A,** Side one.

Yale S. Pulchick, D.D.S.
3455 Granger Road
Akron, Ohio 44313
(216) 666-0035

Date ____________

Name ____ Phone ______________

Referred by ___________________________________ Phone ______________

SEE PATIENT HISTORY

SHOULDER R L
ILIAC CREST R L
POSTURAL IMBALANCE F B R L
FINGER-NOSE TEST R L NORMAL

MUSCLE AND AREA EXAMINATION –
TENDERNESS AND PAIN ON PALPATION

GASTROCNEMIUS R L SUPRA SCAPULAR R L
SUPRA SPINATUS R L TRAPEZIUS R L
CERVICAL TRAPEZIUS R L
ANTERIOR BORDER TRAPEZIUS R L
LEVATOR SCAPULA
NUCHAL LINE R L
PARIETAL R L
OCCIPITAL R L
VERTEX R L
TEMPORALIS R L
TEMPORAL FOSSA R L
ZYGOMA R L
ANTERIOR TO TRAGUS R L (PREAURICULAR)
ANTERIOR WALL OF AUDITORY MEATUS R L
FRONTAL R L
SUPRA ORBITAL R L
INFRA ORBITAL R L
GLABELLA
LEVATOR LABII R L
ANGLE OF MANDIBLE R L
MENTAL R L
MENTALIS R L
LATERAL BORDER TRAPEZIUS R L
POSTERIOR TRIANGLE R L
STERNO CLEIDOMASTOID R L
SUPRA CLAVICULAR R L
INFRA CLAVICULAR R L
TRIANGLE OF BURNS SPLENUS CAPITUS R L
INTER COSTALS R L
PECTORALIS R L
INFERIOR MAXILLARY NODES L R
SUBMANDIBULAR NODES L R
DEEP CERVICAL NODES L R
ARM R L
FINGERS R L
OTHER
PLAN OF TREATMENT (Rx):
.... TMJ XRAYS
.... FULL SERIES
.... MUSCLE TREATMENTS
.... MUSCLE EXERCISES
.... NEUROMUSCULAR RE-EDUC.
.... MEDICATIONS
.... DIET LIST
.... CERV. PILLOW
.... L R S.L.
.... A.D.L.
.... AUTO RELAX.
.... E.G.S. .... MUSCLE INJ.
.... V.C.S. .... EQUIL.
.... ORTHOTIC .... HOT PACKS

TMJ SYMPTOMS OTHER THAN PAIN

NOISES (stethoscopic)
a. CREPITATION R L
b. RUBBING R L
c. SAGITTAL OPENING CLICK:
IMMEDIATE R L
INTERMEDIATE R L
FULL OPENING R L
d. SAGITTAL CLOSING CLICK.
IMMEDIATE R L
INTERMEDIATE R L
TERMINAL CLOSURE R L
e. CLICKING IN EXCENTRIC RANGES LATERAL R L TMJ R L
AUDIBLE CLICK R L
ABNORMAL MOVEMENT OF CONDYLE ON PALPATION R L
SUBLUXATION R L
TMJ SWELLING R L

SAGITTAL PATTERN OF MANDIBULAR MOVEMENT

DEVIATION FROM STRAIGHT–VERTICAL–OPENING–AND–CLOSING MOVEMENTS

WIDEST INTERINCISAL OPENING ________ mm.

WIDEST INTERINCISAL OPENING ________ mm. AFTER VAPOCOOLANT SPRAY

INTERFERING OCCLUSAL CONTACTS

CENTRIC RELATION ....
RIGHT FUNTIONING RANGE.................................
LEFT NONFUNCTIONING RANGE..........................
LEFT FUNCTIONING RANGE................................
RIGHT NONFUNCTIONING RANGE.................
PROTRUSIVE RANGE..

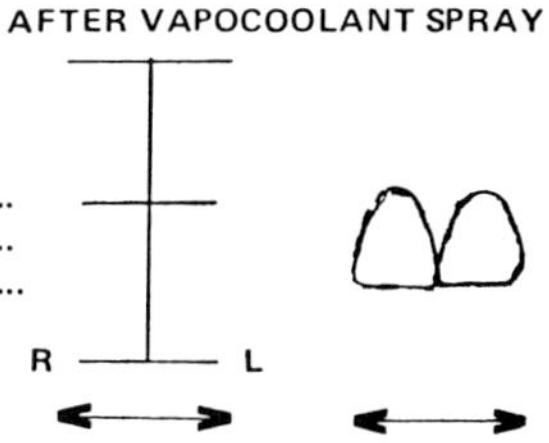

TISSUE CHANGES
CHEEK R L
LIPS R L
CORNER OF MOUTH R L
PALATE – HARD
SOFT
TONGUE– SCALLOPED
TONGUE– GEOGRAPHIC
PERIODONTAL

MASSETER R L
INTERNAL PTERYGOID R L
EXTERNAL PTERYGOID R L
LEVATOR PALATINI R L
CORONOID PROCESS R L
OUTSIDE ANGLE R L
INSIDE ANGLE R L
ANTERIORS WORN & CRAZED ....

TEETH MISSING

1 2 3 4 5 6 7 8 9 10 11 12 13 14 15 16
32 31 30 29 28 27 26 25 24 23 22 21 20 19 18 17

TEETH TENDER TO PERCUSSION

1 2 3 4 5 6 7 8 9 10 11 12 13 14 15 16
32 31 30 29 28 27 26 25 24 23 22 21 20 19 18 17

side 2

YSP 25 ● 1977

B

Fig. 17-1, cont'd. B, Side two.

helps in planning the treatment approach and evaluating the prognosis.

Simple neurological problems may be ruled out by asking the patient to extend the arms alternately to the side and then bring the index finger to the nose, again while standing with feet and toes together, eyes closed.

Each muscle or area listed on the examination sheet is subjected to digital pressure to determine if tenderness exists (Figs. 17-5 to 17-8). Signs and/or symptoms of the TMJ problem are noted, as outlined on the examination sheet. Excessively large masseters, for example, may be a clue to how long the patient has been clenching and to whether there is TMJ displacement. The sagittal pattern of mandibular movement is measured in deviation from both the vertical opening and closing movements. The maximum interincisal opening is noted and sketched on the examination sheet (Fig.

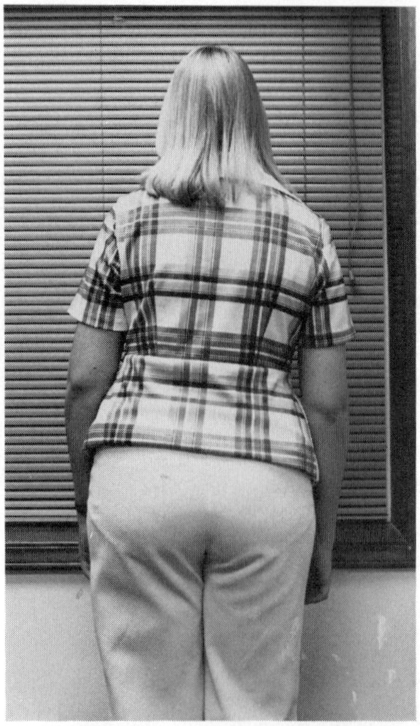

Fig. 17-2. Stance observation.

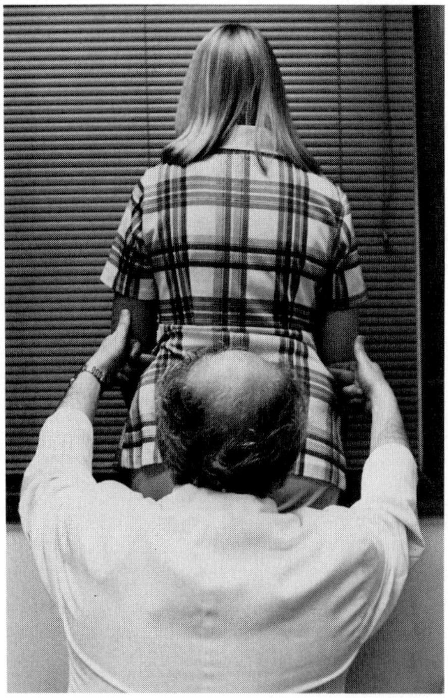

Fig. 17-3. Iliac crest observation.

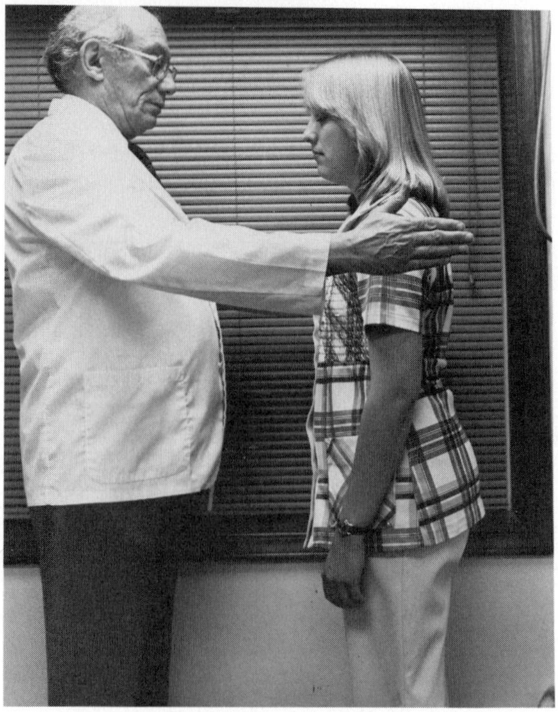

Fig. 17-4. Imbalance observation.

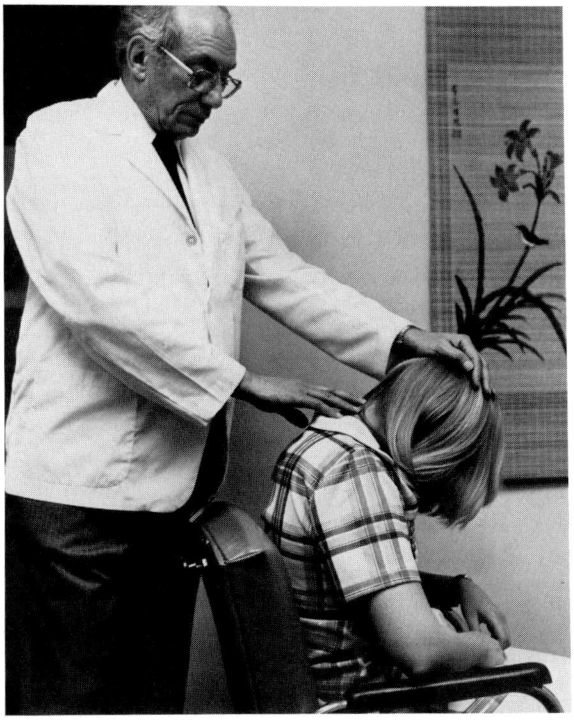

Fig. 17-5. Cervical trapezius observation.

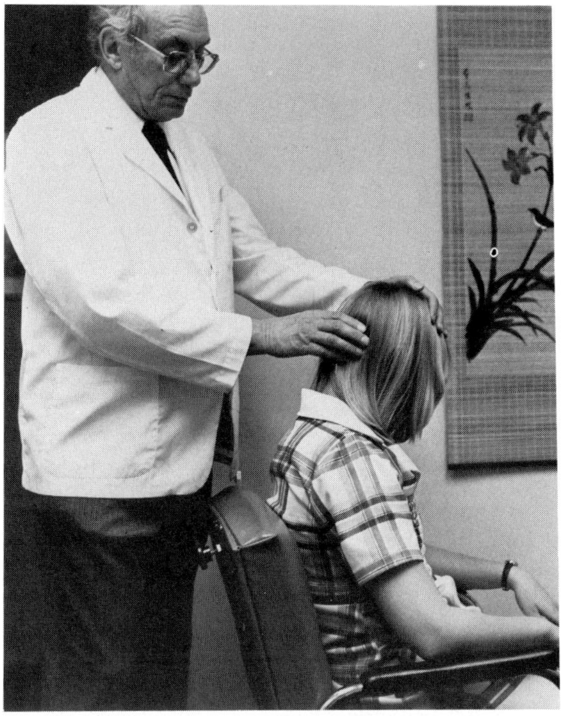

Fig. 17-6. Occipital area examination.

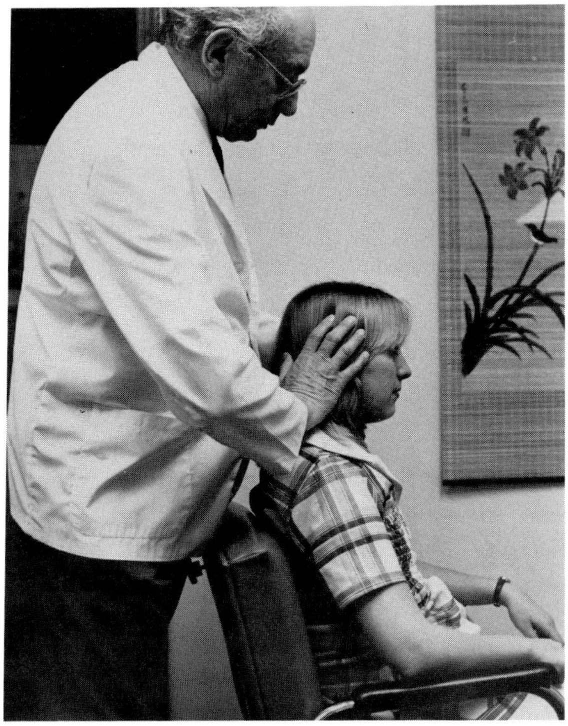

Fig. 17-7. Temporal muscle examination.

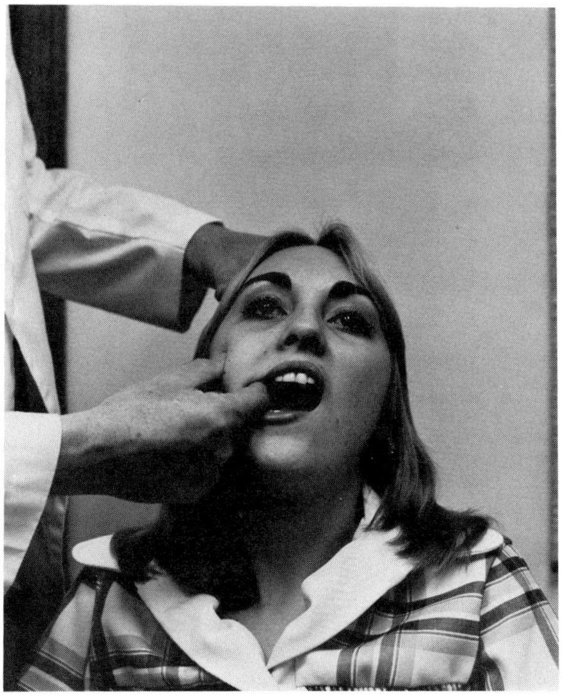

Fig. 17-8. Masseter muscle examination.

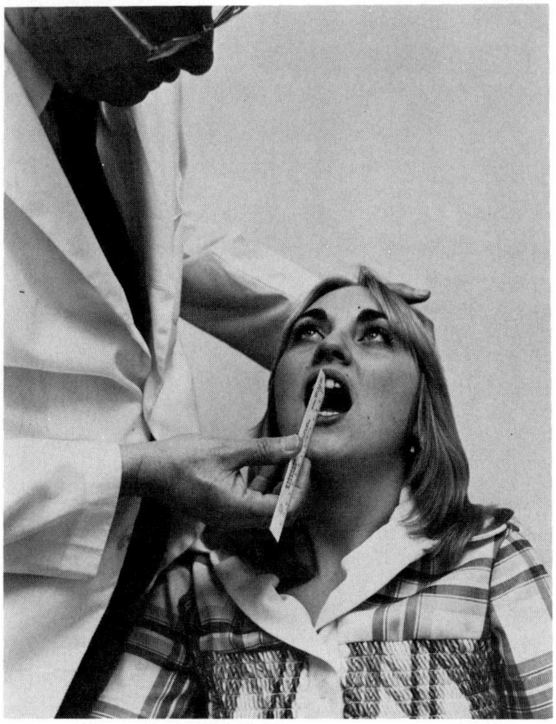

Fig. 17-9. Interincisal opening.

17-9). The mandibular anterior teeth in relation to the maxillary central teeth are sketched (Fig. 17-10). The deviation is marked between the arrows for both the sagittal opening path and the centric-relation position. With the aid of a stethoscope, noises of occlusal discrepancies are noted (Fig. 17-11).

Our style of living and learning often adversely affects our body position so as to enhance head and neck pain. A large proportion of the population holds the head forward with the cervical spine flexed. To maintain the face in a vertical plane, the head is held in extension. This sequela of head and neck position results in acute and chronic disorders of the craniomandibular apparatus because of the narrowing or closing of the space between occiput and atlas and a consequent entrapment of nerves and blood vessels in that area. The anterior neck muscles also are affected by this anatomical malposition. With the head in extension, swallowing difficulties can be encountered, which provides a physiological explanation for some of those unfortunate patients formerly considered merely neurotic when complaining of chronic sore throat and difficult swallowing without observable organic disease.

To rule out spasms of trigger areas in this vicinity, press the cricoid cartilage laterally with the first two fingers extended and locked. Push the soft tissue back against the spine in the space created by this lateral

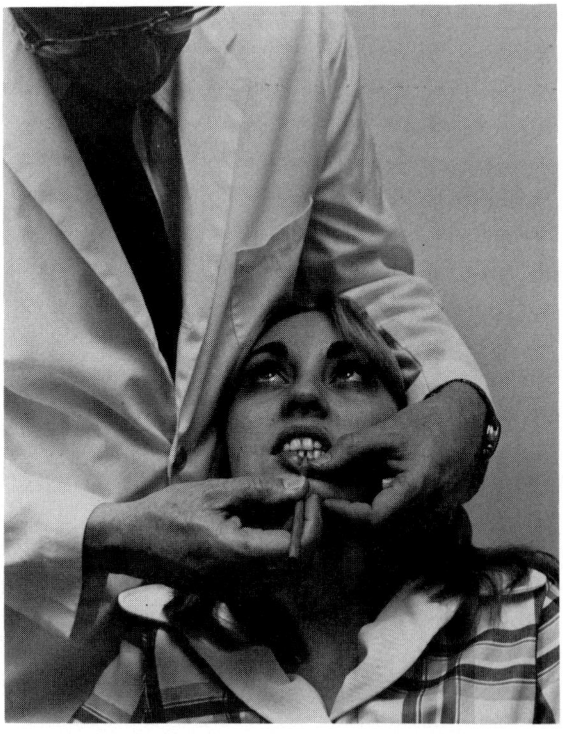

Fig. 17-10. Relationship of anterior teeth.

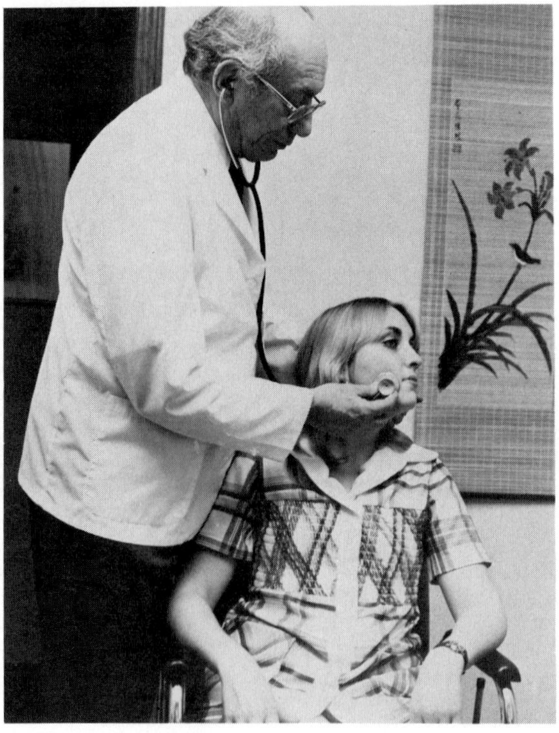

Fig. 17-11. Occlusal sounds.

displacement. With this approach one can palpate the longissimus cervicis and the longus colli muscles. If the muscles are tender on palpation and recreate the clinical symptoms as related by the patient, it can be assumed that treatment will reduce or eliminate these symptoms for a long period. The clinical use of ultrasound (of 1 W or less) moving along the direction of the fibers for several minutes in a number of different appointments is often beneficial.

The transverse processes of the atlas also should be palpated below the mastoid process and next to the ramus of the mandible to detect pain. There are 13 muscle attachments in this area, and more than half of all the rotation of the head is between the axis and atlas. The clinician should become familiar with the muscles of the head and of the anterior and posterior cervical spine and knowledgeable about what radiographs can contribute to a diagnosis of head and neck pain. For example, the patient may have a pain in the mandible and the neck that is caused by a bilateral compression of the paravertebral muscles. Another example of mandibular pain is that which arises from an abnormality between the facets of the C2 and C1 vertebrae.

Peripheral entrapment neuropathy as a result of muscular involvement is quite common and should be explored. Abnormal stresses that affect body position more often than not will be referred to the mandible. As early as biblical times, references to the jaw in relation to stress were made; and as recently as the development of oral contraceptives, connections were being discovered between endocrine changes (in the chemistry of the woman who is either taking birth control pills or is pregnant) and effects on the TMJ capsular fibers, which can result in hypomobile joints. The work of Rocabado,[7] which relates the position of the fibers to the condyle and the TMJ, is excellent.

In addition to these observations, other items such as missing teeth, teeth that are sensitive to percussion, tissue abnormalities, and swelling are noted (Figs. 17-12 and 17-13). Even mouth breathing should be noted to see if it might be a reaction to an orthopedic problem. The orthopedist should also note if any treatment appliances make the patient's tongue drop enough so that he or she is forced to bring the head forward and slightly up to get a better airway. If nasal breathing can be accomplished, it will reduce the strain on the anterior neck muscles.

After the examination the lateral neck and head muscles are sprayed with Fluori-Methane, a vapocoolant, and the interincisal opening is remeasured and noted (Fig. 17-14). The plan of treatment is indicated, and other needed items not printed are listed to the right on the form. (See Fig. 17-1, *B*.) Space does not permit discussion of treatment of the individual muscles

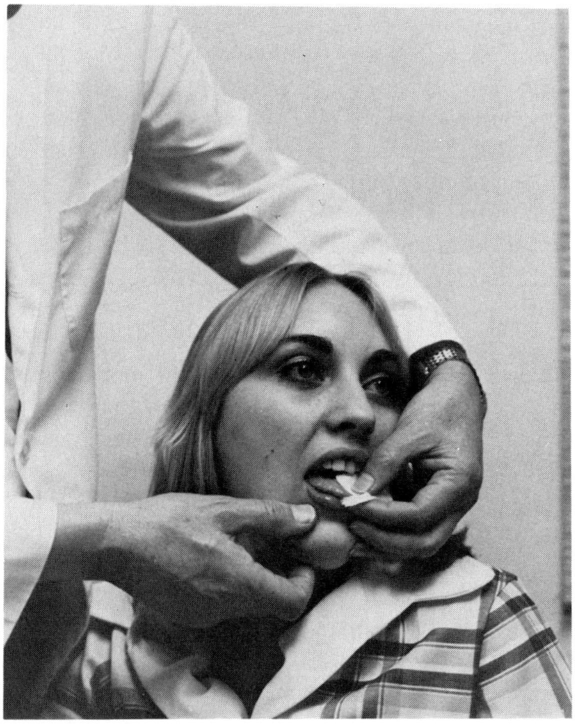

Fig. 17-12. Examination of tongue (scalloped edge).

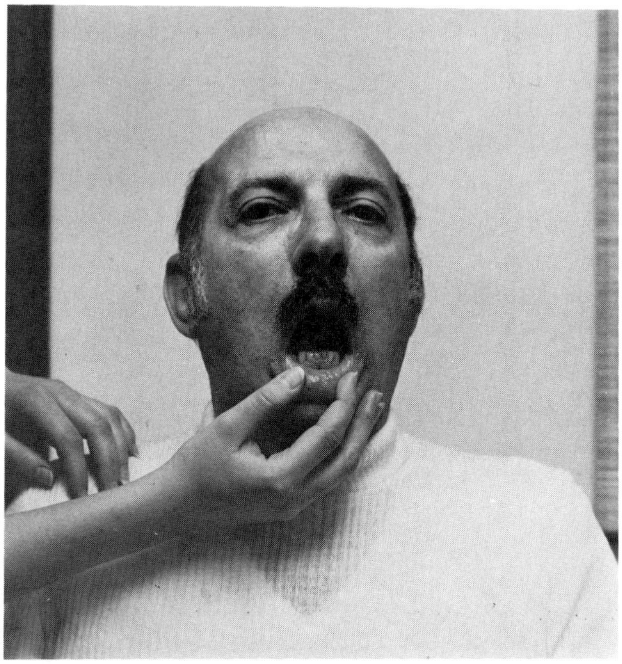

Fig. 17-13. Anterior teeth worn and crazed.

involved in the craniomandibular apparatus, but it must be kept in mind that the major goal is to teach the patient a normal basis for head and neck positions and muscle tonus. The restoration of rest position of the mandible and proper positioning of the tongue are paramount. For long-term effects, postural factors must be corrected. And in addition, the patient should be instructed by the therapist how to work toward abolishing traumatic habits.

By the time this book is published, a new system of checking and recording occlusal contacts will have been brought to the marketplace. This system will enable the clinician to record, note the prematurities, evaluate the stresses, strains, and the occlusal contacts, file them in the patient's folder, and compare pretreatment and posttreatment occlusion in 3 months, a year, or whatever time frame is needed. This permanent record of occlusion over a period will not only enable the dentist or staff to record occlusal relationships but also will equip physicians with a method of registering jaw relationships to evaluate abnormalities and decide on referrals.

This method for recording the pressure relationship between the teeth or the distance between them uses materials designed by the Medical Systems Group of the Vishay Company (Malvern, Penn.) in cooperation with the Technion in Israel.[3] A plastic medium is used to register the patient's bite. The patient may have to make one or two trials to get the idea of what it means

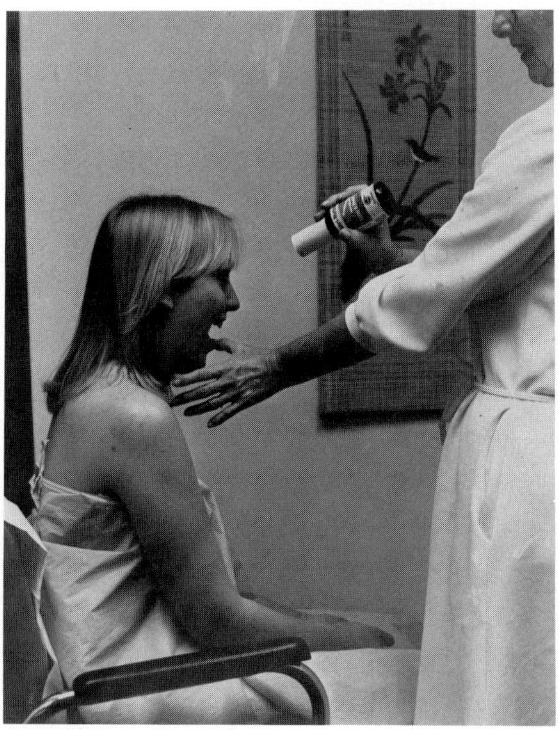

Fig. 17-14. Stretch and spray of masseter and temporal muscles (also used in treatment).

to bite down with the appropriate force to approximate swallowing so that there is no undue stress. The plastic medium memorizes any load instantly, registering the load and then maintaining the memory so that it can be kept for reference over an extended period.

A light source—a ray of light of random or different lengths—is put through first a vertical polarizer lens and then a second horizontal polarizer lens. By the time the light comes through the second lens, the rays change. The optical qualities of the plastic medium (on which the patient is biting) are such that the more load applied, the more colors appear in sequence. This strain-color phenomenon is caused by residual birefringence resulting from permanent local deformation of the plastic during tooth contact. This local permanent deformation is directly related to the in vivo contact, and the pattern appears in colors, with each color corresponding to a different strain intensity.

A color-calibration chart is used to provide strain-intensity values, which begin at zero (0.00), or black, and continue to gray, white, yellow, orange, and finally red. A tint of passage going from one area to another is registered as purple and then continues to blue, blue-green, green-yellow, orange, and red, where a strain intensity of 2.00 is reached. Again, a purple band can be noted as one intensity leads to another. Eventually a strain intensity of 2.67 is reached and displayed as pink. The fringe passage of going from one intensity to another can be measured as accurately as 15 μ. Normal articulating paper is approximately 100 μ, so these thin films which can register as little as 15 μ are another advantage of this system.

Thus the percentage of penetration of the medium can be registered in terms of microns and colors produced, enabling the clinician to tell the pressure between teeth, the primary contact, and the intensity of contact. Each color that appears in the pattern corresponds to a different strain intensity, so that comparisons of the various contact areas can be made with the help of the color-calibration chart. This view from the patient's tongue looks very much like a topographical map or a view from an airplane of the terrain below. Some of the color lines appear quite close together, others far apart, just as though the view were of gentle slopes and steep ridges.

Yet another advantage of this equipment is that the image can be enlarged 10 times on a screen for a better view of the intensity of the primary contacts in centric occlusion or centric relation. As the original impression of the arch is studied, it can be seen if there is symmetry between the right and left sides, if there is a grading front to back, and if there is a prematurity of occlusal contact. Each individual tooth contact can be told and cusp height ascertained by the light-colored rings or lines produced. This viewing system gives the clinician an accurate record of the prematurities in the patient's dentition to compare pretreatment and post-treatment effects. It has relativity, reproducibility, and permanence.

TREATMENT

In beginning treatment it must be emphasized that no promise of the degree of improvement should be made to the patient. The patient can only be assured that other persons exhibiting similar signs and symptoms have received some degree of relief after treatment.

Therapeutic appliance

At the first appointment upper and lower impressions are taken of the maxillary arch and mandibular arch and subsequently are poured in hard dental stone. If the patient wears full dentures, then impressions are taken of the dentures. Should some of the anterior teeth be missing, obtain a tooth shade, and add teeth to the appliance. The upper model is surveyed, and the undercuts are waxed out. The upper model then is duplicated and articulated with the lower model, and a flat-plane upper therapeutic appliance is waxed and prepared for processing. The appliance is designed with a flat plane to help eradicate pathological factors caused by clenching that prohibits normal isotonic contractions. Using this procedure will help minimize the distortion that occurs with appliances that are pulled on a Vacu-Form apparatus.

As soon as the therapeutic appliance is completed, it should be inserted in the maxillary arch and adjusted so that the mandibular teeth are touching the flat plane. The appliance should be worn at all times for 10 days to 2 weeks, after which the occlusion should be equilibrated in centric. The lateral and protrusive movements should follow at weekly intervals. The rationale behind the waiting period before equilibration is to reduce muscle memory. After equilibration has been completed, the patient is instructed to wear the appliance while sleeping and during times of stress (both physical and emotional).

Six temporomandibular joint x-ray views are taken, three on either side in each of three positions: with teeth clenched, with the mandible at rest and the teeth separated, and with the mouth propped wide open. Do *not* remove the prop while obtaining this transcranial film of both sides. This procedure will enable a comparison of the translation of one side to another. The amount of the incisal opening with the mouth prop in place is put on the x-ray holder so that the opening is recorded on the film. Frequently the transcranial films will indicate the need for laminagraphs.

Therapy

The therapist's first session with the patient consists of taking the blood pressure, draping the patient to expose the shoulders, locating the trigger areas as determined from the history and examination, and then working very lightly with the muscles plus using a stretch-spray-stretch pattern, preferably using the nonflammable, nontoxic Fluori-Methane spray (Fig. 17-15).

A

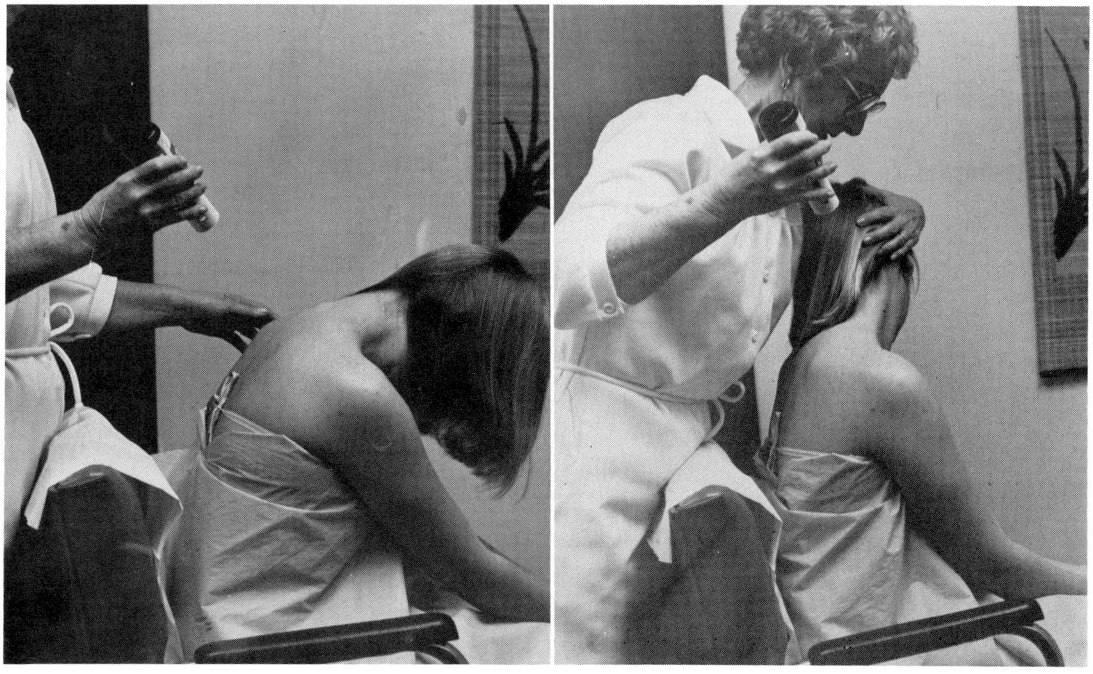

B

Fig. 17-15. Stretch and spray of trapezius **(A)** and lateral neck muscles **(B)**.

A

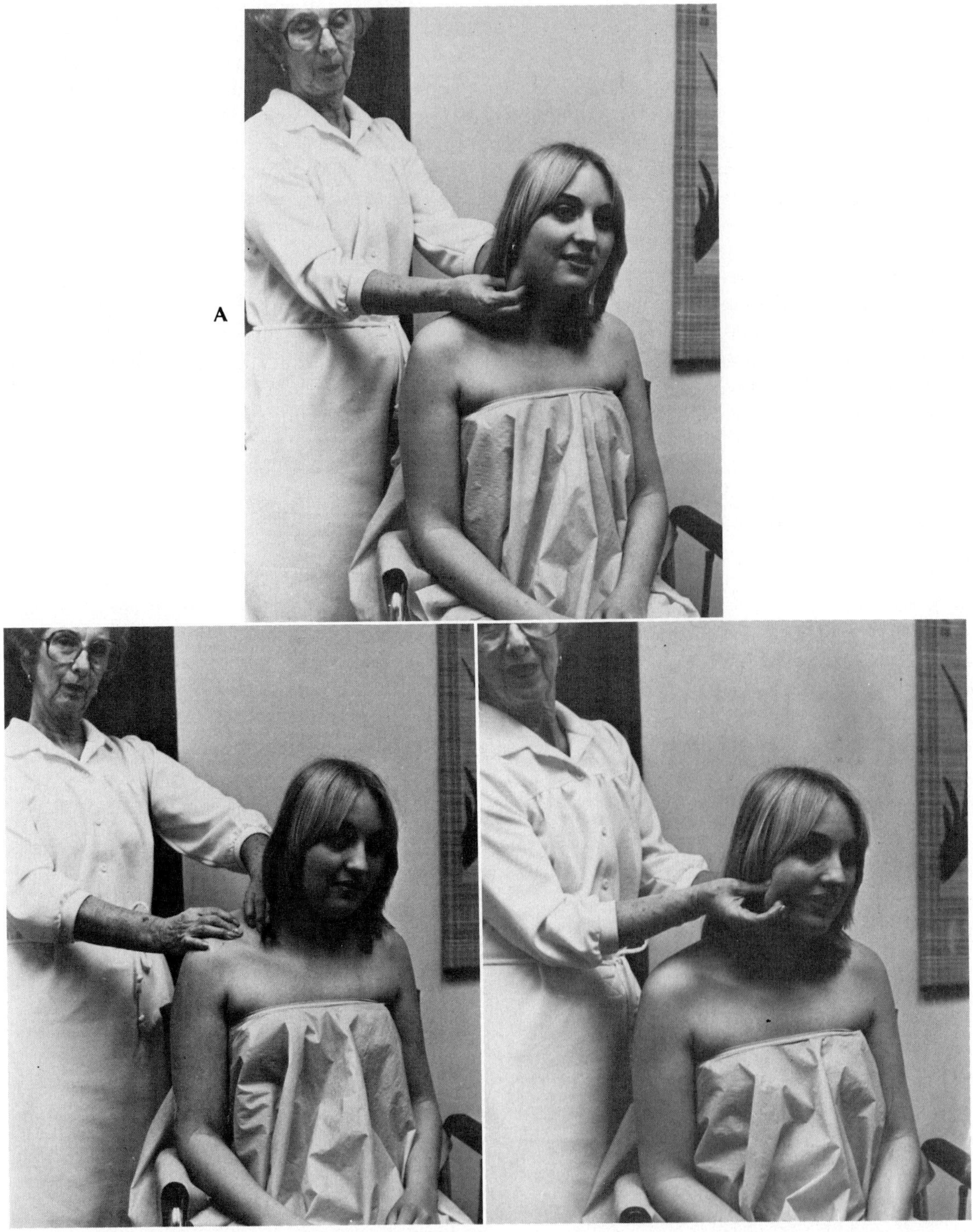

B C

Fig. 17-16. Rolling muscle knots. **A,** Sternocleidomastoid muscle. **B,** Anterior border of trapezius muscle. **C,** Masseter muscle.

Muscle knots are gently rolled between the fingers using talcum powder as a lubricant. The muscles inside the mouth usually are not treated at this particular point (Fig. 17-16). Follow with wet heat, using a hydrocollator pack that has been carefully insulated, and apply this to the area of the cervical portion of the trapezius and the lateral neck muscles for about 20 minutes. A face pack also is applied to each side of the face (Fig. 17-17). Fig. 17-18 shows the heating unit for hot packs and a bottle of Gebauer Fluori-Methane spray. U.S.P. talc is used as a lubricant when working with muscle knots to reduce surface irritation. (See Fig. 17-21.)

While the patient is under the heat, some informative material on stress headaches, muscle tension, joint pain, or diet may be given to the patient to read. Patients' prognoses improve when they are aware that their condition is known and that others have been treated and described in the literature.

Diet

When the heat is removed, the patient is instructed in the use of the V.I.V. shrug (see Fig. 17-21) and given directions to keep track of all foods ingested for 1 week. This diet compilation will be reviewed with the patient later. If the patient has vascular problems in addition to muscle spasms, care should be taken to instruct the patient to avoid eating chocolates, aged cheeses, red wines, ham, corned beef, hot dogs, and any other foods that are made or preserved with nitrites. The therapist should tell the patient to note if pain seems to be triggered by any of these foods. The patient's diet will be evaluated in regard to protein intake and excessive carbohydrates. The effects of hypoglycemia are discussed. It is important that the patient have an understanding of how the diet may relate to some of the problems or pain being experienced.

Evaluation of work and sleep habits

The patient's work and sleep habits are evaluated. All patients are issued a Cervi-Pillow and instructed in its usage. Suggestions may be offered to correct work habits that are felt to be possible contributing factors to the pain. An interesting note here is that occupations such as keypunch operators offer the most difficulty in correcting work habits, since the job necessitates reaching forward for long periods with no support for the arms.

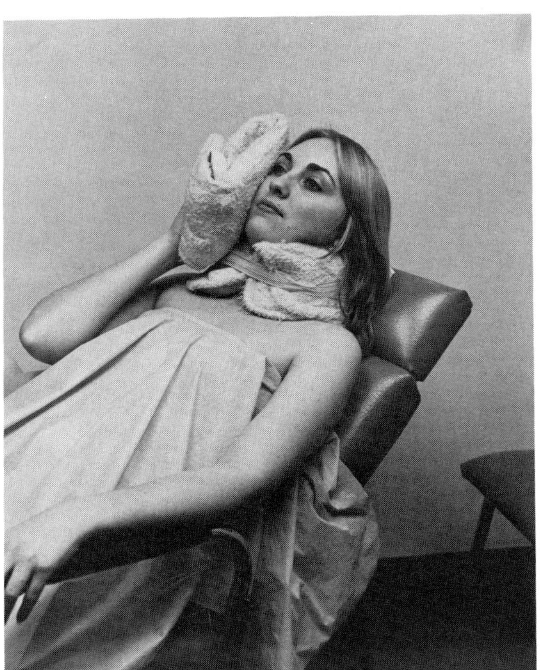

Fig.17-17. Application of wet heat.

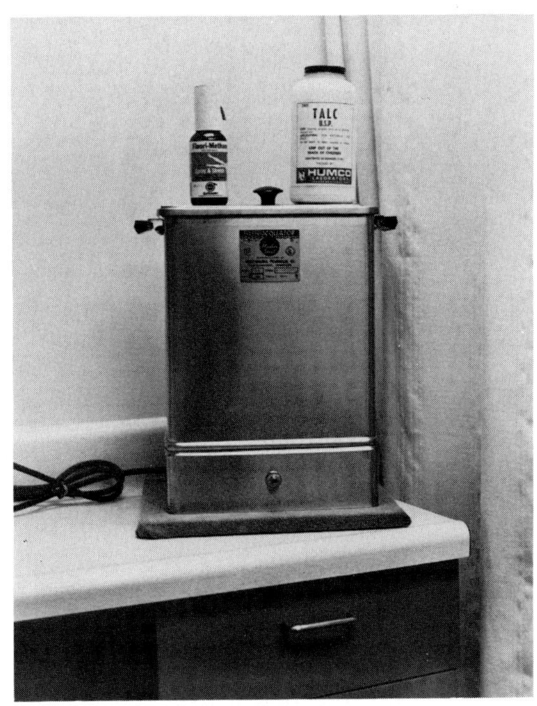

Fig. 17-18. Accessories: heating unit for hot packs, Gebauer Fluori-Methane, and U.S.P. talc.

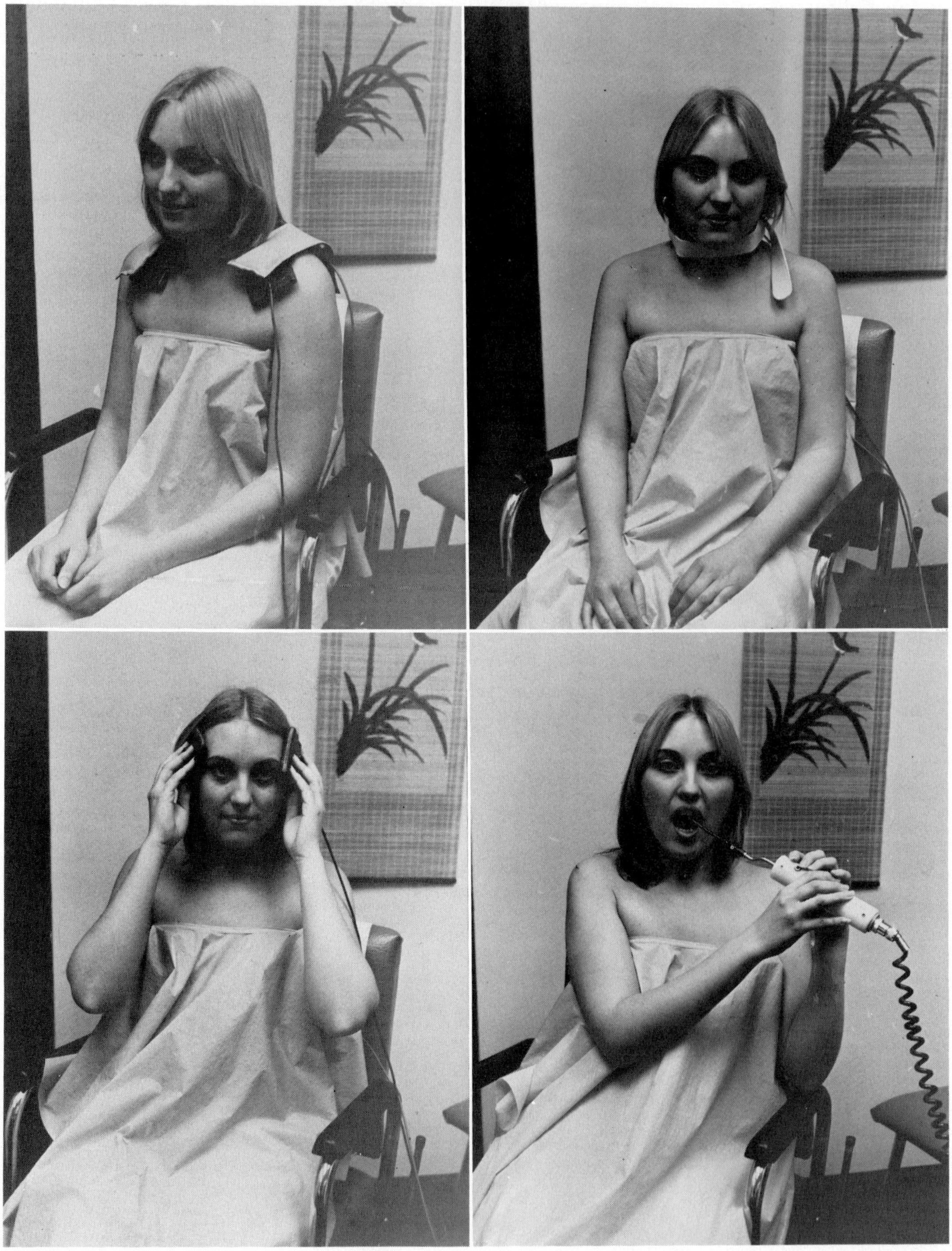

Fig. 17-19. Electrical stimulation of shoulder area **(A)**, sternocleidomastoid muscle **(B)**, and temporal area **(C)**. **D,** Electrogalvanic stimulation of intraoral muscles.

Additional therapy sessions

It is highly desirable that the patient be seen the next day for the second therapy appointment, at which time the therapist can work with the patient's muscles as before, only a little more extensively. At each appointment the results of the therapy are evaluated, and the activities of daily living are reviewed. An additional exercise may be introduced. (See section on exercises.) Patients should be advised that some discomfort may occur when doing the exercises and that relief can be sought by applying wet heat, either by taking a hot shower or by applying wet hot packs.

Starting with the fourth appointment, electrical stimulation is applied for 8 to 10 minutes at each trigger area (Fig. 17-19). Ultrasound is frequently used (Fig. 17-20). For muscles inside the mouth, have the patient hold warm water in the mouth while ultrasound is applied externally. Ultrasound also is used for some areas that are more resistant to therapy before the decision to use injections is made.

Injections in the muscles may be necessary. If so, 0.5% procaine hydrochloride in saline solution is the preferred medication. If local anesthetics are used, they should be used without vasoconstrictors to prevent ischemia of the muscles. Occasionally injections to the TMJ itself will be necessary. The type of medication used depends on the condition being treated (Table 17-1). The advantage of the vapocoolant spray (Fluori-Methane) is that it does not produce other pains as do the injections. However, both techniques are needed and used.

Treatments should continue two or three times per week for a period of 2 to 3 months, with gradual reduction in frequency as the patient experiences improvement. More and more attention is directed to exercises and home care. It is important for the patient to recognize that the signs and symptoms usually are of long standing and that the period of treatment is of necessity rather lengthy, although not necessarily commensurate with that of the causes. The patient should clearly understand that the symptoms experienced are frequently dissipated rather early in the treatment, but that to be effective the treatment must continue until the practitioner or therapist feels that all the trigger areas have been eliminated or reduced and that most of the patterns of living have been corrected to minimize future causative factors. The patient must accept that successful therapy can accomplish a reversal of the trend rather than a quick cure and therefore must continue with home care, relaxing methods, and exercises to help keep the symptoms either eliminated or at a very low level.

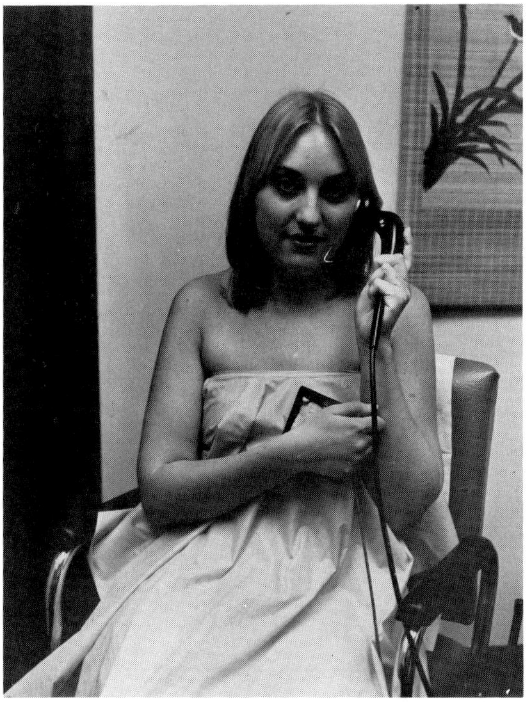

Fig. 17-20. Ultrasound application.

Table 17-1. Prescribed medications

Medication*	Dose (mg)	Number	Directions
Chlordiazepoxide (Libritabs)	10	50	tid and hs
Methocarbamol (Robaxin)	750	50	tid and hs
Z-BEC or Berocca	—	100	bid first week, qd thereafter
Vitamin E	400	100	Capsule tid with meals
Vitamin C or ascorbic acid powder	500	100	Tablet or 1/4 tsp powder tid with meals; may be reduced
Citrus bioflavonoids	500	100	Tablet tid with meals
Multiple vitamins (e.g., Theragran-M)	—	100	qd at opposite time Z-BEC or Berocca is taken

*All medications are noted *non repetatur* on the written order.

Corrective exercises

The following tables describe some of the corrective exercises that are used in the treatment of the patient (Table 17-2 to 17-4). In instructing the patient in these exercises, the therapist must be certain that the patient understands that these exercises are strictly for relaxation and gentle stretching of the muscles, not muscle building; therefore it is extremely important that the number of repetitions of the exercise be strictly adhered to and that the action of these exercises be kept fluid.

The positions in the resistive exercises must not be held for more than 5 seconds, and the amount of resistance/pressure should not exceed 5 pounds. The most important aspect of these exercises is that a regular regimen must be maintained. The ideal regimen would consist of two exercise sessions, one in the morning and one in the evening. The exercises that follow refer to this ideal when the patient is instructed to do them twice daily at the onset of treatment. The number of repetitions, unless otherwise specified, should be gradually increased at the discretion of the therapist.

It is not sufficient for the therapist to simply describe or demonstrate the exercise. The execution of the exercise must be carefully supervised by the therapist. It is important that the exercises be introduced at reasonable intervals rather than immediately at the beginning of treatment.

Autoprogressive relaxation. Autoprogressive relaxation is taught to the patient by the therapist in a comfortable room. The noise should be low level or nonexistent. Directions from the therapist should be evenly modulated in both tone quality and word delivery. The hand-on-arm position discussed previously is frequently effective with women. The therapist and the patient should both be seated, with the therapist to the side of and facing the patient.

The object of autoprogressive relaxation is to keep the mind actively engaged in the execution of muscle relaxation. However, the patient should be "given permission," if the mind should wander, to return to thinking about the last muscle just relaxed. Some patients feel an "itch"; the therapist should reassure them it is normal to "scratch."

There are several exercises in autoprogressive relaxation. For example, the patient is instructed, step by step, to sit relaxed with hands on thighs, feet flat on the floor, mouth slightly open so that the jaw is relaxed with the teeth not touching, and the eyes closed. The patient is reassured, statement by statement, that being aware of outside noises and feeling the urge to scratch or swallow is perfectly normal. Then, beginning with the top of the head, the therapist leads the patient in picturing how it will feel when each area or group of muscles is relaxed. The patient may need a reminder to keep the mouth open and the jaw relaxed. The patient then should be instructed to feel if any muscle is still tense. If so, the patient should repicture that muscle in a relaxed state. Finally, the patient should be told to count silently with the therapist from five to one, thinking these thoughts as the therapist counts:

5. I am feeling relaxed.
4. I am feeling relaxed and refreshed.
3. I am feeling more relaxed and refreshed.

Table 17-2. Relaxing and active exercises

Name—type	Preliminary position	Action	Directions
V.I.V. shrug—relaxing (Fig. 17-21)		1. Raise shoulders as close to ears as possible 2. Drop shoulders back into relaxed position 3. Take one long deep breath 4. Repeat	Do frequently throughout day (office workers might be instructed to do this exercise each time they arise from desk); do as preliminary exercise to all other exercises
Elbow touch/release—active (Fig. 17-22)	Fingers are interlocked behind head with elbows extended to side	1. Using slight resistance on back of head, move elbows gradually together until touching in front of head (fingers slide through each other) 2. Return elbows to original position, forced back as far as possible 3. Then move elbows slightly downward	Do twice, twice daily

Table 17-2. Relaxing and active exercises—cont'd

Name—type	Preliminary position	Action	Directions
Neck bend—active	Right hand is placed on right side of head	1. Maintaining smooth movement at all times and using no more than 5 pounds pressure, bend head to left as far as possible 2. As soon as maximum extension is reached, bring head back to upright position 3. Reverse hands; repeat action to right NOTE: It is important to emphasize that movement must be kept smooth and that reversal must begin as soon as maximum extension is gained. Care must be taken that patients do not pull head too hard while bending it	Do twice each direction, twice daily
Arm extension—active (Fig. 17-23)	1. Bend body over (forward) as far as possible 2. Extend arms as far as possible with hands clasped 3. Mouth is open, jaw relaxed; open mouth prevents patient's bracing by clenching teeth	1. Bring body smoothly into upright position 2. Raise arms, still extended, to position above head 3. Then release hands, moving arms in opposite directions and describing large circles to sides 4. Conclude with body bent slightly forward, arms dangling toward rear	Do once, twice daily
Elbow circle—active (Fig. 17-24)	1. Place fingers on shoulders 2. Keep elbows together in front of body	1. Keeping elbows together and hands on shoulders, raise elbows as far as possible 2. After maximum position has been reached, break contact and continue movement in opposite directions, describing circle 3. Continue until elbows come to sides of body 4. Slip fingers off shoulders, extending arms backward while bending forward 5. Conclude with arms dangling	Do once, twice daily
Arm rotation—active (Fig. 17-25)	Arms are extended to side of body parallel to floor	1. Rotate arms by describing 30-cm (1-foot) diameter circles with finger tips 10 times in one direction 2. Reverse direction. Repeat exercise	Do once or twice an hour during working day; this exercise is especially beneficial for persons who spend long periods in one position
Raggedy Ann/Andy—active and relaxing (Fig. 17-26)	Stand with body erect; when possible, women should be braless	1. Bend forward at waist as far as possible 2. Alternately raise one shoulder while lowering other	Done as closing for other exercises at each session, 5 to 10 times; may also be done during working day for relaxation

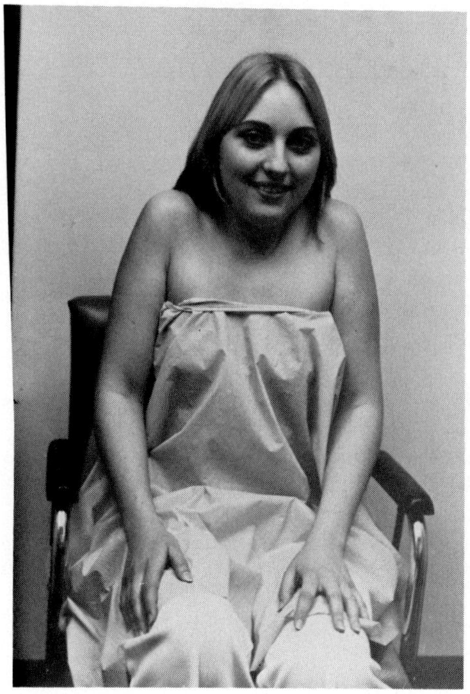

Fig. 17-21. V.I.V. shrug.

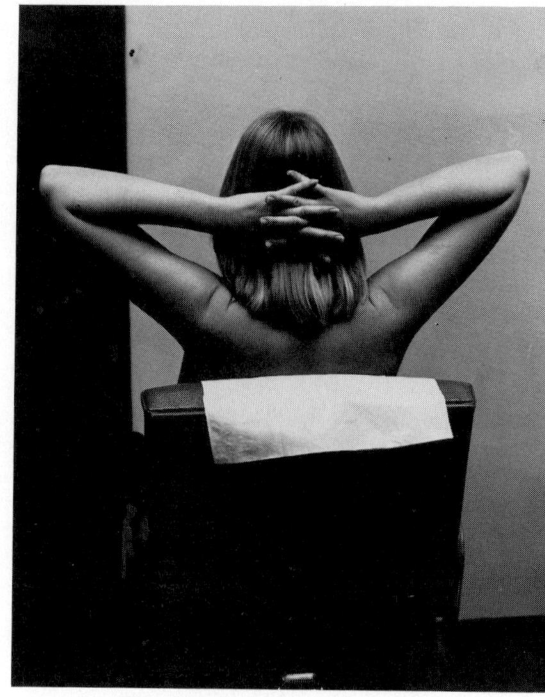

Fig. 17-22. Elbow touch/release.

A 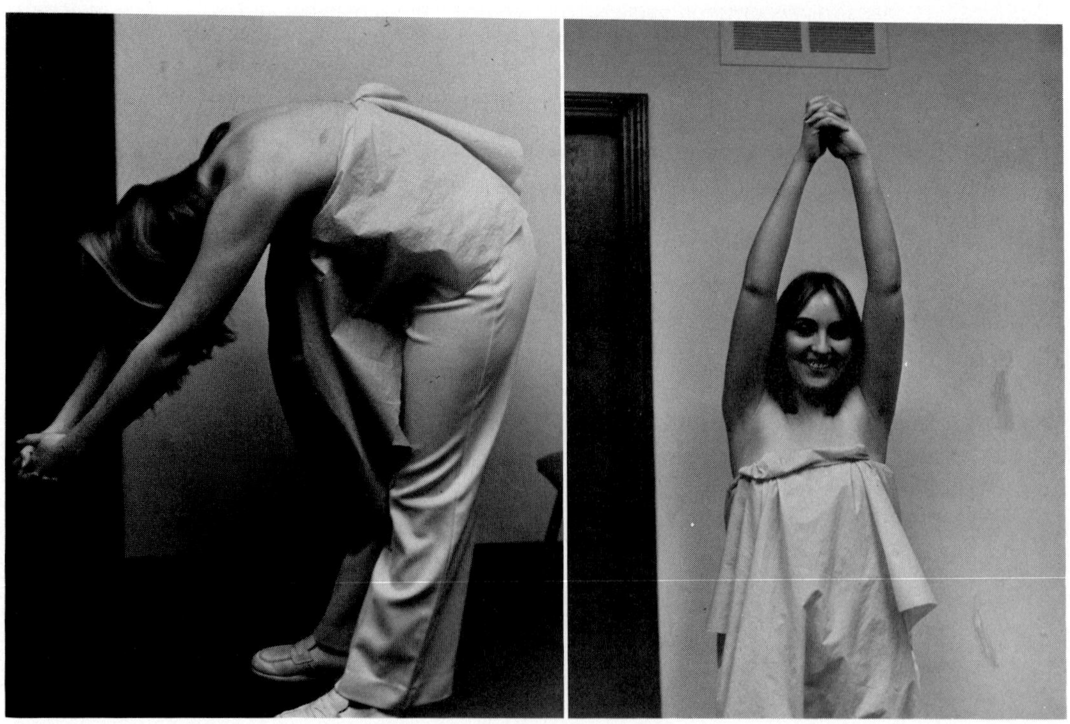 B

Fig. 17-23. Arm extension. **A,** Body bent forward. **B,** Body in upright position.

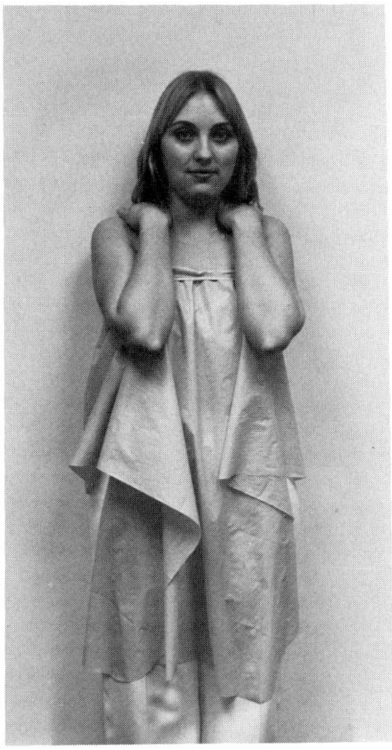

Fig. 17-24. Elbow circle, beginning with fingers on shoulders.

2. I am feeling much more relaxed and refreshed.
1. I feel very refreshed and will now open my eyes.

After this exercise the patient should be questioned as to how he or she now feels.

Another exercise in autoprogressive relaxation is done before retiring. The patient is instructed to press the fingers gently against the mattress or the thighs, counting from the little finger to the thumb across each hand, twice, repeating with each pressure, "Progressive relaxation will help me achieve the things I desire."

The first exercise should be practiced three times per day for about 1 week, and then the therapist may wish to introduce another exercise. Once comfortably seated with feet flat on the floor and hands on thighs, the patient should fix some distant spot in mind. The therapist should count from one to five and ask the patient to close the eyes. Again the patient should be reassured about noises, swallowing and itching. Then the therapist should give directions, asking the patient to count from 50 to 1 very slowly (with the therapist setting the pace), picturing each number as though it were coming from the distant spot that has been fixed in mind. (Should the count be lost or the mind wander, the patient should be instructed to return to the last number remembered.) On reaching the number one, the patient goes back to five and counts down, repeating the instructions given in the first exercise, including a discussion of awareness of feeling in the body. It is

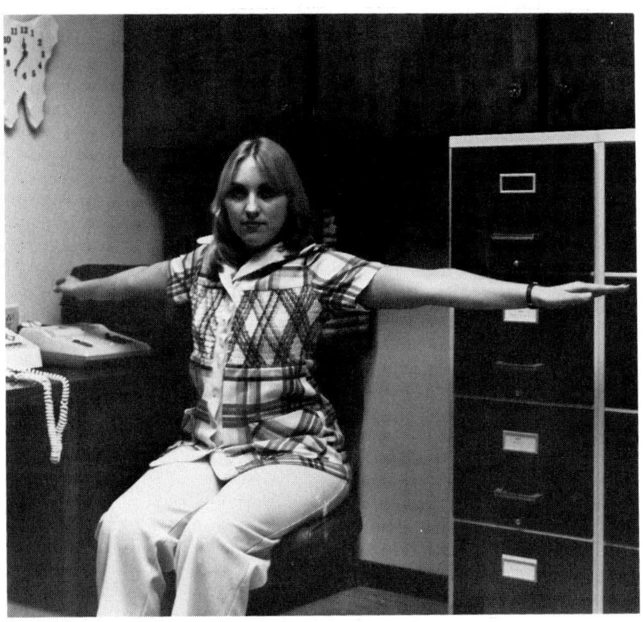

Fig. 17-25. Arm rotation.

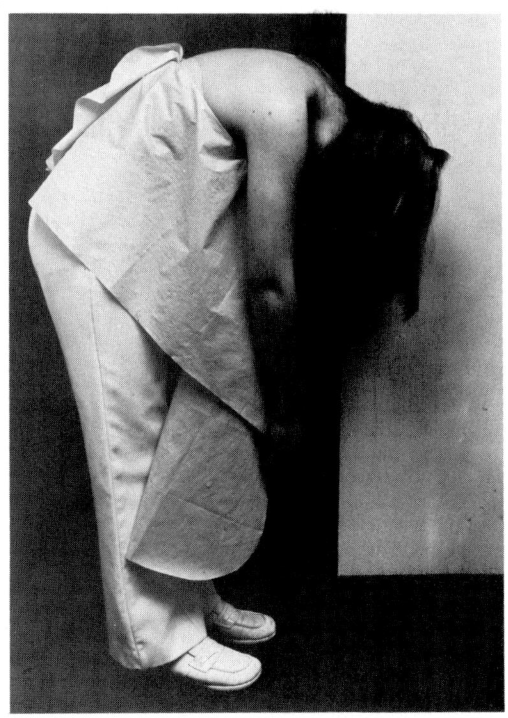

Fig. 17-26. Raggedy Ann/Andy exercise.

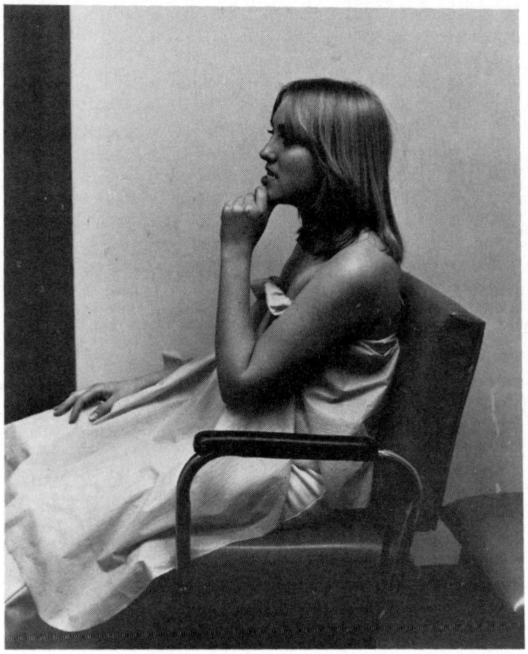

Fig. 17-27. Jaw jut.

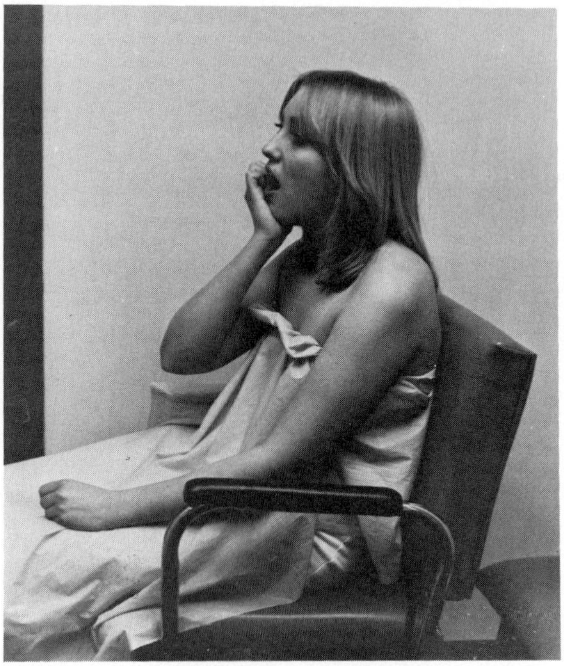

Fig. 17-28. Chin depression.

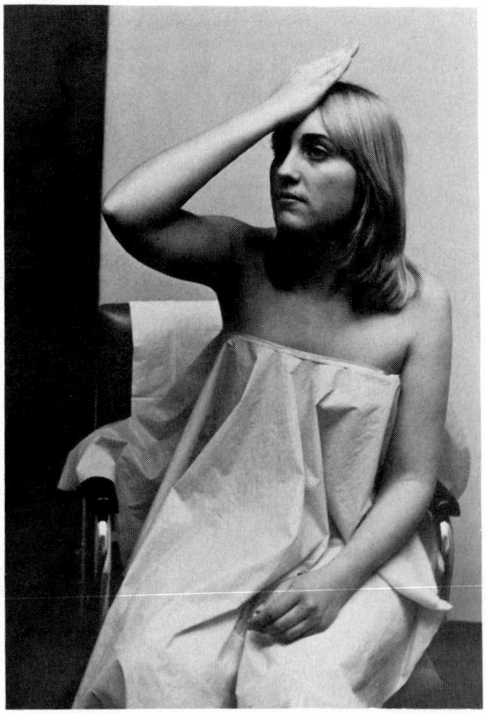

Fig. 17-29. Forehead resistive exercise.

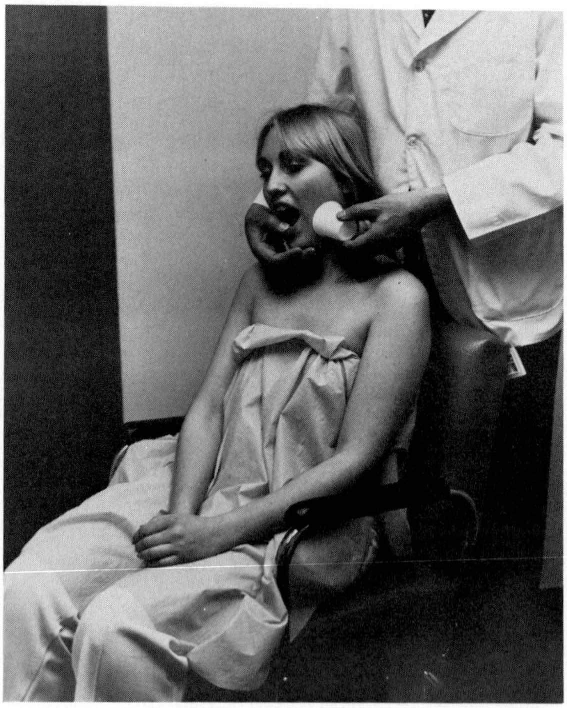

Fig. 17-30. Ice massage.

Table 17-3. Resistive exercises*

Name	Preliminary position	Action	Directions
Jaw jut (Fig. 17-27)	Thumb and forefinger are placed over lower jaw	1. Push thumb and forefinger against jaw 2. Jut jaw forward and retrude	Do once, twice daily
Chin depression (Fig. 17-28)	1. Open mouth 2. Place heel of hand under tip of chin	Push heel of hand upward against chin, resist with mouth open	Do once, twice daily
Jaw deviation	Right hand is placed on right side of jaw	1. Push jaw against hand 2. Reverse hands; repeat in opposite direction	Do once, twice daily
Forehead (Fig. 17-29)	Either hand is placed on forehead	Push head forward against hand	Do once, twice daily
Back of head	Either hand is placed on back of head	Push head backward against hand	Do once, twice daily
Temple	Flat of right hand is placed against right temple	1. Push head against hand 2. Reverse hands and repeat in opposite direction	Do once, twice daily

*All exercises use 5 pounds of resistance.

Table 17-4. Faciliatory and passive exercises

Name—type	Preliminary position	Action	Directions
Tongue cluck—faciliatory	Tongue is placed against hard palate	Cluck tongue 10 times	Do three times daily
Gargle—faciliatory		Gargle with warm water	Do three times daily
Diaphragmatic/intercostal breathing—faciliatory	1. One hand of patient is placed on midline of patient's body 2. Therapist places hand on top of patient's hand 3. One hand of therapist is placed on midline of therapist's body 4. Patient places one hand on top of therapist's hand	1. Expand waistline while inhaling over a count of 5 seconds 2. Hold air momentarily and inhale, raising shoulders and filling upper half of lungs 3. Exhale with hissing sound to count of 10 4. Relax 5. Repeat exercise, gradually extending exhale to count of 25; increase waiting period between each part by 1 second	Do whenever possible in series of 5
Electrogalvanic stimulator; ultrasound; ultrasound with water in mouth—faciliatory		Applied by therapist	
Ice massage (Fig. 17-30)	Keep ready 30 to 90 ml frozen water	1. Used as home treatment 2. When muscle spasms begin, rub ice along length of muscle fiber in one direction only, with muscle in stretched position *only* when ice is applied 3. Make five or six passes 4. Dry with towel 5. Apply warm hand over area 25 seconds	Repeat series five times
Example: neck stretch—passive (Fig. 17-31)	1. Patient is placed as horizontally as possible 2. Therapist sits behind patient with hands supporting head and neck of patient	1. Applied by therapist 2. Head is rotated to one side with gentle stretch along long axis of body 3. Repeat with intermittent stretching of neck to other side and with head parallel to long axis	Stretch minimum of 20 seconds
Autoprogressive relaxation: see p. 320			

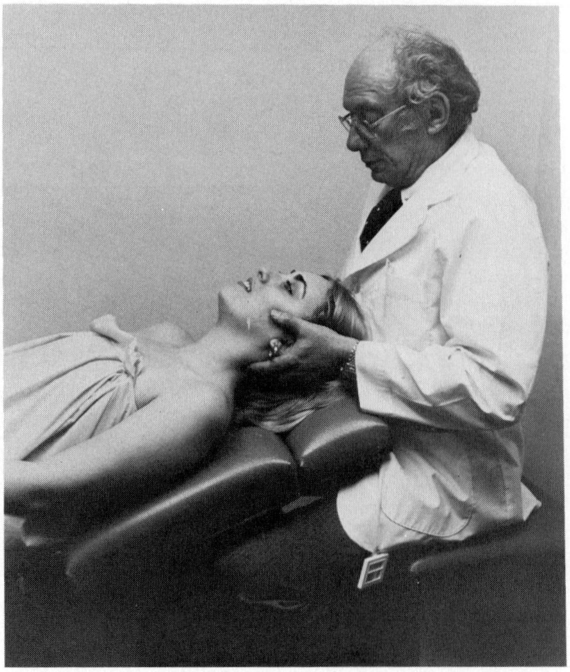

Fig. 17-31. Passive neck stretch exercise.

recommended that the patient repeat this procedure three times daily for a period of 1 week; thereafter it is repeated whenever necessary at least twice daily.

As the muscles become conditioned, it may be possible to reduce the number of counts, possibly beginning with 25. It will be found that this exercise will be able to be used in any surroundings.

REFERENCES

1. Bonica, J.: The relation of injury to pain (letter), Pain **7**:203, 1979.
2. Cheraskin, E., Ringsdorf, W., Jr., and Brecher, A.: Psychodietetics, New York, 1974, Stein & Day Publishers.
3. Harrington, R.W.: Personal communication, 1981.
4. Jackson, R.: The cervical syndrome, Springfield, Ill., 1966, Charles C Thomas, Publisher.
5. Kraus, H.: Therapeutic exercise, ed. 2, Springfield, Ill., 1963, Charles C Thomas, Publisher.
6. Palchick, Y.S.: Stress headaches, 1961, Summit Co. Medical Soc.
7. Rocabado, M.: Personal communication, Chile, 1980.
8. Shore, N.A.: Temporomandibular joint dysfunction and occlusal equilibration, ed. 2, Philadelphia, 1976, J.B. Lippincott Co.
9. Travell, J.G.: Personal communication, 1958.

18 Biofeedback

MURRAY GROSSAN, M.D.

Schwartz,[15] in *Disorders of the Temporomandibular Joint*, states that "Our investigations have demonstrated that although 'occlusal interferences' or 'premature contacts' may contribute to the onset of muscle spasm, muscle spasm can and does create 'interferences' . . . .We feel that treatment should not be undertaken until both the patient and his muscles are relaxed. . . ." He also used electromyography to show that with the temporomandibular joint syndrome there was marked increase of muscle electrical output.

Schwartz[15] described various methods of achieving muscle relaxation, including that of Jacobson,[8] called *progressive relaxation*. This is a method whereby the physician trains a patient to relax all the muscles progressively from the tips of the toes, up through the abdomen and chest, and finally the muscles of the eyes. Jacobson used electromyographic recordings to demonstrate the effectiveness of this relaxation training. Schwartz achieved significant results using this method.

Recently a rapid method of achieving muscle relaxation has become available—biofeedback.[2] *Biofeedback* is the use of special equipment to isolate and identify certain physiological parameters and to display them to the patient so that these parameters can be modified. Almost any physiological process in the body can be displayed if sensors can be introduced to the area and extraneous impulses sifted out.

VARIOUS BIOFEEDBACK PARAMETERS

The most commonly used biofeedback device is the electromyographic (EMG) biofeedback machine.[1] This device senses cutaneous electrical outputs. Every time a muscle contracts, an electrical current is given off, which diffuses outward and may reach the skin. Current from muscles near the skin is much easier to detect than current from the deeper muscles. Muscles give off specific frequencies of electrical output. The amperage and voltage vary with the amount of muscle activity. The biofeedback device elaborately filters out nonmuscle frequencies and accurately gauges the amount of amperage and voltage. Cutaneous electromyography has the advantage of being noninvasive and painless and can be repeated frequently.

Temperature biofeedback consists of placing a delicate thermistor on the skin. The temperature is measured in tenths of a degree centigrade. The temperature can be variously displayed as a digital readout, a sound, or a color. Thus the higher the temperature, the higher the pitch of sound. For limbs with poor circulation, as in Raynaud's disease, an individual can increase the temperature as well as the circulation.

For migraine, Green and co-workers[5] have reported training individuals to raise the temperature of their hands at the onset of a migraine attack, thereby shifting the blood out of the dural vessels into the hands.

Gastrointestinal hypermotility can be displayed as a sound or as a visual digital reading. The individual learns to reduce the digital reading, thereby reducing hypermotility.

Heart rate can be displayed, and individuals have been taught to slow their heart. Diastolic pressure also can be reduced in this manner.[16]

Brain waves have been arbitrarily divided into alpha waves (8 to 13 Hz), beta waves (14 Hz or greater), and theta waves (4 to 7 Hz). It is suggested that alpha waves are associated with relaxation and creativity, and electroencephalographic (EEG) biofeedback has been used to teach people to make alpha waves. Epileptics have been trained to modify their brain waves to help them avoid seizures.[18] Individuals have been trained to specifically make the type of waves that will help them sleep.[10]

One device is available to treat impotency. A simple strain gauge is placed on the penis of the individual. He learns what to do to achieve erection.

A psychogalvanometer detects minute sweating, which is associated with anxiety. This reading can be demonstrated as a digital or meter readout, so that the individual learns to reduce anxiety, whatever the cause.

Dizziness with nystagmus has been treated by converting the nystagmus into a quantitative output, so that the greater the nystagmus, the greater the sound. Patients have been taught thereby to suppress the sound and to learn to suppress dizziness.[6]

Most applications of biofeedback are perfectly safe, with the exception of circulation biofeedback. Some patients have learned to slow the heart rate excessively or to drop their blood pressure excessively, and this type of therapy requires expert monitoring.

ANIMAL RESEARCH

The earliest work on biofeedback was done on animals. They were rewarded with food or with stimulation of the pleasure center when they learned to control their physiological parameters. Rats have been taught to raise the temperature of one ear and to lower the temperature of the other ear. Rats quickly learn to make alpha waves or whatever wave for which the experimenter rewards them. Rats have been taught to slow their heart to the point of death.[12]

ADVANTAGES OF BIOFEEDBACK

Objectivity

Objectivity is the outstanding advantage of biofeedback.[4] Thus an individual specifically changes the electromyographic output when he or she relaxes from a 30 to a 5 μV output. Using the same machine, the same results are obtained consistently. These biofeedback results can be recorded, graphed, and analyzed. The results of biofeedback training are durable. Various studies have shown that 6 months or longer after cessation of training the individual retains most of what has been learned.[1] Biofeedback training is noninvasive, and much of it is simple. Treatment can be administered by assistants. Often results can be obtained in a few treatment sessions.

Safety

An excellent safety feature of many EMG biofeedback machines is that they operate off a few D-cell batteries. It is reassuring to know that there is no possibility of electricity passing through a patient.

Simplicity

The biofeedback device need not be a complicated machine. A girl learning to put on lipstick for the first time, in a dark room without a mirror, is without visual cues as to how to do it right. Even though she has seen pictures explaining how to apply lipstick, she may have difficulty. With good lighting and a good mirror, she gets visual biofeedback and learns how to put on her lipstick correctly.

When someone is having difficulty parking a car, the addition of curb feelers that make a noise as they scrape against the curb will aid him in parking. With the curb feelers, he learns to do it correctly; suddenly, one day something clicks, and he is able to do it properly from then on even without the curb feelers.

Simple home use

New crystal papers are available in strips that can be placed on a limb with poor circulation. These strips turn color with 0.2°F change in temperature. They can be used to train patients to increase temperature in that limb. Through practice, the patient learns to change the color of the paper, thereby increasing circulation.

Another simple mechanism is the steering wheel biofeedback device.[6] This mechanism is worn on the hand, somewhat like a glove. It is turned on and programmed to buzz when the individual squeezes the steering wheel of the automobile at any predetermined pressure, such as 5 psi (Fig. 18-1). For a driver who normally drives squeezing the steering wheel until the knuckles are white, this device reminds him or her to relax his grip whenever exceeding 5 psi of pressure. Thus the individual learns to drive relaxed by hearing how to do it correctly and can then increase the sensitivity to 4 psi or lower. Since driving consumes a large portion of the average individual's time, this steering wheel device can be used every day for learning purposes. Once the individual learns to loosen the grip while driving, relaxation can be learned for most of the muscles. This same device can be used in the dental chair for persons who grip the chair hard as a manifestation of their anxiety. The buzzing reminds them to relax. Anxiety while flying also may be treated in this manner.

Complex devices

Biofeedback devices also may be complicated. To teach a child to make alpha waves, a machine is used so that a toy electrical train runs in proportion to the amount of alpha waves generated. Thus, the more alpha waves a child makes, the faster the train goes. Either correct electromyographic or correct brain waves will cause a slide projecter to change, flashing a sequence of interesting slides. The subject matter is selected in accordance with the subject's taste. A light behind a picture can become bright enough to see the picture, or it can dim out. Music played through a tape device can become loud enough to hear or too soft to hear in proportion to the desired physiological output.

In the earlier experiments subjects were paid money when they performed in the correct physiological manner.

HYPNOSIS

Biofeedback is not hypnosis! Hypnosis requires the individual to cooperate consciously and to follow suggestions. It is the individual's belief that aids him or

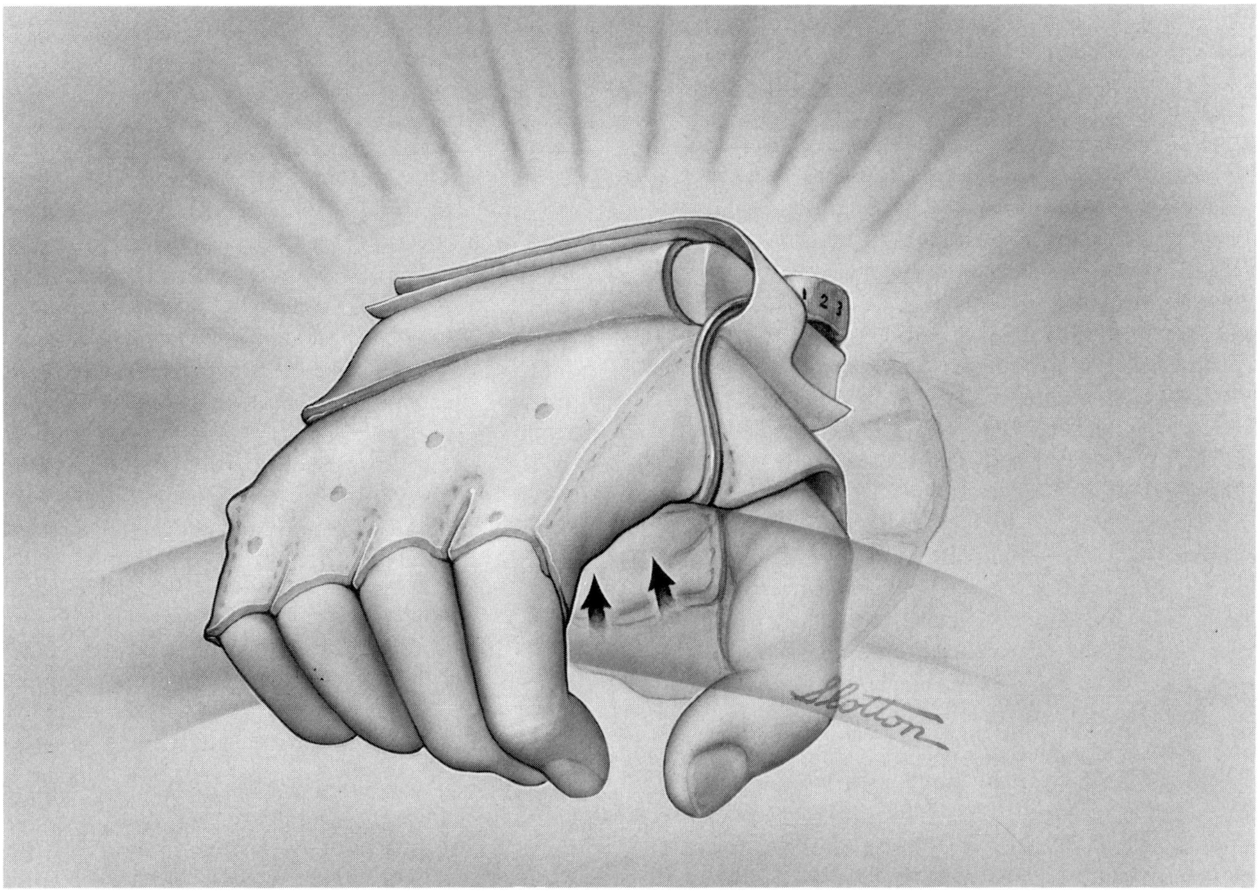

Fig. 18-1. Biofeedback steering wheel device.

her in following the suggestions of the hypnotist. On the other hand, with biofeedback the individual is doing it completely alone. Just like rats, humans do not do a specific, conscious act. Rather, they automatically follow sensory clues given back to them by the auditory or visual display.

APPLICATION OF ELECTROMYOGRAPHIC BIOFEEDBACK

Tension headache

A major application of biofeedback is the treatment of tension headache.[3] Normally, individuals maintain muscle pull to hold the head erect. This muscle pull may be in excess of that required. The head is perfectly balanced, and it makes no difference whether the anterior and posterior muscle pull is minimum or strong. Since only a miminum amount of anterior and posterior tension is required to hold the head balanced, excessive tension is wasted, causing decreased circulation to the muscle and helping to build up toxins. In other words, an individual who maintains a state of constant tension and anxiety will have a headache.

Wolpe and Lazaras[20] have shown that muscle relaxation is physiologically incompatible with an anxiety response. Anyone who has relaxed on the beach, comfortable in the warm sun, has been aware of anxiety leaving the body as he or she becomes more and more relaxed. Thus tension headache is relieved with muscle relaxation. Biofeedback has been found to be an excellent way of reeducating the muscles to maintain the proper tension pull, thereby relieving tension headache. In addition, biofeedback muscle relaxation allows the individual to substitute a relaxation response when ordinarily there would be an anxiety response. Anxiety often is manifested by wrinkling the eyebrows as well as by gnashing the teeth, so that the sensors placed on the frontal muscle can be used to train the individual to have muscle relaxation and reduced anxiety.

Other applications

After stroke or paralytic injury, EMG biofeedback is used to reeducate partially denervated muscles. Here, biofeedback is used to strengthen a muscle: the more contracture and movement, the better the sound or readout. This is of value in Bell's palsy.

Temporomandibular joint disorders

Biofeedback in temporomandibular joint disorders is applied as in tension headache. In the presence of anxiety there may be bruxism, teeth clenching, and subluxation.[19] By relaxing muscles, according to Wolpe and Lazaras,[20] anxiety must be reduced.

For various reasons there may be an imbalance of the muscles' elastication—one set causing more spasm and thus causing both joints to be thrown off balance. Biofeedback is ideal for restoring the balance. With marked muscle spasm, circulation to the muscle is decreased, with resultant pain. The more the spasm, the less the circulation and the more the anxiety. After overly long or painful dental treatment, the muscles may be easily pulled to the point of pain, with resultant spasm or splinting.[11] Biofeedback electromyography works to reduce this muscle spasm.

When one set of muscles starts to relax, this spreads to other muscles as well. Thus electromyographic relaxation learned at the frontal muscle immediately can be applied elsewhere by the patient. For example, in the condition of tensor tympani muscle spasm, the patient complains of severe and distressing fluttering because of a persistent spasm of the tensor tympani muscle. Biofeedback relaxation at the frontal muscle has been quickly effective for this condition, usually requiring only one 20-minute treatment.

This relaxation of one set of body muscles spreading in a nonspecific manner to other sets of muscles is most helpful for temporomandibular joint disorders.

Good candidates. Patients who are good candidates for biofeedback treatment of temporomandibular joint disease are those who have an absence of obvious anatomical deformity. Younger patients seem to do better than older patients. Those associated with a high anxiety level, especially where there is a cycle of anxiety-muscle spasm-pain-anxiety, do well because biofeedback muscle relaxation breaks this cycle. Patients who have undergone trauma, either through whiplash or lengthy dental work, are good candidates. Those who have heard of biofeedback and who come with the expectation of being helped also do well. Patients with simple clicking, bruxism, subluxation, or grinding associated with temporomandibular joint symptoms also respond.

Poor candidates. Poor candidates are those who are older; those who have had the condition for such a long time that fibrosis has replaced muscle tissue; those who have a psychological displacement of their emotional dysfunction onto an organ, which happens to be the temporomandibular joint; or those individuals who, because of language or intellectual barriers, are unable to fully comprehend what biofeedback is supposed to do.

METHODS OF TREATMENT

All patients are given an explanation of how muscles are responsible for the temporomandibular joint pain syndrome. It should be explained how the head is perfectly balanced and that this balance can be achieved with minimum or maximum muscle contracture. Similarly, the muscles of mastication and the muscles of the temporomandibular joint can perform their actions with minimum or maximum contracture. An example is how the fist is clenched so that the knuckles are white, indicating decreased circulation. This analogy refers to how the temporomandibular joint muscles, by achieving constant contracture, have poor circulation with resulting pain and development of anxiety, which causes even further contracture.

Office procedures

Three office procedures may be followed:

1. The patient is seated in a comfortable chair, like a television lounge chair. The sensors are placed over the frontal muscle. Two sensors are placed over each frontal with a central ground. Earphones are placed on the patient so that muscles contractions can be heard. The patient is placed with the voltmeter in view, which indicates how much amperage is produced. The machine used* detects surface electrical output between 120 and 1000 Hz and filters out the 60-cycle current. By using the frontal muscle region, the practitioner is attacking the basic area that reflects anxiety when a person is tense, anxious, frowning, or using the eyes to look and pay attention. When the frontal muscle is relaxed, there is generally a spread of learning that indirectly affects the temporomandibular joint muscles.
2. A method recommended by many physicians consists of starting with the sensors on the dorsal portion of the forearem. Now the patient can learn precisely what contraction of the muscle means. The patient can see the muscles, and it is easier to understand the meaning of the high bleeps that are heard and what the needle pointing to "high" means. After the dorsal forearm muscles are learned perfectly, then the next pickup points can be the frontal or masseter muscle.
3. Another method is to start directly with the masseter muscle or the temporal muscle, whichever appears to be the muscle at fault.[17]

*Model PE-2 Biofeedback Systems, Inc., 2736 47th St., Boulder, Colo. 80301.

Home treatment

Temporomandibular joint disorder can be treated outside the office by using the biofeedback steering wheel device. This is performed while the patient drives back and forth to work.

Suggestions for relaxation

Whichever method is used, patients are given various suggestions for learning musculature relaxation, such as the following:

1. Visualize yourself floating on clouds or on the ocean, and try to capture that relaxed sensation.
2. Think of the Hering-Breuer reflex; that is, inhalation is a contracture, and exhalation is a relaxation. Think of the relaxation, and every time you exhale, consider this a signal to relax all the muscles. Since there is actually such a signal being transmitted through normal physiological breathing, thinking about this reflex and spreading it to voluntary muscles can be highly effective.
3. Raise the index finger, count to three, then drop the finger. When the finger drops, let that be a signal to relax.
4. Let the jaw sag forward and also let the head roll forward. Take a deep breath and let every muscle relax during exhalation.

The patient monitors the response, both through the use of earphones, through which are heard the muscle contractures, and by viewing the voltmeter. Thus, the patient is able to determine which of these methods, or combinations of these methods, is more effective. Patients individually will find some picture or method among these four that is effective for them. Once they learn the correct mechanism, they can then be ensured of proper relaxation by repeating the same activity at will, without the aid of the machine.

Biofeedback need not be used by itself. Biofeedback treatment may be accompanied by instructions to stay on a soft diet and to wear an Ace bandage as a splint when at home, coupled with the suggestion that this treatment will be effective.

Disadvantage

One disadvantage of using specific masseter muscle biofeedback is that if the right muscle is the diseased muscle and is treated, it can become too relaxed and, instead of being hyperactive, is now seriously hypoactive; whereas the opposite muscle, which was normal, now assumes the hyperactive state and tends to pull the jaw to the opposite side. Now the left jaw muscle is painful instead of the right.

Nasal obstruction

Nasal congestion or obstruction may cause temporomandibular joint symptoms, especially in children. Chronic sinusitis, of itself, may cause bruxism, or it may cause a secondary hypertrophy of adenoidal tissue with mouth breathing and bruxism. An excellent treatment for chronic sinusitis is the use of the pulsatile irrigator device* with isotonic saline at 5 psi.

FINDINGS

Forty-eight patients with no obvious anatomical deformities were treated. Of these 48 patients, 23 were relieved of their symptoms and did not find it necessary to return after two visits. One explanation for biofeedback working so fast is that, in a state of nearly constant contracture, circulation to the muscles is impaired. This causes buildup of toxic products within the muscles without removal of these products. As the muscles remain in constant spasm, the normal movement of muscles that enables them to function as a lymphatic and venous pump is markedly reduced, causing further buildup of toxins. Through biofeedback treatment the muscles are relaxed, circulation is increased, and the muscles are used so that they can function as a lymphatic and venous pump and remove toxins. With relief of pain, the cycle of pain-spasm-anxiety-reduced circulation-spasm is broken. Similarly, when the temporomandibular joint syndrome is brought on by a purely physical act of trauma to the joint such as an overlong dental appointment, a blow to the jaw, or excessive cervical traction, a spastic splinting effect may take place among the masseter and pterygoid muscles. Once this spasm has ended, circulation increases, and the cycle is again broken. With relaxation of muscles, anxiety becomes reduced.[20]

CASE HISTORIES

Case 1

A 23-year-old woman presented with the complaint of left ear pain. She showed crepitation and localized tenderness. Gross malocclusion was not evident. Initially, she showed high frontal muscle output of 30 μV. On her third visit she was more relaxed, had more acceptance of the treatment, and was able to bring her frontal activity down to 10 μV. At her fourth visit she had fewer symptoms. After her fifth visit she remained symptom free for a week, and when seen 2 weeks later for her sixth and last visit, she was asymptomatic.

She had no specific history of trauma, and no etiological factor was established for her temporomandibular joint pain-dysfunction syndrome.

Case 2

An 18-year-old woman had been undergoing extensive dental repair. After two visits to the dentist, each of which was unusually lengthy, she developed aching in both jaws. She complained of this to the dentist, but it was necessary to

*Available from Hydro Med, Inc., P.O. Box 91273, Los Angeles, Calif. 90009.

continue another lengthy session. Her jaws ached so that she refused to return for a fourth visit. She was given muscle relaxants and 1/2 grain Empirin codeine with poor results.

On examination there was no evidence of gross malocclusion, but both temporomandibular joints were markedly tender, and both external and internal pterygoid muscles were markedly spastic. Localized tenderness of the right sternocleidomastoid muscle insertion area was noted but was not seen on the left.

On biofeedback she showed a maximum output of the frontal muscle. Considerable time was spent explaining and reassuring this patient about how, since her initial visit to the dentist, she was reinforcing muscle spasm. After her second biofeedback treatment she was asymptomatic.

Case 3

A divorced 35-year-old woman, who had been a patient for 5 years with various problems, including recurrent nasal symptoms, sore throat, difficulty in swallowing, and vague headaches, was seen for left otalgia, which had been present for 6 months. She gave a voluminous history of family and personal problems and various etiological factors to explain her symptoms. She was aware that she was grinding her teeth but did not think that this was the cause of her symptoms. Biofeedback treatment was started, and she immediatley was able to relax her frontal musculature. After 20 minutes of treatment she showed 3 μV of output and, indeed, fell asleep. She was asked to practice this at home daily. She was seen again a week later, but showed no improvement. Her earache was still bothersome, and even though an explanation was given that her pain was coming from her temporomandibular joint, she insisted that the pain must be from her ear itself and demanded some type of eardrops. An anesthetic eardrop was prescribed. With biofeedback she was able to easily achieve a relaxed frontal muscle. She canceled her third visit with the excuse that the eardrops were giving her adequate relief, and she did not think that further biofeedback treatments would be beneficial to her.

This patient apparently was leading the practitioner into treating her as she wished. She may have needed psychotherapy and would not benefit from occipital frontal muscle relaxation. Indeed, she could relax her muscles nicely, without difficulty, and already knew how to do so. This patient did not have a temporomandibular joint pain-dysfunction syndrome; rather, she probably had psychogenic headaches with psychogenic referred pain. The fact that anesthetic eardrops benefited her was probably a result of the value of receiving attention and care from her physician.

Case 4

A 35-year-old man complained of pain behind the left ear. There was some pain on chewing but more of a vague left earache. Recently he had been forced to sell his house and move an additional 25 miles away from his work. His pain was worse at the end of the day, and in addition, on close questioning he was found to feel tired, which he attributed to the longer drive. He was found to have localized trapezius and sternocleidomastoid insertion pain, with pain in the left internal pterygoid. He could open his jaw without difficulty or specific pain. He admitted gripping the steering wheel too tightly when driving and therefore was given a trial of the biofeedback steering wheel device.

He used the device for 10 minutes daily for a week and found that he could reduce the pressure from a setting of severe pressure on the first day to a setting of very light pressure by the end of the first week. He was proud of this achievement and was completely conscious of how he previously squeezed the steering wheel too tightly, thereby causing muscle spasm. He returned the steering wheel device, saying that he had learned correct handling and would be aware of any tightening of his grip in the future. He noticed a considerable increase in energy in the evening; he no longer felt tired and dragged out when he arrived home. He commented that before he could achieve good relaxation of his hands while driving, he had to experiment a bit with the proper height of his seat and various seat positions until he found the exact height and position that offered him the most opportunity for relaxing his arms while driving.

COSTEN'S SYNDROME

Costen described tinnitus as accompanying temporomandibular joint disease. I have personally not seen a case of Costen's syndrome but have used frontal electromyographic muscle relaxation as a treatment for tinnitus since 1970. In many patients tinnitus results in an anxiety-muscle spasm-tinnitus cycle. With muscle biofeedback, muscle tension is reduced, anxiety can be relieved, and patients generally report a reduction in tinnitus.[7a]

OTHER APPLICATIONS OF EMG BIOFEEDBACK

Professionals who use biofeedback in temporomandibular joint disease will find many other uses for this technique.[14] For example, patients with dentures that are troublesome because of splinting, biting down, and general anxeity level will respond well to muscle biofeedback. When a patient is unaccountably dissatisfied with the dental treatment received, reasons may be anxiety and mucle spasm.[13] Biofeedback is most useful in breaking this anxiety cycle. As a means of relaxing the patient before dental work, muscle biofeedback is at least as good as preoperative sedation.

For the patient who has violent reactions to every drug taken and in whom every treatment causes a most unusual response, the element of anxiety should be considered and reduced with muscle biofeedback.

Patients who learn EMG biofeedback may reap a whole host of unexpected, beneficial side effects. For example, once the individual learns good muscle relaxation, often allergy symptoms are reduced, especially when the allergic symptoms are compounded by anxiety. Relief of the temporomandibular joint symptoms also will help the patient's tension headaches. Backache often may be improved. For arthritics who have an undue amount of muscle spasm accompanying their arthritis, biofeedback has been of help. An individual who has learned good muscle relaxation then is able to give autosuggestions while in a state of relaxation. Thus the person can suggest to himself or herself to reduce smoking or to reduce the desire for apple pie. This same learned muscle relaxation can be remembered in the midst of a tough sales meeting to bring on proper relaxation.

In addition to allergic nasal conditions that fail to respond to standard treatment, symptomatic postnasal drip has been found to be relieved. A series of 300 patients who complained of postnasal drip was studied. These patients were found to have markedly impaired nasal mucociliary flow. They were tested with the saccharin test, which consists of placing a particle of saccharin on the inferior nasal turbinate and then determining the speed with which the saccharin particle is moved by the nasal cilia to the back of the throat, where it is then swallowed and tasted on the tongue.[7] These patients then were treated for slowed cilia by using pulsating saline irrigation at 5 psi daily for 2 weeks. On retest, 82% were found to have speeded or normal nasal cilia. After a month approximately 24 patients were found to have nasal cilia that did not respond to this or other treatment. The element of anxiety was suspected, and 15 patients were given a course of biofeedback. After four biofeedback treatments, 12 of the 15 patients had restoration to normal of their nasal mucociliary flow with full or partial relief of symptoms. Thus biofeedback appears to be applicable in many situations in which anxiety influences the presence of symptoms.

Biofeedback for exhaustion

There are many disease entities that can be described as states of exhaustion, including emotional and allergic conditions. The patient who is not getting enough sleep is exhausted, and anxiety reinforces this condition. The patient who has been sneezing for 6 weeks or the patient who scratches the skin or rubs the eyes excessively is also reinforcing these conditions. The patient who has completely failed allergy managment and has had exacerbation of the symptoms for weeks is especially susceptible to exhaustion.

These patients may respond dramatically to biofeedback, which breaks the anxiety-reinforcement cycle and at the same time allows (in a state of relaxation) the body to rest. Nearly all patients, even those who fail to have their symptoms relieved through biofeedback, report that they sleep better.

MUSCLE DISORDER NOT CAUSED BY ANXIETY

Not all tension headaches or temporomandibular joint syndromes are caused by anxiety. The cause of tension headache may be purely physical, as in trying to type while seated in a chair that encourages poor posture or trying to read in dim light with inadequate glasses. A common type of headache may be seen among individuals who purchase a low-slung sports car and then drive crouched extremely low while trying to force the head out of the cockpit to see where they are going. The cure for this is simply a seat cushion. Similarly, bruxism can be brought on by a splinting caused by poor occlusion, a raised bone spicule, a draft to the ear, or other physically caused muscle spasm. An easy way to bring on bruxism is to drive all night with the window open so that cold air blows on the muscles. Indeed, this same cold air can also cause Bell's palsy. Without anxiety, biofeedback can benefit the patient by showing how to use the muscles properly.

CAUTIONS

In using biofeedback, close monitoring is necessary for patients who are hypertensive, diabetic, hyperthyroid, or hypothyroid. These patients may inadvertently improve so that their medication is too strong for them. For example, a hypertensive patient being treated for bruxism may be currently taking 25 mg, hydralazine (Apresoline) and 15 mg hydrochlorothiazide (Esidrix), both tid. The initial blood pressure may be 150/90. After biofeedback treatment the blood pressure may revert toward normal, and then the hypertension medication will become excessive for this patient.

This is particularly true of the newer beta-blocking agents. With biofeedback the autonomic nervous system imbalance tends to become better balanced, and former dosages may become excessive.

CONCLUSION

Since biofeedback is so easy to administer, is noninvasive, and has marked side benefits, this can be recommended as a useful adjunct in the treatment of temporomandibular joint disorders in which an obvious anatomical deformity is not present.

REFERENCES

1. Budzynski, T.H., and Stoyva, J.M.: Feedback-induced relaxation: application to tension headaches, J. Behav. Ther. Psych. **1**:205, 1970.
2. Budzynski, T.H., and Stoyva, J.M.: An electromyographic feedback techinque for teaching voluntary relaxation of the masseter muscle, J. Dent. Res. **52**:116, 1973.
3. Dohrmann, R.J., and Laskin, D.M.: An evaluation of electromyographic biofeedback in the treatment of myofascial pain-dysfuncton syndrome, J. Am. Dent. Assoc. **96**:656, 1978.
4. Gessel, A.H., and Aldeman, M.: Managment of myofascial pain dysfunction syndrome of the temporomandibular joint, Psychosomatics **12**:302, 1971.
5. Green, E.E., et al: Self regulation of internal states. In Rose, J., editor: Progress of cybernetics, London, 1969, Gordon & Breach Science Publishers, Ltd.
6. Grossan, M.: A brief introduction to biofeedback for otolaryngologists, ORL Digest **37**:15, 1975.

7. Grossan, M.: The saccharin test of nasal mucociliary function, Eye Ear Nose Throat Mon. **54**:415, 1975.
7a. Grossan, M.: Treatment of subjective tinnitus with biofeedback, Ear Nose Throat J. **55**:10, 1976.
8. Jacobson, E.: Progressive relaxation, ed. 2, Chicago, 1938, University of Chicago Press.
9. Jacobson, E.: Modern treatment of tense patients: including the neurotic and depressed with case illustrations, follow-ups, and EMG measurements, Springfield, Ill. 1970, Charles C Thomas, Publisher.
10. Kimiya, J.: Biofeedback, Psychol, Today **1**:57, 1968.
11. Laskin, D.: Etiology of the pain dysfunction syndrome, J. Am. Dent. Assoc. **79**:147, 1969.
12. Miller, N.E., et al.: Circulation changes, Circ. Res. (Suppl.) **27**:3, 1970.
13. Moulton, R.D.: Emotional factors in nonorganic temporomandibular joint pain, Dent. Clin. North Am., p. 609, Nov., 1966.
14. Principato, J.J., and Barwell, D.R.: Biofeedback training and relaxation exercises for treamtent of temporomandibular joint dysfunction, Otolaryngology **86**:766, 1978.
15. Schwartz, L.: Disorders of the temporomandibular joint, Philadelphia, 1960, W.B. Saunders Co.
16. Silver, B.V., and Blanchard, E.B.: Biofeedback and relaxation training in the treatment of psychophysiological disorders: or, are the machines really necessary? J. Behav. Med. **1**:217, 1978.
17. Solberg, W.H., and Rugh, J.D.: The use of biofeedback devices in the treatment of bruxism, J. South. Calif. State Dent. Assoc. **40**:852, 1972.
18. Sterman, M.B.: Suppression of seizures in an epileptic following EEG feedback training, Electroencephalogr. Clin. Neurophysiol. **33**:89, 1972.
19. Travell, J.: Temporomandibular joint pain referred from muscles of the head and neck, J. Prosthet. Dent. **10**:745, 1960.
20. Wolpe, J., and Lazaras, A.: Behavior therapy techniques, New York, 1966, Pergamon Press.

19 Acupuncture

HARRY QUINT, Jr., D.D.S., F.A.C.D., F.I.C.D.

If one studies temporomandibular joint dysfunction at all, one observes that there may be a myriad of causes of this problem in the human being. However, the outstanding concern and the priority of treatment procedures are generally the same.

It is traditional procedure for the therapist to discover the cause of the pain and dysfunction of the temporomandibular mechanism and then to correct it. This is easier said than done most times because, unless the pain associated with the dysfunction can be relieved, it is difficult to discover the underlying cause. Often pain and muscle spasm create such a variety of biomechanical and psychological signs and symptoms that one cannot easily remove the screen that obscures the original cause of the problem. When this is the case, there is no question that the first step in treatment is to relieve the pain. Once this is done, the dysfunction phase of the diagnosis and treatment is easier to deal with. Acupuncture is a simple, effective, and conservative pain-control modality recently introduced to Western medicine. It is so effective and simple to use in temporomandibular joint pain control that one would be, in my opinion, unwise not to use it if one knew how. The purpose of this chapter is not to discuss and teach the fundamentals of Chinese acupuncture but to translate the traditional acupuncture treatment into a Western rationale.

It is hoped that by studying this chapter one can learn and use the simple procedures that have been found effective for eliminating some types of temporomandibular mechanism pain.

METHOD OF ADMINISTRATION

Acupuncture treatment is accomplished by inserting needles into appropriate points on appropriate so-called meridians. These meridian points of the Chinese are generally associated with major nerve and arterial pathways, joints, and fascial planes and are described here in Western anatomical terms as well as identified by Chinese acupuncture meridian point nomenclature. This is to help those who have access to traditional acupuncture charts to find and identify these points on the charts, and if one does not have these charts, *Gray's Anatomy* may be helpful.

If one does not have access to acupuncture needles, local anesthetic disposable needles are equally applicable. The 30-gauge 1-inch needle is generally available and adequate for this treatment. It is inexpensive, sterile, small, sharp, and penetrates with little discomfort.

METHOD OF INSERTING THE NEEDLE

Rotating a sharp, small needle between the fingers rapidly and pressing it through the skin rapidly usually results in little or no discomfort to the patient in the acupuncture points used for temporomandibular joint pain. One should practice on one's self first to develop the skill of quick penetration of the skin and to recognize the sensation that indicates when one has reached the proper point with the needle.

SENSATION OF THE NEEDLE

In the area of the needle the patient may feel soreness, distension, heaviness, or numbness if it is placed into the so-called acupuncture point. These sensations may vary from one patient to another. Since thresholds of pain also vary from one person to another, the amount of stimulation used will depend on whom one needles. One should strive for a slight amount of discomfort but avoid causing pain to the patient if possible. If the patient feels no sensation or a great deal of pain, you probably have missed the point. Withdrawal and reinsertion in a slightly different location then should be done.

METHOD OF STIMULATING THE NEEDLE MANUALLY

Increased movement of the needle will cause increased stimulation of the acupuncture point and a quicker result than if it is simply inserted and left immobile in the tissue. The type of stimulation is described for each acupuncture point illustrated.

Acupuncture points used in temporomandibular

joint pain are identified first by their traditional acupuncture meridian number and then anatomically. The innervation and blood supply are identified, and the depth and direction of needle insertion and the type of stimulation are suggested.

LARGE INTESTINE MERIDIAN NO. 4

Anatomically, large intestine meridian no. 4 is in the first dorsal interosseous muscle (Fig. 19-1). It is located by having the patient bring the thumb and forefinger together, then inserting the needle into the highest point of the mound of that muscle. This point is located about 1 cm ulnar to the proximal end of the crease between the thumb and forefinger. Since the point is approximately 1 cm in diameter, it is not difficult to locate and needle. Large intestine meridian no. 4 should be stimulated bilaterally, since often the contralateral site is more effective than the ipsilateral.

Blood supply to area: Branches of radial artery and arterial network on back of hand
Nerve supply to area: Branches of radial, median, and ulnar nerves
Direction of insertion: Perpendicular to skin surface
Depth of insertion: 1/2 to 3/4 inch (or about halfway between back and palm of hand)
Type of stimulation: 1/4 inch up-and-down or in-and-out movement; rotating movement may be used as well
Length of stimulation: 2 minutes if strong, 20 to 30 minutes if weak

Results are notably better if the patient experiences a mild electric shock–like sensation, accompanied by a reflex jerk of the forefinger.

Notes

1. The radial nerve arises from the cervical spinal nerves VI, VII, and VIII. The median nerve arises from cervical spinal nerves V, VI, VII, and VIII. The ulnar nerve arises from cervical spinal nerves VII and VIII and thoracic nerve I.
2. The point is traditionally used for many ailments in Chinese acupuncture treatment, and I have found it to be effective for many head and neck pain problems.
3. If the temporomandibular joint mechanism pain is eliminated by stimulation of this point, there is no need to proceed to the points that are subsequently identified and discussed.
4. If a residue of pain in the joint area exists after this hand point is stimulated, points anterior to the ear and posterior to the TMJ are stimulated.

If pain persists in the area of the temporomandibular joint, the next point to stimulate is small intestine no. 19.

SMALL INTESTINE MERIDIAN NO. 19

Location: Depression behind condyle and anterior to tragus of ear when mouth is opened slightly
Blood supply to area: Branches of temporal artery and vein
Nerve supply to area: Auriculotemporal branch of mandibular division (V3) of cranial nerve V (trigeminal); also possibly zygomatic branches of the cranial nerve VII (facial)
Direction of insertion: Perpendicular to skin
Depth of insertion: 1/4 to 1/2 inch, depending on thickness of skin; it is not important to penetrate into capsule of joint
Type of stimulation: In and out and rotation of needle
Length of stimulation: 2 minutes if strong, 20 to 30 minutes if mild

The patient should experience a mild electric shock–like sensation. If pain still persists in the area immediately surrounding the condyle, needle triple warmer no. 21.

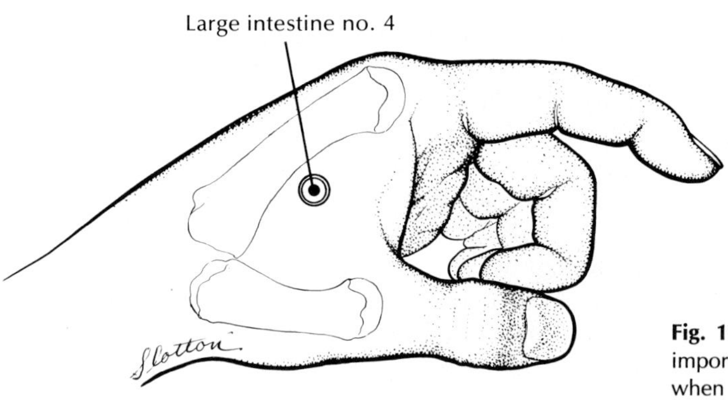

Fig. 19-1. Location of large intestine no. 4 acupuncture point. This is an important point for all head and neck pain. Usually best results are obtained when this point is stimulated bilaterally.

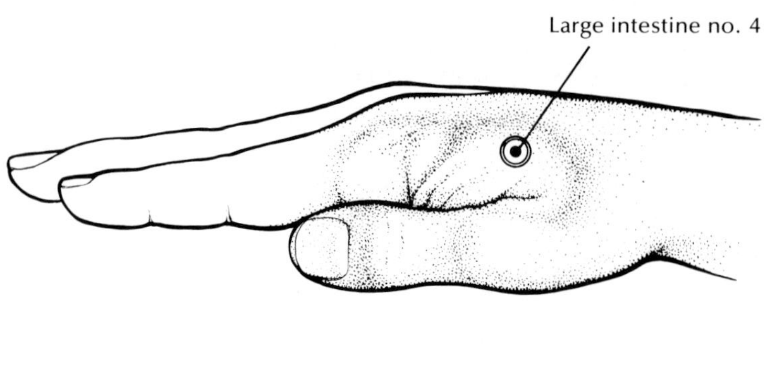

TRIPLE WARMER MERIDIAN NO. 21

Location: In front of ear, at depression between top of tragus and end of helix of ear (Fig. 19-2)
Blood supply to area: Branches of temporal artery and vein
Nerve supply to area: Auriculotemporal branch of mandibular division of the cranial nerve V
Direction of insertion: Perpendicular to skin
Depth of insertion: $^1/_4$ to $^1/_2$ inch, depending on thickness of skin
Type of stimulation: In and out and rotation of needle
Length of stimulation: 2 minutes if strong, 20 to 30 minutes if mild

The patient should experience a mild electric shock–like sensation. If pain still persists in the area immediately surrounding the condyle, needle gallbladder no. 2.

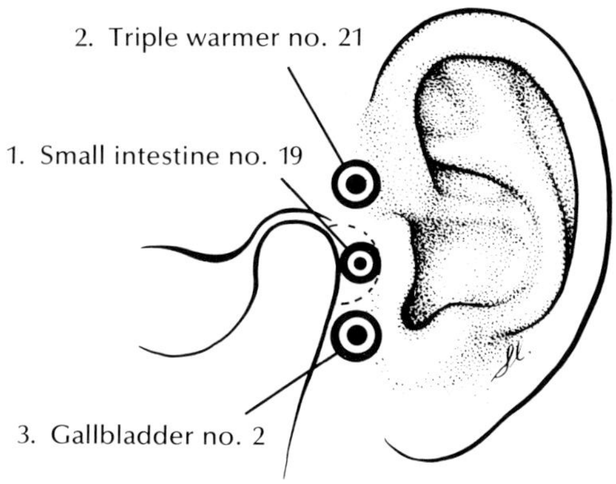

Fig. 19-2. Location of the three acupuncture points in condyle and TMJ area anterior to ear. They should be used in order numbered.

GALLBLADDER MERIDIAN NO. 2

Location: Just below head of condyle, anterior and inferior to tragus and just anterior to tragal notch (Fig. 19-2)
Blood supply to area: Branches of temporal artery and vein
Nerve supply to area: Auriculotemporal branch of mandibular division of the cranial nerve V; also branches of the cranial nerve VII
Direction of insertion: Perpendicular to skin
Depth of insertion: $^1/_4$ to $^1/_2$ inch, depending on skin thickness
Type of stimulation: In and out and rotation of needle
Length of stimulation: 2 minutes if strong, 20 to 30 minutes if mild

The patient should experience a mild electric shock–like sensation. If pain still persists in the area, needle stomach no. 6.

STOMACH MERIDIAN NO. 6

Location: In depression of masseter muscle, a finger's width anterior and superior to angle of mandible; this depression is sensitive to firm finger pressure (Fig. 19-3)

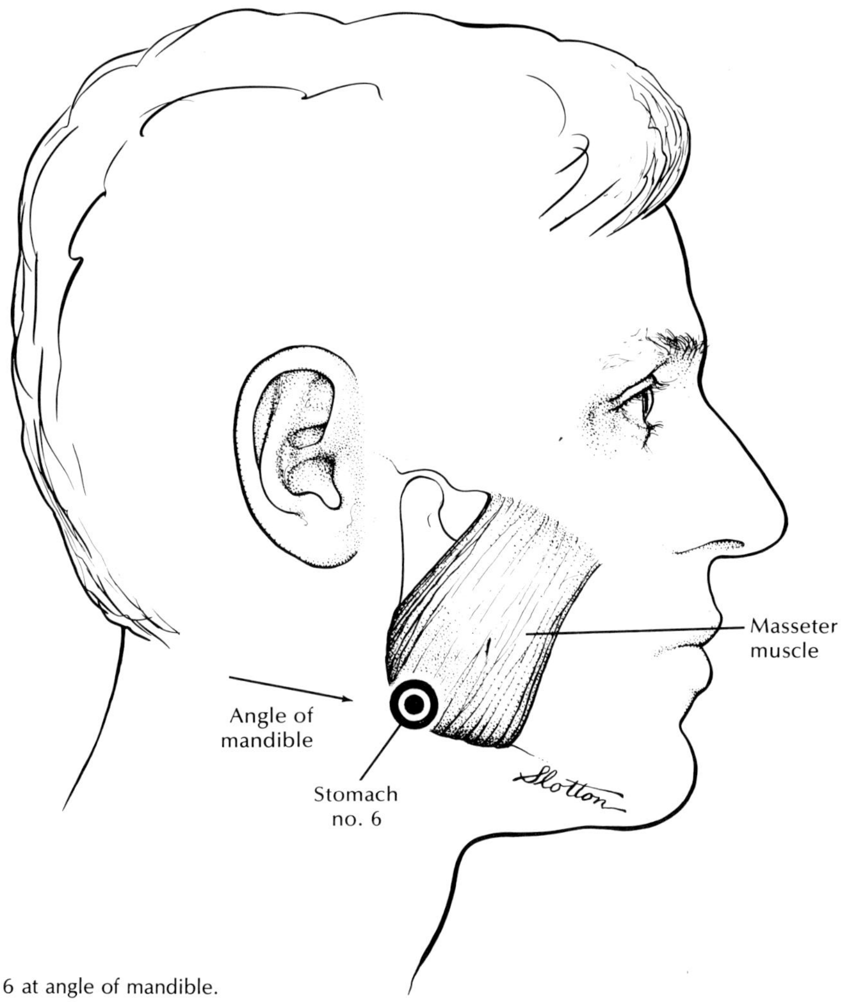

Fig. 19-3. Location of acupuncture point stomach no. 6 at angle of mandible.

Blood supply to area: A branch of internal maxillary artery
Nerve supply to area: Auriculotemporal branch of the mandibular division of the cranial nerve V; also branches of the cranial nerve VII
Direction of insertion: Perpendicular to skin
Depth of insertion: $^1/_4$ to $^1/_2$ inch, depending on thickness of skin
Type of stimulation: In and out and rotation
Length of stimulation: 2 minutes if strong, 20 to 30 minutes if mild

The patient should experience a mild electric shock–like sensation. If pain continues subsequent to the foregoing treatment, needle stomach no. 7.

STOMACH MERIDIAN NO. 7

Location: In mandibular notch area below zygomatic arch and $1^1/_2$ cm anterior to condyle (Fig. 19-4)
Blood supply to area: Facial artery and vein
Nerve supply to area: Auriculotemporal branches of mandibular division of the cranial nerve V; also muscular branches of V3 to the masseter and pterygoid muscles and possibly zygomatic branches of the cranial nerve VII
Direction of insertion: Perpendicular to skin surface
Depth of insertion: $^1/_4$ to $^1/_2$ inch, depending on thickness of skin
Type of stimulation: In and out and rotation of needle
Length of stimulation: 2 minutes if strong, 20 to 30 minutes if mild

The patient should experience a mild electric shock–like sensation or perhaps a hot, burning sensation around the point of the needle.

DISCUSSION

Relief of temporomandibular joint pain with acupuncture has been found to be effective. In some cases relief will be dramatic with perhaps unilateral needling in only the hand point (large intestine no. 4). Generally

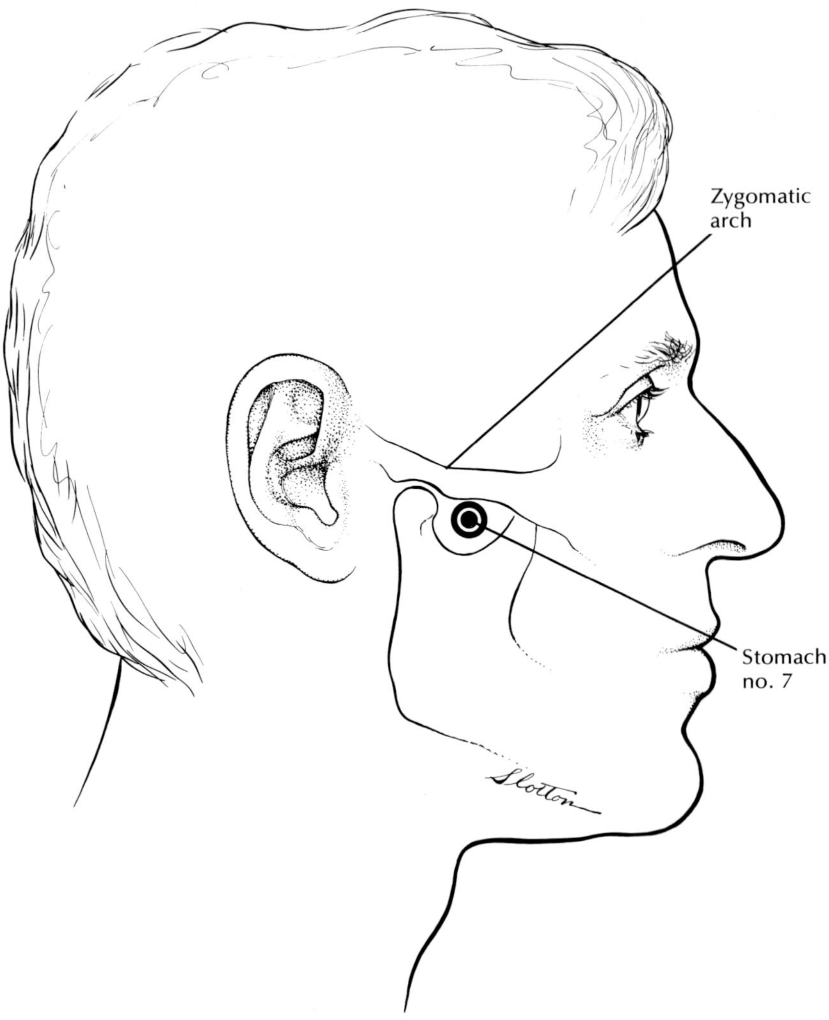

Fig. 19-4. Location of acupuncture point stomach no. 7 below zygomatic arch in mandibular notch.

one or two other points are added, but only if there is some residual pain. Usually the small intestine no. 19 in addition to large intestine no. 4 is all that is needed. If trigger points are detected in the bellies of the masseter in the sternocleidomastoid, temporal, or upper areas of the trapezius muscles, needling of these pressure-sensitive areas is indicated and is often productive.

Relief of pain does not always eliminate the trismus when it is associated in the syndrome. However, relief of pain allows one to prescribe and use stretching exercises or other means to diagnose and treat the problem.

Pain may disappear and not reappear, but one should explain to the patient that it may return and that further treatment might be required. Generally, in the case of recurrent problems one can expect to have the episodes grow further and further apart.

If the pain does not recur, there is no need to routinely continue the acupuncture treatments. If one can detect the cause of the problem after pain relief, one should proceed with appropriate therapy.

Since acupuncture is simple, conservative, and so economical of time, it should be the palliative treatment of choice in most instances.

Not much can be accomplished in TMJ diagnosis and corrective therapy until the crippling effects of pain and muscle spasm can be relieved. Acupuncture is not a panacea for TMJ problems, but it should be incorporated in the modern Western therapeutic repertoire.

RECOMMENDED READINGS

Academy of Traditional Chinese Medicine: An outline of Chinese acupuncture, Peking, 1975, China Books.

Choi, Y.W.: The topography of meridians, Alhambra, Calif., 1973, Cunningham Press.

Goss, C.M., editor: Gray's anatomy of the human body, ed. 29, Philadelphia, 1973, Lea & Febiger.

Koa, F.F., and Koa, J.J.: Acupuncture therapeutics, New Haven, 1973, Eastern Press.

Tan, L.T., et al.: Acupuncture therapy: current Chinese practice, Philadelphia, 1973, Temple University Press.

20 Electrical acupoint therapy for temporomandibular joint–myofacial pain

ROBERT J. PESHEK, D.D.S.

This chapter deals with the treatment of temporomandibular joint–myofacial pain using electrical acupoint procedures. The treatments are painless.

TREATING TEMPOROMANDIBULAR JOINT–MYOFACIAL PAIN WITH AURICULAR ELECTROACUPUNCTURE

The theory of treatment with auricular electroacupuncture was developed as a result of applying the principles of Oriental medicine related to acupuncture and nutrition. No explanation can be given of how the treatment works; however, it seems logical to assume that membrane potentials of cells are put into balance, which eliminates pain. Recent studies[1] have shown the release of druglike chemicals from the central nervous system that are capable of preventing pain.

Acupuncture is essentially based on various energy balances or imbalances in the body. This energy is said to be flowing through 12 channels, called meridians.[6] The 12 meridians are named after organs of the body: (1) liver, (2) gallbladder, (3) heart, (4) small intestine, (5) heart constrictor (blood vessels), (6) triple heater (lymph), (7) spleen-pancreas, (8) stomach, (9) lung, (10) large intestine, (11) kidney, and (12) bladder. When the energy flow through these 12 meridians is out of balance, symptoms occur in the body, such as headaches, dizziness, insomnia, lack of energy, and pain in muscles.

Imbalances of meridians are "recorded" in various areas of the ear.[5] The ear is a minicomputer that records problem areas throughout the body. Other areas such as the hands, feet, and skull also are minicomputers that record meridian imbalances, and these areas frequently are used for treating imbalances of meridians. However, because of the compact, easy accessibility of points in the ear, the ear is the organ of first choice in treating the pains associated with the temporomandibular area which are usually associated with the muscles of mastication. The foot is the second choice, and the hand is the third.

When a patient comes to the office with pain in a temporomandibular joint or muscle, the occlusion is examined for malfunction. If occlusal problems exist, they are corrected, and the patient is released for several weeks. If pain continues, or if there are no occlusal problems, the patient is examined for imbalances in body chemistry.[7-9] I try to determine if the pain is caused by (1) a muscle-tendon-ligament condition, (2) a biological nutritional condition, (3) bone dysfunction, (4) referral from another organ system, causing imbalances in the 12 meridians, or (5) a neurological condition.

It has been my observation, based on clinical experience, that most of the pain associated with the temporomandibular joint area is not caused by the bony parts of the joint itself but rather by the imbalance of the muscles, ligaments, and neurological structures associated with this area. Many pains found in the temporomandibular area are referred pains from the cervical neck area, usually as a result of an old known or unknown injury. Prolotherapy (the injecting of ligaments and tendons with a solution of a dextrose proliferate stock solution containing 2.5% phenol, 25% glucose, and 25% propylene glycol in sterile water, diluted 1:2 with 1% aqueous lidocaine [Xylocaine] or 0.15% tetracaine [Pontocaine]) is used as a treatment to eliminate many referred pains to the temporomandibular joint area from the cervical neck area.[4]

The management of temporomandibular joint problems usually is approached through occlusal adjustment of the teeth by the dentist. There is a well-known direct relationship between malfunctioning occlusion and muscle function associated with the temporomandibular joints. Many such oral-related pains can be corrected by the dentist; however, there are many patients who do not obtain relief from pain in the temporomandibular joint area on completion of occlusal corrections. These are the patients who are candidates for electroacupuncture therapy.

No matter what the cause, there is usually a biochemical nutritional imbalance associated with this pain, and biological nutritional supplementation needs to be given. This is determined by a series of nutritional kinesiology tests, nutritional endocardiograph[8] tests, blood chemistry tests, and the use of auricular electrodiagnosis.[7-9]

Auricular electroacupuncture without needles is used to treat most meridian imbalances and muscle, tendon, or ligament conditions.

Procedure of treatment

1. An electrotranscutaneous stimulator is used to treat the ear points. The Accu-O-Matic or the Mini-O-Matic electrotranscutaneous stimulators* are recommended (Figs. 20-1 to 20-3).
2. An ear chart is used to locate the ear points (Fig. 20-4).
3. The Accu-O-Matic instrument is set on 20 Hz for 20 seconds, until the patient feels just a slight stinging sensation with the general purpose probe. The treatment is painless if a cotton tip wetted with saline water is used as the probe.
4. Clean the patient's ear with alcohol to remove hair spray and oil.
5. Treat the gallbladder point first, that is, no. 96 in the right ear (according to *The Ear Meridian Points Form*[2]; other charts have different numbering systems), for 2 to 4 or more minutes. The majority of temporomandibular joint-muscle-meridian imbalances are caused by an imbalance in the gallbladder. This statement is based on results of my 9 years of clinical nutritional research. *Gallbladder* refers to the bile system of the body. There is only one gallbladder point, which is located in the right ear (Fig. 20-4).
6. Treat each of the following points for 2 to 4 minutes *or* until no more relief from pain is obtained on that point. Always ask the patient to check for the percentage of relief from each point. Write this information on *The Ear Meridian Points Form*[2] so you can use the major relief points for any future treatments.
   a. Small intestine point nos. 88 and 89
   b. Triple heater point no. 104
   c. Stomach point no. 87
   d. Bladder point no. 92
   e. Large intestine point no. 91
   f. Kidney point no. 95
7. Treat the right ear for pain on the right side. The patient often will receive up to 50% relief on the left side when the right side is being treated, and vice versa.
8. Treat the left ear. If the pain is only on one side, treat only the ear on that side.
9. By the time you treat the kidney point, all or 98% of the pain in the TMJ is gone if the pain is caused by an imbalance of energy in the 12 meridians. The remaining 2% of pain can be eliminated by treating two points in the toes (gallbladder no. 43 and liver no. 2) with the Accu-O-Matic set on the same readings (Fig. 20-5).[10] Treat each toe point until maximum relief from pain is obtained. If there is still some pain remaining, needle acupuncture can be used in the hand point large intestine no. 4 and the foot point stomach no. 44 on the right and left sides (Figs. 20-6 and 20-7). Regular disposable 30-gauge dental needles are used. These points should be learned by the practitioner, since various phantom pains of the head and neck often can be eliminated when needled. The needles are left in for 1 hour.

*Distributed by Color Coded Systems, 7759 California Ave., Riverside, Calif. 92504. The Accu-O-Matic is now known as the My-O-Matic, and the Mini-O-Matic is now known as the Mini-My-O-Matic.

Clinical conclusions of treatment

The pain associated with the temporomandibular joint can be eliminated with the treatment of the first ear point, gallbladder no. 96, within seconds, or there may be a gradual dissipation of pain as treatment progresses to each point.

One to three appointments lasting from 30 to 40 minutes each usually are required to relieve pain and/or to correct the range of restricted mandibular motion. There are numerous case histories in my records of patients who were treated 5 years ago without recurrence of pain and/or restriction of mandibular motion. Some patients' pain will come back from a few hours to several weeks after treatment. Many of these patients have biological nutritional imbalances, and these imbalances have to be corrected.

If there is a simple biological nutritional imbalance in the patient, often there will be pain over the temporomandibular joint when palpated. This pain often can be eliminated by treating the toe point gallbladder no. 43 with the Accu-O-Matic or the Mini-O-Matic for

A

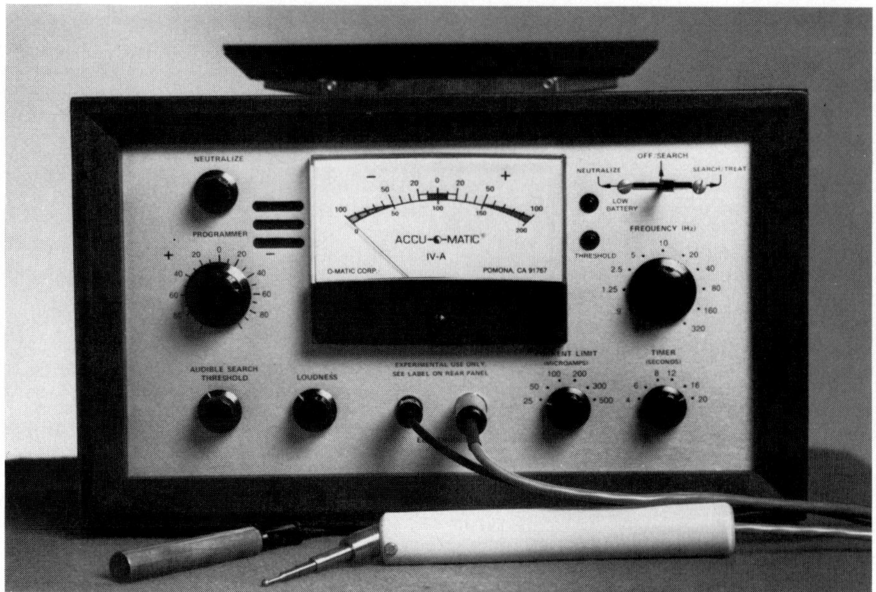

B

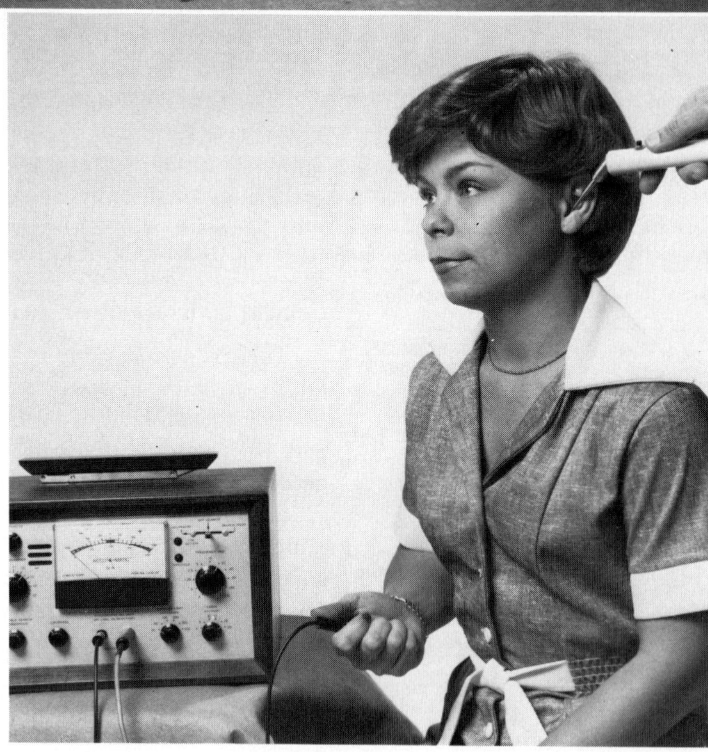

Fig. 20-1. A, Accu-O-Matic instrument used for electrotranscutaneous stimulation of acupuncture and electrical points; it is also a point finder. **B,** Treating ear points with Accu-O-Matic instrument.

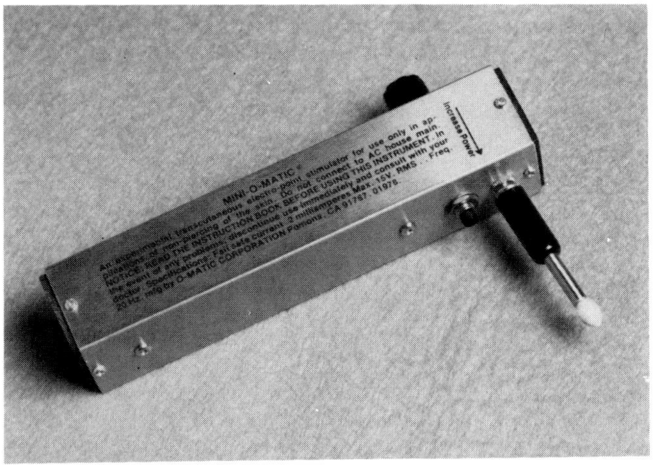

Fig. 20-2. Mini-O-Matic instrument used for electrotranscutaneous stimulation of acupuncture and electrical points. It cannot locate points.

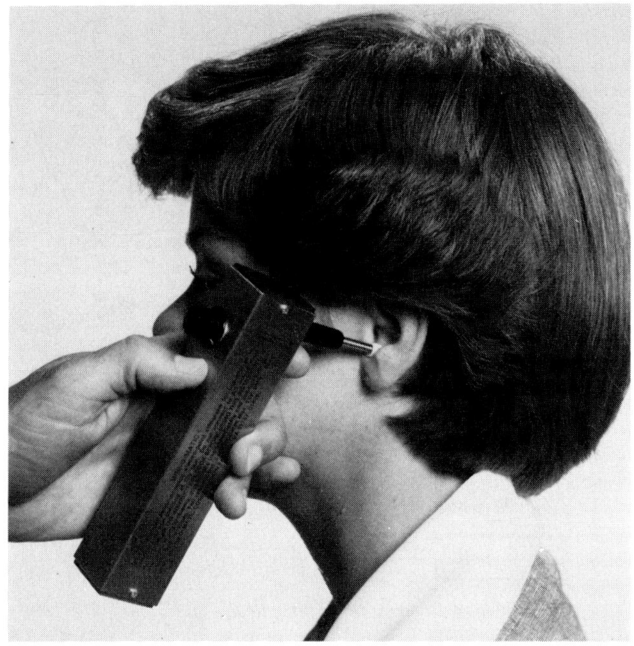

Fig. 20-3. Mini-O-Matic instrument treating ear points.

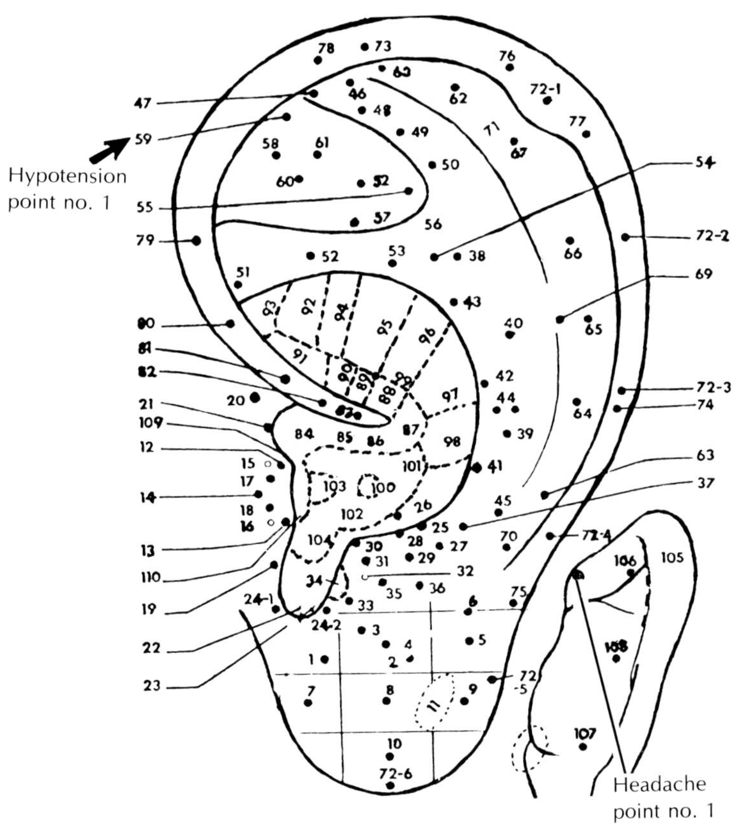

Fig. 20-4. Wong's ear points representing areas of body. (From Peshek, R.J.: Balancing body chemistry with nutrition, Riverside, Calif., 1979, Color Coded Systems.)

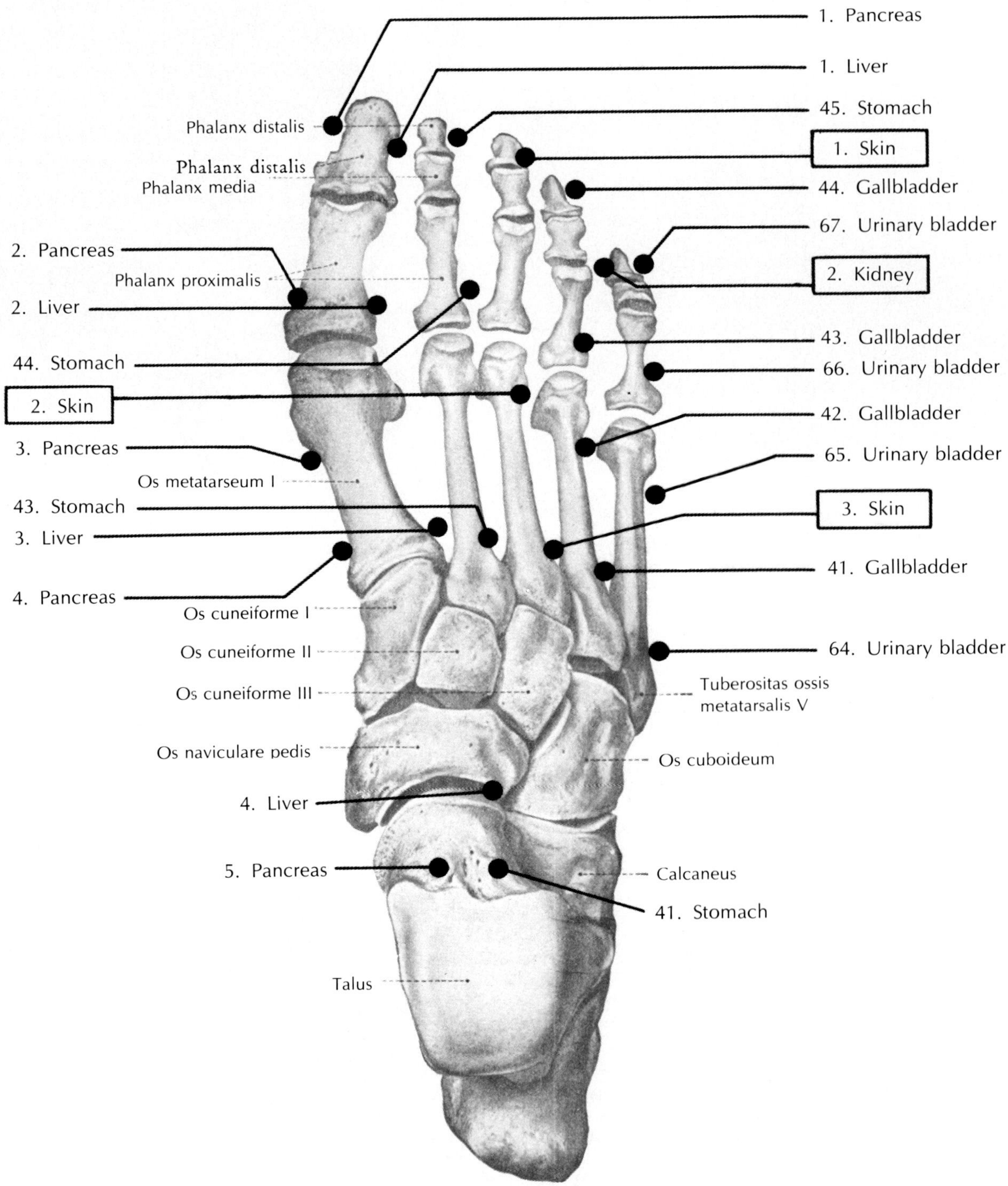

Fig. 20-5. Voll's foot points. (From Voll, R.H.: Topographic positions of the measurement points in electroacupuncture, vol. 1, Uelzen, 1976, Medizinisch Literarische Verlagsgesellschaft.)

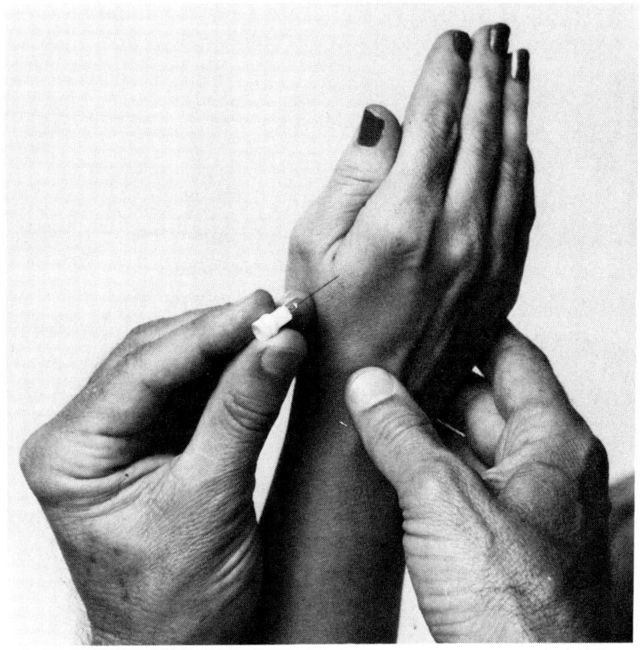

Fig. 20-6. Acupuncture point large intestine no. 4; locate with Accu-O-Matic instrument. Put index finger close to thumb. There is a fold that forms. Go 1/4 inch toward top of hand from tip of fold. Insert needle 1/4 to 1/2 inch and move up and down and around until a shock sensation is felt by patient.

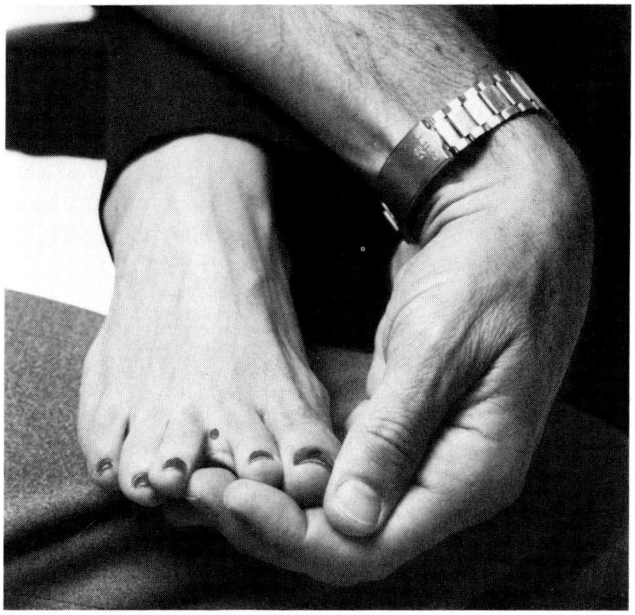

Fig. 20-7. Acupuncture point stomach no. 44, located in between second and third toe; locate with Accu-O-Matic instrument. No shock sensation is felt in this point.

several minutes or until the pressure pain is gone. No other treatment is required.

Palpation pain of the temporomandibular joint will come and go, and I believe this to be a reflex or referred pain to this area as a result of biological nutritional imbalance that occurs constantly within muscles. The muscle involved can be located any place in the body.[3]

TREATING PERIPHERAL EAR POINTS

Myofacial pain also can be treated through the peripheral areas of the ear that correspond to the local structures of the muscles, tendons, and ligaments as they relate to the temporomandibular joint. The ear chart in Fig. 20-4 and the Accu-O-Matic are used for this treatment procedure.

Locating sensitive ear points

1. Put the Accu-O-Matic programmer on −60.
2. Put the off/search switch to search/treat.
3. Put the ball probe into the hand probe. The small pointed probe can be used to be more accurate and precise.
4. Clean the ear with alcohol and let it dry thoroughly.
5. Have the patient hold the hand probe in either hand.
6. Explore the area of the ear around nos. 37, 27, 32, 6, and 5. Locate the points in this area that are more sensitive. This area corresponds locally to the temporomandibular joint and related tissues of muscles, tendons, and ligaments. The most sensitive points will activate the neurometer dial on the Accu-O-Matic toward the red zone. As you reduce the programmer (closer to zero), only the most sensitive ear points will register a reading of various degrees on the neurometer. The object is to find the most sensitive points in this area of the ear, which may be one or several points. If the temporomandibular joint pain is in the right ear, locate only those points in the right ear; if it is in the left ear, locate only those points in the left ear. The peripheral ear points seem to relate to therapy only on the side of pain, even though in organ treatment there can be an overlapping of treatment results from

the opposite ear. When treating the gallbladder point found only in the right ear, pain in the left temporomandibular joint can be corrected up to 100% from the right ear. However, when treating peripheral points (nonorgan points) of the ear, always try the opposite ear, since in some patients relief from pain is obtained. I find this true more often in cases other then temporomandibular joint pain. Put an ink mark on points so you can refer back to them quickly. Turn the programmer dial down, or closer to zero, and explore again. When you have found the most sensitive one to four points, stop exploring. You are now ready to start treatment.

Treatment of ear points

1. Set the Accu-O-Matic frequency dial to 20 Hz.
2. Set the time to 20 seconds.
3. Set the current microamperage dial to a setting that is comfortable for the patient.
4. Use the ball metal probe for treatment. If the patient feels uncomfortable pain with the lowest current setting, use the cotton tip probe for treatment. This will enable you to use more current without pain. However, you cannot be as precise with the treatment area.
5. Set the off/search to search/treat.
6. Put the treatment probe on the first ear point that you want to treat, and set the button on the hand probe on treat.
7. The other hand probe can be held in either hand by the patient.
8. Treat the point until no more relief from temporomandibular joint pain is obtained. Then move on to the next ear point.
9. Repeat this procedure until maximum temporomandibular joint pain results are obtained. Often the temporomandibular joint pain will get worse as a point of the ear is being treated. If this occurs, treat the same ear point area on the back of the ear. This usually reverses this action. Some patients' temporomandibular joint pain will dissipate by treating only the back of the ear that corresponds to the located ear points on the front of the ear.

Results of treatment

The results of treating just the peripheral ear points will range from no relief to 100% relief from all temporomandibular joint–related pain and from no relief to 100% relief from functional jaw problems. The lasting effects of such treatment vary with patients. Many patients will experience greater relief of pain after a few days. This is especially true if there is any inflammation present in the involved area of discomfort.

TREATING GOLGI ORGANS, SPINDLE CELLS, AND MISCELLANEOUS ELECTROACUPUNCTURE POINTS

If the treatment of auricular organs and peripheral auricular points does not give optimum relief of temporomandibular joint pain, often the pain can be eliminated or the range of motion of the jaw improved by treating the area of pain directly with a Golgi organ treatment, spindle cell treatment, or various electrosensitive acupuncture point (trigger points) treatments on the involved muscle.[11,12]

Setting on the Accu-O-Matic

Set the frequency to 0.6 Hz for 0.6 seconds with a current of 100 or more μA. The cotton swab probe or the ball metal probe can be used. If the swab is used, wet it with saline water. Put the off/search switch to search/treat.

Golgi organ treatment

Place the treatment swab probe or ball metal probe on the origin area of the masseter muscle and the hand-held probe (with the probe removed, just use the metal clip) held also by the clinician on the insertion area of the masseter muscle (Fig. 20-8). Press the treatment button. Repeat several times along the path of origin and insertion. Better results may be obtained if the muscle is put into function and the two probes are pushed apart with a gentle pressure. Treat until no more results are obtained.

Spindle cell treatment

Place the two probes about 12 mm apart in the belly of the masseter muscle, and press the muscle together gently with both probes (Fig. 20-9). Press the treatment button and treat the muscle in several areas until no more relief from pain is obtained. The muscle does not have to be in function.

Miscellaneous electroacupuncture points

Treat just like with the spindle cell procedure but treat the area of pain only. Circle the area with several treatment cycles or until no more relief from pain is obtained.

Place the hand-held probe in the patient's hand. Put the off/search switch to search/treat. Place the progammer on about −60 (higher or lower as needed). Explore the area posterior and anterior to the angle of the jaw for any sensitive points (Fig. 20-10). The ball metal probe is used. The neurometer on the Accu-O-Matic

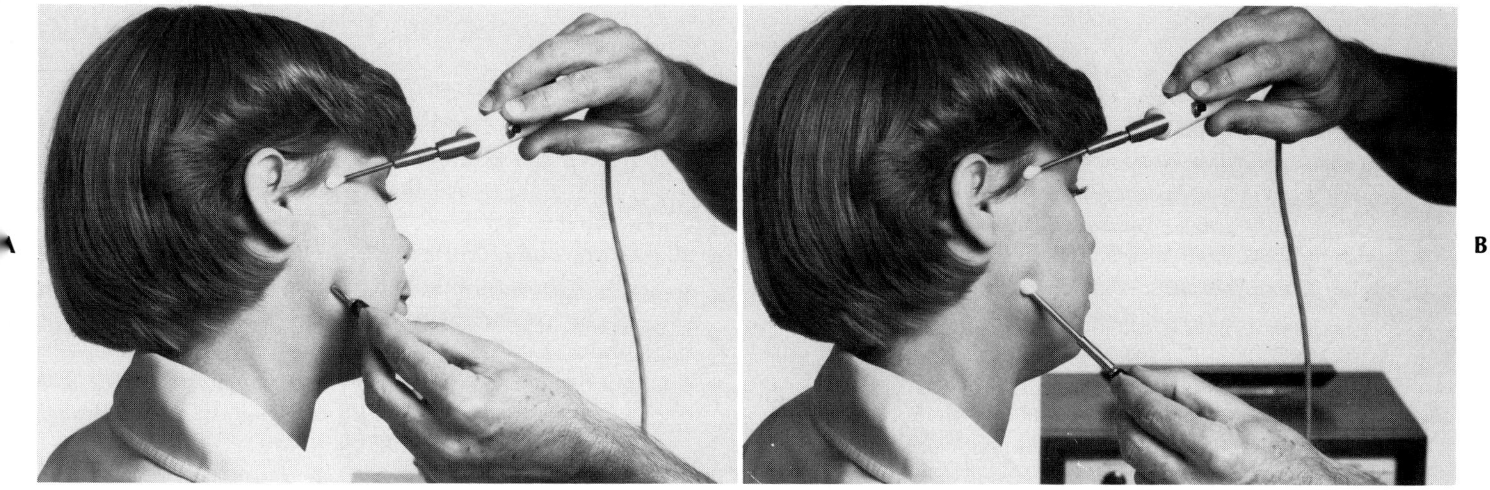

Fig. 20-8. Using Accu-O-Matic instrument to treat Golgi points **(A)** and muscle Golgi points **(B)**.

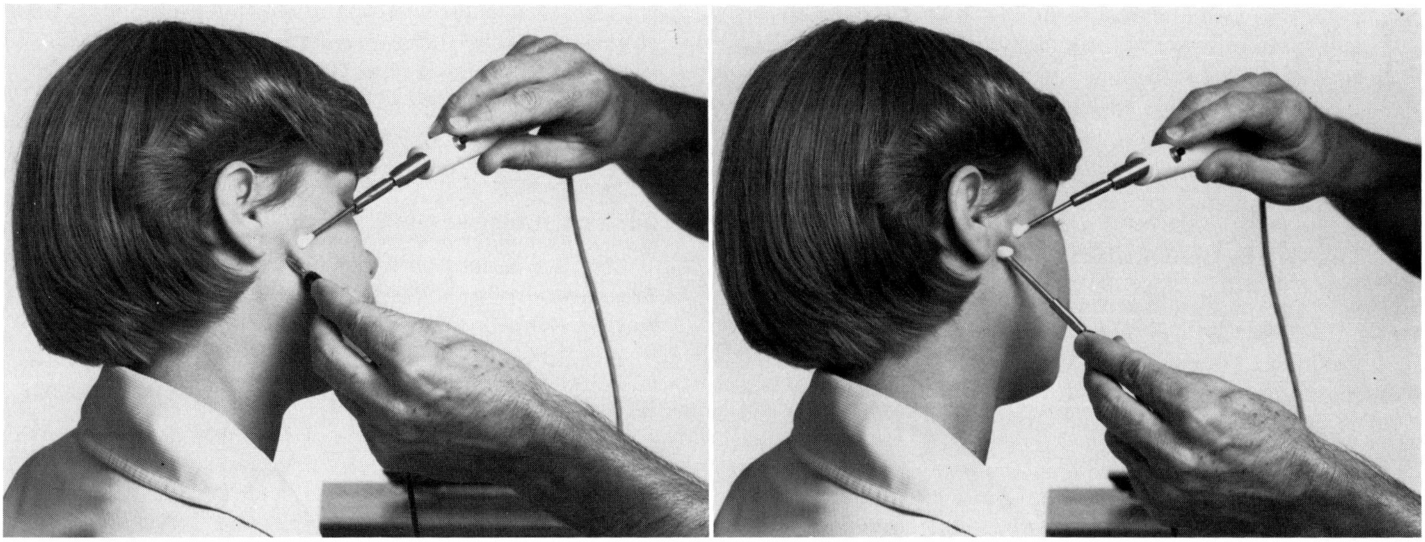

Fig. 20-9. Treating spindle cells with Accu-O-Matic instrument.

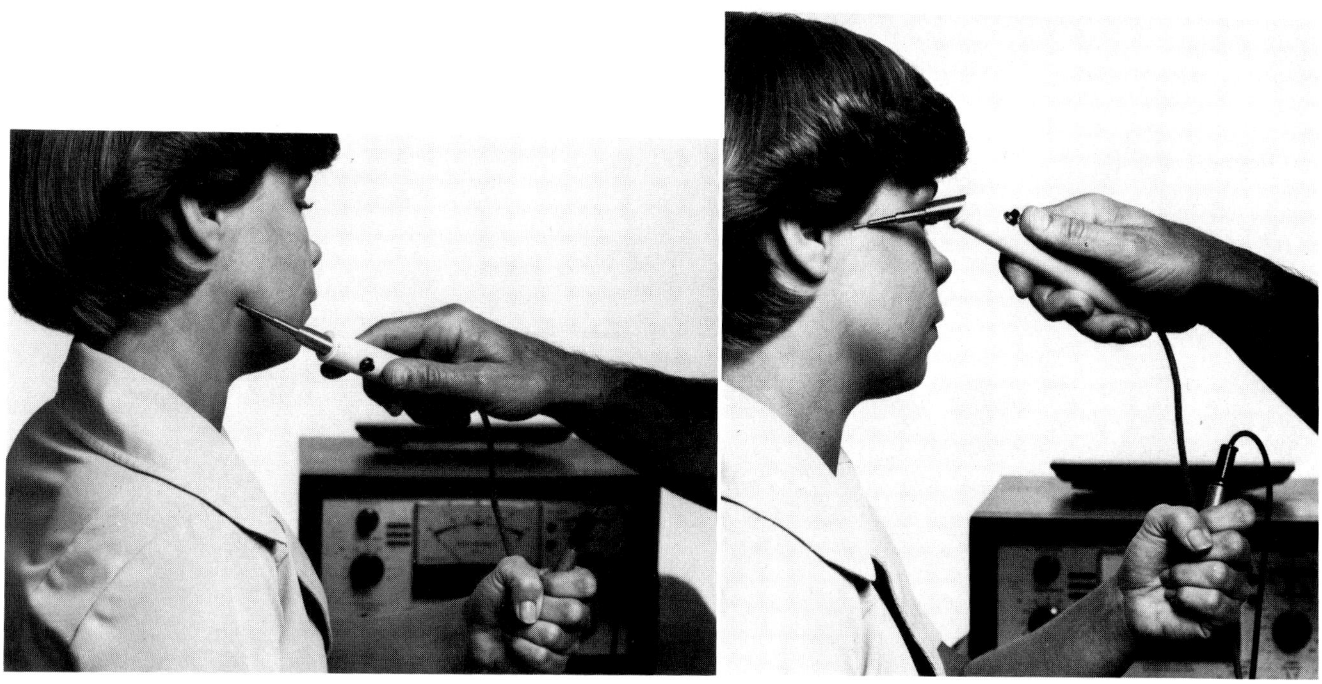

Fig. 20-10. Locating and treating hot spots, or trigger areas, with Accu-O-Matic instrument.

will indicate "hot spots" by a swing of the needle toward the red zone. Explore the body of the masseter muscle upward to just above the temporomandibular joint socket area. When you have discovered sensitive points, mark them with an ink pen. Check the sternocleidomastoid and upper trapezius muscles for hot spots. Treat the most sensitive areas, with the handheld probe being held by the patient. Treat until no more relief from pain is obtained. There are two points that seem to be common for most patients, one just anterior and under the angle of the mandibular bone and one over or near the temporomandibular joint socket; the former gives more relief from temporomandibular joint pain than does the latter.

Results of treatment vary from 100% relief from temporomandibular pain to no relief from pain. The pain often will be less a few days after the treatment and often will not return. Some patients' pain will return after a few days to several months. Several treatments spread over several days to several weeks give lasting results. Some patients may have to return monthly for treatment to maintain relief. Treatment schedules vary with each patient.

TREATING HEADACHES WITH ELECTROACUPUNCTURE

Either the Accu-O-Matic or Mini-O-Matic instrument can be used to treat headaches using electroacupuncture points. The setting for the Accu-O-Matic instrument is 20 Hz, 20 seconds, search/treat, with the current set to where the patient feels just a slight sting when the metal probe is used. If the cotton tip is being used, no feeling is usually experienced.

In the Mini-O-Matic instrument there is a built-in 20 Hz adjustable current. Make sure when you treat with the Mini-O-Matic instrument that you touch the skin of the patient with your free hand to ground the instrument. Otherwise you will be treating yourself.

Three electroacupuncture points are used:

1. Pituitary forehead point, or the Peshek antiheadache point (Figs. 20-11 and 20-12)
2. Ear point no. 59, or the hypotension point (see Fig. 20-4)
3. On the back of the ear, headache point no. 1 (see Fig. 20-4)

The headache that responds to this treatment probably is caused by imbalances in membrane potentials of various types of muscles. Headaches that do not respond to electroacupuncture therapy can often be corrected by balancing the body chemistry with nutrition.[7,8,10]

Pituitary forehead point

Set the patient on a chair in front of you. To locate the pituitary forehead point, place the fingers of both hands on the protuberance of the frontal bone. Move down until your fingers fall onto the base of this protuberance. Mentally draw a horizontal line that bisects

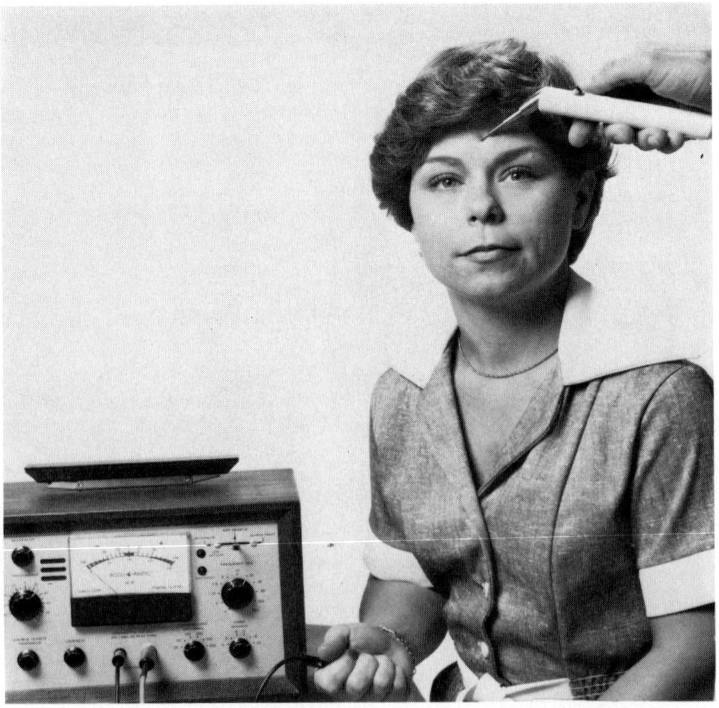

Fig. 20-11. Peshek antiheadache point being treated with Accu-O-Matic transcutaneous stimulator.

the vertical midline (governing vessel). Where the two lines bisect is where the pituitary forehead point is.

Stimulate this point until the patient starts to get relief from the headache. This may require from a few to 4 or more minutes. Instruct the patient to tell you when he or she is not getting any more relief from the headache. If relief continues, keep stimulating the point until no more relief is obtained (this may take 5 to 10 minutes) or until the headache is gone.

If the headache disappears, no further treatment is required. I have had many patients with chronic headaches every day of their life be treated on this one point and experience complete relief with no reccurrence.

If there is a certain percentage of the headache still remaining after treating the pituitary point, continue with the next point.

Headache point no. 1

On the back of the ear, just a few millimeters distal to where the top of the ear meets the skull, is where headache point no. 1 is located. Treat it until no more relief from pain is obtained, which may be from a few to several minutes. If the headache stops, no more treatment is necessary.

If you have obtained relief with this point but there is still some pain, continue to the next point.

Ear point no. 59

Ear point no. 59 is on the front of the ear and is also known as the depressing point or the hypotension point.

By the time you get to this point, most of the headache is gone. Often the only area that still needs relief is in the upper back, shoulder, or neck area. Treatment of point no. 59 will relax these muscles and relieve the headache. Care must be taken not to stimulate this point too much, since the pain in these areas can come back, which will then contribute to another headache. Treat both ears.

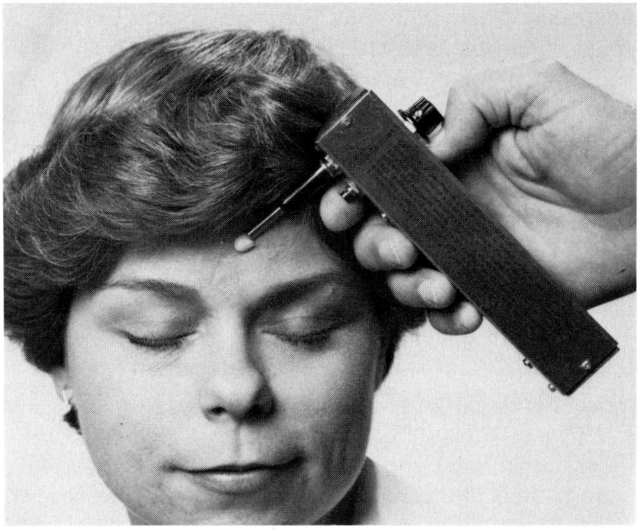

Fig. 20-12. Peshek antiheadache point being treated with Mini-O-Matic transcutaneous stimulator.

SUMMARY

Electrical acupoint therapy for the treatment of temporomandibular joint and/or myofacial pain provides another dimension in eliminating symptoms for patients. This type of therapy is in its infancy; however, the results seen over the last 10 years have been outstanding.

Although this chapter discusses only the electrical therapy of the temporomandibular joint–myofacial pain, one should be acutely aware that many patients' symptoms are caused by biochemical nutritional imbalances. (I estimate the figure to be as high as 75%.) References have been given for continued studies in the area of biochemical nutrition.[7,8,10]

Electrical acupoint therapy, when used in conjunction with occlusal equilibration, orthopedic repositioning appliances, biochemical nutrition, needle acupuncture, and possibly surgery, will give the treating clinician a well-rounded armamentarium in the treatment of temporomandibular joint–myofacial pain.

REFERENCES

1. Chinese connect acupuncture and brain chemistry, Medical Tribune, Feb. 19, 1975.
2. The ear meridian points form, Riverside, Calif., Color Coded Systems.
3. Houston, F.M.: The healing benefits of acupressure, New Canaan, Conn., 1974, Keats Publishing, Inc.
4. Kayfetz, D.O., et al.: Whiplash injury and other ligamentous headache—its management with prolotherapy, Headache **3**:21, 1963.
5. Lu, H.C.: A complete textbook of auricular acupuncture, Vancouver, British Columbia, Canada, 1973, The Academy of Oriental Heritage.
6. Mann, F.: Acupuncture, the ancient Chinese art of healing and how it works scientifically, New York, 1971, Random House, Inc.
7. Peshek, R.J.: Balancing body chemistry with nutrition, Riverside, Calif., 1977, Color Coded Systems.
8. Peshek, R.J.: Nutrition for a healthy heart—for the treatment of pain TMJ-myofacial and angina, Riverside, Calif., 1979, Color Coded Systems.
9. Peshek, R.J.: Clinical nutrition—using the seven lines of defense against disease, Riverside, Calif., 1980, Color Coded Systems.
10. Voll, R.: Topographic positions of the measurement points in electro-acupuncture, vol. 1, Riverside, Calif., 1979, Color Coded Systems.
11. Wing, C.: See-Do, Lower Lake, Calif., 1980, See-Do.
12. Wing, T.: The theory of applied electro-acupuncture and technique of non-needle acupoint therapy, Lower Lake, Calif., 1980, See-Do.

21 Pharmacological methods

WILLIAM P. HALL, M.D.

The role of pharmaceutical agents in the treatment of temporomandibular joint disorders is one of considerable controversy. Opinions vary from, "Drugs have no place in the management of TMJ problems," to "Give them all diazepam, and no other treatment is needed." The naive thinking expressed by both of these viewpoints has led to increasing patient dissatisfaction with and distrust of the medical and dental professions and reinforces the growing tendency of patients to seek unconventional methods and to self-medicate and self-treat, often with disastrous results.

Only after taking a careful history, performing a physical examination, and establishing a rapport with the patient, based on an understanding of the problem and a willingness to help, should medications be prescribed. Pharmaceutical methods used in this context enhance the art as well as the science of medicine. Before diagnostic procedures have been performed to delineate the problem, drugs may not only help to alleviate symptoms, but response may actually shed considerable light on establishing a proper diagnosis.

Physical, psychological, mechanical, and surgical modalities are available in the treatment of TMJ disorders, and the reader is referred to other chapters in this book for descriptions of these methods and their application. Drugs rarely are used as primary therapeutic agents but can and should be employed as adjunctive therapy. Specific categories of available pharmaceutical agents are discussed here as well as their place in the management of TMJ problems.

ANALGESICS AND ANTIINFLAMMATORY AGENTS

Humans have searched the world for the perfect drug to relieve pain. In *Paradise Lost* Milton declared, "Pain is perfect misery, the worst of evils; and excessive, overturns all patience." Cases have been reported by Morgan and others in which the pain in TMJ disease has driven the suffering patient to suicide. The use of analgesics is a double-edged sword, and addiction may be a major problem in patients suffering from chronic pain. The practitioner must not only be familiar with the actions of analgesics but also must diagnose and relieve the underlying causative disorder as expeditiously as possible to prevent drug abuse.

Salicylic acid and its derivatives, the most commonly used being acetylsalicylic acid, or aspirin, are analgesics that also have antipyretic and antiinflammatory actions. The type of pain amenable to relief by salicylates is low intensity, particularly myalgia, headache, and arthralgia, rather than visceral pain.[4] For years it was believed that the main analgesic action of the salicylates was on the central nervous system; however, recent research[8a] has revealed that peripheral mechanisms also are operative. The central analgesic effect is at the subcortical level but is poorly understood. Analgesia and antiinflammatory activity have been found to be on the basis of inhibition of prostaglandin synthetase activity. This action is shared by a number of newer drugs referred to collectively as nonsteroid antiinflammatory drugs, or NSAIDs.

Prostaglandins, so named because originally demonstrated in seminal fluid, are formed in nearly all tissues whenever cells are damaged. Their release is responsible for pain and inflammation both directly and by potentiating the effects of pain-producing kinins, sensitizing the peripheral pain receptors. Prostaglandins are synthesized from fatty acids, chiefly arachidonic acid, derived from the phospholipids of cell membranes. The cyclooxygenase enzyme system converts arachidonic acid to intermediates called endoperoxides, which in turn are converted to prostaglandins. The NSAIDs act by inhibiting the cyclooxygenase system.[5,14] Fig. 21-1 summarizes the present concept of the mode of action of the NSAIDs.[12]

Aspirin and other salicylic acid derivatives increase bleeding time by inhibiting platelet aggregation. Gastrointestinal intolerance is common, largely as a result of inhibition of a prostaglandin prostacyclin, which is generated by the gastric mucosa and is a potent mucosal vasodilator and inhibitor of ulcer formation. These

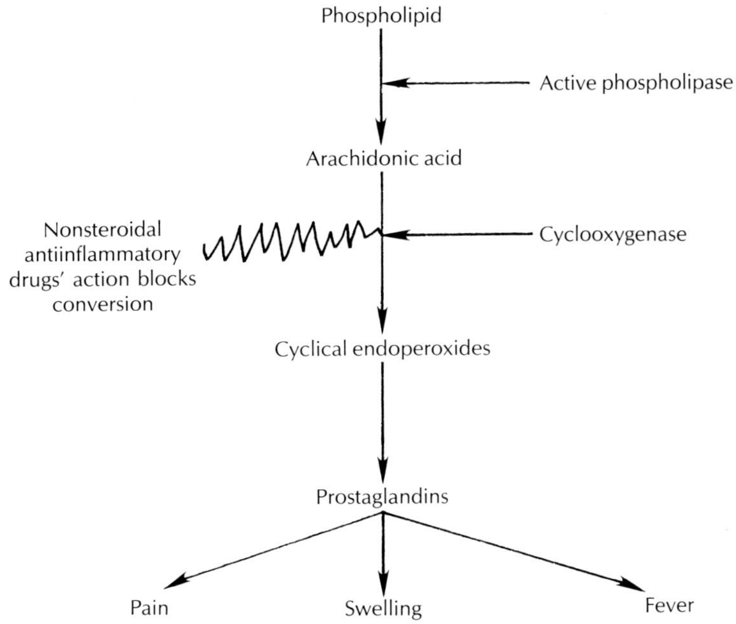

Fig. 21-1. Present concept of mode of action of NSAIDs.[12]

and other side effects are present to a greater or lesser extent with other NSAIDs, which limits usage of some.[1,6,7] The following is a classification of NSAIDs (prostaglandin synthetase inhibitors); for spectrum of usage, dosage, and side effects, the reader is referred to the *Physician's Desk Reference*.

1. Aryl carboxylic acids
   a. Salicylic acids
      (1) Acetylsalicylic acid
      (2) Diflunisal
   b. Anthranilic acids
      (1) Flufenamic acid
      (2) Mefenamic acid
      (3) Meclofenamic acid
      (4) Clofenamic acid
2. Aryl alkanoic acids
   a. Arylacetic acids
      (1) Alclofenac
      (2) Diclofenac (Volterol 50)
      (3) Naproxen (Naprosyn)
   b. Aryl propionic acids
      (1) Ibuprofen (Motrin)
      (2) Ketoprofen (Orudis)
      (3) Fenoprofen (Nalfon)
   c. Hetero arylacetic acids
      (1) Tolmetin (Tolectin, Zomax)
      (2) Fenclogic acid
   d. Indoleacetic and indene acetic acids*
      (1) Indomethacin (Indocin, Indocid)
      (2) Sulindac (Clinoril)
3. Enolic acids*
      (1) Phenylbutazone (Butazolidin)
      (2) Oxyphenbutazone (Tandearil)
      (3) Ozopropazone

As of this writing, some are only used for rheumatoid arthritis. No long-term controlled studies of their use in TMJ osteoarthritis or myofascial pain-dysfunction syndrome have been published.

Acetaminophen (Tylenol, Phenaphen) and phenacetin are paraaminophenol derivatives that have an analgesic and antipyretic action without antiinflammatory activity. Their central analgesic action is raising the threshold of pain in the same manner and degree as salicylates. The duration of action is 3 to 4 hours. The usual dosage is identical to that of aspirin—300 to 600 mg q 3 to 4 hours.

Dextropropoxyphene (Darvon) is a pure analgesic of intermediate strength; however, its use may lead to tolerance and habituation and must be carefully supervised in chronic pain problems.

Narcotic analgesics have limited use in the management of pain in temporomandibular joint disease. Too

*Produce more side effects.

frequently patients are seen who already have developed tolerance, habituation, or even dependence on drugs, and the diagnosis of the disease process and causative factors as well as treatment plan is clouded by the patient's insistence on medication for relief from pain. The term *opioid*, synonymous with narcotic analgesic, refers to any natural or synthetic drug with opium-like action. Opium is one of the oldest drugs known to humans, the ancient Greeks and Egyptians having used it to obtund pain. Paracelsus (1493-1541) carried opium in the pommel of his sword.[8] Sydenham wrote "Medicine would be a one-armed man without Opium," and Sir William Osler referred to morphine as "God's own medicine." Morphine remains the standard against which new opioids are measured. The analgesic effects of morphine and other opioids are a result of their action on the central nervous system. In addition to analgesia, morphine produces drowsiness, changes in mood, and mental clouding, so that even when pain is still perceived, the patient feels more comfortable. The rare use of morphine in TMJ disease is limited to hospitalized patients with severe pain and contributing factors. Meperidine (Demerol) is a synthetic opioid with similar action and usage to morphine. Codeine, an alkaloid with antitussive properties as well as analgesic action, is effective orally and is usually prescribed in combined form with aspirin or acetaminophen. The usual dosage is 30 mg q 4 hours. Other opioids include hydromorphone (Dilaudid), nalbuphine (Nubain), oxycodone (Percodan), and phenazocine (Prinadol). Pentazocine (Talwin), a synthetic compound developed in an effort to find an effective analgesic with little or no abuse potential, has proven to be an effective analgesic in doses of 30 mg parenterally or 50 mg orally. Dependence with parenteral administration has been reported but not with oral use.

MUSCLE RELAXANTS AND ANTIANXIETY DRUGS

Muscle spasm may be the pathological entity in the spasm-pain-spasm cycle, and relief of spasm by pharmacological methods in some cases of myofascial pain-dysfunction syndrome, along with explanation of the diagnosis and counseling to relieve tensional habits, may result in complete relief of severe symptoms. In other patients with occlusal problems, trauma, degenerative osteoarthritis, or other entities, muscle spasm is a secondary but nonetheless major pathological process requiring treatment. Often proper diagnosis cannot be made without breaking the spasm. Therefore the proper use and dosage of the pharmacological agents available are extremely important in diagnostic and therapeutic modalities of a wide and varied nature. When splinting is indicated to alter occlusion, fabrication of the proper appliance is often impossible because of trismus. Proper equilibration may not be possible for the same reason.

The spasm in the pain-spasm-pain cycle is treated by physical and psychological modalities, as well as by systemic and local pharmacological methods. Chapter 16 reviews the total treatment of muscle spasm. The benzodiazepines have a spectrum of effects, ranging from relief of skeletal muscle spasm to a hypnotic effect, with relief of anxiety in the center and carrying over the entire spectrum (Fig. 21-2).

Experimentally, diazepam has been found to directly combat muscle spasm in animals, and Engle,[3] among others, has proven the efficacy of diazepam as a skeletal muscle relaxant in a double-blind controlled study. Such controlled studies, however, are rare, and it is difficult to separate the antianxiety effect from the skeletal muscle effect in clinical practice. It has been my experience and that of co-workers that diazepam, as well as the newer analogues, lorazepam (Ativan) and clorazepate dipotassium (Tranxene), has been extremely useful in the treatment of muscle spasm. In employing the Mandibular Kinesiograph of Jankelson, a single dose of 22.5 mg clorazepate dipotassium has succeeded in eliminating muscle spasm where other measures had been ineffective. The usual dosage of diazepam is 2 to 5 mg three to four times daily or as needed. A single larger dose of diazepam or clorazepate dipotassium at bedtime may be effective in relieving bruxism while asleep.

Meprobamate (Equanil, Miltown) is a safe and effec-

← ANTIANXIETY →

MUSCLE RELAXANT — HYPNOTIC

Diazepam (Valium)	Oxazepam (Serax)	Nitrazepam (Mogodon)
Lorazepam (Ativan)	Chlordiazepoxide (Librium)	Flurazepam (Dalmane)
Clorazepate dipotassium (Tranxene)		

Fig. 21-2. Benzodiazepines.

tive minor tranquilizer useful in relieving anxiety and, either directly or indirectly, muscle spasm. In the medical treatment of bruxism, 400 mg is often prescribed at night. Tybamate (Solacen, Tybatran) is related to meprobamate but is shorter acting.

Phenothiazines and other major tranquilizers have no place in the management of TMJ disease, and the use of barbituates and other hypnotics is to be discouraged except in rare and complicated situations.

Methocarbamol (Robaxin), a skeletal muscle relaxant, occasionally has been effective in treating acute muscle spasms of TMJ disorders, in oral dosages of 0.75 to 1.5 g qid, although long-term usage in chronic problems is not recommended. It is extremely effective intravenously (1 to 3 g of 10% solution) but has limited application in this dosage form. Carisoprodol (Soma, Rela) and chlorzoxazone (Paraflex) are other skeletal muscle relaxants with some analgesic properties.

Cyclobenzaprine (Flexeril) is a newer skeletal muscle relaxant, related chemically but not pharmacologically to the tricyclic antidepressants. Given in 10-mg doses tid, it is effective in acute muscle spasm of local origin but should be used only for short-term therapy.

The injection of local anesthetics into painful trigger zones in the muscles surrounding the TMJ may permanently relieve the pain-spasm-pain cycle in the myofascial pain-dysfunction syndrome.[13] Intraarticular injection of 1% lidocaine (Xylocaine) into the TMJ may be an effective diagnostic as well as therapeutic method.[10] One percent procaine or 1% lidocaine without epinephrine is used for this procedure. Fluori-Methane spray is also an effective method of treatment to localized areas of muscle spasm. Its application is described in Chapter 16.

STEROIDS

Systemic adrenocorticosteroid therapy is seldom advised in temporomandibular joint disease except for short-term usage in complicated cases. Formerly, intraarticular steroids were frequently injected into the joint. However, repeated injections have been found to produce osteoporosis in the joint so that this treatment must be employed cautiously and as an adjunct to other definitive therapeutic procedures. The reader is referred to standard texts, the *Physician's Desk Reference*, or manufacturers for details on products and dosages.

PROTEOLYTIC ENZYMES

Proteolytic enzymes are used as adjunctive therapy for reduction of inflammation and edema and to ease pain, speed healing, and accelerate tissue repair. Their application to temporomandibular joint disorders therefore may be as part of the medical regimen in severe or acutely painful syndromes, particularly where edema is associated, in traumatic cases, and postoperatively. Their effectiveness has not been substantially demonstrated experimentally. Although the mode of action of proteolytic enzymes has not been fully established, depolymerization of fibrin and permeability modification of venules and lymphatics underlie the action. Bromelain (Ananase) is a proteolytic enzyme derived from the pineapple plant. Usual dosage is 50,000 to 100,000 units qid. Papain (Papase), derived from *Carica papaya*, is an alternate preparation usually prescribed 20,000 units orally or buccally qid. Chymotrypsin with trypsin (Chymoral) is an animal enzyme prescribed orally, 100,000 units qid.

ANTIVERTIGINOUS DRUGS

Vertigo may be the most distressing symptom of the patient with TMJ disease, and specific medication for symptomatic relief of vertigo is effective and inexpensive and rarely produces side effects. The most commonly prescribed preparation is meclizine (Antivert, Bonine), which is an antihistamine, recommended in dosages of 12.5 to 25 mg bid or tid or as needed. Dimenhydrinate (Dramamine) is the chlorotheophylline salt of the antihistamine agent diphenhydramine. It is given in 50-mg oral dosages tid or as needed and is available in tablet or liquid form as well as parenterally or as a suppository. Cyclizine (Marezine) is another antihistamine with antivertiginous activity, available in 50-mg tablets, suppositories, or by injection. Anticholinergics, such as scopolamine, may be of benefit.[9]

TINNITUS

Until recently there has been no effective pharmacological agent for the relief of tinnitus—the symptom of noises in the ear, common in TMJ disease as well as a variety of other entities. As is pointed out in Chapter 11, tinnitus is a symptom of otological as well as nonotological diseases, and treatment should be directed toward the underlying cause. If decreased circulation to the inner ear is thought to be a factor, a vasodilator regimen along with avoidance of tobacco, coffee, and other vasoconstrictors is employed.[11] When associated with TMJ disease, the cause of tinnitus is obscure. Nicotinic acid, 50 mg tid, 20 minutes ac, and thiamine, 50 to 100 mg tid, may be used in these cases. The variable response and the efficacy of other therapy make one wonder whether any positive subjective benefits might be a result of placebo effect. It has been established, however, that intravenous lidocaine has completely relieved tinnitus in the majority of cases. The effect, however, is transient and as such is impractical for therapeutic purposes. Tocainide hydrochloride, a primary analogue of lidocaine, has been given experimentally in high dosages (600 mg orally qid), and a short-term double-blind study by Emmett and Shea[2] produced evidence of therapeutic promise at this dosage level. More intensive studies are underway, and the authors state, "Tocainide Hcl may well prove to be the ideal medication in the treatment of tinnitus in that it is oral, has a long half-life, and has little or no side effects."

VITAMINS AND MINERALS

Proper nutrition, including adequate vitamins, is essential in both healthy individuals and TMJ patients. Where tissue damage is present, supplemental vitamins are encouraged. The current fad for "megavitamin" therapy is to be discouraged, since not only is it ineffective and wasteful, but also overdoses of fat-soluble vitamins may be harmful. Calcium, essential for muscle contraction, is routinely given when muscle spasm is a factor. Many forms are available, although particularly recommended is Os-Cal Forte, one tablet tid, a multiple vitamin and mineral supplement containing 250 mg of calcium carbonate.

SUMMARY

A review of pharmaceutical agents available at this time in the treatment of temporomandibular joint disorders and related symptoms has been presented. Their use does not preclude standard diagnostic and therapeutic methods, but when the drugs are used with discretion and selectivity, the patient's response may have an important diagnostic function, and the alleviation of distressing symptoms is aided. The more "arrows one has in the quiver," the more one is able to cope with diagnostic as well as therapeutic problems; however, "shotgun" therapy is to be avoided. Advances are continually being made in pharmaceutical research, and it behooves the practitioner to constantly reassess his or her prescribing habits. Enthusiasm must be balanced by caution; Pope's adage, "Be not the first by whom the new are tried nor yet the last to lay the old aside," has just as much application today as when written in the eighteenth century.

REFERENCES

1. Bowers, D., Dyer, H.R., Fosdick, W.M., Keller, K.E., Rosenberg, A.L., Sussman, P., and Vancil, M.E.: Naproxen in rheumatoid arthritis: a controlled trial, Ann. Intern. Med. **88**:470, 1975.
2. Emmett, J.R., and Shea, J.J.: Treatment of tinnitus with tocainide hydrochloride, Otolaryngol. Head Neck Surg. **88**:442, 1980.
3. Engle, H.A.: The effect of diazepam (Valium) in children with cerebral palsy: a double-blind study, Dev. Med. Child Neurol. **8**:661, 1966.
4. Goodman, L., and Gilman, A.: The pharmacological basis of therapeutics, ed. 5, New York, 1975, Macmillan Publishing Co., Inc.
5. Granstrom, E.: Prostaglandin chemistry, Acta Obstet. Gynecol. Scand. (Suppl.) **87**:13, 1979.
6. Huskisson, E.C., Wojtulewski, J.A., Berry, H., Scott, H., Hart, F., Duddley, and Balme, H.W.: Treatment of rheumatoid arthritis with fenoprofen: comparison with aspirin, Br. Med. J. **1**:176, 1974.
7. Huskisson, E.C., Woolf, D.L., Balme, H.W., Scott, J., and Franklyn, S.: Four new anti-inflammatory drugs: responses and variations, Br. Med. J. **1**:1048, 1976.
8. Krantz, J.C., and Carr, C.J.: Pharmacologic principles of medical practice, ed. 4, Baltimore, 1958, Williams & Wilkins Co.

8a. Lim, R.K.S.: Salicylate analgesia. In Smith, M.J.H., and Smith, P.K., editors: The salicylates: a critical bibliographic review, New York, 1966, John Wiley & Sons, Inc.

9. Mattox, D.E.: Medical management of vertigo, Ear Nose Throat J. **59**:383, 1980.
10. Norris, C.W., and Eakins, K.: Head and neck pain: TMJ syndrome, Laryngoscope **84**:1466, 1974.
11. Pulec, J.L.: Treatment of tinnitus, ORL Allergy Digest **41**:15, 1979.
12. Sharma, I.N., and Buchanau, W.W.: Some modern aspects of the mode of action of non-steroidal anti-inflammatory drugs, Pharmatherapeutica **2**:387, 1980.
13. Travell, J., and Rinyler, S.H.: The myofascial genesis of pain, Post. Grad. Med. **11**:425, 1952.
14. Whittle, B.J.R.: Prostaglandin synthetase inhibitors, Acta Obstet. Gynecol. Scand. (Suppl.) **87**:21, 1979.

22 Surgery of the temporomandibular joint

DOUGLAS H. MORGAN, D.D.S., LELAND R. HOUSE, M.D., WILLIAM P. HALL, M.D., and S. JAMES VAMVAS, D.D.S., F.A.C.D.

HISTORICAL BACKGROUND

Oral and maxillofacial surgeons, otolaryngologists, and other clinicians through the years have been challenged by the temporomandibular joint. This area, because of the closeness to other structures and the variety of pain symptoms, has been of interest to the orthopedist, the neurosurgeon, the neurologist, the plastic surgeon, the head and neck surgeon, as well as the general dentist and other dental specialists. The purpose of this chapter is to increase the understanding of the subject based on experience and new concepts that have been developed over recent years.

Costen[12] did much to shed light on the subject. He believed that the basic cause of these problems was faulty occlusion. We have since come to realize the causes are more complicated than occlusal disharmony. One of the major factors, as it is now understood, is psychophysiological conditions, which cause muscle spasms in the muscles involving the joint.[26] This in turn can cause synovitis in the capsule, which can cause malocclusion of the teeth on the affected side. Malocclusion can cause temporomandibular joint problems. However, temporomandibular joint inflammation can distract the teeth on the side affected and cause a faulty occlusion.

Bell[3] accurately put temporomandibular joint problems into five major categories: (1) spontaneous dislocation, (2) traumatic joint, (3) chronic mandibular hypomobility, meaning fibrous and osseous ankylosis, (4) temporomandibular arthritis, and (5) temporomandibular myofascial pain-dysfunction syndrome.

Surgical treatment of this joint dates back as far as 1934, when Risdon[35] discussed his work of placing gold foil in the glenoid fossa to prevent reankylosis of the temporomandibular joint. In 1946 Eggers[15] wrote of success in placing tantalum foil into the fossa and over the head of the condyle after an arthroplasty of the joint. In 1957 Smith and Robinson[40] wrote of a surgical procedure for the creation of a false temporomandibular joint, in cases of ankylosis, by means of a nonelectrolytic metal. In 1958 Walker[43] did a significant paper on arthroplasty of the ankylosed temporomandibular joint. He advocated fascia and, later, Silastic as an interposing material in the joint space to prevent reankylosis, emphasizing the necessity of thorough physiotherapy after surgery.

In 1960 Robinson[36] wrote an important paper reporting the new procedure of correcting temporomandibular ankylosis by creating a false stainless steel fossa. In the report he showed the excellent results obtained by placing his metal fossa against the floor of the skull, using screws in the zygoma to retain it in place (Fig. 22-1). Robinson stated:

> Previous attempts in interposing the stainless steel had been to attach the metal to the mandible; and, therefore, the metal moves when the mandible moves. This has resulted in the metal migrating from between the bones in some patients. This new procedure is offered as a method of correcting temporomandibular joint ankylosis by introducing a stainless steel, cup-like fossa, which remains stationary, and inhibits new bone formation between the mandible and the temporal bone.

With this pioneering device developed, Christensen[10] in 1963 reported three cases for correction of ankylosis of the temporomandibular joint by insertion of a cast Vitallium glenoid fossa. Christensen stated in essence that attempts have been made to cover the condylar stump with some type of nonanatomical barrier. A better approach would be to put a metallic barrier against the base of the skull, since there would be less tendency for it to loosen. This is essentially the same idea as that presented by Robinson,[36] but this method endeavors to make the appliance more anatomical.

Henny and Baldridge[19] accomplished excellent results in selected patients with a high condylectomy,

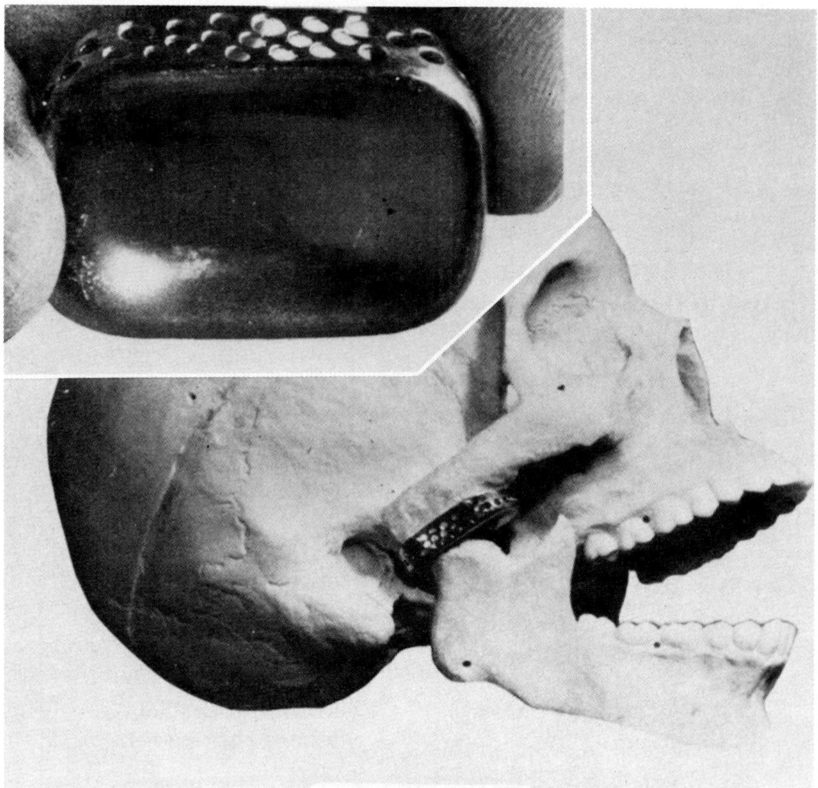

Fig. 22-1. Robinson metallic fossa prosthesis secured to zygoma by metallic screws. (From Robinson, M.: J. South. Calif. State Dent. Assoc. **6:**186, 1960.)

maintaining the meniscus. In a later paper[18] Henny states*:

> Proliferative changes in the mandibular condyle are relatively common in patients with rheumatoid arthritis. Many patients continue to function well despite this, and it is only when joint pathology has progressed to the point of functional impairment that surgical intervention is indicated. When proliferative changes occur in the condyle, the meniscus is subject to gradually increasing damage so that it finally becomes perforated, and eventually, is destroyed. In view of this progression of pathology, it is wise to interfere surgically before the meniscus is irreversibly damaged. In some instances, even when the meniscus appears radiographically to be almost destroyed, it can still be preserved at surgery by means of a high condylectomy. A perforation, if not too extensive, can be repaired by careful suturing. If the perforation is too extensive for suturing, a sheet of Silastic can be inserted.

The work of Henny substantiates the belief in maintaining a functional disc or disc substitute between the head of the condyle and the articular eminence. Henny also believes that surgery is indicated before perforation of the disc is complete, bringing about the possibility of a true fibrous or bony ankylosis.

*From Henny, F.A.: Surgical treatment of the painful temporomandibular joint, J. Am. Dent. Assoc. **79:**171, 1969. Copyright by the American Dental Association. Reprinted by permission.

DIAGNOSTIC CRITERIA

First, the diagnostic part of this problem is considered. All rational treatment is based on understanding the causes and pathological consequences of disease, and any surgical technique that does not take these into consideration is only an exercise.

Many have experienced the symptom of a snapping or popping sound when the mouth is opened or closed. These sounds may or may not be indicative of serious disease. Although they are not normal, the seriousness depends on their frequency and the type of sound, as well as on other symptoms developing. The snapping or popping sound is in itself not necessarily a precursor of joint disease, although it can indicate this.

Several explanations have been given for this phenomenon. In 1918 Pringle's dissections[32] led him to disagree with the then classic description of the meniscus as being of oval form, transversely broad, thickest in the posterior portion, and thinnest at its center. Pringle found that there was a decided central thickening of the meniscus situated in the coronal plane over the head of the condyle. In front of this ridge was a distinct depression fitting the articular eminence below, anterior to which was a second thickening, forming the anterior border. The external pterygoid muscle is attached to this lowest part of the disc. Therefore the two thickenings with the intervening depression gave the superior aspect of the disc, from a lateral view, the typical concavoconvex outline, fitting accurately to the articular surface of the temporal bone. According to Pringle, when the disc is dragged askew, it is pulled forward and inward, so that the fixed central ridge becomes displaced obliquely instead of lying in the coronal plane. Pringle believed that when this occurs, the disc acts as a foreign body in the joint, either getting caught between the rolling condylar head and the articular eminence or moving with the condyle. He believed that in the normal joint any abnormality of the relationship between the condylar head, articular eminence, and disc must be caused by this displacement.

Rees,[33] on the other hand, held that the meniscus does not move with the condyle, but that each moves separately at a different rate. The forward excursion of the condyle, for example, is greater than that of the disc as they both move forward. Rees held that there is a correlation between the structure he found and the function he describes. The inner position of a thin zone between two thicker zones makes the disc more flexible and enables it to alter its shape more easily from concave to convex as it slides forward from the fossa to the articular eminence. Since the condyle is separated in its retrusive position from the temporal bone by the thickest part of the disc, as it moves onto the articular eminence by the thinnest part, the opening movement does not have to follow the sinuous contours of the temporal bone but can become a straightforward arc of a circle with its center near the lingula. Rees' observation led to the hypothesis that clicking may be produced any time the ridge jumps over a band or when a band slips over the ridge. Alteration of function because of increased muscle tension or spasms may conceivably change the relationship of the meniscus cartilage to the articulating surface of the condyle and to the articular eminence of the temporal bone. If the meniscus is not brought forward fully, the click during the extreme opening movement may occur earlier. If the meniscus is not permitted to go back, a click may be heard as the mandible closes from extreme opening.

In a cinephotographic study of temporomandibular movements in 1956 Berry and Hofmann[6] observed with a microphone that a click occurred during the initial phase of the closing movement, and a slight posterior movement was seen as the click was heard. A similar mechanism may be postulated to explain the clicking toward the end of the closing movement, as well as after the beginning of the opening one. The problem during protrusion and retrusion is much like that during opening and closing. Clicking during lateral movements may be explained by Pringle's concept[32] of the meniscus being pulled askew.

Sicher's explanation[38] in 1955 is more physiological. He states*:

> Two facets in regard to the articular disc must be remembered; namely, the attachment of muscle fibers on the anterior rim, and the loose attachment to the capsule at its posterior edge. If the muscles of the mandible fall into spastic contraction or contracture, the unilateral muscle attachment eventually will cause a displacement of the disc with relation to the condyle. In the "fight" of the irritated muscles against each other, the disc may be held in place while the mandible is displaced posterior, or the mandible may be stabilized where the disc is displaced anterior; or, more probably, a combination of these possibilities becomes reality.

The final word related to this phenomenon is yet to be written.

The next symptom of consequence is pain, which can be classified as arthralgic or myalgic. After analyzing many hundreds of patients with this disorder since 1960, we have come to the conclusion that the pain consequence of this syndrome is great. There is the obvious arthralgic pain in the ear and joint itself. Other pain areas involve the angle of the mandible, the temporal region, the supraorbital and occipital regions, and occasionally the cervical region, shoulders, and arms. Myalgia involves the external pterygoid, temporal, internal pterygoid, and masseter muscles.

The symptom of crepitation can appear in this joint. This occurs when the disc is perforated and there is bone-to-bone contact of the condylar head and articular eminence during functional movements.

Another symptom is dysmasesis—the inability to open one's mouth and masticate food without significant pain. The fact that an individual cannot open the mouth does not necessarily mean there is ankylosis. This inability to open the mouth wide or at all most of the time is the body's way of relieving irritation to this area. Limitation of motion can be the result of a neuromuscular reflex. Myalgia can cause muscular spasm, particularly, as Vaughan[42] explained, if the external pterygoid muscle is involved. We believe that most people with temporomandibular joint problems that involve limited jaw motion have chronic muscle spasm and not a true fibrous or bony ankylosis.

It has been our experience that pain in the joint is most severe when the individual is able to open the mouth wide and chew normally. When the individual uses the mandibular joint very little by not masticating heavy foods or opening wide, this tends to diminish the pain to a tolerable level. Many cures have been claimed that are nothing more than the person existing on a soft diet, using the mandibular joint moderately.

---

*From Sicher, H.: Structural and functional basis for disorders of the temporomandibular articulation, J. Oral Surg. **13**:275, 1955. Copyright by the American Dental Association. Reprinted by permission.

We also have observed a number of patients complaining of tinnitus, vertigo, parotitis, and pain symptoms similar to tic douloureux. One patient had been given the diagnosis of both Meniere's disease and tic douloureux. She also had a ringing sound in her ear. It proved to be a temporomandibular joint arthritis that masked itself as these other entities. It is important in individuals suffering from these symptoms to have pathological conditions of the temporomandibular joint ruled out. To illustrate the range of symptoms, Tables 22-1 and 22-2 present the initial symptoms and pain locations in 90 patients suffering from temporomandibular joint dysfunction.

Table 22-1. Initial symptoms of TMJ dysfunction in 90 patients presented to the TMJ team

Symptoms	Number of patients	Percent
Pain: head, neck, shoulder	80	88
Grating sound in joint (crepitus)	68	76
Tinnitus and pain	59	66
Functional disorders of mouth—partial or total inability to open	54	60
Vertigo and pain	46	51
Weakness of facial muscles and pain	2	2+
Vertigo and tinnitus, no pain	1	1+

From Morgan, D.H.: Surgical correction of temporomandibular joint arthritis, J. Oral Surg. **33:**766, 1975. Copyright by the American Dental Association. Reprinted by permission.

Table 22-2. Location of subjective pain in 90 patients with TMJ arthritis

Location	Number of patients
Ear, TMJ, temple, mandible, maxilla, teeth, mastoid, zygoma, eye, tongue, neck, and shoulder	42
TMJ, ear, and temporal area	15
Maxilla and teeth	7
Mandible and teeth	6
Posterior cervical area, shoulder, arms, hands	6
Ear, tongue area	4
Ear alone	3
Ear, mastoid area	3
TMJ alone	2
Zygoma-cheek area	1
TOTAL	89*

From Morgan, D.H.: Surgical correction of temporomandibular joint arthritis, J. Oral Surg. **33:**766, 1975. Copyright by the American Dental Association. Reprinted by permission.

*One patient had no pain but had only vertigo and tinnitus.

Bernstein, Mohl, and Spiller[5] state:

> Perhaps the most important idea to convey is that this syndrome of pain and dysfunction can masquerade as acute or chronic disease of the ear, nose, and throat. . . . TMJ dysfunction produces symptoms of recurrent temporal pain initially diagnosed as migraine; ear and mastoid pain diagnosed as acute mastoiditis; fullness, tinnitus, and vertigo diagnosed as labyrinthine disease; fullness and subjective hearing loss diagnosed as eustachian tube malfunction or secretory otitis media; pain in the zygomatic arch and fullness in the cheek diagnosed as acute sinusitis; pain in the preauricular area and gonial angle diagnosed as acute parotitis.

There has been much discussion as to the source of pain in this area. Bernick[4] claims to have found nerve tissue in the disc of the rat. Clark[11] also states that there are nerve fibers entering into the capsule of the meniscus from the muscles of mastication. This work also has been verified by Schmid[37] in his dissection on infants less than a year old. Schmid also found that this joint receives various branches from the fifth nerve and autonomic fibers from the otic ganglion, and a branch of the facial nerve could be found entering the capsule.

The articulation of the mandible is governed by the temporomandibular joint, the occlusion of the teeth, and the neuromuscular mechanism. The function is controlled by sensory and motor branches of the third division of the trigeminal nerve and perhaps by a few fibers of the facial nerve. The posterior part of the capsule is innervated by separate branches from the auriculotemporal nerve. The anterior part of the capsule is supplied by sensory branches emanating from the masseteric, deep temporal, and external pterygoid muscles. According to Hromada[21] these nerves supply the sensory function that allows the muscle control of the joint to respond promptly and precisely to the changes of pressure within the joint. Pressure in the capsule caused by meniscitis or osteogenic changes is registered by these nerve fibers and referred to other areas of the head and neck. This, we believe, accounts for many of the pain symptoms. Pressure on the anterior malleolar ligament that also attaches to the capsule and disc of the joint can account for symptoms of the middle and inner ear. Costen[13] in an earlier article, spoke of temporomandibular joint problems causing ear symptoms.

The work of Goodfriend[16] and Pinto[31] has been most important in helping the understanding of the probable mechanisms of vertigo, tinnitus, and related phenomena. Goodfriend states*:

> Dizziness and related auditory, vagal, and ocular symptoms may be predisposed and caused by traumatic malrela-

*From Goodfriend, D.J.: Odontogenic dizziness and related symptoms. In Spector, M., editor: Dizziness and vertigo: diagnosis and treatment, New York, 1967, Grune & Stratton, Inc. By permission.

tionships of the temporomandibular joints as the result of abnormalities of the masticatory system. The temporomandibular joints are situated in a critical part of the head in close anatomic relation with the auditory and vestibular conduction systems. The fossa of the temporomandibular joint is in the temporal bone, separated from the pars tympani by the pterotympanic or glacerian fissure. The fissure is an opening between the middle ear or tympanic cavity and the temporomandibular joint. It is traversed by the anterior tympanic artery, the chorda tympani nerve, and the malleus-mandibular ligament. The malleus-mandibular ligament (or anterior malleolar ligament) extends from the anterior process of the malleus to the capsule and meniscus of the temporomandibular joint.

Pinto[31] states:

> A structure was found which seems to be absent in textbooks of anatomy. This structure resembles a fibroelastic tissue with ligamentous qualities. It was found inserted into the neck of the malleus immediately above the anterior process and lying laterally to the chorda tympani nerve. The "tiny ligament" spread from this point in a cone-shaped form forward, downward, and laterally to insert into the medioposterosuperior part of the capsule and meniscus of the temporomandibular joint. Movement of the capsule by grasping the exposed part of its posterosuperior border or movement of the meniscus of the temporomandibular joint seemingly caused this tiny ligament, the chain of ossicles, and the tympanic membrane to move.
>
> All specimens dissected disclosed this tiny ligament. It appeared clearly in the six postmortem specimens. In all instances, this structure connected to the temporomandibular joint region and passed through the iter chordae anterius (canal of Huguier) together with the chorda tympani nerve.

Pinto[31] concludes:

> An investigation was made of the existing relationship between the temporomandibular articulation and the middle ear. Twenty joints were carefully dissected from a superior approach. One joint was serially sectioned for microscopic study.
>
> A tiny ligament was found connecting the neck and anterior process of the malleus to the medioposterosuperior part of the capsule, the interarticular disc, and the sphenomandibular ligament. The fibrous layer of the tympanic membrane seemed to be continuous with this structure. The tiny ligament has an embryologic origin common with that of the malleus and incus.

Removal of the meniscus has been advised to alleviate pain.[14] This operation is being done less frequently, which coincides with our increased understanding of this area. Antoni,[2] in a close follow-up study of nine cases of meniscectomies, discovered that six patients complained again of varying degrees of discomfort within 2 months after surgery. Removal of the meniscus may be helpful, however, provided that a TMJ prosthesis is emplaced at the same time.

The function of the disc, or meniscus cartilage, is next to be discussed. This anatomical structure in essence acts as a separating medium between the articular eminence and the head of the condyle. The anterior portion of the disc is continuously being used as a buffer between the condyle and the articular eminence. The only functioning area of a normal joint is between the anterior head of the condyle and the descending and ascending slopes of the articular eminence. This is better understood when a skull is held to the light and the thinness of the bone in the concave portion of the mandibular fossa is observed. The muscle pull on the joint is primarily in an anterior and superior direction. It is only because of unusual trauma that one sees the head of the condyle pushed into the intercranial fossa. (A prizefighter is susceptible to this type of injury.) This has been referred to as a non–stress-bearing joint. This refers to the joint only when the teeth are lightly in occlusion. When the mandible is opening or closing, it *is* a stress-bearing joint. The stress occurs between the anterior portion of the head of the condyle and the descending slope (and, on occasion, the ascending slope) of the articular eminence. The disc acts as a separating medium with synovial fluid on either side to function as a hydrocushion. When pathological conditions occur, this system is disrupted. Accurate radiographs, as discussed in an article by Morgan,[29] show that this disc can be worn down or perforated. When this occurs, the space that normally appears in TMJ radiographs representing a functioning disc is drastically diminished or not present. What appears to be bone-on-bone contact between the head of the condyle and the articular eminence can be seen.

Bruxism can wear down and/or perforate a meniscus cartilage through the years. Tensional habits involving the masticatory apparatus are one of the major causes of this occurring. Early diagnosis and treatment can eliminate much pain for the patient and ensure, when surgery is necessary, improved function of the joint.

The disc does not actually have to be perforated to result in osteoarthritis or degenerative arthritis. Compression of the disc can bring the bony surfaces of the articular eminence and anterior head of the condyle close together where osteogenic changes can occur. These changes can set up an inflammatory reaction within the capsule, causing synovitis, ear symptoms, and muscle spasms.

Degenerative joint disease is not well known to dental clinicians. Ricketts[34] has described how in osteoarthritis the cartilage disappears, and the surface becomes irregular. The exposed bone becomes osteosclerotic, and lipping may occur as a result of proliferation of the perichondrium. Recurring trauma continues the process. For this discussion of clinical implications in orthodontics, traumatic arthritis is particularly significant, especially in the young. Older patients may voice no clinical complaints, but they may have episodes of pain with clicking or be in chronic discomfort with many bizarre symptoms of the referred type.

Irby[22] has stated:

Unfortunately, however, there have developed in the dental profession several schools of thought relative to the cause of this syndrome. Certainly the most common of these views attribute occlusal disharmony to be the primary factor and believe that muscle spasm and joint pain follow in sequence. Another group places special emphasis on emotional factors, fatigue, and psychotic disturbances as the primary factor, and a third group includes both the occlusal disturbances and the various emotional factors as possible precipitating factors. Little consideration by any of these groups is given to pathologic or functional disturbances arising within the joint as causative factors. Although conceding that changes do occur within the joint, it is generally agreed that these changes are secondary to prolonged occlusal disharmony or muscle spasm.

The temporomandibular articulation is a delicately balanced mechanism functioning under neuromuscular dictation. It is subject to many extrinsic influences including occlusal disharmony (especially those recently induced), and, through hypertonicity and spasm, the muscles of mastication most certainly reflect the impact of severe emotional or psychogenic disturbances. Aside from this circumstance, *one must be aware that the joint itself is subject to both pathologic and functional disturbances just as is any other joint in the body. This may serve as the focus of pain, which in turn initiates muscle spasm. Therefore when the entire spectrum of etiologic factors is considered, one must consider both extrinsic and intrinsic factors, the latter being those which arise within the joint itself.* [Italics added.]

The joint in which irreversible changes have occurred and which does not respond to conservative treatment is the one for which surgery offers hope of relief. . . .

Pain arising within the joint may be due to a number of factors, among which are (1) severance of the meniscus from the anterior portion of the capsule as a result of trauma, (2) tearing or perforation of the meniscus, (3) impingement on the meniscus and synovia on the anterior periphery due to incoordination of movement between the meniscus and condyle head, (4) erosion of the head of the condyle, (5) spurs on the condyle head, (6) systemic diseases such as rheumatoid arthritis or gout, (7) infectious arthritis, and (8) tumors.

In a question-and-answer epilogue[22] it was asked how long the delay should be referring a patient to an oral surgeon after all conservative methods for the treatment of a severe temporomandibular joint pain have failed. The conclusion by F. Michael Gardner was:

We might use 2 or 3 weeks of the previously mentioned palliative treatments to rule out acute injury to the joint. Once the splint phase of therapy has been instituted, assuming that the splint is properly made to do the job attempted, improvement is usually seen in 2 to 3 weeks. Occasionally total recovery is not accomplished, but some improvement is seen. In these cases, with continuing adjustment of the splint, recovery should occur in 4 to 6 weeks. As I stated earlier, I would not attempt a total equilibration or reconstruction in the face of continuing pain. I believe that it is rare to see a patient who does not respond to the outlined treatment in as little as 2 to 6 weeks, but if there were no improvement at the end of 2 months after insertion of a correctly adjusted splint, I would consider referral to an oral surgeon for evaluating the possibility of surgical or injection treatment of what could probably be considered an intrinsic joint problem.

TYPES OF SURGERIES

Eminectomy

Irby[22] has rationalized that when injury to the anterior portion of the disc or uncoordinated movement between the condyle and the meniscus exists, pain is triggered when the condylar head reaches the posterior slope of the eminence. If the articular eminence were removed (Fig. 22-2), the pain then could be alleviated. Five patients, who had experienced prolonged and severe pain associated with clicking, grating, and locking of the condylar head and who had been unresponsive to all conservative methods, were operated on. All patients experienced relief from pain extending up to 2 years, with a disappearance of the clicking or crepitus. Irby has now operated on over 30 patients using this procedure in the treatment of (1) recurrent dislocations, (2) chronic hypermobility associated with pain, and (3) irreversible temporomandibular joint pain associated with clicking or grating. Consistently good results have been obtained by him with this relatively simple procedure.

Zygomectomy

A new procedure has been advocated by Boudreau and Tideman[7] for chronic subluxation. This involves a vertical cut through the ascending slope of the eminence and fracturing the distal section of the zygoma through the zygomatic frontal suture. The bone is placed downward, and a small wedge of bone is used to hold it in position. The procedure in essence increases the size of the articular eminence and prevents the condyle from subluxating (Fig. 22-3).

This procedure does seem to have merit. It has been found that placing the articular eminence prosthesis to increase the contour of the eminence also has the same helpful effect.

Meniscectomy

In the middle 1950s procedures involving removal of the disc (Fig. 22-4) were popular, predicated on the idea that an injured or defective disc will cause pain

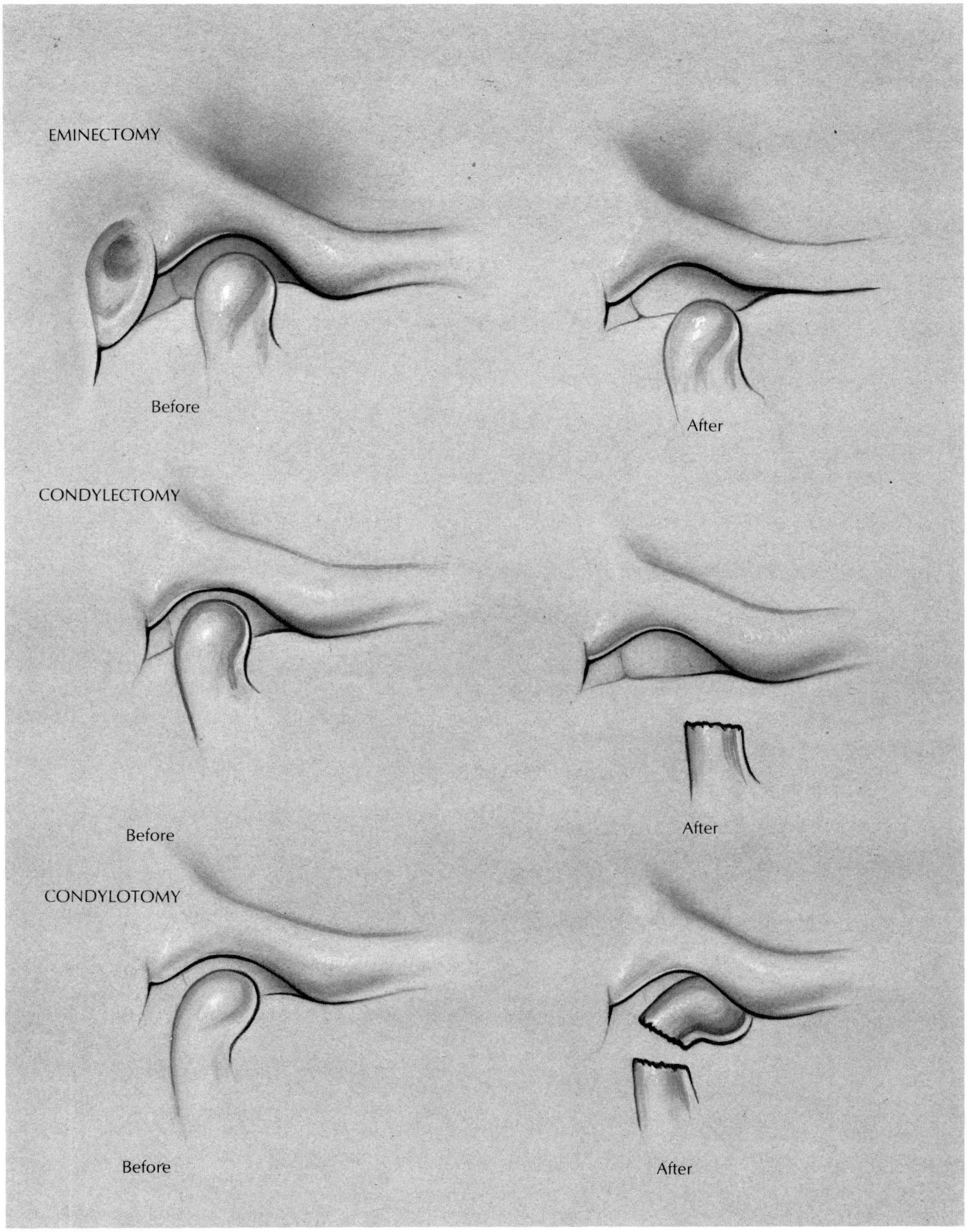

Fig. 22-2. Surgical procedures performed on TMJ: eminectomy, condylectomy, and condylotomy.

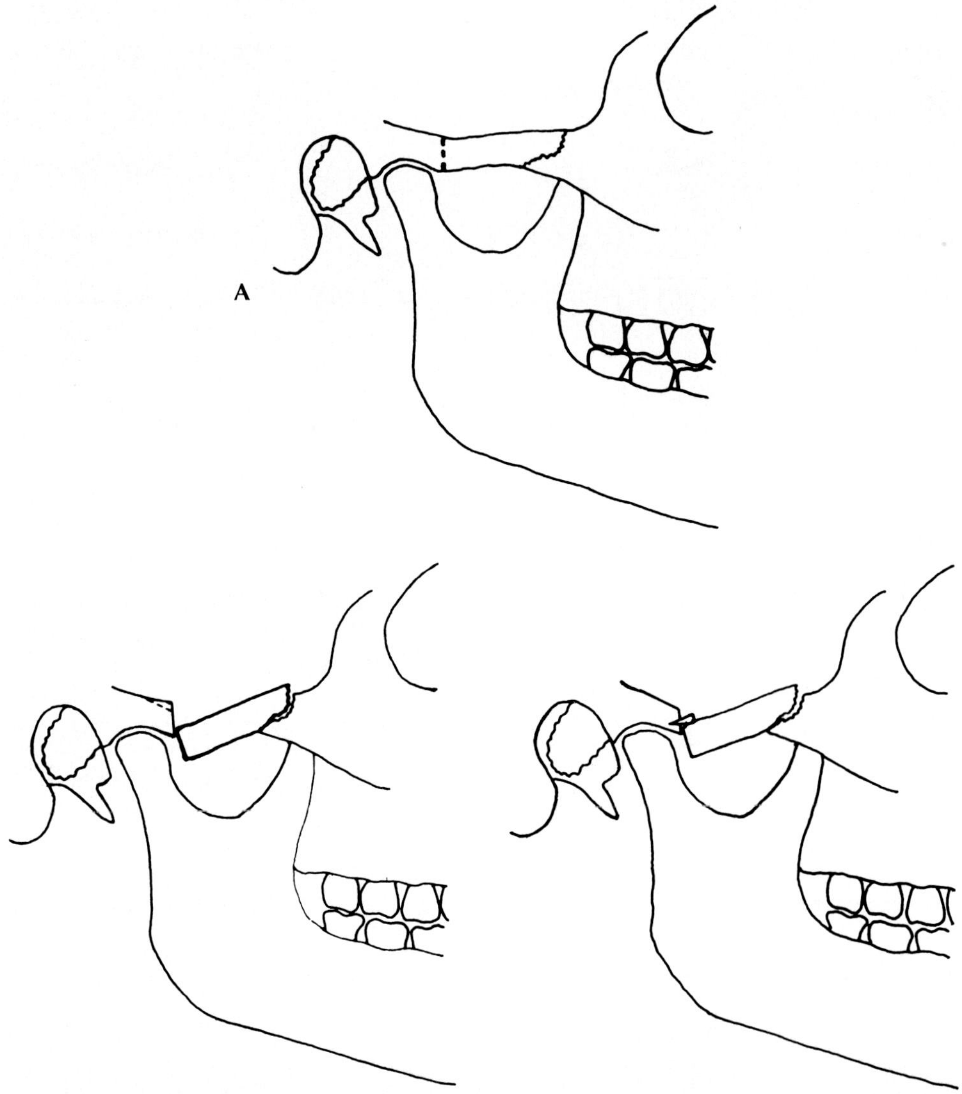

A B C

Fig. 22-3. A, Vertical osteotomy in region of articular wedge. **B,** Zygomatic arch depressed and horizontal wedge removed. **C,** Wedge inserted in place. (From Boudreau, R.G., and Tideman, H.: Treatment of chronic mandibular dislocation, Oral Surg. **41:**169, 1976.)

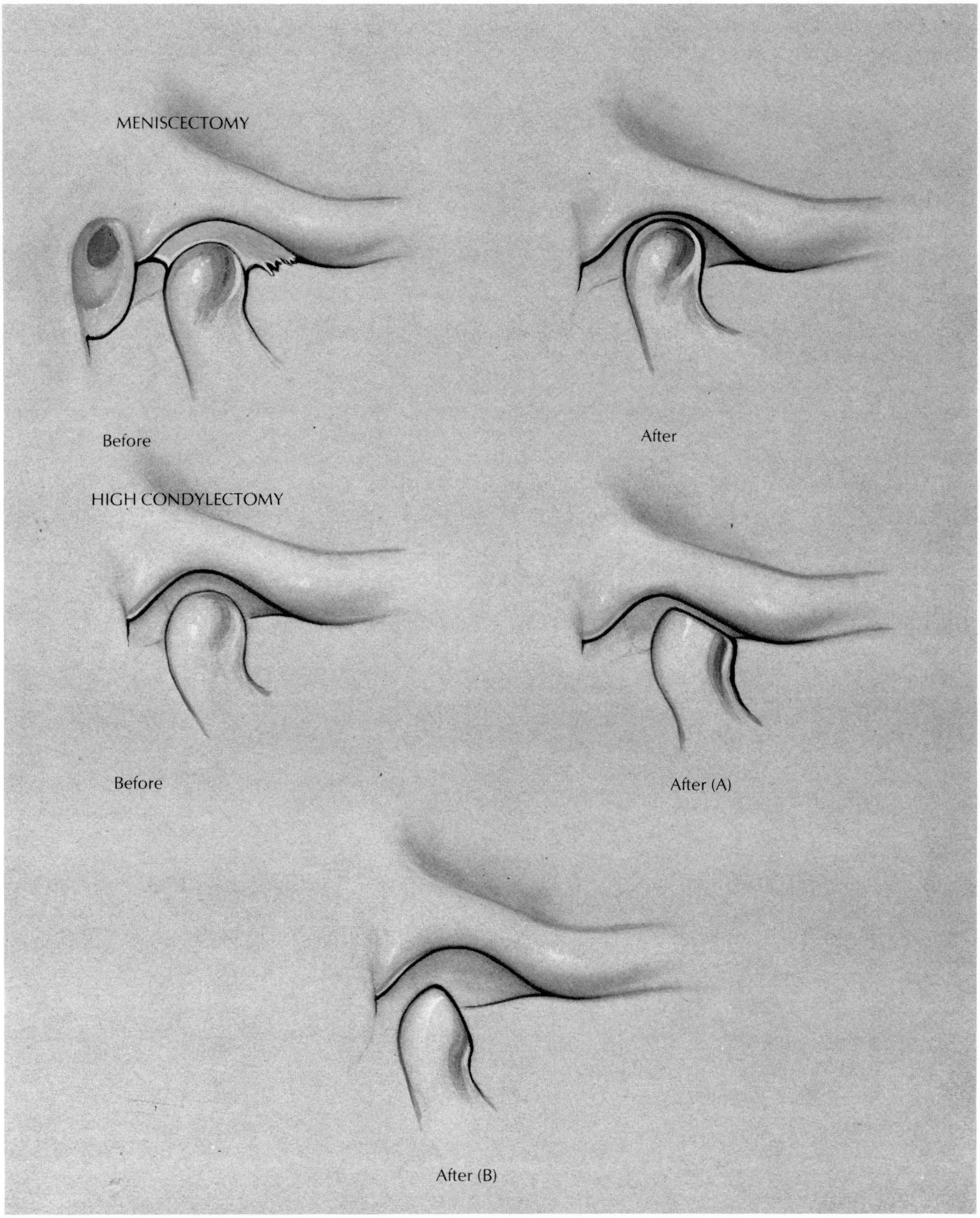

Fig. 22-4. Surgical procedures performed on TMJ: meniscectomy and high condylectomy. After high condylectomy, disc space may be extremely diminished as in *A*, or space may be three to four times normal because of synovial pressure, as in *B*. Henny[19] advocates suturing torn disc or placing sheet of Silastic in joint after high condylectomy.

and that its removal would effect relief of pain.[24]

Agerberg and Lundberg's findings,[1] which are borne out by clinical observations, show that many patients complained of a return of discomfort in the joint area. It became evident that meniscectomies alone without prosthesis placement possess definite limitations.

High condylectomy

The high condylectomy has been advocated by Henny and Baldridge[19] and by others. This usually involves removing the anterior aspect of the head of the condyle. Originally they also recommended removing the disc, but they now advocate suturing of the disc if it is torn or inserting a sheet of Silastic to compensate for a torn disc. The high condylectomy is done so that no fibrous attachment of the external pterygoid muscles is affected (Fig. 22-5).

Repositioning of the head of the condyle

It was observed in England that several patients who had suffered from temporomandibular joint pain and who had later incurred displaced fractures of the neck of the condyle were subsequently free from the joint pain. This observation lent further credence to the concept that pressure on the anterior periphery of the disc may cause pain in certain patients and that an altered position of the condylar head could relieve this pressure and relieve the pain. The procedure is done by blind approach using a Gigli saw, with which the condylar neck is severed at its base. It is faster than the open technique for the high condylotomy, but there is always the slight chance of severing the facial nerve or internal maxillary artery.[22]

Condylectomy

Irby[22] describes the condylectomy procedure as follows:

> It has been demonstrated repeatedly through both animal research and clinical experience that the removal of the condyle head, including the attachment of the lateral pterygoid muscle, is an injurious and deforming procedure. In both humans and animals, this operation invariably results in hyperocclusion on the operated side with deviation of the mandible toward the operated side. However, if the portion of the condyle head located above the attachment of the lateral pterygoid muscle is removed, none of these disturbing factors occurs with any degree of significance. Removal of the articular surface of the condyle head above the muscle attachment is a gratifyingly effective procedure for relief of certain types of temporomandibular joint pain. In contrast, the removal of the entire condyle head with its muscle attachment is a surgical catastrophe. . . .
>
> To remove the condyle and neck without replacement in some manner is almost certain to condemn the patient to a

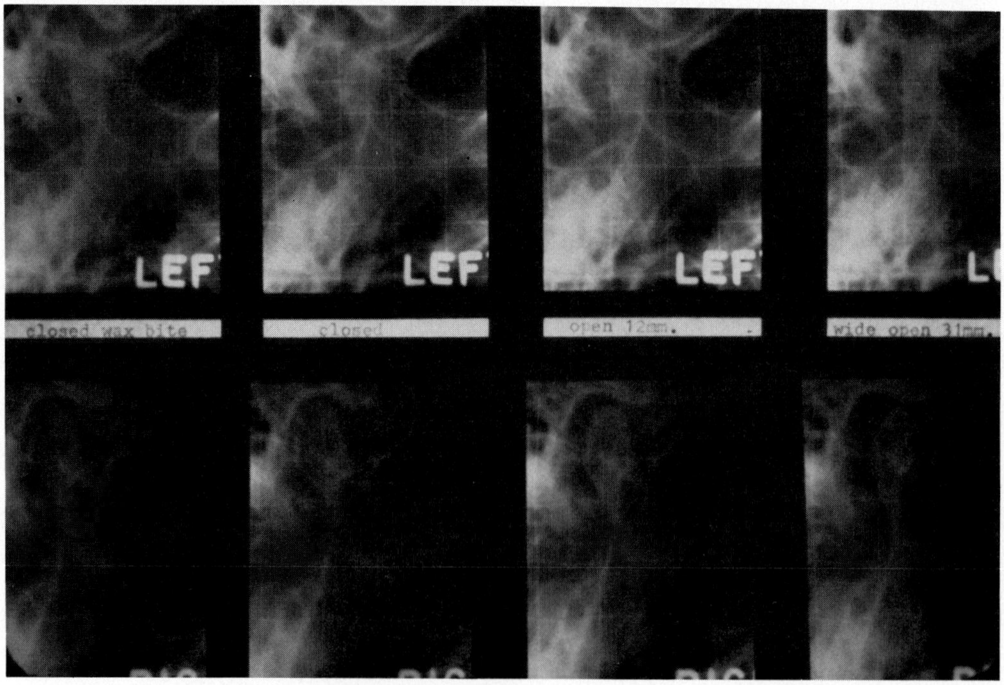

Fig. 22-5. TMJ radiographs showing high condylectomy affecting left joint.

life of altered mandibular function and occlusal disharmony. Removal of the condyle deprives the joint of the two factors essential to normal jaw relationship and function: the condyle head and the attachment of the lateral pterygoid muscle.

However, there is a difference of opinion regarding condylectomy procedures. Silver, Simon, and Litchman[39] summarize their surgical treatments of arthritic temporomandibular joints using condylectomies and meniscectomies as follows*:

> Arthritis of the temporomandibular joint is not an uncommon disorder. Its symptoms are often attributed incorrectly to diseases of the ear or teeth because of unfamiliarity with this condition.
>
> Conservative therapy may give temporary relief. Ultimately, symptoms and disability will recur since the arthritic process is invariably progressive.
>
> Condylectomy of the mandible and excision of the damaged meniscus is an effective procedure for arthritis of the temporomandibular joint. Convalescence is rapid and the period of hospitalization is short. One hundred and eleven condylectomies of the temporomandibular joint in 100 patients were performed between 1954 and 1971. Thirty-six patients have undergone follow-up studies for more than 5 years, and 76 patients for more than 2 years postcondylectomy. One hundred and six patients had free, painless opening of the mouth postoperatively, were eating regular food, and were classified as having good results. Eleven patients had bilateral condylectomies. Of these, seven had good results. Four patients had retrusion of the mandible with an anterior open bite and were classified as having poor results. Bilateral condylectomy should be reserved for patients with rheumatoid arthritis and congenital fibrous ankylosis of the jaws.
>
> No wound infections of the temporomandibular joint area occurred in this series. One death, due to infection at the tracheotomy incision which resulted in erosion of the carotid artery, occurred 15 days after condylectomy for bilateral bony ankylosis.

Surgery for derangements of the disc

Using arthrography, as well as other criteria, McCarty and Farrar,[28] Wilkes,[44,45] and Ireland[23] have described the internal derangement of the disc in reciprocal clicking or locking or degenerative arthritis. They conclude that when the disc is displaced anteriorly and the teeth are closed in the intercuspal position, the condyle is displaced upward and/or backward.

The surgical technique for reconstructive arthroplasty and disc repositioning designed by McCarty and Farrar[28] corrects the intercapsular derangements of the disc and condyle while affording a high degree of safety. They report their technique as neither adversely modifying the relationship of the patient's occlusion, injuring the facial nerve, nor causing many of the other problems sometimes associated with TMJ surgeries such as meniscectomy and condylectomy.

In this surgical approach the initial preauricular incision, 2 to 3 mm deep, begins with a hockey stick–shaped incision above and in front of the ear, extending downward to the lobule. The incision is deepened to the temporal fascia. Using the fascia as a base, the flap is swung downward and forward, exposing the capsular ligaments. The parotid gland is reflected forward and downward.

The articular capsule is entered through a horizontal incision, made approximately 2 mm below the zygomatic process of the temporal bone. The incision extends anterior to the eminence and posterior along the border of the capsule (Fig. 22-6, *A*). The capsular ligaments are reflected to expose the superior joint space and the superior surface of the disc. A horizontal incision is made through the collateral ligament, which is reflected downward to expose the inferior joint space and the articular surface of the condyle.

The herniated posterior ligament of the disc is transected lateral to medial (Fig. 22-6, *B*). The disc now may be displaced anteriorly toward the eminence to see the entire condyle. A predetermined amount of bone is removed from the posterosuperior portion of the condyle, and the cut surface of the condyle is contoured with a small, round diamond stone (Fig. 22-6, *C*). The disc is returned to its normal position, and after the amount of bone reduction and function are tested, the herniated posterior ligament (usually a 2-mm section) is incised and removed. The disc is then sutured to the posterior attachment, medial to lateral (Fig. 22-6, *D*).

ARTHROPLASTY

Restoration of the joint to a more anatomical and functional level should be accomplished by arthroplasty and prosthetic replacement of the damaged parts of the joint.

Over the years, working with many individuals exhibiting mandibular joint difficulties and studying carefully the radiographic and clinical symptoms, we have made these observations:

1. The area most significant in interpreting symptoms of the temporomandibular joint is the area between the anterior portion of the head of the condyle and the articular eminence portion of the temporal bone—primarily the lateral half of the eminence and condyle (Fig. 22-7).[7]
2. The disc-space relationship between the head of the condyle and the articular eminence, denoting a thinning or perforation of the meniscus, can be

*From Silver, C.M., Simon, S.D., and Litchman, H.M.: The surgical treatment of the arthritic temporomandibular joint, Surg. Gynecol. Obstet. **136**:251, 1973. By permission of Surgery, Gynecology & Obstetrics.

A

B

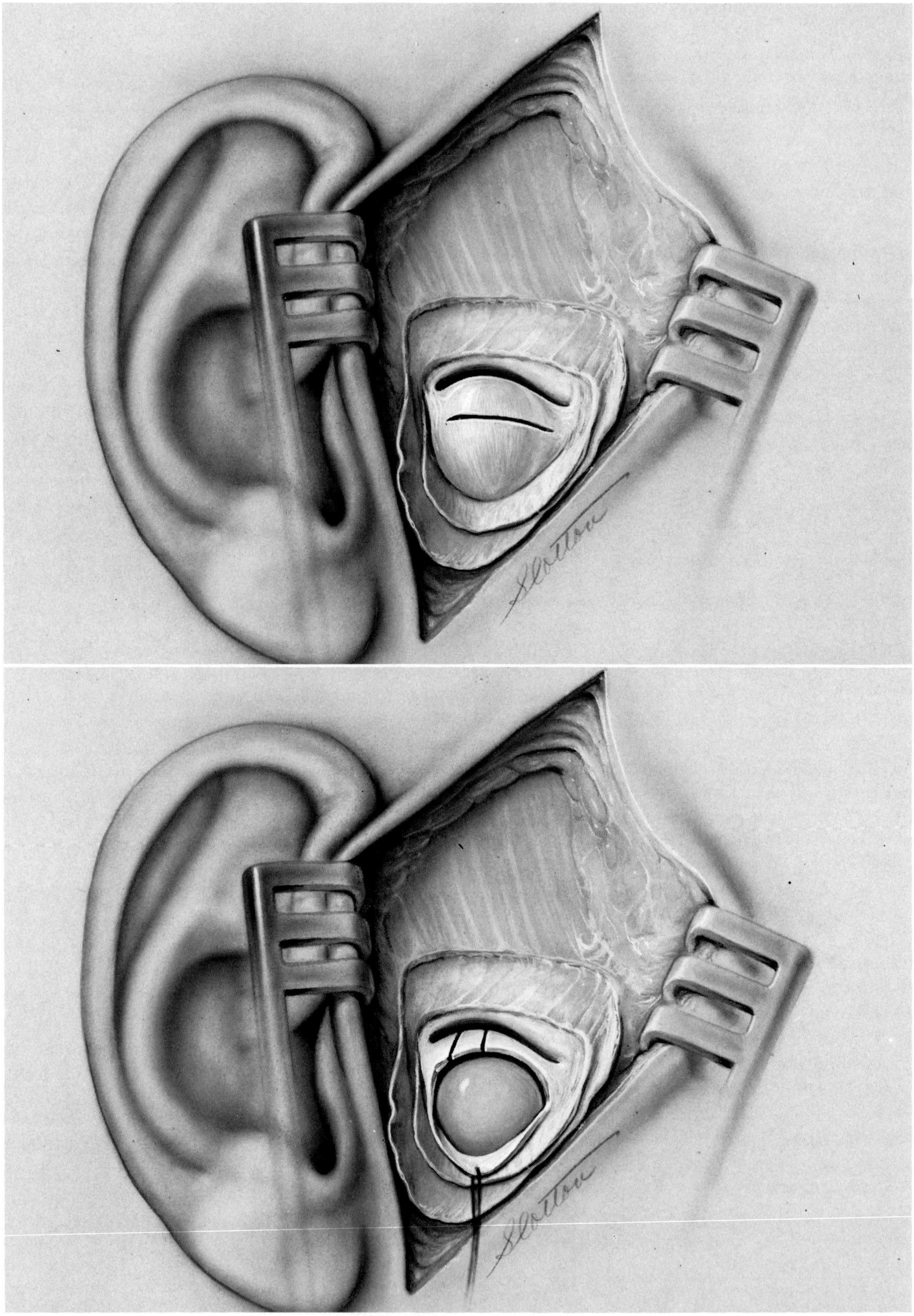

Fig. 22-6. A, Horizontal incision of approximately 2 mm is made below zygomatic process of temporal bone. **B,** This incision is extended anteriorly to the eminence and posteriorly downward to border of capsular ligament. Capsular ligaments are reflected downward, exposing superior joint space. Incisions are made through herniated section of bilaminar zone.

C

D

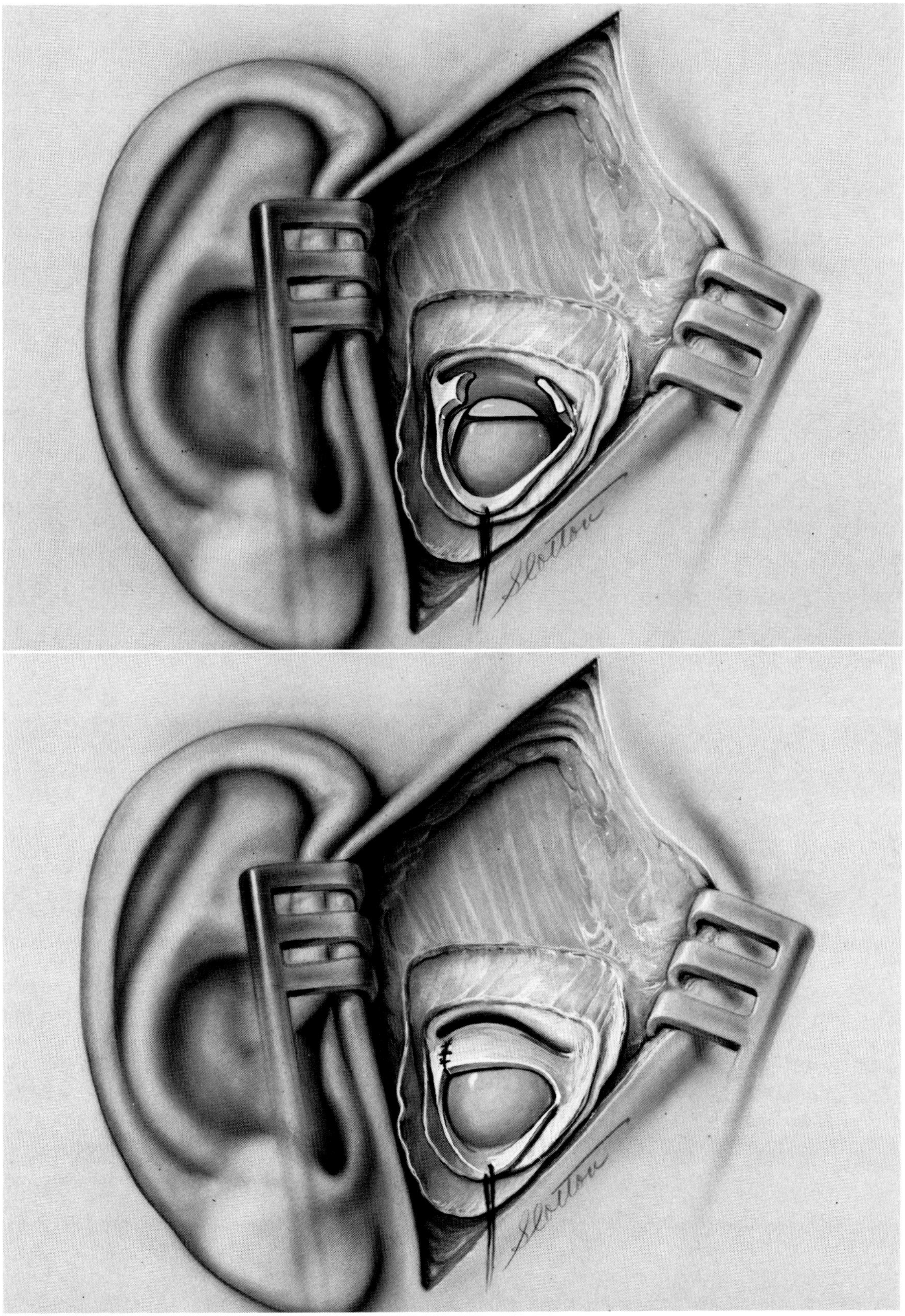

Fig. 22-6, cont'd. C, Capsular ligament is reflected downward and maintained with stay suture. Posterior ligament of disc that is herniated is transected lateral to medial. Measured amount of bone is removed from posterosuperior head of condyle. **D,** Disc is sutured posteriorly. Sutures are placed every 2 mm, medial to lateral. Joint capsule and ligaments are closed in usual manner.

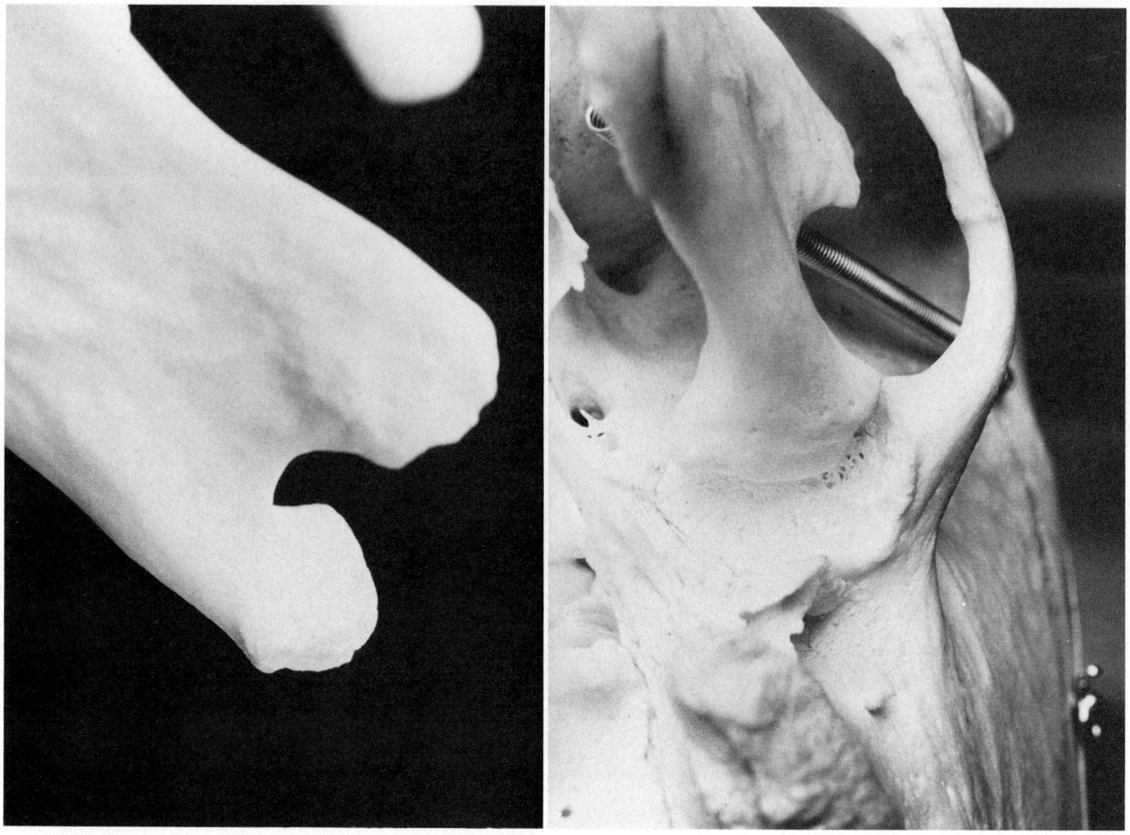

A B

Fig. 22-7. A, Disarticulate condyle shows effect of degenerative osteoarthritis on lateral pole of condyle. **B,** Erosion of cortical layer of bone on lateral aspect of eminence and flattening of lateral pole of condyle.

studied and measured and is important in the diagnosis of pathological conditions.

3. The articular eminence is significant as a flattening of the surface, which can be seen radiographically.
4. The pattern of the bone trabecula in the head of the condyle and articular eminence is significant. An osteophytic or mottling effect, as in arthritis, is clearly visible. In many radiographs of this area osteophytes (small bony protruberances) as well as arthroliths (broken-off osteophytes) can be seen on the condyle. There also can be erosive changes in the postmandibular fossa area and the posterior head of the condyle.
5. Bony and fibrous ankylosis should be treated by surgery; osteoarthritis and/or arthrosis, under certain conditions, also can be treated surgically.
6. Fibrous ankylosis limits motion, but more frequently a pseudoankylosis is present. Pseudoankylosis is related primarily to muscle spasms of the internal pterygoid muscle plus spasms of the masseter, external pterygoid, and temporal muscles.

Many individuals with significant temporomandibular joint problems suffer from arthrosis, which Thoma[41] defines as consisting of "arthralgia, myalgia, dysmasesis, and clicking." However, thinning of the disc usually occurs and can be detected radiographically. Rheumatoid arthritis should be differentiated from osteoarthritis by the severity of the radiographic bone pathological condition of the condylar head and articular eminence and by blood studies. According to Thoma, arthritis is probably "more often the cause of temporomandibular dysfunction than would appear from a study of the literature. . . ."

According to Mayne and Hatch,[27] nonspecific inflammatory arthritis radiographically would show a narrowed joint space, evidence of destructive lesions of the condyle, and limited temporomandibular joint motion as seen in the views taken with the mouth open and closed. Hatch[17] concludes from this study that the temporomandibular joint is involved in rheumatoid arthritis much more commonly than is generally reported.

It is our belief that people suffering from rheumatoid arthritis and osteoarthritis of the temporomandibular joint can be helped first by accurate radiographs

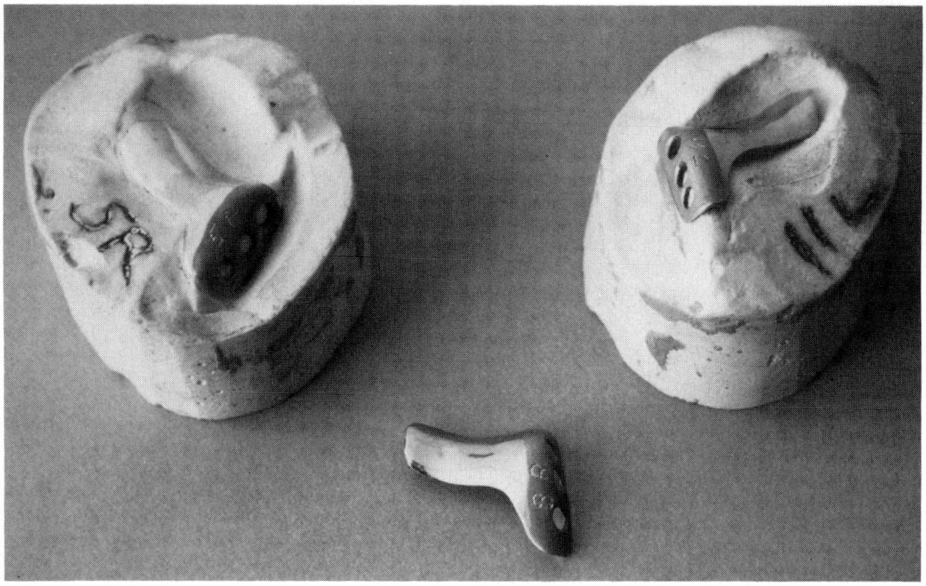

Fig. 22-8. Articular eminence prosthesis with dies.

and diagnosis and then by surgical intervention when necessary. This recognizes that the great majority of mandibular joint problems should be treated nonsurgically.

Most of the surgeries were not performed for true ankylosis, bony or fibrous, but for other pathological conditions of this joint. Prostheses have been developed for bony and fibrous ankylosis where it is necessary to cover the entire mandibular fossa to prevent reankylosis. Christensen[10] has explained in detail his experience in placing a metal barrier between the two bone surfaces as a possible means of preventing future ankylosis; a cast Vitallium glenoid fossa prosthesis was chosen from 60 appliances that had been previously prepared.

Since we are not surgically treating bony or fibrous ankylosis in most cases, we are not concerned with a reankylosis and the necessity of total coverage of the fossa. In designing the new prosthesis (an artificial metallic articular eminence with modifications) 50 skulls were used. Impressions of the right and the left articular eminences were made. A hundred castings were fabricated. Experimentally, these castings were tried on the 50 skulls until five appliances for each side were selected that fit all eminences uniformly well (Fig. 22-8).

Surgery time is minimized by this technique. There is no disturbance of occlusion after surgery, since the relationship of the condyle in the fossa has not changed. The condyle contacts the appliance only on opening or closing movements (Fig. 22-9). In other appliances the condylar head is of necessity continuously in contact with the metallic fossa.

Fig. 22-10 shows a kit of 10 articular eminence prostheses: five for the right articular eminence and five for the left. The size and form of these implants were determined by one of us (D.H.M.) by having dies and castings made for 50 right and 50 left articular eminences. The various castings were tried on all the eminence dies until five varieties of right and five varieties of left were found that would fit all the 50 varying shapes of the eminences. These 10 forms also were clinically checked on a number of patients at the time of surgery. These forms prevent the necessity of having 50 sizes for one joint and 50 sizes for the other, which helps cut down the surgery time.

Silastic insert in articular eminence prosthesis

In some individuals it is found that the condyle is jammed, not only anteriorly against the articular eminence but also superiorly against the fossa and posteriorly against the postglenoid fossa. When this condition occurs, a Silastic insert is secured to the articular eminence prosthesis by sutures (Fig. 22-11) or bonding.

The Silastic insert is reinforced with nylon mesh. When it is secured to the zygoma, the screw penetrates the Silastic and mesh and holds it to the zygoma. Also, pressure holds the Silastic insert in a mediolateral direction against the bone. There is little possibility of the Silastic becoming loose. It acts as a buffer in the superior and posterior directions.

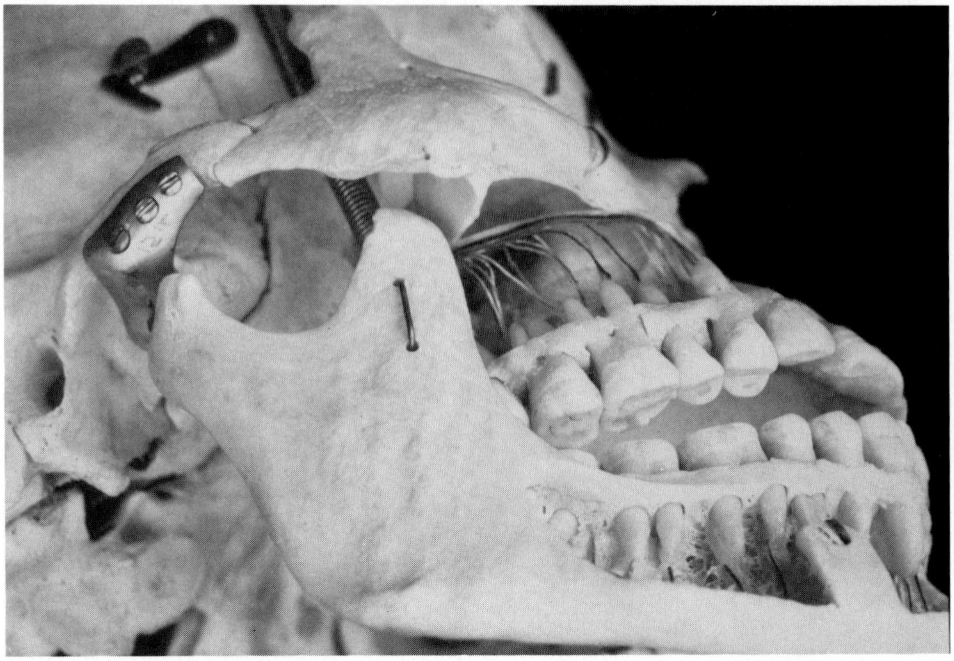

Fig. 22-9. Articular eminence prosthesis showing condyle functioning against prosthesis.

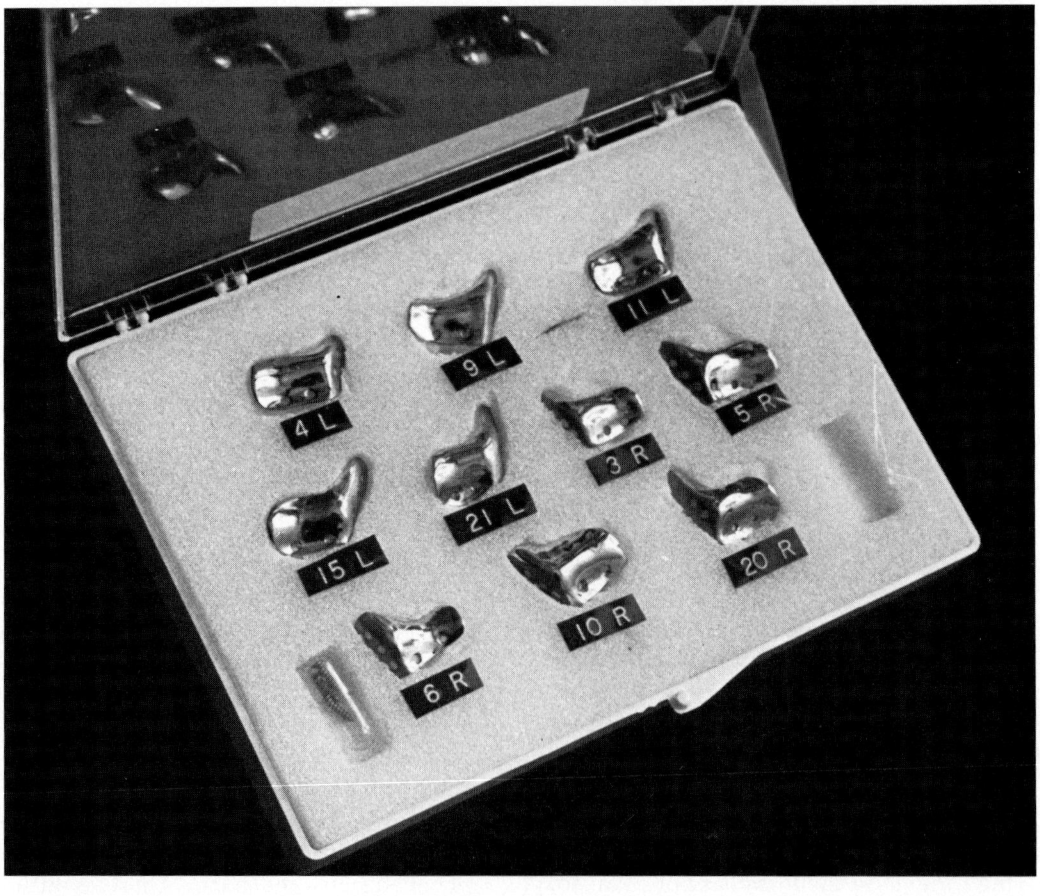

Fig. 22-10. Articular eminence prostheses in kit form with appropriate screws produced by Howmedica, Inc. (Rutherford, N.J.). There are five prostheses for right side and five for left.

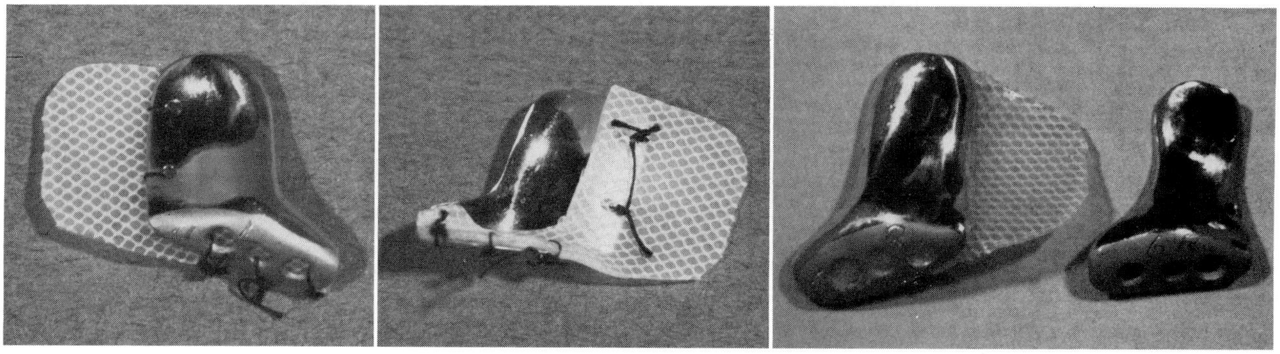

A B C

Fig. 22-11. A, Silastic insert sutured to prosthesis with nonabsorbable suture material. B, Internal view of Silastic insert. C, Silastic insert secured to prosthesis using Silastic glue.

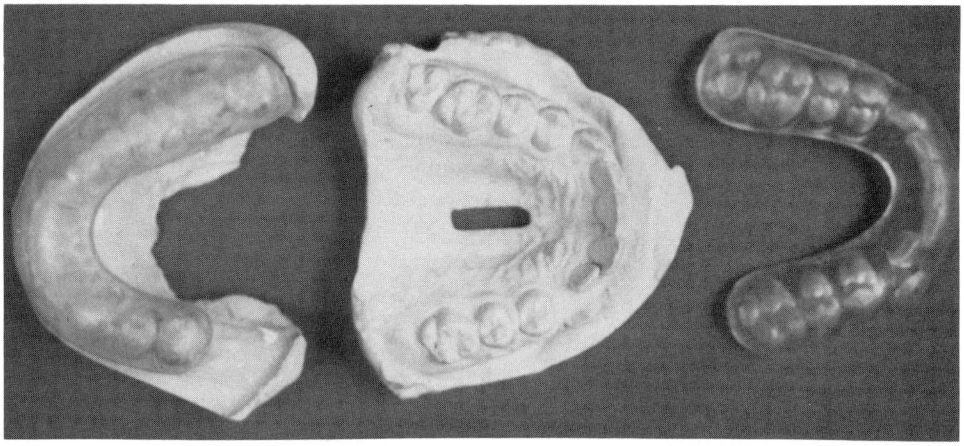

Fig. 22-12. Temporary resilient dental splints.

Preoperative evaluation

1. Specialized radiographs
   a. TMJ radiographs, wax bite, fourth view
   b. Intracanthus films
   c. Cephalometric films
   d. Full-face, right and left profile, and teeth views of patient
2. Evaluation on a Mandibular Kinesiograph
3. Dental evaluation
   a. Full-mouth dental films
   b. Models of teeth and jaws mounted on articulator
4. ENT evaluation
   a. Audiometry (when indicated)
   b. Electronystagmography (when indicated)
5. Neurological evaluation (when indicated)
6. Medical examination (general physician or internist)
7. Psychological evaluation
   a. Minnesota Multiphasic Personality Inventory (MMPI) given by psychologist
   b. Refer to psychiatrist or clinical psychologist when necessary for therapy before or after TMJ treatment; stress reduction therapy
8. Myofunctional therapy evaluation
9. Muscle and physiotherapy examination

Postoperative management

1. Dental (occlusal) splints
   a. Resilient (Fig. 22-12)
   b. Other
2. Equilibration
3. Restore missing teeth
4. Myotherapy
   a. Muscle therapy
   b. Dry needling techniques

   c. Physiotherapy
   d. Myo-Monitor
   e. Myofunctional therapy
5. Acupuncture
6. Emotional support
   a. Stress reduction therapy
   b. Psychotherapy, group or individual
7. Follow-up results every 6 months when possible
   a. Postoperative radiographs
   b. Postoperative questionnaire
   c. Clinical examination

Medical regimen for TMJ treatment

1. Hydrocollator (moist heat), neck type, 30 minutes a day to both joints
2. Os-Cal 40, two tablets tid
3. Soft diet
4. Myo-Monitor stimulation treatment—electronically restores fatigued muscles (See Chapter 31.)
5. Resilient splint, maxillary or mandibular type
6. Meprobamate (Equanil, Miltown), 400 mg hs
7. Diazepam (Valium), 5 mg, one tablet tid
8. Bromelain (Ananase), 100,000 units qid for 2 weeks
9. Psychological support, psychotherapy when necessary; personal interest of practitioner
10. Have missing teeth restored or replaced; check for uneven occlusion; check for closed bite with special TMJ radiographs
11. Eliminate gum chewing and any unusual oral habits
12. Continue regimen at least 2 months

Surgical techniques[30]

Insertion of the prosthesis is accomplished by a modified preauricular incision approximately 5 cm long. The superior portion of the incision has a hockey-stick appearance to hide part of the incision in the hairline and to allow better access to the site. The skin is undermined approximately 3 cm anteriorly and secured to the cheek with 3-0 silk sutures (Fig. 22-13, *A*). By sharp and blunt dissection, the superior portion of the incision is first extended to the level of the temporal muscle fascia. It is easier to locate this layer of fascia in the upper portion of the incision. Bleeding vessels are electrocoagulated or tied with 3-0 chromic sutures. The dissection is then extended along the plane of the fascia in an anterior and inferior direction to expose the zygomatic arch. At this point a 3-cm horizontal incision is made over the zygoma superior and medial to branches of the facial nerve (Fig. 22-13, *B*). The periosteal elevator is used to retract the capsular ligament from its at-

A

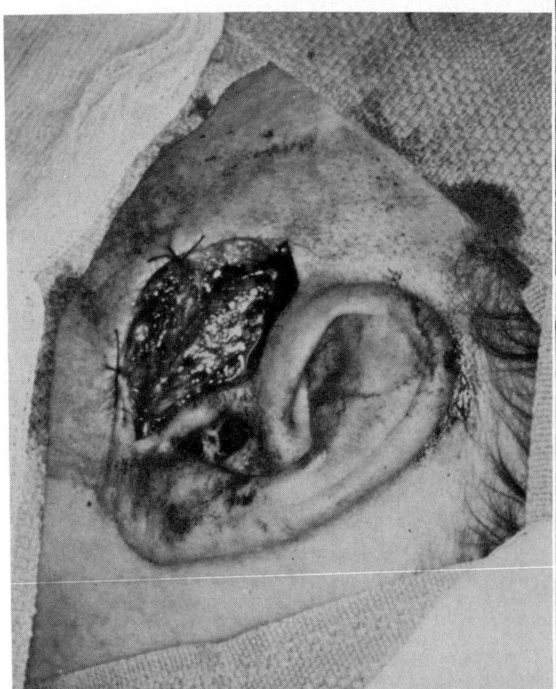

B

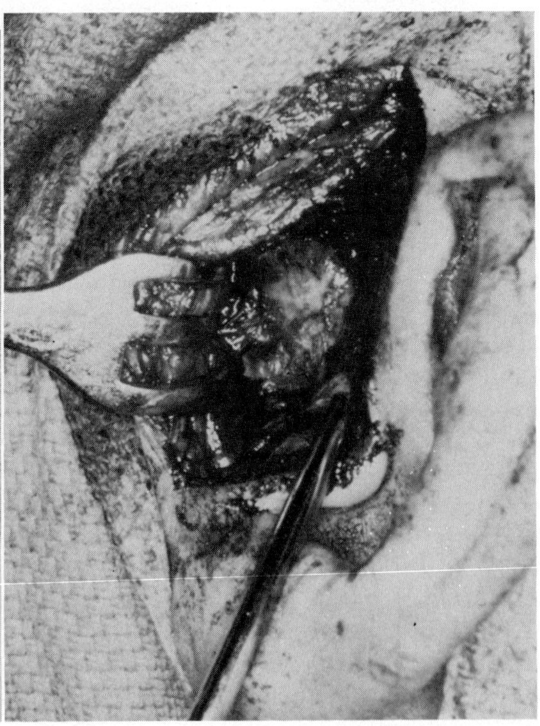

Fig. 22-13. A, Skin flap sutured to cheek. **B,** A 3-cm horizontal incision made over zygoma.

tachment to the zygoma in an inferior direction. The lateral surface of the articular eminence, the posterior part of the zygomatic arch, the mandibular fossa, the superior surface of the meniscus, and the underlying condyle are exposed (Fig. 22-14, *A*). The eminence and zygomatic arch are denuded of periosteum in preparation for receiving the appliance (Fig. 22-14, *B*).

There are three considerations for selection of the proper prosthesis. The first is the height of the articular eminence. Some eminences are flat, and some are relatively steep. It is necessary to select the proper appliance from the five varieties for each side. Another consideration is the relationship of the angle of the eminence to the zygomatic arch in the horizontal plane. In some individuals this is a right angle; in others it is an acute or obtuse angle. The last consideration is the mediolateral contour of the eminence. Some eminences are straight across, whereas others have a vaulting or concave effect. When placing the prosthesis into position, it is necessary that the metal fit closely to the eminence at its junction with the fossa. It is not so crucial that the portion overlying the zygomatic arch fits precisely, since this portion has no direct stress placed on it. The portion overlying the eminence has the condyle translating over it, so it must fit correctly, or the prosthesis could become loose.

Once the proper prosthesis is in position, it is secured by two or three 5-mm cast Vitallium screws (Fig. 22-15). The capsular ligament is repositioned and sutured using 3-0 Dexon or Dermalon sutures. The deep vertical incision is closed with the same material. The skin flap is closed using numerous subcuticular sutures of 3-0 Dexon. The skin margin is closed with either 5-0 or 6-0 Dermalon mattress or interrupted sutures.

For total TMJ replacement plus reconstruction of the entire mandible following ablative surgery for neoplasia or trauma such as massive gunshot wounds a titanium mesh is used (Fig. 22-16). The appliance is overfilled with particulate cancellous marrow grafts to restore jaw form and function. In Fig. 22-17 a surgical view is seen of the condyle and glenoid fossa with a thin sheet of Silastic affixed via wiring through the lateral rim. A condyloplasty and meniscectomy also were performed for treating an osteophyte that caused a perforation of the disc.*

*Case courtesy Charles D. Hasse, D.D.S.

A

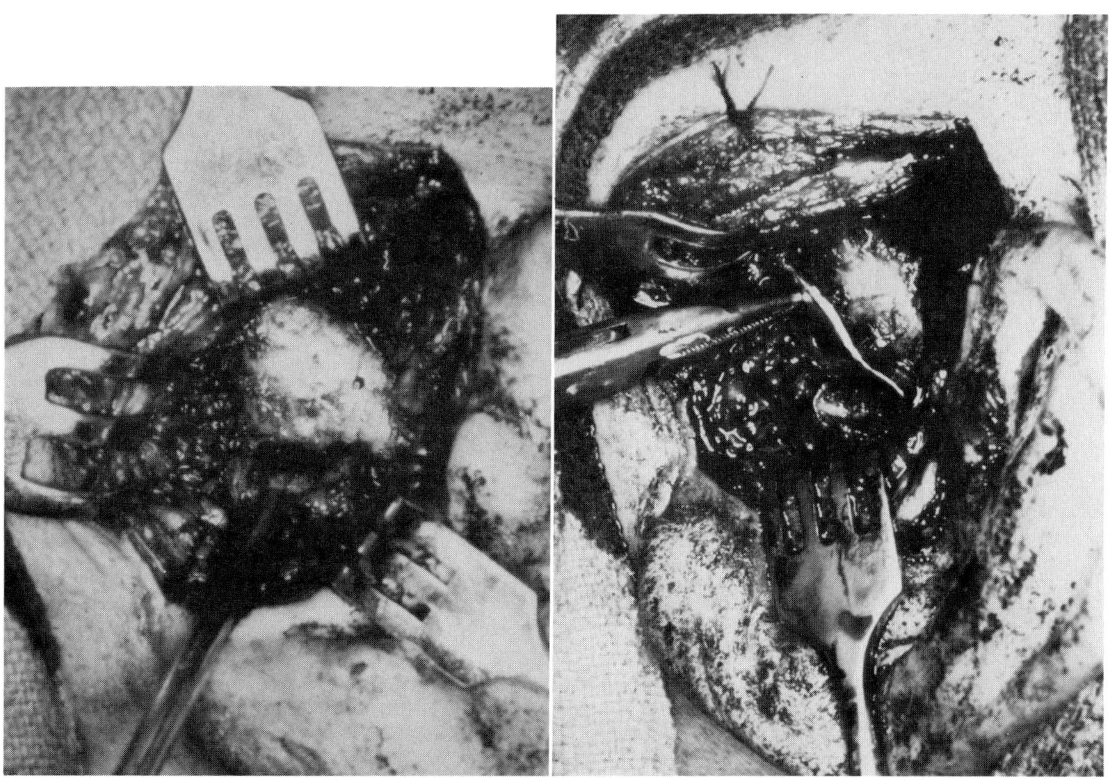

B

Fig. 22-14. A, Exposure of condylar head and articular eminence. **B,** Placement of prosthesis.

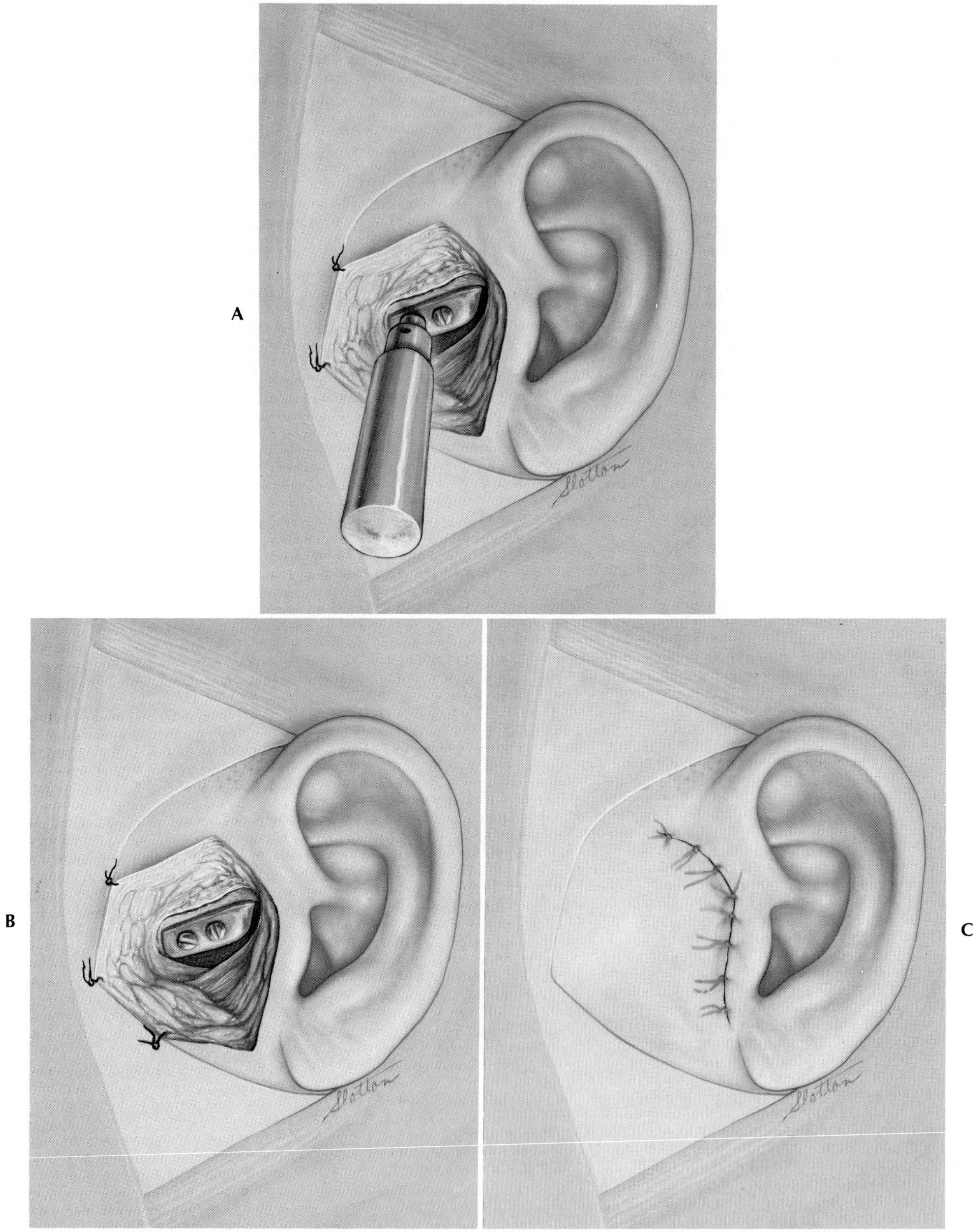

Fig. 22-15. A, Specialized screwdriver (designed by Morgan-Atwood) securing prosthesis to zygoma. **B,** Prosthesis in position. **C,** Wound area closed and sutured with 5-0 or 6-0 Dermalon.

Complications

Allergic reaction to implant material: Prior to surgery tests with Vitallium, tantalum, Silastic, and stainless steel are recommended.

Loosening of prosthesis: Extra screws are used for stabilizing the prosthesis.

Psychogenic factors: All patients are evaluated with the MMPI before any therapy is started.

Weakness of zygomatic-frontal nerve: Obtain an informed consent signed by patient and witnessed as to this possibility.

Infection: There is always a possibility of infection or delayed infection. Any postoperative surgical procedures in the mouth should be preceded by appropriate antibiotic therapy. Obtain an informed consent signed by patient and witnessed as to this possibility, even a year after surgery.

Spasm of external pterygoid muscle: Because this is often caused by oral intubation, nasal intubation is used whenever possible. With nasal intubation you can determine if occlusion is correct after placing implant.

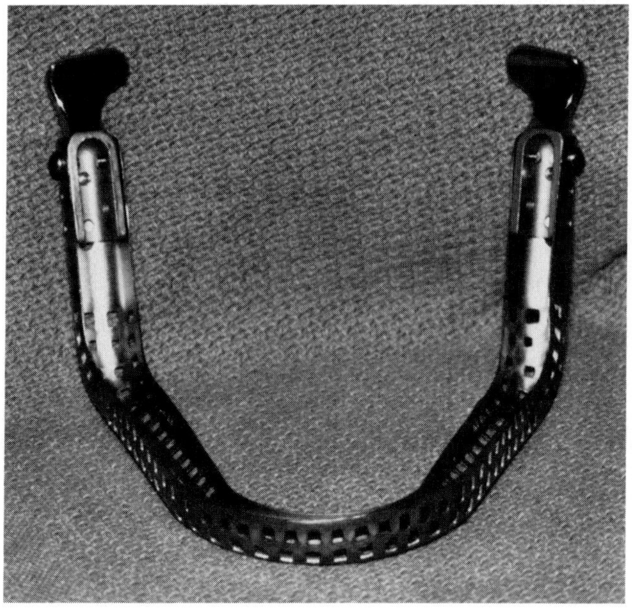

Fig. 22-16. Appliance for replacement of entire mandible and TMJ. (Courtesy Charles D. Hasse, D.D.S.)

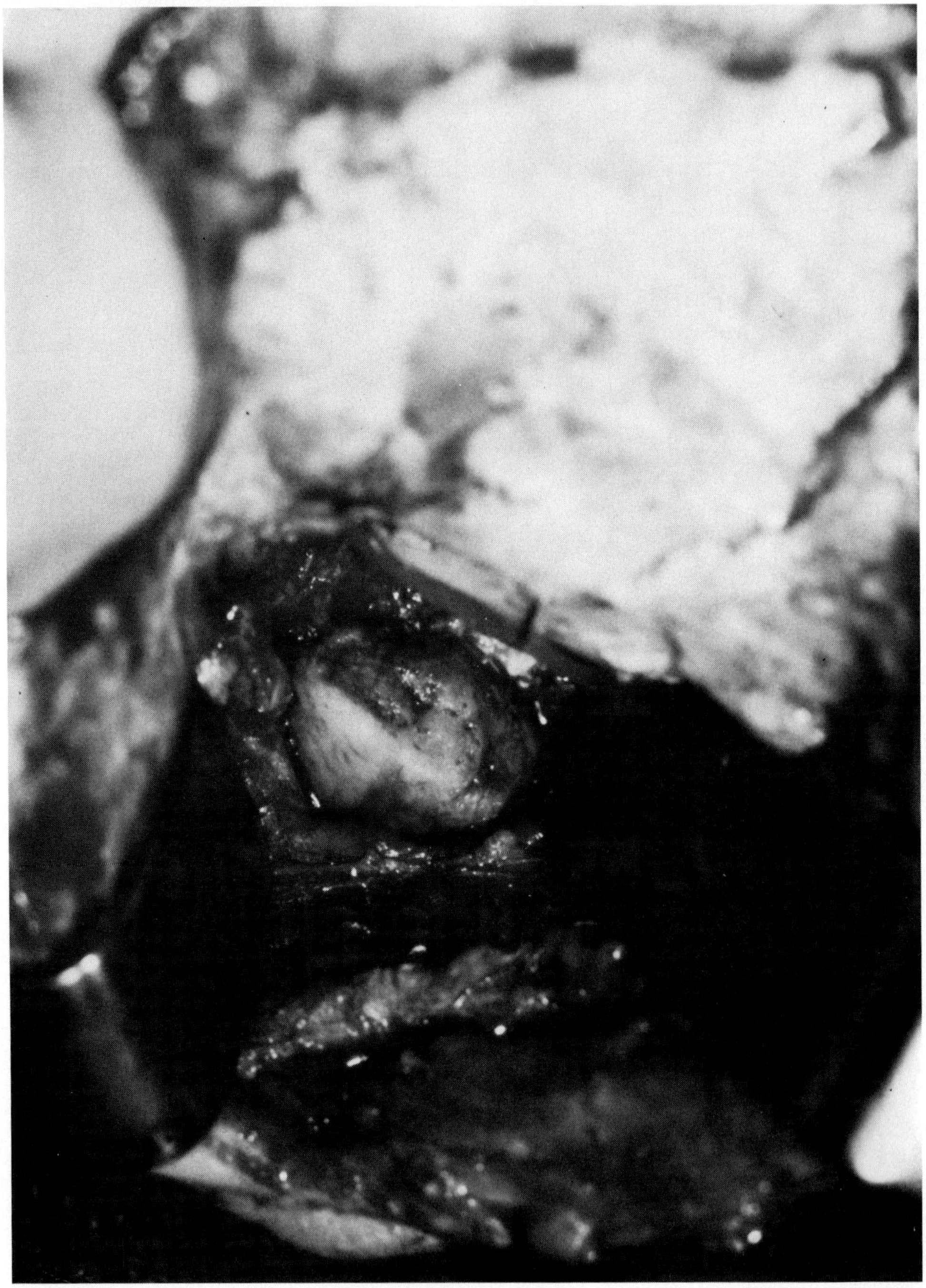

Fig. 22-17. Surgical view of condyle and glenoid fossa with thin sheet of Silastic affixed via wiring through lateral rim. (Courtesy Charles D. Hasse, D.D.S.)

RECENT DEVELOPMENTS: ARTHROPLASTY PLUS MENISCECTOMY

Tables 22-3 and 22-4 show the initial diagnosis made on 90 patients with TMJ dysfunction and the postoperative results of their 132 temporomandibular joints operated on over an 8-year period. These patients were selected from nearly 1000 patients presenting with TMJ symptoms. The other patients were helped by nonsurgical methods. We have performed a meniscectomy on 12 patients who had a previous arthroplasty with insertion of an articular eminence prosthesis. These were those 14% (8% showing no improvement in pain symptoms in Table 22-4 and 6% showing more discomfort than before surgery) in the group who had not been helped by this process. To date, 8 of the 12 patients have had improvement of their pain symptoms.

In these individuals apparently the disc has been so damaged and displaced that it has continued to irritate the joint, creating chronic synovitis. It has been stated by Dingman and Moorman[14] and by Kochan[25] that the disc has synovial tissue at its periphery, where it attaches to the capsular ligament, and lining the surface of the disc.

Pathological studies of our specimens also confirm

Table 22-3. Initial diagnosis of 90 patients with TMJ dysfunction (osteoarthritis or rheumatoid arthritis)

Diagnosis	Symptoms	Number of patients
Labyrinthine disease	Fullness, tinnitus, vertigo	17
Migraine	Recurrent temporal pain	15
Psychogenic disorders	Variety of symptoms with no apparent organic basis	12
Eustachian tube malfunction or secretory otitis media	Fullness, subjective hearing loss	9
Functional disorders of TMJ, pseudoankylosis, chronic subluxation	Inability to open or close mouth	8
Acute sinusitis	Pain in zygomatic arch, fullness in cheek	7
Tic douloureux	Fifth nerve trigger zones	6
Odontitis	Toothache	5
Suspected brain lesions, acoustic neuroma	Ear, deep head pains	4
Bell's palsy	Earache, weakness in facial muscles	2
Acute mastoiditis	Ear and mastoid pain	2
Acute parotitis and/or mixed cell tumor of parotid gland	Pain in preauricular area, gonial angle, swelling	2
Rheumatoid arthritis	Resorption of condyles	1

From Morgan, D.H.: Surgical correction of temporomandibular joint arthritis, J. Oral Surg. **33**:766, 1975. Copyright by the American Dental Association. Reprinted by permission.

Table 22-4. Postoperative results of 90 patients with 132 temporomandibular joints operated on over 8-year period, from questionnaire and clinical and radiographic examinations*

Symptoms	Elimination of symptoms (%)	Improvement of symptoms (%)	No improvement (%)	More discomfort and/or symptoms than before surgery (%)
Pain: head, neck, shoulder, arm	62	24	8	6
Grating sound in joint	63	28	6	3
Tinnitus	49	32	13	6
Functional disorders	66	20	9	5
Vertigo	63	34	3	—
Weakness in facial muscles	100	—	—	—

From Morgan, D.H.: Surgical correction of temporomandibular joint arthritis, J. Oral Surg. **33**:766, 1975. Copyright by the American Dental Association. Reprinted by permission.

*Unilateral operation, 58 joints; bilateral operation, 32 joints (including unilateral to bilateral operation, six joints); 10 joints reoperated (four allergic reactions, four loose screws, one external pterygoid muscle spasm, one because of psychogenic factors).

this. In the future it may be more frequently considered to perform a combined procedure of an arthroplasty with insertion of an articular eminence prosthesis and a meniscectomy.

PATHOLOGICAL CONDITIONS OF THE TMJ

Carlsson, Kopp, and Oberg[8] have described their pathological findings and have concluded that lesions are most frequent in the lateral part of the disc and temporal eminence (Figs. 22-18 and 22-19). In our clinical and surgical practice at the White Memorial Medical Center most specimens that have been available for microscopic tissue examination for determining the histological changes from disease have come almost exclusively from the menisci removed at surgery. Gross disease of the joint capsule, the menisci, the condyles, the joint cartilage, and articulating surfaces is visualized and palpated during surgery. But the microscopic studies have been limited to the fibrocartilage and capsular tissues removed at surgery. Several of these cases are described here.

Case 1

C.B. is a 32-year-old woman. After we exposed the right temporomandibular joint, a tear in the lateral aspect of the meniscus was identified. The lateral aspect of the articular eminence was roughened and could be palpated with the thin end of an elevator. As the joint was widened with a lamina spreader, the anterior aspect of the condylar head presented roughness. The meniscus appeared thin from compression and was very friable and torn. Microscopic study of the removed meniscus showed fibrocartilage with some dense fibrous connective tissue. No specific disease changes were identified microscopically. In this case the findings on the left were very similar grossly and microscopically to those on the right, but the meniscus was not quite as thin and friable as on the left.

Case 2

J.H. is a 32-year-old man. There was clinical limitation of joint mobility on the left side and audible and palpable clicking on opening of the mouth. The radiographs showed the principle pathosis to be on the left side, with erosion, absorption, tearing and flattening of the eminence, and some in-

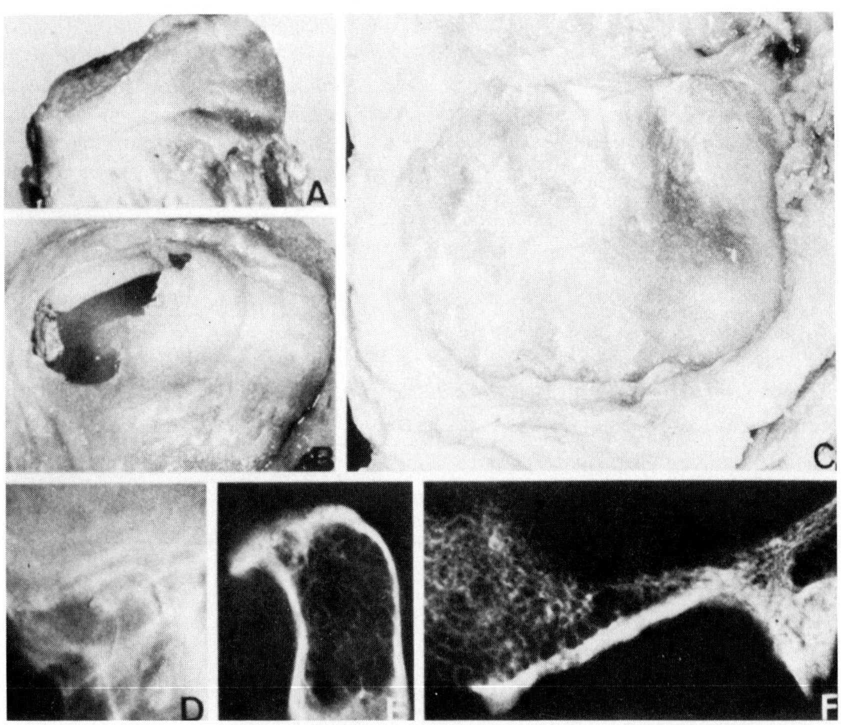

Fig. 22-18. Series of photographs depicting area of organic disease most frequently found in TMJ. (From Carlsson, G.E., Kopp, S., and Oberg, T.: Arthritis and allied diseases of the temporomandibular joint. In Zarb, G.A., and Carlsson, G.E., editors: Temporomandibular joint function and dysfunction, St. Louis, 1979, The C.V. Mosby Co. © 1979, Munksgaard International Publishers Ltd., Copenhagen, Denmark.)

creased bone density. The condyle showed flattening and surface irregularity with a small nodular lipping posteriorly. The point space behind the condyle was widened. Gross findings in the left joint at surgery revealed deficiency or flattening of the eminence, which was crepitant and roughened when palpated with the elevator. The meniscus was thin, friable, and perforated—almost nonexistent. The condylar head was irregular with slight exostosis posteriorly. Microscopic examination showed fraying, fragmentation, and degenerative changes of fibrous connective tissue.

Case 3

A third patient (C.U.), a 15-year-old girl, had an onset of problems when her jaw was dislocated while she was vigorously chewing gum. X-ray examination indicated limitation of translation of the condyle. There was marked atrophy of the left condyle, presenting as a narrow bar or post without a head. With her mouth wide open the condyle moved poorly and was widely separated from the eminence. After surgical exposure the eminence was found to be quite flat with a sandpaper-like roughness of its surface. The meniscus was quite redundant and loose, with a tear in the lateral portion. The meniscus was also thin and atrophic. The gross findings on the right side were similar, but there were significant adhesions in the lateral portion. The looseness of the meniscus led to the belief that it could roll up in layers, perhaps interfering with normal opening of the mouth and creating crepitus or a clicking sound. Microscopic study revealed it to be like fibrocartilage with some fibrous connective tissue partly covered by synovium.

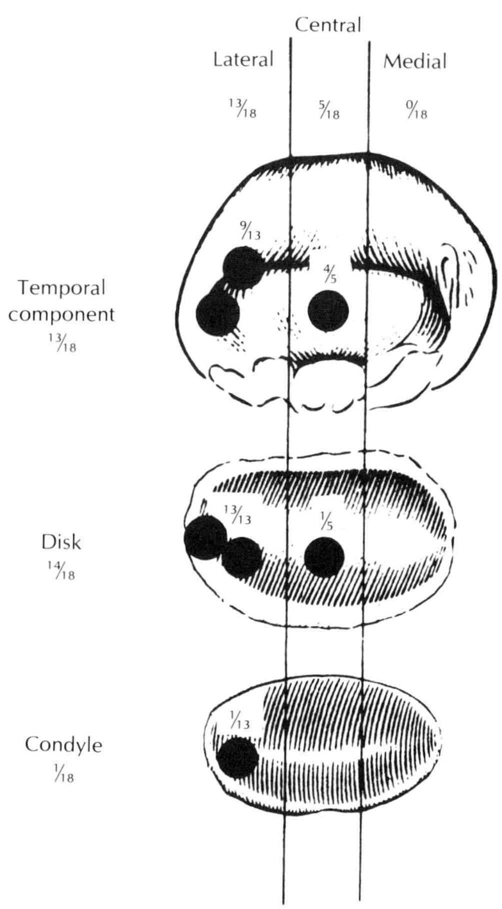

Fig. 22-19. Analysis of lesions in temporomandibular joints from autopsy material of 102 adult joints from Swedish hospital, showing lesions most frequently found in lateral part of disc and temporal eminence. (From Oberg, T., Carlsson, G.E., and Fojers, C.M.: Acta Odontol. Scand. **29:**349, 1971.)

Case 4

A woman age 27 (G.K.) with a bilateral arthroplasty presented with gross roughness in both articular eminences. The right condyle also showed some roughness and erosion on the lateral aspect. Microscopic tissue studies showed fibrocartilage with loose and dense fibrous connective tissue attached.[28] A considerable amount of synovium covered the meniscus, and some of this showed necrotic and papillary changes.

Case 5

A woman age 20 (M.B.) had an automobile accident 3 years prior to surgery. She also had a right-sided concussion 9 months later associated with torticollis, which required a brace and later surgery. Chewing difficulty pointed to a TMJ problem. There was fairly good occlusion, but the right TMJ was tender, and chewing movements produced crepitation. X-ray films showed excess motion of the condyle in the wide-open position. Increased radiodensity of the disc area suggested calcification on one side. Gross findings at surgery revealed the common findings of roughness of the articular eminence and a lateral tear in the meniscus and hypertrophy. There was a prominent spicule of hypertrophic bone on the lateral portion of the condyle on both sides. These were removed. Microscopic sections of the meniscus showed only fibrocartilage and connective tissue.

Case 6

L.F., a 55-year-old-woman, had symptoms and unilateral surgery on the left side. Grossly, there were osteoporotic changes in the eminence and in the condyle. Both were smoothed with a curette. Microscopic examination of the meniscus again revealed fibrocartilage and connective tissue partially covered with synovium.

Case 7

A 39-year-old woman had undergone secondary surgery, at which time the previously placed prostheses were removed. It was noted that a thickened capsule of connective tissue had been produced to cover the condyle almost as completely as the normal meniscus. This was noted in more than one instance, leading us to be impressed at how the body compensates for removal of the meniscus by forming a substitute.

TOTAL TEMPOROMANDIBULAR JOINT

We have had the opportunity to reoperate on several patients who have had the combined procedure of arthroplasty and meniscectomy. In each case it was found that after approximately 3 to 6 months a fibrous connective tissue covered the head of the condyle and also the metallic implant. Consequently, it appears that the body recovers these surfaces after the combined procedure in which a damaged and malfunctioning disc is removed and an implant inserted. This does not occur when the disc or its remnants are left in the joint. A furthur consequence is that, if for any reason the implant were to be removed later, there would be a fibrous connective tissue barrier resembling a disc between the upper and lower portions of the joint.

An independent medical research group evaluated our TMJ patients for a 14-year-period. In January 1978, 205 TMJ questionnaires were mailed to patients who had undergone TMJ implant surgery. The population surveyed, representing 314 TMJ procedures, was asked (1) to make a subjective overall assessment of the surgical result, and (2) to rate the improvement, elimina-

Table 22-5. TMJ surgical population: by survey and response

	Surgical population surveyed		Surgical population response	
Year of first TMJ surgery	**Number of joints involved**	**Number of patients**	**Number of joints involved**	**Number of patients**
1965	1	1	1	1
1967	3	3	2	2
1968	2	2	1	1
1969	3	2	—	—
1970	9	9	4	4
1971	29	21	17	13
1972	46	28	20	13
1973	46	31	18	13
1974	49	32	29	17
1975	51	30	30	16
1976	40	22	25	15
1977	31	20	20	12
Unknown	4	4	—	—
TOTAL	314	205	167	107

Table 22-6. Patient ratings of pain symptoms after TMJ surgery (1965 to 1977)

	Patient rating (%)				
Pain location	**Eliminated**	**Improved**	**No change**	**Worse**	**Not applicable**
Joint	35.4	35.4	9.2	9.2	10.8
Headache	18.6	42.9	19.3	1.4	17.9
Facial muscles	33.6	34.4	9.9	3.8	18.3
Lower jaw	38.1	27.8	8.7	6.4	19.1
Upper jaw	37.7	27.7	7.7	6.9	20.0
Ear	29.5	27.1	9.3	5.4	28.7
Neck	23.7	29.0	11.5	3.8	32.1
Forehead	24.2	32.0	9.4	1.6	32.8
Around eyes	29.6	22.4	6.4	4.0	37.6
Shoulder	22.1	22.9	8.4	0.8	45.8
Tongue	17.4	9.9	5.8	3.3	63.6

tion, or worsening of each of 22 surgical indications (whenever such indications were applicable).

The overall results are shown in Tables 22-5 to 22-8. The overall group assessment results were 41.7% excellent, 28.8% good, 14.1% fair, and 15.3% poor. The five most frequent symptoms indicating TMJ surgery were a grating sound in the joint, partial inability to open the mouth, pain in the joint, clicking in the joint, and headaches.

For a number of years orthopedists have been operating on hip joints and performing in essence a total restoration of that joint by placing a prosthesis not only in the lower portion of the joint but in the upper portion as well. These same principles apply to the temporomandibular joint. We had previously operated on a patient (G.M.) for whom we had contemplated placing a prosthesis in the upper portion of the joint. Because of the length of the surgery, however, it was elected not to do so. In a more recent surgery it was thought that the patient would be helped by a total restoration of the joint. This was done with a Vitallium and acrylic condylar prosthesis and by restoration of the up-

Table 22-7. Patient ratings of symptoms other than pain after TMJ surgery (1965 to 1977)

Symptom	Patient rating (%)				
	Eliminated	Improved	No change	Worse	Not applicable
Grating sound in joint	39.2	29.2	10.0	11.5	10.0
Partial inability to open mouth	25.9	31.1	4.4	23.7	14.8
Clicking sound in joint	32.8	31.2	12.0	6.4	17.6
Snapping sound in joint	38.2	22.1	8.4	11.5	19.9
Popping sound in joint	38.2	25.2	6.1	7.6	22.9
Vertigo	30.0	31.4	10.0	0.7	27.9
Fullness, pressure, blockage in ear	19.1	29.4	8.1	8.1	35.3
Ringing in ears	21.7	17.1	19.4	6.2	35.7
Nausea	26.5	12.9	7.6	0.8	52.3
Subjective hearing loss	19.0	10.7	12.4	3.3	54.6
Total inability to open mouth	21.3	4.6	1.9	2.8	69.4

Table 22-8. Patient's subjective overall assessment of surgical results

Year of surgery	Number of joints involved	Number of responses	Patient rating (%)			
			Excellent	Good	Fair	Poor
1965	1	—	100.0	—	—	—
1967	2	—	100.0	—	—	—
1968	1	—	100.0	—	—	—
1970	4	—	50.0	50.0	—	—
1971	17	—	70.6	11.8	11.8	5.9
1972	20	—	25.0	45.0	—	30.0
1973	18	—	33.3	44.4	5.6	16.7
1974	29	—	34.5	24.1	—	41.4
1975	30	2	50.0	21.4	21.4	7.1
1976	25	2	39.1	13.0	43.5	4.4
1977	20	—	30.0	50.0	20.0	—
TOTAL	167	4	41.7	28.8	14.1	15.3

per portion of the joint with an articular eminence prosthesis and a Silastic insert. This procedure went well, and it is anticipated that this approach could be helpful to many individuals. Fig. 22-20 shows a condition where a total TMJ replacement could be beneficial.

CASE HISTORIES

Case 8

D.G., a 55-year-old woman with rheumatoid arthritis of her spine and, to a lesser degree, her hands, noticed that only her back teeth were contacting when chewing. There was pain primarily in the area of the right joint. She had attacks of dizziness on occasion. The patient was anxious about her condition and her inability to chew. Her facial muscles tired easily, and she was unable to completely open or close her mouth.

The patient's mouth was forced open with a mechanical mouth device. Specialized TMJ radiographs showed that there was resorption of the condyles in both the right and left joints (Fig. 22-21). The articular eminences in both the right and left joints were flattened, and the intraarticular space was diminished. There appeared to be more of a hinge action than a translatory movement. Pain was noted in the right and left joints on palpation. An anterior open bite was present, and the mandible appeared to be receding. Cephalometric radiographs confirmed this change (Fig. 22-22).

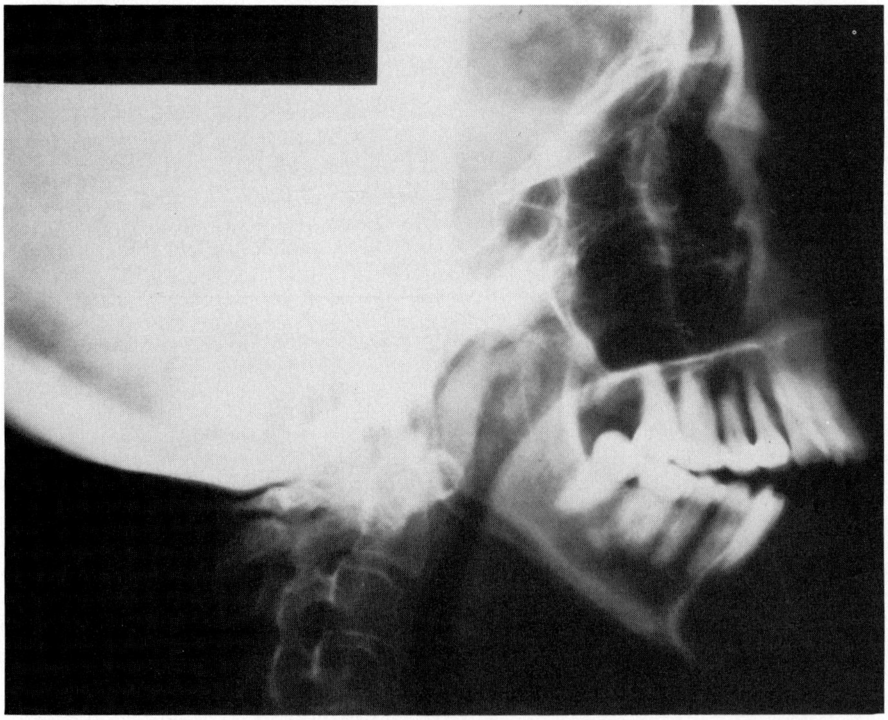

Fig. 22-20. Severe rheumatoid arthritis showing resorption of condyle, retrusion of mandible, and open bite.

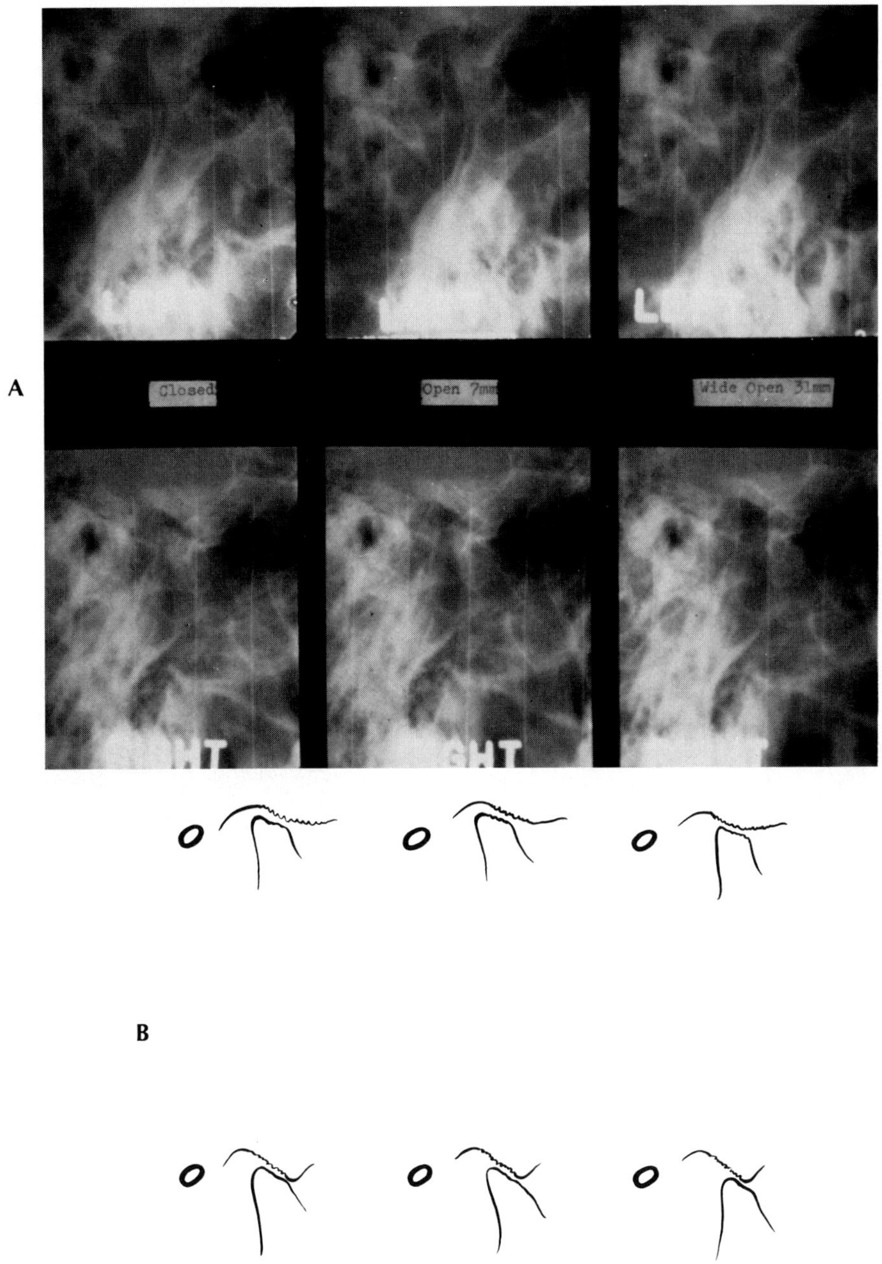

Fig. 22-21. A, Transcranial lateral oblique films showing flattening of left eminence and diminished intraarticular space. **B,** Line drawings also show flattening of eminences and erosion and flattening of condylar heads.

Because of the rheumatoid arthritis, both condyles were resorbing. The muscles were pulling the resorbed joint surfaces against the articular eminence (Fig. 22-23). This had the effect of retruding the mandible and creating an anterior open bite. There was a possibility that this would lead to ankylosis. Procedures done in the past had consisted of building new condyles bilaterally (Fig. 22-24).

However, securing a prosthesis depends on healthy bone. Since rheumatoid arthritis can continue to affect the bone supporting the prosthesis, it can loosen and permit the mandible to regress to its previous state (Fig. 22-25). Consequently, a new approach was applied. James Nethery, a maxillofacial prosthodontist, constructed a prosthesis for the articular eminence that had a Silastic portion extending into the fossa (Fig. 22-26). The Silastic was mechanically attached to the metal prosthesis. In essence, instead of building a new condyle, the floor of the fossa was lowered (Fig. 22-27). This had the effect of moving the mandible forward and placing the teeth in their proper relationship. The prosthesis is nonmovable, with less possibility of loosening.

Surgery was performed on December 14, 1971. On entering the joints, we noticed both eminences were to rough and flattened. The prostheses were fitted into the joints. The Silastic portions of the prostheses were contoured so they could be adjusted at the time of surgery with a Bard-Parker blade. After insertion of the prostheses, we noticed that the mandible tilted forward and upward and that the teeth were in their proper position. Arch bars previously had been placed so that elastic traction could be used at the time of surgery (Fig. 22-28). The patient has maintained good function to the present.[30]

Text continued on p. 390.

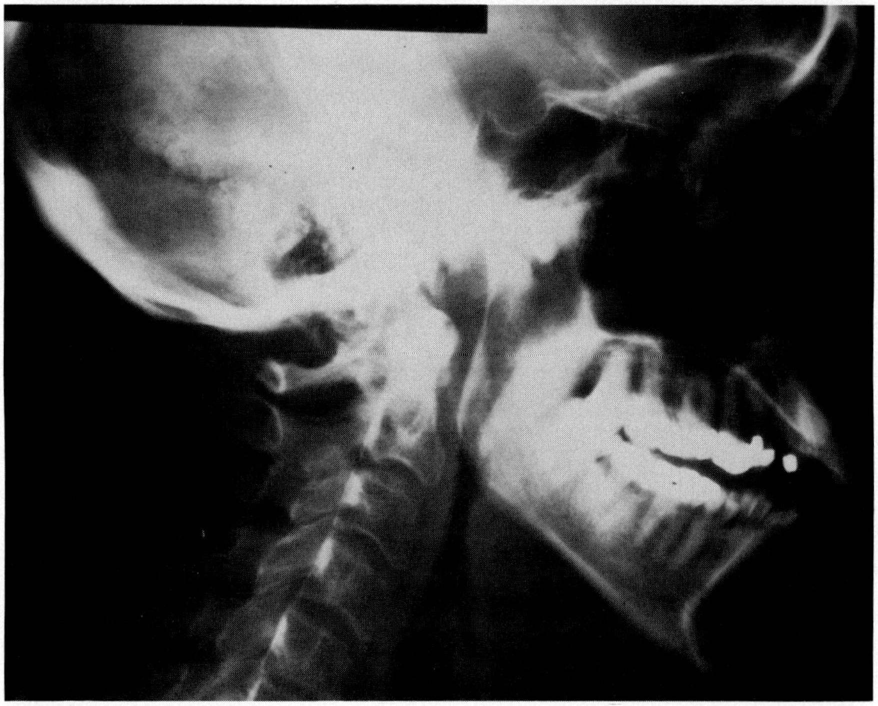

Fig. 22-22. Cephalometric film of D.G. showing open bite and retrusion of mandible.

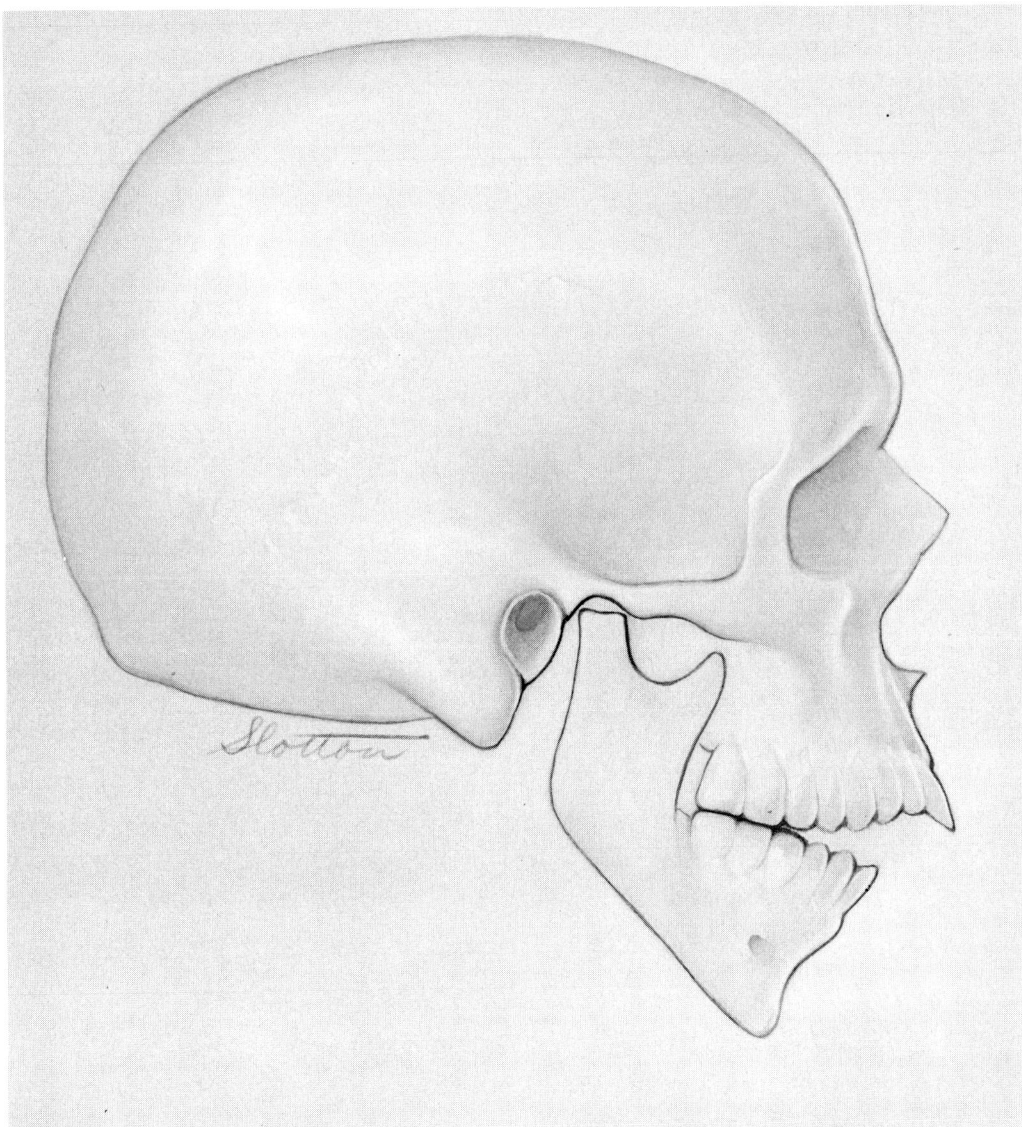

Fig. 22-23. Drawing of D.G. showing retrusion of mandible and open bite.

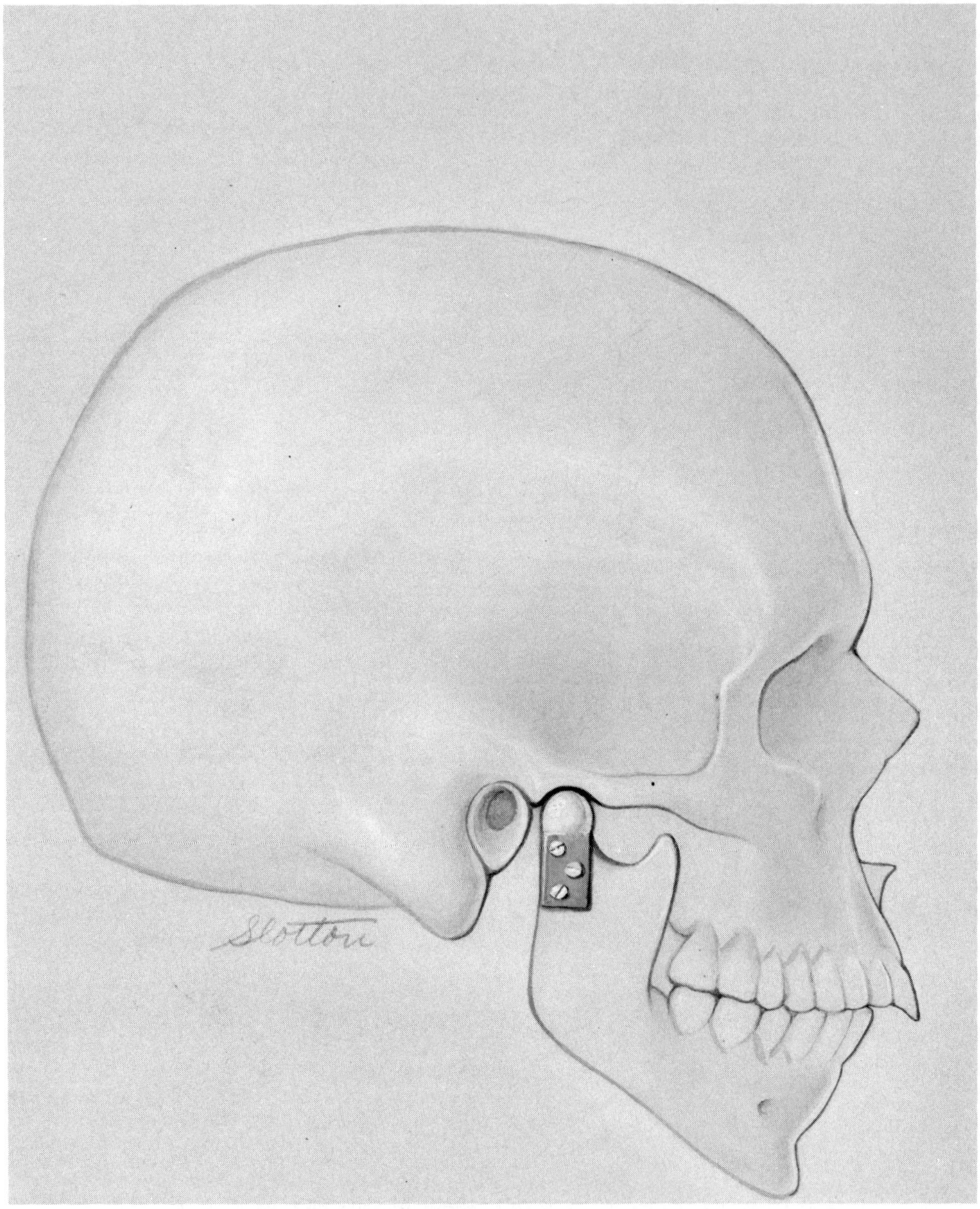

Fig. 22-24. Metal and plastic condylar prosthesis.

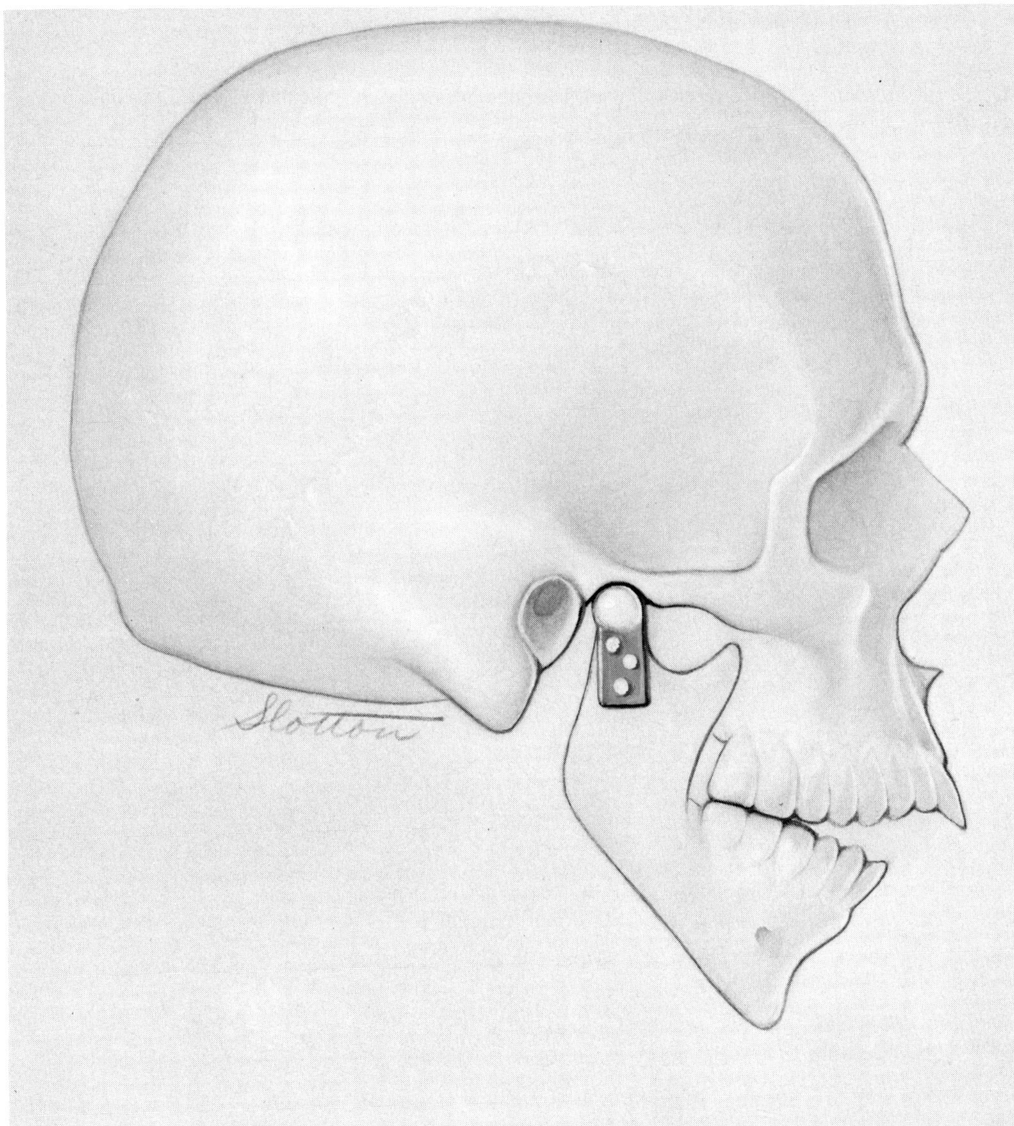

Fig. 22-25. Loosened condylar prothesis.

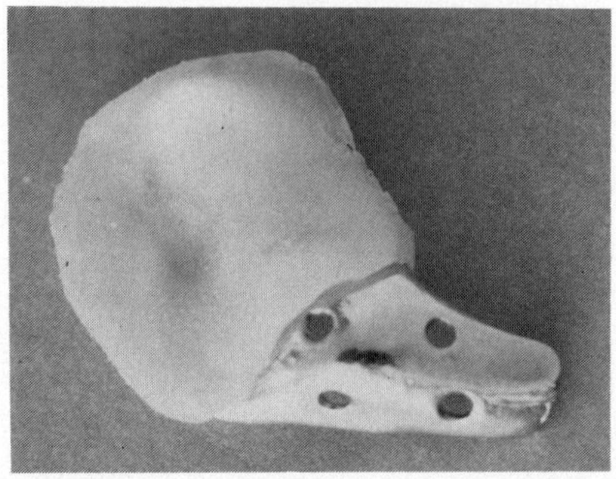

Fig. 22-26. Articular eminence prosthesis with thickened Silastic insert (designed by D.H. Morgan and constructed by J. Nethery).

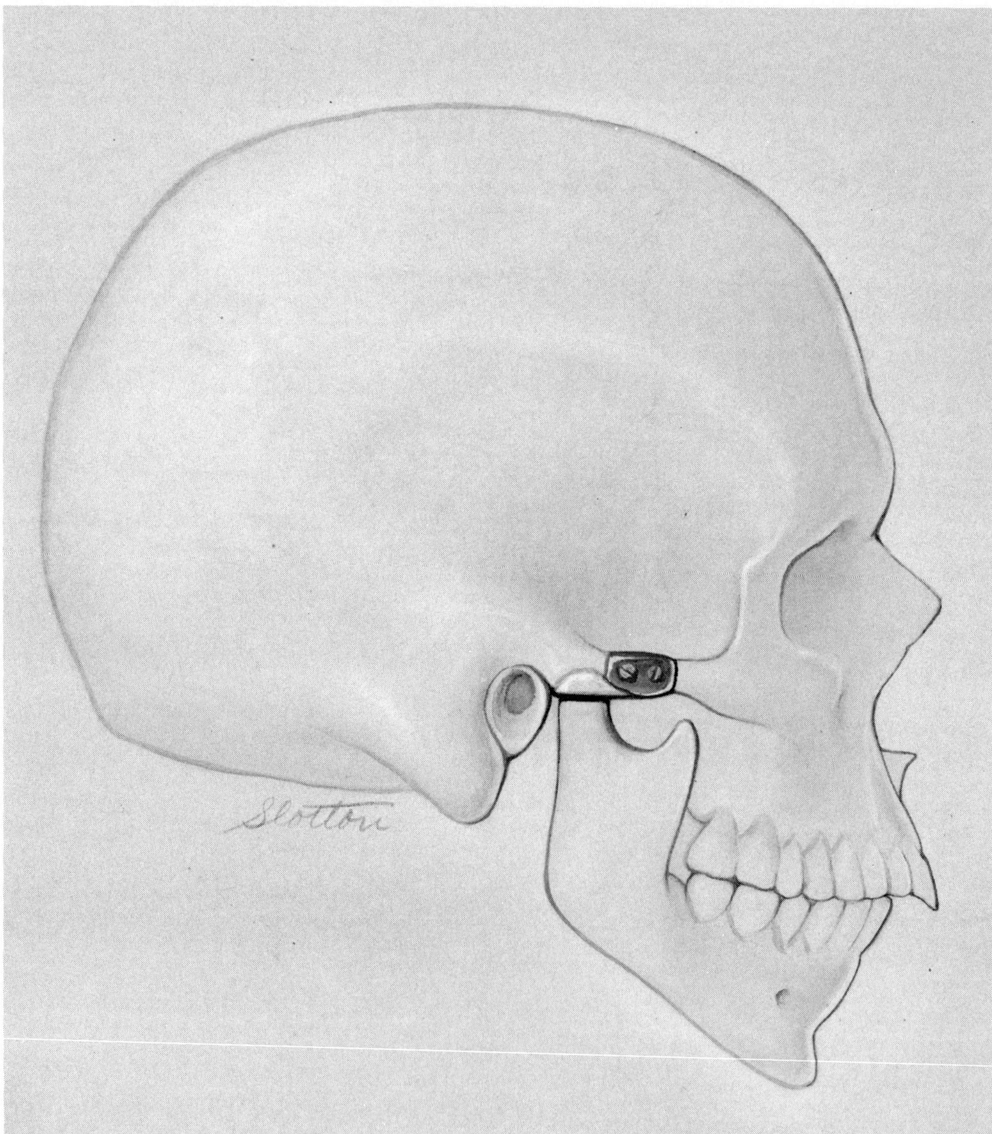

Fig. 22-27. New prosthesis showing lowering of floor of fossa.

A

B

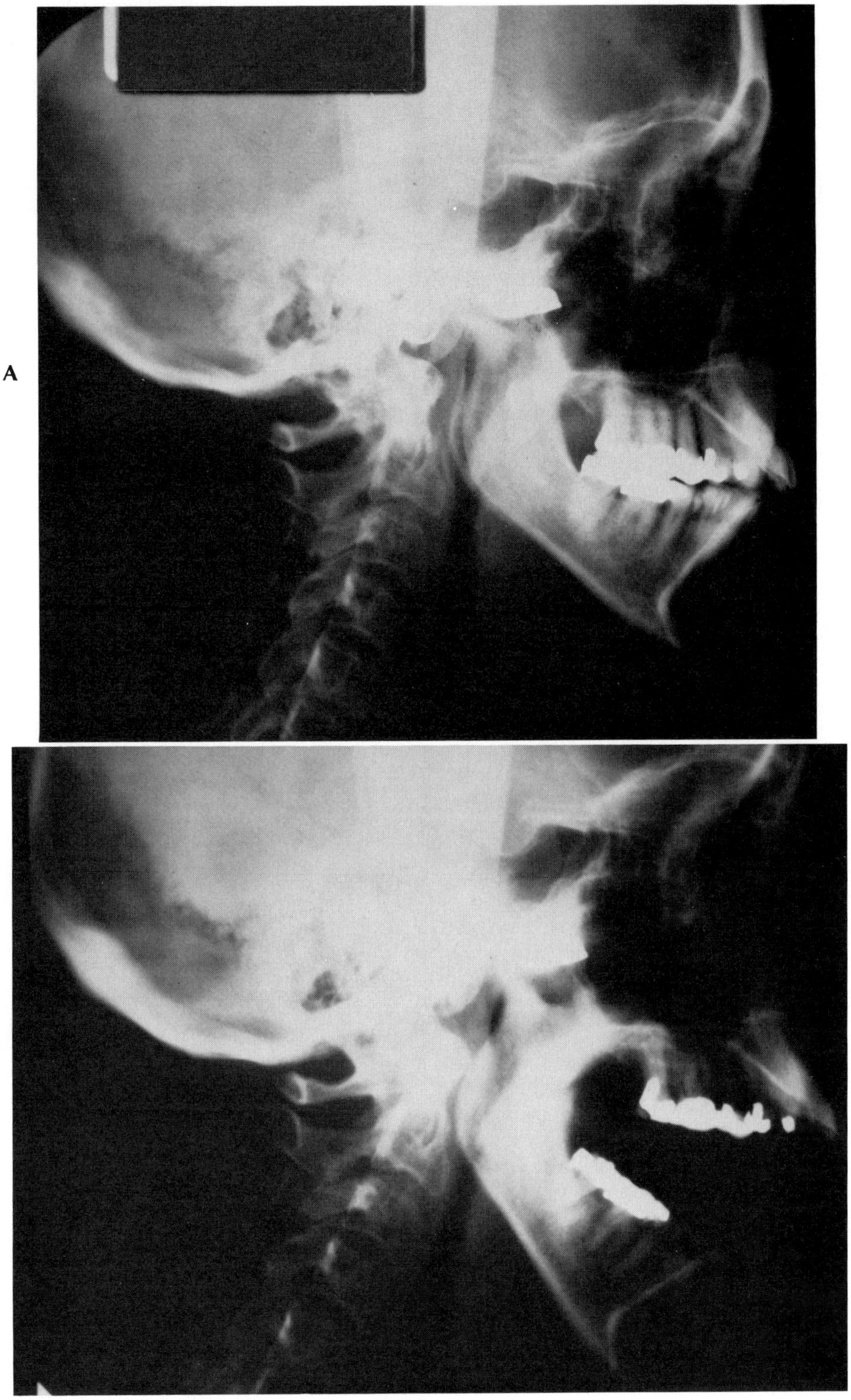

Fig. 22-28. A, Postoperative cephalometric film of D.G. showing normal jaw relationship. **B,** Cephalometric film showing good functional movement.

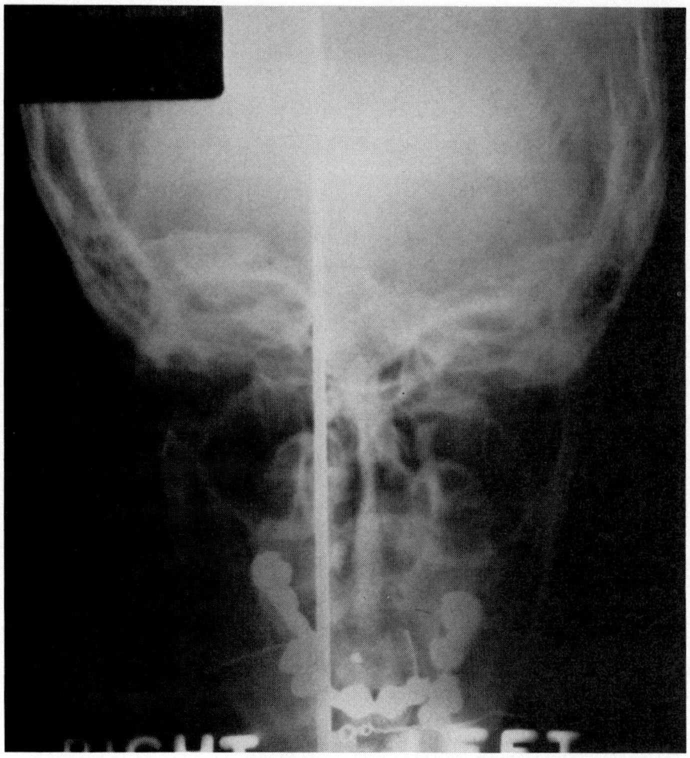

Fig. 22-29. Anteroposterior view of G.M. showing Silastic cap wired to right condyle.

Case 9

G.M., a 30-year-old woman, complained of severe pain in the left side of her face and some pain on the right. She also had dizziness and ear sounds. Three years previously she had a condylectomy and a Silastic cap placed over the condyle of her right joint (Fig. 22-29). This was done for severe pain on the right side of her head and neck after conservative measures were of no avail. The patient stated that since her condylectomy she had some moderate pain, but there was an improvment. However, she was unable to exert any pressure in chewing on the right side of her mouth and ate only on the left. An arthroplasty of the left temporomandibular joint with insertion of an articular eminence prosthesis was advised.

The clinical examination revealed that she was able to open her mouth only 12 mm. There was pain on palpation of both right and left joints and a grating sound, or crepitus, in the left joint. When she opened her mouth, the mandible moved to the right.

The radiographic examination revealed stainless steel ligatures attached to the stump of the condyle in the right joint. In the left joint there appeared to be bone-to-bone contact of the condyle as it translated over the eminence (Fig. 22-30).

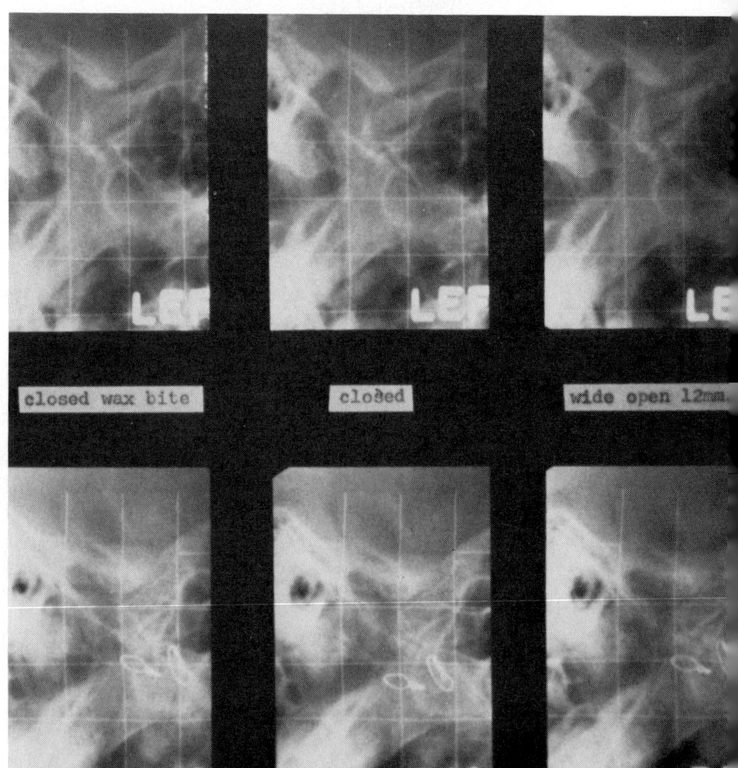

Fig. 22-30. Transcranial lateral oblique films showing bone-to-bone contact of left condyle to eminence and condylar stump in right temporomandibular joint with interosseous wires securing Silastic cap to condylar stump.

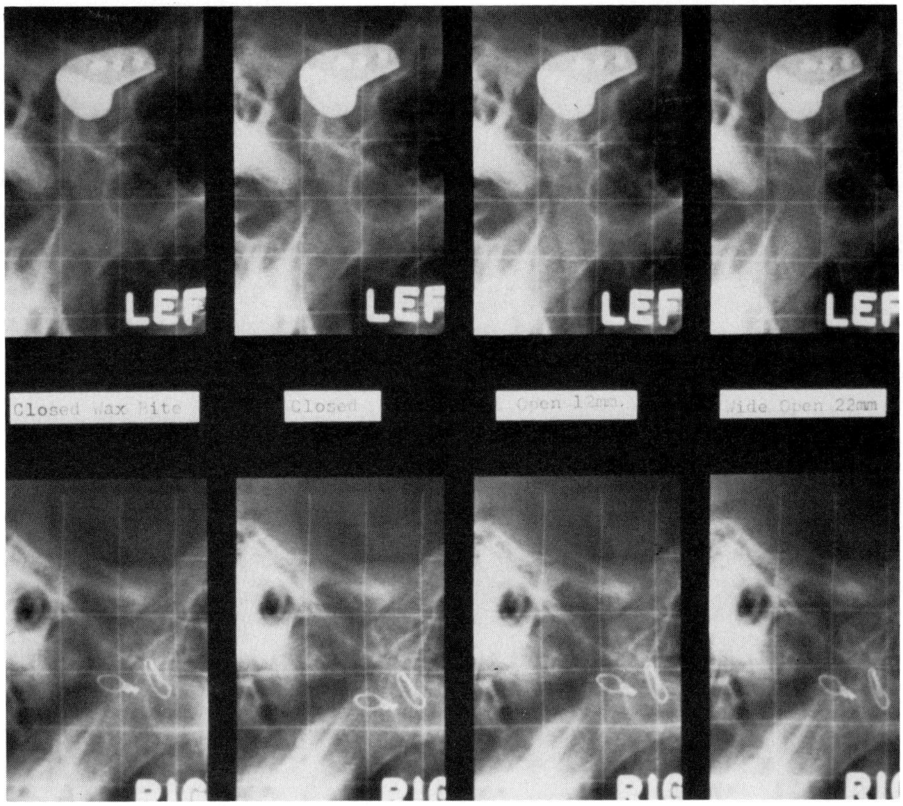

Fig. 22-31. Transcranial lateral oblique films taken a week after surgery showing good translation in left joint with articular eminence prosthesis in position.

Treatment. Surgery was performed August 15, 1973. On opening into the left temporomandibular joint, we found roughness of the articular eminence on palpation with a periosteal elevator, and a tear in the disc was noted. The first prosthesis went well into position. It was secured in the usual manner, and the wound area was closed in the usual way.

The next day the patient commented that her pain symptoms were significantly better, and she was able to chew soft foods. At the end of the fifth postoperative day she stated that there were no pains in the left side of her head. She still had some residual pain in the right joint from the high condylectomy (Figs. 22-31 and 22-32).

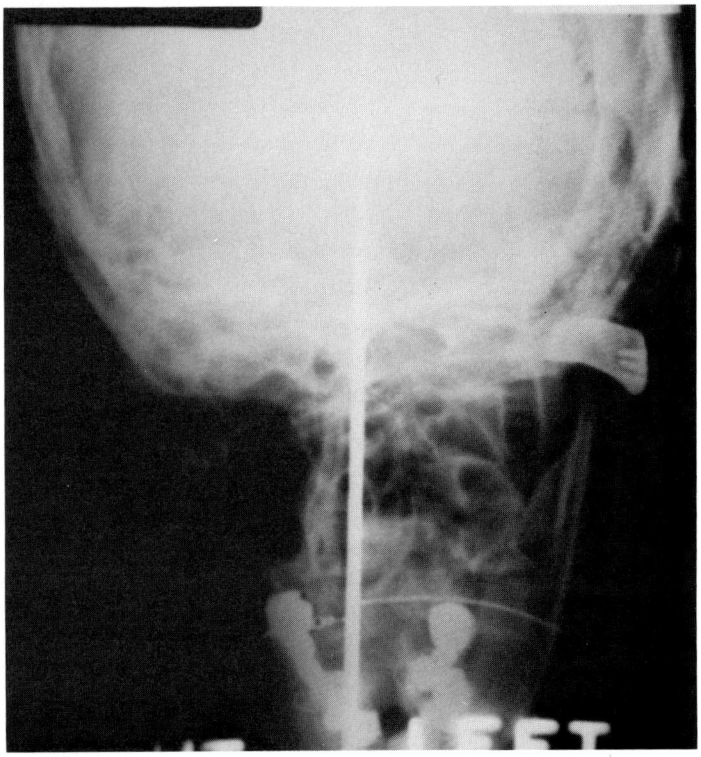

Fig. 22-32. Anteroposterior view showing prosthesis in position.

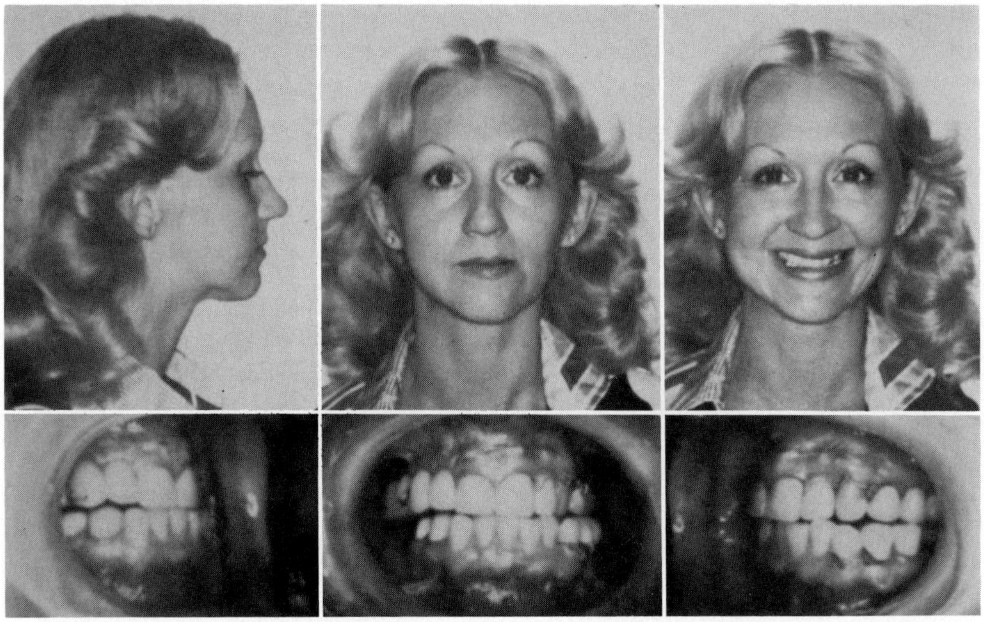

Fig. 22-33. Full-face view showing shift of mandible to left and nonocclusion of teeth on right side.

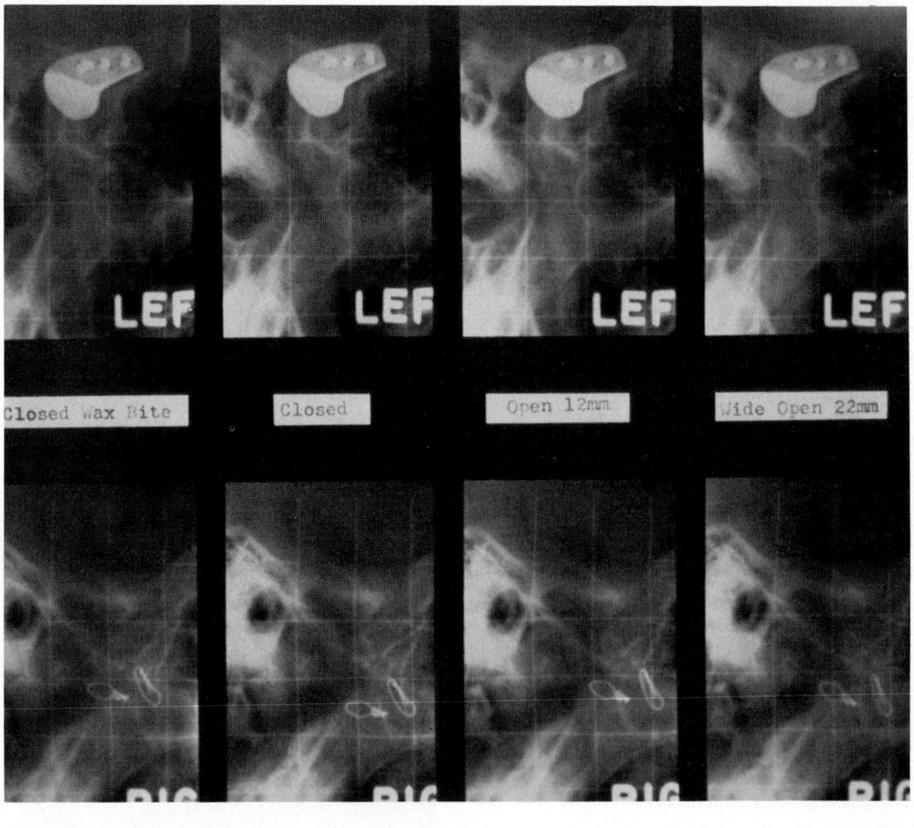

Fig. 22-34. Transcranial lateral oblique film showing functioning left condyle and spasm of muscle affecting right joint area.

On July 16, 1975, the patient was seen again. She stated that a month previously while having dental work done, her jaw had shifted to the left, and her teeth did not meet. She was in great pain and unable to chew food. Her teeth were wired together to try to bring the occlusion back to normal. This had been done at an air force facility. They were unable to help her, and a note was made on her medical chart that her problem was primarily psychosomatic (Fig. 22-33).

New radiographs were taken. They revealed that the prosthesis in the left joint was functioning properly (Fig. 22-34). However, muscle spasms in the right joint had forced the condyle into a more anterior and medial position. It was elected that the joint be operated on and a new condyle built.

Surgery was performed August 24, 1975, with a preauricular and a Risdon approach. The dissection was done in the usual manner in the Risdon approach, until the lower border of the mandible was located. The incision was made through the previous incision site. A preauricular incision was made, and the joint area was exposed. There was no condyle in the fossa.

Maxillary and mandibular Winter arch bars were placed, as well as rubber-band traction to bring her occlusion into normal relation. Her muscles were temporarily paralyzed to bring this about. The Silastic cap and stainless steel ligatures supporting it could be seen. The wires were cut, and the Silastic cap was removed. Two types of acrylic and metallic condyles were tried (Fig. 22-35). These prostheses fit on either side of the ramus to give a more stable fit of the prosthesis to the bone.

After considerable manipulation the largest prosthesis was placed. It was secured to the ramus by eight 5-mm screws. The acrylic condyle fit nicely into the fossa. It was debated whether a prosthesis should be placed into the upper portion of the joint. Because of the lengthy surgical time, this was not done. The wound area was then closed in the usual fashion.

The elastic traction was removed a week after surgery. The patient was able to open her mouth immediately approximately 21 mm. The mandible did not deviate on opening. She now comments that she can put pressure on the right side of her jaw whiile chewing. He pain symptoms have also gradually subsided. Follow-up pictures were taken a year postoperatively (Fig. 22-36). The patient is pain free. She is able to chew vigoriously on the right side.

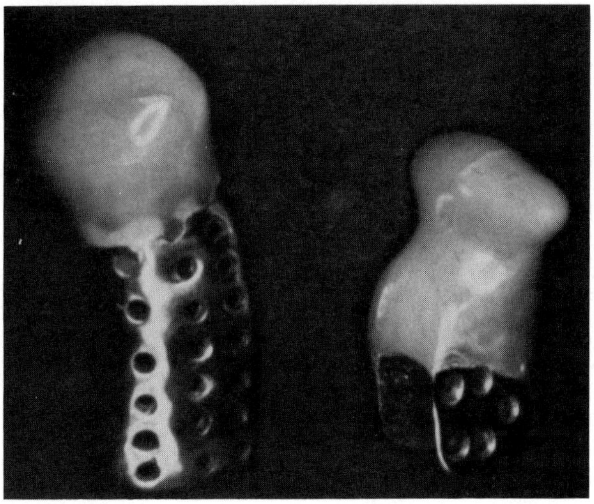

Fig. 22-35. Two varieties of metallic and acrylic condylar prostheses. Prosthesis on left has greater coverage of ramus by metal and more holes for bone screws to be placed.

A

B

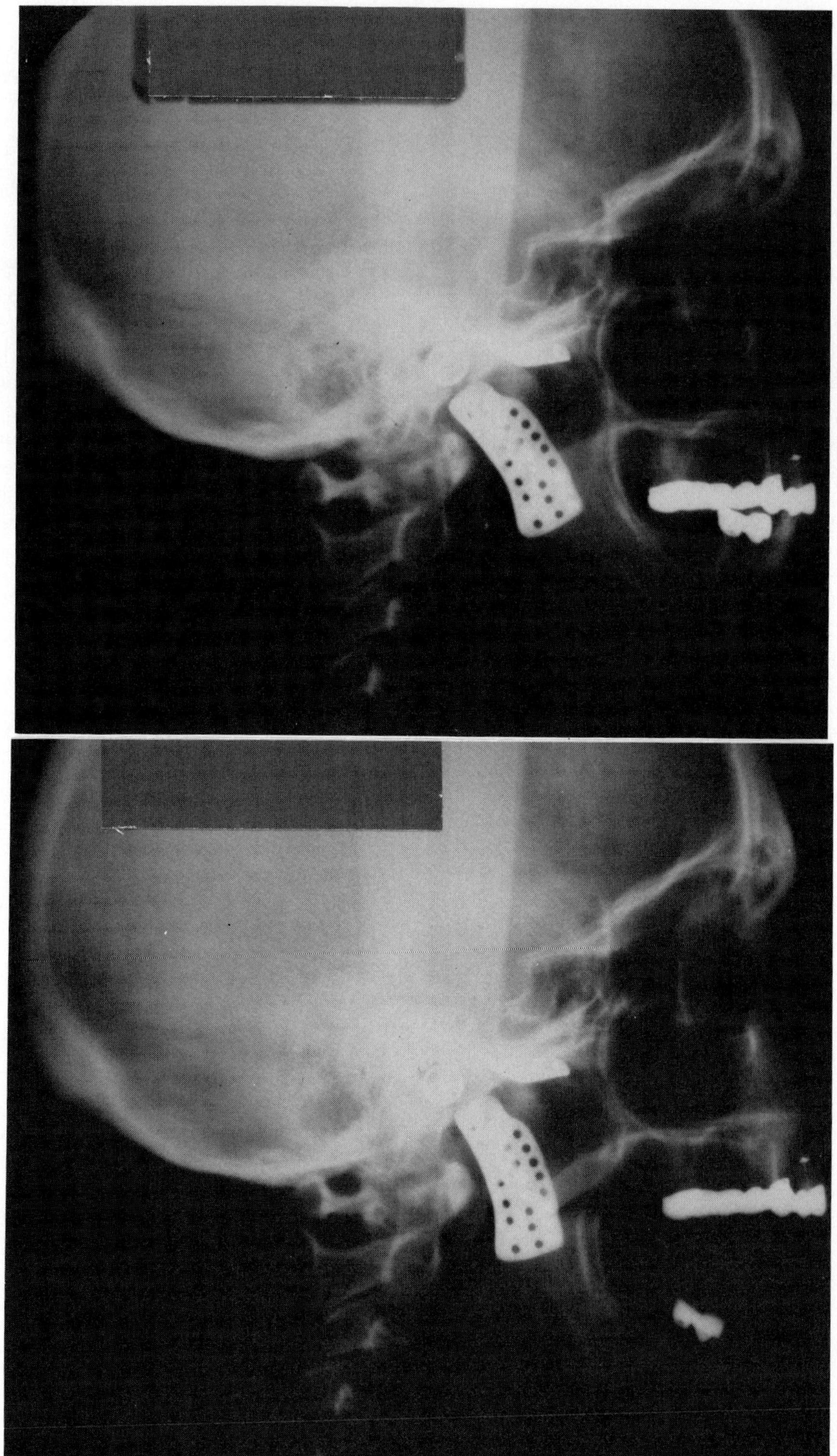

Fig. 22-36. Postoperative films of G.M. taken a year after surgery. **A,** Cephalometric closed view with condylar replacement in place. **B,** Cephalometric open view with condylar replacement in place.

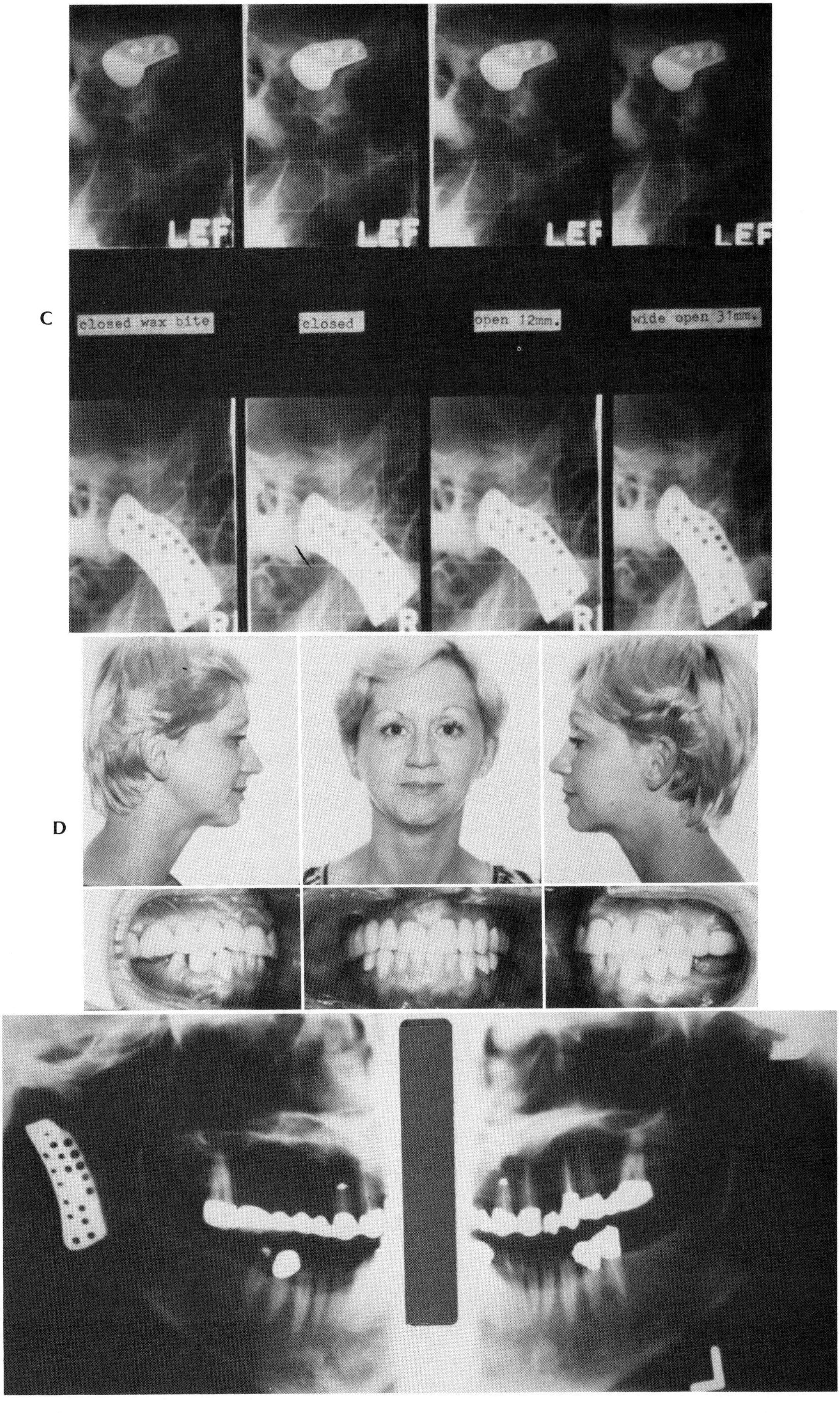

Fig. 22-36, cont'd. C, Transcranial lateral oblique films (four views) showing condylar prosthesis in right joint area and articular eminence prosthesis in left joint. **D,** Profile and full-face views showing minimum scarring from surgery on right side of face and normal occlusion. **E,** Panorex radiograph showing prosthesis in place.

Case 10

R.K., a 41-year-old woman, was referred for pain, more severe on the right side of her head than the left. The affected areas were the upper and lower jaws, the shoulders, facial muscles, and ears. She experienced a subjective hearing loss in both ears, tinnitus, a popping sound, and pressure blockage. She had difficulty opening her mouth widely, and her mouth would move off to one side when opening. She also had difficulty chewing and felt her teeth were not meeting properly. The patient's history dated back to approximately 4 years before, when she was involved in an automobile accident in which she received multiple fractures of the mandible and a fracture of the right condyle. Because of the multitude of other fractures, the attending oral surgeon at that time elected to leave alone the right condylar fracture. Since that time the patient had had a second wiring of her teeth to bring the occlusion into a better relationship, root canals on several teeth, and occlusal equilibrations.

Clinical examination revealed soreness of both joints on palpation and soreness of the muscles of mastication on both sides. Dental x-ray films revealed a well cared for mouth. The right mandibular canine was missing, and root canals had been performed on the mandibular left first and scond premolars. Cephalometric films showed what appeared to be a slight open bite (Fig. 22-37). Specialized TMJ films revealed that the eminence fossa was void of a condyle in the right joint, and there appeared to be a condyle in a condylar stump in an anterior direction. There appeared to be flattening of the anterior head of the condyle in the left joint and some lipping (Fig. 22-38). Intracanthus views revealed the right condyle had been pulled anteriorly and medially (Fig. 22-39).

Treatment. The patient was seen first on April 22, 1976. A number of nonsurgical treatments, including dental splints, equilibration, moist heat, and other medications, were used first, but these treatments gave her no relief. Instead she noticed that the pain on the left side, which had not been too severe, was becoming more so. It was decided that the right joint should be restored with a total TMJ prosthesis, and the left joint with an articular eminence prosthesis.

Surgery was performed on May 9. On the right side a preauricular incision was made and the dissection carried down to the area of the joint proper. A Risdon approach was then used, and the mandible was explored. These two incision sites were tied in, and it was noted that the mandible was slightly forward of its normal position, and the stump of the condylar head was pulled forward. It was possible to pal-

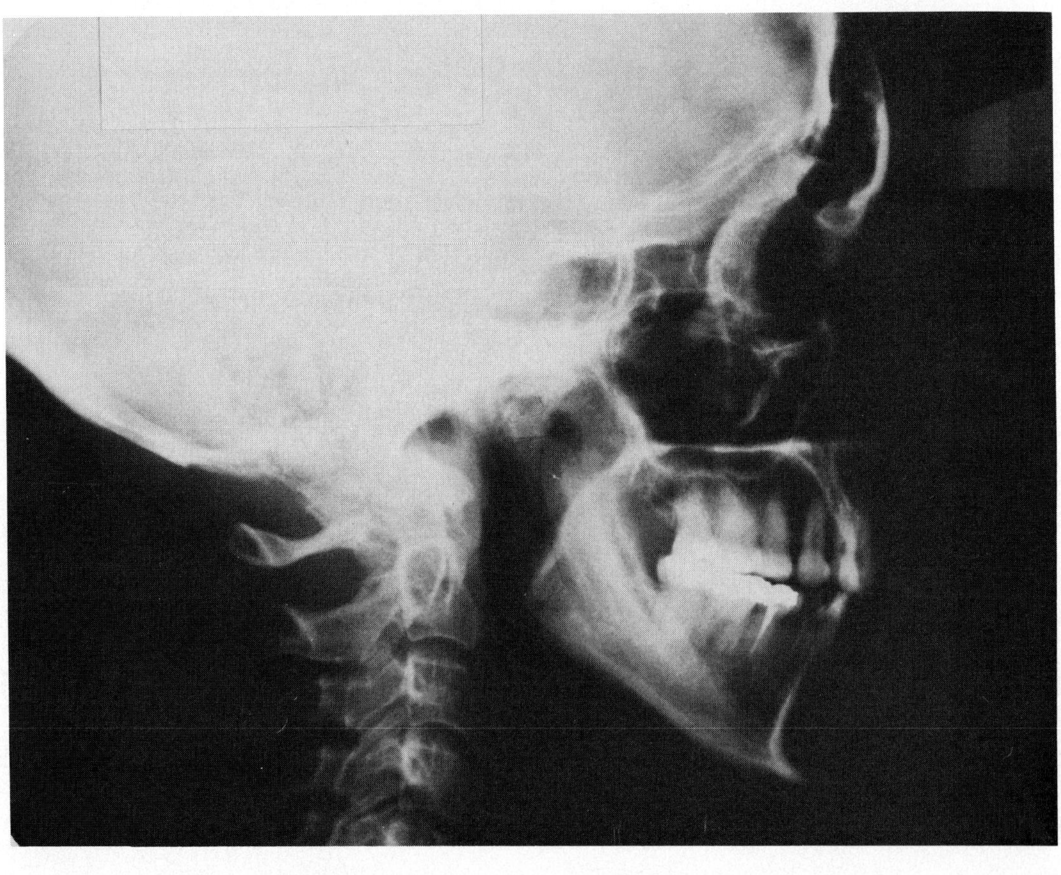

Fig. 22-37. Cephalometric film showing slight open bite.

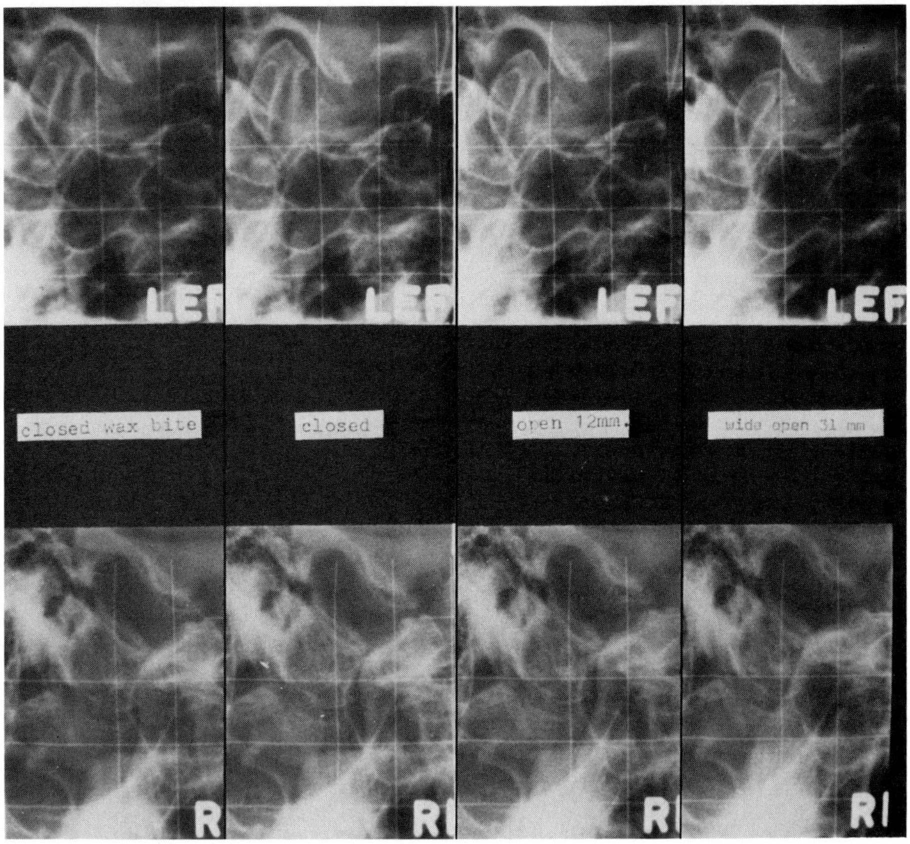

Fig. 22-38. Specialized TMJ films showing void in right condylar fossa area and flattening of anterior head of condyle in left area.

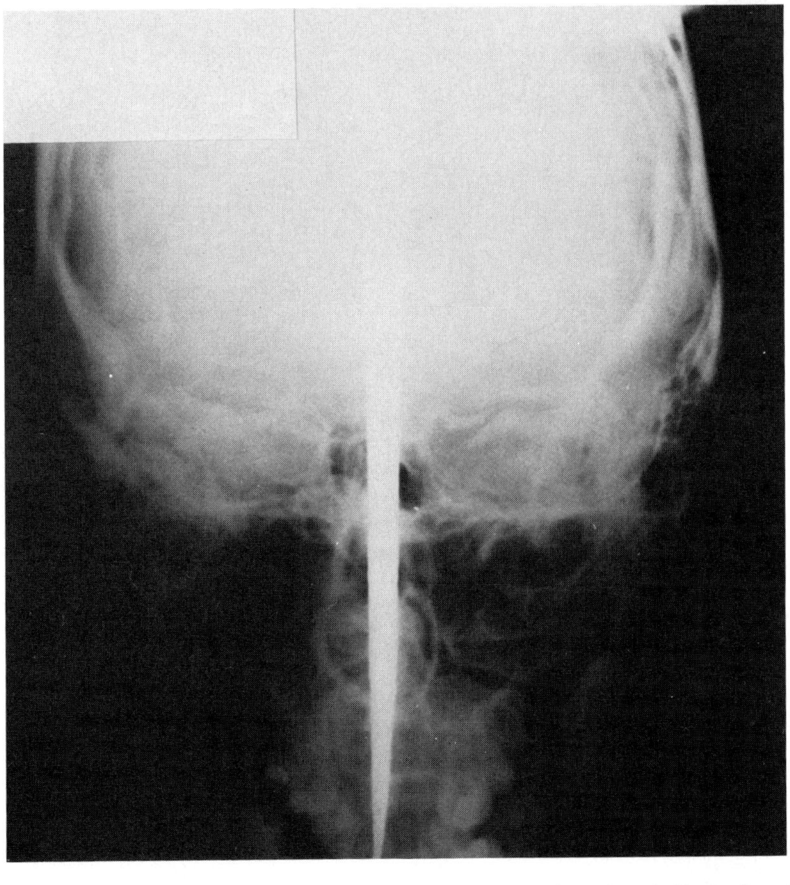

Fig. 22-39. Intracanthus view shows right condyle anteriorly and medially displaced.

pate this stump. The prosthesis was placed through the Risdon approach; it fit well on the body of the ramus, and the condylar portion fit well into the fossa. It was not necessary to remove the remnant of the condylar head, since it was anterior and out of the way of the prosthesis. Several articular eminence protheses with Silastic inserts were tried for fit. The Silastic portion was then trimmed to fit well into the eminence fossa. The metal and Silastic prosthesis was placed into the upper joint surface. At this time the patient's teeth, which had previously had arch bars applied, were occluded by use of rubber-band traction. The appliance fit well, and it was secured to the lateral border of the ramus by the use of seven cast Vitallium screws. The wound area was closed in the usual manner. Postoperative x-ray films taken 5 days after surgery showed a properly fitting *total prosthesis* in the right joint and an articular eminence prosthesis in the left joint (Figs. 22-40 to 22-45).

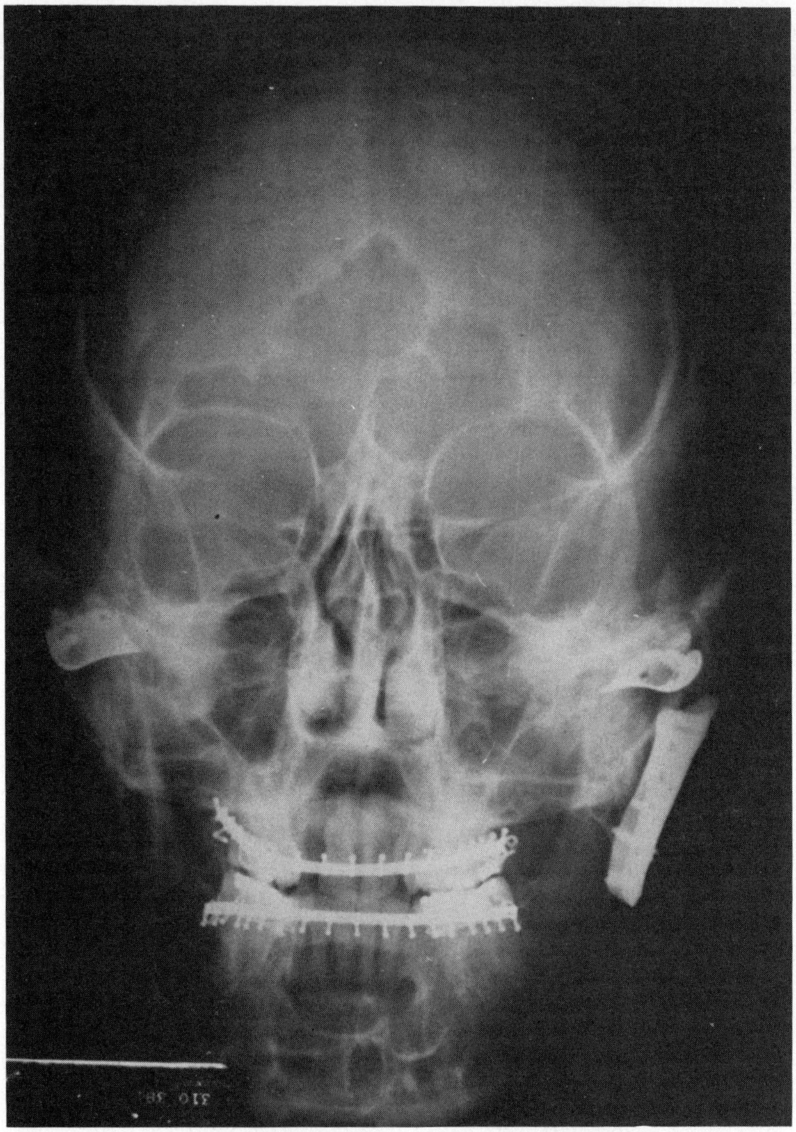

Fig. 22-40. Anteroposterior view showing proper position of right total TMJ prosthesis and left articular eminence prosthesis. (Prosthesis designed by D.H. Morgan and constructed by Joseph Costello, C.D.T.)

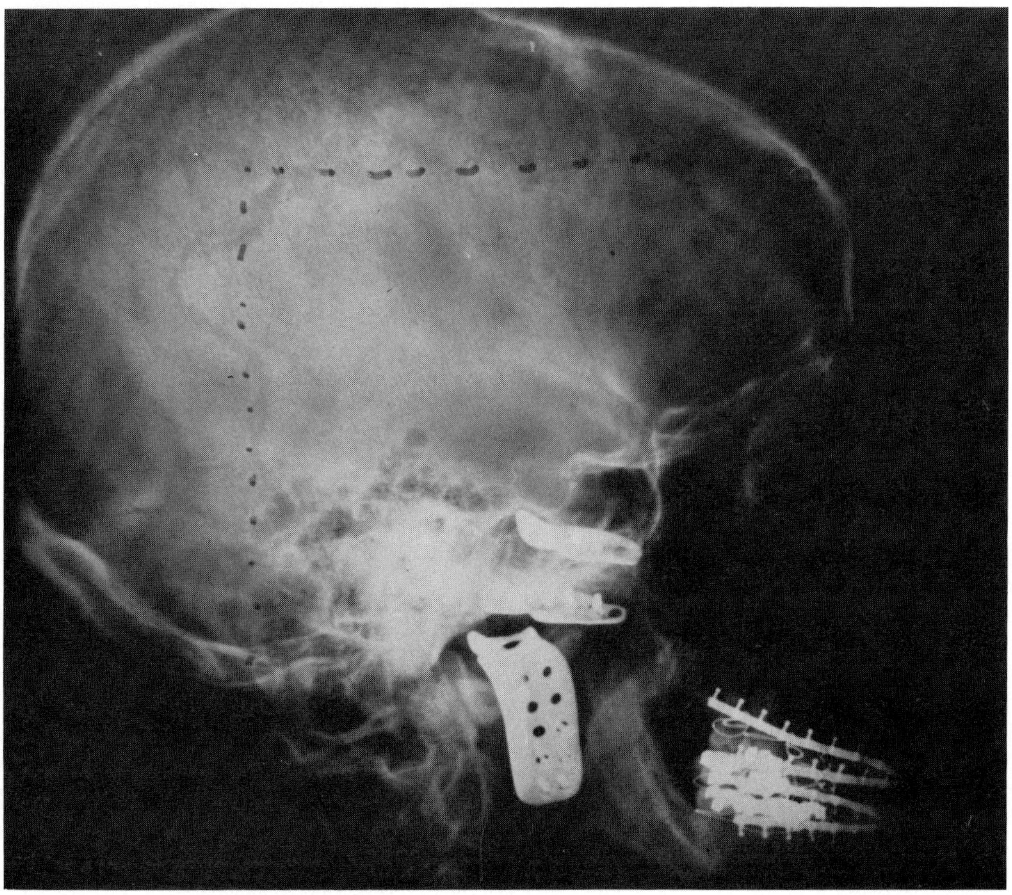

Fig. 22-41. Lateral view showing properly positioned prosthesis. Condylar head not seen because acrylic material is radiopaque.

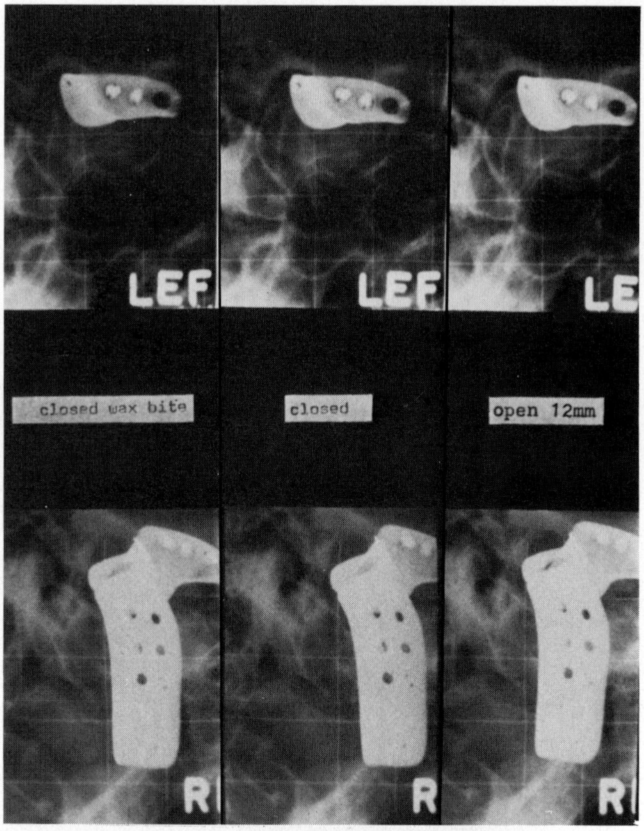

Fig. 22-42. Special TMJ x-ray films taken approximately 3 weeks after surgery showing position of total TMJ prosthesis in right joint and articular eminence prosthesis in left joint.

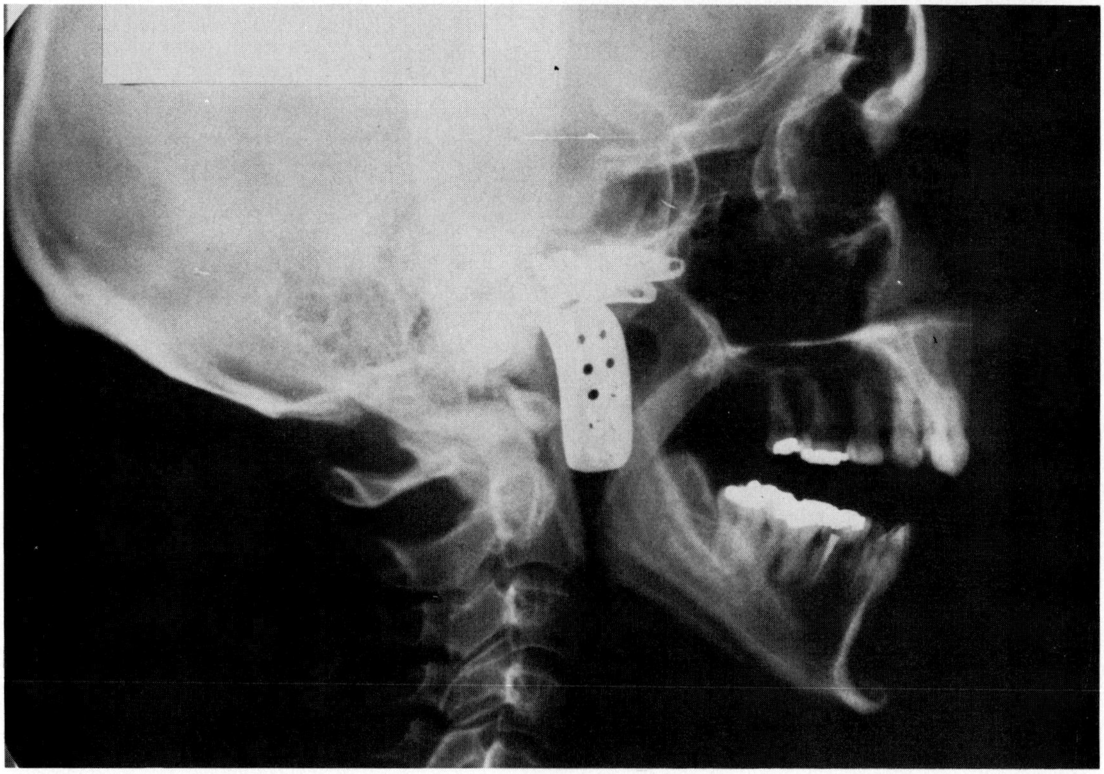

Fig. 22-43. Cephalometric film taken 3 weeks after surgery showing patient able to open mouth 30 mm. She is able to chew moderately.

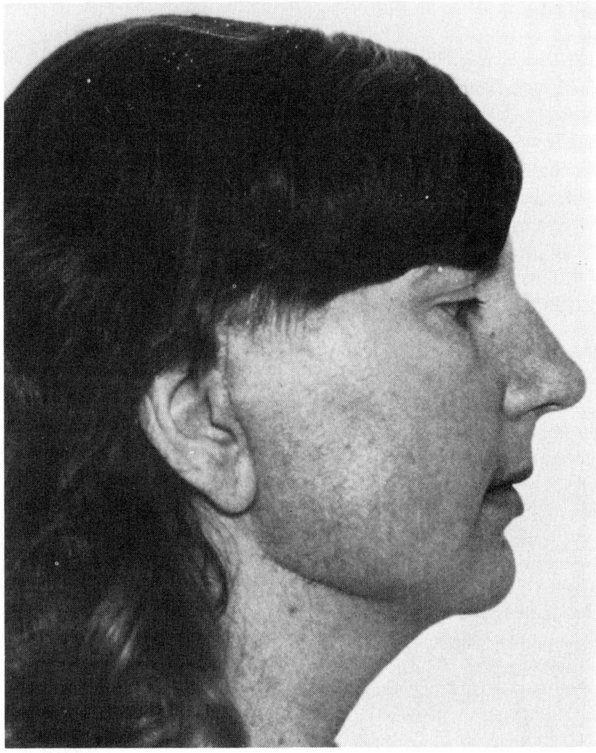

Fig. 22-44. Three-week postoperative photograph showing preauricular and submandibular Risdon incision healing well on right side.

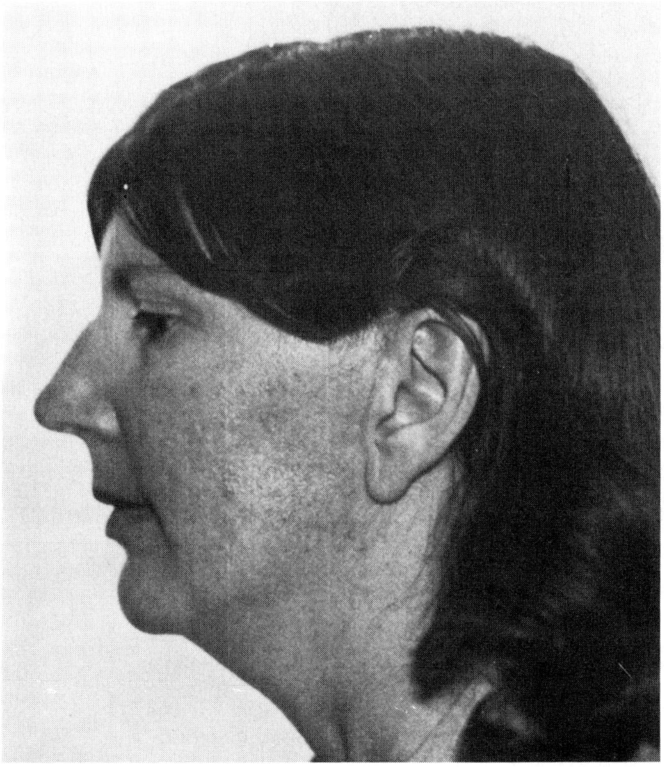

Fig. 22-45. Postoperative photograph showing healing of preauricular incision of left side.

Case 11

F.M., a 46-year-old woman, had been suffering for the previous 6 years from severe pain, primarily affecting the right side of her head. She had been to numerous practitioners in her home state and had received several kinds of treatment, including cortisone injections, but had not been relieved. Eventually the problem was diagnosed as relating to the TMJ, with osteoarthritic degeneration. In January 1977 an oral surgeon performed a high condylectomy on the right TMJ and placed a cap of Silastic over the condylar stump, wiring it into place. The specialized TMJ x-ray films show the right condyle with the wire in place and the left condyle with minor movement (Fig. 22-46, *A*). She was able to open only 12 mm. The full-face, profile, and teeth views show the mandible shifting to the right in an upward direction and an open bite in the left mandible (Fig. 22-46, *B*).

The patient had no occlusion in the left premolar-molar area and poor occlusion in the right area. Since the condylec-

A

B

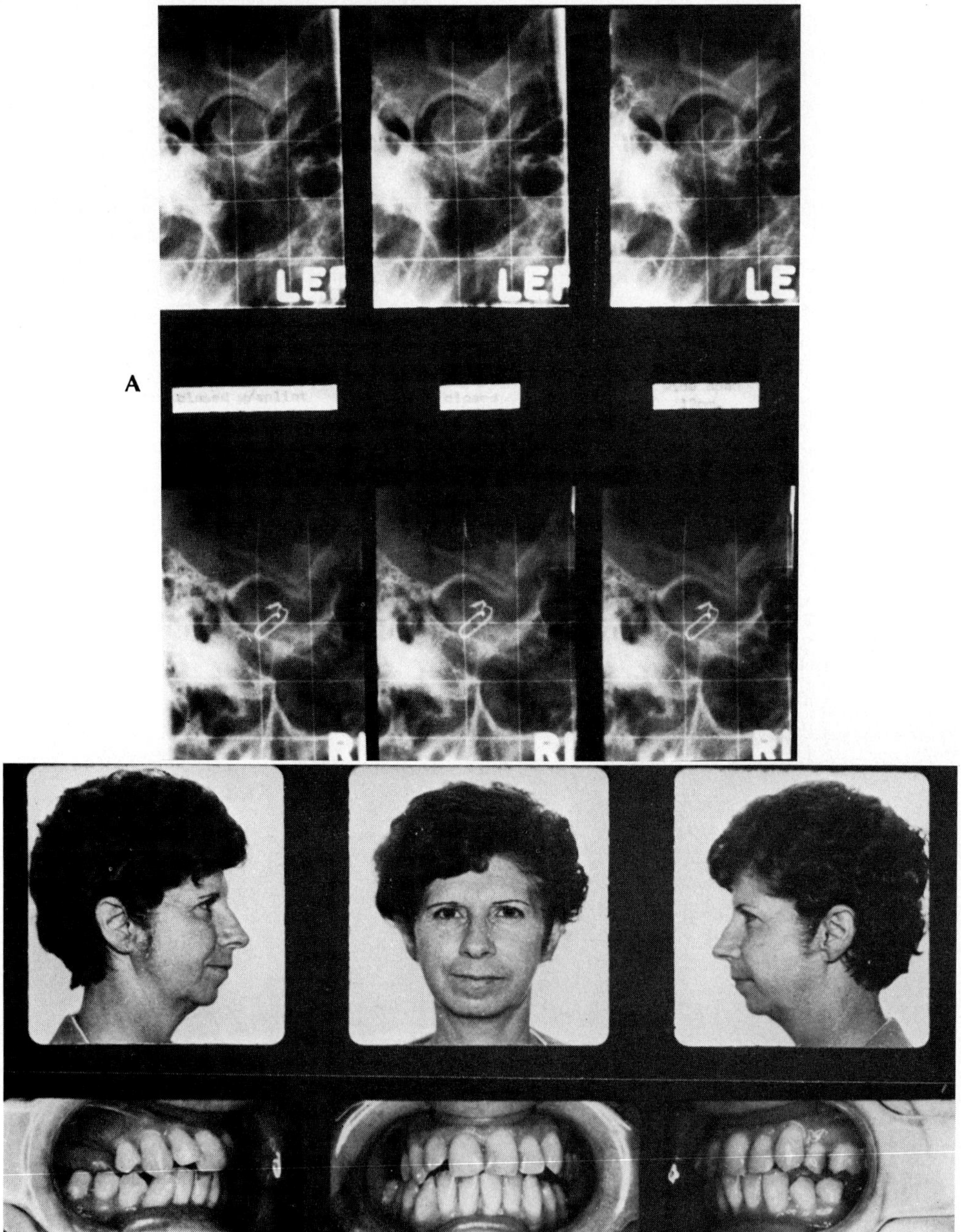

Fig. 22-46. A, Specialized TMJ x-ray films showing stainless steel ligatures through stump of right condyle securing Silastic cap to condylar stump. In left side can be seen some slight translational movement on maximum 12-mm opening. **B,** Full-face, profile, and teeth views showing mandible shifting to right and open bite in left mandible.

C

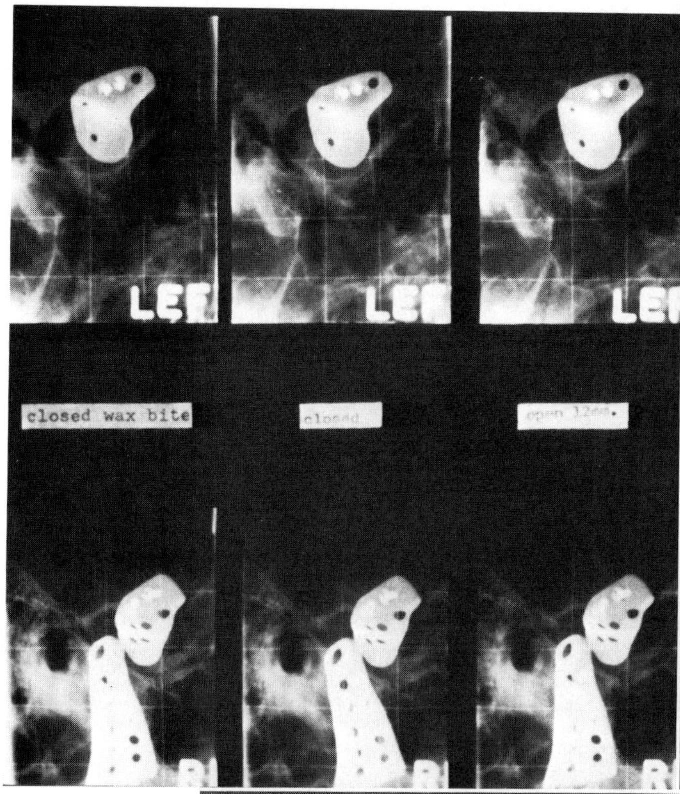

D

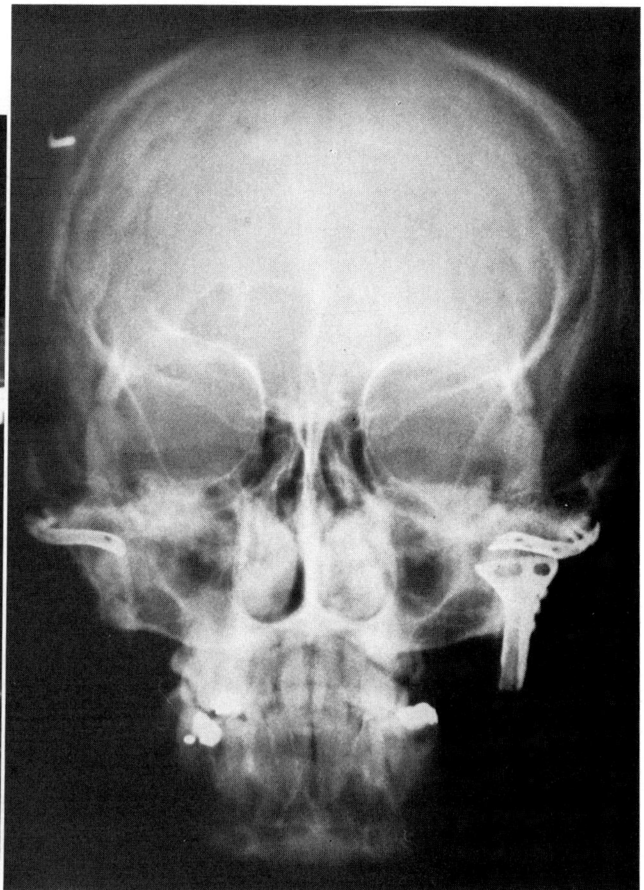

E

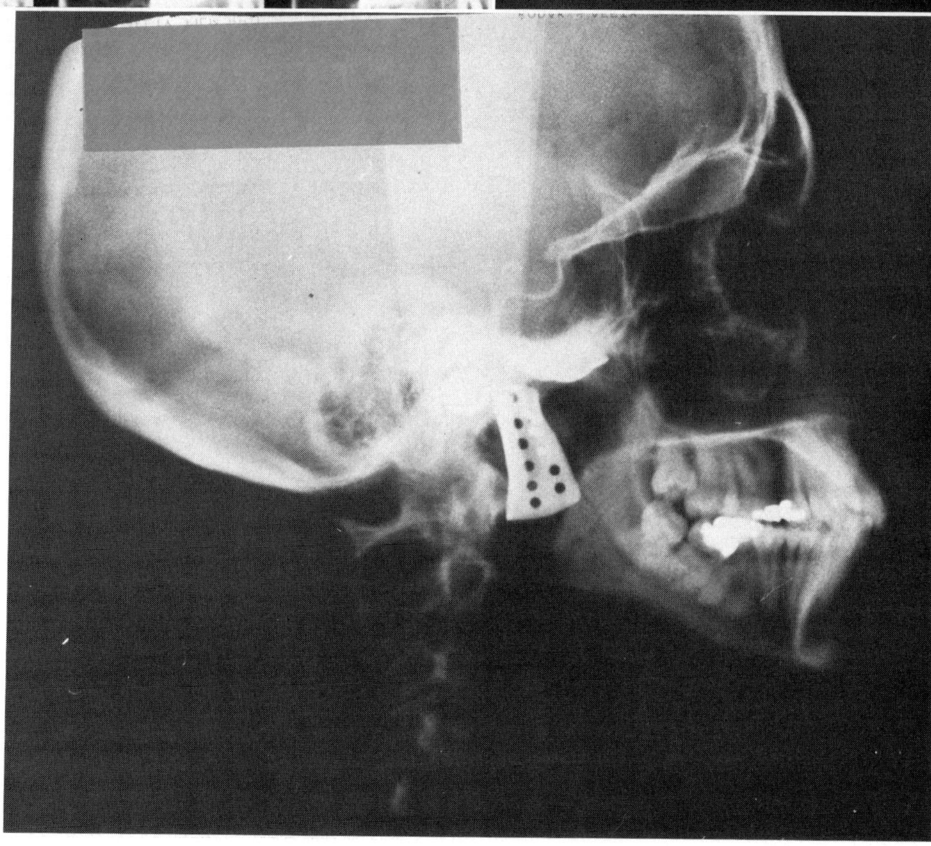

Fig. 22-46, cont'd. C, Specialized TMJ films showing total TMJ prosthesis in right joint. Acrylic and Silastic portion of implant cannot be seen, since they are radiopaque. In left joint, articular eminence prosthesis is in good position. **D,** Anteroposterior view shows prosthesis in good position with proper interdental relationship. **E,** Lateral view shows teeth in normal occlusion.

Continued.

tomy, she had noticed severe pain now affecting the left jaw joint and an inability to open her mouth more than 12 mm. Additionally, there was crepitus in the left joint, denoting a tear in the disc. She was treated at a local dental school with splints for 6 months and then referred to us in September 1977.

Treatment. Following the examination of this patient it was decided that the right joint should be restored via a total TMJ replacement and the left joint treated via meniscectomy with placement of an articular eminence prosthesis. At the time of surgery maxillo-mandibular arch bars were placed with elastic traction that moved the teeth to the correct interdental position. On the right side a preauricular incision was made and the dissection carried down to the area of the joint proper. A

F

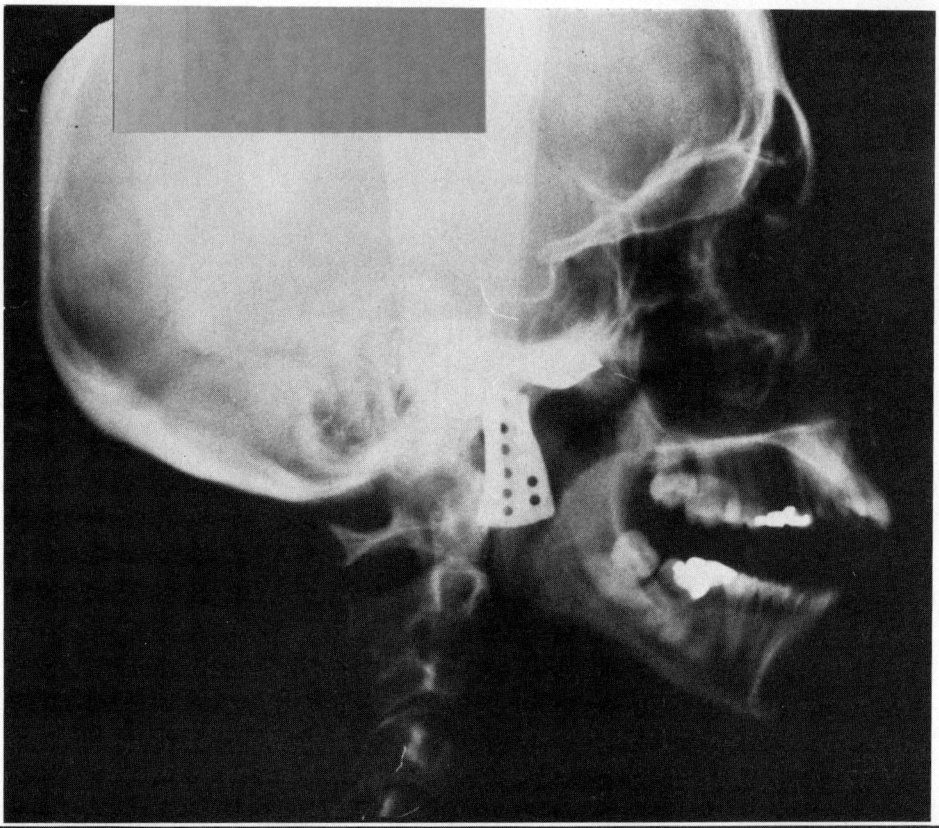

G

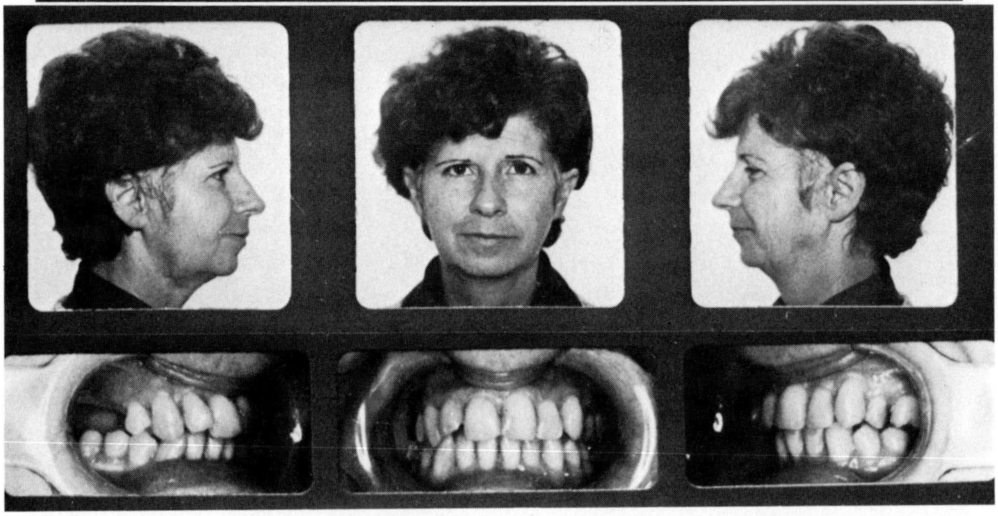

Fig. 22-46, cont'd. F, Patient can now open over 20 mm, as confirmed by lateral x-ray view. **G,** Full-face, profile, and teeth views shows normal occlusal relationship with mandible shifted back to the left, closing the open bite.

Risdon approach was then used, and a condylar prosthesis was placed, chosen from a number that had been previously constructed for best fit. A specially prepared metal and Silastic prosthesis was placed through the incision and secured to the body of the ramus by a number of metal screws. On the left side a preauricular incison also was made in the usual manner. A perforated disc was noted and removed in several pieces. A number of articular eminence prostheses were tried; one fit well. The wounds were closed in the usual fashion.

The patient did well and was discharged 5 days postoperatively. The elastic traction remained for 10 days after surgery. The postoperative TMJ films show the total TMJ prosthesis in the right joint (Fig. 22-46, *C*). Because they are radiopaque, the acrylic condylar head and the Silastic portion extending into the fossa cannot be seen. The patient was able to open 12 mm after surgery. The anteroposterior view shows the prosthesis with normal interdental relationship (Fig. 22-46, *D*). Lateral views show the prosthesis with the teeth in normal occlusion (Fig. 22-46, *E*). She is able to masticate food, and she can now open over 20 mm (Fig. 22-46, *F*). Full-face, profile, and teeth views show the normal occlusal relationship (Fig. 22-46, *G*). She is now having some missing teeth replaced to complete her treatment.

Case 12

A 49-year-old woman from Canada had a 7-year history of pain to both jaw joints, the ears, and around the eyes, necks, shoulders, face, and even arms. She was edentulous and dated her pain symptoms back to the multiple extractions she had had 7 years previously. After seeing a number of physicians and dentists without results she underwent surgery in 1974. Using a Gigli saw, the oral surgeon had cut through the neck of the right condyle and detached it. After the procedure, however, she developed more pain and a deviation of her mandible to the right side as she opened her mouth. A dentist in Toronto, Ontario, who had heard of our work then referred her to us.

The clinical examination revealed that the patient had soreness of both joints on palpation, with more on the left. There was also a grating sound in the left jaw joint area, and a Mandibular Kinesiograph evaluation was made. Most of the muscles of mastication were sore, and the patient could hardly chew. She could open 31 mm, and her jaw deviated to the right approximately 3 mm.

Specialized TMJ x-ray films revealed in the right joint that the condyle was totally displaced and pulled medial and forward because of the previous surgical procedure. In the left joint the films reveal compression of the disc (Fig. 22-47, *A*). The intracanthus view shows the right condylar stump and remnant of the condylar head, medially and anteriorly displaced (Fig. 22-47, *B*). The Panorex shows the displacement of the condylar head (Fig. 22-47, *C*). The cephalometric view shows the loss of vertical dimension on the right side (Fig. 22-47, *D*). Full-face, profile, and teeth views also show the loss of vertical dimension, affecting the right side of the face (Fig. 22-47, *E*).

Treatment. The patient was operated on in March 1979. The beginning part of the procedure involved placing three wires in the mandible and securing the lower denture by the circumferential wires. The maxillary denture was secured by the used of two Steinmann pins, which secured it to the hard palate. Elastic traction then was used to close the mandible and hold it in a more normal relationship.

A preauricular incision was made on the right side. It was thought that if the condylar fragment could be found, it might be placed in a functional position and secured by use of a Roger Anderson–type appliance, as though it were a fracture being reduced. On entering the joint proper, however, it was noted that there had been too much resorption of the condyle for use of this technique. The stump of the condyle was located and found to be displaced medially and anteriorly by the pull of the external pterygoid muscle. It was carefully removed from the joint and examined. Because of the resorption and the way the condyle was sectioned, there was no way to mechanically secure the condylar head to the stump of the ramal neck. It was elected to do a total TMJ replacement. The remnants of the meniscus were removed, and a Risdon approach was made on the mandible. On reaching the mandible, we explored the ramus and achieved contact with the stump. Several condylar prostheses were tried until one fit on well. An articular eminence prosthesis with a Silastic portion in the fossa also was secured in the upper portion of the joint. The condylar prosthesis (of Vitallium and acrylic) was secured to the ramus of the mandible by a number of 7-mm cast Vitallium screws.

On the right side a preauricular incision was made. On entering the joint proper, a tear in the lateral portion of the meniscus was noted, and the condylar head could be seen through this tear. The disc was removed and the roughness of the articular eminence and lateral pole of the condyle noted. Several prostheses were tried; one fit well. The wounds were closed in the usual manner.

The patient did well and was discharged 5 days postoperatively. Postoperative TMJ x-ray films show the prostheses properly placed (Fig. 22-47, *F*). Closed cephalometric x-ray films also show the prostheses properly placed (Fig. 22-47, *G*). Open cephalometric x-ray films show the patient opening 25 mm (Fig. 22-47, *H*). The Panorex x-ray film shows the properly placed total TMJ implant in the right joint and an articular eminence implant in the left joint (Fig. 22-47, *I*). Full-face, profile, and teeth views show increased vertical dimension on the right side of the face (Fig. 22-47, *J*). The patient has had significant relief from symptoms, particularly on the left side, and is now able to apply equal pressure as she chews food. She also has had new dentures constructed.

Text continued on p. 410.

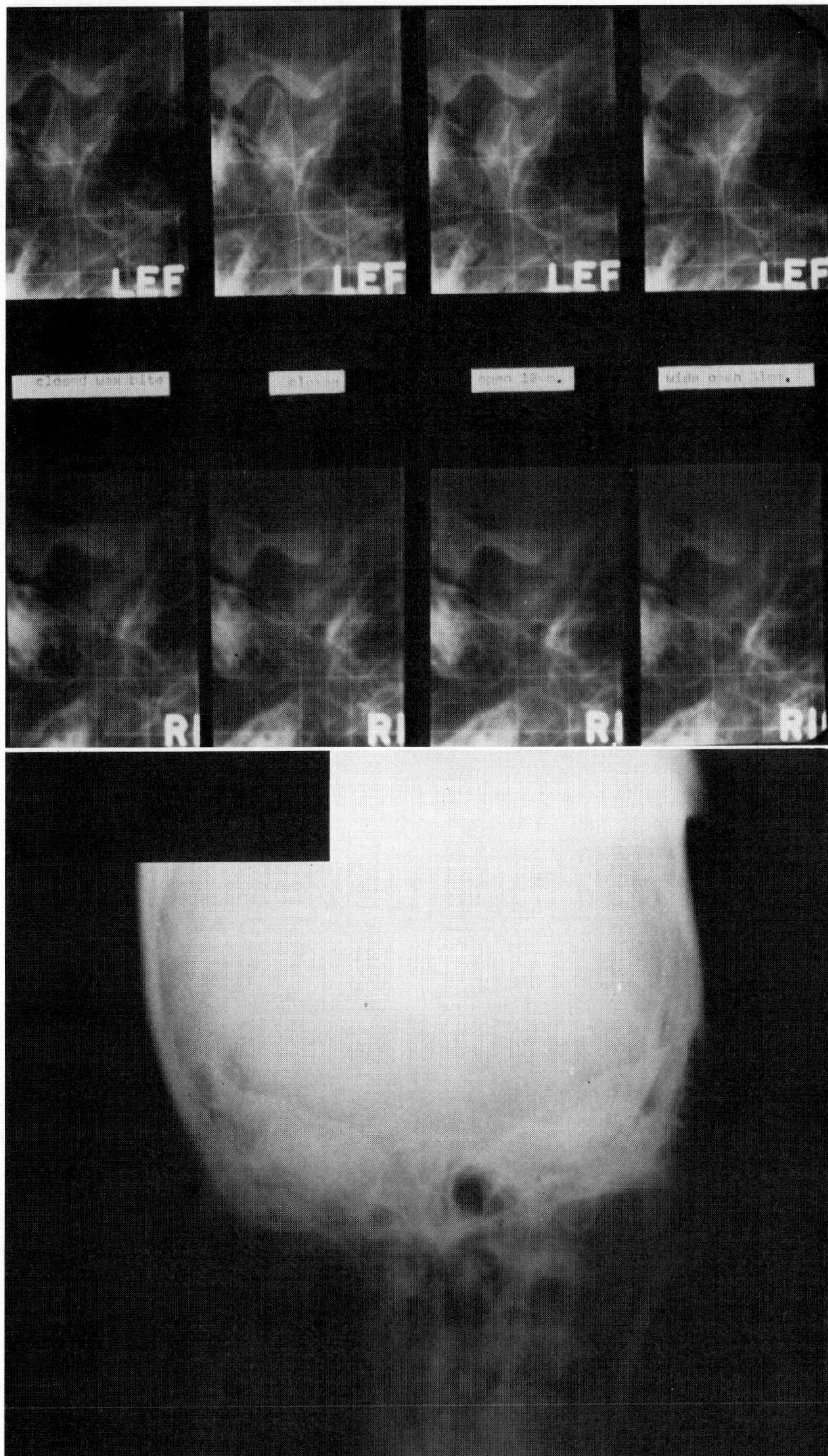

A

B

Fig. 22-47. A, Specialized TMJ x-ray films showing condylar head displaced anteriorly and medially in fossa of right joint. In left joint there is some lessening of disc space in closed view. **B,** Intracanthus view showing right condylar stump and remnant of condylar head, medially and anteriorly displaced.

C

D

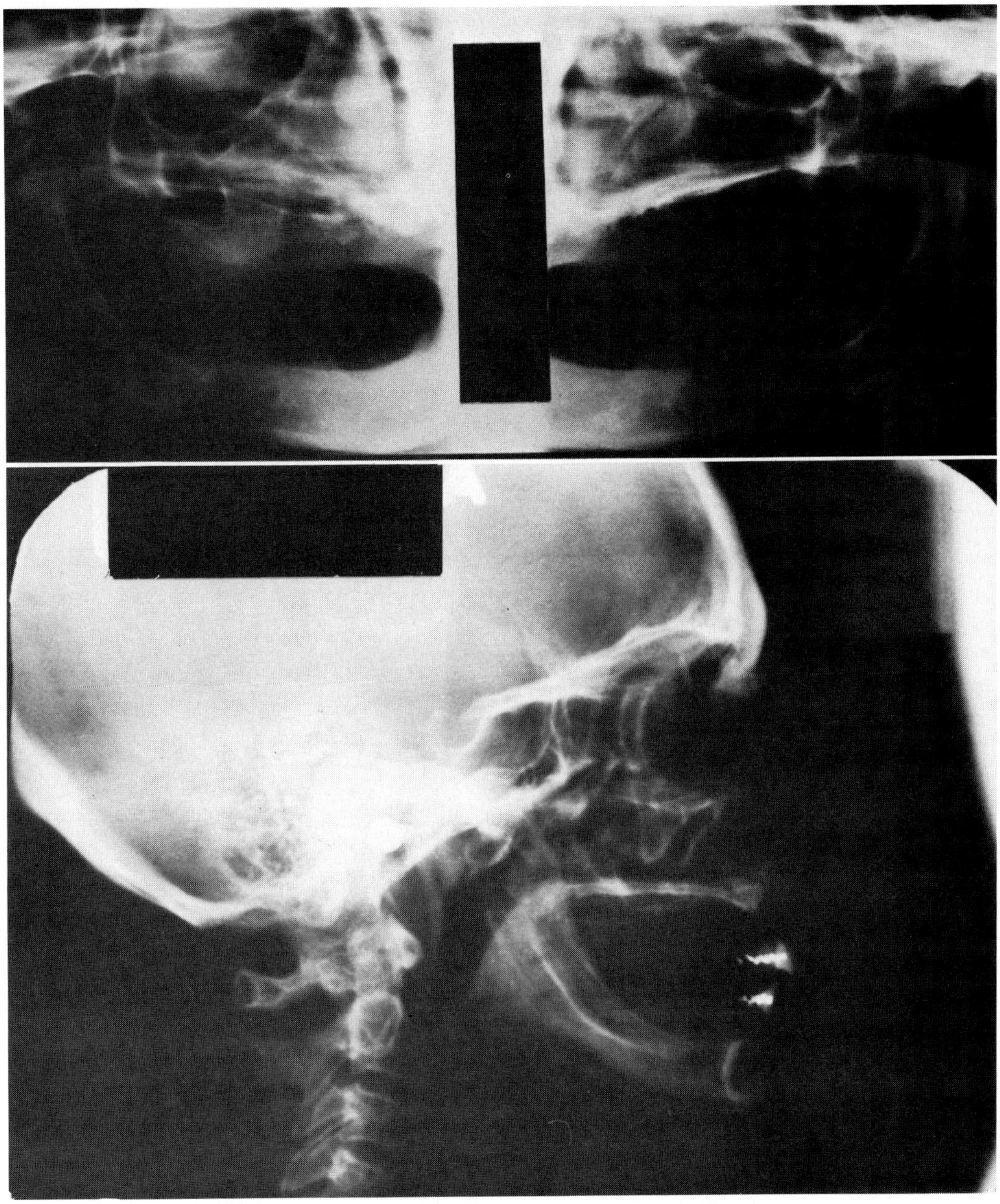

Fig. 22-47, cont'd. C, Panorex view showing displacement of condylar head. **D,** Note border of right mandible is approximately 5 mm superior to left mandible.

Continued.

E

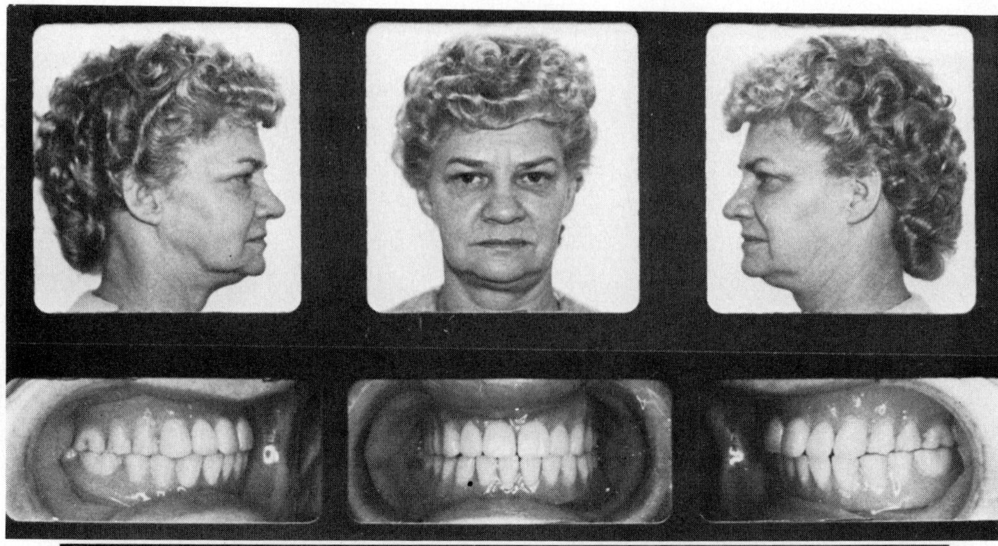

F

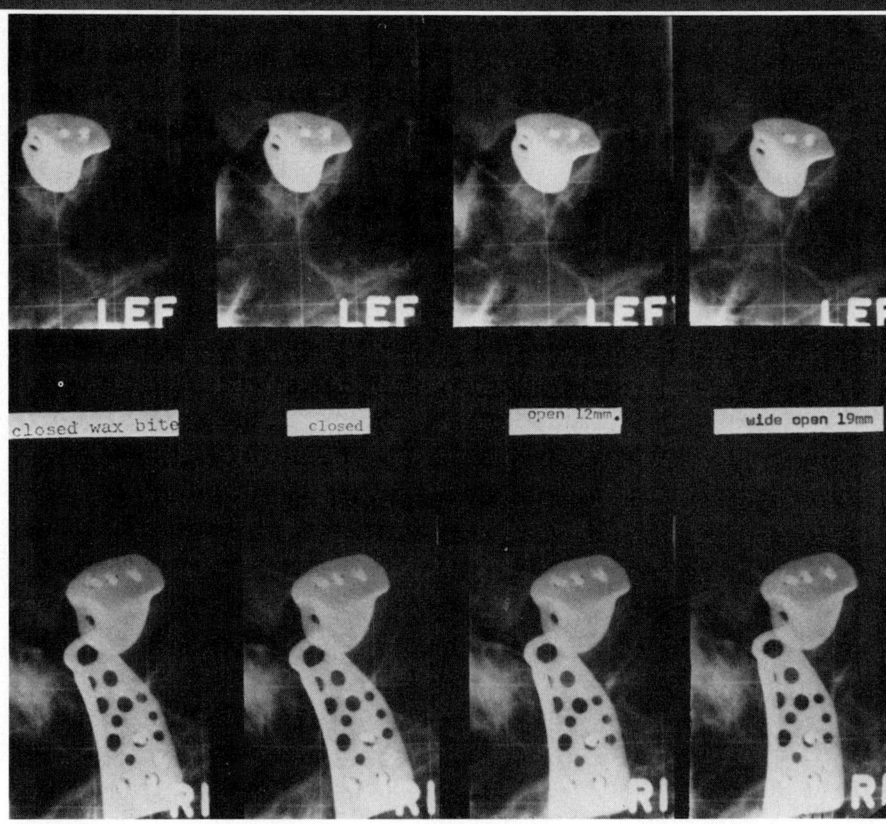

Fig. 22-47, cont'd. E, Full-face, profile, and teeth views showing loss of vertical dimension affecting right side of face. **F,** Specialized TMJ x-ray films showing in right joint the ramal and condylar implant articulating properly with upper metallic and Silastic implant. Condylar head cannot be seen, since material is radiopaque.

G

H

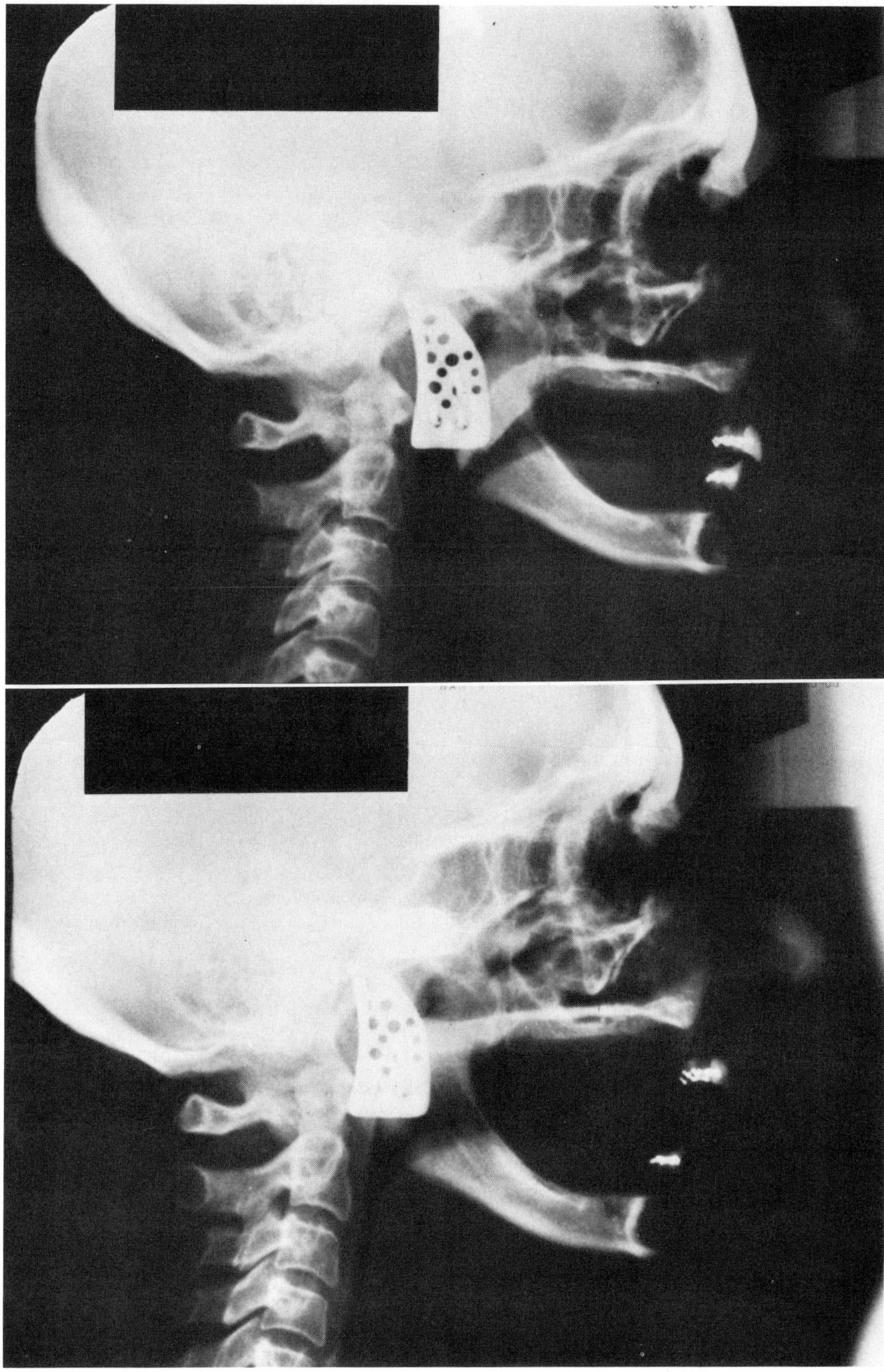

Fig. 22-47, cont'd. G, Closed cephalometric x-ray films showing properly placed prosthesis. **H,** Open cephalometric x-ray film taken approximately 1 month after surgery, showing patient able to open 25 mm.

Continued.

I

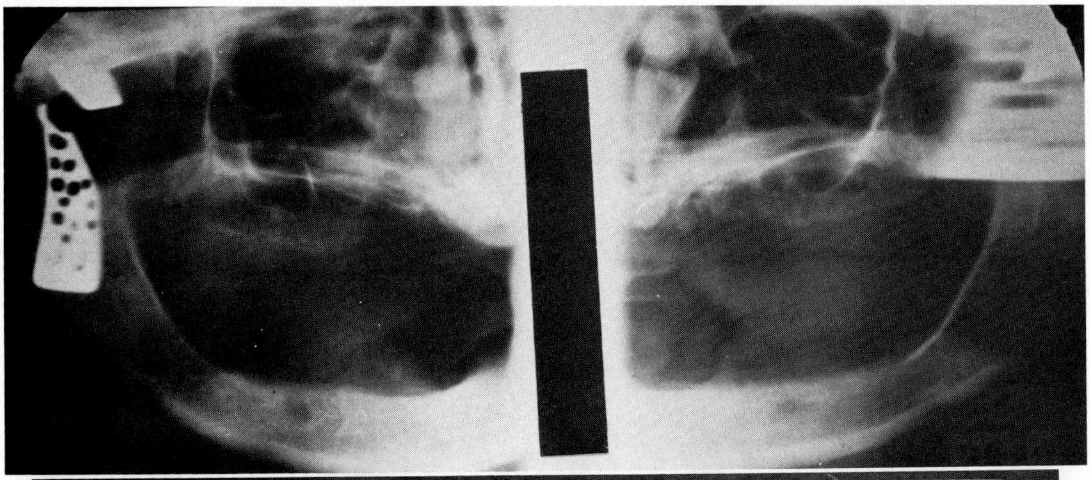

J

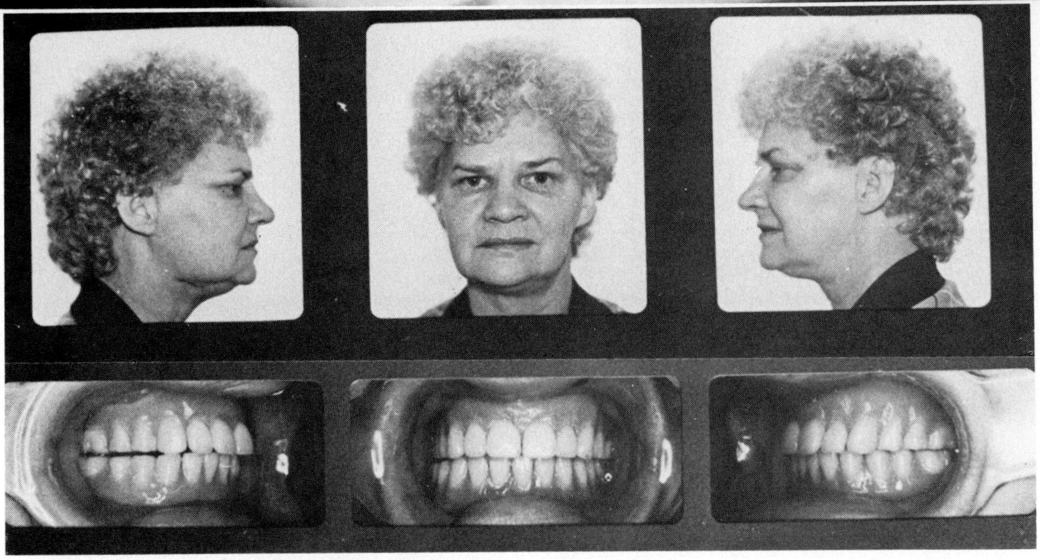

Fig. 22-47, cont'd. I, Panorex x-ray film shows properly placed total TMJ implant in right joint and articular eminance implant in left joint. **J,** Full-face, profile, and teeth views show that bite is open approximately 2 mm on right side because vertical dimension on right side was increased by that amount. Her new dentures have since brought her teeth into proper occlusion.

Case 13

K.L., a 33-year-old woman, had fallen onto cement on the right side of her face when she was 7 years old. After that her jaw always would seem to lock on the right side if she chewed gum or ate foods such as steak or French bread. She kept the problem fairly well under control for years by only eating easy to chew foods and seeing numerous dentists who precribed conservative treatments such as jaw straps while sleeping. By the time she was 30 years old, the pain in her right jaw, as well as her left, had become severe. He jaw chronically would slip back and lock closed on the right side and would have to be forced back into place manually, loudly cracking each time she did so. There would be a sharp pain if a finger was pressed on the right joint or if she tried to eat anything that was not soft. She tried splints, cortisone injections, acupuncture, compresses, and pain medications. Finally she was referred to us by a prosthodontist who was familiar with TMJ syndrome.

The clinical examination revealed pain in both joints on palpation. Her mouth opened asynchronously with a grating sound in both joints. She was able to open 31 mm, and her jaw deviated 4 mm to the right. There was no pain in the muscles of mastication. She also exhibited an anterior open bite of approximately 3 mm, and her bite came together only on the first and second molars.

Specialized TMJ x-ray films revealed in the left joint significant flattening of the eminence and some flattening of the anterior condylar head. In the right joint the condylar head was tightly placed posteriorly within the fossa, and there was flattening of the anterior portion of the condylar head and erosion of the cortical bone (Fig. 22-48, *A*). Cephalometric x-ray films show the anterior open bite (Fig. 22-48, *B*). Full-

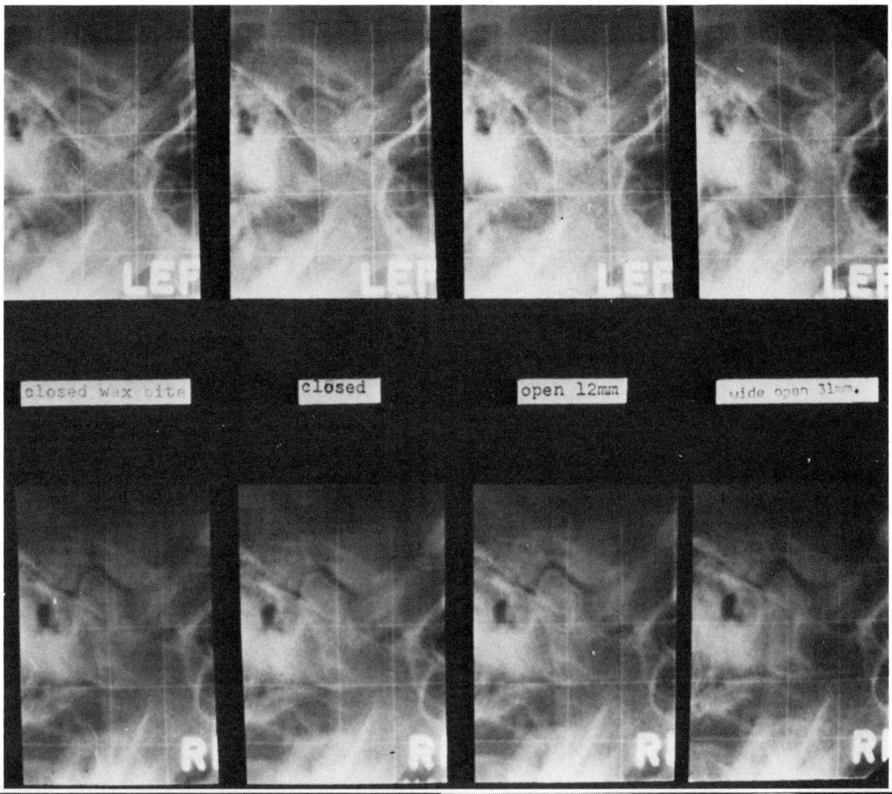

A

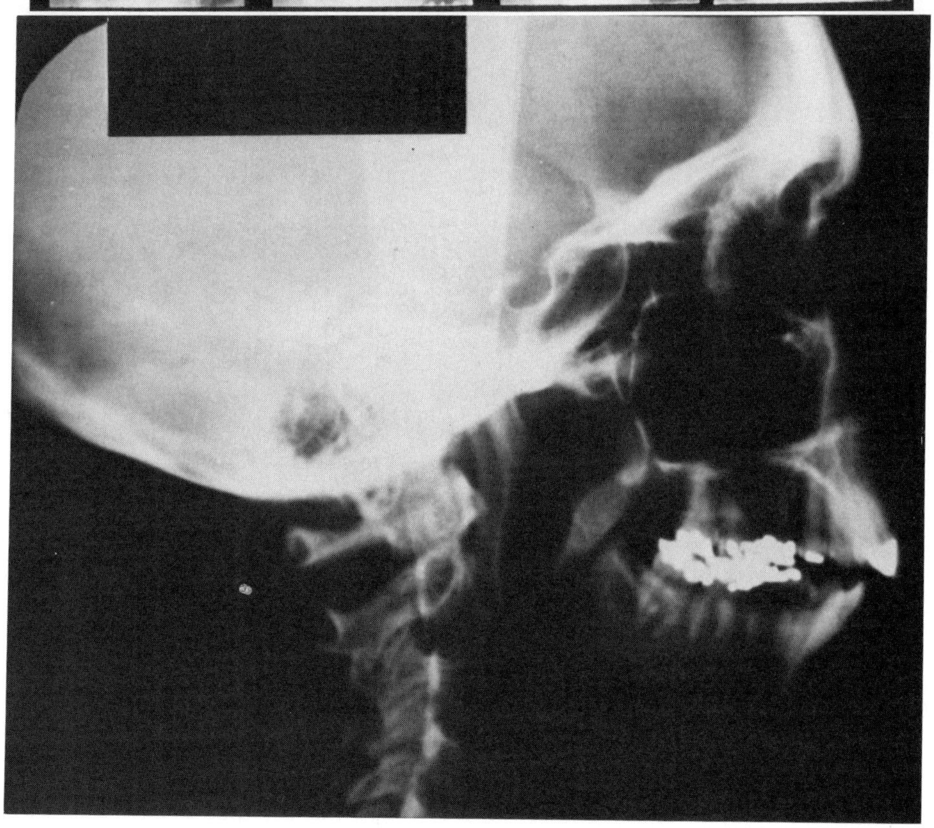

B

Fig. 22-48. A, Specialized TMJ x-ray films showing flattening and dishing out of right condylar head with minimum movement of condyle over eminence. In left joint there is anterior displacement of condyle. In closed views flattening of eminence can be seen. There is asymmetrical condylar function between right and left joints. **B,** Cephalometric x-ray films show the anterior open bite.

Continued.

C

D

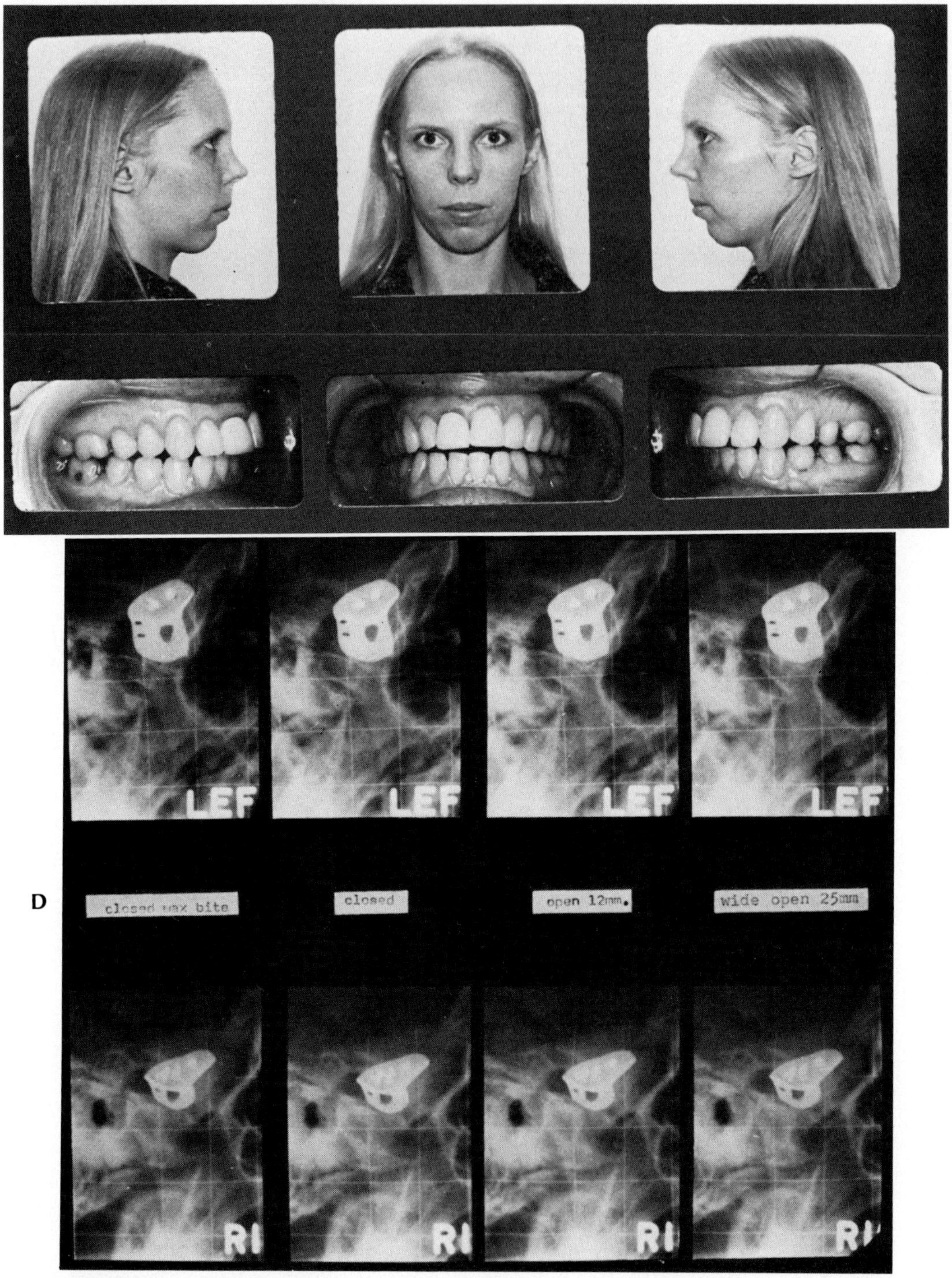

Fig. 22-48, cont'd. C, Full-face, profile, and teeth views show anterior open bite and teeth contacting only on molars. **D,** Postoperative TMJ film shows properly placed articular eminence prosthesis with Silastic insert. Silastic material is radiopaque and cannot be seen. In right and left sides, lowered position of condylar head with relation to fossa can be noted.

face, profile, and teeth views show an anterior open bite and teeth contacting only on the molars (Fig. 22-48, *C*).

Treatment. Surgery was performed in March 1978. Prior to the incision Winter's arch bars were placed with elastic traction between the arch bars to bring the mandible to a more normal position and to close the anterior open bite.

On the right side a preauricular incision was made. When we entered the joint, the roughness of the bone could be seen, as well as damage to the disc. A sharp lip of bone that projected from the lateral portion of the eminence was removed, as was the disc. Several special metal and Silastic prostheses were then placed to lower the floor of the fossa and give the condylar head an articulating surface. One fit well and was secured to the zygomatic arch.

On the left side a preauricular incision was made. Roughness of the eminence was seen in this joint also, as well as a torn disc. Several prostheses were tried until one fit well over the eminence and lowered the floor of the fossa to the point where the condyle made contact with it. Wound areas were closed in the usual manner.

The patient was discharged from the hospital 3 days postoperatively. The arch bars and elastic traction were removed 10 days postoperatively. Postoperative TMJ films show a properly placed prosthesis (Fig. 22-48, *D*). Full-face, profile, and teeth views show normal occlusion postoperatively (Fig. 22-48, *E*). The patient is free from pain and is now able to eat and chew normally.

E

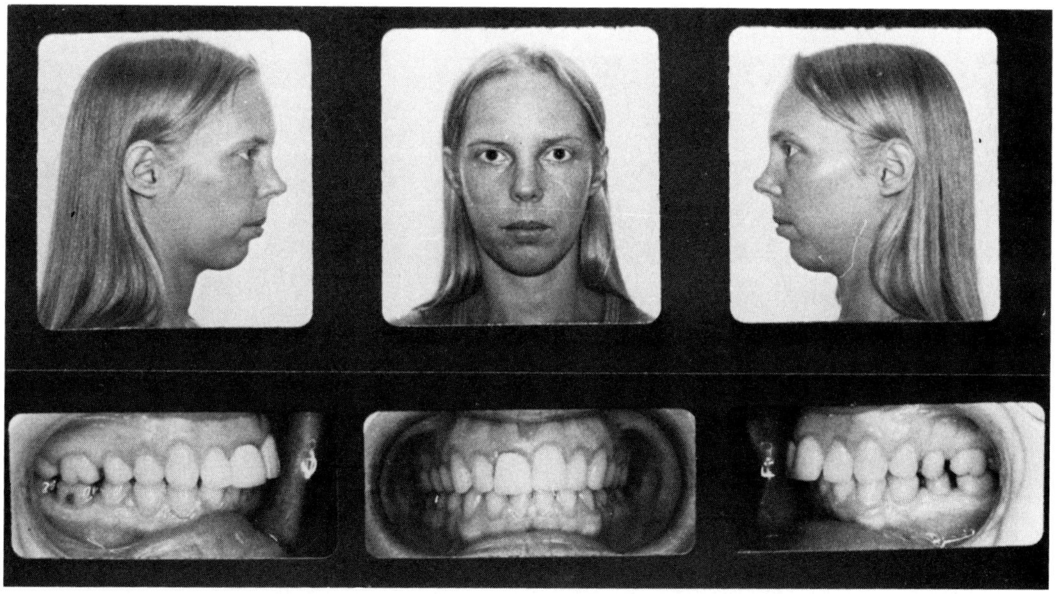

Fig. 22-48, cont'd. E, With teeth in normal occlusion, relaxed appearance of patient's face can be compared with her preoperative condition.

Case 14

B.L., a 36-year-old woman, had a long-standing problem with her bite. As a child, she kept trying to push her jaw forward to make up for what she felt was a shortening of the jaw. In 1973, when she was 30 years old, she began having headaches. Eye examinations, neurological testing, a routine physical examination, and psychological evaluation were done, with no significant findings. In 1974 she went for an evaluation at a university dental school where her sister was a student. She was diagnosed as having a Class II retrognathia and an acquired bite in which her mandible was protruded in an effort to compensate. Habitual bruxing and clenching were also determined, and it was noted that three extracted molars had not been replaced. She was then treated for about a year with bite planes, soft diet, moist heat, muscle exercises, and a removable partial denture to replace the missing molars.

After this year severe pain continued, so additional evaluations were made, and several different bite appliances were tried. Blood tests were done and further psychological counseling given. The following year the jaws were wired together for 2 weeks with only temporary relief. A series of osteopathic manipulations were no help. She was then sent to another medical university, where an oral surgeon diagnosed degenerative joint disease and arranged for surgery in October 1977. She was to have bilateral eminectomies, a high condylectomy on the left side, with a nylon-reinforced Silastic sheet secured to the upper part of the joint with stainless steel ligatures, and suturing of a tear in the meniscus.

After this surgery recovery seemed normal for about 6 weeks, and then soreness began to return, particularly on the left side. A year later the pain had worsened, particularly in the left joint area. At this point her sister, by now a dentist, referred the patient to us.

The clinical examination revealed soreness of both joints on palpation and a grating sound on both sides, denoting bone-on-bone contact and a tear in the meniscus. The masseter and external pterygoid muscles, as well as the left neck and shoulder muscles, were sensitive on palpation. She was also evaluated on a Mandibular Kinesiograph, which confirmed that the damage was primarily in the joints. She could open her mouth 31 mm with difficulty, and her jaw deviated 1 mm to the left.

Specialized TMJ x-ray films revealed flattening of the eminences and erosion in both joints and, in the left joint, two small wires where a sheet of Silastic had been secured to the zygomatic arch. Also, in the left joint bone-on-bone contact of the condyle to the eminence could be seen in the 12-mm view (Fig. 22-49, *A*). Cephalometric x-ray films show the pa-

A

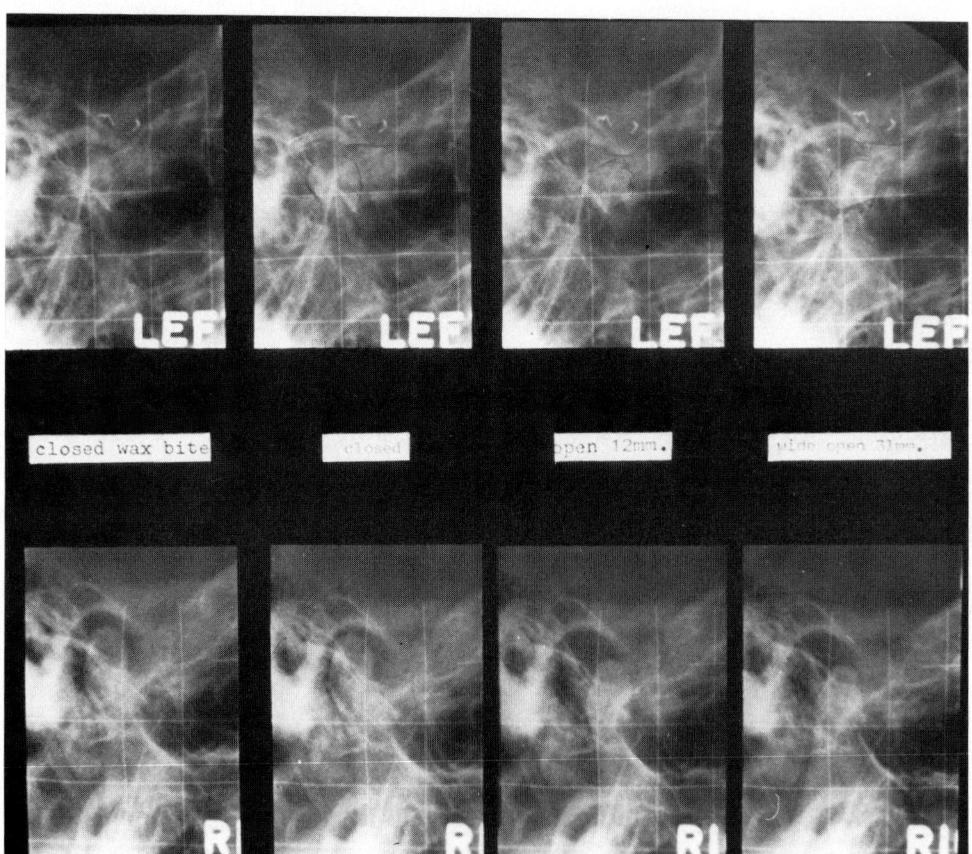

Fig. 22-49. A, Specialized TMJ films showing bilateral eminectomies. On left side can be seen high condylectomy and placement of Silastic sheet in upper portion of joint.

B

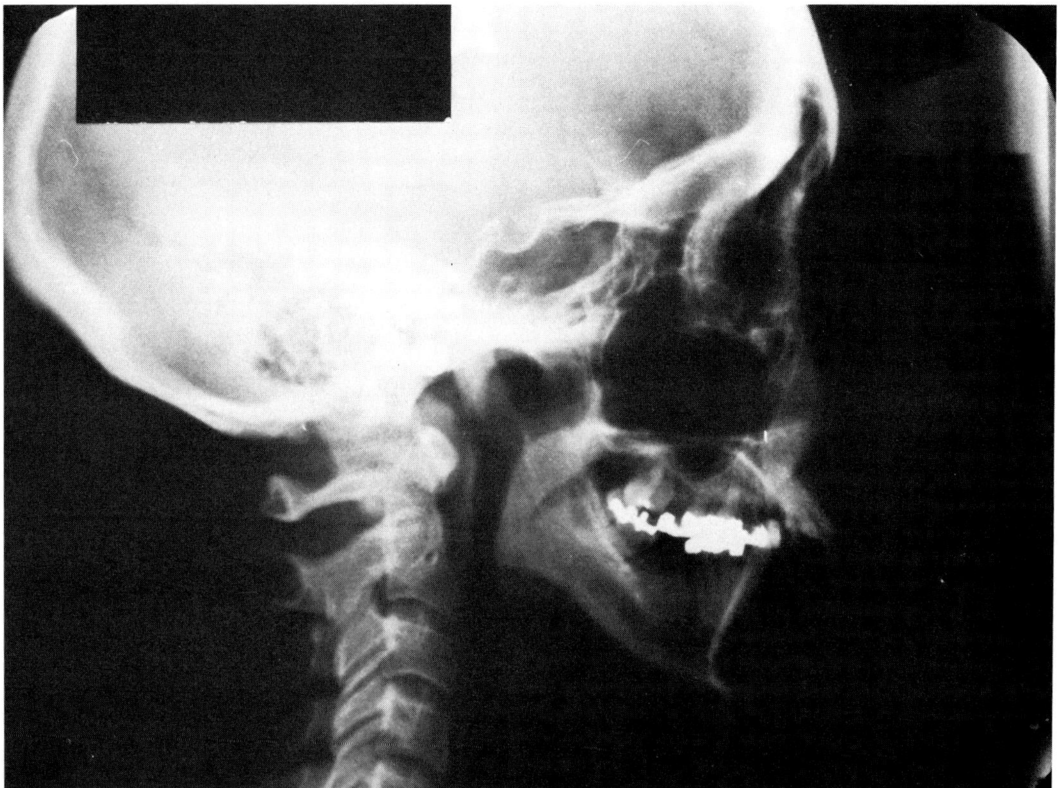

C

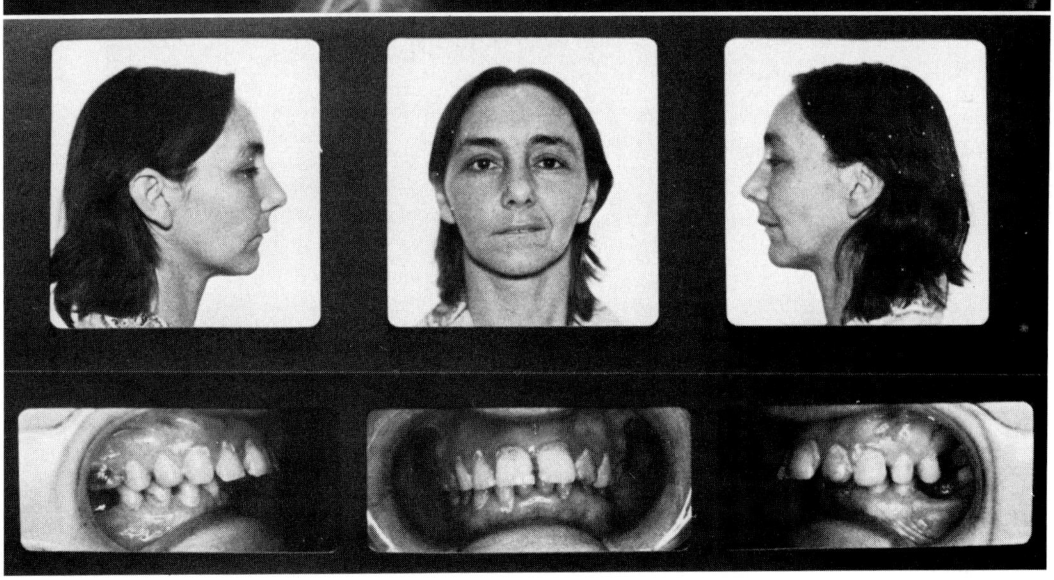

Fig. 22-49, cont'd. B, Cephalometric x-ray films showing that patient has Class II occlusion and protrusion of maxillary teeth. **C,** Full-face view showing loss of vertical dimension on left side of face and muscular asymmetry between left and right sides of face.

Continued.

tient had a Class II occlusion and protrusion of the maxillary teeth (Fig. 22-49, *B*). Full-face, profile, and teeth views show a loss of vertical dimension on the left side of the face (Fig. 22-49, *C*).

Treatment. It was decided that the joint should be restored by removal of the sheet of Silastic and the wire, bilateral arthroplasty, meniscectomy, and insertion of an articular eminence prosthesis with a metal and Silastic implant on the left side.

The patient was operated on in April 1979. On the right side a preauricular incision was made. On entering the joint proper, we found significant fibrous adhesions in the joint, and it was noted that the eminence had been surgically flattened. The disc tissue was removed and the roughened condylar head located and smoothed. Several prostheses were tried to find the best fit to restore the shape of the eminence to a more normal contour.

On the left side a preauricular incision also was made, and

D

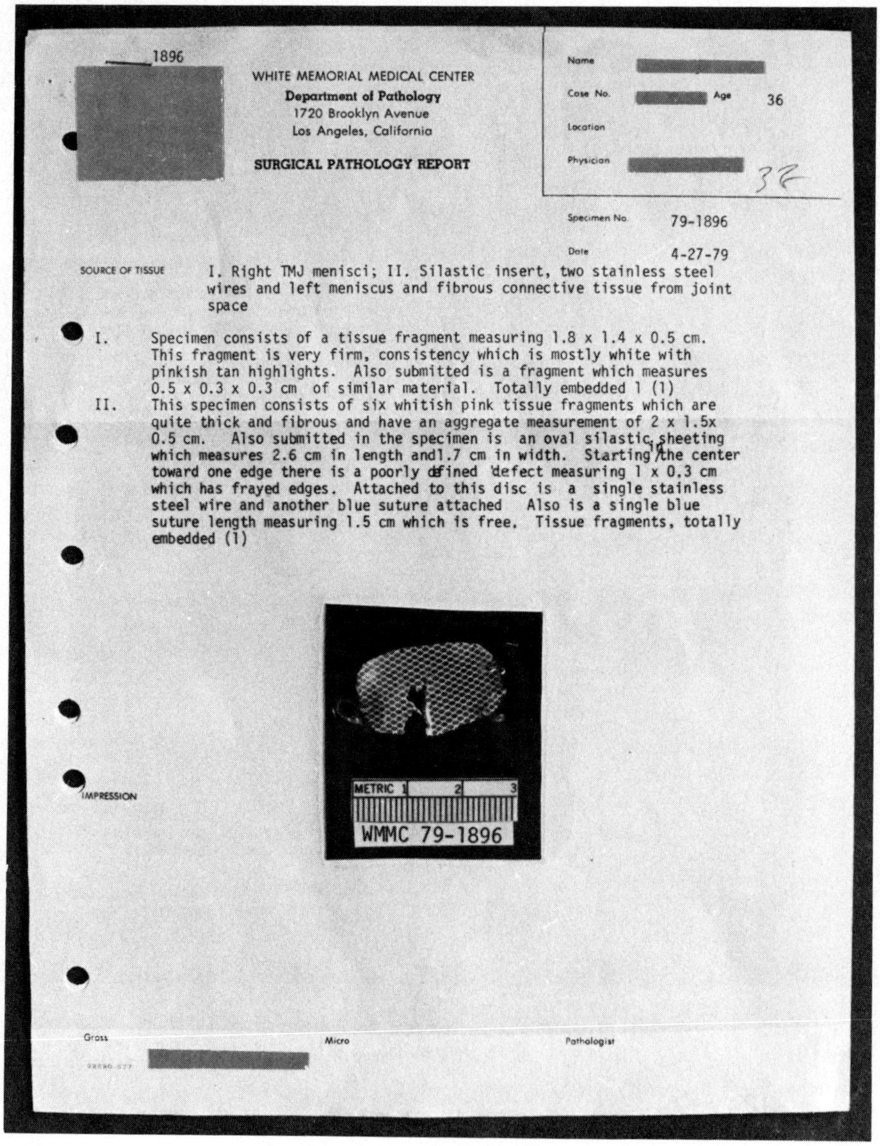

1896

WHITE MEMORIAL MEDICAL CENTER
Department of Pathology
1720 Brooklyn Avenue
Los Angeles, California

SURGICAL PATHOLOGY REPORT

Name
Case No. Age 36
Location
Physician

Specimen No. 79-1896

Date 4-27-79

SOURCE OF TISSUE I. Right TMJ menisci; II. Silastic insert, two stainless steel wires and left meniscus and fibrous connective tissue from joint space

I. Specimen consists of a tissue fragment measuring 1.8 x 1.4 x 0.5 cm. This fragment is very firm, consistency which is mostly white with pinkish tan highlights. Also submitted is a fragment which measures 0.5 x 0.3 x 0.3 cm of similar material. Totally embedded 1 (1)

II. This specimen consists of six whitish pink tissue fragments which are quite thick and fibrous and have an aggregate measurement of 2 x 1.5x 0.5 cm. Also submitted in the specimen is an oval silastic sheeting which measures 2.6 cm in length and1.7 cm in width. Starting in the center toward one edge there is a poorly defined defect measuring 1 x 0.3 cm which has frayed edges. Attached to this disc is a single stainless steel wire and another blue suture attached Also is a single blue suture length measuring 1.5 cm which is free. Tissue fragments, totally embedded (1)

METRIC 1 2 3
WMMC 79-1896

IMPRESSION

Gross Micro Pathologist

Fig. 22-49, cont'd. D, Surgical Pathology Report. Picture of Silastic insert showing tear and resorption of reinforced Silastic.

in this joint it also was noted that it was filled with fibrous adhesions. A small stainless steel ligature was found to be securing a sheet of Silastic to the upper portion of the joint, and this wire was cut and the sheet removed. Examination showed there had been erosion and dissolution of a large segment of the nylon-reinforced Silastic because of the condyle pushing against it (Fig. 22-49, *D* and *E*). It was difficult to identify the condyle until most of the fibrous tissue had been removed from the joint. The condyle, which had had a high condylectomy performed on it previously, was identified and its sharp edges rounded. The eminence had been surgically flattened, and a number of metal and Silastic prostheses were tried until a proper fit was found. The wounds were closed in the usual manner.

The patient did well postoperatively. She was discharged in 4 days. She has had relief of most of her symptoms and currently is having her teeth restored and her bite opened 3mm.

E

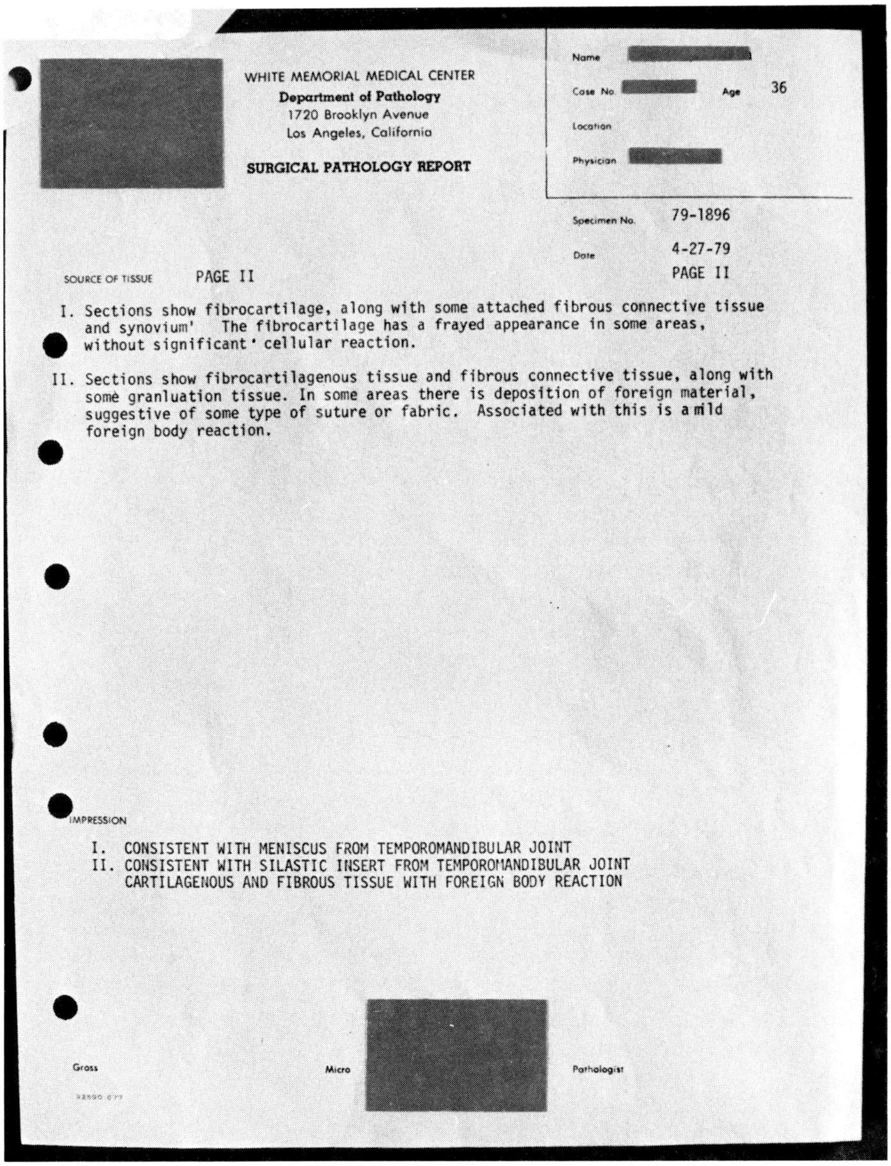

WHITE MEMORIAL MEDICAL CENTER
Department of Pathology
1720 Brooklyn Avenue
Los Angeles, California

SURGICAL PATHOLOGY REPORT

Name

Case No. Age 36

Location

Physician

Specimen No. 79-1896

Date 4-27-79

PAGE II

SOURCE OF TISSUE PAGE II

I. Sections show fibrocartilage, along with some attached fibrous connective tissue and synovium' The fibrocartilage has a frayed appearance in some areas, without significant' cellular reaction.

II. Sections show fibrocartilagenous tissue and fibrous connective tissue, along with some granluation tissue. In some areas there is deposition of foreign material, suggestive of some type of suture or fabric. Associated with this is a mild foreign body reaction.

IMPRESSION

I. CONSISTENT WITH MENISCUS FROM TEMPOROMANDIBULAR JOINT
II. CONSISTENT WITH SILASTIC INSERT FROM TEMPOROMANDIBULAR JOINT
CARTILAGENOUS AND FIBROUS TISSUE WITH FOREIGN BODY REACTION

Gross Micro Pathologist

Fig. 22-49, cont'd. E, Second page of report.

Case 15

V.M., a 40-year-old woman, had a 2-year history of pain and discomfort in her joints, both jaw areas, neck, shoulders, face, and additional right-sided symptoms of subjective hearing loss, fullness in the ear, tongue pain, and ringing in the ear. After a year an oral surgeon performed a high condylectomy and an eminectomy in the right joint and placed a fascia insert between the bony surfaces. However, she continued to have symptoms, which included a cold feeling on the left side of the face as well as the nose and eyes. Her throat hurt when she turned her head, she noted it was hard to see at times, and she felt her right ear must in some way be connected to the jaw bone because of the pain. The woman was edentulous in the maxilla, and her dentist did a good job of maintaining occlusion. She had a mandibular partial denture with bar attachment on two remaining mandibular teeth. The cephalometric profile radiograph shows this condition (Fig. 22-50, *A*).

Clinical examination revealed pain in both joints on palpation and a grating sound in the right joint. The patient could open approximately 31 mm, with a deviation of 2 mm to the right on openings. Specialized TMJ x-ray films revealed a high condylectomy and eminectomy in the right joint with fascia secured by wires to the condylar stump. The lateral portion of the eminence was significantly flattened (Fig. 22-50, *B*). In the 31-mm view there appears to be bone-on-bone contact between the condylar stump and the medial portion of the eminence. In the closed view there is some flattening of the anterior head of the condyle and erosion. In the left joint the condyle appears to be slightly posteriorly displaced. Full-face, profile and teeth views show loss of vertical dimension, affecting the right side of the face (Fig. 22-50, *C*).

Treatment. Surgery was performed in February 1980. A preauricular incision was made on the right side, and the joint was opened in the usual fashion. On entering the, we noted significant scar tissue. The upper part of the joint, or eminence, was significantly flattened, and the area was rough on palpation. In the lower compartment of the joint, wires were holding tissue over the condylar head. The condylar head could be seen through a tear in the disc, or fascia-like tissue. This tissue was removed in segments, as was the small wire-like suture material. Some type of high condylectomy appears to have been performed on the condylar head, which by this time was burnished smooth. A specialized articular eminence prosthesis with Silastic was tried on the joint proper. It was difficult to secure the prosthesis because of the eminence being cut down, but eventually this was accomplished. The stump of the condylar head was seen to function smoothly in the new fossa and eminence. The sound area was closed in layers in the usual fashion.

In the left joint a similar process was accomplished. On entering the joint proper, we could palpate the roughness of the articular eminence. A tear also was noted in the lateral aspect of the meniscus. The meniscus did not seem to be displaced anteriorly. An incision was made in the lower portion of the joint to explore the underpart of the disc. The anterior attachment to the meniscus was freed from the superior fibers of the external pterygoid muscle by sharp dissection. A lamina spreader was placed between the upper and lower portions of the joint to facilitate the removal of the meniscus. Again, a section of this meniscus appeared to be very dense and hypertrophic. The meniscus tissue was removed, using a Beaver no. 66 blade with sharp dissection, and was sent to the laboratory for histological study. When the lower part of the condyle could be seen, a roughness of the anterior head of the condyle was noted. Several prostheses were tried; one fit well to the eminence and was secured by three 5-mm cast Vitallium screws. The condylar head was seen to function smoothly over the prosthesis. The wound area was closed in layers.

Postoperative x-ray films reveal a properly placed metal and Silastic implant in the right joint and, opening wide, the condyle translating over the implant. The left joint also shows a properly placed implant and translational movement of the condyle (Fig. 22-50, *D*). She was helped with all her pain symptoms.

A

B

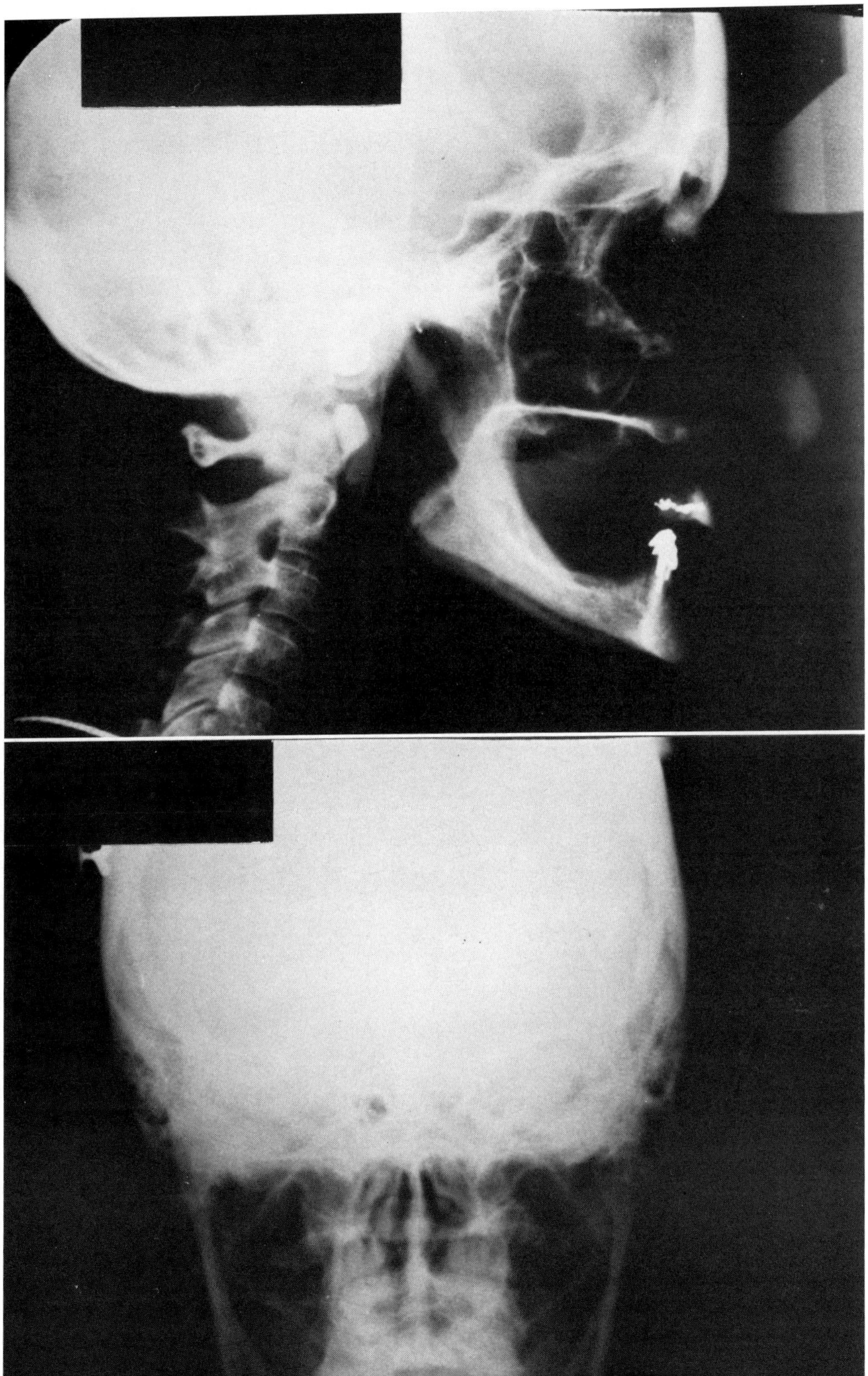

Fig. 22-50. A, Cephalometric profile radiograph showing maxillary denture and mandibular plastic partial denture attached to bar between two remaining mandibular teeth. **B,** Specialized TMJ x-ray films of right joint reveal high condylectomy, eminectomy, and stainless steel ligatures securing fascia to condylar stump.

Continued.

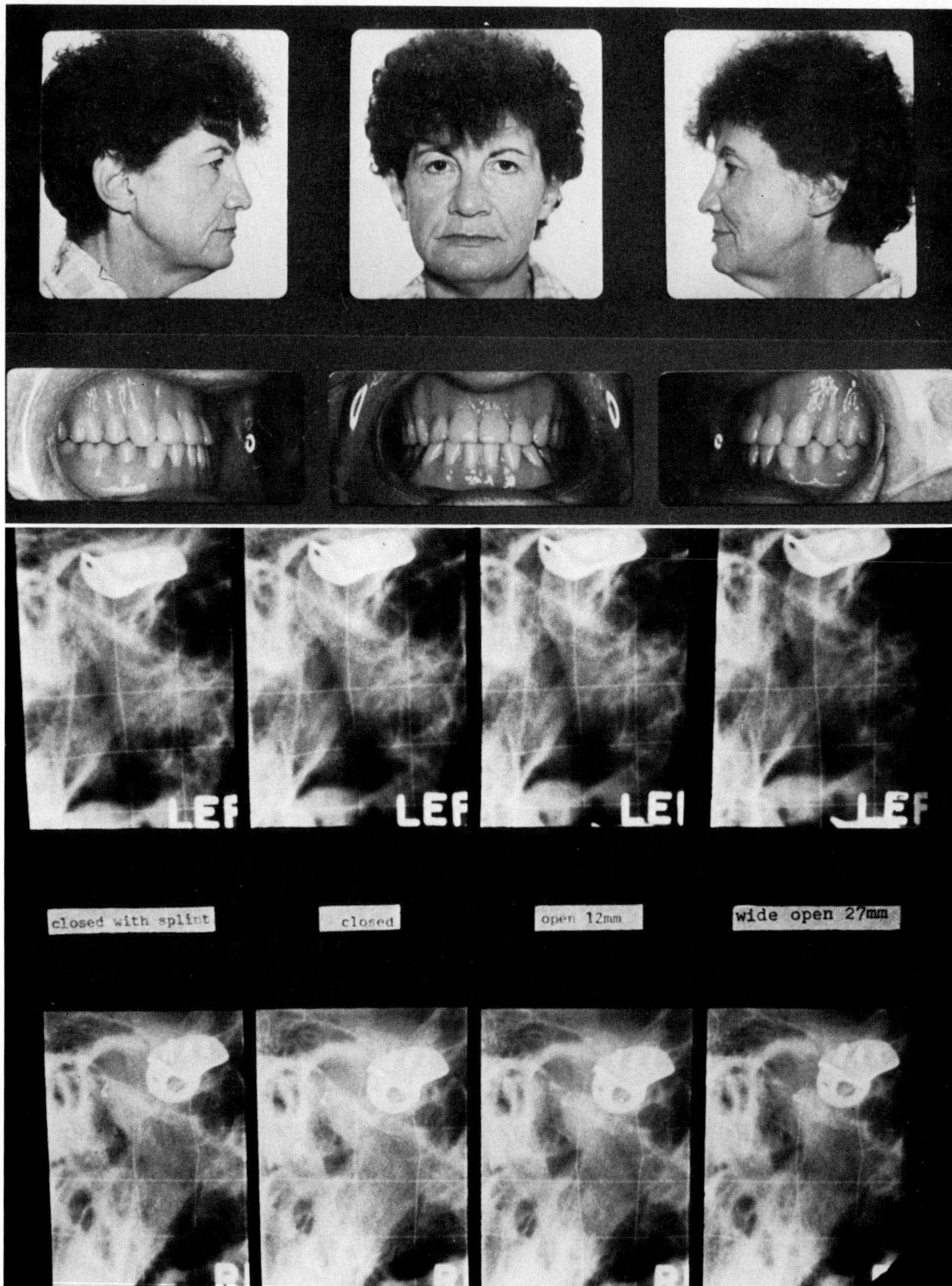

C

D

Fig. 22-50, cont'd. C, Full-face, profile, and teeth views showing loss of vertical dimension affecting right side of face. **D,** Postoperative TMJ films showing implants in position. On the right side, metal and Silastic implant is in place. Note that right condyle is quite far from fossa portion of joint. This is because of the Silastic implant, and it compensates for loss of condylar height by lowering floor of fossa. There is translational movement of both condyles.

Case 16

K.R., a 30-year-old schoolteacher, began to notice over the previous year that she was having difficulty pronouncing words, which significantly affected her work. She also noted that her front teeth were not fitting together and that her bite was no meeting only on her back teeth. There was minor discomfort in her lower jaw, neck, and shoulders and an occasional ringing in her ears. She had been given cortisone and pain medication and had her teeth ground down in August 1977 in an attempt to close her bite. Her family dentist then referred her to us.

Specialized TMJ x-ray films revealed significant osteoarthritis of both joints (Fig. 22-51, *A*). In the left joint there was significant flattening of the condylar head and some flattening of the eminence. In the right joint there was lessflattening of the eminence, but the anterior condylar head was significantly flattened. There was a loss of vertical dimension of both condyles. This loss was the main factor in the anterior open bite, since the muscle pull on the mandible is always in a superior and anterior direction. The cephalometric view shows the anterior open bite (Fig. 22-51, *B*). The full-face, profile, and teeth views also shows the open bite (Fig. 22-51, *C*).

Treatment. It was decided that the joints would be restored with metal and Silastic prostheses. This would have the effect of lowering the fossa to compensate for the loss of condylar height and would rotate the mandible downward and upward, also preventing further osteoarthritic degeneration of the joint.

Surgery was performed in December 1977. Before the surgery, arch bars with interdental traction were placed to close the bite and to hold the teeth in the normal position. A preauricular incision was made on the left side. On entering the joint proper, severe damage was noted within the joint itself. The left eminence was nearly flat and the disc tissue abnormal in appearance. The disc was removed, and the lateral portion of the condylar head was carefully smoothed. Several specialized prostheses, which had been specifically made for this problem of filling in and compensating for the loss of the condylar head, were tried until a good fit was obtained.

A preauricular incision was also made on the right side. The disc tissue was abraded, roughened, and abnormal looking. It was removed. The rough condylar head was smoothed over with a special instrument. Several special prostheses were tried on the joint proper until one fit well. The wound areas were closed in the usual manner.

The patient was discharged 3 days postoperatively, and

A

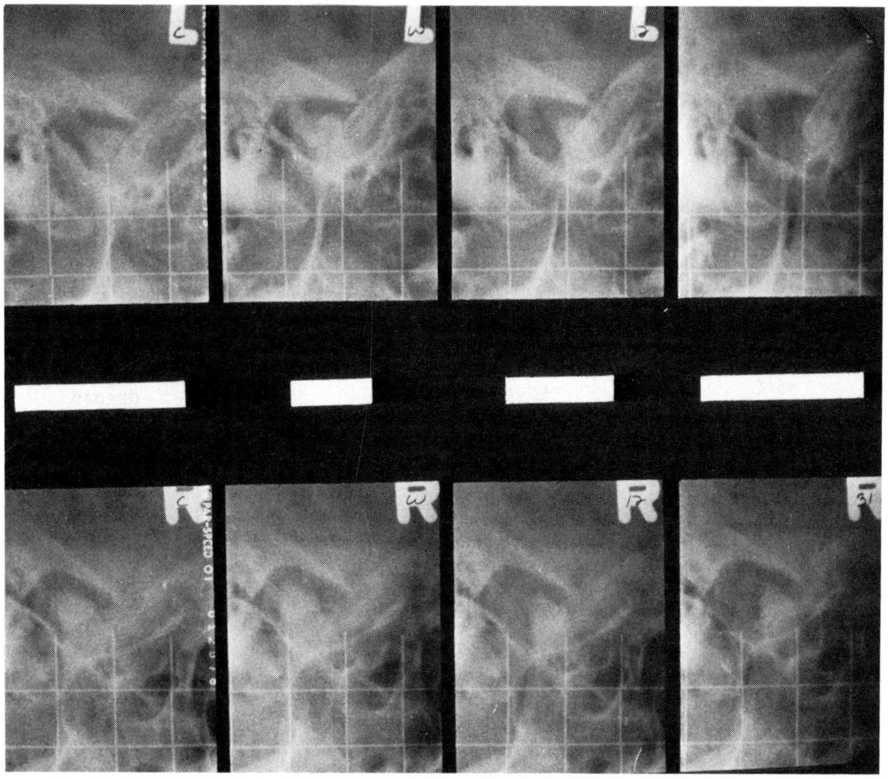

Fig. 22-51. A, Specialized TMJ film showing severe flattening of left articular eminence, as well as flattening of both right and left condyles and loss of vertical dimension.

Continued.

the arch bars were removed 10 days postoperatively. Postoperative TMJ films show the prosthesis in place (Fig. 22-51, *D*). Postoperative cephalometric films show the proper bite (Fig. 22-51, *E*). Postoperative intracanthus films show the two prostheses in place (Fig. 22-51, *F*). Postoperative full-face, profile, and teeth views show normal occlusion (Fig. 22-51, *G*). The patient has since returned to work. Her speech is normal, and she has had no further symptoms or discomfort.

B

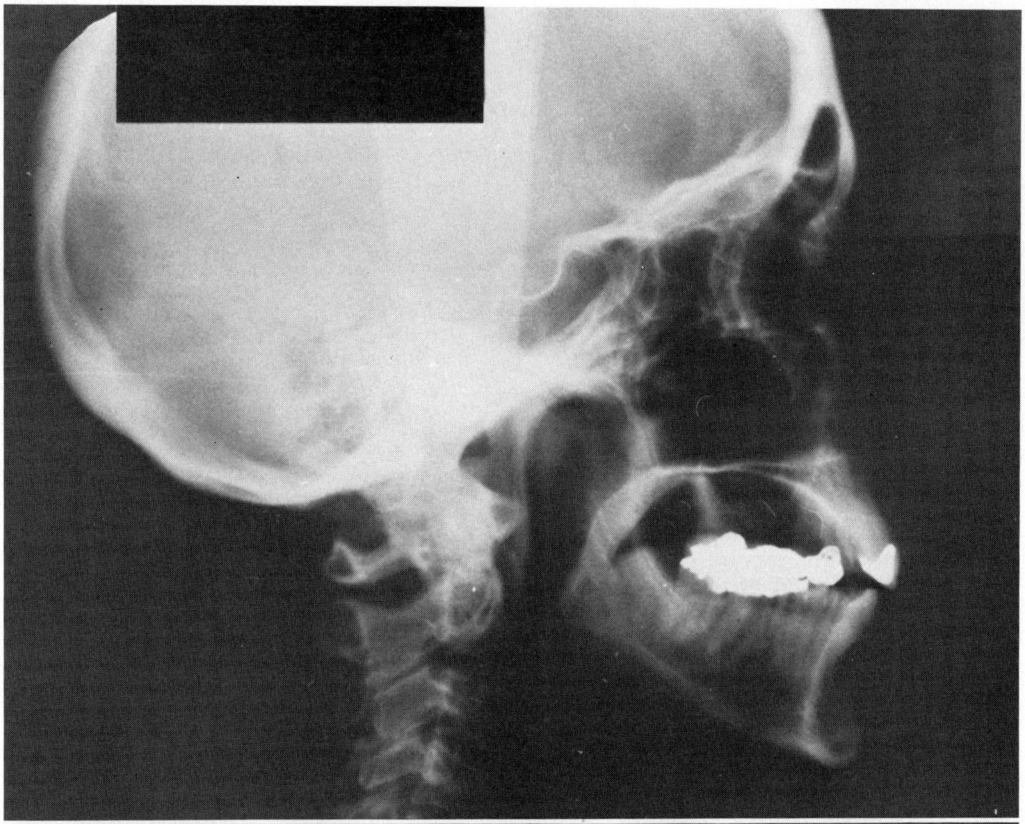

C

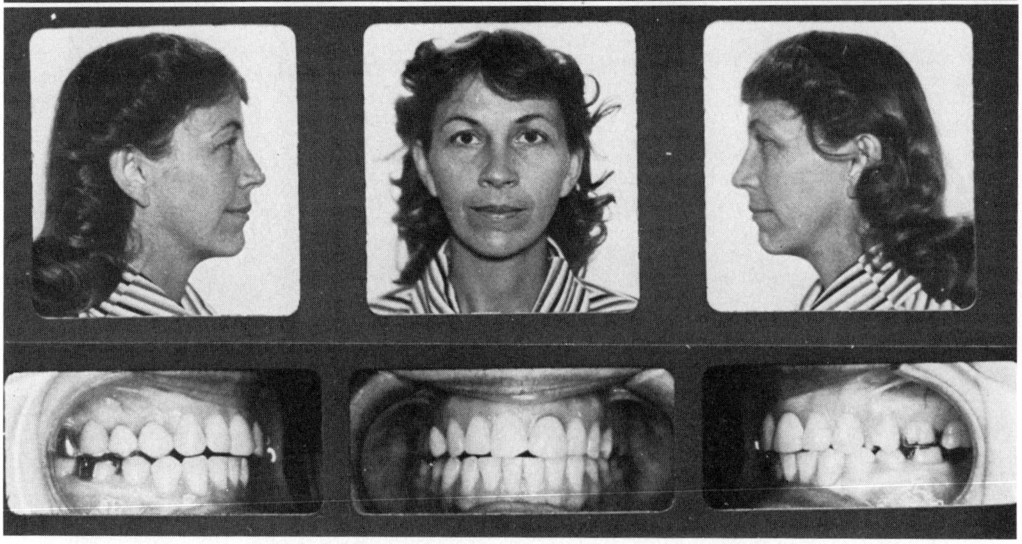

Fig. 22-51, cont'd. B, Cephalometric film showing anterior open bite. **C,** Full-face, profile, and teeth views also showing anterior open bite. Note tension of facial muscles caused by skeletal malrelationships.

D

E

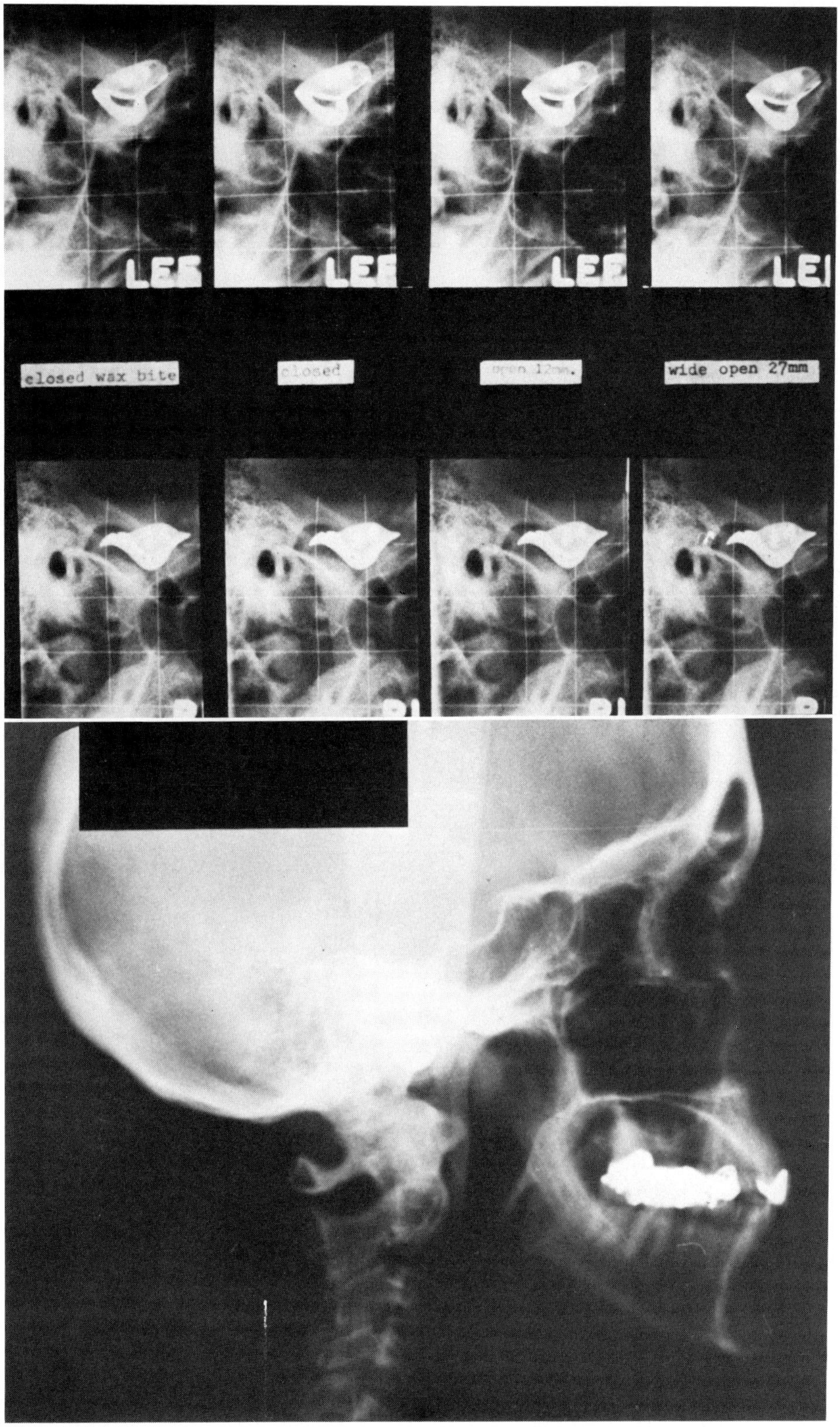

Fig. 22-51, cont'd. D, Postoperative TMJ film showing metal and Silastic implants in position. This also shows effect of lowered fossa floor which enabled damaged condyles to function more normally. **E,** Postoperative cephalometric film showing the condylar head has been moved downward and anterior teeth rotated upward to restore normal occlusion.

Continued.

F

G

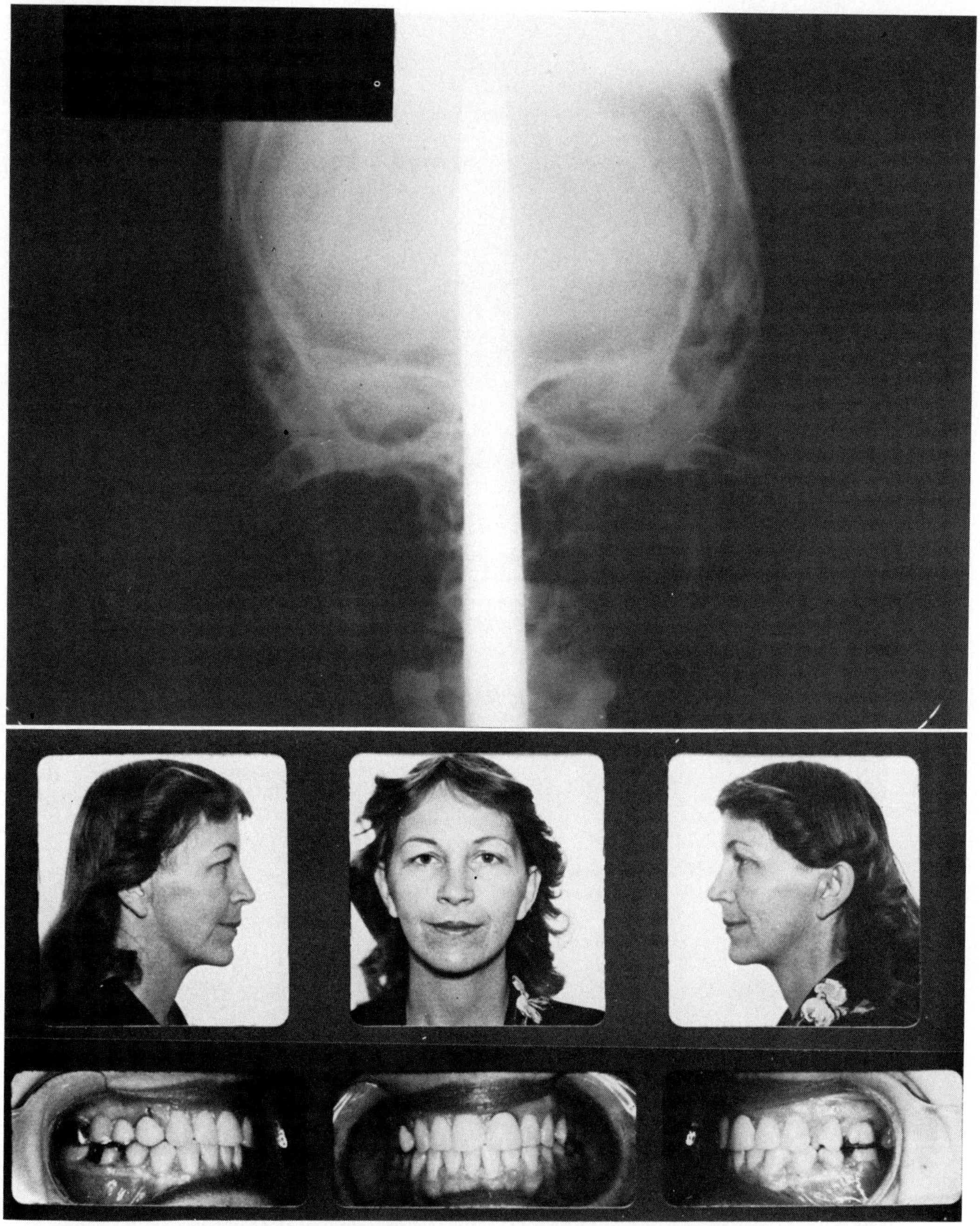

Fig. 22-51, cont'd. F, Postoperative intracanthus film showing two prostheses in place. **G,** Full-face, profile, and teeth views showing teeth in normal occlusion. Note relaxed appearance of facial musculature in full-face view and improvement of profile with mandible in its normal position.

Case 17

M.G., a 29-year-old woman, had had severe pain on the right side of her head for over 3 years, as well as a ringing in her ears, dizziness, and an inability to open her mouth more than 3 mm. A background history revealed that she had fallen on the playground, hitting the side of her head, when she was 8 years old. A more recent fall had perhaps involved a whiplash injury. During the previous 3 years, as the pain worsened, she had been to many physicians and dentists and had tried various treatments, including procaine (Novocain) injections, muscle relaxants, cortisone, naproxen (Naprosyn), indomethacin (Indocin), the removal of a third molar, ultrasound, hot packs, coolant sprays, neck brace, acetaminophen (Tylenol), codeine, biofeedback, swallowing exercises, myofunctional therapy, bite splint, isometric exercises, acupuncture, and a final suggestion that full-mouth orthodontic appliances be tried. She was eventually referred to us by a prosthodontist who suspected a TMJ problem.

The full-face, profile, and teeth views show that her teeth were hitting only on the right side, with no occlusion on the left (Fig. 22-52, *A*). Specialized TMJ x-ray films revealed in the left joint a slight posterior displacement of the condyle in the closed view and erosion of the eminence. In the right joint there is an erosion of the cortical layer of bone over the eminence and a significant flattening and erosion of the anterior head of the condyle (Fig. 22-52, *B*). The cephalometric x-ray view shows a unilateral open bite (Fig. 22-52, *C*).

In addition to the other symptoms, the patient had crepitus or a popping sound in both joints, denoting tears in the meniscus. As the problem was analyzed, it was felt that the loss of condylar height in the right joint had the effect of pulling the body of the mandible upward, distracting and rotating the body of the mandible on the opposite side. Consequently, the use of a specialized metallic and Silastic prosthesis in the right joint would compensate for the lack of condylar height and would have the effect of closing the open bite and rotating the mandible to the left.

Treatment. The patient was operated on in September 1979. Arch bars were placed between the mandible and maxilla, and elastic traction was placed between them to close the bite defect and to overcome the muscle pull. A preauricular incision was made on the right side. At the lateral pole of the condylar head was a bony growth. This was excised. The disc had a tear and was removed. Several prostheses were tried. One was seen to fit well over the eminence, and it compensated for the loss of height caused by the resorption of the condyle from the arthritic process.

The left side also was operated on through a preauricular incision, and a tear could be seen in the lateral portion of the meniscus. The meniscus was removed, and the rough edge of the eminence could be palpated with a periosteal elevator. A number of previously prepared prostheses were tried over the eminence, and one was seen to fit well and was secured to the zygomatic arch in the usual manner.

The patient was discharged 4 days postoperatively, and the arch bars were removed 10 days postoperatively. Specialized TMJ film shows properly placed metal and Silastic implants. Full-face, profile, and teeth views show a more normal occlusion (Fig. 22-52, *D*). The cephalometric view shows a normal jaw relation (Fig. 22-52, *E*). The open view shows the patient opening 40 mm (Fig. 22-52, *F*). The right condylar head is positioned downward and rotated slightly to compensate for loss of vertical dimension from the arthritic disease (Fig. 22-52, *G*). The patient's pain symptoms all have improved. She will have orthodontic treatment to complete normal occlusion in the left area.

A

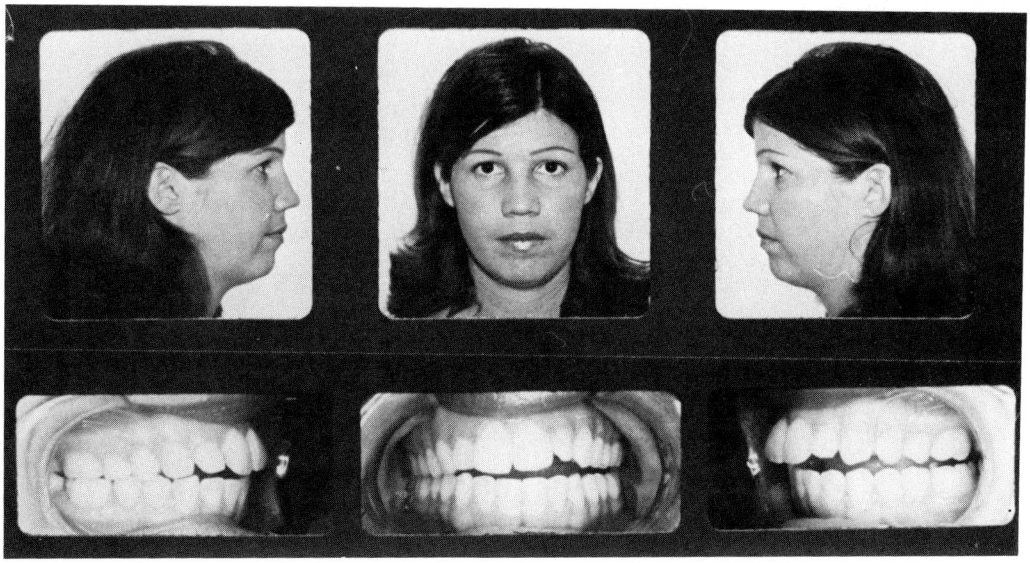

Fig. 22-52. A, Full-face, profile, and teeth views showing mandible rotated to right with anterior open bite and open bite on left with teeth separated approximately 3 to 5 mm.

Continued.

B

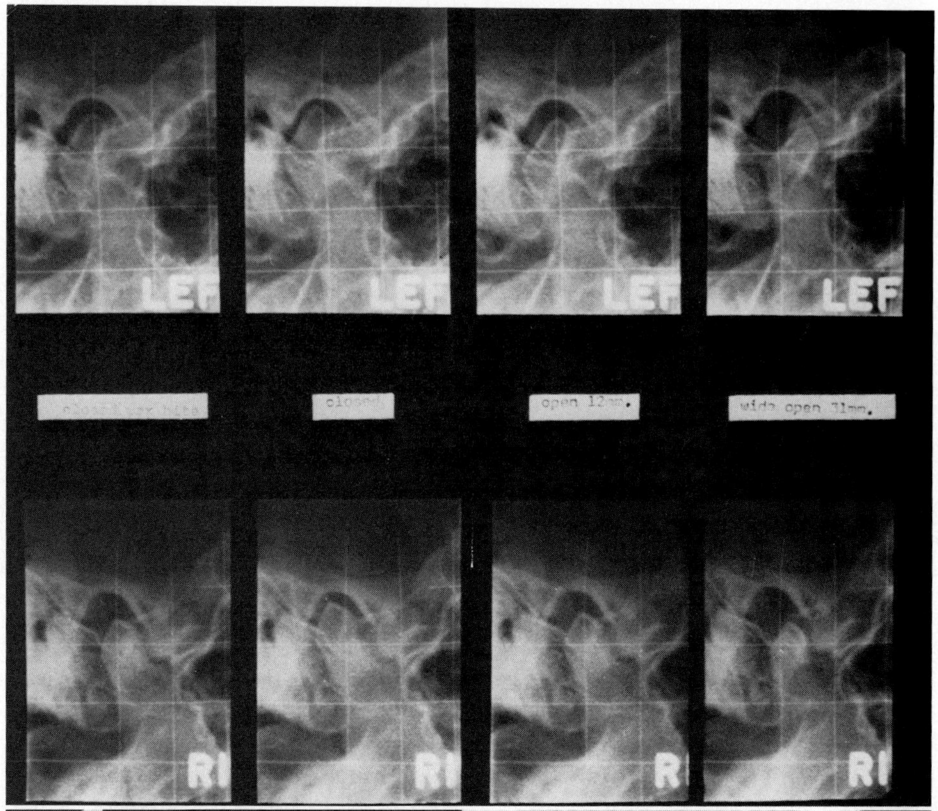

C

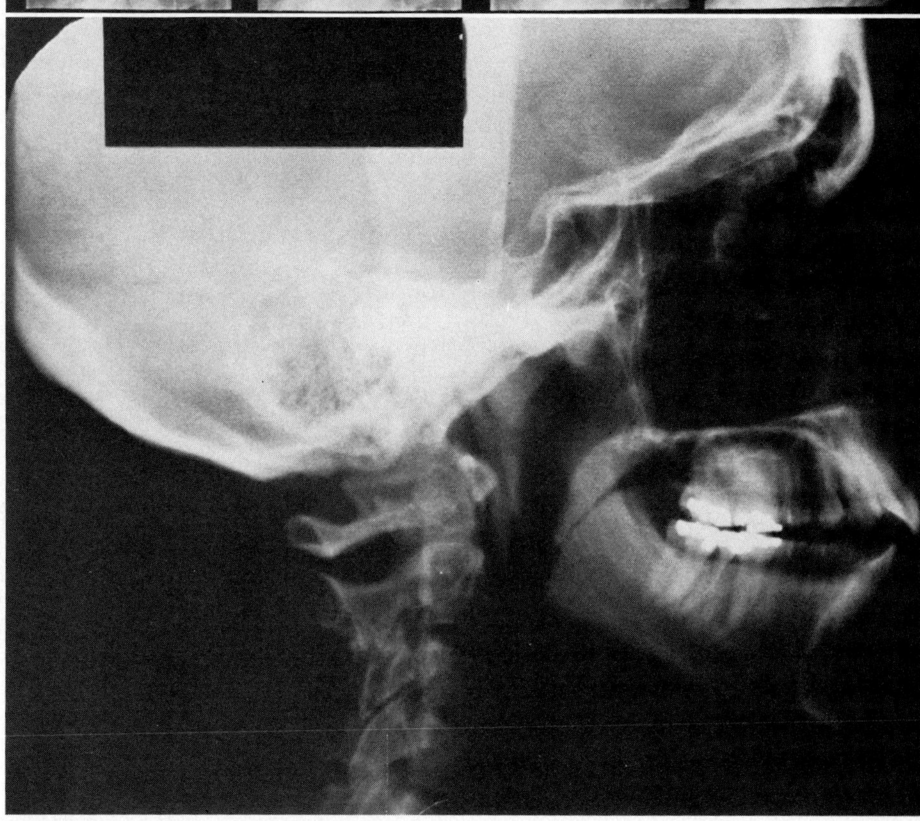

Fig. 22-52, cont'd. B, TMJ x-ray films reveal erosion of eminences in right and left joints, flattening of right condylar head, and asymmetry of condylar movement. **C,** Cephalometric x-ray film showing teeth contacting only on right molar area and anterior open bite of 5 mm.

D

E

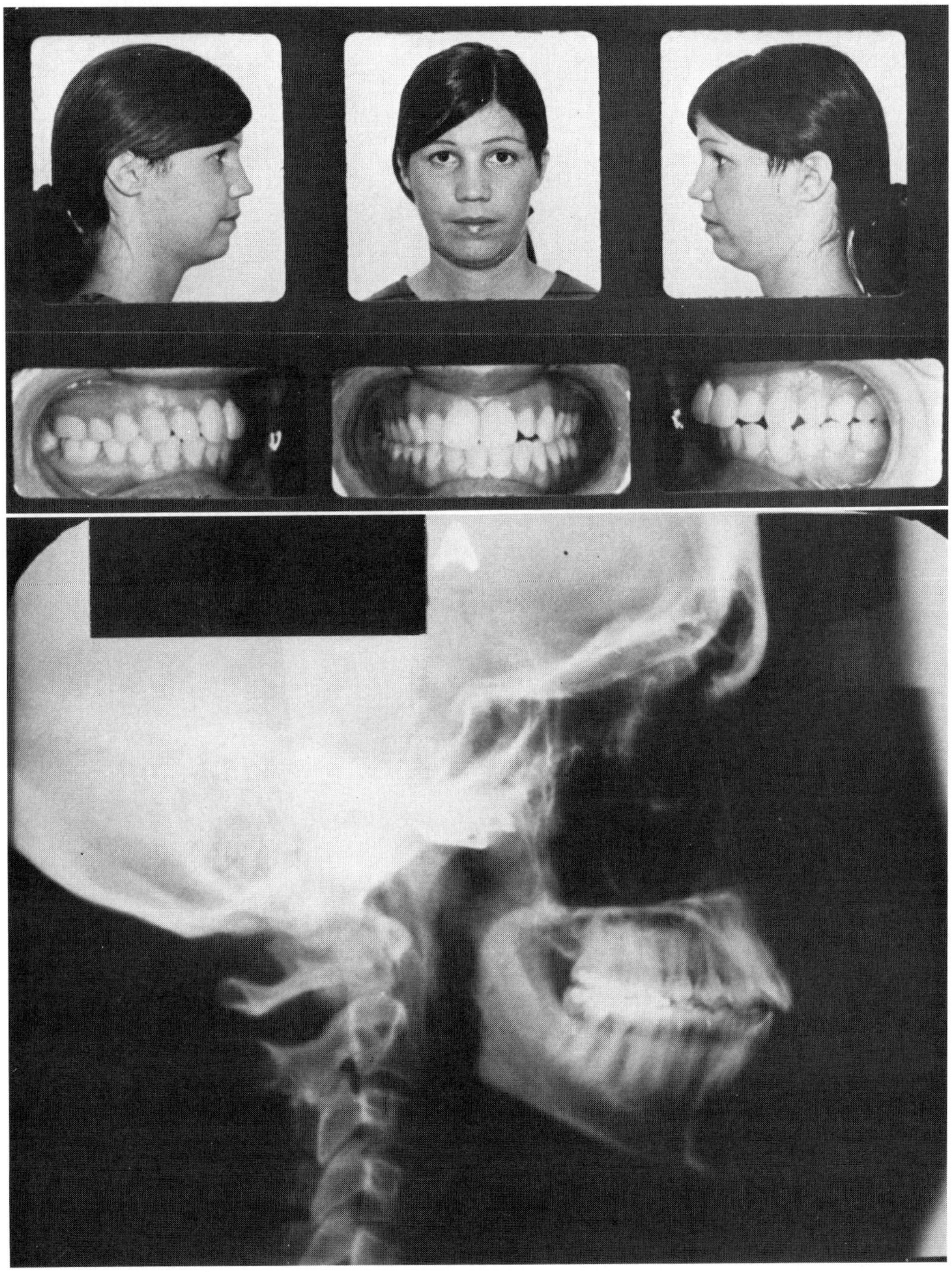

Fig. 22-52, cont'd. D, Full-face, profile, and teeth views showing body of mandible has rotated to left and also anteriorly rotated, closing the bite. **E,** Cephalometric view showing normal relation and proper overbite and overjet.

Continued.

F

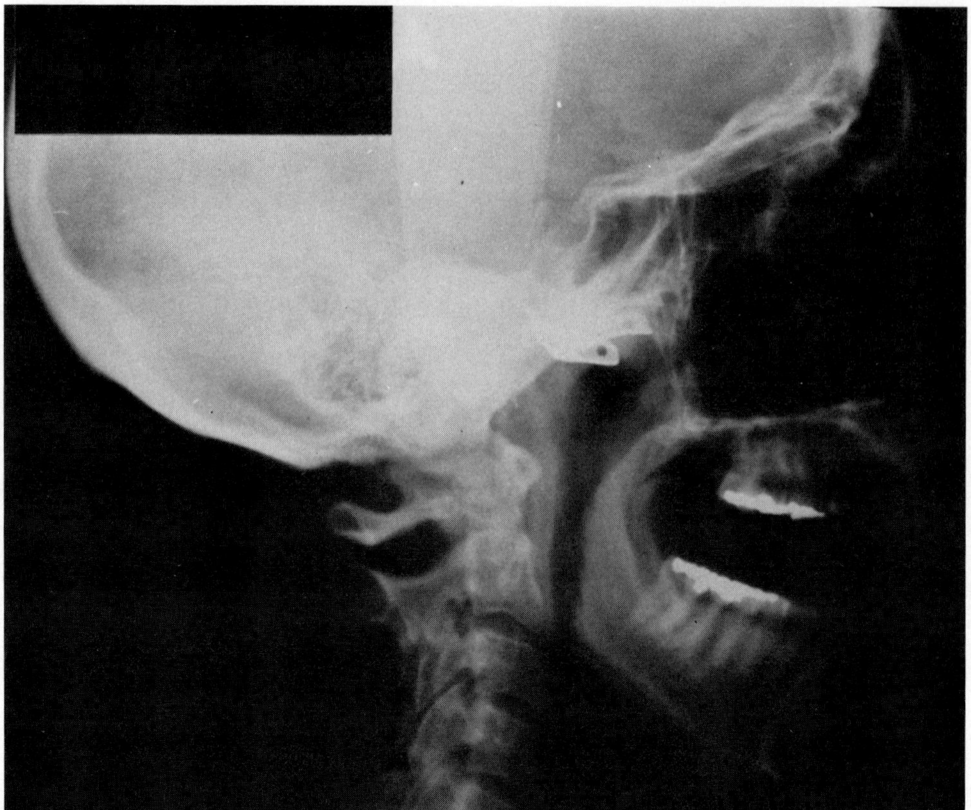

G

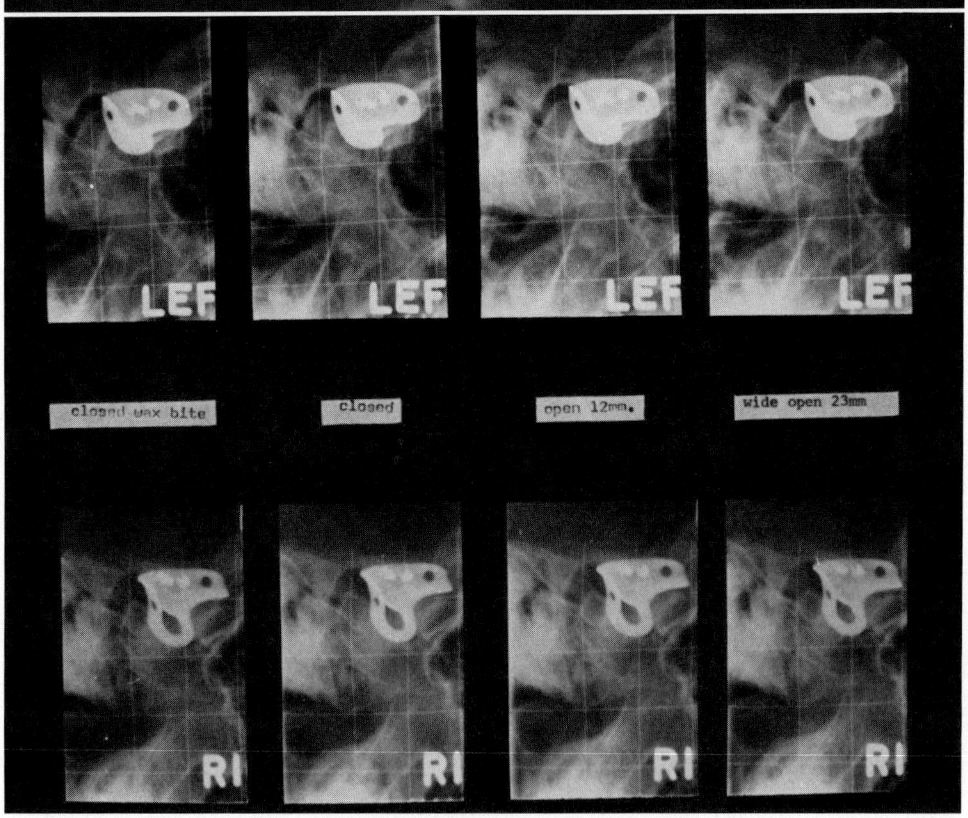

Fig. 22-52, cont'd. F, Cephalometric open view showing patient now able to open 40 mm incisally, compared with 3 mm preoperatively. **G,** Specialized TMJ film showing properly placed metal and Silastic implants. Right condylar head is positioned downward and rotated slightly to compensate for loss of vertical dimension from arthritic disease.

Case 18

B.C., a 19-year-old man, had been treated by a number of physicians and dentists for problems affecting his jaw, which began approximately 10 years previously when he fell off a bicycle, hitting the right side of his jaw. Since then, the mandible had been slowly moving to the left, and the right side of his face appeared to be more developed than the left. His orthodontist had done a good job of maintaining some type of occlusion. However, he had no control over the abnormal growth. The patient was referred to us for evaluation in June 1979.

The patient did not present with pain symptoms but only a clicking sound in the right joint. It could not be immediately ascertained if the abnormal development was the result of overdevelopment of the right side of the jaw, underdevelopment of the left, or a combination of both.

The full-face, profile and teeth views shows this condition of the mandible deviating to the left. Orthodontic appliances are apparent on his teeth (Fig. 22-53, *A*). Cephalometric views show the relation of his maxilla to mandible (Fig. 22-53, *B*). Anteroposterior views show the abnormal mandible (Fig. 22-53, *C*). Another cephalometric view shows the mouth closed (Fig. 22-53, *E*). Specialized TMJ x-ray films reveal in the right joint, closed view, a compression of the disc and some osteoarthritic erosion of the eminence. In the left closed view the condyle and eminence appear normal but with a widened disc space. In the 31-mm view this disc space appears to be three times normal (Fig. 22-53, *F*).

Treatment. In analyzing the problem, it seemed most probable that the accident to the right side of the face had caused the right condyle to overdevelop. This had the effect of moving the jaw downward and to the left. There appeared to be two problems: one relating to the condyle and the other regarding the facial asymmetry that in the future might require some surgical procedure to the body of the mandible.

The best approach seemed to be to diminish the vertical height of the right condyle, as well as the posterior portion of the condylar head, so that the mandible could be returned to a more normal position with relation to the fossa. This would require the right condyle to be moved posteriorly and superiorly. In the left joint this would have the effect of moving the left condyle inferiorly and anteriorly to balance the joint relation.

Surgery was performed in August 1979. A preauricular incision on the right side was made in the usual manner. The mandible was moved to its more normal position with the teeth in better occlusion. The vertical height and posterior width of the condyle were diminished by the used of a diamond stone. The damaged meniscus was removed and an articular eminence prosthesis emplaced and secured in the usual manner. The maxilla and mandible were then held in the proper relation via a dental splint, which had been constructed previously, and stainless steel ligatures were placed between the maxillary and mandibular arch bars.

On entering the left joint, we noted the increased space between the condylar head and the upper portion of the joint. A specialized metal and Silastic prosthesis was emplaced, which lowered the floor of the fossa to provide an articular surface for the condyle. It was secured in the usual manner, and the wound was closed. The patient was discharged 5 days postoperatively, and the arch bars and ligatures were removed 10 days postoperatively.

Postoperative x-ray films, three views, show the teeth now in a more normal position and the mandible moved to the right (Fig. 22-53, *G*). The orthodontist will endeavor to have the teeth in the left maxilla retrude so they will be even with the right side. The mandible is now in a normal horizontal plane (Figs. 22-53, *H* and *I*). A cephalometric postoperative film, open and closed views, shows the patient able to open his mouth 40 mm (Fig. 22-53, *J*). Specialized TMJ x-ray films show properly placed prostheses in both joints (Fig. 22-53, *K* and *L*). The anteroposterior view shows normal mandibular relation with prostheses in position (Fig. 22-53, *M*).

The patient is pain free. Since this procedure his appearance has improved. It may not be necessary to do further corrective surgery on the body of the mandible.

Text continued on p. 436.

A

B

C

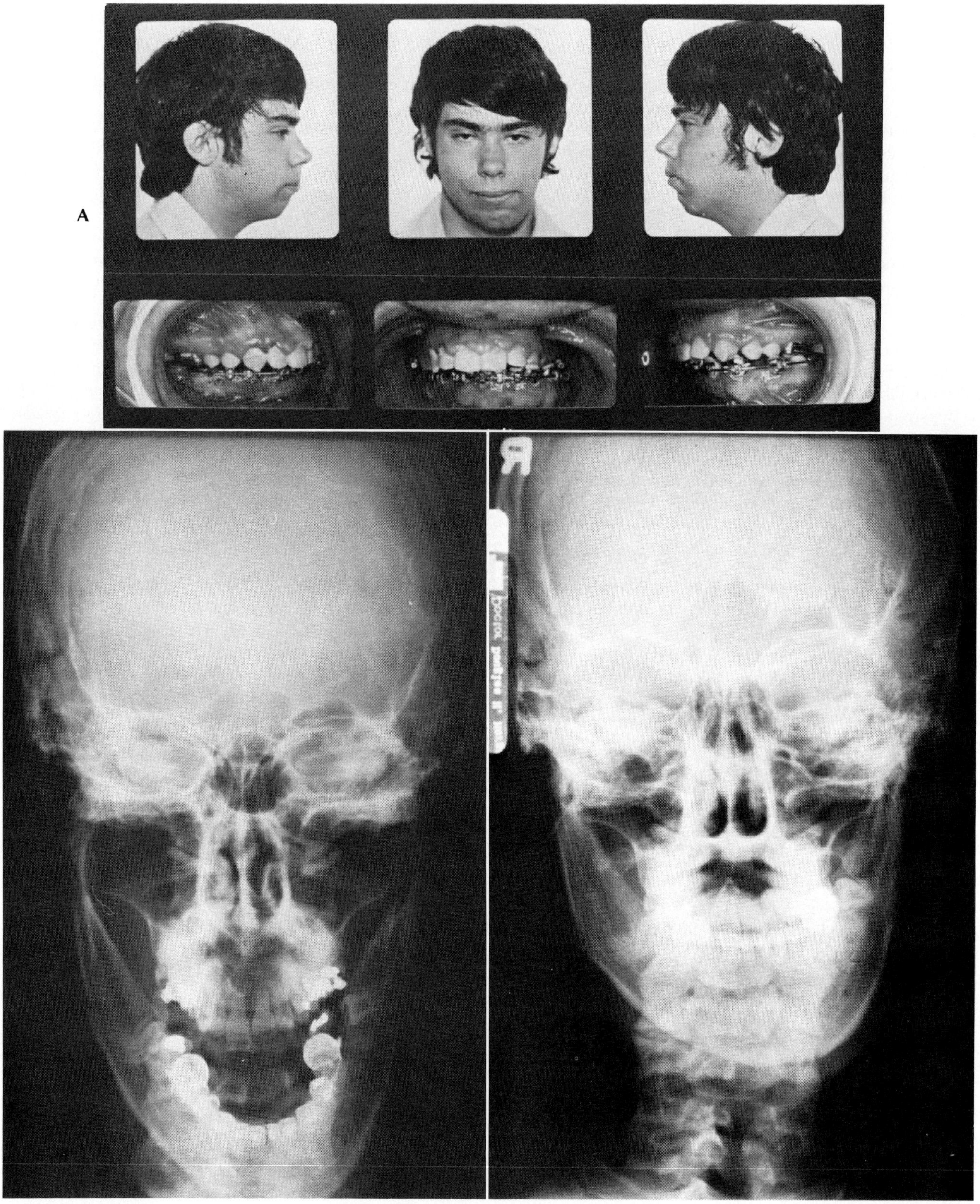

Fig. 22-53. A, Full-face, profile, and teeth view shows mandible deviating to left and orthodontic appliances on teeth. Plane of left maxilla and mandible is approximately 15 degrees off horizontal plane. **B,** Anteroposterior view with mouth open showing abnormal maxillomandibular relationship. **C,** Anteroposterior view shows overgrowth of right mandible and shifting of jaw to left.

D

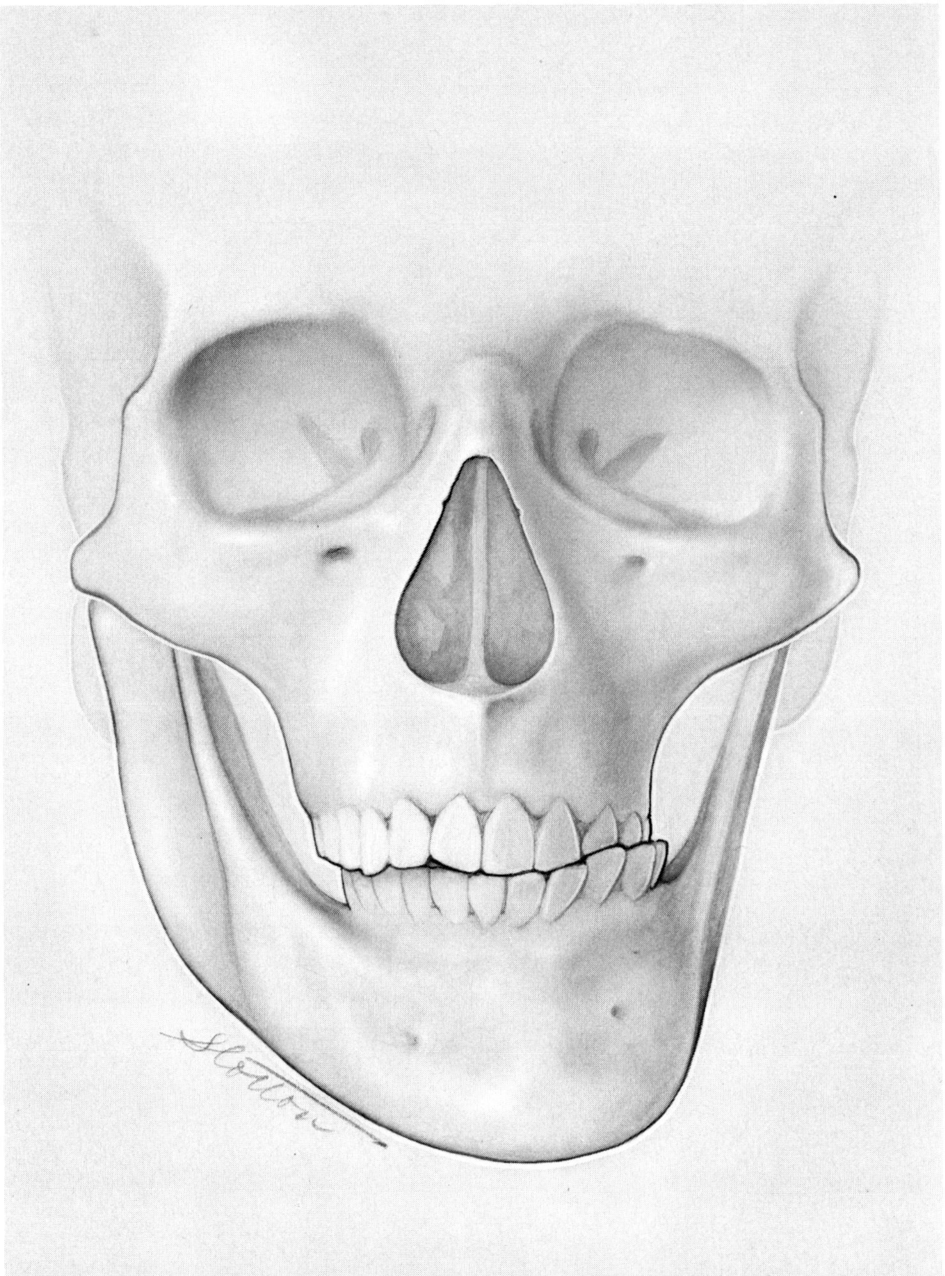

Fig. 22-53, cont'd. D, Maxillary and mandibular teeth on left side are at 15-degree angle from horizontal plane because of shifting of mandible to that side.

Continued.

E

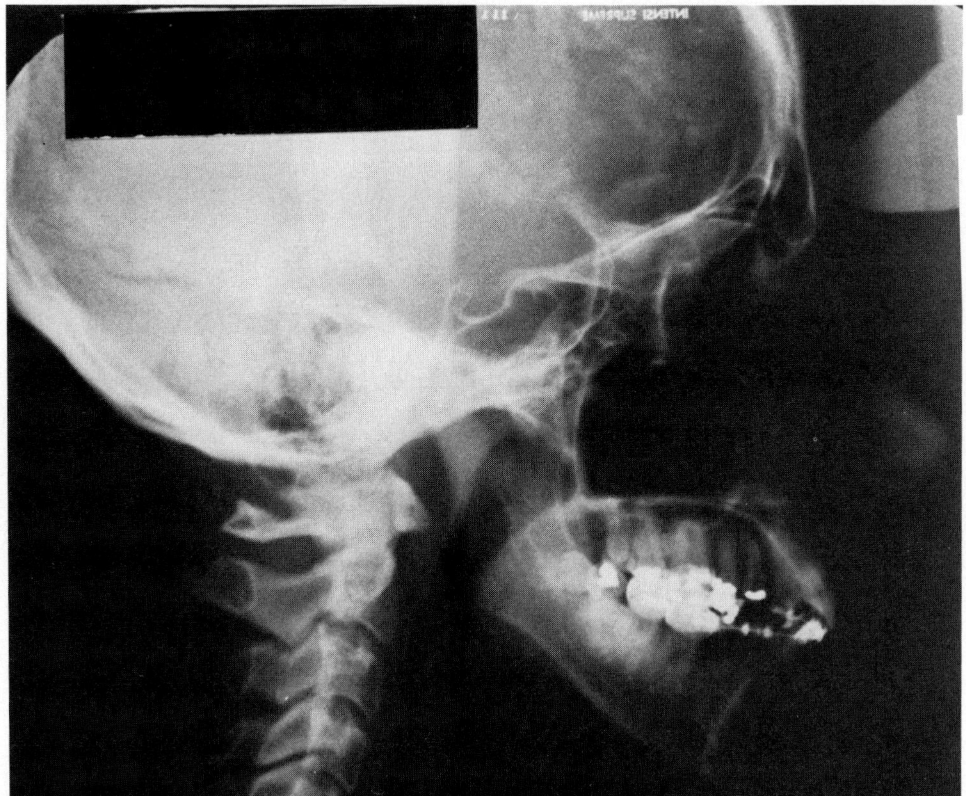

F

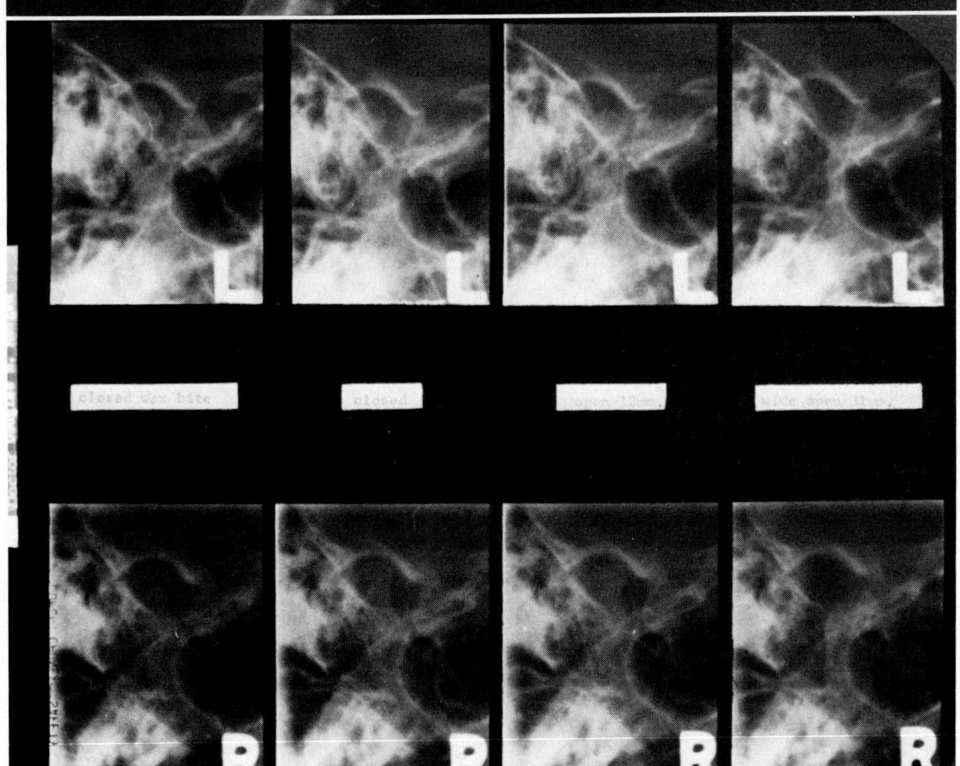

Fig. 22-53, cont'd. E, Cephalometric view shows mouth closed. **F,** Specialized TMJ film in right closed view shows compression of disc and some osteoarthritic erosion of eminence. In left closed view, condyle and eminence appear normal but with widened disc space. In 31-mm view this disc space appears to be three times normal.

G

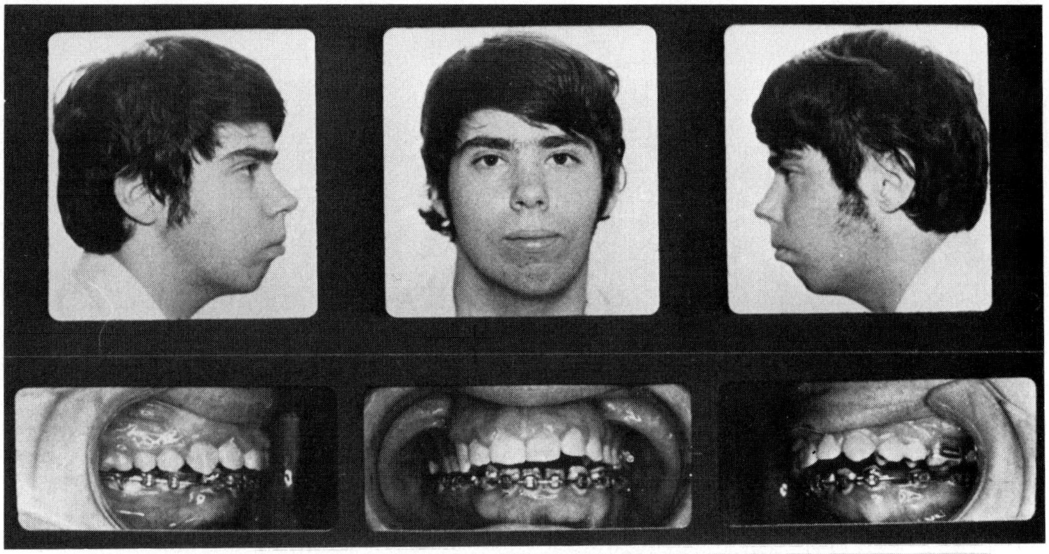

H

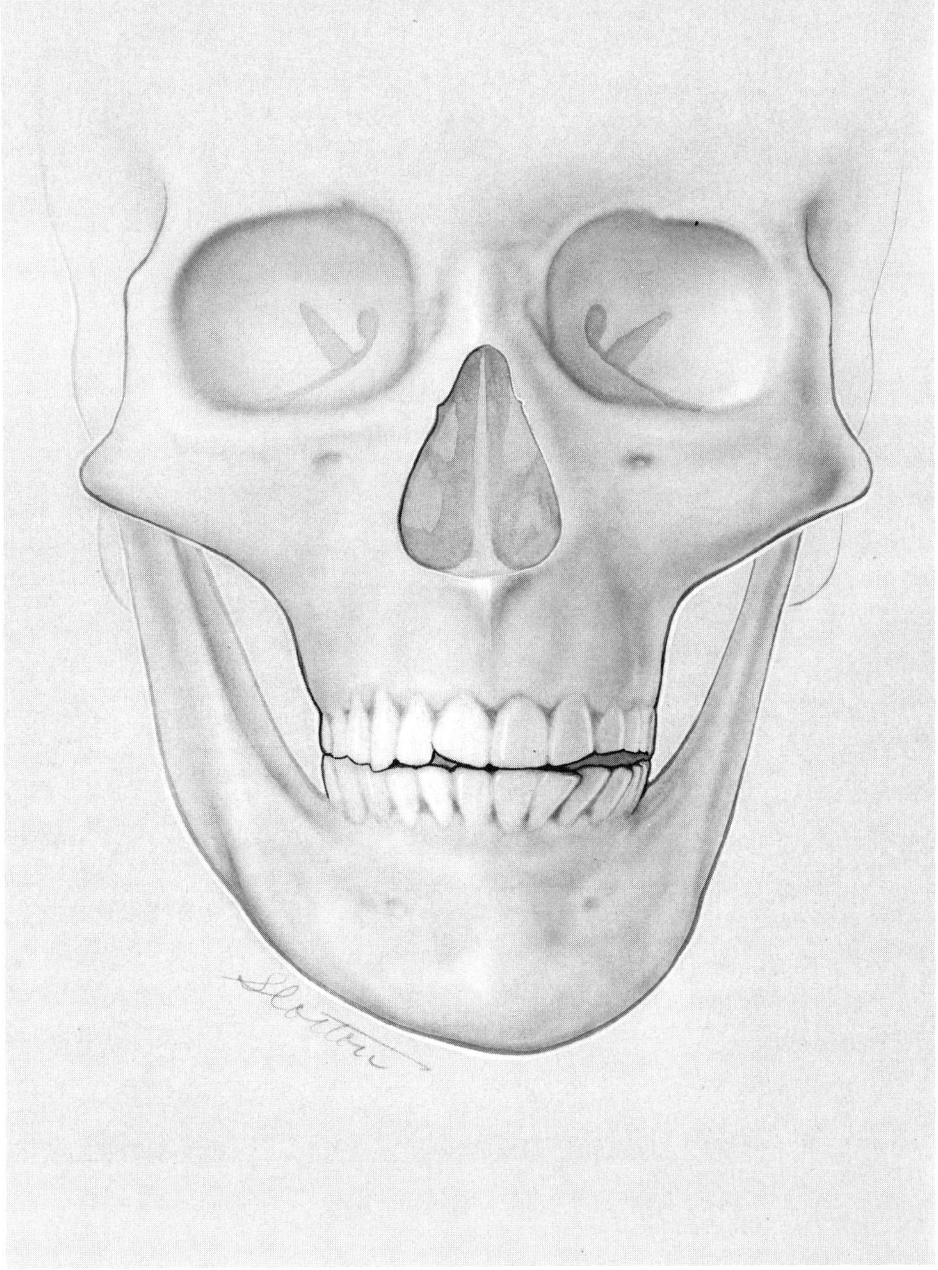

Fig. 22-53, cont'd. G, Three postoperative views show mandible has been moved to right. Plane of mandible is now in normal horizontal position. **H,** Drawing depicts more normal relationship of mandible to skull and horizontal plane. Left maxillary teeth will be orthodontically moved to coincide with mandibular teeth.

Continued.

I

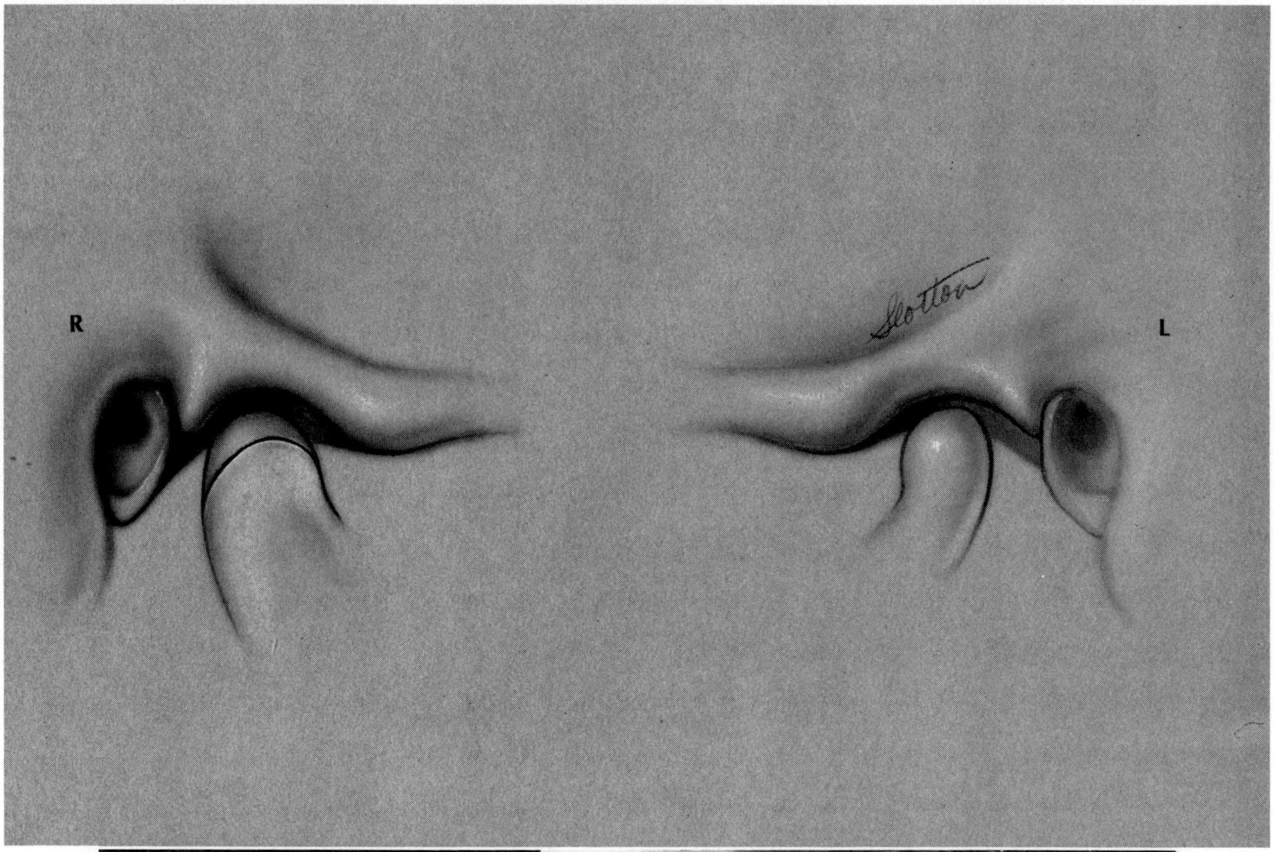

J

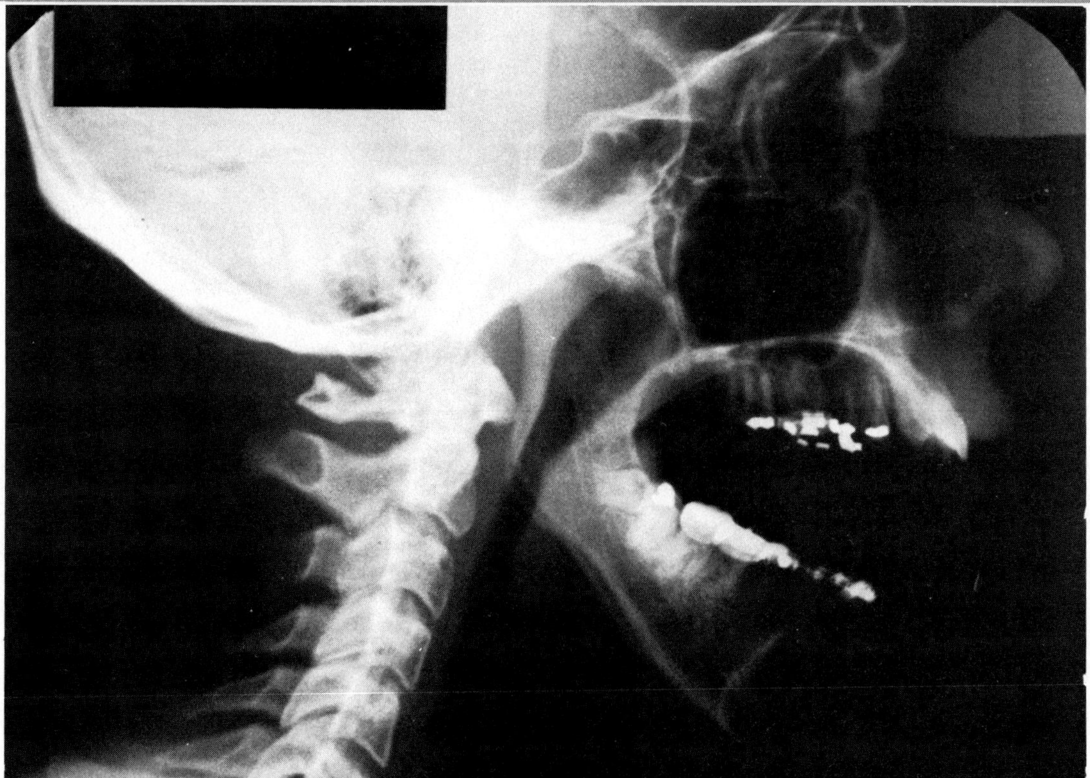

Fig. 22-53, cont'd. I, Drawing depicting in right joint the removal of bone from condyle, superiorly and posteriorly. **J,** Postoperative cephalometric film shows patient able to open 40 mm.

K

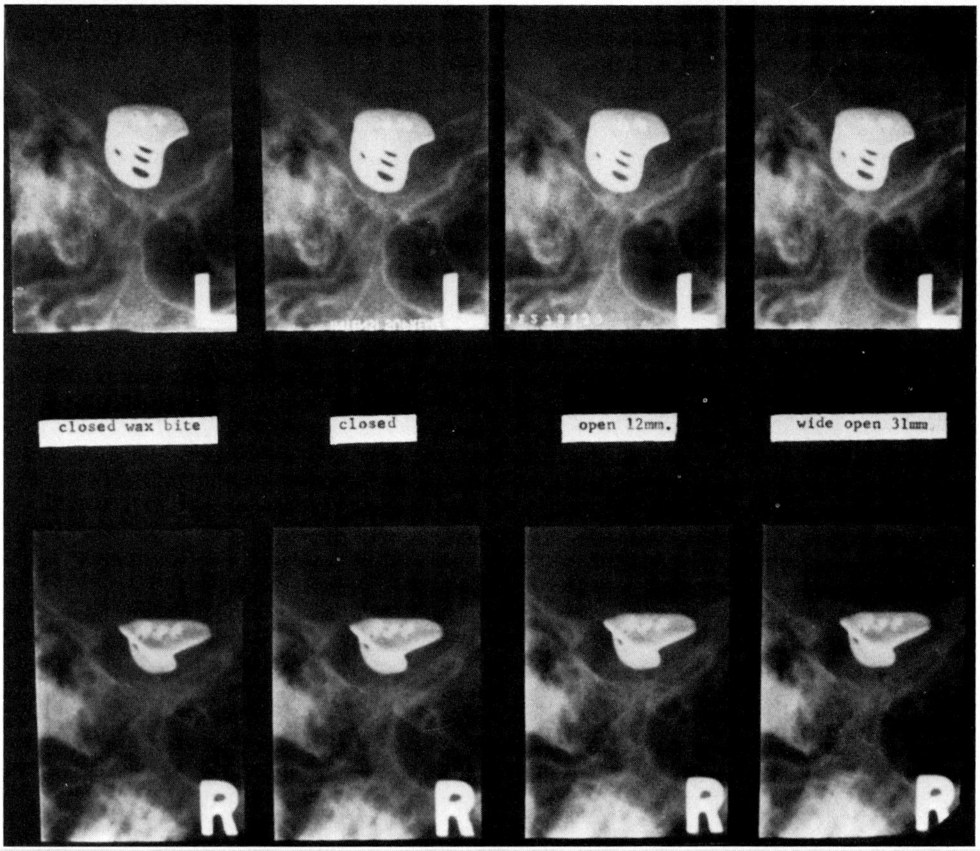

L

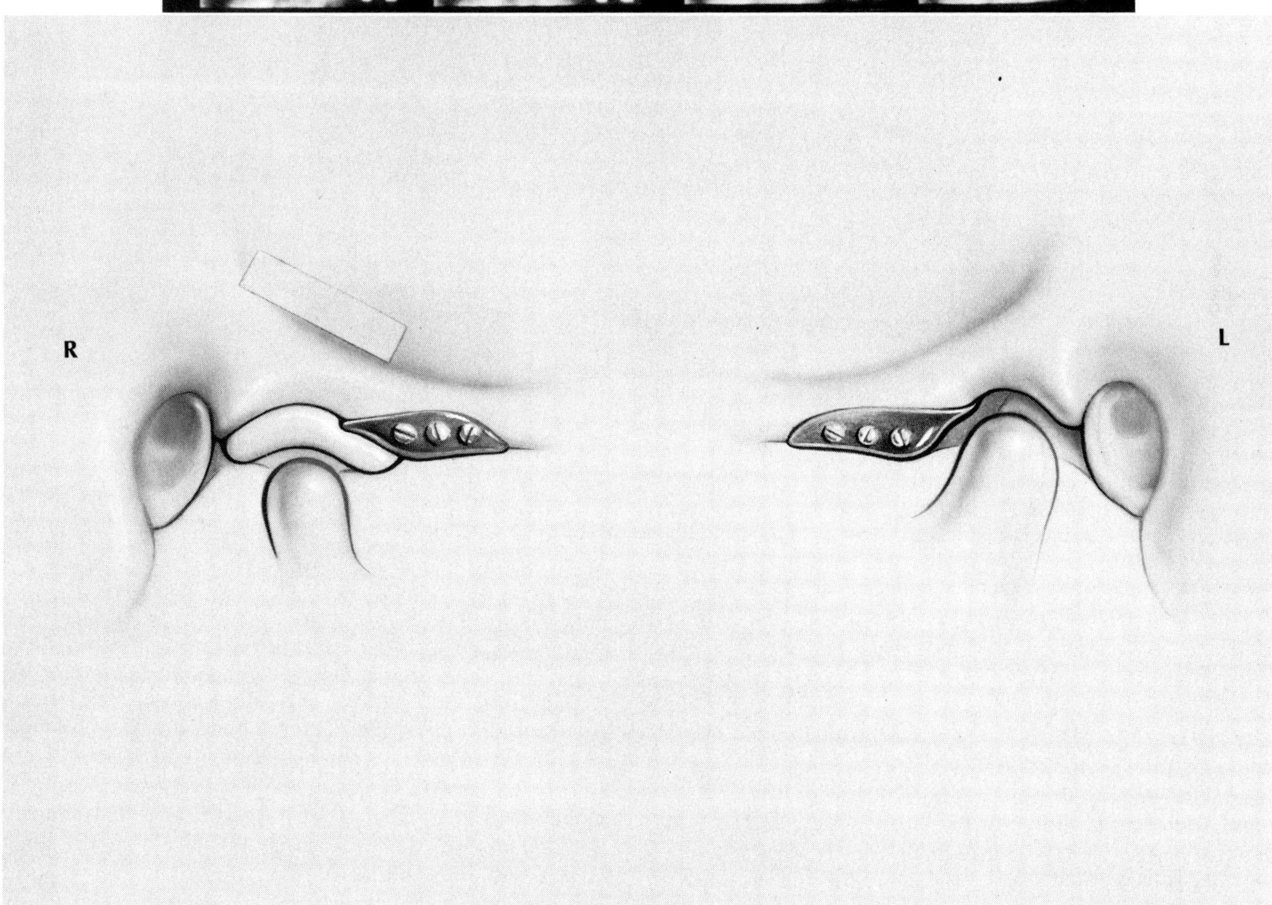

Fig. 22-53, cont'd. K, Specialized TMJ x-ray films show properly placed prostheses. **L,** Drawing depicts in left joint metal and Silastic prosthesis lowering floor of fossa and compensating for new vertical relationship of mandible to maxilla. In right joint is shown new position of right condyle and implant in which reduced size of condylar head permits condyle to move superiorly and posteriorly for new postion of mandible to maxilla.

Continued.

M

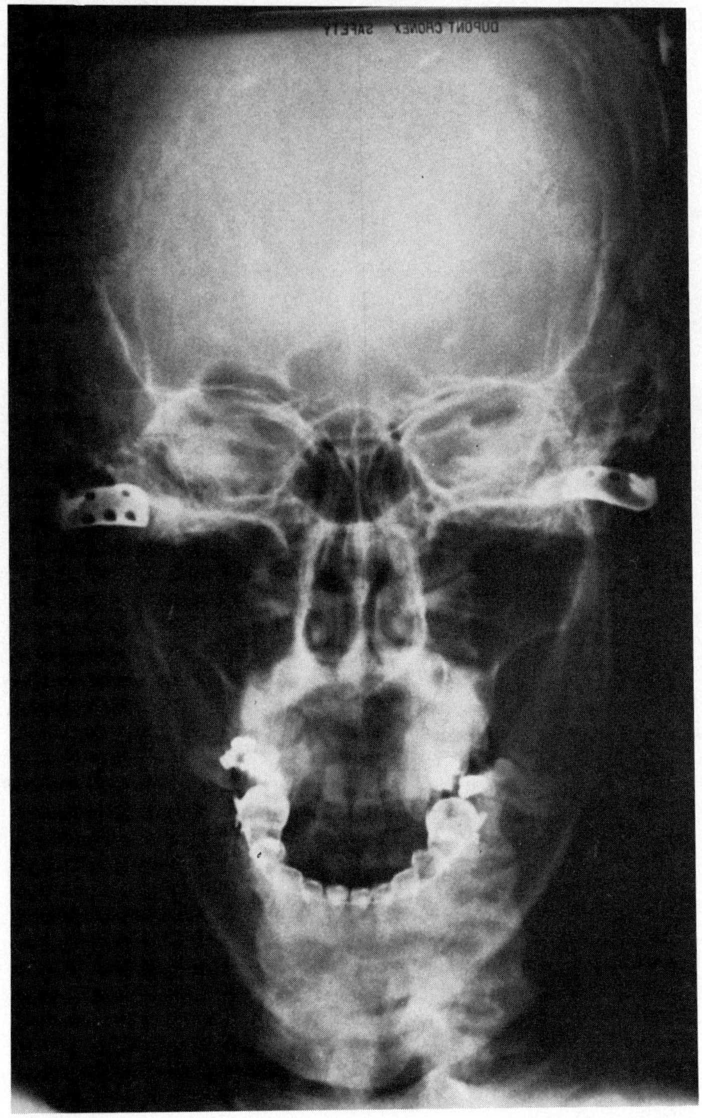

Fig. 22-53, cont'd. M, Anteroposterior view shows normal mandibular relation with prostheses in position.

Case 19*

This 22-year-old patient had ankylosing spondylitis (Fig. 22-54, *A*). As seen from his full-face photograph, his presurgical interincisal opening was limited to 4 mm (Fig. 22-54, *B*). A modification of the Howe technique was used for treatment.[20] After arthroplasty, medical-grade Silastic was injected into the glenoid fossa and allowed to polymerize, thus forming a customized TMJ implant. The implant was then trimmed and secured in place (Fig. 22-54, *C* and *D*). The postsurgical occlusion's interincisal opening increased to 32 mm (Fig. 22-54, *E*). Fig. 22-54, *F*, shows the medical-grade Silastic elastomer material used to fabricate customized TMJ implants. The implant may be preformed and affixed in the glenoid fossa, as described by Howe (Fig. 22-54, *G*). Frontal and lateral views show the implant affixed to the head of the condyles and secured in the glenoid fossa (Fig. 22-54, *H* and *I*).

*Courtesy Charles D. Hasse, D.D.S.

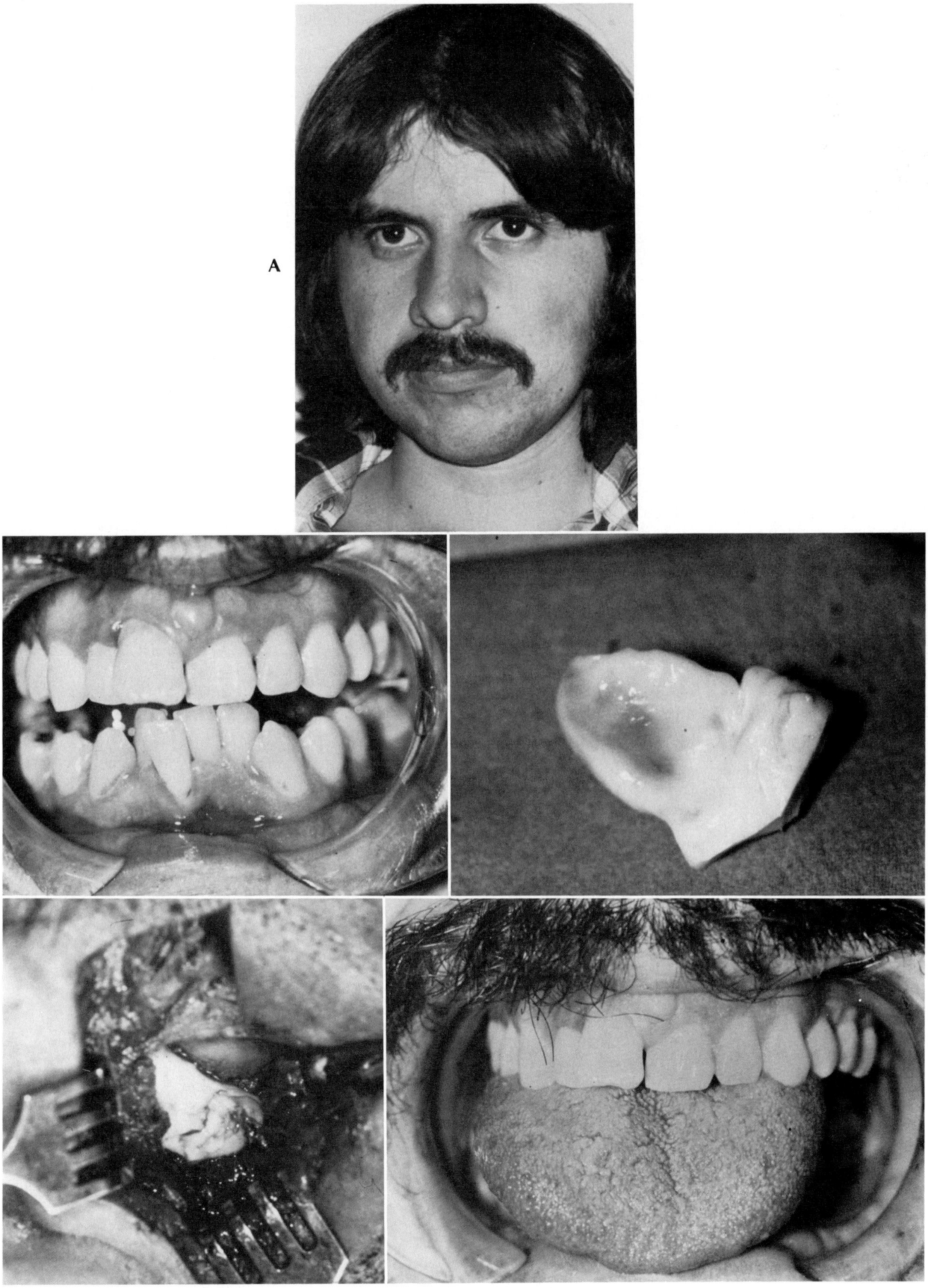

Fig. 22-54. A, Patient with ankylosing spondylitis. **B,** Presurgical interincisal opening limited to 4 mm. **C,** Trimmed customized TMJ implant. **D,** Implant secured in place. **E,** Postsurgical occlusion with interincisal opening increased to 32 mm.

Continued.

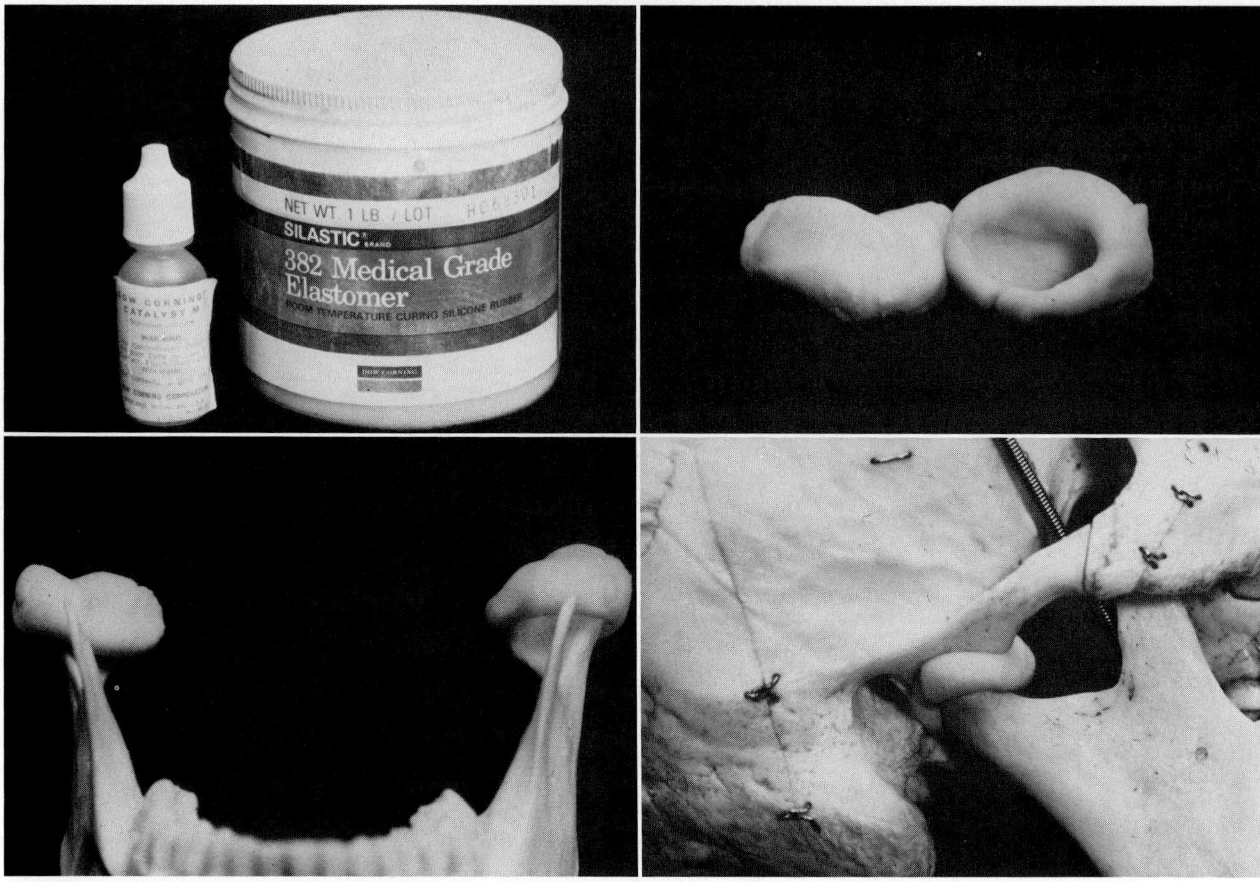

Fig. 22-54, cont'd. F, Medical-grade Silastic elastomer material used to fabricate customized TMJ implants. **G,** Implant preformed and affixed in glenoid fossa. **H,** Frontal and, **I,** lateral views showing implant affixed to head of condyles and secured in glenoid fossa. (Courtesy Charles D. Hasse, D.D.S.)

Case 20*

Morgan[30] has reported a case of chronic subluxation in which the articular eminence was flattened. This permitted the external pterygoid muscle to go into spasm, holding the condyle in an anterior position. By restoring the height of the eminence, further chronic dislocation was prevented.

*Courtesy Charles D. Hasse, D.D.S.

In another case of chronic dislocation a 22-year-old patient was treated by emplacement of a TMJ restrictive device developed at Long Beach Veterans Administration Hospital by Sam J. Poidmore, D.D.S., and Paul D. Braun, D.D.S. (Fig. 22-55, *A* and *B*). This placement is demonstrated in Fig. 22-55, *C* to *F*, and Fig. 22-55, *G*, shows the panographic view of the patient with the restrictive device in place.

A

B

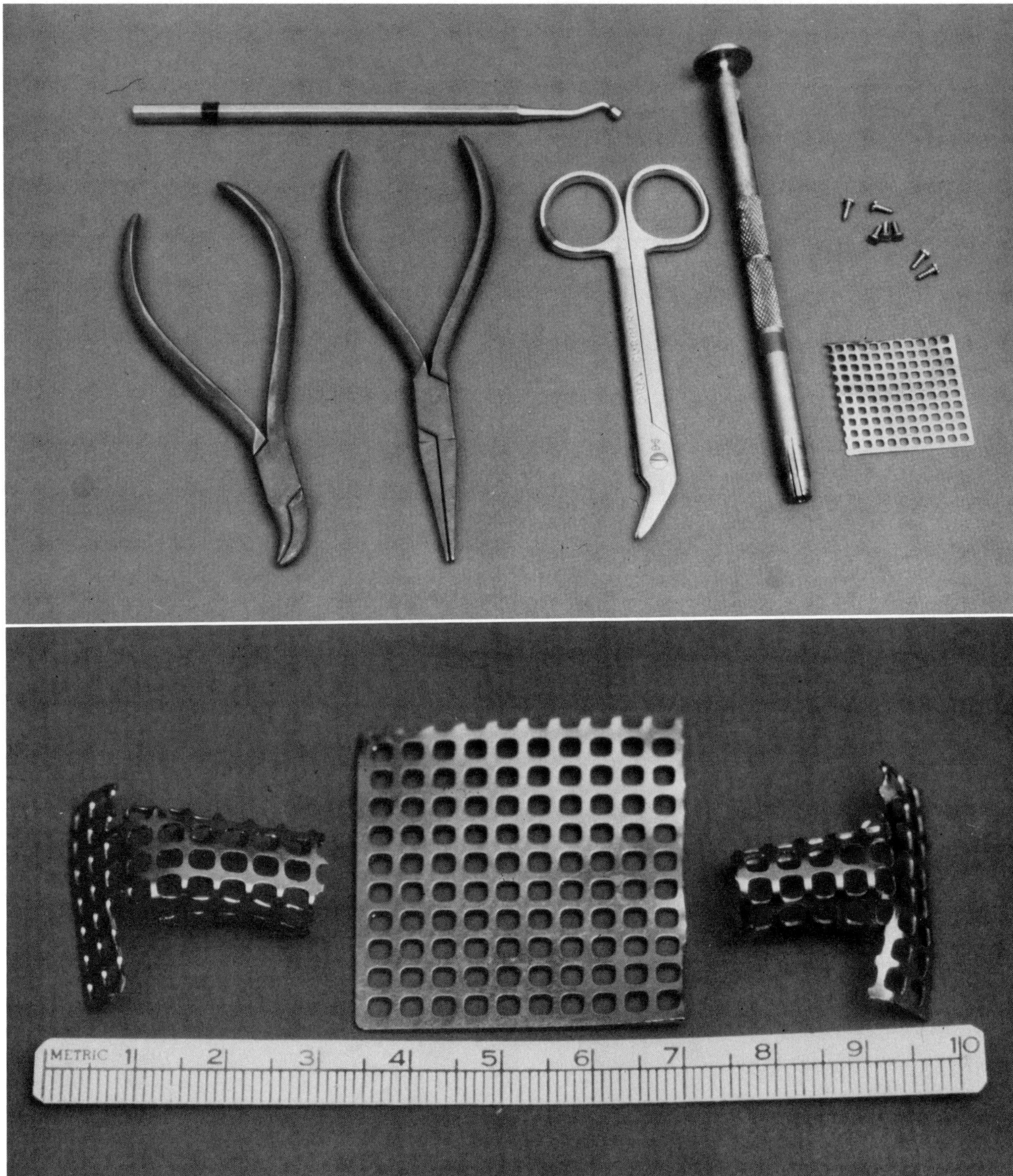

Fig. 22-55. A, and **B,** Vitallium TMJ restrictive device developed by Poidmore and Braun. Appliance is used to treat chronic dislocation of TMJ by acting as mechanical barrier.

Continued.

C

D

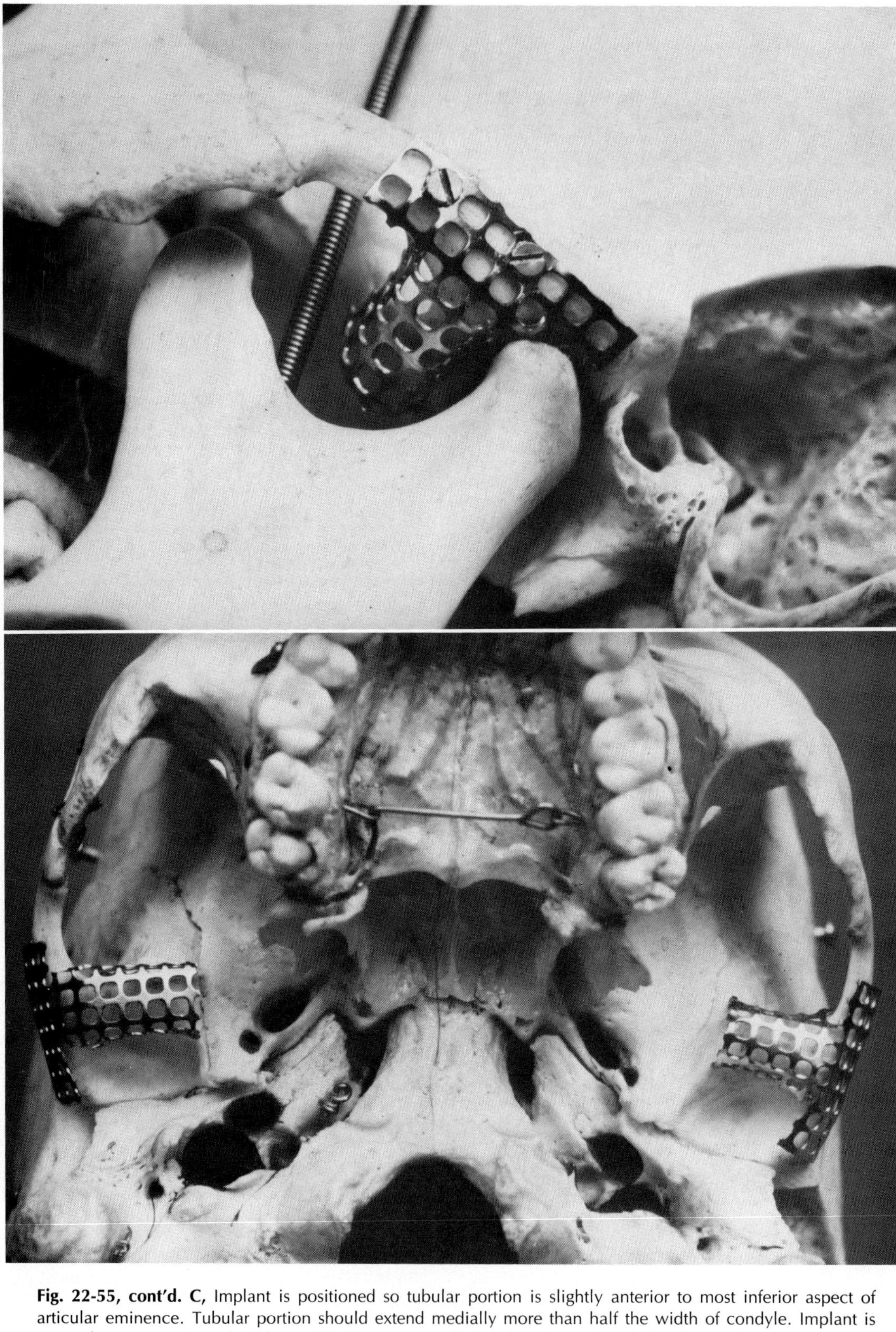

Fig. 22-55, cont'd. C, Implant is positioned so tubular portion is slightly anterior to most inferior aspect of articular eminence. Tubular portion should extend medially more than half the width of condyle. Implant is secured to zygomatic arch with two Vitallium screws. **D,** Inferior view of restrictive devices in place.

E F G

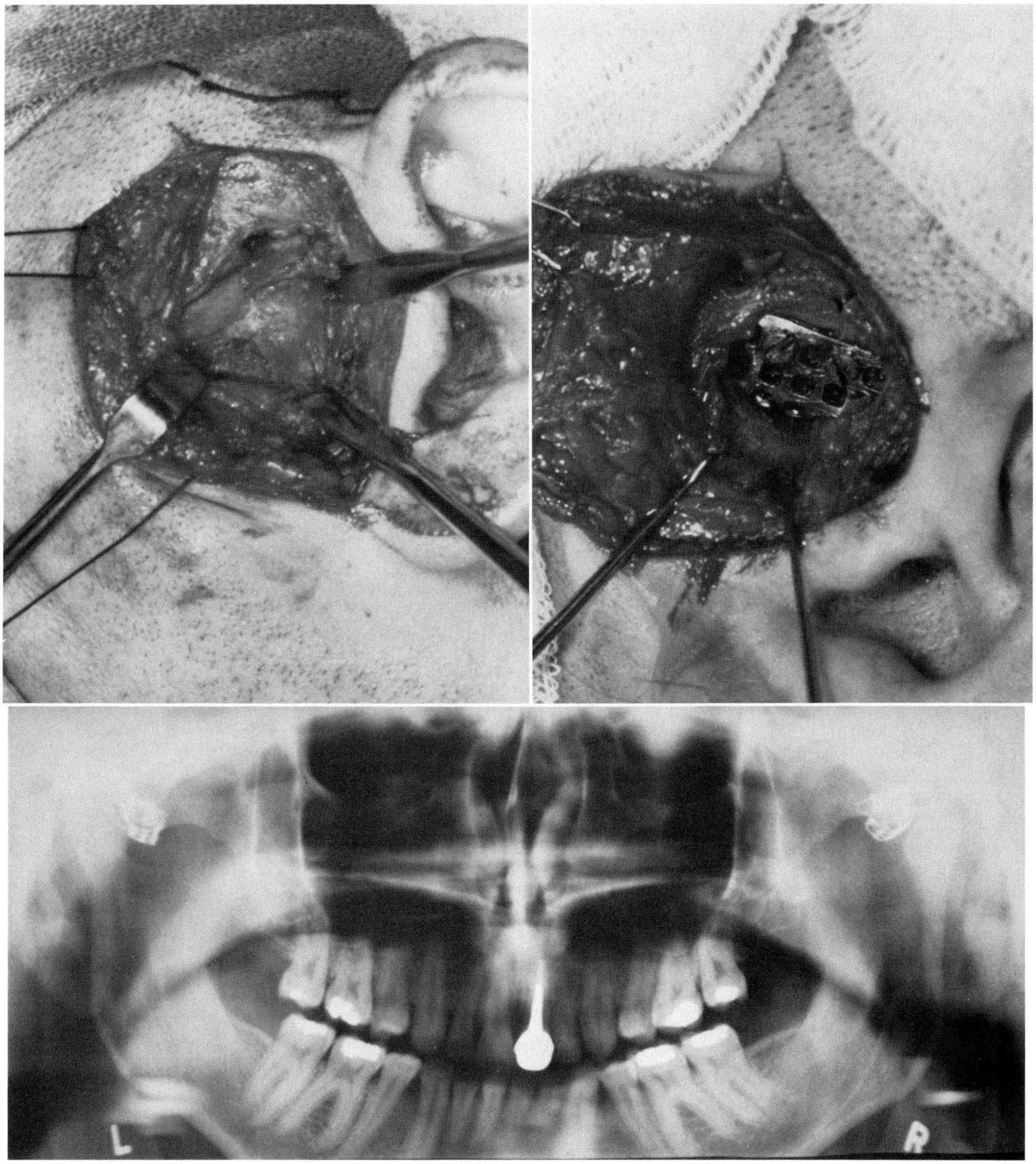

Fig. 22-55, cont'd. E, Cut down on temporomandibular joint prior to placement of restrictive device. **F,** Clinical appearance of restrictive device fixed in position. **G,** Panographic view illustrating application of TMJ restrictive device used in treating 22-year-old patient with history of chronic dislocation. (Photographs courtesy Charles D. Hasse, D.D.S.)

REFERENCES

1. Agerberg, G., and Lundberg, M.: Changes in the temporomandibular joint after surgical treatment, Oral Surg. **32**:865, 1971.
2. Antoni, A.A.: Temporomandibular joint, J. Can. Dent. Assoc. **21**:90, 1966.
3. Bell, W.E.: Clinical diagnosis of the pain-dysfunction syndrome, J. Am. Dent. Assoc. **79**:154, 1969.
4. Bernick, S.: Vascular and nerve supply to the temporomandibular joint of the rat, Oral Surg. **15**:488, 1962.
5. Bernstein, J., Mohl, N., and Spiller, H.: Temporomandibular joint dysfunction masquerading as disease of the ear, nose, and throat, Trans. Am. Acad. Ophthalmol. Otolaryngol. **73**:1210, 1969.
6. Berry and Hofmann. In Schwartz, L., editor: Disorders of the temporomandibular joint, Philadelphia, 1959, W.B. Saunders Co.
7. Boudreau, R.G., and Tideman, H.: Treatment of chronic mandibular dislocation, Oral Surg. **41**:169, 1976.
8. Carlsson, G.E., Kopp, S., and Oberg, T.: Arthritis and allied diseases of the temporomandibular joint. In, Zarb, G.A., and Carlsson, G.E., editors: Temporomandibular joint function and dysfunction, St. Louis, 1979, The C.V. Mosby Co.
9. Carlsson, G.E., Oberg, T., Bergman, F., and Fajers, C.M.: Morphological changes in the mandibular joint disk in temporomandibular joint pain dysfunction syndrome, Acta Odontol. Scand. **25**:163, 1967.
10. Christensen, R.W.: The correction of mandibular ankylosis by arthroplasty and the insertion of a cast Vitallium glenoid fossa, J. South. Calif. State Dent. Assoc. **31**:4, 1963.
11. Clark, W.E.L.: The tissues of the body, Oxford, England, 1946, Clarendon Press.
12. Costen, J.B.: Syndrome of ear and sinus symptoms dependent upon disturbed function of the temporomandibular joint, Ann. Otol. Rhinol. Laryngol. **43**:1, March 1934.
13. Costen, J.B.: Neuralgia and ear symptoms associated with distrubed function of the temporomandibular joint, J.A.M.A. **107**:252, 1936.
14. Dingman, R.O., and Moorman, W.C.: Meniscectomy in the treatment of the temporomandibular joint, J. Oral Surg. **9**:214, 1951.
15. Eggers, G.W.N.: Arthroplasty of the temporomandibular joint in children with interposition of tantalum foil: preliminary report, J. Bone Joint Surg. **28**:603, 1946.
16. Goodfriend, D.J.: Odontogenic dizziness and related symptoms. In Spector, M., editor: Dizziness and vertigo: diagnosis and treatment, New York, 1967, Grune & Stratton, Inc.
17. Hatch, G.S.: Clinical and radiographic findings of the temporomandibular joint in patients with rheumatoid arthritis, Master's thesis, Rochester, Minn., 1967, Mayo Graduate School of Medicine.
18. Henny, F.A.: Surgical treatment of the painful temporomandibular joint, J. Am. Dent. Assoc. **79**:171, 1969.
19. Henny, F.A., and Baldridge, O.L.: Condylectomy for the persistently painful temporomandibular joint, J. Oral Surg. **15**:24, 1957.
20. Howe, D.J.: Preformed Silastic temporomandibular joint implant, J. Oral Surg. **37**:59, 1979.
21. Hromada, J.: Die Innervation des Kiefergelenks, und einige anatomischklinische Bemerkungen, Dtsch. Zahn. Mund. Kieferheilkd. **34**:19, 1960.
22. Irby, W.B.: Surgery of the temporomandibular joint. In Irby, W.B., editor: Current advances in oral surgery, St. Louis, 1974, The C.V. Mosby Co.
23. Ireland, V.E.: The problem of the clicking jaw, Proc. R. Soc. Med. **44**:363, 1951.
24. Kiehn, C.L.: Meniscectomy for internal derangement of the temporomandibular joint, Ann. J. Surg. **83**:365, 1948.
25. Kochan, E.J.: Treatment of temporomandibular joint disturbance with hyaluronidase, Oral Surg. **9**:513, 1956.
26. Laskin, D.M.: Etiology of the pain-dysfunction syndrome, J. Am. Dent. Assoc. **79**:147, 1969.
27. Mayne, J.G., and Hatch, G.S.: Arthritis of the temporomandibular joint, J. Am. Dent. Assoc. **79**:129, 1969.
28. McCarty, W.L., and Farrar, W.B.: Surgery for internal derangements of the temporomandibular joint, J. Prosthet. Dent. **42**:2, 1979.
29. Morgan, D.H.: Diagnosis of temporomandibular joint problems, J. South. Calif. State Dent. Assoc. **33**:523, 1965.
30. Morgan, D.H.: Surgical correction of temporomandibular joint arthritis. J. Oral Surg. **33**:766, 1975.
31. Pinto, O.F.: A new structure related to the temporomandibular joint and middle ear, J. Prosthet. Dent. **12**:95, 1962.
32. Pringle, J.H.: Displacement of the mandibular meniscus and its treatment, Br. J. Surg. **6**:385, 1918.
33. Rees, L.A.: Structure and function of the mandibular joint, Br. Dent. J. **96**:125, 1954.
34. Ricketts, R.: Clinical implications of the temporomandibular joint, Am. J. Orthod. **52**:416, 1966.
35. Risdon, F.E.: Ankylosis of the temporomandibular joint, J. Am. Dent. Assoc. **21**:1933, 1934.
36. Robinson, M.: Temporomandibular ankylosis corrected by creating a false stainless steel fossa, J. South. Calif. State Dent. Assoc. **6**:186, 1960.
37. Schmid, F.: On the nerve distribution of the temporomandibular joint capsule, Oral Surg. **28**:63, 1969.
38. Sicher, H.: Structural and functional basis for disorders of the temporomandibular articulation, J. Oral Surg. **13**:275, 1955.
39. Silver, C.M., Simon, S.D., and Litchman, H.M.: The surgical treatment of the arthritic temporomandibular joint, Surg. Gynecol. Obstet. **136**:251, 1973.
40. Smith, A.E., and Robinson, M.A.: A new surgical procedure for the creation of a false temporomandibular joint in cases of ankylosis by means of a non-electrolytic metal, Am. J. Surg. **94**:837, 1957.
41. Thoma, K.H.: Oral surgery, vol. 2, ed. 5, St. Louis, 1969, The C.V.Mosby Co.
42. Vaughan, H.C.: Temporomandibular joint pain, the external pterygoid mechanism, J. Prosthet. Dent. **5**:80, 1955.
43. Walker, R.V.: Arthroplasty of the ankylosed temporomandibular joint, Am. Surg. **24**:(6), 1958.
44. Wilkes, C.H.: Arthrography of the temporomandibular joint, Minn. Med. **61**:654, 1978.
45. Wilkes, C.H.: Structural and functional alterations of the temporomandibular joint, N.W. Dent. **57**:287, 1978.

23 Treatment of fractures and ankylosis

CARY B. SIMONDS, D.D.S., M.S. with case histories by
DOUGLAS H. MORGAN, D.D.S.

Trauma to the temporomandibular region presents a special problem to the oral surgeon because of the frequent involvement of the temporomandibular joint complex. Management of trauma in this region has varied widely through the years. Until adequate x-ray techniques were established that could properly illustrate the temporomandibular region to the surgeon, management of trauma in this region often was not well understood and then many times founded on false concepts. However, with anteroposterior views (such as the Towne, Parma, and exaggerated Waters) along with various lateral views (such as transorbital)[11] available at most hospitals, as well as the invaluable panoramic radiograph (used routinely in many oral and maxillofacial surgical offices today), we may obtain a nearly complete and accurate assessment of bony and foreign body trauma to the temporomandibular region.[35,47,48,71]

We will concern ourselves with trauma in the temporomandibular area as it relates to condylar and associated fractures, since these fractures account for over 99% of all acute trauma to the temporomandibular joint.[13,21] That condylar fractures will take care of themselves with only the simple application of intermaxillary fixation (IMF) is an opinion expressed frequently by many authors, both historically and in the current literature.[13,42,45] By far the majority of the literature (especially that by surgeons lacking dental training), when referring to treatment of condylar fractures, concludes with a generalizing statement regarding their success in treating condylar fractures by so-called conservative means.[13,42,45]

However, careful follow-up studies of the final postoperative results of many of these "conservatively" treated patients does not give one a satisfied feeling regarding a single mode of treatment for all condylar fractures. Dissatisfaction was shown as far back as 1934 and earlier in the literature when Risdon[40] reported complete ankylosis in 5% of his cases. Federspiel[10] pointed out that there was limitation of motion to some degree in every case of fracture—dislocation that he treated. Gruber and Lyford[17] examined 10 patients, all of whom had been treated for 6 weeks with intermaxiallary fixation. Their results showed that five patients had minimum loss of function, three patients had appreciable loss of function with malocclusion and deviation of the mandible on opening, and two patients had ankylosis of their joints that required secondary surgical arthroplasties.

For a surgeon to consider a single mode of treatment as a universally acceptable one with regard to a particular fracture entity (especially when the fracture region involves the most complicated, intricate, and delicate neuromuscular apparatus governing any joint in the body) could not possibly be the patient's best interest consistently. Having a basic concept of normal occlusal relations is not at all adequate in treating patients with condylar fractures, particularly when each and every fracture, without exception, is a potentially debilitating injury. Understanding fully the concepts of gnathology, including mandibular movements (hinge, axis, centric occlusion versus centric relation, and protrusive and Bennett movements) and balanced dental occlusion, as well as the concept and technology of occlusal equilibration, is essential to providing patients with the quality of care they deserve.

A thorough review of the literature reveals numerous conflicting articles with regard to effectiveness of various modes of treatment of condylar fractures.* These conflicting reports in the literature, along with numerous modes of treatment being advocated by various clinicians, indicate a mood of dissatisfaction within surgical circles as to their present management of condylar fractures.[13, 15, 20] With this in mind, this chapter will merely propose a few guidelines regarding treatment of some of these frequently misunderstood and mishandled fractures.

*References 5, 6, 13, 15, 20, 24, 26, 33.

CLASSIFICATION

Comprehensive studies of condylar fractures were done as early as 1928 by Ruedi and 1929 by Dufourmentel. Numerous methods of classification of these fractures have been offered.[30] However, the following classification may be preferred, since it relates more directly to the mode of treatment to be instituted for management of that fracture:

1. Intracapsular condylar head fractures
   a. Nondisplaced intracapsular fractures
   b. Nondisplaced bony lacerations of condylar head
   c. Displaced fractures not interfering with full intercuspation of existing dentition or mandibular movement
   d. Displaced fractures with fractured segment avulsed from articular capsule and not interfering with full intercuspation of dentition or mandibular movement
   e. Displaced fractures with fractured segment preventing full intercuspation of dentition or mandibular movement on affected side
2. High and midcondylar neck fractures
   a. Nondisplaced and greenstick fractures
   b. Displaced fractures in which condylar head remains in glenoid fossa
   c. Displaced fractures in which condyle is dislocated from glenoid fossa, but proximal segment does not infringe on distal mandibular segment or interfere in any way with its movement or full intercuspation of dentition
   d. Displaced fractures that impinge on mandibular movement and/or interfere with full intercuspation of dentition
3. Subcondylar or condyloramal fractures
   a. Nondisplaced and greenstick fractures
   b. Displaced fractures with vertical overriding of fracture segments
   c. Displaced fractures in which proximal fracture site has been displaced medially, so that fracture margins are not in bony contact

It should be kept in mind that any of the traumatic injuries just listed (and many less traumatic injuries) may or may not be associated with significant trauma (usually of a compressive, crushing, or tearing nature) to the articular disc.[16,23,36] Considering that the temporomandibular articular disc is the single most avascular piece of tissue in the entire body, it is not hard to understand that traumatic perforation and/or necrosis (because of crushing trauma) resulting in perforation of this disc is not an uncommon sequela of temporomandibular trauma.

Disc perforation and resulting bone-on-bone contact of the articulating surfaces (or tearing of the anterior third of the disc or the anterior attachment of the meniscus to the capsule) may then lead to chronic TMJ disease with resulting clicking or popping with pain and dysfunction.* It is impossible to assess acute damage to the articular disc unless it is decided that an open reduction through a preauricular incision is necessary for treatment of the case, at which time the disc may be examined easily.

In light of this, it is considered prudent and proper to always inform the patient with TMJ trauma of the potential future complications secondary to traumatic injury of this important structure.†

CLINICAL EXAMINATION

Physical findings vary greatly according to type or classification of the fracture. First of all, keeping in mind that many such fractures go undiagnosed and untreated, the surgeon should approach the examination suspecting such a fracture in any patient who has sustained significant mandibular and/or other facial trauma. Clinical signs and symptoms of such temporomandibular fractures include the following:

1. Extraoral
   a. Preauricular tenderness
   b. Preauricular palpation of bony stump or fragments
   c. Tenderness of joint on palpation through external auditory meatus
   d. Crepitus on palpation through meatus or preauricularly
   e. Crepitus on auscultation of joint on opening
   f. Slight deviation of midline of mental region to affected side on opening
   g. Swelling, ecchymosis, and edema in temporomandibular region
   h. Complete or partial occlusion of external auditory canal from subperiosteal hematoma secondary to fracture of tympanic plate
   i. Bleeding from affected ear canal
2. Intraoral
   a. Slight unilateral open bite (last molar on same side may or may not be occluding)
   b. Bilateral crossbite, as commonly seen in unilaterally displaced condylar neck fracture
   c. Slight deviation of midline when beginning to open mouth and gross deviation to affected side during translatory stage of opening in unaffected side
   d. Anterior displacement of entire mandible, usually accompanied by slight open bite
   e. Posterior displacement of entire mandible, usually associated with gross open bite

*References 9, 23, 31, 38, 39, 46.
†References 4, 8, 11, 18, 30, 37, 43.

f. Tenderness on opening or in lateral excursions with some significant malocclusion

It has been established by da Fonseca[14] of Brazil that blunt trauma applied to the symphysis region of the mandible which is insufficient in magnitude to produce mandibular fractures will in many instances produce bony lacerations of the condylar head.[1] The ramifications of this are obvious. If there are bony lacerations of the condylar head, then there is intracapsular bleeding with its potential complications of fibrosis and ankylosis. If this injury can be sustained from trauma insufficient to fracture the condylar complex, then it most certainly should be suspected in any case where these fractures are incurred.

The treatment for this type of intracapsular injury is physiological function, instituted as soon as possible. Adults will tolerate 3 weeks on intermaxillary fixation, when other fractures necessitate it, before instituting joint physiotherapy. In children this period is held to 2 weeks.

CONSIDERATIONS IN OPEN REDUCTION OF A COMPLEX CONDYLAR FRACTURE

One important and basic orthopedic principle should be brought out at this time, but it should be remembered that it is a principle and not a hard-and-fast rule. As a principle, it should be considered and weighed against all other factors involved when determining the best treatment for the patient. It is that *the proper treatment of a displaced fracture involving a joint is to align that fractured segment into its original position*.

In treating displaced fractures involving the temporomandibular joint, however, there are certain factors to be considered that in many instances may outweigh the advantages attained by realignment of the fractured segments surgical intervention.[21]

First consideration

Can the condylar fracture be reduced by simple application of intermaxillary fixation (either active or passive) in tight occlusion? Many displaced condylar fractures may be reduced nicely by this means, especially those fractures displaying vertical overlapping of the fractured segments. Elastic intermaxillary fixation may be helpful in achieving adequate intercuspation. However, elastic intermaxillary fixation should not remain on longer than 3 to 7 days, at which time static wire intermaxillary traction should be placed.

Second consideration

The temporomandibular joint is not a weightbearing joint,[23] and an overwhelming number of case reports have shown that it can continue to function acceptably in an altered anatomical relation.[12,13,19,23] The term *altered anatomical relation* and its limits cannot be fully described in brief terms, and clinical judgment must be used.

Third consideration

According to Irby,[23] maxillomandibular relationship and resulting mandibular function depend on a delicately balanced neuromuscular mechanism controlling the muscles of mastication and the suprahyoid complex of muscles. The head of a condyle with a healed fracture of the condylar neck may be out of the fossa, but it still retains its external pterygoid muscle attachment. Thus, after certain compensatory changes of the external pterygoid muscle fibers it may regain its neuromuscular balance resulting in acceptable function and occlusal relationships in a high percentage of these cases.[13,19,23,45]

Fourth consideration

Is the potential morbidity of the surgical procedure (necessary to reestablish anatomical relations) significant? Although the submandibular and retroangular surgical approaches are safe and postoperative complications are few, the restrictions they place on the surgeon's access (especially in high–condylar neck fractures) are considerable and indeed make this approach to some condylar fractures completely inadequate.[5] The preauricular approach to the joint space, as used to reach the articular eminence and upper condylar head, is itself a safe surgical procedure. However, with the extension of the surgical field both medially and inferiorly, as is necessary to adequately expose high fractures of the condylar neck and, especially, fracture-dislocations, the surgical risk is increased (especially risk of damage to the facial nerve trunk, internal maxillary artery, and retromaxillary venous plexus).[5,25] For this reason this extensive type of preauricular surgery usually is avoided. However, when this approach has been necessary, it has proved to be an invaluable aid to the surgeon in providing the appropriate care for the patient.[21]

Fifth consideration

Is the patient a child? If so, all possible attempts to avoid an open reduction should be made. It is well established that pediatric patients suffering displaced fractures of the mandibular condyle in a high percentage of cases will completely re-form another articulating condyle; in many cases they will actually resorb the previously displaced condylar fragment.* If physiological function can be established within 2 weeks of the initial fracture, the patient's prognosis is good with regard to mandibular growth potential, mandibular function, and future joint pain.[34]

---

*References 19, 20, 22, 24, 28.

Sixth consideration

Do the age and health of the patient permit an open surgical procedure?

Situations justifying open reduction

Only after weighing these considerations against the potential complications of leaving the displaced condylar fracture unreduced should an open reduction of a condylar complex fracture be done. Those condylar fractures requiring open reduction (with internal or external fixation) are limited. We consider the following five situations justification for open reduction*:

1. Displaced condylar head and neck fractures that interfere with mandibular movement and/or full intercuspation of dentition
2. Severe midface trauma involving maxillary and mandibular fractures and complicated by displaced condylar fractures[22]
3. Displaced condylar neck and subcondylar (condyloramal) fractures, so that there is no bony contact of fracture segments and nonunion is imminent
4. Displaced condylar fractures in patients who are bilaterally edentulous posterior to the premolars and who do not have functioning partial dentures; in lieu of open reduction of these fractures a posterior condylar reduction applicance may be used in some of these patients[44]
5. Edentulous patients with displaced condylar fractures and no dentures (which could help the surgeon reestablish vertical dimension of the patient's face)[2,7,27,44]

It should be emphasized once again that all factors must be considered and that, when speaking of surgery, there is never a hard-and-fast rule. Because of the complex nature of condylar fractures and the desirability of early physiological function, treatment of these fractures is considerably more challenging than that of any other facial fracture. The use of numerous treatment modalities will be necessary when treating condylar fractures complicated by other facial fractures, particularly mandibular fractures.

BASIC COURSE OF TREATMENT

For the closed treatment of condylar fractures (displaced and nondisplaced) that are not complicated by any other mandibular fractures, intermaxillary fixation is applied for a period of 3 weeks. The patient is seen at least once a week during the fixation period. After removal of intermaxillary fixation the patient is allowed to open freely (with only two to four intermaxillary elastics) during waking hours, kept on a strict liquid diet, and instructed to apply numerous intermaxillary elastics at bedtime (ensuring maximum intercuspation of teeth during sleep). The patient returns 2 days after removal of intermaxillary fixation for a check and light exercising instructions.

At the end of 4 weeks postoperatively the intermaxillary elastics may be removed during waking hours, but use of night elastics is continued for 6 weeks. The patient should be thoroughly examined every week to ensure early detection of any developing problem with mandibular movement or occlusion. At the end of 6 weeks the patient is told to stop applying intermaxillary elastics altogether and is given an appointment to return in 3 days for a thorough occlusal evaluation. The results of this examination should be compared closely with previously taken records. If a functional discrepancy has developed since night elastics were removed, then appropriate elastic guidance should be applied.

On the seventh week postoperative visit (a week after removal of all intermaxillary tension), assuming intermaxillary relations and mandibular movement are satisfactory, the patient's arch bars are removed, and the patient is appointed to return on the ninth and twelfth postoperative weeks for follow-up checks. Should minor occlusal equilibration be necessary, it may be done at this time but not before the twelfth postoperative week because of the potential for slight settling of the dentition.[29]

ADDITIONAL COMMONLY USED TREATMENT MODALITIES

Frequently patients with condylar complex fractures have suffered other mandibular fractures as well. Usually fabrication and placement of an acrylic lingual splint, when secured firmly to the dentition or the mandibule by circummandibular wires, will substantially increase stabilization of the mandibular body and symphysis (regardless of whether they themselves needed open reduction) to allow institution of early physiotherapy.

Another excellent means of stabilizing other mandibular fractures to facilitate early physiotherapy is the biphasic extraskeletal pin fixation system. For mandibular angle and ramal fractures a Vitallium mesh sheet offers excellent stabilization of the fracture through the physiotherapy period, when adequately secured across a fracture site.[3,29,33,]

CONCLUSION

It is not sufficient to restore an acceptable facial contour if at the same time the patient is crippled from a functional standpoint. Unfortunately this is all too of-

*EDITOR'S NOTE: In my (D.H.M.) experience, there may be two other situations in which an open reduction should be considered: (1) bilateral displaced fractures with an open bite and (2) displaced fractures or severely macerated joint and meniscus accompanied by other multiple maxillary or mandibular fractures requiring 6 to 8 weeks of interdental traction.

ten the case because emphasis has been placed on appearance and bony contour, and insufficient attention has been paid to restoration of function. In most instances condylar fractures can be managed to produce both esthetic and satisfactory functional results.

CASE HISTORIES

When an individual has a high condylar fracture and it is totally displaced from fossa by the pull of the external pterygoid muscle, it is helpful to restore the condyle to its anatomical position if possible. An open reduction is accomplished through either a Risdon or a preauricular approach. It is difficult to prevent the condyle from being pulled from its anatomical position by spasm of the external pterygoid muscle unless there is adequate fixation. Interosseous fixation with a stainless steel ligature is difficult. Sometimes the trauma of accomplishing this will later bring about a fibrous or bony ankylosis. The clinician understandably believes that it is better to have an abnormal joint than one that does not move. Two techniques may be suggested that may solve these problems. One technique involves a simpler way of holding the fragment in position. The other technique prevents the possibility of an ankylosis developing after surgical reduction.

The first technique involves the use of pins to stabilize the fragment. A Roger Anderson pin is drilled into the condylar head. Another pin is placed in the mandible. External fixation is then used to tie the two segments together and prevent movement of the condylar fragment. This usually takes considerably less time than drilling holes through the condyle and neck for placement of interosseous wires, and there is less trauma.

The next technique involves placement of an articular eminence prosthesis with or without the Silastic insert, depending on the severity and damage to the joint. The prosthesis has the effect of preventing an ankylosis from occurring.

Case 1

C.B., a young woman, was kicked by a horse. She had a total displaced fracture of the right condyle. Her occlusion was affected, with her mandible pulled to one side. Arch bars and elastic used interdental traction were placed to hold the teeth in proper centric relation. A preauricular approach was then used to perform an open reduction of the condyle using a Roger Anderson pin to hold the fragment in the proper position (Figs. 23-1 and 23-2). She had a good postoperative result with normal occlusion and function. Some years later she did develop some pain on that side. If the symptoms should become more severe, it is anticipated that an articular eminence prosthesis would be emplaced. In retrospect, it would have been wise to have placed an articular eminence prosthesis at the time to prevent future problems.

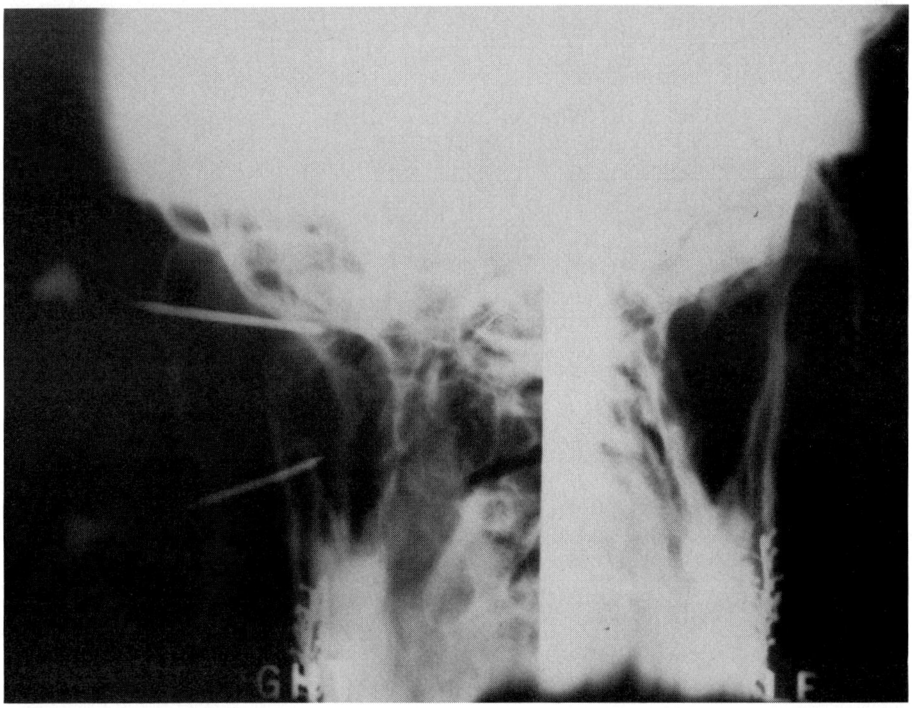

Fig. 23-1. Radiograph of C.B. showing Roger Anderson pin inserted in condyle in mandible to prevent displacement of condyle caused by spasm of external pterygoid muscle.

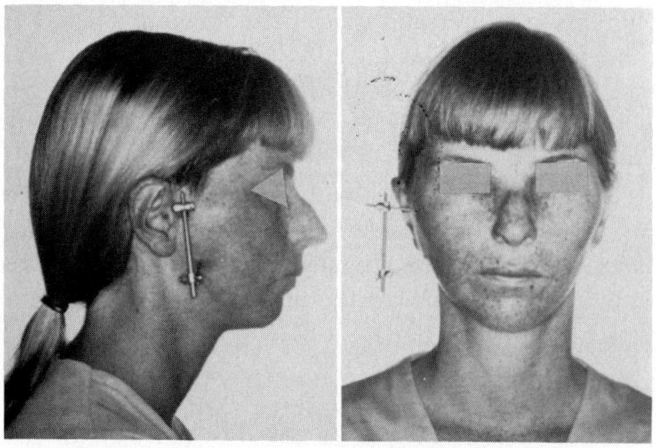

Fig. 23-2. Full-face view showing pins in position.

Case 2

B.C. was thrown with his son from a motorcycle. He sustained severe head injuries as well as a broken arm and leg. He had multiple fractures of the body of the mandible and a segmental fracture of the anterior maxilla. He had nondisplaced fractures of both condyles with severe maceration of the condyle and compression and tearing of the meniscus discs. The maxillary and mandibular fractures were reduced with combined open and closed procedures. He had arch bars and elastic traction placed. Because of the many fractures, we thought he should have the maxillary and mandibular traction sustained for 8 weeks. There was concern about a fibrous ankylosis occurring to the joints during this time. Consequently, an articular eminence prosthesis was placed in both joints. Surgery confirmed that both menisci were severely torn. Postoperatively he did well. He was able, after removal of this traction, to open his mouth wide (Figs. 23-3 and 23-4). He has had no functional or pain problems since surgery (Fig. 23-5). It was not necessary to institute physiotherapy in this case.

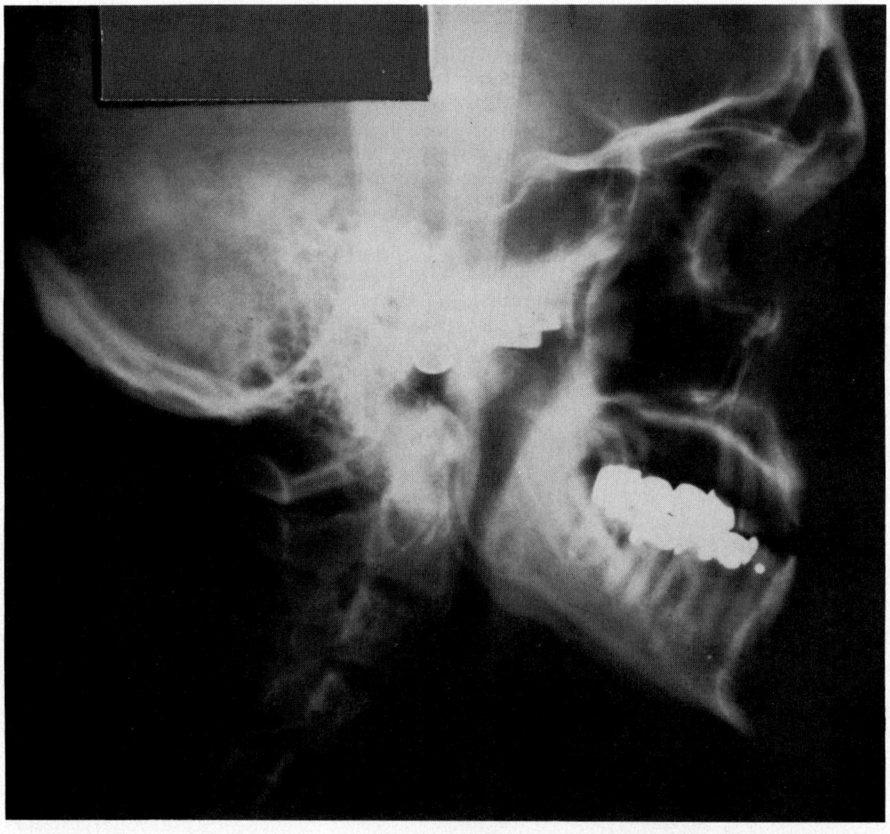

Fig. 23-3. Cephalometric radiograph of B.C. showing prosthesis in position, closed-mouth view.

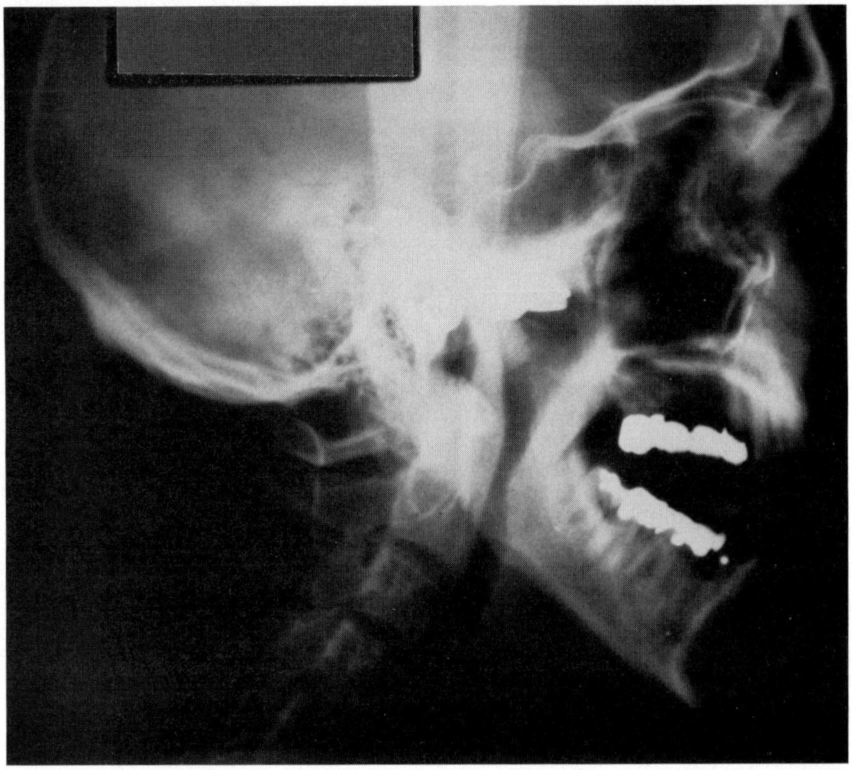

Fig. 23-4. Prosthesis in position, open-mouth view.

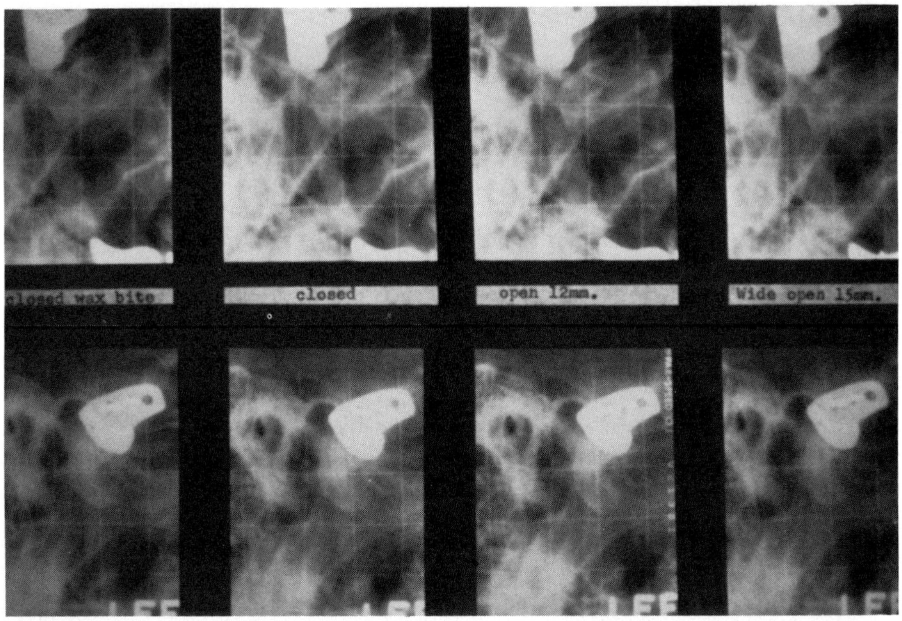

Fig. 23-5. Postoperative transcranial lateral oblique films of B.C. showing normal functioning of condyles over articular eminence prosthesis.

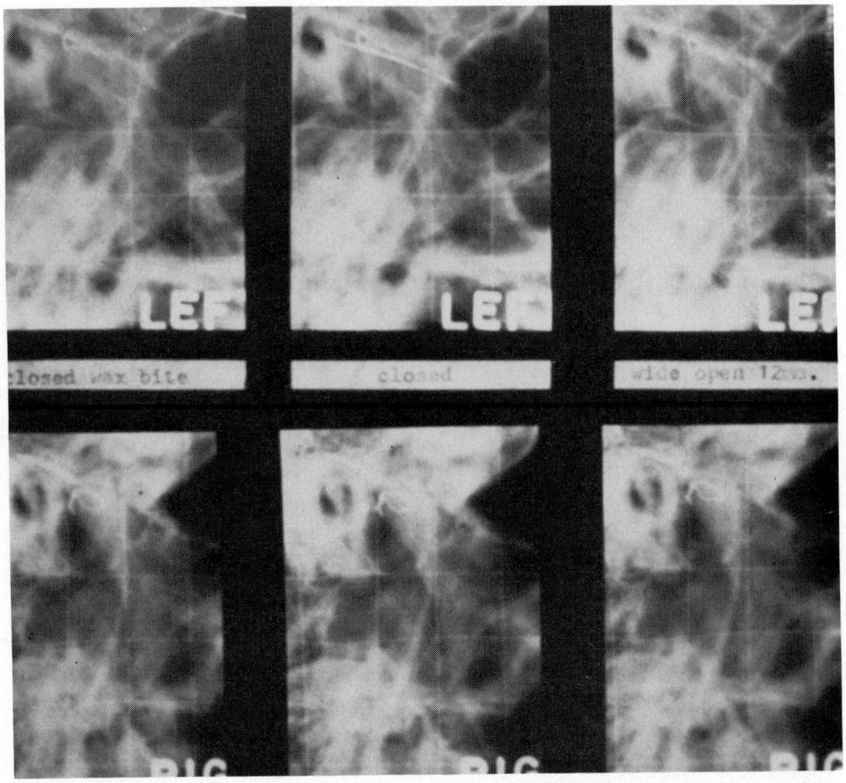

Fig. 23-6. Transcranial lateral oblique films showing joints.

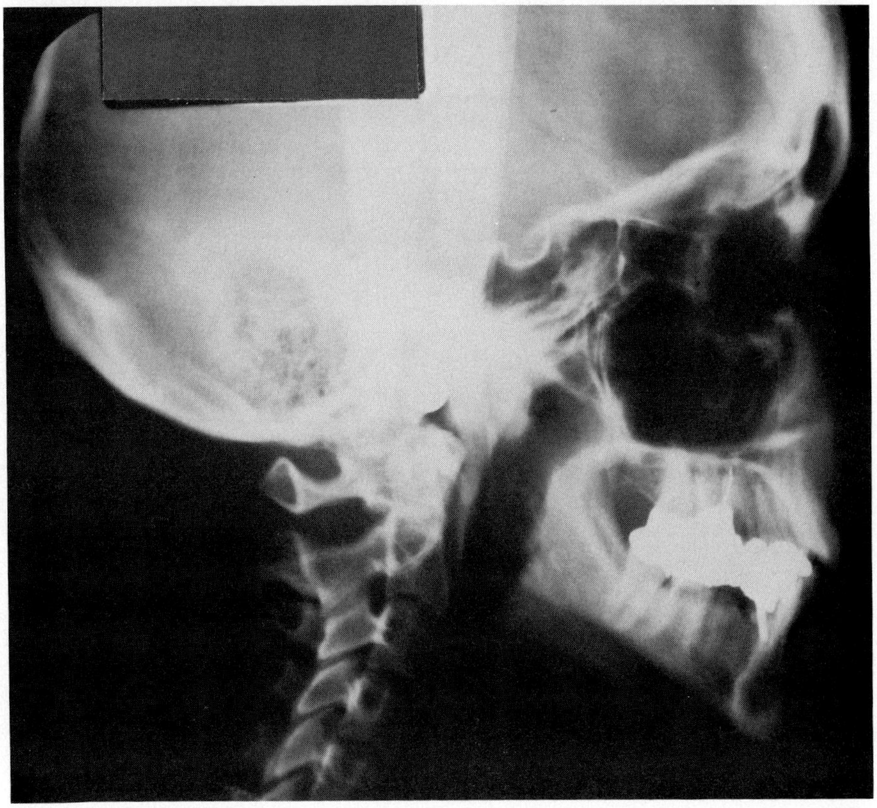

Fig. 23-7. Cephalometric film showing patient able to open only 5 mm.

Case 3

D.R., a young woman, was involved in a severe automobile accident in Hawaii. She had multiple fractures of her maxilla and mandible, and individual teeth were displaced. Both condyles were fractured and totally displaced. She had an open bite. The ENT surgeon and her dentist reduced her fractures well. The dentist constructed metallic splints to which he wired her teeth, ensuring proper relationships. She had both fractured condyles reduced by open reduction and use of interosseous wires. Gradually, over the next $2^1/_2$ years, she developed a bony ankylosis in one joint and a fibrous ankylosis in another. She was able to open 5 mm with difficulty (Figs. 23-6 and 23-7).

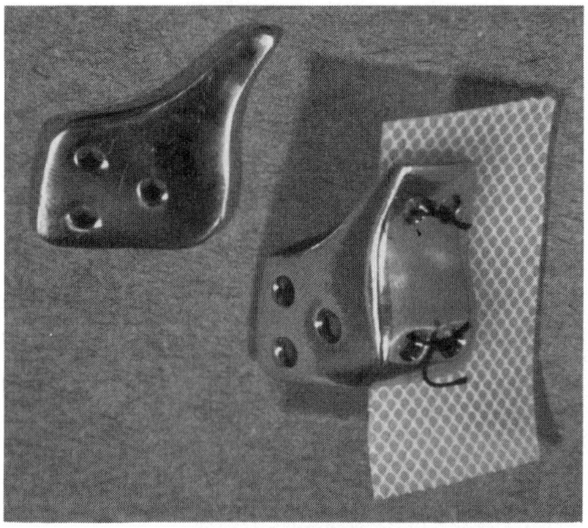

Fig. 23-8. TMJ right-angle prosthesis with template and Silastic insert.

Then she was referred for temporomandibular joint surgery. Two distinct procedures were performed. On the side with the bony ankylosis a template was constructed, which was secured to the ankylosed joint. This template then was used as a guide for cutting free the bone and making a new joint below the normal joint area. This was necessary to avoid accidentally opening into the intracranial fossa, with all the concurrent dangers. Once the joint was free, a right-angle prosthesis identical to the template was placed with a Silastic insert to prevent reankylosis (Fig. 23-8). Then the opposite side was operated on. Since it was a fibrous ankylosis, an articular eminence prosthesis with a Silastic insert was used. The patient has had physiotherapy and is now opening 31 mm (Figs. 23-9 to 23-11).

An important point must be made: bony and/or fibrous ankylosis is a serious problem. It is difficult to correct. Normal function is rarely achieved. With increased understanding, it is better to prevent this possibility from happening. Placing a prosthesis in the joint after reducing a severely displaced condyle is not difficult or time consuming. This surgical procedure is less traumatic than a later osteoarthrotomy and offers the likelihood of more normal function as well as avoidance of future pain and other symptoms.

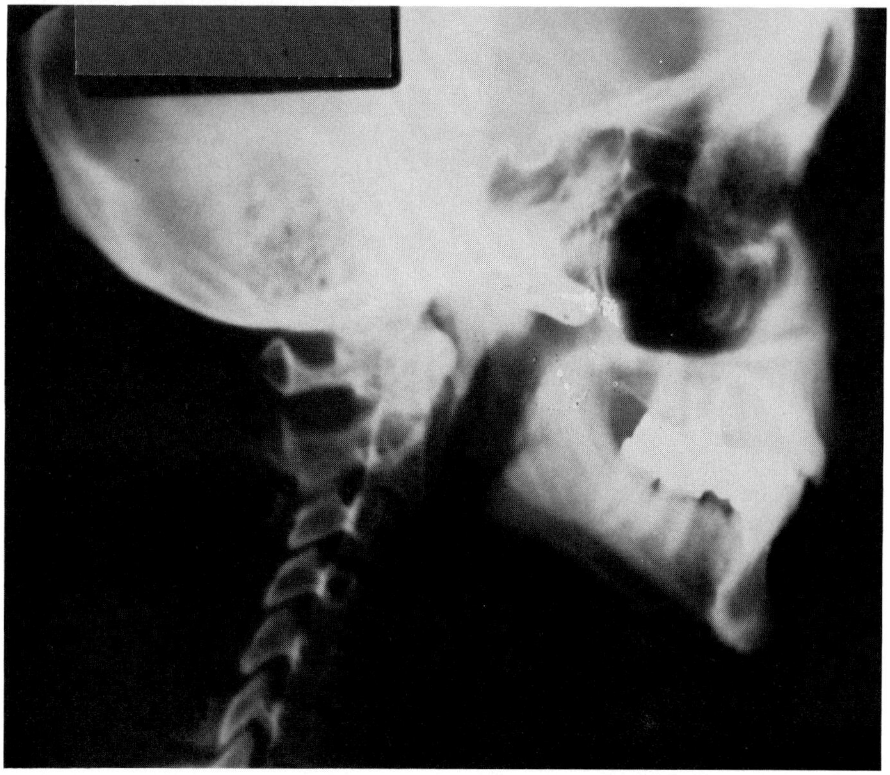

Fig. 23-9. Cephalometric view, closed position.

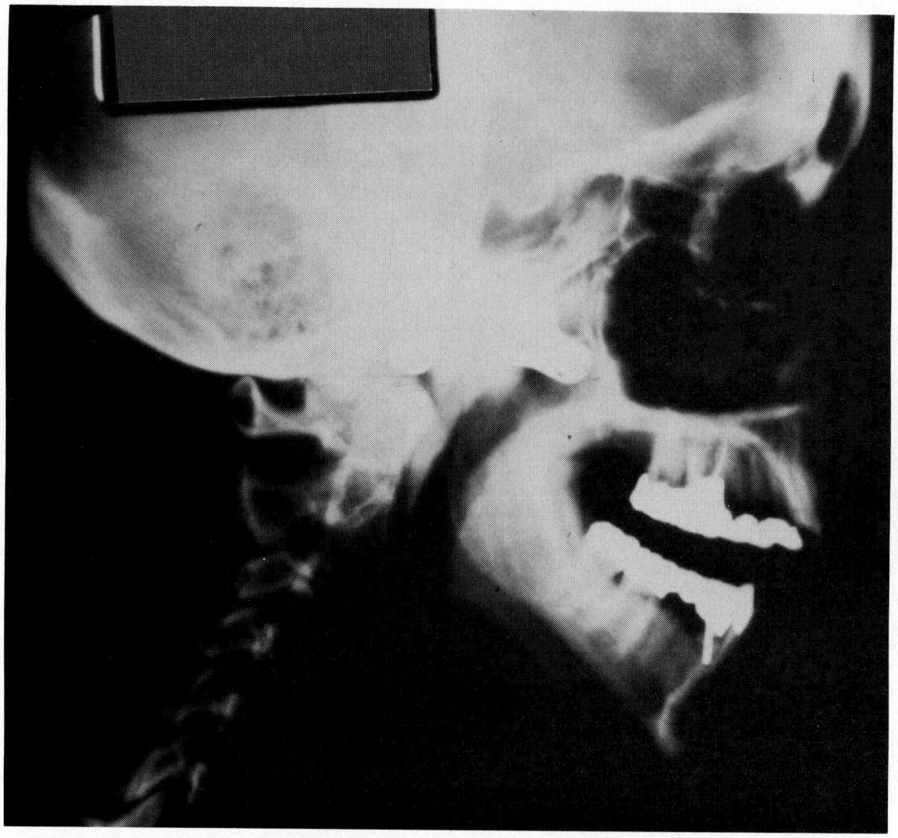

Fig. 23-10. Cephalometric view, open position.

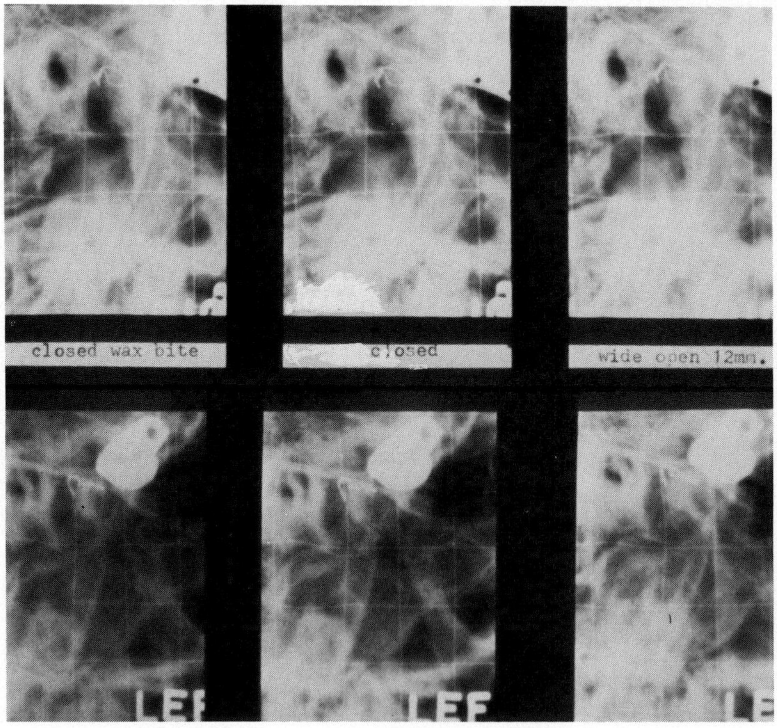

Fig. 23-11. Transcranial lateral oblique films showing some translational movement of left condyle.

Case 4

D.G., a 19-year-old man, was admitted to a county hospital with acute temporomandibular trauma received in a motorcycle accident. Radiographs and physical examination revealed (1) nondisplaced fractures of two ribs requiring only palliative treatment and (2) a high fracture-dislocation of the left mandibular condylar neck with anteromedial distraction of the condylar head. Anteroposterior views confirmed that there was no bony contact between these fracture segments. A decision was made to openly reduce the condylar segments using a preauricular approach. After exposure of the joint space it was found that the articular eminence had sustained multiple fractures, resulting in comminution of that articulating process.

An articular eminence prosthesis was placed over the comminuted structures, thus ensuring an anatomical and smooth articulating surface for the condylar head to function against. After reduction of the condylar neck fracture and proper positioning of the condylar head within the glenoid fossa, the fracture segments were stabilized by extraskeletal pin fixation. Functional exercises were begun at 3 weeks. His postoperative course was uneventful, and he was discharged from care 5 months after the operation. On discharge, he showed an interincisal opening of 37 mm with a slight (2 mm) shift of his mandibular midline to the left on extreme opening (Fig. 23-12).

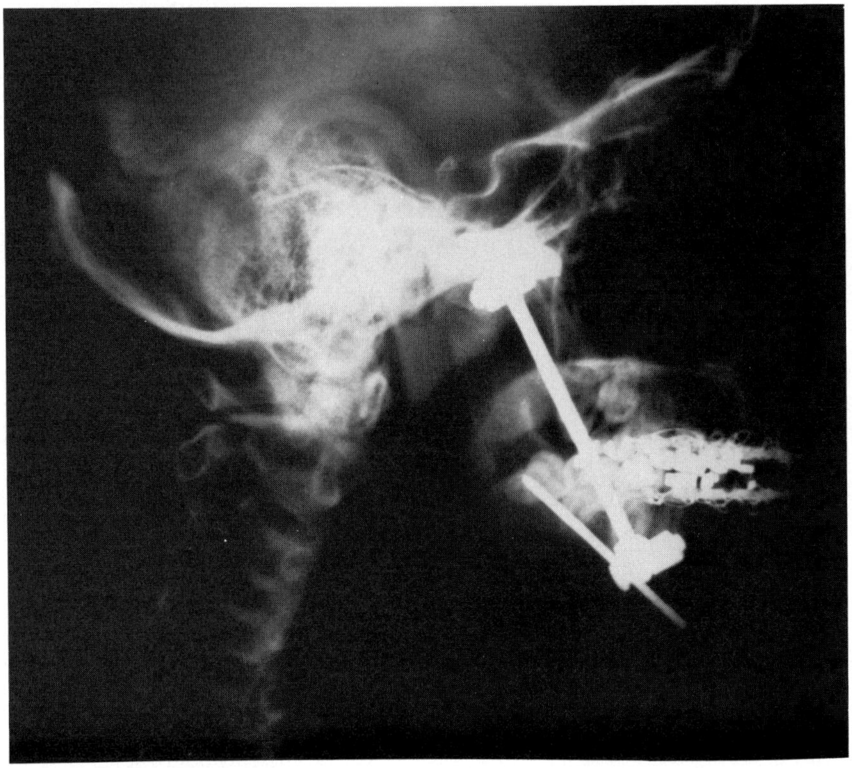

Fig. 23-12. Cephalometric radiograph showing Roger Anderson pins in condyle in body of mandible, with articular eminence prosthesis in position.

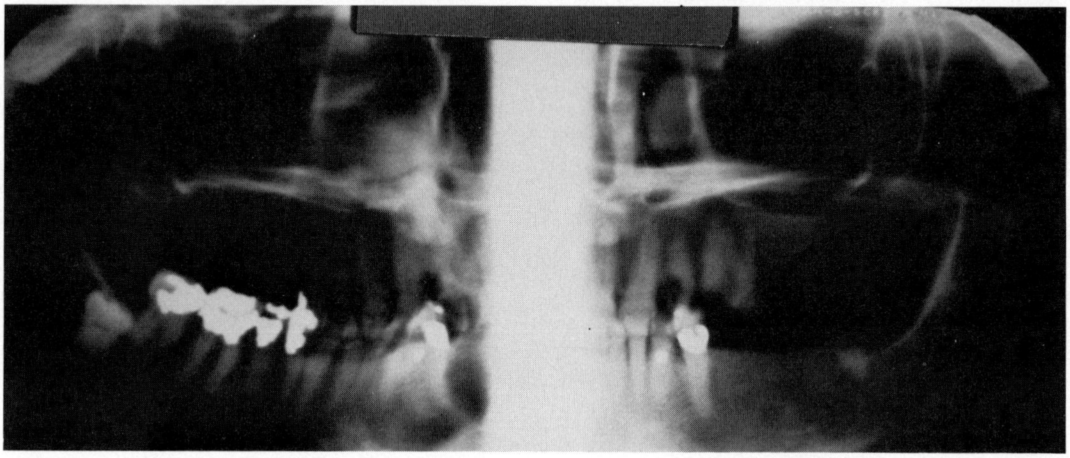

Fig. 23-13. Panorex radiograph showing decayed teeth and root tips in N.A.'s mandible and maxilla and abscessed teeth.

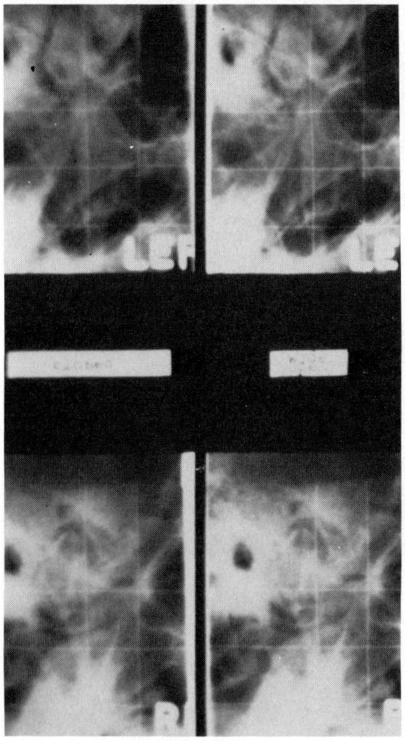

Fig. 23-14. TMJ preoperative transcranial lateral oblique films showing bony ankylosis in left TMJ and fibrous ankylosis in right.

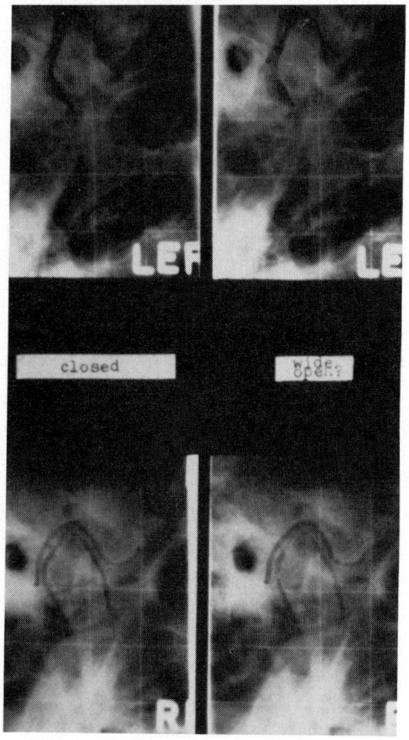

Fig. 23-15. TMJ line drawings overlying radiographs depicting bone-to-bone contact of condyle to eminence in left and showing some disc space remaining between condylar head and upper portion of joint.

Case 5

N.A., a physician's wife, had been unable to open her mouth for 9 years. She had blended or cut up her food in small pieces and pushed them between two back teeth that had decayed and broken off (Fig. 23-13). Her history dates back 12 years when she had cervical neck disease. She was placed on cervical traction and other devices for a long time, which helped the neck problem but had the effect of irritating her jaw joint.

She eventually had cervical laminectomies. After this her mouth would subluxate whenever she had a dental appointment. It was forced closed. Over the next 2 years this subluxation became more and more frequent. She could not drink or eat with her mouth open. It was decided that a blocking operation should be done. This was performed at a large medical center in the Midwest in 1967. After this operation she then had the opposite problem of not being able to open her mouth. The plastic surgeon who performed the operation advised her that this was a cosmetic result. If a condylectomy were done, she might then have a return of the other problem. She elected to live with this difficulty.

TMJ radiographs taken April 7, 1976, revealed what appeared to be nonfunctioning joints (Fig. 23-14). From the outline of the condyle and the articular eminence fossa, it looked as though there was bone-on-bone contact in the left joint (Fig. 23-15). Her operation was performed on April 12, 1976. In surgery there was a complete bony ankylosis. It was necessary to do an osteoarthrotomy and to emplace a right-angle prosthesis, as was previously described.

In the right joint there was a fibrous ankylosis. A combined articular eminence and Silastic prosthesis was emplaced (Fig. 23-16). At the end of surgery her mouth could be opened by surgeons 40 mm. Radiographs taken a week after surgery show her able to open her mouth without physiotherapy approximately 7 mm (Fig. 23-17). She is able to chew food in small pieces. With physiotherapy it is expected that she will be able to open her mouth approximately 30 to 49 mm over the next 6 months (Fig. 23-18).

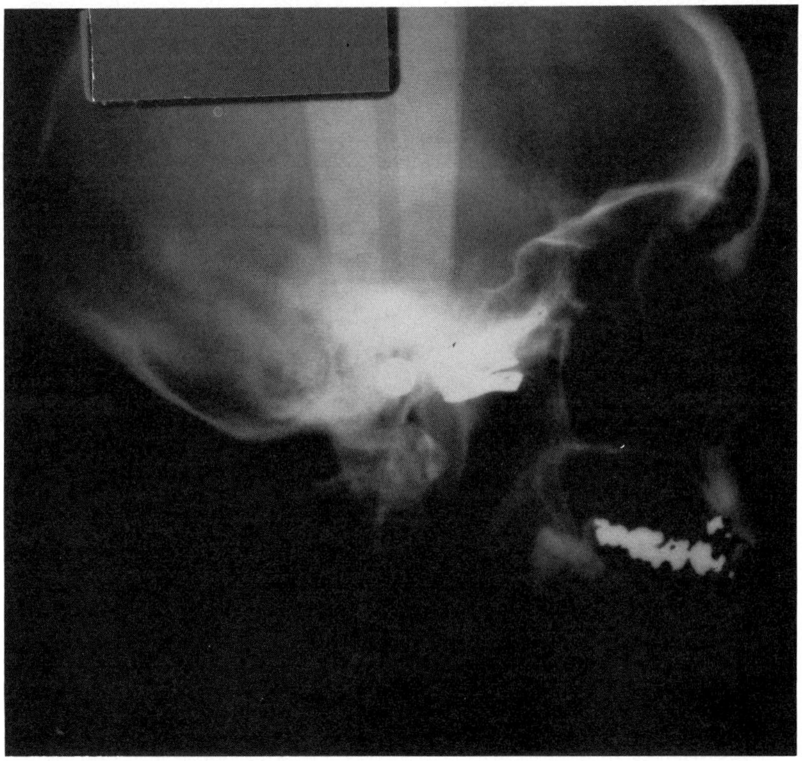

Fig. 23-16. Cephalometric radiograph of N.A. a week after operation, showing prosthesis in position.

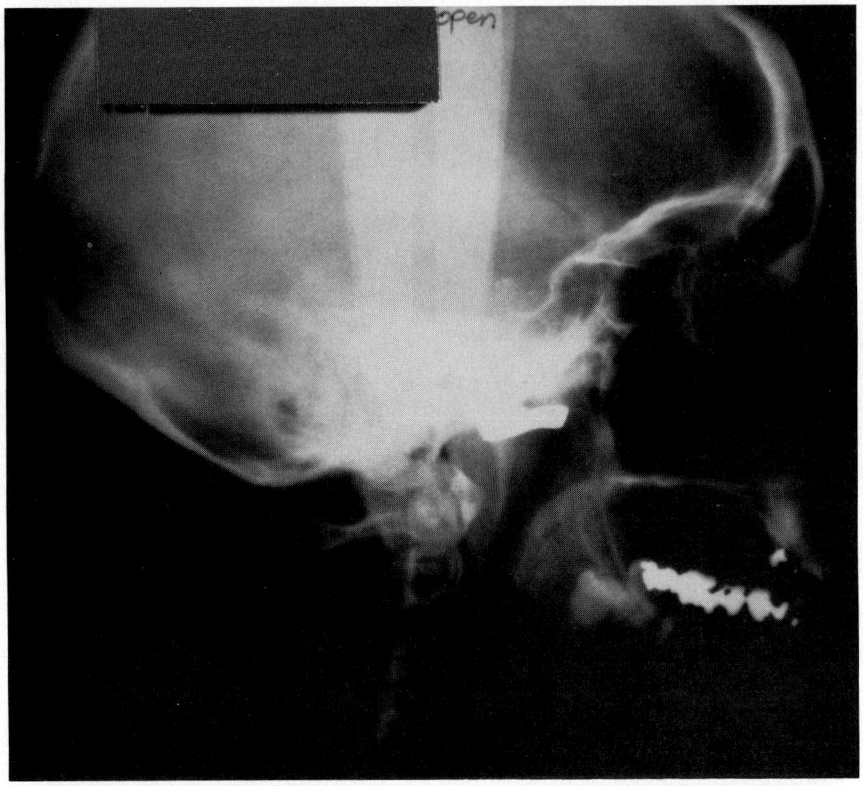

Fig. 23-17. Postoperative cephalometric radiograph showing N.A. opening approximately 7 mm without any physiotherapy or exercises.

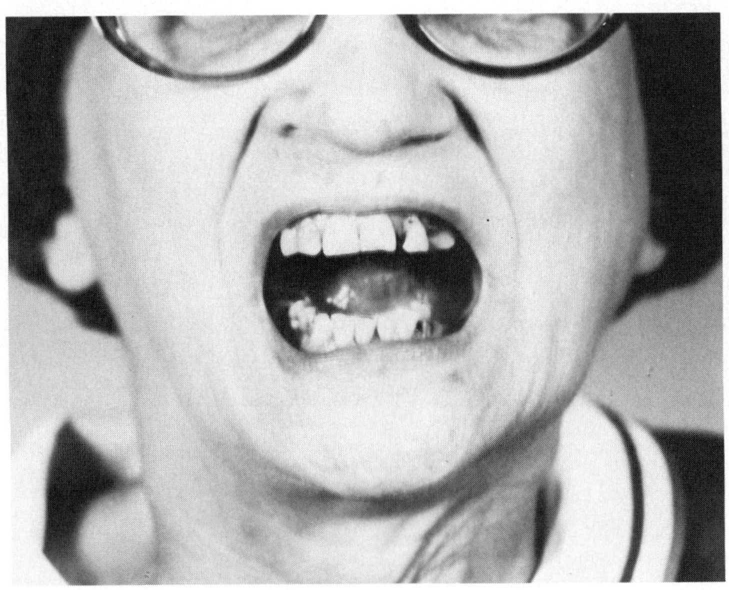

Fig. 23-18. N.A. opening 30 mm interincisally 2 months after surgery.

Case 6*

This patient with ankylosis was originally treated by placement of a hinge-axis prosthesis in the ramus of the mandible. The appliance failed, necessitating its removal. Large segments of fused bone also were removed and an arthroplasty performed, with the placement of a Kent TMJ appliance (Figs. 23-19 to 23-22).

*Courtesy Charles D. Hasse, D.D.S., and Dean L. Duncan, D.D.S.

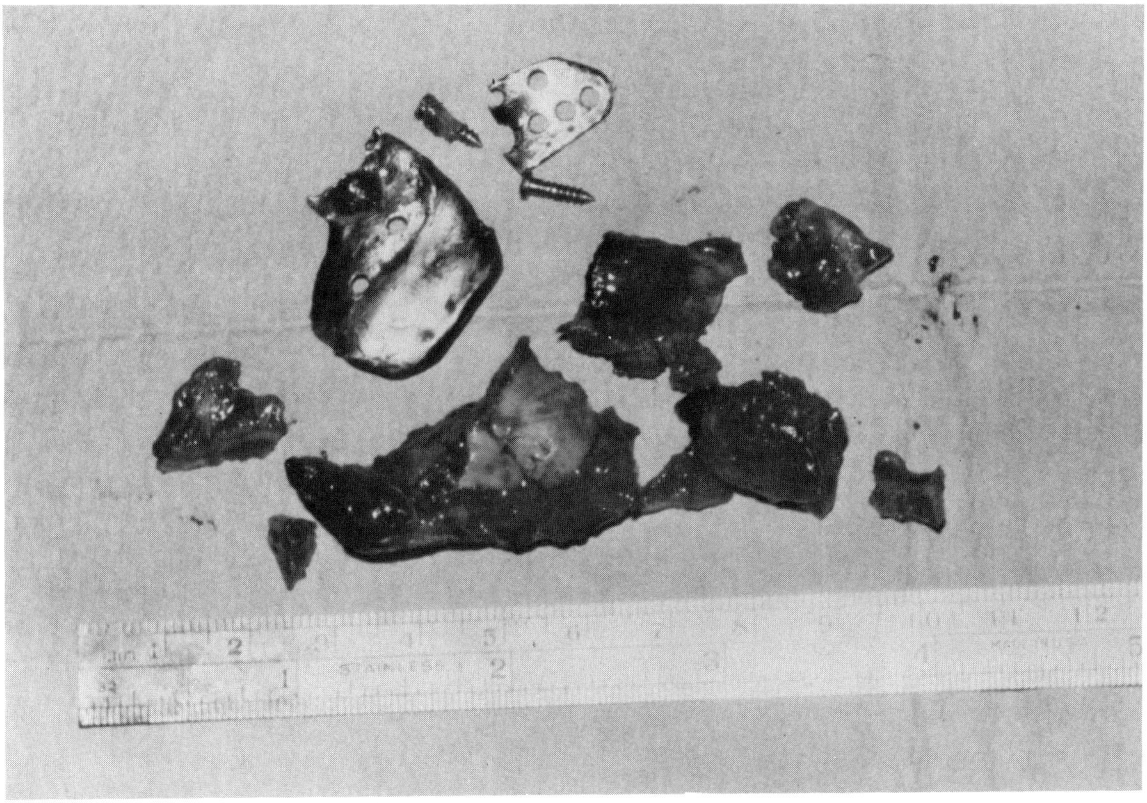

Fig. 23-19. Removed appliance with ankylosed bone segments.

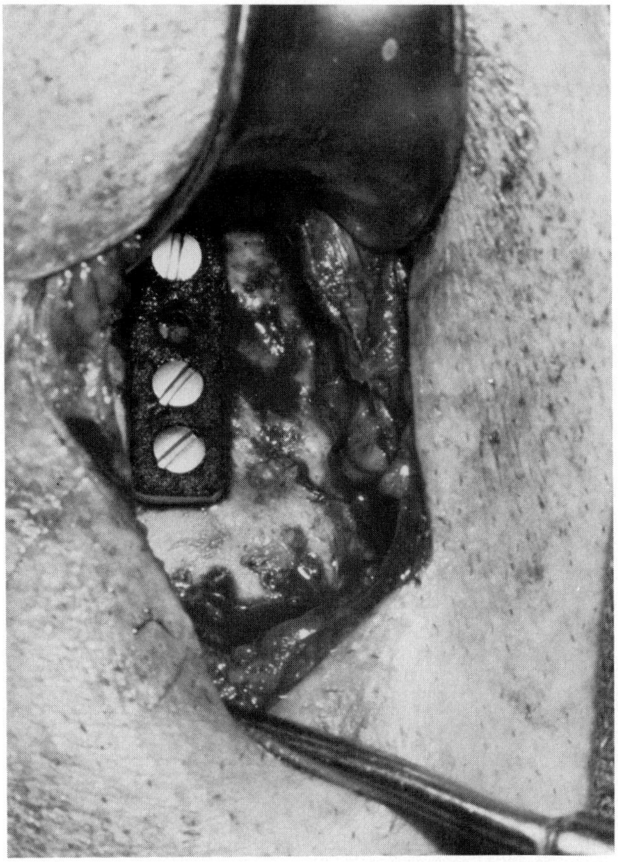

Fig. 23-20. Kent appliance with Proplast artificial ramus affixed via Risdon approach.

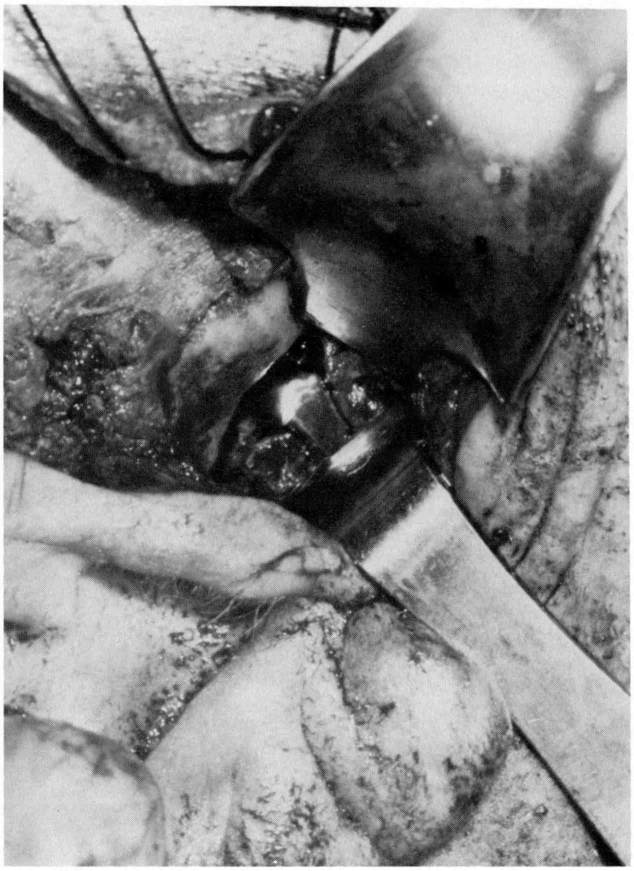

Fig. 23-21. Recontoured fossa with artificial condyle of Kent appliance in view.

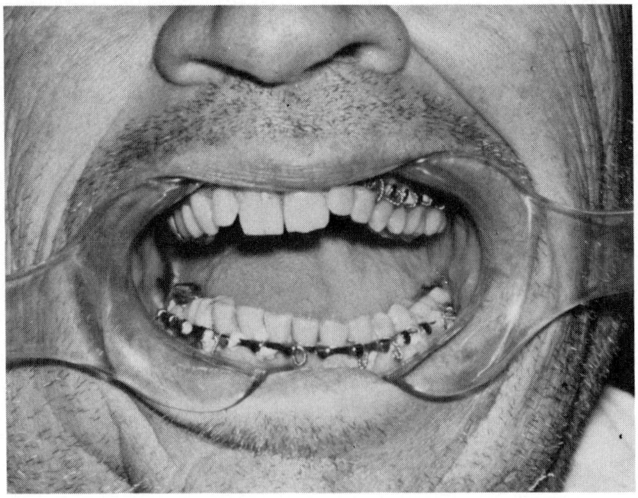

Fig. 23-22. Immediate postoperative opening increased from 6 to 25 mm. With postsurgical exercise patient eventually achieved opening of 38 mm.

REFERENCES

1. Alling, C.C., Rawson, D.W., Staats, O.J., and Middleton, R.A.: Synovial chondromatosis of the temporomandibular joint, case 2, part 2, J. Oral Surg. **31**:691, 1973.
2. Archer, W.H.: Oral surgery, ed. 4, Philadelphia, 1966, W.B. Saunders Co.
3. Bear, S.E., Green, R.K., and Wentz, W.W.: Stainless steel wire mesh—an aid in difficult oral surgery problems, J. Oral Surg. **29**:27, 1971.
4. Boyne, P.J.: Osseous repair and mandibular growth after subcondylar fractures, J. Oral Surg. **25**:300, 1967.
5. Canniff, J.P.: Longstanding bilateral intracapsular fracture dislocation on the condyles treated by closed condulotomy, Trans. Congr. Int. Assoc. Oral Surg. **4**:336, 1973.
6. Cook, R.M., and MacFarlane, W.I.: Subcondylar fracture of the mandible, Oral Surg. **3**:297, 1969.
7. Dingman, R.O., and Natvig, P.: Surgery of facial fractures, Philadelphia, 1964, W.B. Saunders Co.
8. Donoff, R.B., and Roser, S.M.: Management of condylar fractures in patients with cervical spine injury: report of cases, J. Oral Surg. **31**:130, 1973.
9. Farrar, W.B.: Diagnosis and treatment of anterior dislocation of the articular disc, N.Y.J. Dent. **41**:348, 1971.
10. Federspiel, M.N.: Incomplete and complete jaw ankylosis, J. Am. Dent. Assoc. **26**:585, 1939.
11. Findlay, I.A.: Ankylosis of the coronoid to the zygomatic bone, Br. J. Oral Surg. **10**:30, 1972.
12. Fitzpatrick, B.: Indications for surgery on the painful temporomandibular joint, Aust. Dent. J. **16**:355, 1971.
13. Fluur, E., Haverling, M., and Molin, C.: Unusual complication following surgically treated fracture of the mandibular condyle, Int. J. Oral Surg. **2**:297, 1973.
14. Fonseca, G.D.da: Experimental study on fractures of the mandibular condylar process (mandibular condylar process fractures), Int. J. Oral Surg. **3**:89, 1974.
15. Frer, A.A., Friedman, A.L., and Jarrett, W.J.: Intraoral osteotomy of mandibular symphysis to correct bilateral lingual crossbite: report of case, J. Oral Surg. **30**:754, 1972.
16. Goode, R.L., Linehan, J.W., and Shorago, G.: Recurrent mandibular dislocation relieved by removal of articular eminence, Arch. Otolaryngol. **98**:97, 1973.
17. Gruber, L.W., and Lyford, J., III: Care of military and civilian injuries: the conservative treatment of simultaneous fractures through the necks of both mandibular condyles associated with multiple fractures of other parts of the mandible, Am. J. Orthod. **28**:258, 1942.
18. Hale, R.H.: Treatment of recurrent dislocation of the mandible: review of literature and report of cases, J. Oral Surg. **30**:527, 1972.
19. Hall, R.K.: Injuries of the face and jaws in children, Int. J. Oral Surg. **1**:65, 1972.
20. Henny, R.A.: Fractures of the jaws, Semin. Roentgenol. **6**:397, 1971.
21. Hunter, K.J.: Midline and condylar fracture in an 18 month old child, a case report, Aust. Dent. J. **17**:373, 1972.
22. Irby, W.B.: Facial trauma and concomitant problems: evaluation and treatment, St. Louis, 1974, The C.V. Mosby Co.
23. Irby, W.B.: Current advances in oral surgery, St. Louis, 1975, The C.V. Mosby Co.
24. Jacobsen, P.U., and Lund, K.: Unilateral overgrowth and remodeling processes after fracture of the mandibular condyle: a longitudinal radiographic study, Scand. J. Dent. Res. **80**:68, 1972.
25. James, P.: The surgical treatment of mandibular joint disorders, Ann. R. Coll. Surg. Engl. **49**:310, 1971.
26. Kohn, M.W., Chase, D.C., and Marciani, R.D.: Surgical misadventures, Dent. Clin. North Am. **17**:533, 1973.
27. Kruger, G.O.: Textbook of oral surgery, ed. 4, St. Louis, 1974, The C.V. Mosby Co.
28. Kwapis, B.W., Dryer, M.H., and Knox, J.E.: Surgical correction of a malunited condylar fracture in a child, J. Oral Surg. **31**:465, 1973.
29. Lund, K.: Unusual fracture dislocation of the mandibular condyle in a 6 year old child, Int. J. Oral Surg. **1**:53, 1972.
30. Lundin, K., Ridell, A., Sandberg, N., and Ohman, A.: Complications after jaw fractures, Acta Otolaryngol. (Stockh.) **75**:362, 1973.
31. MacAlister, A.D.: The dislocating jaw, Trans. Congr. Int. Assoc. Oral Surg. **4**:259, 1973.
32. Maw, R.B., and McKean, R.W.: Scarification of the temporal tendon for treatment of chronic subluxation of the temporomandibular joint, J. Oral Surg. **31**:22, 1973.
33. Messer, E.J.: A simplified method for fixation of the fractured mandibular condyle, J. Oral Surg. **30**:442, 1972.
34. Moffett, B.C., Jr.: Alterations in craniofacial growth resulting from unilateral fracture of the mandibular condyle in a young rhesus monkey, J. Dent. Res. **50**:1486, 1971.
35. Muldoon, C.J.: Bilateral coronoid hyperplasia, J. Ir. Dent. Assoc. **17**:121, 1971.
36. Myrhaug, H.: A surgical technique for treatment of habitual luxation of the temporomandibular joint (application in an instance of indurated temporomandibular joint luxation), Quintessence Int. **3**:9, 1972.
37. Pirok, D.J., and Merrill, R.G.: Dislocation of the mandibular condyle into the middle cranial fossa: report of a case, Oral Surg. **29**:13, 1970.
38. Ranta, R., and Ylipaavalniemi, P.: The effect of jaw fractures in children on the development of permanent teeth and the occlusion, Proc. Finn. Dent. Soc. **36**:99, 1973.
39. Rehrmann, A., and Kreidler, J.: Late results after arthroereisis of the temporo-mandibular joint by autoplastic bone graft, J. Maxillofac. Surg. **1**:99, 1973.
40. Risdon, F.: Ankylosis of temporomaxillary joint, J. Am. Dent. Assoc. **21**:1933, 1934.
41. Rowe, N.L.: The history of the treatment of maxillo-facial trauma, Ann. R. Coll. Surg. Engl. **49**:329, 1971.
42. Russell, D., Nosti, J.C., and Reavis, C.: Treatment of fractures of the mandibular condyle, J. Trauma **12**:704, 1972.
43. Storrs, T.J.: A variation of the auriculotemporal syndrome, Br. J. Oral Surg. **11**:236, 1974.
44. Thoma, K.H.: Oral surgery, ed. 5, St. Louis, 1969, The C.V. Mosby Co.
45. Waite, D.E.: Pediatric fractures of jaw and facial bones, Pediatrics **57**:551, 1973.
46. Warren, R.E., Winberg, S., and van de Mark, T.B.: Prolonged traumatic dislocation of the mandible, J. Oral Surg. **32**:535, 1974.
47. Yule, A.: Two aspects of a road traffic accident, Radiography **38**:145, 1972.
48. Yune, H.Y., Hall, J.R., Hutton, C.E., and Klatte, E.C.: Roentgenologic diagnosis in chronic temporomandibular joint dysfunction syndrome, Am. J. Roentgenol. Radium Ther. Nucl. Med. **118**:401, 1973.

RECOMMENDED READINGS

Azaz, B., and Lustmann, J.: Anatomical configurations in dry mandibles, Br. J. Oral Surg. **11**:1, 1973.

Chasens, A.I.: Facial pain with dysfunction, J. Oral Med. **27**:59, 1972.

Coccaro, P.J.: Growth in mandibular deformities (ten year study of two cases), J. Dent. Res. **50**:1497, 1971.

Converse, J.M., Coccaro, P.J., Becker, M., and Wood-Smith, D.: On hemifacial microsomia: the first and second brachial arch syndrome, Plast. Reconstr. Surg. **51**:268, 1973.

Homsy, C.A., Kent, J.N., and Hinds, E.C.: Materials for oral implantation—biological and functional criteria, J.Am. Dent. Assoc. **86**:817, 1973.

Leake, D.L., Leake, R.D., Davee, J.S., and Hansen, R.W.: Definitive treatment of mandibular fractures in young children, Oral Surg. **36**:164, 1973.

Rawls, H.C., Bruni, A., and Hamilton, M.K.: Surgical correction of the permanently dislocated mandible, J. Oral Surg. **31**:385, 1973.

Sperling, A.L.: Limitation of mandibular movement secondary to coronoid impingement, J. Oral Surg. **31**:780, 1973.

24 Oral myofunctional therapy

BARBARA J. GREENE, M.F.T., and RICHARD S. SHEPPARD, D.D.S.

PART I*

Myofunctional therapy

Let us suppose that we are seated in choice seats for a performance of a Philharmonic orchestra esteemed to be the most excellent in the world. The anticipation of this event has been with you for many days, and your heart is pounding as the conductor raises the baton to begin another masterpiece. Your ears welcome the sound of such finely balanced chords of music, expertly played by musicians dedicated to excellence. As you rest, lost in a world of balance and harmony, you are suddenly jolted back to reality with your nerves screeching you to a bolt upright position. The lead violinist is playing off key and out of rhythm with the rest of the orchestra and seems totally unaware of his plight. Not even the frenzied conductor can immediately regain control of the situation. Soon every other musician is showing signs of stress. They are nervously fidgeting in their seats while trying their best to continue following the lead of their conductor and somehow regain composure and restore harmony. You are distinctly aware that your $50 seat is not as comfortable as it was a few moments ago. Unless the situation changes, it is debatable what will happen to everyone who is seated in this magnificent auditorium.

And so it is with the body, which is truly a Philharmonic orchestra of the finest caliber. The human body is a masterpiece performance of harmony and balance with the unique ability of functioning with many systems coming into play. However, if one group in this finely tuned organ becomes out of sync with the rest of the body, the entire body is set on edge. Stress results, with every other organ and system having to rally around to cope with the situation, doing their best to maintain control and continue existence. Balance and harmony are so easy to understand. Let us then view them in relation to the delicate balance of the muscle system of the oral-facial-head complex as it interplays with the rest of the body.

*This section was contributed by Barbara J. Greene, M.F.T.

Imbalanced oral musculature

Imbalanced oral musculature is the use of muscles in a stressful, tense environment. Imbalanced muscles are adverse pulling forces on the bony framework of the head, with a rippling effect from the head throughout the entire body. This pull is diverse and may be (1) forward, (2) lateral (either unilateral or bilateral), or (3) a combination of forward and lateral pulls. In the presence of these forces there is a variety of symptoms. Generally, combinations of the following will exist:

1. Imbalanced facial symmetry
2. Respiratory difficulty with associated mouth breathing
3. Allergic tendencies
4. Imbalanced occlusal relationships
5. Poorly developed oral structure
6. Postural weakness and imbalance
7. Eating and drinking abnormalities
8. Stressful use of facial muscles during function
9. Digestive imbalances
10. Poor habits in and around the mouth and face
11. Temporomandibular joint symptoms
12. Pain

By and large these produce effects on (1) appearance, (2) physical and mental health, (3) growth and development, (4) effectiveness in daily activities, including learning capabilities, and (5) the ability of the body to cope.

Factors affecting development of the muscular system

To the best of our current knowledge, the following areas appear to affect the way that the muscles will develop and ultimately be used by the body. The difficulty is in determining just what combination of these situations brought about the imbalance or problems seen in the patient and the most judicious way of bringing harmony back to the musculoskeletal system.

Trauma to the skeletal structure. Trauma to the skeletal structure may occur in the following ways:

1. Pressure to the bony structure during pregnancy
2. Pressure to the bony structure during birth (during long or hard labor, delivery, and/or after delivery)
3. Trauma to the entire musculoskeletal system as a result of falls, blows, and accidents of varied descriptions and degrees of pressure *throughout* the person's life
4. Pulling of the skeletal system out of functional harmony as a result of stress of imbalanced muscles

Further discussion regarding this delicate balance continues in the latter part of this chapter, with reference material indicated. Balance in relation to the muscle system is crucial in many cases, since where the bones are, the muscles attached to them are also. Therefore one could have abnormal muscle function *because* of the position of the bony structure. In other instances, retraining of the muscle framework has facilitated a change in the bony structure. What is important is the regaining of *normal* function, not just *better* function.

Feeding of the infant. The way in which an infant is fed is extremely important. The imbalanced musculature is often directly related to the manner in which a baby has sucked. Basically, proper suckling involves a forward thrusting of the tongue, followed by a posterior pull against the palate with a rhythmic posterior flat-plane pulling of the lips. As a result of this force relationship, the palate is molded and shaped, and the proper tone of the orbicularis oris–masseter-buccinator–posterior temporal muscle framework is established.

Improper feeding or drinking permits the reverse of this, with a forward thrusting of the tongue followed by anterior or anterolateral movement without proper lip and lateral muscle force. Improper shaping and molding of the palate occurs, with an imbalance in the occlusal development. The imbalanced muscle force could continue throughout the patient's life.

Sucking or biting habits. Sucking of the thumb, fingers, knuckles, wrists, lips, blankets, sheets, teddy bear ears, etc. may predispose an individual to an imbalanced muscle framework, allowing the following:

1. Low-forward posturing of the tongue
2. Anterior and/or lateral movement of the tongue
3. Weakness of the lip structure
4. Forward positioning of the mandible (TMJ syndrome)
5. Drooling
6. Poor posture of the head and neck musculature
7. Improper molding forces of the oral structure

Biting and sucking habits often are observed in the adult patient as the following mannerisms: (1) digit sucking or biting, (2) lip, cheek, or tongue biting or sucking, (3) object sucking or biting, and (4) oral fixations.

Diet and nutrition. The diet of the mother and father before conception and before birth influences the overall development of the body of the child, including the muscle framework. The diet of the infant also is critical to growth and development. Much progress currently is being made in the understanding of infant needs as they relate to the establishment of good nutritional balance and diet habits. In the presence of muscles developing in an imbalanced state, it appears that young children will make modifications in the manner in which they eat as well as in the actual choice of foods. They will avoid food difficult to chew or swallow. This is because of the anterior movement of the musculature, producing a gagging feeling. Thus fibrous, coarse foods such as fruits, vegetables, and whole grains may be low on their priority list, whereas soft carbohydrates and sweet foods will be high, since they are easier to consume. In this imbalanced state there could be gas, burping, hiccups, and/or stomachaches caused by air swallowed during food consumption. Noisy, sloppy open-mouth chewing traits might exist. Difficulty in swallowing pills, drooling, and gagging also may be manifested.

All too often the patient exhibits allergic tendencies ranging from general congestion to a major allergic state. A *true* allergy may not exist. Instead we may see an overload on the body from stress conditions. Symptomatic changes occur once these stresses are relieved. Diet modifications, minor or major, are generally necessary.

Genetics. We cannot overlook genetics, since inherited weaknesses, growth and development factors, etc. can play a part in what a person's overall makeup will be. The clinician's abilities and techniques may be strongly affected by the patient's inherited potentials.

Environment. Responding to our surroundings, physical or emotional, influences our growth, development, and sustaining of life in general. How each person responds to his or her own set of circumstances can be greatly influenced by the stresses being placed on the mechanisms of the body. It is also true that a change in circumstances such as a physical accident or a severe emotional shock can dramatically effect a change in a once stable environment. An adequate history of each patient is very important so we may determine just what the environment is now for this patient. In the presence of orofacial muscle imbalance a change in the physical or emotional environment may possibly manifest itself in the following ways:

1. Jaw, facial, head, or neck pain
2. Sudden migration of teeth
3. Periodontal breakdown
4. Tooth loss
5. Inability to cope with prosthetic devices
6. A feeling that the tongue is too big for the mouth
7. Mouth burning
8. A sudden *over*awareness of the mouth

Activities and hobbies. We tend to overlook the area of activities and hobbies all too often. The manner in which we do things throughout our lives can greatly affect the delicate balance of the musculoskeletal framework. Pressures exerted have a strong influence on proper function.

Musical instruments. Several instances could be listed where imbalance was caused or facilitated by the manner in which a musical instrument was used. Do not ever underestimate this force area. The following are three examples:

1. A violinist, 52 years of age, who played 2 to 5 hours per day, presented with an advanced stage of oral dyskinesia. A unilateral swallowing imbalance to the right exaggerated her problem, combined with the pushing force of the violin.
2. A flutist and former saxophone player did not respond to orthodontic correction even after successful myofunctional therapy. The pressure exerted by the lower lip structure during the playing of the flute and the resultant overstrengthening of the musculature is causing relapse of the teeth.
3. An oboe player continued to have breakdown on the lower central incisors, with tooth movement and bone loss. The pressure of the mouthpiece was too great, even after removal of tongue pressures during swallowing.

Leaning habits. Leaning habits can be monumental in their effects. Observe the manner in which the majority of patients lean and the relationship of this to their symptoms. Often you will find that there is a corresponding effect. The pressure during leaning is major, especially when done during prolonged spans of time such as when driving, watching television, reading, and doing schoolwork or office work.

Hobbies. It is very important to find out what hobbies involve a person's time. For example:

1. A policeman with severe TMJ symptoms—ear pain and tinnitus—all on the right side of the head happened to be a champion skeet shooter as well as a champion marksman of powerful rifles and magnum revolvers. All were held and fired on the right side of the body. Much spare time and work time was spent involved in the hobby.
2. A child with beginning TMJ symptoms, in assembling a model toy, was observed to be biting the tongue throughout the entire procedure.
3. A singer enunciates to perfection but has severe TMJ symptoms because of overuse of an already imbalanced musculature. A major lateral shift of the jaw accompanied by a forward thrusting of the mandible occurs each time a sound is uttered. A distortion of the face also is noted.

Abnormally imposed pressures. Gum chewing represents a major misuse of the muscle-jaw structure. Stress, fatigue, torquing, occlusal disharmony, misuse of the tongue musculature, and open-mouth posturing often result.

Prolonged use of the telephone produces pressure, which is magnified if the person holds the phone between the ear and the shoulder. Telephone headsets are recommended when prolonged use is necessary. Many teenagers spend from 4 to 7 hours per day on the telephone, assuming unusual body postures, many of which cause imbalance and stress.

Pressures from improper sleeping postures, such as stomach sleeping, are very detrimental. Back and side sleeping with proper support to the body parts are preferred. We must be sure that the person is not holding an arm, hand, teddy bear, etc. under the face or head. We want *rest* not *stress*.

Chewing on objects, such as sunglasses, toothpicks, pipe stems, pens, pencils, fingernails, cuticles, and knuckles, imbalances the occlusion, sets up incorrect muscle pulls, and places stress on the TMJ apparatus.

Chewing, biting, or sucking habits of the lips, cheeks, tongue, or digits may be done subconsciously. The patient may not be aware of the habits. Helpful information can be gained through observation during the evaluation and from family members. The effects of these habits can be disastrous as they relate to shifting the mandible, imbalancing the occlusion, pulling the muscles, and posturing of the tongue.

It is possible that the body will acquire many of these biting or sucking habits to achieve a semblance of balance, especially in the presence of a lateral pulling muscle force. The habit appears to shift the mandibular joint to the opposite side, possibly to achieve balance of the TMJ apparatus. It is possible that once the muscle system is in harmony with the bony structure, the habits will disappear without further correction. Possibly the body no longer has the need to compensate.

Oral myofunctional therapy

Oral myofunctional therapy is a program to reeducate the muscles of the mouth and face to work in a balanced relationship. The subconscious level must be reached to establish a new muscle activity. Retraining "on command" is not adequate, since the new habit must be substantial enough to be maintained 24 hours per day, during any activity, and without conscious effort.

Diagnostic criteria

A *complete differential diagnosis* is of the utmost importance and has been an area of weakness in the past. Diagnostic criteria could include any combination of the following symptoms, all of which are affected by other circumstances.

1. Breathing through the mouth and poor mouth habits should be noted (Fig. 24-1).
2. Note resting tongue posture, which may be forward (maxillary, mandibular, or between), lateral, or forward and lateral, applying pulling pressure to the musculoskeletal system and/or direct pressure to the teeth (Fig. 24-2). Forward carriage of the mandible or forward/lateral carriage is often observed. Through instrumentation with the Myoscanner accurate measurements can be made of the force the tongue is exerting.
3. Imbalanced lip pressures should be noted. The strength of the lips can be determined through use of the lip force gauge and with the Myoscanner. Diagnostic signs include the following:
   a. Flaccidity and weakness (Fig. 24-3)
   b. Tenseness with overdevelopment of facial muscles (Fig. 24-4)
   c. Lip conditions such as cold sores, dryness and cracking, swelling, puffiness, lack of color or contour, and lip licking
4. Imbalanced forces of the tongue during swallowing should be noted, but we must be careful not to rely on just visual observation of the swallow. With the use of the Payne black light technique, using Orabase and florescene dye or a quick method using Orabase with zinc oxide powder, these pastes on the tongue will facilitate observations of where the tongue is applying pressure. This force could represent many combinations:
   a. Anterior, between the teeth (Fig. 24-5)
   b. Posterior unilateral flare to the right or left (Fig. 24-6)
   c. Posterior bilateral flare to both the right and left (Fig. 24-7)
   d. Anterior, against the teeth but not visible, with pressure either maxillary, mandibular, or against both the maxillary and mandibular teeth (Fig. 24-8)
   e. Anterior, with flaring lateral forces between the posterior teeth
   f. Complete posterior molar-to-molar flare with separation of the entire bite (Fig. 24-9)
5. Imbalanced masseter and posterior temporal muscle activity may be present; both areas could be overdeveloped or underdeveloped. In either case it could indicate the presence of improper tongue use and mandibular carriage. For example, if the mandible is being carried forward, the most posterior portion of the temporal muscle could be weak and/or imbalanced. In this instance the masseter muscle could be overdeveloped. Bruxing tendencies might be obvious. In normal function the posterior temporal muscle is strong, with activation of the masseters during swallowing.
6. Abnormal facial muscle use could be manifested as the following:
   a. Grimace, activation of the facial muscles surrounding the lip structure, and tightening of the lips during swallowing (Fig. 24-10)
   b. Lip crease
   c. Mentalis muscle activity during swallowing and/or overdevelopment of the mentalis muscle (Fig. 24-11)
7. Indications of abnormal intraoral pressures include the following:
   a. Tongue scalloping, indicating a pushing force of the tongue on the teeth, leaving a scalloped effect along the borders of the tongue (Fig. 24-12)
   b. Lateral ridges on the tongue, indicating biting of the tongue between the tooth surfaces (Fig. 24-13)
   c. Cheek ridges, indicating biting or sucking of the cheeks
   d. Lip scalloping anteriorly, indicating a suctionlike effect of the lips against the dentition
   e. Tongue sores on the tongue surface, indicating biting of the tongue by accident or as a habit
8. The presence of ankylotic muscle tissue should be noted (Fig. 24-14).
   a. Ankylotic tongue, preventing a seal of the tongue within the palate
   b. Ankylotic labial frenum, creating tension against the lower dentition
   c. Ankylotic maxillary frenum, possibly creat-

ing a shortness of the upper lip and tooth spacing

9. Enlarged tonsillar tissue should be noted, since removal of tonsils that are fibrous and engorged generally is recommended (Fig. 24-15). Proper tongue function is impaired, and poor respiratory function is observed. Often tonsils are enlarged and edematous in a mouth breather with oral muscle imbalance; however, a decrease in size of the tonsillar tissue is generally noted once proper breathing is established, diet modifications are made, and proper muscle function is facilitated. The presence of enlarged adenoid tissue, a deviated septum, enlarged turbinates, and/or polyps also must be determined. Sufficient airway is essential.
10. Palatal arch width should be measured (Fig. 24-16). The neurological input of the relationship between the tongue and its placement in the palate directly against the bones of the maxilla is being found to be of paramount importance to the motor-sensory-neurological system of the whole body. Where there is restricted arch width or a vaulted arch that does not permit a complete tongue seal, the patient may manifest the following:
    a. Overall body weakness
    b. Poor development of the entire oral cavity
    c. Forward muscle activity
    d. Mouth-breathing tendencies
    e. Allergic tendencies
11. Imbalanced facial symmetry should be noted; imbalanced pull by the muscle framework on the bony structure results in an imbalance of the facial structure.
12. Speech difficulties may occur in the presence of muscle imbalance.
    a. Articulation with poor tongue placement, with or without associated sound distortion
    b. Movement of the mandible forward, lateral, or both
    c. Maintenance of a poor tongue and jaw posture following sound production
13. Bruxing and/or clenching activity is often observed in the presence of imbalanced musculature. Once harmony is restored, the habit generally is altered.
14. Bony interferences, or tori, should be noted; if the bony prominence is large enough, proper muscle function could be interrupted (Fig. 24-17).
15. Biting and sucking habits of the lips, cheeks, tongue, or digits can cause improper placement of the jaw and imbalancing forces of the muscles (Figs. 24-18 and 24-19).
16. TMJ symptoms are the following:
    a. Jaw sounds
    b. Jaw pain
    c. Jaw deviation (Fig. 24-20)
    d. Dysfunction
17. Ear symptoms are the following:
    a. Ringing or buzzing
    b. Fullness or blockage
    c. Pain
18. Pain symptoms may be intraoral or of the face, head, neck, or a combination of these areas. It is important to note that symptoms listed in 16 and 17 are often found in the young child. Reestablishing balance often alleviates the symptoms
19. Tooth migration, periodontal weakness, and/or tooth loss may occur in varied degrees as a result of constant imbalanced stress (Figs. 24-21 and 24-22). This area is often overlooked in its relationship to the pressures of the tongue, lips, cheeks, or objects. Surgical, orthodontic, or prosthetic attempts to solve the problems often will be unsuccessful without correction of the muscle forces.
20. Inability to maintain prosthetic devices should be noted (Fig. 24-23). A patient who is having difficulty adjusting to or is unable to use a partial or complete prosthesis is often the patient with oral muscle imbalance. In the presence of a lateral muscle force, even the placement of a fixed bridge can bring on many complaints and lack of acceptance. The problem may be manifested as the following:
    a. The tongue seeming *too big* for the mouth
    b. Burning of the mouth
    c. Abnormal mouth movements
    d. Difficulty in eating or drinking
    e. Impairment of speech
    f. Movement or suction breakage in the prosthesis
    g. Patient feeling as though he or she is gagging
    h. A general increase of orofacial habits
21. Poor eating and drinking habits may be manifested as the following:
    a. Noise while eating
    b. Sloppiness and "too fast" a speed during eating
    c. Open-mouth chewing
    d. Poor selection of foods
    e. Gas, burping, hiccups, stomach pain
    f. Gulping, drooling, or visibility of tongue during drinking
    g. Difficulty in swallowing

22. Occlusal disharmony should be noted, since occlusal harmony is impossible in the presence of muscle dysfunction. Loss of vertical dimension appears to be an ever-increasing problem.
23. Habits, activities, and hobbies should be determined (Fig. 24-24). It is important to determine their relationship to the overall picture of symptoms and to deal with them as necessary to achieve balance.
24. Past history should be determined in regard to the following:
    a. Prebirth and birth
    b. Injuries and accidents
    c. Medical and dental health
    d. Basic life style

Is therapy beneficial?

The *earlier* we treat, the *more* successful we can be. Then the imbalances are not as major, and establishing normal function is a much easier task, with the clinicians working together. No one person is able to do the job. The adult as well as the child can be treated successfully. Patients ranging in age from 4 to 84 (or higher) have achieved the varied goals that we have set. The therapy program requires a high degree of motivation on the part of the clinician, the patient, and the family. This is a critical factor. The continued positive changes that occur throughout therapy aid in keeping the patients' attention and further progress. A daily routine of exercise is the key in training muscles. The only difference between this type of therapy and a tennis lesson is that we are teaching a subconscious act, and therefore we must establish a pattern for a 24-hour day, not just for a short time.

Much negativity has been generated during the past several years as a result of incomplete diagnosis, poorly trained clinicians, and lack of pertinent data. That day is passing. We are now able to diagnose with more accuracy, measuring actual muscle strength with a compilation of data throughout therapy. Biofeedback units aid in visual and sensory retraining. Study and work seminars with the patients increase their understanding of the goals they have set out to achieve and help them establish the subconscious patterns. With combined efforts, just as in a Philharmonic orchestra, we build, blend, and create harmony. We now face a future of success, not failure. It is an exciting time. The pieces of the puzzle are fitting together, with the patient the recipient and success the result.

Text continued on p. 472.

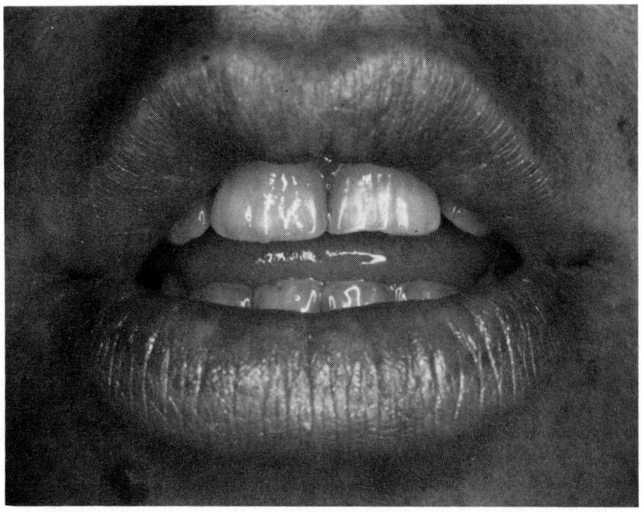

Fig. 24-1. Mouth breather. Note lip puffiness, tissue irritation at lip corners, and poor resting posture of tongue.

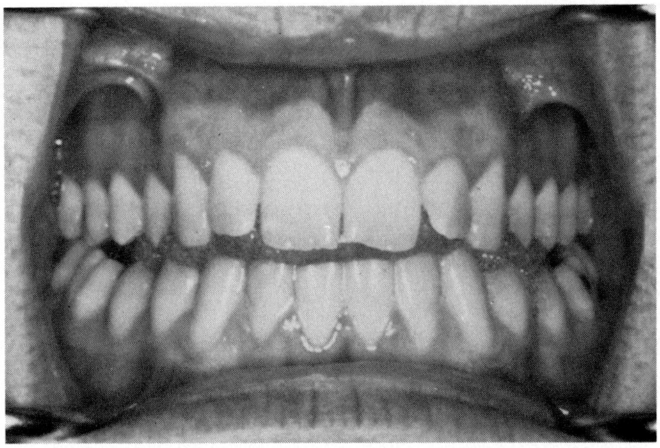

Fig. 24-2. Poor resting tongue posture.

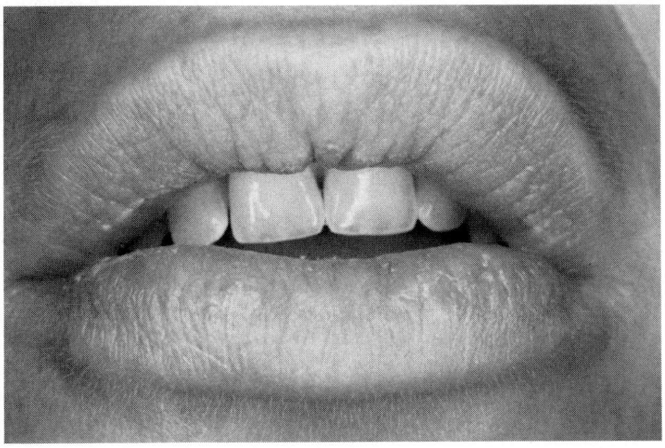

Fig. 24-3. Imbalanced lip structure. Note lip flaccidity, dryness, puffiness, and poor tissue tone.

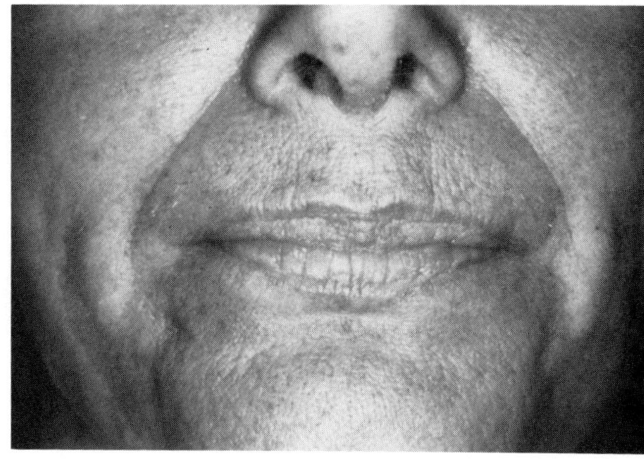

Fig. 24-4. Lip tension at rest with facial muscle tightening. Note facial "age" lines.

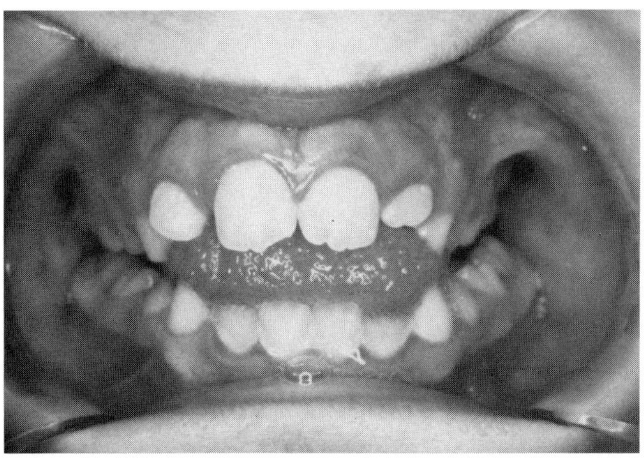

Fig. 24-5. Swallowing imbalance: anterior force.

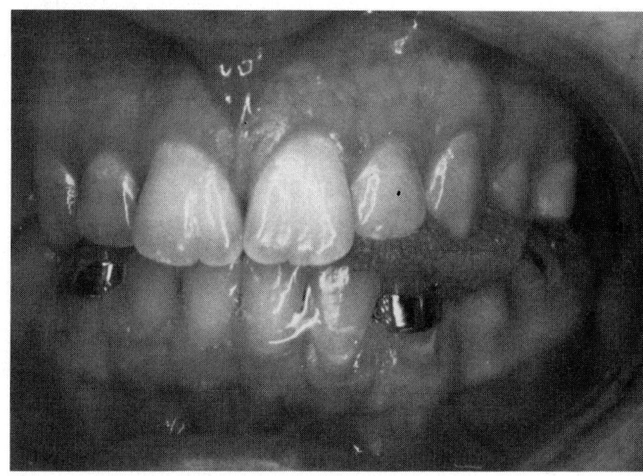

Fig. 24-6. Swallowing imbalance: unilateral force.

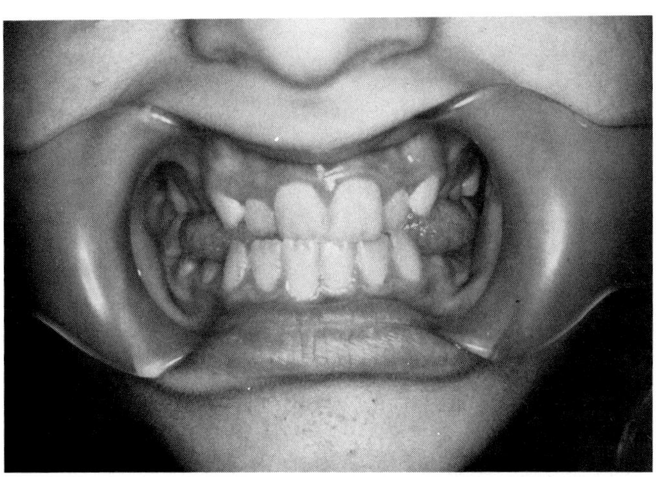

Fig. 24-7. Swallowing imbalance: bilateral force.

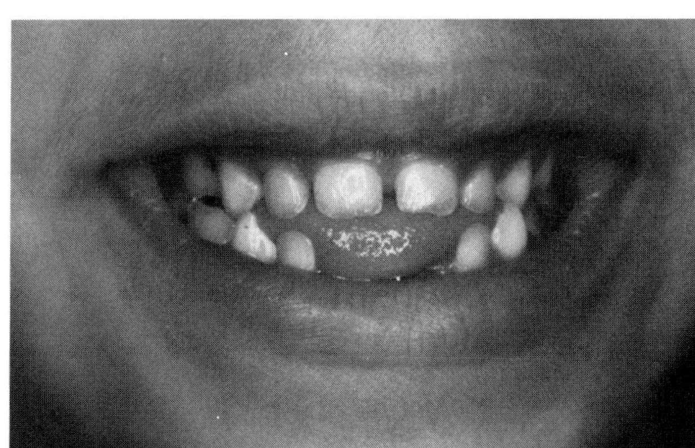

Fig. 24-8. Swallowing imbalance: mandibular force.

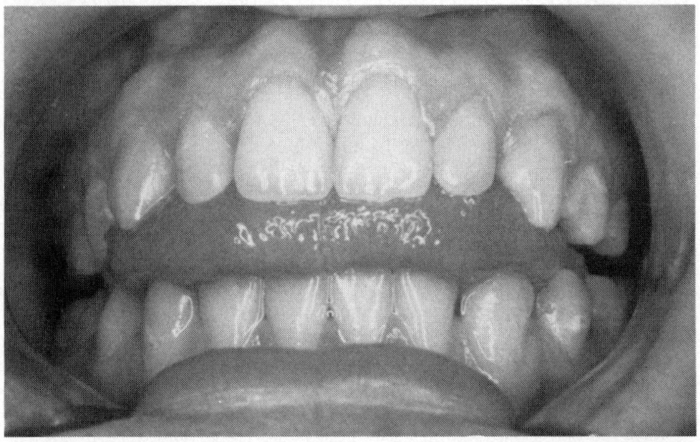

Fig. 24-9. Swallowing imbalance: molar-to-molar force.

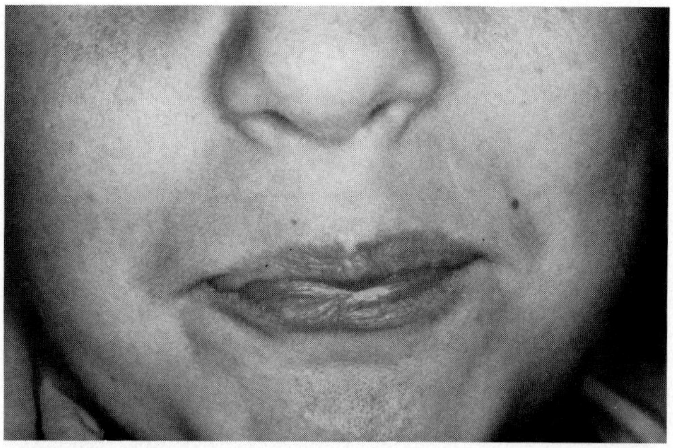

Fig. 24-10. Facial muscle activity during swallowing (grimace).

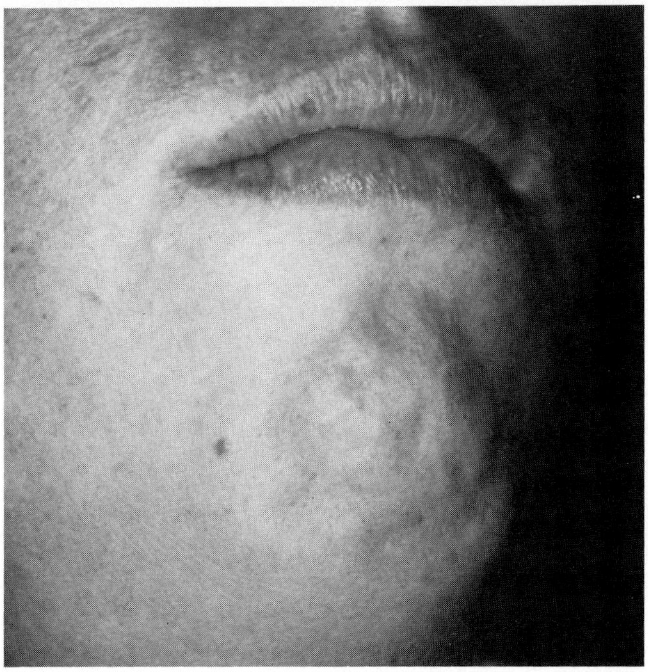

Fig. 24-11. Mentalis muscle activity during swallowing.

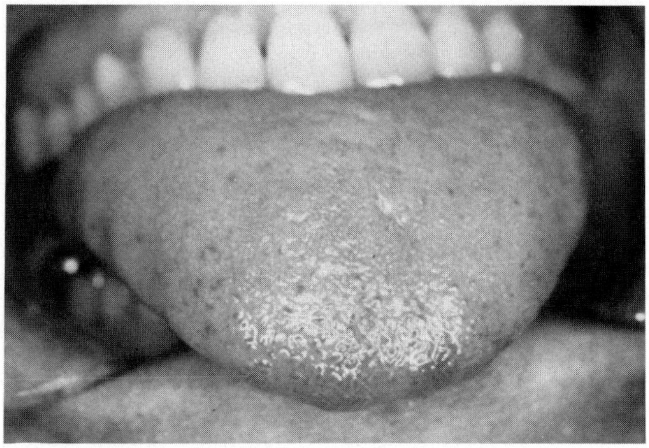

Fig. 24-12. Tongue scalloping indentations.

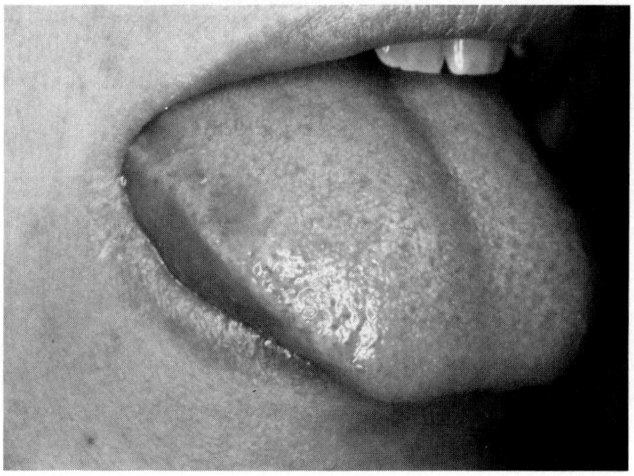

Fig. 24-13. Lateral border tongue ridge.

A 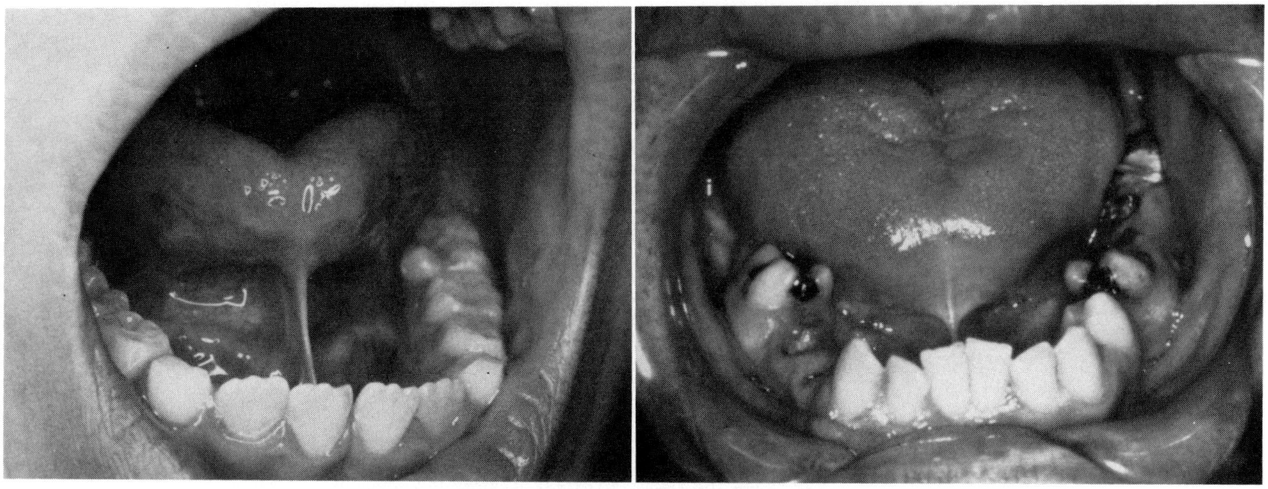 B

Fig. 24-14. A, Ankylotic tongue in child. **B,** Ankylotic tongue in adult.

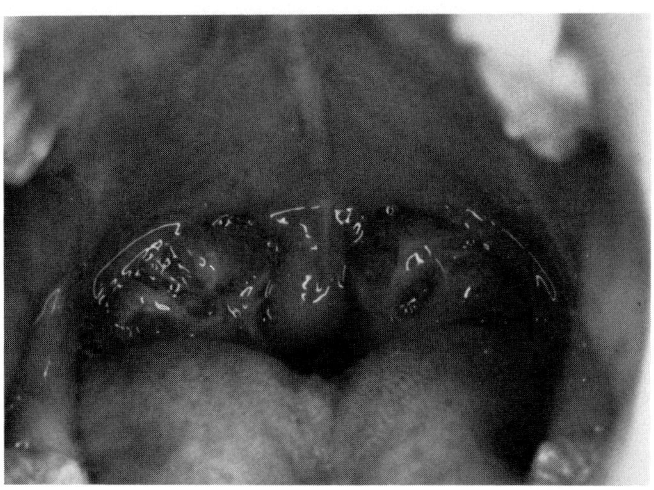

Fig. 24-15. Enlarged tonsillar tissue.

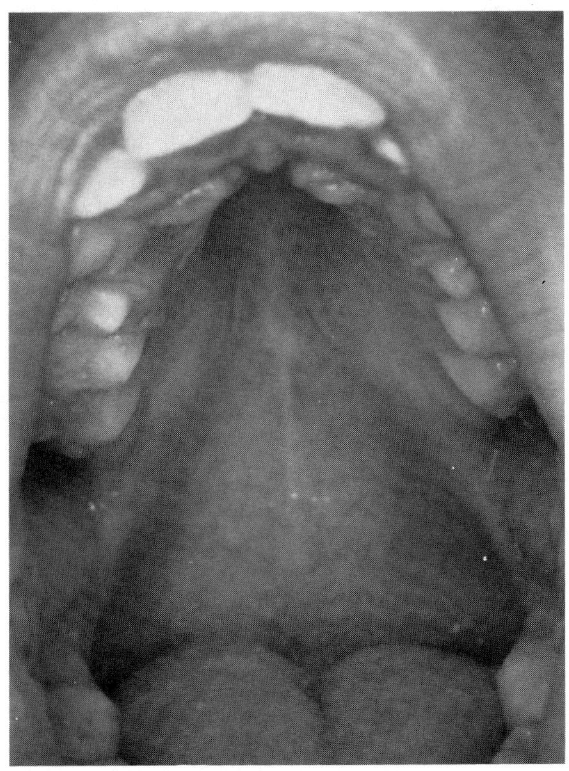

Fig. 24-16. Restricted, vaulted palatal arch.

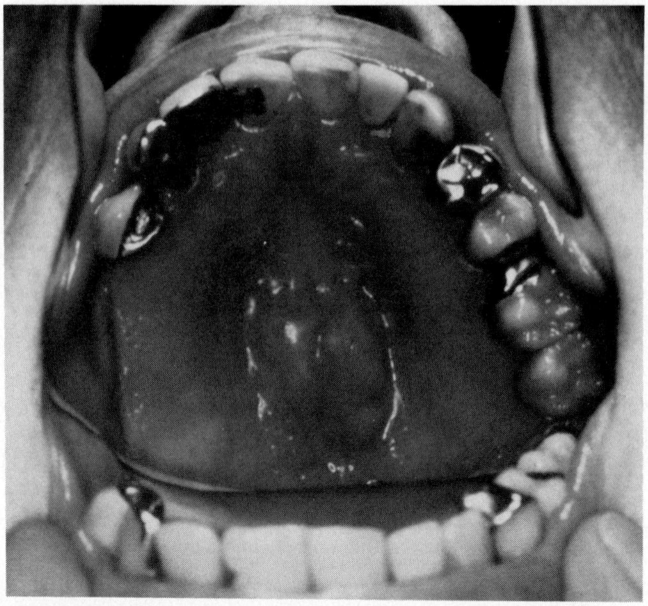

Fig. 24-17. Palatal tori.

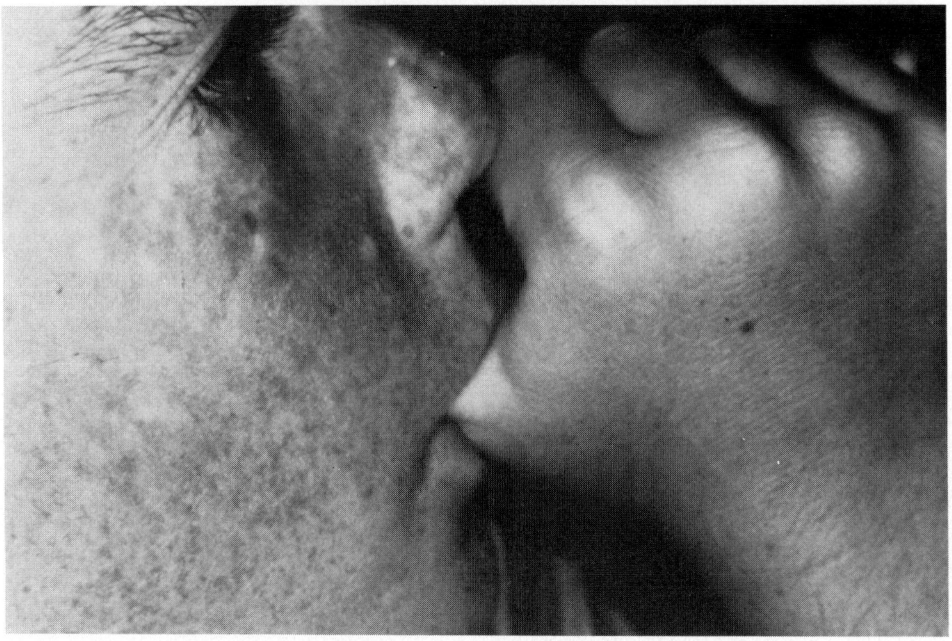

Fig. 24-18. Digit, thumb sucking.

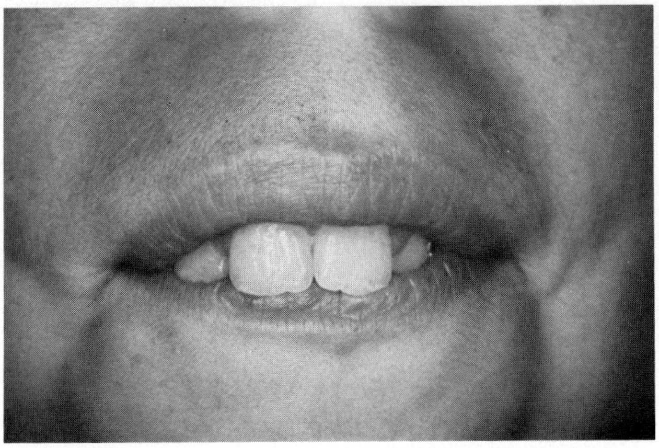

Fig. 24-19. Lip biting and sucking habit.

A

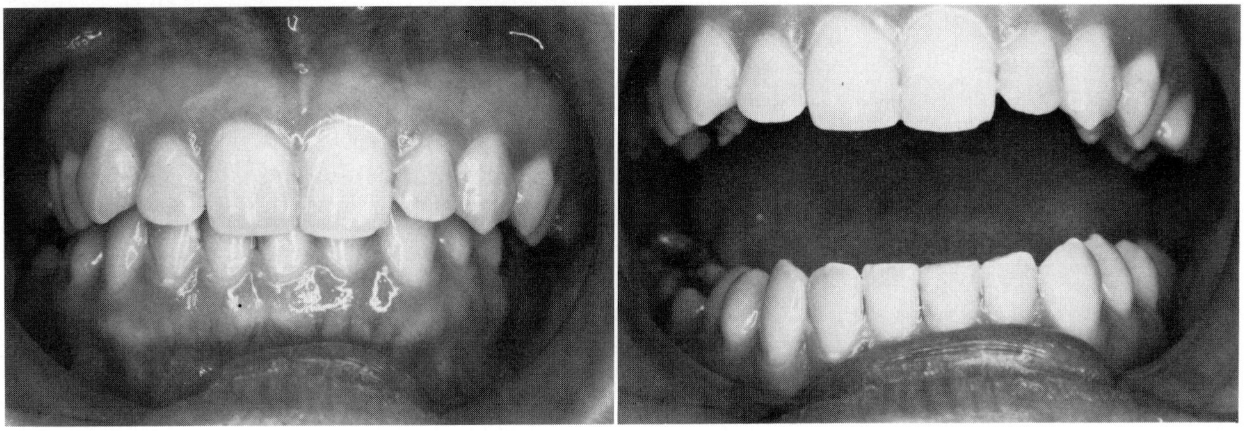

B

Fig. 24-20. A, Posture of jaw prior to opening. **B,** Jaw deviation after opening.

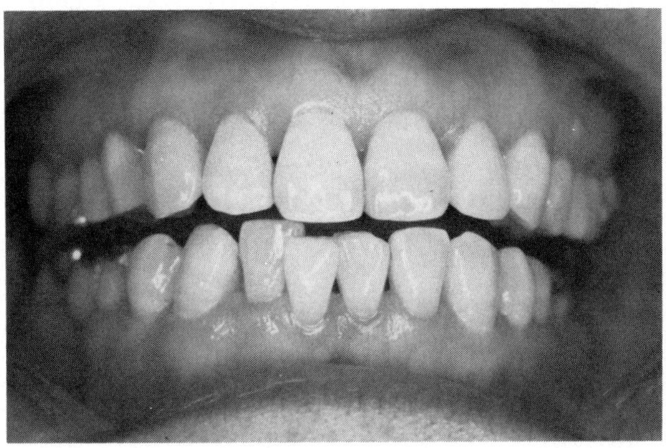

Fig. 24-21. Tooth migration.

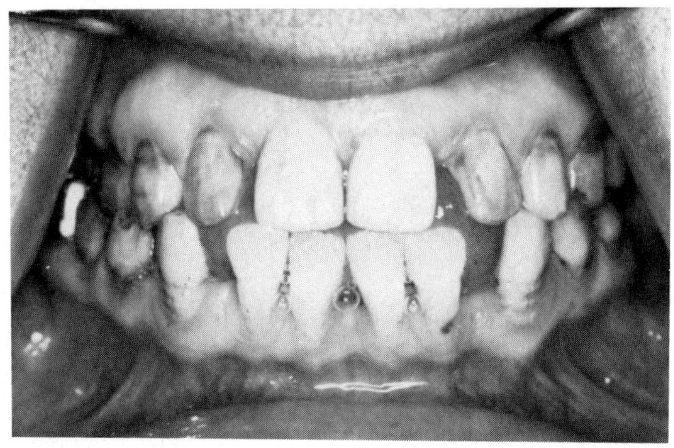

Fig. 24-22. Periodontal breakdown.

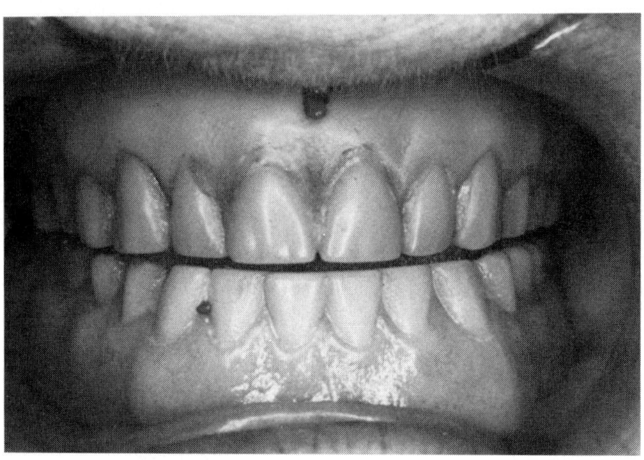

Fig. 24-23. Difficult denture retention.

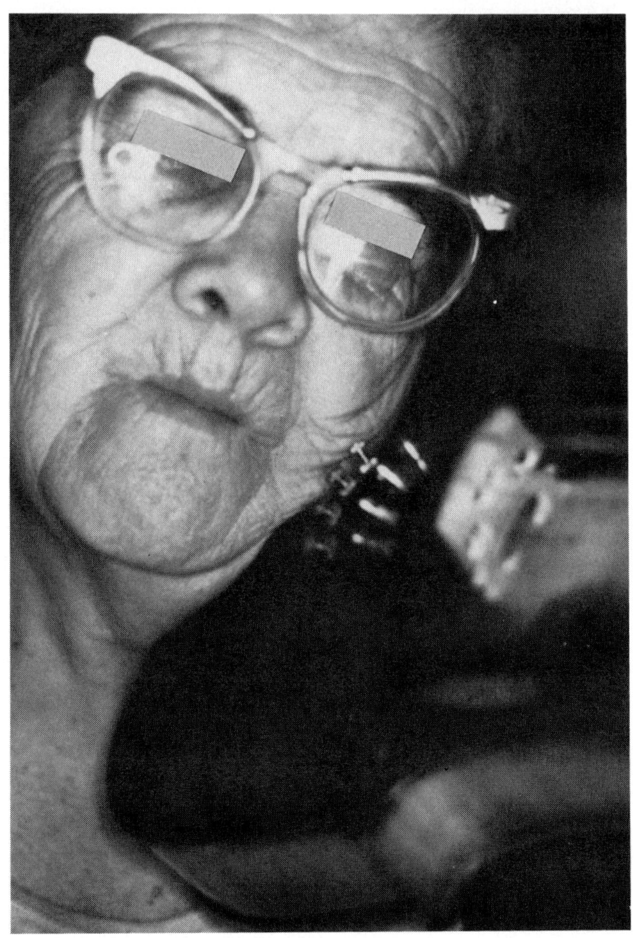

Fig. 24-24. Imbalancing muscle force because of position of musical instrument.

Case histories

Case 1. At the evaluation this 9-year-old boy presented as a thumb-sucker. He was a noncommunicative and very sickly child. He had continual nasal stuffiness, exhibited mouth breathing day and night, and had allergic tendencies as well as a history of colds, flu, ear infections, etc. There were the beginnings of speech distortions, with anterior lisping and visible tongue placement. Other symptoms noted were imbalanced facial symmetry, head held to the right, poor facial profile, lip weakness with a developing lip crease and mentalis muscle tension, ankylotic tongue, enlarged tonsillar tissue, poor developing dentition (open bite with Class II occlusion

A B C D

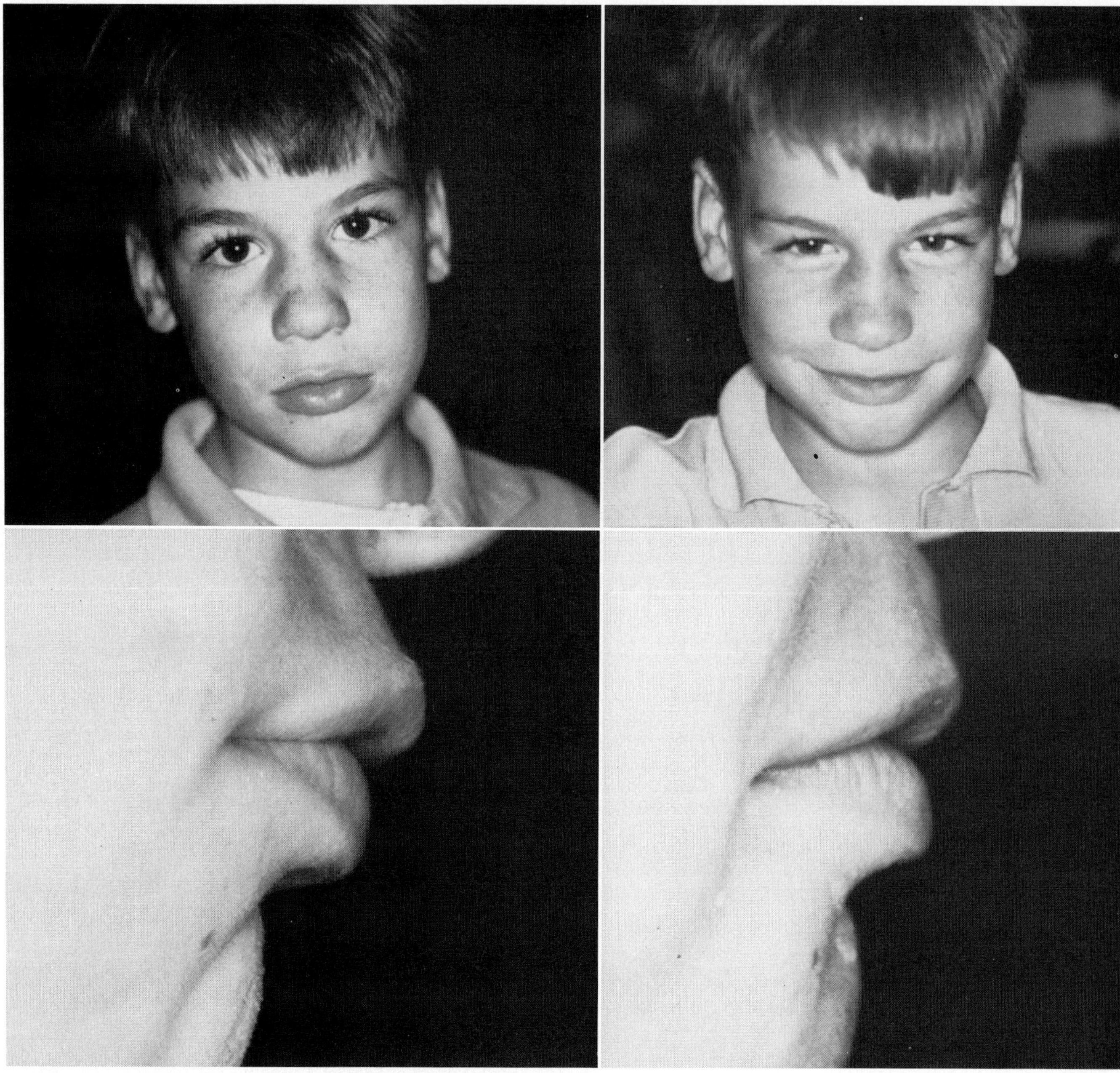

Fig. 24-25. A, Patient before therapy. **B,** Patient after therapy. **C,** Facial profile before therapy. **D,** Facial profile after therapy.

tendency), poor eating and drinking habits, and frequently poor habits such as leaning and stomach sleeping.

Following therapy (approximately 1 year later) there was a significant change in the health of the patient; he became a much happier, outgoing child; there was marked change in the facial contours and occlusal balance; and the speech distortion was altered (Fig. 24-25). The following therapy regimen was applied:

1. Surgery to correct the ankylotic tongue
2. Surgery to remove fibrous, engorged tonsillar mass
3. Corrective thumb therapy to stop the thumb sucking
4. Oral myofunctional therapy

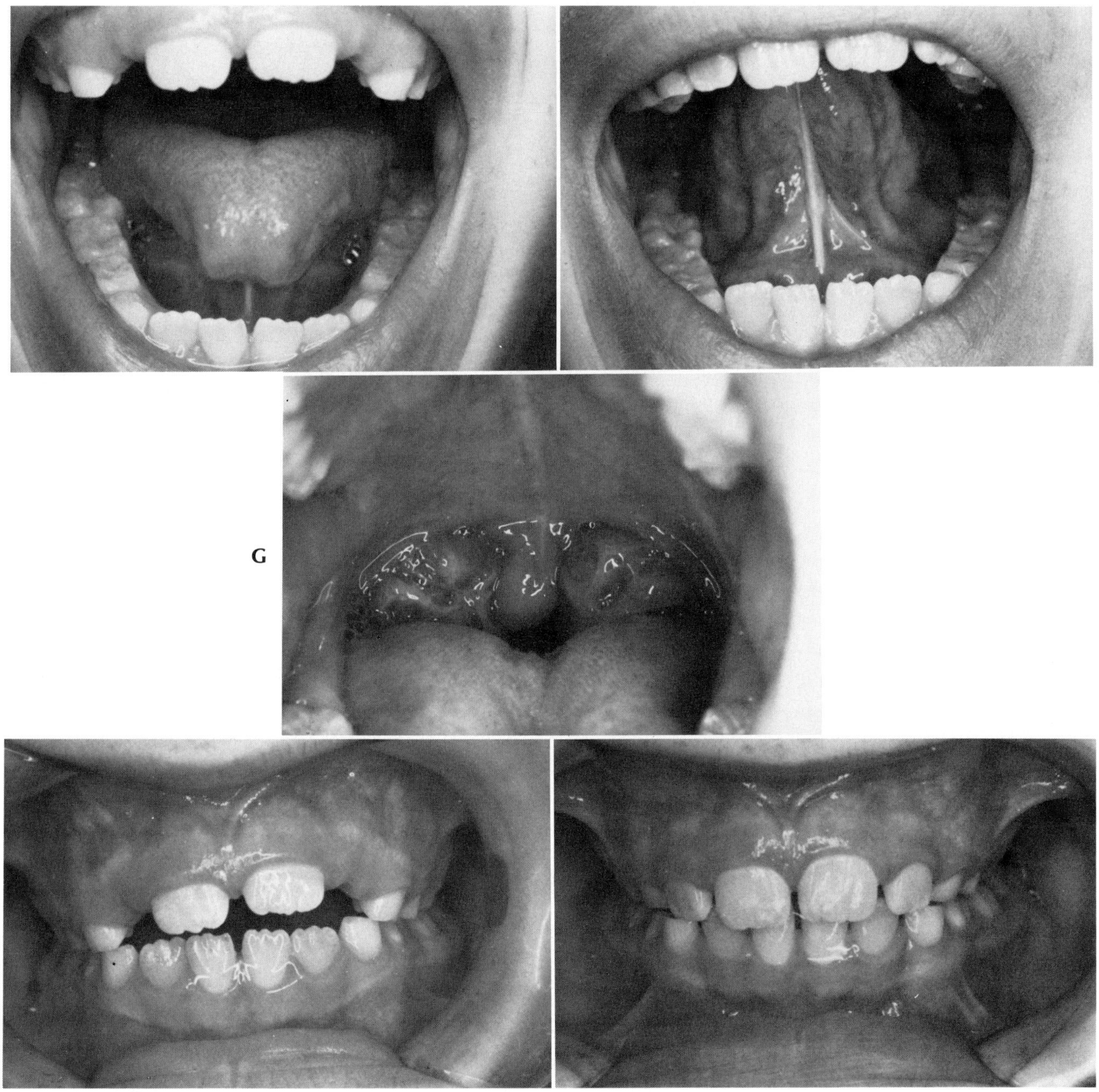

Fig. 24-25, cont'd. E, Ankylotic tongue before surgery. **F,** Tongue mobility after surgery. NOTE: Tongue should be able to touch palate with 38-mm stretch at least. **G,** Enlarged tonsillar mass prior to surgery. **H,** Occlusal relationship before therapy. **I,** Occlusal relationship after therapy.

Case 2. This young woman, age 23, presented at the evaluation with periodontal involvement of the lower anterior tooth quadrant. Periodontal surgery and home-care techniques had not been able to stop the progress of the bone loss and tissue inflammation. Tooth mobility was present, with anticipated tooth loss. Anterior bridgework was the next treatment planned if therapy failed to stop the periodontal breakdown.

The patient had a combination of the following muscle force imbalances:

1. A low-forward swallowing force
2. A restrictive labial frenum, causing tightness and pressure from the lower lip
3. Forward muscle activity during swallowing with mentalis muscle activity
4. A continuation of obvious facial tension during stressful periods with developing facial lines, a developing lip crease, and visible indentations on the inside lower lip tissue from the suction created between the tongue and lip
5. Tongue scalloping both anteriorly and posteriorly

After 9 months of therapy the patient looked much more relaxed, facial tension was markedly lessened with a decrease in facial "age" lines, and the lower anterior teeth were stable. There appeared to be a stabilizaton of the periodontal situation, and no dental treatment was necessary (Fig. 24-26).

The therapy regimen included the following:

1. Surgery to the labial frenum
2. Oral myofunctional therapy

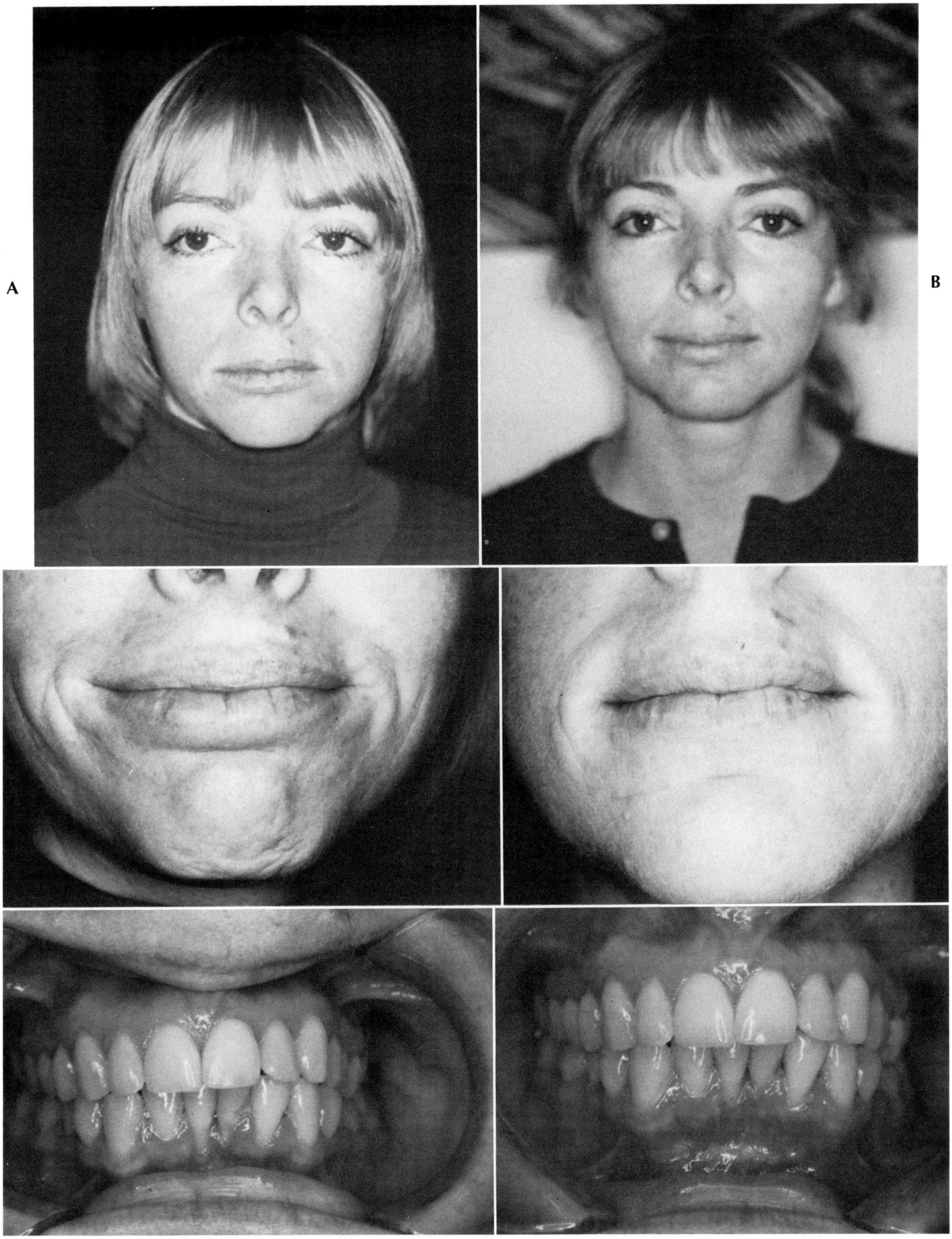

A B C D E F

Fig. 24-26. A, Patient before therapy. **B,** Patient after therapy. **C,** Facial tension before therapy. **D,** Freedom from stress evident in changed facial expression. **E,** Periodontal involvement of lower anterior tooth area. **F,** Stabilization after therapy.

Case 3. This young woman, 21 years old, presented with TMJ symptoms on the right side. Pain was present 24 hours a day, with pain symptoms in the entire right side of the head, face, neck, and shoulder areas. Ear pain, tinnitus, and fullness existed. Other observations were an imbalanced facial symmetry, carriage of the head to the right side, poor habits, fatigue, a unilateral swallowing, and resting tongue posture to the right side.

After therapy, pain symptoms disappeared totally except during stressful periods such as college examinations (when the splint was not worn). Facial symmetry and body contour changed dramatically. There was a marked change in the position in which the mandible was carried during swallowing and while at rest.

The therapy regimen included the following:

1. Oral myofunctional therapy was undertaken.
2. Splint therapy was initiated with an oral surgeon. The new bite registration was stabilized with the splint. This was worn all day at first and later just during the sleeping hours.
3. Orthodontic correction was instituted following oral myofunctional therapy and splint therapy (Fig. 24-27).

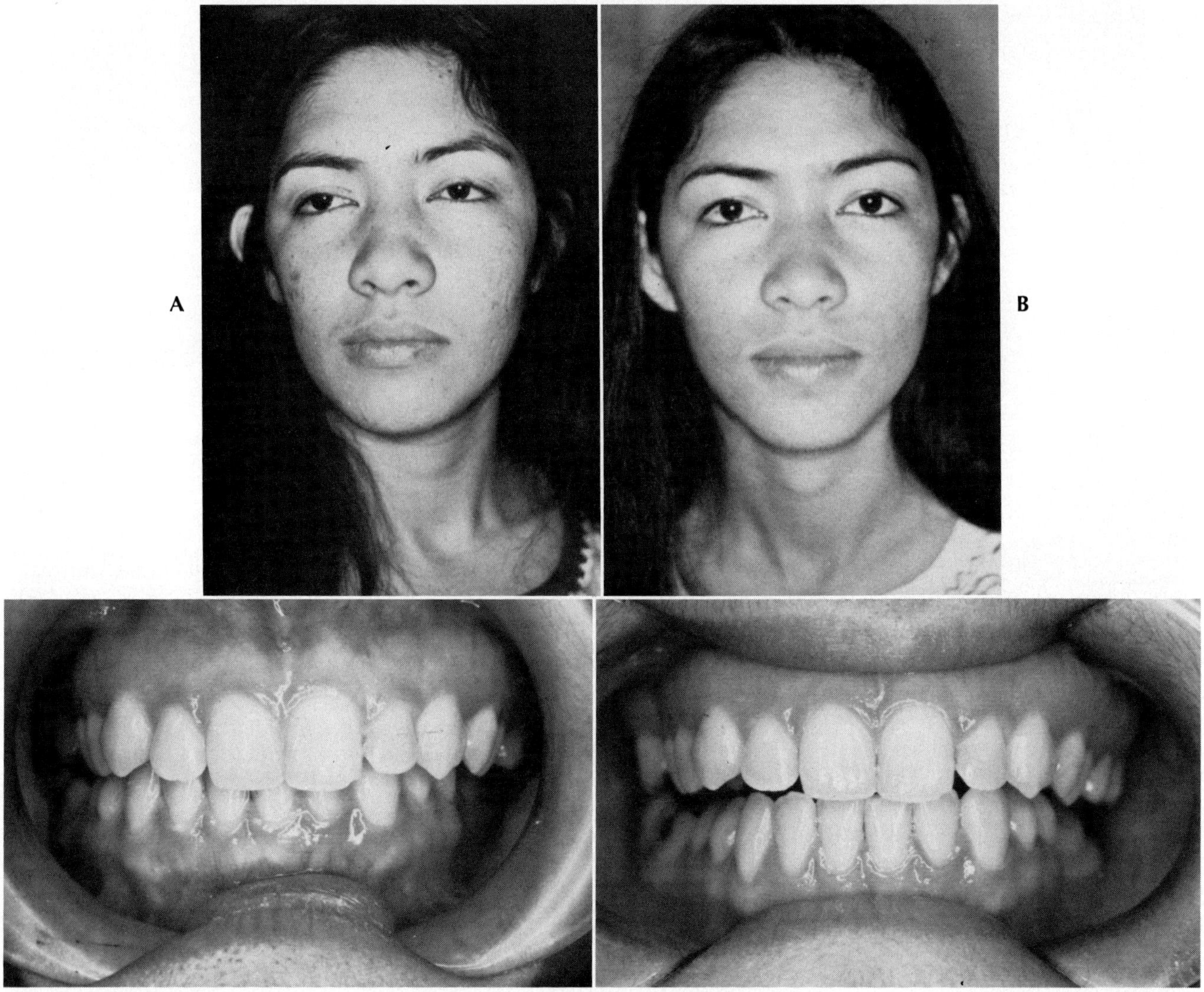

A B C D

Fig. 24-27. A, Patient before therapy. **B,** Patient after therapy. **C,** Occlusal relationship before therapy. **D,** Occlusal relationship after therapy.

Case 4. This 50-year-old woman presented with migration of the upper left central and lateral teeth. Following jacketing of the upper anterior centrals and laterals, the teeth on the patient's left began to migrate. An upper retainer was placed, and the teeth moved back into alignment. Within a short time migration once again occurred. Oral myofunctional therapy was recommended.

After 4 months of therapy an upper retainer was once again placed, with the teeth again moving into alignment. This time the teeth remained in place (Fig. 24-28).

The therapy regimen included the following:

1. Oral myofunctional therapy
2. Correction of imbalance habits
3. Orthodontic retainer

A B C D

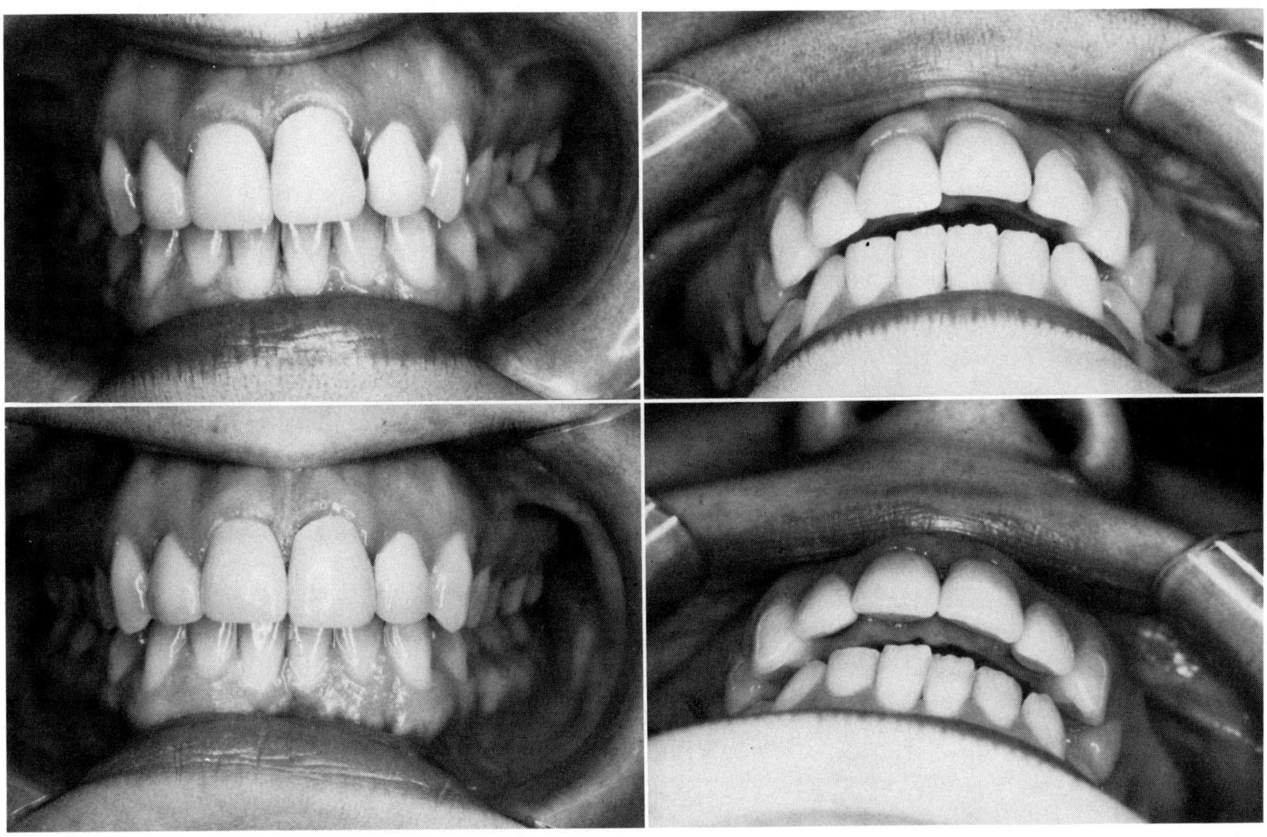

Fig. 24-28. A and **B,** Patient before therapy. **C,** Patient following therapy of muscle imbalance and tooth movement with retainer. **D,** Patient after therapy.

Case 5. This 10-year-old girl presented with an orthodontic cross-bite, diagnosed by her orthodontist as a muscular cross-bite rather than a true orthodontic cross-bite. She was a mouth breather, resting tongue posture was forward and visible with a right lateral flare, swallowing pressures were forward and to the right, touching the cheek tissue, lips were weak, constant nasal congestion with allergic tendencies were present, frequent colds existed, and there was a severe lisp on all *s* sounds with a right lateral flare and lateral sound distortion. Many habits existed, such as biting the right lip area and right cheek, holding the tongue to the left, leaning on the right side, stomach sleeping, and improper eating habits.

Following therapy there was a marked change in the allergic tendencies. Nasal congestion still occurred but only infrequently. The facial asymmetry, previously full on the right and flat on the left, changed to an equal balance following therapy. Poor habit patterns ceased. The occlusal relationship changed dramatically, with the patient being observed by her orthodontist at this time. Speech therapy following oral muscle reeducation facilitated correction of the speech defect (Fig. 24-29).

The therapy regimen included the following:

1. Oral myofunctional therapy
2. Speech therapy
3. Orthodontic observation with orthodontic correction in the future, if necessary
4. Diet modifications

A

B

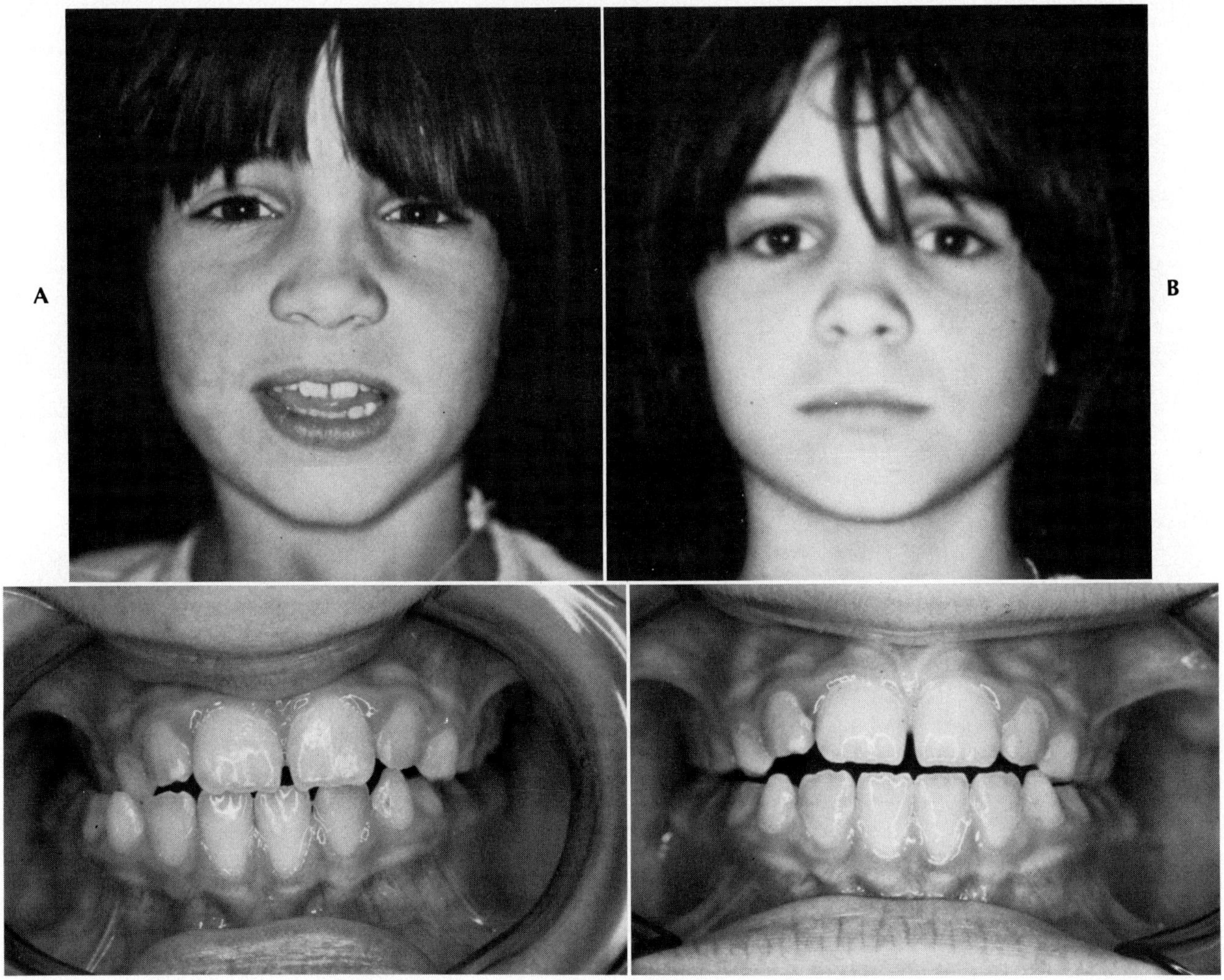

C

D

Fig. 24-29. A, Patient before therapy. **B,** Patient after therapy. **C,** Occlusal relationship before therapy. **D,** Occlusal relationship after therapy.

PART II*

Other therapy regimens

Oral myofunctional therapy has had many failures and unfortunately continues to do so. There are perhaps two reasons why this plethora of unsuccessfully treated patients has and continues to exist. First, there has been insufficient understanding of the interactions of the *entire* body; and second, there has been inadequate background and training of many, if not most, of those practitioners who provide oral myofunctional therapy.

Selection of a treatment modality

Once it is recognized that a problem of muscle imbalance, improper nasal respiration, or abnormal deglutition exists (or any combination of these problems), the next step is the selection of the mode(s) of therapy indicated. When more than one treatment discipline is indicated (and this is the case more often than not), it is extremely important that the sequence in which the modalities are instituted be programmed in the correct order. Maintaining a high level of motivation in patients undergoing oral myofunctional therapy is a never-ending problem for therapists, and if the treatment is unnecessarily protracted because of attempts to solve the problem without building the proper foundation, the case may end in dismal failure. Examples of therapy out of sequence would be the attempt to correct mouth breathing without first establishing a patent nasal airway, or attempting to teach a patient to swallow with the tongue raised to the roof of the mouth with a narrow constricted arch that will not accommodate the tongue's width.

Modalities available. At our disposal we have an impressive number and variety of treatment modalities that can be used to help solve the sometimes involved problems that occur in the field of oral myology. An incomplete list of disciplines that can be used includes acupuncture (both classic and electroacupuncture), biofeedback, cranial osteopathy, and the sacral-occipital technique (SOT) of chiropractic, homeopathy, applied kinesiology, physical therapy faciliatation, nutrition (including detoxification), behavior modification techniques, mandibular repositioning therapy, orthodontics, and of course the exercise and muscle development programs that work specifically with oral musculature.

A short description of these newer disciplines and their application, clinically, to oral myofunctional therapy will perhaps demonstrate the necessity of using care in the treatment-planning sequence for patients requiring aid. An attempt is made to consider the disciplines in a logical order of priority, as would be done in the evaluation of an actual case.

*This section was contributed by Richard S. Sheppard, D.D.S.

Structural considerations

The most basic consideration that must be evaluated when planning a treatment sequence for a patient requiring oral myofunctional therapy is the structures involved with the muscles to be therapeutically treated. The term *structures* is used in deference to the term *form*. The ongoing controversy of what determines what in discussion of *form* versus *function* is not considered here. Regardless of how one may feel about this controversy, the structures are still of paramount importance and must be evaluated first. Most of the inobvious structural deformation occurs during prenatal life and the trauma associated with the act of birth. This cranial bone malalignment, or *cranial faults*, result in loss of correct function in the cerebrospinal mechanism.[6] How critical the proper relationship of the cranial bones can be is demonstrated by consideration of the temporal bones, containing the mandibular fossa and eminence. If one of or both the temporal bones are locked in a rotated position, the resultant malpositioning of the mandibular fossa will cause the mandible to be displaced in one of four ways. If both the temporals happen to be locked in external rotation, the mandible will be forced into a more retruded position and will carry the associated musculature, including the tongue, with it. The result of a retruded or distal positioning of the mandible is encroachment by the tongue in the area of the tonsillar fauces. If the temporals are both locked in internal rotation, the effect on the mandible through the mandibular fossae relationship will be a protruded position, therefore causing encroachment by the tongue in the area of the anterior maxillary teeth. A third condition can arise where one of the temporal bones is functioning normally, and the other is locked. This will result in a twist of the mandible and a stretching effect on the associated musculature on one side. The final condition that may be present is where one temporal bone is locked in internal rotation, and the other is locked in external rotation. The net effect of this situation is a parallelogram effect, which again causes a twisting of the mandible and stretching of musculature and ligaments.

In any of the situations just described the resulting muscle function during deglutition and speech to some degree will be abnormal or compensatory in nature. When abnormal or compensatory function is continued for an extended period, there are several possible areas that may be adversely affected. The first of these is the temporomandibular joint itself. The condylar disc may become perforated, resulting in crepitus. The capsular ligaments may become stretched, which may result in cracking or popping as the mandible opens and closes. Or degenerative changes may occur in the bony structure of the head of the condyle, the eminence or mandibular fossa of the temporal bone, or all three. Muscles, such as the external pterygoid or temporal, may either go into spasm or become extremely tender from prolonged stretching. Deformations of the dental arches and occlusion may result from the continuous unbalanced muscle pull and abnormal function. One additional symptom that may occur as a result of locked rotations of the temporal bones is tinnitus.

It seems obvious that attempting to teach muscles to function properly in the face of malfunctioning or distorted structures is to court failure for the patient and discouragement for the therapist. Through evaluations by the techniques used in cranial osteopathy and the sacral-occipital techniques of chiropractic,[2] structural disharmonies in both cranial structure and function can be discovered and in most cases successfully reduced. It also will be found in a great many cases that when cranial faults and malfunctions are eliminated, a number of the patient's symptoms improve or disappear. Allergic rhinitis, chronic sinusitis, chronic tonsillitis, and ear problems are a few of the conditions that may clear with the successful use of cranial techniques. A reduction in symptoms in any of these areas is an obvious benefit to oral myofunctional therapy.

The four *obvious* structural deformations that must be corrected before actual muscle therapy can be successfully instituted are the following:

1. Incorrect mandibular position
2. Insufficient width of the maxillary arch to accommodate the width of the tongue
3. Deviations in the nasal septum that result in the loss of a patent nasal airway
4. A tongue overly limited in its excursions because of restrictions by the lingual frenum

Orthopedic repositioning therapy is needed in cases of mandibular malposition. Orthodontic corrections are usually indicated in cases of constricted maxillary arches, and surgical corrections are required in cases of severely deviated nasal septums and tongue ties.

Evaluation of allergic and toxic conditions

Next in the order of importance is an evaluation of the allergic and toxic conditions of the patient. A complete evaluation of these conditions by necessity requires the overlapping and interplay of several individual disciplines. However, an attempt is made here to show how this may be accomplished effectively. Starting with history forms, such as *Symptom Survey Form* published by Standard Process Laboratories and the *Cornell Medical Index*, an excellent insight can be obtained as to the patient's nutritional status and as to what systems or organs of the body are being adversely affected. These forms, together with their appropriate keys, provide the basis for a nutritional program designed for detoxification and nutritional support for the patient, based on that person's individual needs. The basic program may be refined through the use of hair analysis and other laboratory procedures.

Another very common finding in patients is that they are suffering from toxic-allergic reactions to dental materials that have been used for restorative procedures in their mouths. The allergic reactions to dental materials cannot be controlled nutritionally, and many times it is impractical to replace the materials involved with alternate choices. Fortunately developments in the field of homeopathy[8] can now provide a means of neutralizing the negative effects the patient may be experiencing from dental materials.

The science of homeopathy[4] was first discovered by Samuel Hahnemann, a German physician who lived in the latter part of the eighteenth and first part of the nineteenth century. The principle of homeopathic treatment is that "similar cures similar," and this principle currently is used by all physicians working in the field of immunization. A common example of this principle is the treatment of an allergy to ragweed by giving the allergic patient a ragweed substance in diluted form. Homeopathic medications of dental materials, or for that matter any material, are made by taking a small amount of the substance to be "potenized," diluting it with either alcohol or distilled water, and then "succussing," that is, shaking, the solution a few times. Then a quantity of this solution is diluted again, usually on a 10:1 basis, and again succussed. This process is continued until the desired potency or dilution is obtained. The material thus potenized, in this case dental material, is then administered to the patient, and a "cure," or neutralization of the detrimental effects of the material in the mouth, takes place.

Other common findings are adverse reactions to pesticides, herbicides, and the heavy metals, plus noxious gases that occur in polluted air. The reactions of these materials in the body commonly affect the nervous system, including the cranial nerves. Many nervous tics of the face can be effectively treated through the use of homeopathic medications made from the material(s) causing the problem. The obvious question that arises is how to determine which material or materials are responsible for the toxic-allergic response. This can now be accomplished in one of two ways: first, by using the muscle testing techniques of applied kinesiology[3,5,9] and matching materials, both homeopathic and nutritional, to the patient's needs. The second way that medications and nutritional supplements may be matched with the patient's requirements is

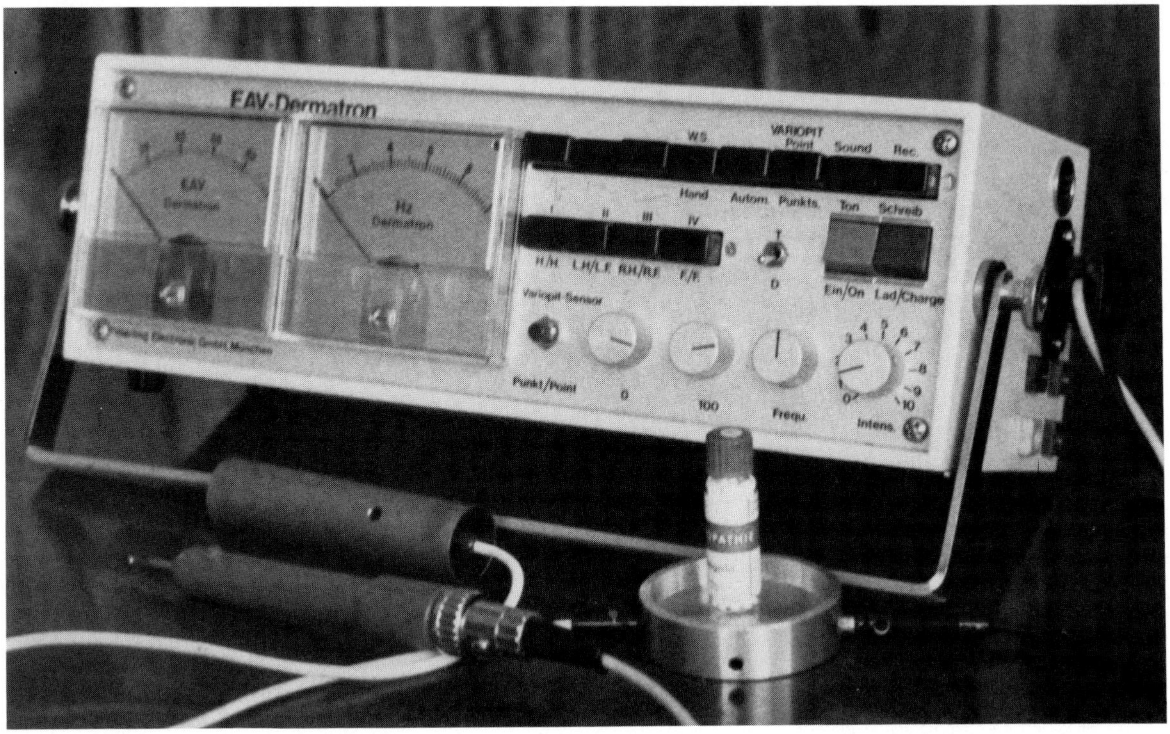

Fig. 24-30. Dermatron, electroacupuncture instrument used for acupuncture meridian diagnosis and determination of proper medication.

through the use of the Dermatron instrument and EAV (as described in *Electroacupuncture According to Voll*[7]). Each of these techniques is briefly discussed, and the reader is encouraged to more fully explore these disciplines through the references given.

Reinhold Voll,[7,8] a German physician, has developed a technique and an instrument—the Dermatron—that enable the operator to "match" homeopathic medications and other materials on the patient's acupuncture points (Fig. 24-30). The correct medication will normalize the acupuncture points' energy and will alleviate or cure the patient's problem. The Dermatron also correctly measures the potencies of medicines the patient should take, whether they are homeopathic medications, food supplements, or even raw herbs. A knowledge of acupuncture and meridian therapy is a prerequisite for effective use of the Dermatron and EAV. At the time of this writing the Dermatron is still considered experimental in the United States, but it has been extensively used in Europe for some years. Voll has been developing the technique and expanding its range of usefulness for over 20 years.

Applied kinesiology has been developed to its present state largely through the efforts and insight of a chiropractor, George Goodheart, D.C., of Detroit. Briefly, applied kinesiology is a technique that involves testing muscles of the body and correlating the strength and weaknesses of these muscles with organs, systems, and structures. Through a vast amount of clinical trial and error it has been shown that one given muscle can relate to (1) a particular tooth, (2) a particular organ, (3) a particular acupuncture meridian, (4) a particular food supplement, and (5) a particular structure. If any one of these relating items is malfunctioning, the muscle will test weak. The efficacy of treatment therapy therefore can be easily evaluated by retesting the muscle after the corrections have been made, because if the muscle then tests strong, the proper treatment has been given. The objection to the muscle testing procedures of applied kinesiology is that the results are measured completely on a subjective basis rather than objectively. Several instruments now have been developed to objectively measure the differences in muscle resistance, so that now muscle strength can be measured both before and after therapy (Fig. 24-31). As documentation using these instruments is accumulated to support the subjective clinical results, this objection to applied kinesiology should be overcome.

Muscle functional training

After the forgoing procedures the patient should be structurally sound, have his or her allergic and toxic conditions controlled or neutralized, and be nutritionally programmed to maintain optimum conditions so that the actual muscle functional training or retraining can begin with a high expectation for success. The sequence of events required for successful myofunctional therapy can be likened to a piano, a piano tuner, a piano teacher, and a music student. Regardless of the skill of the teacher and the highly motivated efforts of the student, the music produced will sound terrible if the piano is badly out of tune. But if the piano tuner first properly tunes the piano, then the efforts of the piano teacher, with the motivated student, will produce music that is pleasant to the ear, or at least as the composer intended.

Oral myofunctional therapy (the actual muscle training) can be viewed as being of two types—passive and active. The passive type of therapy in most cases will be the first to be indicated. In passive therapy functional appliances such as Bionators, Activators, Frankel, and some TMJ repositioning appliances are used to guide the tongue and strengthen the musculature. All these functional appliances will develop oral structures as well as establish correct mandibular position. The second type of therapy, the active type, will be needed at times to supplement the passive therapy and at other times will be primarily indicated. If passive therapy was indicated (for example, additional palatal width was required for correct tongue placement) and the patient has worn the appliance until the required development has been obtained but correct muscle action is still lacking during swallowing, then active therapy must be started. Active therapy would be primarily indicated in those cases where neither arch development nor changes are required and there is correct mandibular position. Active therapy refers to the various exercises and habit-forming techniques that are used to strengthen muscles and retrain them in correct patterns of deglutition, speech, and resting posture.

Appliances have long been used to discourage the tongue, in its excursions within the mouth, from traveling to areas where the pressure exerted produces deleterious effects. The appliances are of the removable type as well as those cemented to the teeth with orthodontic bands. Barbed rakes, palatal traps, and variously designed fences have been used with only poor to limited results. Inasmuch as swallowing is a subconscious neuromuscular action, it is not surprising that when these inhibiting appliances are removed, the patient returns to the subconscious pattern that has always been used. Some removable appliances that are

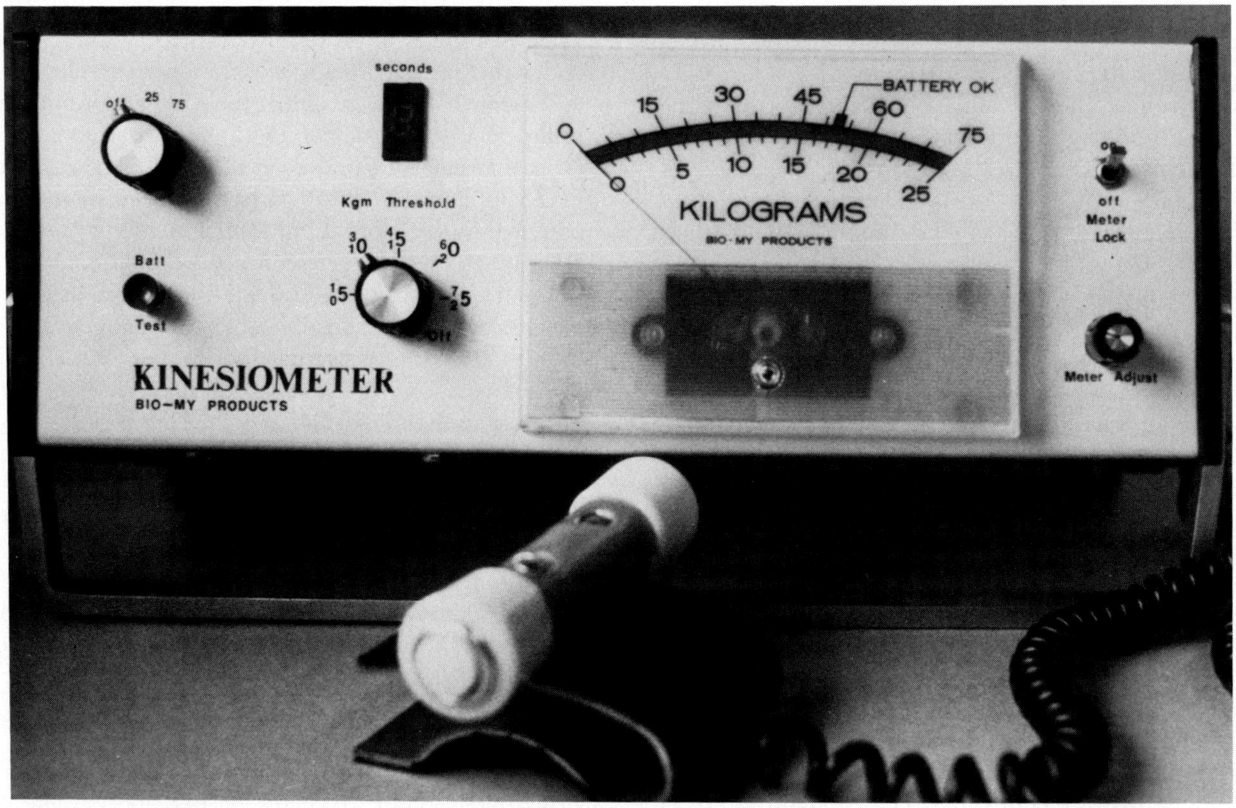

Fig. 24-31. Kinesiometer, tension-measuring instrument used to obtain objective values in applied kinesiology techniques.

used in conjunction with functional orthodontics and temporomandibular joint repositioning have shown promise in training tongue movement by guiding it to correct positions (Fig. 24-32). It would appear that the guidance appliance affirmatively influences the neuromuscular reflexes, whereas the inhibitory types—the rakes and fences—have little if any effect on the subconscious patterns.

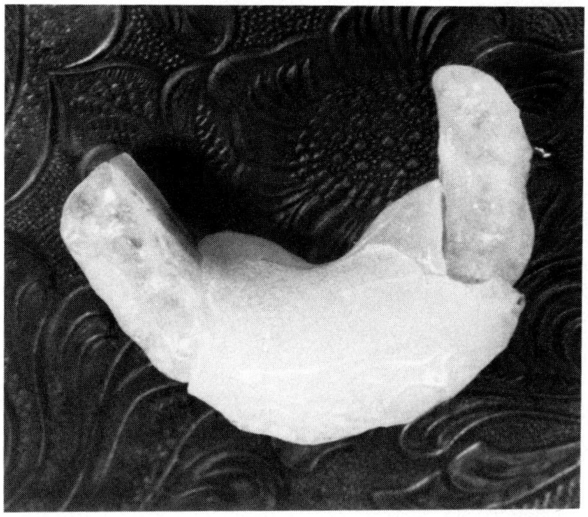

Fig. 24-32. Mandibular intraoral appliance used to guide tongue to proper location in oral cavity.

Numerous exercises (ably described in the writings of Barrett and Hanson[1] and Garliner[4]) have been developed to strengthen weak muscles that through disuse have suffered atrophy and therefore cannot perform the swallowing act correctly. This muscle weakness may be either bilateral or unilateral. other exercises have been designed to teach the proper oral locations and correct sequential order the tongue and associated oral musculature must use to effect a normal or correct act of deglutition. These exercises must be repeated frequently for a rather extensive period to be effective, and therefore the ability of the therapist to maintain motivation in the patient is all important. Behavior modification techniques are used by some therapists with excellent results as an aid in maintaining the necessary level of motivation.

Various instruments and devices are available for obtaining both a more accurate diagnosis and a basis on which to measure results. Some of these instruments also may be used as teaching aids. Biofeedback for monitoring the tongue's movements in the mouth (Fig. 24-33), habit-breaking devices for chronic mouth

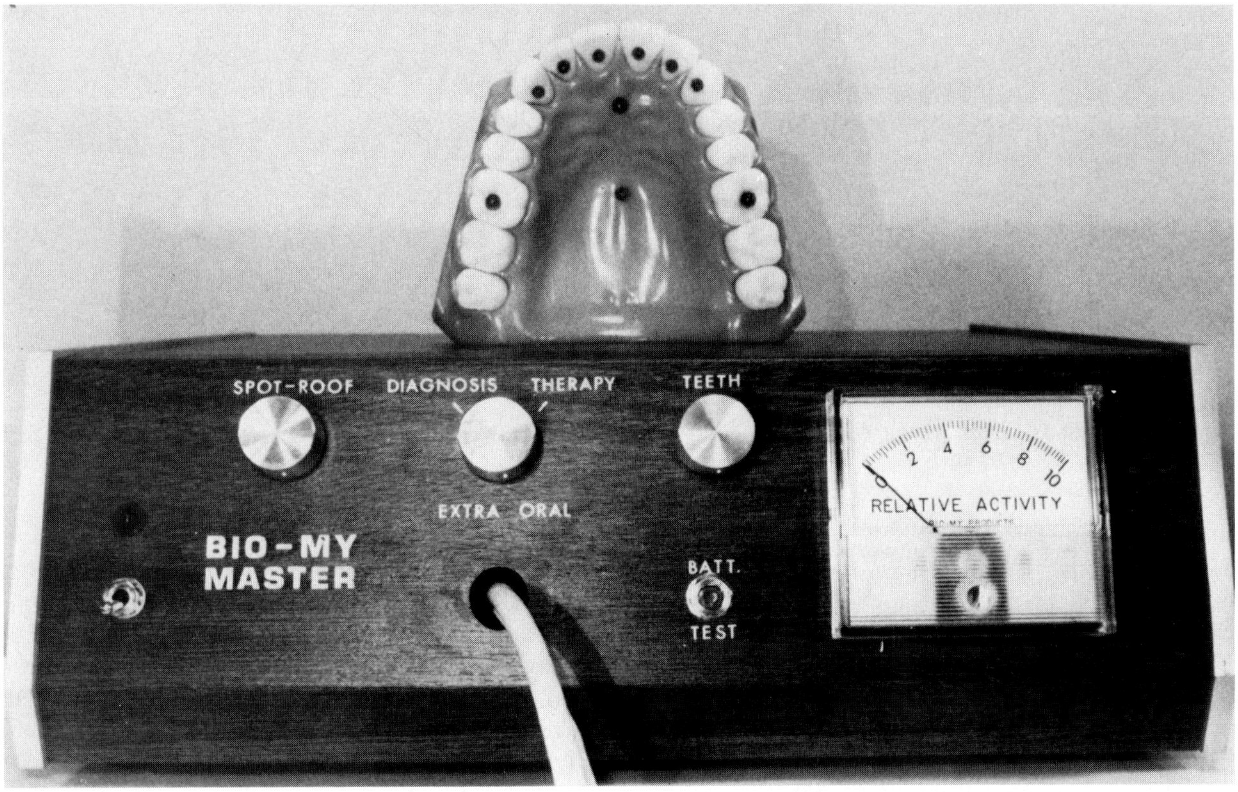

Fig. 24-33. Bio-My Master, six-channel biofeedback instrument used in diagnosis and therapy in oral muscle retraining.

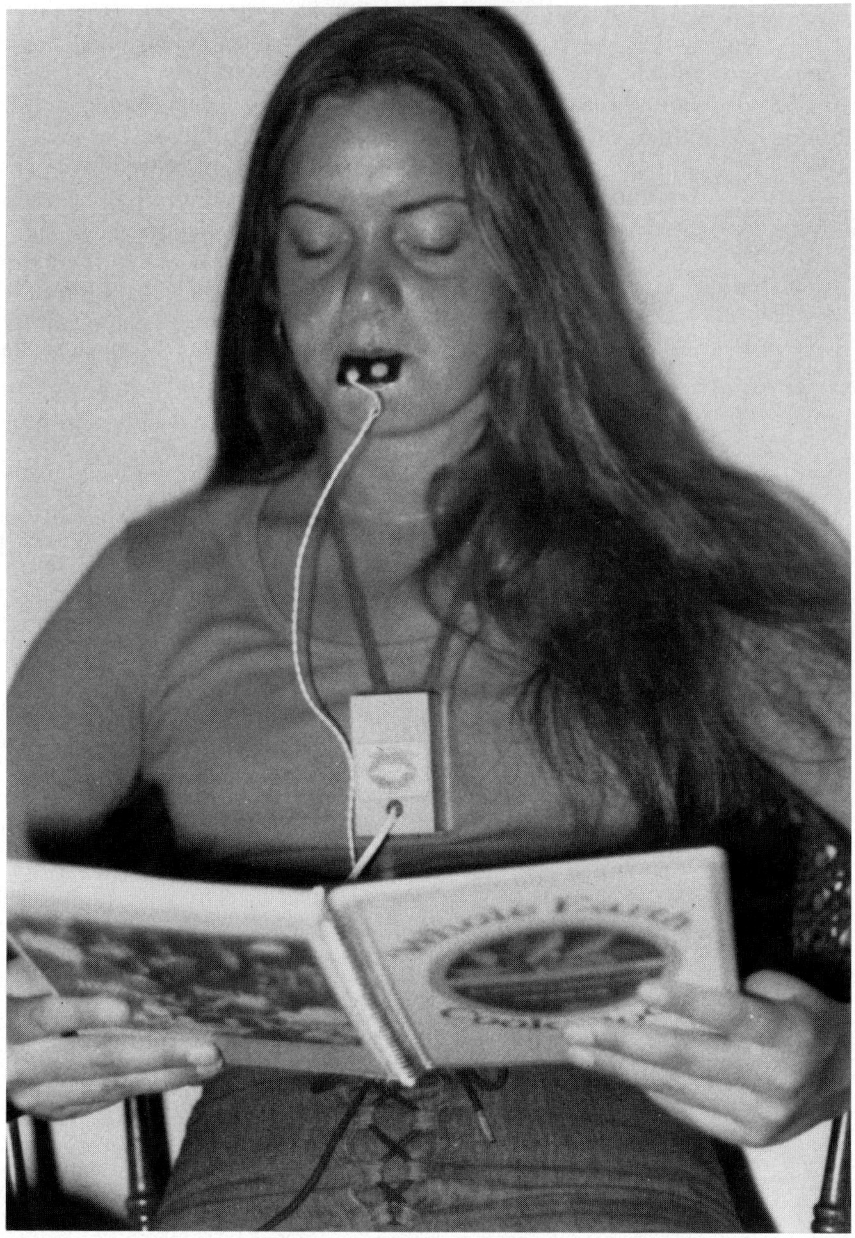

Fig. 24-34. Patient using LIP-EX, device used in breaking habitual mouth breathing. When lips are not held together, buzzer sounds.

breathing (Fig. 24-34), and tension-measuring instruments for ascertaining muscle strengths are some of the equipment used to facilitate therapy. Another most useful technique is the use of subconscious reminders; these may be either drawings, pictures, small objects, or cards. With one of these reminders placed in an obvious location, such as in front of the dinner plate, the patient receives a nonverbal cue to swallow correctly, breathe nasally, or any other lesson that he or she is learning.

Conclusion

We have shown that there are numerous disciplines and techniques available to correct muscle imbalances, neuromuscular reflexes, and the peripheral discrepancies that are present within the overall field of oral myofunctional therapy. Many of the "failures" in therapy and the sometimes high rate of recidivism of treated patients are the result of an incomplete differential diagnosis or the implementation of procedures in the incorrect order. Unfortunately most oral myology therapists and dentists do not have the required background in all the various subjects involved to adequately diagnose, much less treat, a patient *completely*. In most cases it becomes necessary for several practitioners to be involved to achieve overall success. The disenchantment that many people have with oral myofunctional therapy is not the fault of the therapist, since most therapists perform a conscientious, thorough effort to correct their patient's problem. The problem lies in lack of sufficient background and training to fully understand and appreciate the difficulties of the situation they are treating. It would appear at this time that what is needed in the field of oral myology is a reevaluation of the overall problem and decisions as to what disciplines must be taught as background and what licensure should be required so patients can receive adequate therapy that is economically feasible.

An example of how the problem of overall therapy can be minimized is found in conservative (nonsurgical) treatment of TMJ cases. It is becoming common practice for a dentist to work in cooperation with a cranial chiropractor or cranial osteopath. While the dentist is performing splint therapy to establish vertical and anteroposterior occlusion, the cranial practitioner is eliminating faults and establishing proper function of the cerebrospinal mechanism. At the same time one or the other is detoxifying the patient, nutritionally balancing the diet, and perhaps providing tension-control therapy. With only two practitioners involved, the patient receives complete treatment. This concept must be embraced to broaden the therapeutic base of oral myofunctional therapy, as it is employed both in the treatment of TMJ cases as well as in routine abnormal muscle function during deglutition and speech.

REFERENCES

1. Barrett, R.H., and Hanson, M.L.: Oral myofunctional disorders, ed. 2, St. Louis, 1978, The C.V. Mosby Co.
2. DeJarnette, B.: Sacral-occipital technic, Nebraska City, 1979.
3. Eversaul, G.A.: Dental kinesiology, Las Vegas, 1978, George A. Eversaul.
4. Garliner, D.: Myofunctional therapy in dental practice, ed. 2, Brooklyn, 1978, Bartel Dental Book Co.
5. Kendall, H.O., et al.: Muscles: testing and functions, ed. 2, Baltimore, 1971, Williams & Wilkins Co.
6. Magoun, H.I.: Osteopathy in the cranial field, ed. 3, Kirksville, Mo., 1976, Journal Printing Co.
7. Voll, R.: Electroacupuncture according to Voll, English ed. 1, Vols. 1 to 4, Uelzen, W. Germany, 1978, C. Beckers Buchdruckerei.
8. Voll, R.: Interrelationships of odontons and tonsils, English ed. 1, Uelzen, W. Germany, 1978, C. Beckers Buchdruckerei.
9. Walther, D.S.: Applied kinesiology, Pueblo, Colo., 1976, Systems DC.

25 Psychological treatment

WARREN L. JONES, M.D., Ph.D.

The title of this book promises a multidisciplinary approach to the diseases of the temporomandibular apparatus, necessitated by the multiplicity of factors involved in both the causes and effects of this disease. The physiological ramifications have prompted chapters by specialists of not only the mouth but also the ear, nose, and throat and descriptions of involvement of not only teeth but also muscles, nerves, bones, and discs. The complexities do not end there. There are, in addition, several psychological factors that must be considered for the successful diagnosis and treatment of TMJ disorders.

There are times in practice when a psychiatrist or psychologist may come in contact with TMJ disease. If aware of its existence and signs, this clinician could spot the syndrome in its progressive states: at its beginning in the bruxing and clenching of a potential TMJ sufferer, during its progression in the pain of a present TMJ victim or in its aftereffects in the stress of a former TMJ patient.

Each of these stages of TMJ trouble—the beginnings, progression, and aftereffects—is a definite stress impasse stage of the TMJ patient, each stage having its characteristic physical *and* emotional parameters. The focus and techniques of the psychological/psychiatric clinician working with such a patient then will likewise depend on the stage of stress impasse. As the TMJ disorder advances, the clinician will find it necessary to move from a short-term preventive counseling approach, to a longer term in-depth analysis plus appropriate medical referral, and possibly to a final role as analytic supervisor to the primary physician who has relieved the physical pain. Each of these stages, in terms of both symptoms and analytic strategies, is discussed in this chapter.

RELEVANT RESEARCH

In a series of 30 psychiatric interviews with nonorganic TMJ dysfunction patients Lefer[3] (a psychiatrist and dentist) found that jaw symptoms provided a distraction or defense from focusing on unbearable problems in living. It seemed to be a way of keeping unacceptable needs for dependence, aggressiveness, or depression out of awareness. When McCall, Szmyd, and Ritter[5] administered the MMPI to patients with TMJ dysfunction, as well as to two control groups—one healthy and the other scheduled for oral surgery—they found the TMJ patients to be clearly distinguishable from the others. The TMJ patients, described themselves as fighting their hardest battles with themselves, being frequently worried and indecisive, easily angered, restless, more nervous than most people, continually anxious, suspicious, and "about to go to pieces."

Other studies profiling patients with atypical facial neuralgia give a picture much different from that of the TMJ syndrome personality. Engel[2] described this neuralgia group as shy, flirtatious, exhibitionist, childlike, and often given to masochism and self-punishment. The findings of Lessee[4] with a similar group indicate that their pain was entirely psychogenic or represented a gross overreaction to a minor organic deficit that had long since been corrected. The significance of these studies is the indication that although TMJ disease may have many symptoms in common with atypical facial neuralgia, both the causes of each and the typical personality type afflicted with each are different.

Sufferers from TMJ disease do not show the typical hypochondriacal pattern, in which complaining tends to bring about secondary gains. The more typical TMJ syndrome personality achieves secondary gains by *not* complaining, at least in the early stages of pain. The fantasy of being loved or admired because of the physical or emotional suffering they can endure with gritted teeth and sealed lips is more their style. This form of stoicism is usually coupled with an anxiety that releasing emotions may break down the floodgate they have dammed up behind those clenched teeth, causing the ensuring tide to sweep over them in an emotionally devastating way.

Moulton's[6] interviews with and investigations of patients suffering from a "tensional charley horse of the jaw"[6] revealed that most of them were involved in long-existing life problems or stresses that had gradually built up to intolerable dimensions. These patients fell into two categories: (1) an overtly dependent group who had suffered the loss of an individual on whom they had leaned for support, and (2) a group who tended to be obsessive, perfectionistic, demanding people who were highly effective—several had held interesting, high-pressure jobs.

TMJ SYNDROME PSYCHODYNAMICS

These two categories from Moulton's study[6] bear a strong resemblance to a description of the two major class divisions of the oral personality, as defined in classic psychoanalytical terms. The two modes of oral activity, *incorporation* (or swallowing) and *biting*, are the prototypes for many later character traits that develop. Gullible persons, for example, are those said to be fixated on the oral incorporative level of personality: they will swallow anything they are told. This personality type tends to have strong feelings of dependency, wishing to symbolically swallow up all the significant people in the environment. Or they may be so threatened by their feelings of utter dependence that they develop counterreaction tendencies and deny all their needs (even the rational ones) from others. The second type of oral character is typified more by biting, or oral aggressiveness, displaced usually in the form of sarcasm and argumentativeness. Phrases such as "biting wit" or "he really chewed me out" recognize (perhaps unconsciously) the oral-aggressive origin of verbal assertiveness that is so characteristic of this group.

The TMJ syndrome patient typically, then, tends to display an oral character defense of either the incorporative or biting prototype or a combination of the two. The combination form is illustrated by the person who can be verbally expressive, assertive, or even aggressive to the point of hostility through deprecation and abusiveness as a means of reducing tension and stress. Once having done so, however, the dependency (incorporative) needs become activated as this person begins to fear that the object of the anger (who is also usually the object of many needs) will retaliate or leave him or her. This conflict, plus the guilt often felt for having been so verbally assaultive, may result in the secondary defense of turning the aggressiveness inward—"swallowing the anger" or "biting the bullet," in the stoic terms these patients seem to so much admire. Actual clenching, biting, and grinding occur concomitantly.

Histories of these patients indicate that very often the parent of the same sex has demonstrated a similar pattern in terms of verbal aggressiveness and subsequent conflict or regret concerning that style. In several instances the patient has even recalled that the parent was also a grinder or a clencher. For these patients, beyond the earlier unresolved conflict with at least one parent, there is also a high incidence of interpersonal conflict centered about a significant other in their present lives: often the spouse or, very frequently, the child. These patients tend to subjectively identify with the aggressive acts of their children, even when they are the objects of that aggression. This particular part of the larger pattern was evident from the earliest TMJ patient brought to my attention, prior to a more fully developed TMJ syndrome picture.

Case 1

Patient 1 was a tense, concerned, conscientious woman, a perfectionist about her role as a housewife and mother. As her daughter reached adolescence, the girl began acting out and causing disciplinary problems at school. The mother felt outraged at what she called her daughter's "looseness." She would stay up nights brooding about the situation, clenching her fists and jaws tightly, trying to restrain her angry, unacceptable feelings and to hold back the words she felt like saying to her daughter but that a "good mother" would not say. At this time her husband, already a busy professional man, became more absorbed outside the home in his race for election to the school board and less dependable inside the home for support and involvement.

After some time these problems began to be resolved. The husband lost the election and had more time to spend at home. The daughter passed through the worst of the adolescent phases, and to all intents and purposes things should have been looking brighter. However, the headaches and sore cheeks, which had come on with the tension, did not pass along with their causes. The pain itself began to be a source of tension, which then would cause more pain. The patient went to seven or eight physicians and even had a number of teeth extracted by an oral surgeon, but pain continued on the right side of her head. She became depressed and began using large doses of medication. Finally, she happened to learn of a TMJ center. These physicians were able to diagnose deterioration in the TMJ, whose physical symptoms were so pronounced by that time that one could hear the crackle in the joint. She had surgery with replacement of TMJ disc and subsequent total relief.

STRESS IMPASSE STAGES

The stress impasse stages in the TMJ syndrome are characterized by three distinct steps based on the evolution and progression of the disease. Each step has a defined stress impasse at which point, when further action is taken to reduce the tension overload and the confluence of pressure, results are generally counterproductive. The graph in Fig. 25-1 represents these three stages, described in more detail in the following discussion.

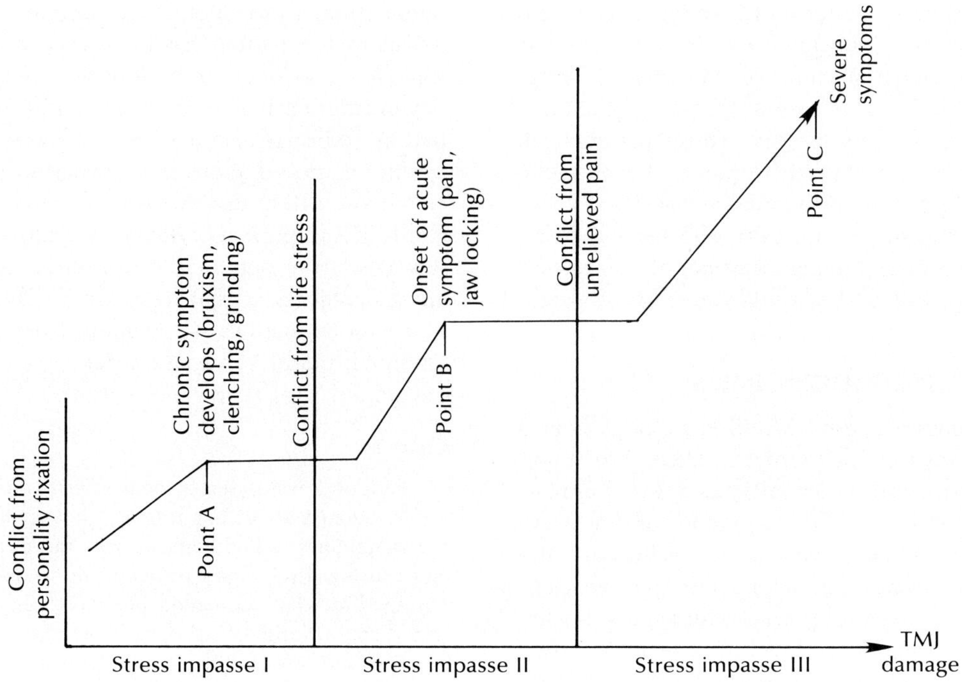

Fig. 25-1. Stress impasse graph.

The conflict from personality fixation reaches a marked peak at a fairly early age (youth or adolescence) during stress impasse I. If this conflict is resolved to a higher psychodynamic level of maturation, this internal conflict will diminish. If not, it tends to plateau for a period, during which time chronic symptoms centering around the oral area and temporomandibular joint may develop. Bruxism, grinding, and teeth clenching are common symptoms.

With the advent of more life stresses, the conflicts from these external stresses will be added to the internal personality tensions, and total stress, including the physiological strain on the TMJ, will rise to the peak of stress impasse II. At this point an acute symptom of TMJ damage will be manifested, such as locked jaw, pain, or loud popping and clicking.

If the TMJ damage is treated and/or the external conflicts resolved, the stress will be relieved. If neither is dealt with, or if treating only one dimension proves inadequate, the situation may tend to plateau for a time. Then the physiological condition of the eroded joint (above and beyond the personality dynamics and external life circumstances), coupled with an inability to find relief from the pain, will result in stress impasse III, which can rise to severe heights.

Stage I

I saw the patient described in Case 1 before I fully recognized the significance of early childhood dynamics in the TMJ syndrome. As I obtained more experience in working with patients suffering from this syndrome, however, it became more apparent that from early childhood there had been a psychophysical oral activity associated with an inability to resolve interpersonal conflicts (usually with significant family members, often the parent of the same sex) by more adequate problem-solving techniques. The emotional frustration and tension would be somewhat relieved by an oral-regressive response against the self through the mechanisms of clenching the jaws and grinding the teeth. This gnashing, grinding, and clenching activity for the most part was done unconsciously, except that the patient could recall frequent complaints of family members in connection with this bruxism. A bed-partner sibling would often be remembered as having complained about the nuisance of sleeping in the same room with a person grinding his teeth throughout the night. The first stress impasse, then, is that early period when an oral-regressive activity has been used to reduce tension as a substitute for more adequate problem-solving behavior. Continuing this tension-reducing response will probably lead to the counterproductive results of (1) stifling some development of better problem-solving techniques and (2) beginning the damage to tissue and anatomical breakdown that may culminate in TMJ erosion.

Stage II

The combination of life stresses (those precipitating events which trigger the trivial and traumatic crises that make up everyday life) and the real tissue damage that has built up over a period of years of oral-regressive bruxing and grinding begins to produce a stress-pain cycle that often commences with the onset of an actue oral symptom. Jaw pain or locking may occur, often during a time of stressful life circumstances. The stress then will be compounded by the pain, the pain will increase the stress, and so on. At this point relief of the acute symptom seems so important that little attention may be paid to the life stress circumstances and probably none to the underlying personality dynamics. Unless the TMJ is given adequate repair at this point, however, or unless the person is treated with a view toward improving the life-coping skills so they are not handled at the expense of the physiological oral apparatus, a continuation of temporary or symptomatic repair work eventually will become counterproductive. For example, one patient who was treated with a splint simply chewed it up. Treating symptoms without realizing their underlying psychological and physiological significance often buys time for the patient to accomplish drastic oral damage.

Stage III

This third level of pain and disability is aggravated by and linked to the variety of diagnostic therapeutic activities that begin to accumulate in the search for relief from symptoms. Even the person who has suffered TMJ damage as the result of a sudden, traumatic injury or accident (and who therefore has not necessarily suffered a prior stressful life situation or developed oral-regressive responses from an early age) may not be immune to stage III. Most TMJ syndrome patients, regardless of whether their injury occurred gradually or suddenly, have suffered numerous misdiagnoses and therapeutic failures, ranging from reflexology to mutilating surgery, in addition to untold dental work. And not to exclude the psychiatric profession, patients also have been treated by analysts who failed to understand that an immense amount of physiological damage has actually occurred, in addition to psychological problems present.

The progressive confusion on the part of the patient, the family, and the clinicians results in further physical and emotional trauma. Even the patient's own referring physician may take umbrage and cast aspersions on the competence and integrity of physician who wishes to perform TMJ surgery, dismissing the technique as a fad and the surgeon as a charlatan. With some degree of suspicion and antagonism to begin with among some clinicians toward surgeons whom they may see as preferring a more lucrative surgical technique to more conservative treatment, this new diagnosis ("replacement of temporomandibular joint disc by articular eminence prosthesis") may evoke extreme hostility toward both TMJ surgeon and the "gullible" patient.

The gradual development of an adversary situation among all concerned parties grows as the multiplicity of opinions involves the patient and the family in concerns regarding the credibility of the treatment programs and the validity of the patient's complaints. The consequent suspicion, mistrust, frustration, and disillusionment may disrupt the family and produce further regression in the patient. This regression may become magnified to psychotic or extreme neurotic manifestations. Psychological examination at this point of extreme crisis will demonstrate the exaggerated psychopathology and eclipse the basic personality characteristics of the premorbid individual.

Case 2, which again describes a patient I saw early in my experience in dealing with TMJ syndrome, does not provide enough background to reveal the complete TMJ personality history but does reveal this third stage very well. There are also subtle suggestions of an oral-regressive mode of dealing with life conflicts.

Case 2

Patient 2 was a handsome black woman who had retired from teaching after a career of 34 years. Her field of specialty was teaching the euphemistically termed Opportunity Classes for Social Adjustment—the behavior problems from all classes. But when asked if such a demanding job could have produced aggravation, she would reply, "I never raise my voice; I never get angry with a child. If I feel myself even begin to, I walk out of the room."

This lady had TMJ surgery after a history of 26 years of severe pain variously diagnosed as trigeminal neuralgia, histamine cephalgia, cluster headaches, and hysteria. She had gone by progressive referral to a long series of physicians, dentists, neurologists, ear, nose, and throat specialists, allergy specialists, a gynecologist, a psychiatrist, and even a reflexologist, who had performed zone therapy on her toes. At one time she had begged her dentist to pull all her teeth. He refused until she was determined that she would have another do it if he did not. He reluctantly pulled a few until she agreed it was no help for the pain. At another frantic time she had begged a physician to remove her right eye for the agony, but he had refused. Relief sometimes came after vomiting so hard that a vessel would burst in her nose or eye.

"Everyone who has this must contemplate suicide!" she emphatically told her oral surgeon. "But I wouldn't do it because of the children, and I've always tried not to complain."

Her TMJ surgery removed her pain and her contemplations of suicide.

EXPANDED CASE HISTORIES

I saw the patients described in the following cases after I had begun to be aware of the more complete picture of the TMJ syndrome patient, including oral psychodynamics, personality clusters, and stress impasse stages.

Case 3

When Patient 3 was only 3 years old, his father was killed in an accident; when he was 5, his mother was killed in another. He was an early teeth grinder in his sleep, clenching his jaw tight at night to keep from crying (stage I). At some level, not even fully verbalized at that age, he felt like he would never dare become dependent on others for vital emotional needs. Early loss is often a characteristic forerunner of the TMJ syndrome. When a person is deprived of vital emotional sustenance, the counterreaction to these unresolved and overwhelming dependency needs is often denial.

Patient 3 was raised by an aunt and uncle in a section of the city in which survival was enhanced, if not actually ensured, by becoming an aggressive street fighter. He learned to severely repress all his tender, soft feelings to cope with the loss he had sustained from his parents' deaths and to become a better street fighter. When he grew up, he became an aggressively competitive real estate salesman. He came to therapy because his marriage was falling apart and he was experiencing jaw pains (stage II). His phrases gave a clue to his oral-regressive coping mechanisms as he spoke of the necessity for "keeping a stiff upper lip," "biting the lip" to keep from being a crybaby, "taking it on the chin," and "keeping your chin up." His wife's complaint was how much distance the patient seemed to want to maintain between the two of them. He insisted that he loved her but had great anxiety about letting anyone get too close. To prove his point, he mentioned how devastating her leaving him would have been had he really let her get "under his skin." His jaw would then clamp shut: he wasn't going to "swallow anybody up."

After several sessions Patient 3 achieved some success in his ability to become less defensive with his feelings, and he was more able to allow his wife to see past some of his barriers. A good deal of his tension was decreased by this therapy. However, the commensurate physical TMJ damage he had by then sustained over the years of gritted teeth and clenched jaw was still there, and this also had to be subsequently treated (stage III).

Case 4

Patient 4 could remember that her sister, who slept in the same room, would often wake her up at night to scold her for the noise she was making grinding her teeth. The most early interpersonal conflict she could recall was with her mother (stage I). The mother was a strict woman, with particular reservations about sex. The patient herself had been ignorant until the time she married about the connection between sexual intercourse and pregnancy. She had once told a younger girl friend that she believed pregnancy was caused orally by French kissing and that one had best keep a tightly clenched mouth on a date to avoid such a consequence. During her courtship she still did not realize the significance of intercourse, which she and her fiancé had a few times—presumably with clenched teeth. She did not realize she was pregnant until nearly her fifth month (The "oral innocent" prototype comes to mind, with wide, round eyes and wide, round mouth saying, "Oh," in naive, gullible amazement.) When the baby, who had been conceived during the courtship, was born 7 months after the wedding, the patient's mother clamped her own mouth shut in tight-lipped fury and refused to speak to her daughter.

The baby had severe colic, and in the patient's words, "We both cried for 8 months." During this time the bruxism in her sleep became noticeable to her husband. On his part, he did try to be supportive and was delighted with the baby's birth but felt frustrated by his mother-in-law's reaction and his wife's unhappiness. The patient felt she was becoming exhausted and at last "had to eat crow," begging her mother to come help her take care of the baby. The mother relented, and the patient began to feel more dependent on her than ever. As time went on, sexual relations with her husband seemed progressively more obnoxious to her, and she began to experience frigidity: a feeling like her vagina was clamping shut, as she had once clenched her teeth to avoid French kissing. She would become angry and verbally abusive, then feel she had gone too far, and "clam up" until the next outburst.

Some time later she and her husband went to a party. She remembered it as being pleasant enough, but when she woke up the next morning, her jaw was locked (stage II). She was not in pain but felt anxiety to the point of panic. The family physician gave her an injection of cortisone, and her jaw released. After this the jaw began to lock more often, always during her sleep. Over the next 11 years she visited 15 specialists, including orthopedists, neurosurgeons, and a psychiatrist. The chronic jaw locks were now accompanied by severe pain (stage III). By now all her most important interpersonal relationships had deteriorated. Her mother and daughter were often allies against her. And her husband had begun to visit a woman friend of the patient on his noon hour. On hearing the latter, the patient drove to her husband's office to confront him and tell him she was leaving. To her surprise, since she had been both cold and verbally abusive for a number of years, he rushed home after her and embraced her. This affirmation of his affection had the effect of bringing forth a resurgence of passion within her which she had not felt toward him in years.

Around this time an orthopedist who noticed a crepitus in her jaw referred her to a TMJ surgeon. After the operation she was completely free from pain and able to eat in a few days. As she began feeling so much better, she gained a more substantial recovery of the relationship with her husband and, eventually, more realistic exchanges with her mother and daughter than bursting out with angry words or holding them back by teeth grinding. Now at age 32 she is an attractive woman who has finally broken through the blockade of the stress impasse system.

Case 5

This 42-year-old patient was a successful director, producer, writer, and technician at a major motion picture and television studio: a man who felt he had to incorporate or "swallow whole" every facet of the tension-producing business at which he spent so many hours daily. When questioned about any habits of bruxism, he could not actually recall any clenching except that so many people through the years, including his wife, had said, "If you don't stop grinding your teeth, it'll drive me crazy!" His father had been a country physician, a voracious worker, and a chain smoker, who died at a relatively early age from heart trouble and "working himself to death." The patient could remember his father grinding his teeth when he got angry and stated, "My brother and I gave him plenty to be angry about." He had much affection for his father but also many conflicts, which apparently both of them had partly handled through teeth grinding (stage I).

In addition to the regular heavy pressures of his job, several life stresses converged on the patient during one period. His oldest daughter, age 13, had become quite obstreperous (the patient admitted she reminded him of himself) and would talk back assertively, or even aggressively, when he "chewed her out" for what he again admitted were often minor infractions. He gave up smoking for his health, which increased his teeth grinding. Then his father-in-law died, necessitating a move in by the mother-in-law. He began going on location more for filming, and his wife complained that he was never home and not meeting any of her needs. When asked if he felt she were too demanding, or he too neglectful or distancing, he maintained that there was no possibility of compromise; they were both simply too different in personality type to be able to change. His wife's neuritis flared up severely, and she had to be hospitalized. A recession in the industry threatened his livelihood. An earthquake did extensive damage to their house. He began to experience severe jaw pains, which would radiate back into his neck, and could hardly chew meat and then bread. If he sneezed or yawned, he would hear a loud popping noise, and his jaw would lock open. He was fitted with a prosthesis to prevent more damage from his grinding, and he chewed it up (stage II).

Patient 5 then began his series of peregrinations from clinician to clinician (stage III). One diagnosed his condition as arthritis; others recommended tooth extractions, massage, and cortisone injections. He was given medication and tranquilizers. A dentist then referred him to a TMJ specialist, and he was placed in a hospital room with another TMJ surgery patient. After his operation he felt completely pain free and was able to reassure his roommate, who was still having some discomfort and fear, that all would soon be well. A few days later the man called to thank him for this assurance, which had proved true. Many others had previously told the roommate the surgery would probably do no good, and it had given him an immense amount of relief to be reassured by a fellow sufferer.

Since that time, this patient has made several changes in his life-style toward being more relaxed at home and less absorbed in work. He spends more time with his wife and is less aggravated by his daughter. He no longer chews out people or chews up prostheses.

Case 6

Patient 6 also had been a grinder and a clencher from an early age. When she was 6 years old, the family separated from the father, who was a violent alcoholic, and moved to the West Coast. She remembered her mother as a quiet, self-effacing, long-suffering woman, who despite all problems would try to carry on with true grit (in the teeth) and no complaints. It was uncomfortable for the girl to be around her saintly mother (stage I). The patient herself cound not stand to be so quiet and had been called bigmouth and loudmouth by a brother, who probably accidentally had hit her in the jaw when she was 13 years old. It had been painful, and she had done more tooth grinding to relieve the irritation, but the incident soon was submerged.

The patient married a man who did building work by contract and was often laid off for long periods between jobs. He was also a quiet person who liked being around the house, an arrangement not equally enjoyed by the patient who would feel the stress of his constant presence, in addition to the tension from the financial strain when he was not working. She would yell at him and often "blow her top," whereas he would calmly refuse to rise to the bait. She decided to become more involved ouside the home in community and school activities and joined the Girl Scouts with her daughter. As she rose through the hierarchy of the Scouts, she came to have more leadership responsibilities. But even though this had helped absorb much of her energy and drive at first, it began to turn to frustration as the five other leaders with whom she was interacting refused to cooperate with her orders. At this same time her husband was in the midst of an 8-month layoff, the finances were becoming stretched, and her mother-in-law came for a protracted stay. Unlike the patient's mother, who had been stoic and long-suffering, the mother-in-law was described as a complainer, difficult, and helpless; the patient had to drive her everywhere. She felt her husband was not interacting with her in any way; he would not go out or even argue. She felt as though she had no impact on anything, even when she gritted her teeth and tried to push it through. Then she had an acute attack of pain with a popping sound in the jaw. The pain seemed to begin in the jaw and radiated down into the shoulders and through the head with a nearly unbearable pressure. She felt as though she literally might be about to blow her top (stage II).

The story of trips to various physicians is nearly too routine to be retold. One told her she should use sex to relieve her tensions, a suggestion she found outrageous. Cortisone treatments and pulled teeth ensued (stage III) until she was finally referred to a TMJ specialist. Since then, her pain has been relieved and her ability to chew restored. She has also seen a pyschiatrist about her tensions and the frustrations in her life situation as well.

STRESS IMPASS STAGE IV?

The primary intent of this chapter is to establish a three-part stress impasse structure evolving from the original oral psychodynamics of the TMJ syndrome patient and progressing through three stages to the completion of successful TMJ surgery. However, at least two recent cases have suggested that a next edition might document a stress impasse stage beyond the successful treatment of the patient—the disbelief they encounter from others afterward. The final two cases illustrate the existence of this impasse.

Case 7

A plaintive letter from a patient who had successfully undergone TMJ surgery illustrates this aspect: "I had the TMJ surgery in February, and since then I can get no one to believe any part of it here in [a town out of state]."

This woman's symptoms had been dizziness, headaches, and frequent jaw locking. She had gone to numerous physicians, a dentist, a neurologist, two internists, a psychiatrist, an ear, nose, and throat specialist, and at last an oral surgeon who had performed the surgery. She had great relief from all the symptoms subsequently. Her next problem began when she applied for a position as a physician's assistant at a clinic. She had excellent references, having worked at three hospitals, and was hired on the spot to begin work the following week after a routine physical examination. But after the examination she was shocked to learn she was no longer acceptable for employment at the clinic. On persistent inquiry, the examining physician told her he had been extremely skeptical of the TMJ surgery she had described on her examination form. After consultation with another physician they had decided that either such surgery had not been performed at all (typically, the TMJ incision heals so well that there is scant indication of it) or that she had had it perfomed just so she could say she had had surgery. Although the woman no longer wanted to work at the clinic, she was outraged and humiliated and had written back to the oral surgeon, asking him to please inform her examining physicians that it was not all a sham.

Case 8

Patient 8, a genteel Southern woman, was another victim of disbelief. A recent marriage to an air force pilot had necessitated several moves over a brief time. She was also rearing a teenage son whom she would attempt to discipline with only a soft word, a raised eyebrow, and clenched teeth. Throughout her life she had had many of the TMJ syndrome stresses.

Her first TMJ surgery, a traumatic high condylectomy requiring months of recuperation and convalescence, had been performed at a large medical center in the Midwest. This operation seemed fairly acceptable and valid to everyone. But her second TMJ surgery, performed on the opposite side, was done by an oral surgeon through far less traumatic measures (replacement of the TMJ disc by an articular eminence prosthesis rather than removal of the bone). She and her husband then moved out of this surgeon's area. After the move the condylectomized side of her jaw began to shoot out severe pains once more. She checked into the hospital at the air force base. Her conviction regarding her second oral surgeon's skill was so fervent and evangelical that it may have aroused jealousy or skepticism among the other physicians. At any rate, the more emphatic she became about the necessity of their contacting her second TMJ surgeon, insisting that her pain was not abating with their treatment and medication, the more hostility and implacability she felt from them.

On the tenth day of her hospitalization she happened to be nearby when her physician accidentally dropped his charts. Helping him pick them up, her eye was caught by her own chart's diagnosis and prescription: "Psychological disorder" and "Placebo." She left the hosptial to travel back to the TMJ surgeon in whom she had confidence. The subsequent surgery he performed was as successful as the first.

TREATMENT APPROACHES

Modern psychiatry is beginning to stress two critical factors in the search for mental health: (1) the importance of preventive, early treatment and (2) the necessity for a holistic approach in an effective treatment program. The psychiatrist who ignores the impact of concomitant physiological damage has perhaps been away from medical school too long and has forgotten that the mind also occupies a body, to which catastrophic things can happen. Preventive treatment is particularly relevant for the TMJ syndrome. Not even the future ulcer patient (whose internal acid secretions cannot be seen or heard by the outside observer) will give as clear a diagnostic symptoms that something is going wrong as will the chronic gnasher, grinder, and clencher of teeth. Prevention in the early stages may preclude a great deal of physiological damage and promote coping through better problem-solving techniques than "eating one's heart (or, more accurately, TMJ) out."

The holistic approach is also vital to the recovery of the TMJ patient. The analyst who deals with such a patient most effectively will be the one who has a broad eclectic background, who understands not only the psychodynamics of what it means to be an "oral personality," but who is also aware of the many behavior modification therapies such as biofeedback training or meditative relaxation. The analyst needs to understand not only the humanistic psychological techniques of working with the life goals of a patient but also the importance of considering dream analysis work for the person who bruxes all night long.

Finally, this clinician may find himself or herself fitting into a team approach with the primary medical or dental physician in one of two ways. In the usual manner the clinician may do psychotherapy with the patient concurrent with or subsequent to the medical treatment. Or he or she may be called on to act in a supervisory role to the primary physician, who is also giving some supportive counseling to the patient.

It has been my experience, particularly with TMJ patients, that unless the patient has already established a relationship with the counseling therapist, he or she will be reluctant to listen to anyone but the primary physician, dentist, or physical therapist who has relieved the terrific, long-standing pain. As has been noted, because of the long-standing trauma of this pain, the person is so relieved of everything from annihilation anxiety to the fear of going mad that he or she often has a nearly evangelical appreciation of the healer and wants to hold on, literally, for dear life (possibly evoking a mental image of little bulldogs holding on with their tight little jaws). These feelings of confidence, or downright salvation, rather than being minimized for the sake of putting things in perspective, can be used by the primary physician (who after all has been working in the primary cavity—the mouth) to get in some basic psychological or emotional counseling as well.

It is certainly not to trivialize psychotherapy to point out that a major part of its effectiveness consists of gaining the patient's complete trust and then using that confidence to promote some basic mental health and stress-management principles. More and more psychiatrists and psychologists are becoming involved in this sort of supervisory or advisory capacity to the person who is the primary interface for or has a direct impact on the patient; thus those therapeutic clinicians who have become part of the TMJ holistic treatment network do so not only in the role of direct counselor but also as consultants to the primary healer, who may be doing the counseling personally.

We are now in the process of developing a stress-management program that can be incorporated into a variety of settings—even as unlikely a place as the dentist's office. A basic three-stage program, this therapeutic procedure will teach basic relaxation exercises, sleep and dream preparation, and containment strategies for worry, grief, and guilt.

Finally, strong emphasis also must be placed on follow-up monitoring of these patients. The typical TMJ syndrome patient may want to discontinue all treatment as soon as the physical pain is relieved. The clinician must make it clear that unless the patient's underlying tensions are worked through, there is no quarantee that the same physical pattern will not be reactivated, with further joint deterioration.

SUMMARY AND CONCLUSION

A 1977 study[1] revealed that the average chronic pain patient (a classification that includes the TMJ syndrome patient) has suffered for 7 years, undergone from three to five major operations, and spent from $50,000 to $100,000 in medical bills. In between the operations the patient has taken countless drugs—from tranquilizers and muscle relaxants to potent narcotics—and there is at least a 50% chance that a drug habit has been acquired along the way.

The need for treatment of chronic pain has become so pressing that a new medical specialty, dolorology, has been developed in response. At least 15 centers are now in operation across the United States, devoted exclusively to chronic pain problems. They employ a wide range of medical disciplines, from anesthesiology to psychiatry, to search for the cause of a patient' problem and to prescribe the most effective treatment. The philosophy that guides these clinics in their treatment programs is the recognition that chronic pain is a complex malady in which physical, psychological, and social factors play a part. As John Loeser of the University of Washington Pain Clinic in Seattle so aptly expresses it, "The overwhelming majority of chronic pain patients need to have their whole lives examined."[1]

This chapter has sought to establish such a holistic concept in terms of the TMJ syndrome patient, recognizing each factor—physical, social, and psychological—as real, interrelated, and critical to the developmental sequence of the temporomandibular joint breakdown. At each point in the stress impasse structure all three factors are operating.

At stress impasse stage I, in the formative years, dynamic characteristics are developed along the lines of an oral-regressive personality style that is accompanied by the physiological component of beginning bruxing habits, in response to a social or interpersonal relationship (often with the parent of the same sex) that has reached a frustrating impasse for the patient.

In stress impasse stage II the environmental and interpersonal/social stresses of later years combine with the personality pattern, which is now more entrenched in its oral-regressive responses (of the dependent or aggressive variety), until buildup of physiological damage to the TMJ reaches the point where an acute symptom (pain, locked jaw) occurs, in addition to the psychosocial stresses.

Stress impasse stage III ensues during the painful and frustrating search for relief from the chronic pain, which now becomes a way of life. Even those people who have suffered TMJ damage through a traumatic injury, rather than the lifetime psychosocial route described, will now find themselves also caught in this stress impasse stage. Almost no chronic pain is well understood, and the TMJ syndrome is certainly no exception, even if the causality is as well defined as a blow to the jaw. Chronic pain, and others' response to it, leads to development of an entire life-style, often destroying the personality in the process.

REFERENCES

1. Clark, M., Gosnell, M., and Shapiro, D.: The new war on pain, Newsweek, April 25, 1977, p. 48.
2. Engel, G.L.: Primary atypical facial neuralgia: hysterical conversion symptom, Psychosom. Med. **13**:375, 1951.
3. Lefer, L.: A psychoanalytic view of a dental phenomenon, Contemp. Psychoanal. **2**:135, 1966.
4. Lessee, S.: Atypical facial pain syndromes of psychogenic origin, J. Nerv. Ment. Dis. **124**:346, 1956.
5. McCall, C.M., Jr., Szmyd, L., and Ritter, R.M.: Personality characteristics in patients with temporomandibular joint symptoms, J. Am. Dent. Assoc. **62**:694, 1961.
6. Moulton, R.D.: Psychiatric considerations in maxillo-facial pain, J. Am. Dent. Assoc. **51**:408, 1955.

PART FOUR

DEVELOPING AREAS

26 Kinesiology

EUEL KING, D.D.S.

DEFINITION

In general, kinesiology, is the science that investigates and analyzes human motion. Dental kinesiology in particular focuses on the motions and functions of the jaw and oral musculature (both smooth and striated), the accompanying neurological, vascular, and other support-system networks, and the impact those muscle functions and neurological dynamics have on dental and systemic health. Dental kinesiology also refers to the use of applied kinesiology techniques in the prevention and treatment of dental and systemic disorders, particularly those problems caused by, or resulting in part from, dysfunctions of the TMJ musculature and/or the TMJ neurological system.

APPLICATIONS OF KINESIOLOGY

The most basic application of dental kinesiology is the reduction and prevention of muscle spasm. Reducing such spasms is helpful for patients who have bruxism problems, jaw clicking pain, or restricted opening capability.

The traditional medical approach to muscle spasm, is to focus on reducing the spasm in the agonist with tools such as muscle relaxants and physical therapy, all directed at the symptom. In Eversaul's kinesiological analysis,[1] however, the muscle spasm is seen to result from a weakening in the spastic muscle's antagonist. Consequently, in the treatment plan from that framework of dental kinesiology, muscles are tested to identify those with a low stress resistance, that is, the "weak" muscles. These will be the muscles most prone to reaching a point of exhaustion with minimum stress, which will then set off a compensating spasm in the agonist. Therefore the clinician uses various dental kinesiology procedures in an attempt to increase the stress resistance of these antagonist muscles to a more optimum level of function. It is understood that *weak* and *strong* are relative terms, varying from individual to individual and from muscle group to muscle group within the same individual.

Additional applications of dental kinesiology therapeutic techniques are as aids in (1) determining the proper vertical dimension necessary for a properly fitted and functional dental appliance, (2) stimulating control over autonomic functions such as the gag reflex, (3) helping control all forms of dental pain, (4) identifying dysfunctioning teeth and tissue, and (5) fine tuning occlusal treatment for the individual's optimum occlusion.

THERAPY LOCALIZATION

In testing for the weaker of dysfunctioning muscles Eversaul[1] uses the technique of *therapy localization,* based on the empirical observation that digital contact with any dysfunctioning area will produce lowered stress resistance in all normally functioning musculature.

The manner of doing this in the office is to first identify a striated muscle group with normal stress resistance, as registered on a kinesiometer. The most commonly used areas for dental office practice are the deltoid and triceps muscles and the fascia lata. After this baseline stress area is identified, the patient touches (preferably with the left middle fingers) the muscle or area the physician wishes to evaluate, usually around the TMJ. The clinician then retests the baseline muscle initially tested, which will then generally demonstrate a *lower* stress resistance than noted previously.

Why touching a muscle or area with kinesiological dysfunction should then also lower the stress resistance of other muscle groups is not well understood. Eversaul[1] speculates that there are electromagnetic dynamics involved. The major advantage of such a therapy localization procedure is that it provides a method for identifying areas of physiological dysfunction. After identifying such an area, however, a differential diagnosis still is needed to ascertain the specific form of dysfunction.

KINESIOLOGICAL CONCEPTS

One of the key concepts of kinesiology is that *muscle* dysfunction is usually only the *symptom;* the *cause* is *neurological* in origin. Whatmore and Kohli's description[3] of the neurodynamics involved in muscle functioning focuses on how *dysponetic signaling,* an inappropriate neurological output, may produce low-grade muscle bracing and lowered stress resistance.

The brain generates output to a muscle, causing it to either relax or contract, and this output is also affected by feedback information sent back to the brain from receptors in the muscles. When the brain perceives, even on a subliminal level, some sort of external distress agent, it sends contracting signals to the muscles, readying them for the classic conditioned "fight or flight" stress response.

But not all distress agents are outside the body. Both dental and dietary stresses, as well as other structural stresses, can cause the same type of fight or flight muscular preparation by stimulating the brain to send inappropriate dysponetic signals to the contracting striated muscles.

Because of the importance of the teeth and head to the organism, Whatmore and Kohli[3] argue that the brain may readily stimulte systemic fight or flight responses to protect the high-priority structures from further threat. In reality, of course, the chronic contracting of the TMJ muscles may promote structural damage. But this damage, in turn, would send more distress signals to the brain, and the dysponetic cycle would continue.

The main forms of dental distress that can send such feedback signals to the brain are improper vertical dimension and improper teeth dynamics. The dietary distress factors that also can stimulate dysponetic signaling are (1) "insufficient fuel" intake, such that the individual is not adequately provided with the essential vitamins, minerals, amino acids, and other necessary nutrients, and (2) "improper fuel" intake, where certain foods (such as refined sugars) are not well tolerated by the individual.

Any of or all these factors—external distress, dental or other structural distress, and dietary distress—therefore may be initiating neurological dynamics that are the cause of the symptomatic muscle bracing and its consequent lowered stress resistance. The importance of this concept is that for successful pain management not only must the symptom of spasm be treated, but also attention must be paid to the possibilities of dental, dietary, and external stresses.

Kinesiological stress analysis therefore is basically concerned with two neurological threshold points: (1) that amount of distress stimulation which produces dysponetic signaling and results in muscle bracing, and (2) that amount of distress reaction which produces physiological exhaustion and results in true muscle spasm (by definition, when the antagonist muscle reaches the point of exhaustion, and the agonist tries to compensate for the exhausted muscle's function).

DIAGNOSIS OF TMJ MUSCLE DYSFUNCTION

Diagnosis of TMJ muscle dysfunction is usually done through (1) palpation, (2) muscle testing for lowered stress resistance, and (3) therapy localization. A fourth method sometimes used is biofeedback via the electromyograph.

In the first portion of muscle examination the clinician palpates the major muscles of mastication: the sternocleidomastoid, digastric, masseter, temporal, and upper trapezius. The clinician instructs the patient to subjectively estimate the amount of pain, if any, that is felt when those muscles are palpated, possibly on a scale from 0 to 5.

The neck flexors, sternocleidomastoid, and upper trapezius muscles should be tested next for lowered stress resistance. If the ears are seen to be in a position in front of the shoulders, TMJ involvement should be suspected as a possible consequence of a weakened upper trapezius.

Therapy localization is sequentially described by Walther.[2] The patient places the hands directly over the TMJs. A previously strong indicator muscle is tested to determine if it weakens. There should be no positive therapy localization to the TMJ when the patient simply puts the hands on it unless there is a pathological condition of the joint, such as arthritis or osteoporosis.

After it has been determined that there is no joint pathosis the patient should rapidly open and close the mouth. Simultaneoulsy test a previously strong indicator muscle. If the muscle weakens, this is an indication of TMJ involvement.

The next step then is to determine if the involvement is on opening or closing. This is accomplished simply by having the patient open the mouth wide and testing the indicator muscle. If it then weakens, the involvement is on opening. If it does not weaken on opening, ask the patient to close the mouth. Test the indicator muscle. Walther[2] believes that most TMJ problems are found on closing.

THERAPIES

In addition to nutritional and meridian therapies (acupuncture is covered in Chapter 19), a basic muscle correction technique used in dental kinesiology is occlusal therapy. Mandibular repositioning appliances, including splints and functional orthodontic appliances such as the Bionator, are the most common tools used to normalize TMJ muscular function.

The amount of vertical dimension used on the splint, one of the most critical aspects of successful splint therapy, is determined via either a swallow reflex or by definitive muscle testing methods. This splint, worn continuously except during eating, is used for several reasons. First, the single-point contact allows significant muscle freedom in repositioning the condyle. Second, the amount of vertical dimension used allows the muscles adequate "vacation" from the proprioceptive memories of premature relationships. And third, the appliance may be quickly balanced, thus making it economically feasible and quick for both patient and therapist. The Bionator is an appliance that should be considered for the patient who is obviously overclosed and will require orthodontic treatment in the long-term occlusal strategy.

During the treatment phase the vertical dimension used is not the maximum kinesiological vertical measurement. Because the patient's TMJ muscle functions may be constantly changing throughout the treatment, it is possible that the vertical dimension may also change. Consequently, for most patients it seems only necessary to construct the appliance at a vertical dimension that is close to the theoretical neurological ideal but that can be determined quickly.

Other treatment procedures to be considered are nutritional therapy, physical therapy, exercise, and applied kinesiological techniques such as the neurolymphatic and neurovascular stimulative techniques described in Walther's text,[2] biofeedback, acupuncture, and structural alterations that may involve restorative surgery.

It is important to realize that the general treatment strategy will vary from patient to patient. Some will need to be seen only a few weeks, others for a more extended period. Some will need only the splint; others will need much attention paid to their diet as well. Some will respond to physical therapy, and others may eventually require surgical intervention for increased stress resistance and complete relief.

The basic concepts of dental kinesiology presented in this chapter may be used as initial or supplementary occlusal therapy in an interdisciplinary approach to TMJ treatment.

REFERENCES

1. Eversaul, G.A.: Dental kinesiology, Las Vegas, 1979, George A. Eversaul.
2. Walther, D.S.: Applied kinesiology, Pueblo, Colo., 1976, Systems DC.
3. Whatmore, G.B., and Kohli, D.R.: The physiopathology and treatment of functional disorders, New York, 1974, Grune & Stratton, Inc.

27 Orthodontic considerations in temporomandibular joint dysfunction: some highlights

JOHN R.J. GAWLEY, D.D.S., M.S.

As indicated by the following quotation from an overview by Bell,[1] the temporomandibular pain-dysfunction syndrome is a multifaceted problem.

> Symptoms associated with the TMJ pain-dysfunction syndrome result principally from dysfunction of the masticatory and cervical muscles. Symptomatic control can be effected in most instances by occlusal disengagement, physiotherapy, myotherapy, myospasm control, drug therapy, relaxation education, and occlusal adjustment. Incomplete understanding of etiologic factors obscures the diagnosis and may necessitate palliative treatment of target symptoms. Treatment of patients with irreparably damaged peri- and intra-articular structures may require surgical intervention.

PURPOSE

The purpose of this chapter is to review some of the areas where a knowledge of orthodontics can help the clinician more fully understand some of the causes and methods of treatment and prevention of the TMJ pain-dysfunction syndrome.

REVIEW OF THE LITERATURE

An excellent article by Ricketts in 1955 reported about laminagraphic studies of 50 normal joints and 200 pathological joints. The normal joints (Fig. 27-1) showed the condyles centered in the fossae, smooth articular surfaces, and no consistent harmony in size, form, or position of the TMJ components (Fig. 27-2). The pathological joints demonstrated "four specific types of joint disturbances caused by conditions of occlusion of the teeth."

Type 1 is excessive function, both in range and position of the condyle. This is characteristic of the Class II, division 1 malocclusion (Fig. 27-3). To incise, the patient may thrust forward as much as five times the normal distance. Dual-bite patients sometimes masticate in the anterior position. These activities can wear the disc and eventually the joint surfaces. Treatment may involve orthodontic correction. Removal of anterior teeth and then the placement of fixed or partial bridgework also has proved effective.

Type 2 is distal displacement, and it is often associated with Class II, division 2 malocclusion (Fig. 27-4). In this malocclusion the upper incisors characteristically demonstrate lingual crown torque, causing them to guide the lower incisors and thus the mandible posteriorly. The ligaments cannot permanently withstand this movement, and the condylar head becomes retruded in the fossa. Thrusting molars also may cause this problem. Opening the bite with an overlay splint or an anterior bite plane usually helps.

With types 1 and 2 it is possible that early orthodontic correction could prevent a future TMJ problem.

Type 3 is characterized by molar and/or premolar interference during chewing and incising. This can be caused by loss and subsequent drifting or posterior teeth. Other possible causes are the destructive balancing interferences that result from lack of canine protection and/or the improper buccolingual axial inclination of the posterior teeth. Spot grinding after acute symptoms have subsided can be helpful. Rehabilitation and/or orthodontic treatment also may be necessary.

Type 4 is loss of posterior support. Loss of posterior teeth may allow the condyle to move higher in the fossa. The joint thereby receives the stresses that the teeth usually bear. Bit blocks and, later, partial dentures may help relieve the TMJ symptoms.

Ricketts[10] makes the point that there are many causes of TMJ symptoms, but that occlusal disharmonies, which cause muscle dysfunction, should be ruled

Text continued on p. 505.

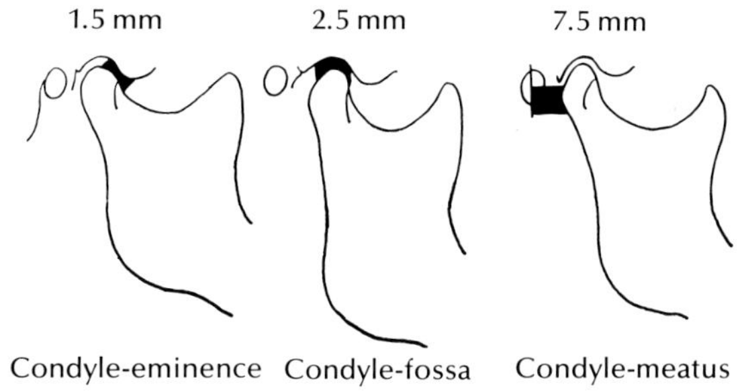

Fig. 27-1. Tracing of three laminagraph sections picked from sample of 100 cases to demonstrate ideal condyle-fossa relationship. Note two common characteristics: well-centered condyle and smooth articular surfaces. *Left,* Average condyle-eminence dimension; *middle,* average condyle-fossa dimension; *right,* average distance from condyle to line through center of external auditory canal. Comparison to strictly perfect relationship demonstrated here would be simple. However, range of natural variation (Fig. 27-2) must be proper yardstick for comparison of abnormal. (From Ricketts, R.M.: Am. J. Orthod. **41**:435, 1955.)

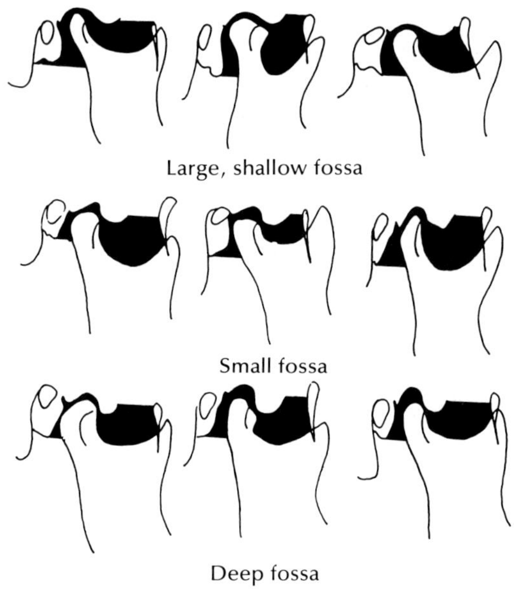

Fig. 27-2. Variation in human temporomandibular joints. Three things account for difference in these joints: (1) *upper* and *lower left,* no harmony in size of condyle and fossa; (2) *left center* and *upper right,* little consistency of form of articulating bodies; (3) *lower right,* variation in condylar position. Natural functional adaptation also must be considered in determining abnormal joints. Note suggested adaptation on condyle in center figure and on eminence in right center figure. (From Ricketts, R.M.: Am. J. Orthod. **41**:435, 1955.)

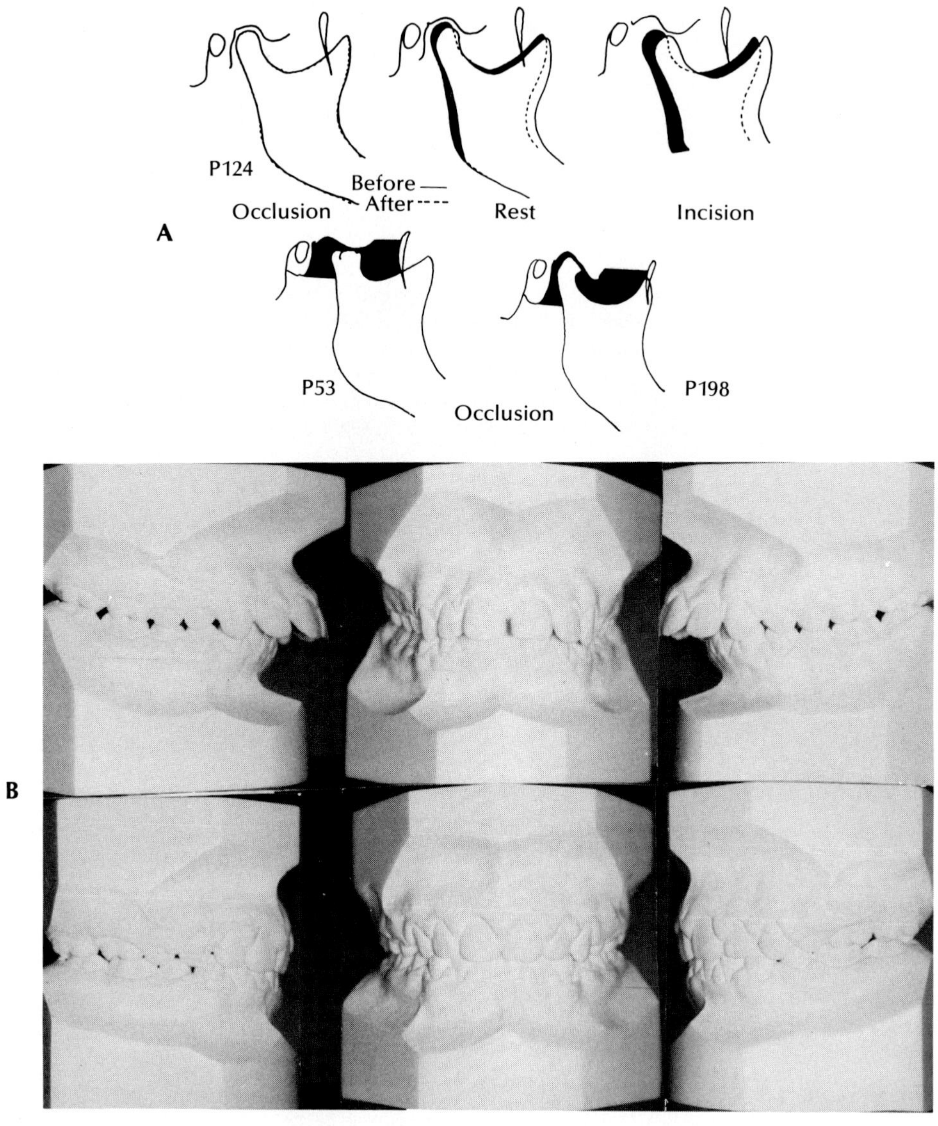

Fig. 27-3. A, Type 1, cases of abnormal function: excessive range of function in Class II division 1. Case P124 shows abnormal range for incision. (Continuous function of condyle on eminence does not appear to be consistent with normal activity.) Note change in rest position after treatment. Cases P53 and P198 demonstrate advanced pathological findings in cases of prolonged function in anterior position. Two such cases observed were postorthodontic patients in whom unsuccessful attempts had been made to position mandible forward. **B,** Example of Class II division 1 malocclusion before and after treatment. (**A** from Ricketts, R.M.: Am. J. Orthod. **41:**435, 1955.)

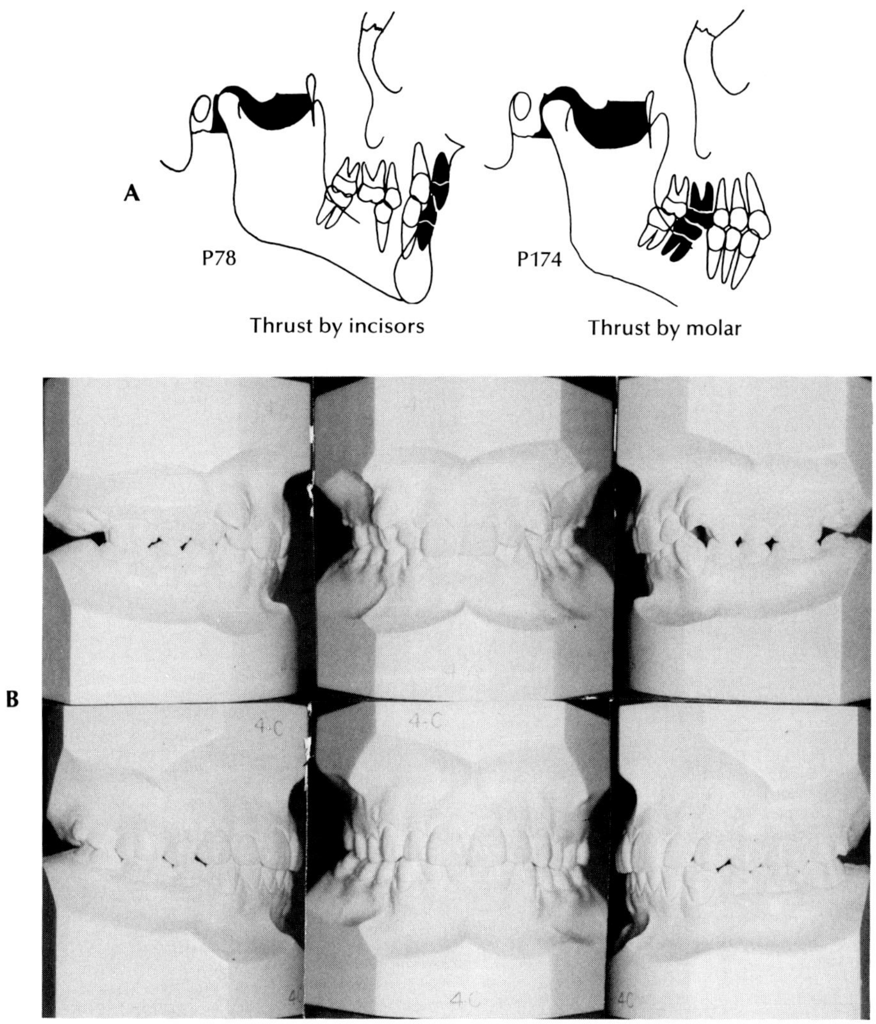

Fig. 27-4. A, Type 2, distal displacement. Note posterior position of condyle in fossa. Dimensions from condyle to eminence outside range. Condition appears to result from Class II division 2 relationship and thrust of mandible because of contact of incisors (Case P78). Displacement also occurs after loss of first molar and drift of teeth (Case P174). **B,** Example of Class II division 2 malocclusion before and after treatment. (**A,** from Ricketts, R.M.: Am. J. Orthod. **41:**435, 1955.)

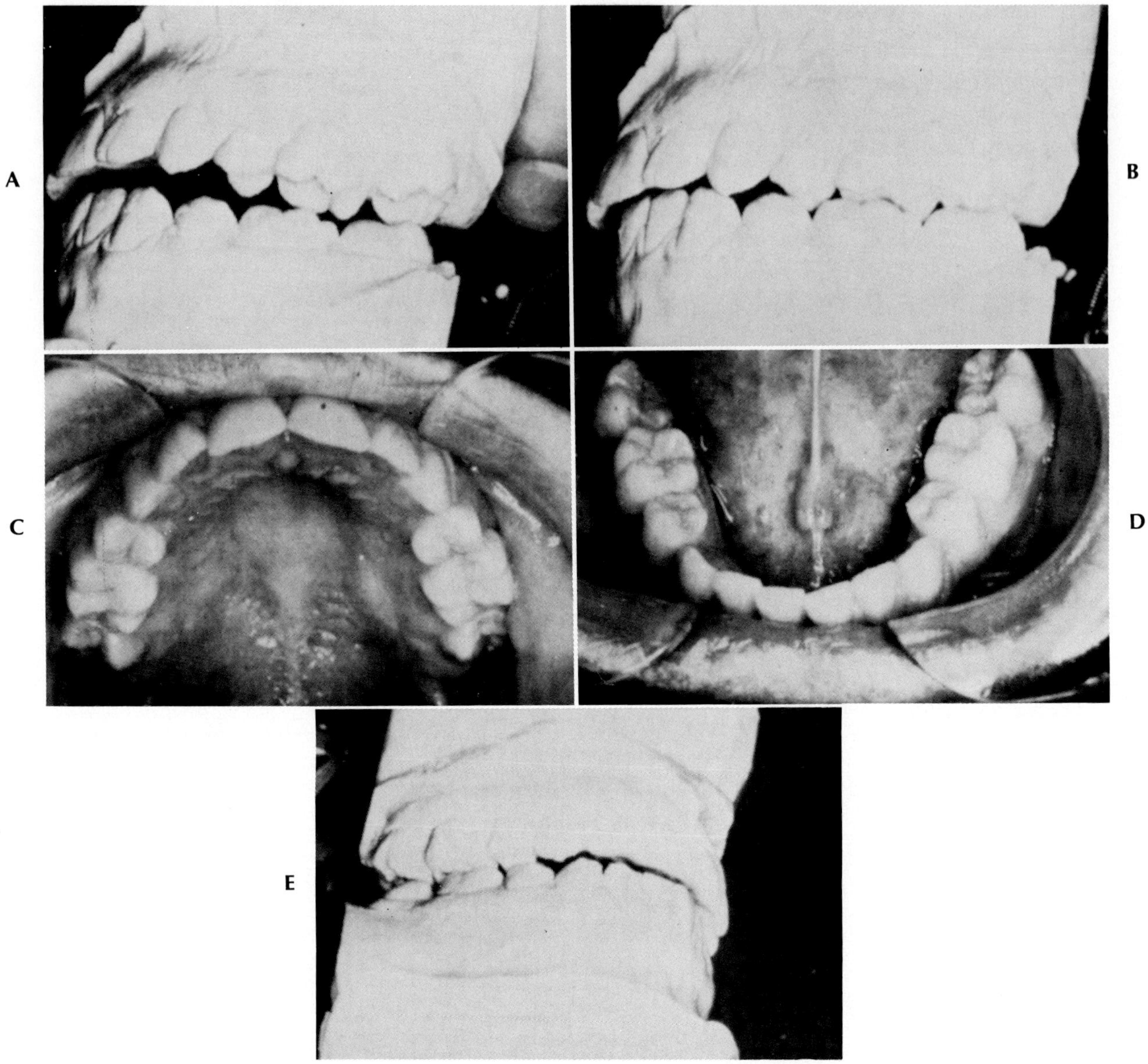

Fig. 27-5. A, Mounted models exhibiting type of balancing interference found on temporomandibular joint pain-dysfunction syndrome subjects. **B,** Posttreatment orthodontic case showing failure to achieve true anteroposterior correction of maxillary to mandibular teeth in centric relation. **C,** Posttreatment orthodontic case showing insufficient lingual crown torque of maxillary molars. **D,** Posttreatment orthodontic case showing too much lingual crown torque of mandibular second molars. **E,** Posttreatment orthodontic case showing arch width incoordination in centric relation.

out before more radical treatment is resorted to. He states:

> Musculature, in the final analysis, is the structure treated in the correction of joint disturbance. It is the damaging effect of musculature that produces trauma to the joint surfaces.

The clinician should apply general orthopedic concepts to joint analysis. This includes the role of stabilization of musculature and the synchronization of muscle activity through the nervous system.

Another study that points out the effects of occlusal disharmonies is by Roth.[13] He set up nine cases from his practice on the Stuart instrument. Seven of the patients had TMJ symptoms of varying severity, and two were selected as control subjects. All nine were successfully treated orthodontic patients.

Roth's hypothesis[13] was that occlusal interferences (Fig. 27-5, *A*) may cause extreme subluxation of the condyles in lateral and/or protrusive excursions and/or closure into maximum interdigitation. This results in stretching of the musculature, which in turn leads to increased muscle tension and muscle splinting to avoid joint trauma. This predisposes the individual toward developing pain-dysfunction symptoms.

Roth[13] further found that the presence of occlusal interferences commonly associated with TMJ pain-dysfunction on postorthodontic cases seemed to be caused by the following:

1. Failure to achieve a true anteroposterior correction of jaw relation (Fig. 27-5, *B*)
2. Insufficent lingual crown torque of maxillary first and second molars (Fig. 27-5, *C*)
3. Too much lingual crown torque of mandibular molars (Fig. 27-5, *D*)
4. Incoordination of arch widths and arch form in terminal-hinge relation (Fig. 27-5, *E*)

Roth[13] states, "The centrically related, mutually protective, occlusal scheme, when accomplished with a high degree of accuracy, is an effective means for correction of the occlusally induced temporomandibular joint pain-dysfunction syndrome."

DISCUSSION

Where does orthodontics fit into the overall treatment picture? Solberg[15] presented the chart shown in Fig. 27-6 to help visualize the interrelationships of many treatment modalities.

If the acute symptoms of pain and dysfunction are overcome, and if it is obvious that an existing malocclusion will predispose the patient to future TMJ problems, then perhaps treatment of the malocclusion to achieve stabilization is indicated. It also might be theorized that early treatment of these conditions may prevent an individual from ever developing those TMJ symptoms.

In the average orthodontic practice TMJ symptoms are not unknown. Perry[9] found in a study of 1146 orthodontic patients ranging in age from 10 to 23 years that 3% had symptoms before treatment, 5.1% developed symptoms during treatment, 7.4% first noticed symptoms after treatment, and 5.1% continued having symptoms after retention.

A more recent study by Williamson[18] showed that 35.2% of *pre*orthodontic patients, 6 to 16 years old, had incipient TMJ dysfunction. This points out the critical circumstances under which the orthodontist begins treatment.

During treatment, TMJ symptoms can be caused by (1) the transient interferences of cusps and marginal ridges of (2) excessive Class II mechanical forces (for example, elastics from the upper canine area to the lower molar area) aggravating an already excessive functional range. After treatment, TMJ symptoms can be caused by (1) continuing tooth interferences, particularly balancing interferences (selective spot grinding in centric and eccentric mandibular movements will minimize this), or (2) undue mechanical stress on the TMJ during certain extraction procedures.

At the White Memorial Hospital TMJ Clinic it has been observed[8] that some patients who have very closed bites also have posterior displacement of the condyles. This observation points out the fact that when the orthodontist treats patients with a closed-bite tendency, an effort should be made to avoid premolar extraction, since this treatment method sometimes exacerbates the closed-bite condition.[5] Obviously it is not possible to avoid extraction in cases with extreme crowding; however, Liddle[4] has shown that the removal of second molars, with subsequent posterior movement of the buccal segments, may be an alternative worth considering.

In orthodontics, cephalometrics are used to help evaluate individuals. The work of Steiner[16] has been particularly helpful. Perhaps Ricketts[11] comes closest to expressing the true value of cephalometric films when he says that the purpose of cephalometric analysis is to describe, compare, classify, and communicate the nature of the orthodontic-orthopedic problem. *I submit that such information would be valuable in evaluating the TMJ patient* to determine conditions such as open- or closed-bite tendency (Fig. 27-7).[17]

The question of whether the postorthodontic patient is more or less prone to TMJ dysfunction was explored by Dorph, Solow, and Carlsen.[2] Their study from the dental school in Copenhagen, Denmark, showed that 28% of the people seen in their TMJ clinic had previously been treated through orthodontics. This study

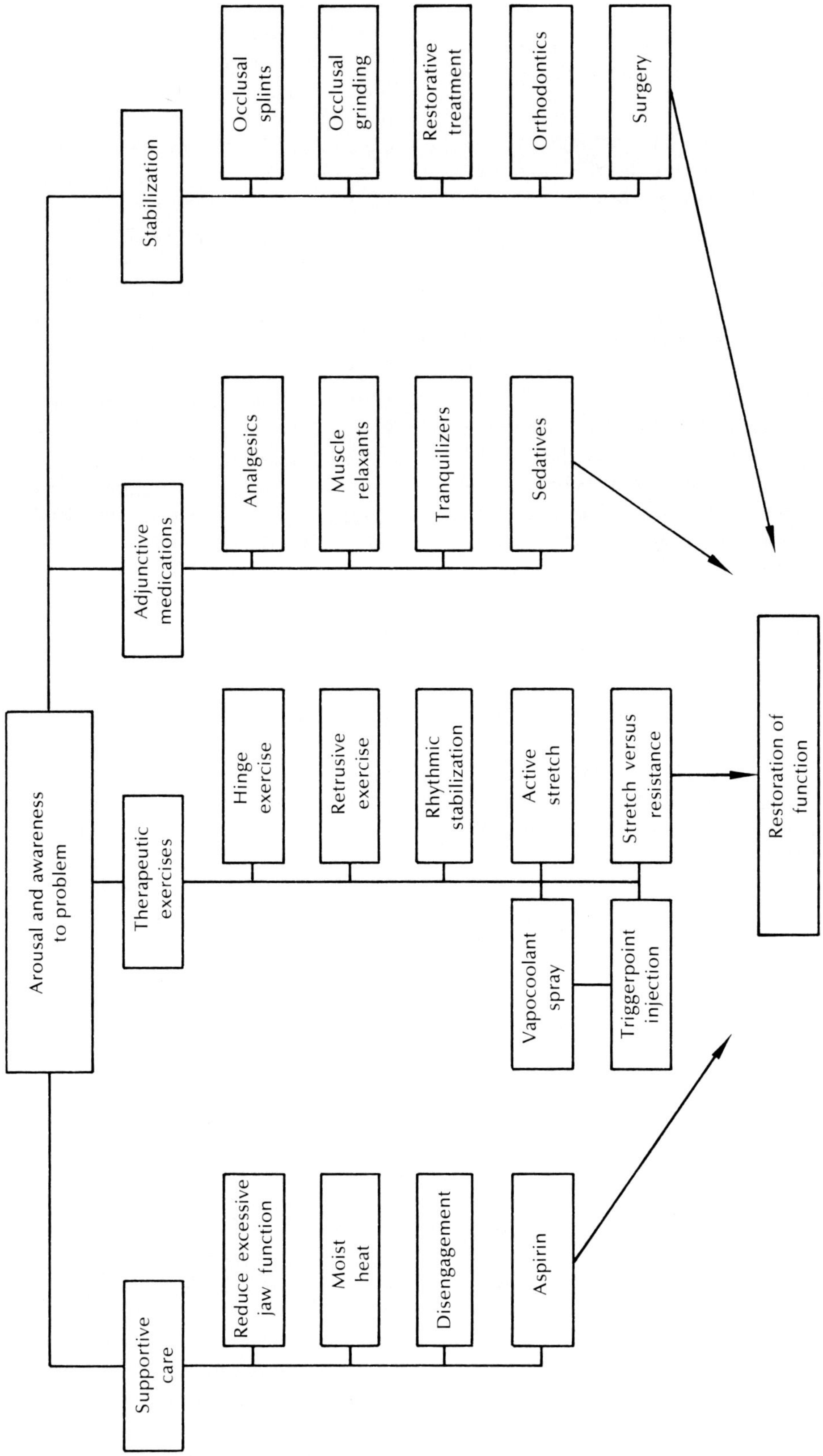

Fig. 27-6. Modalities of muscle relaxation in myofascial pain. (From Solberg, W.K.: Clinical dentistry, vol. 2, New York, 1976, Harper & Row, Publishers.)

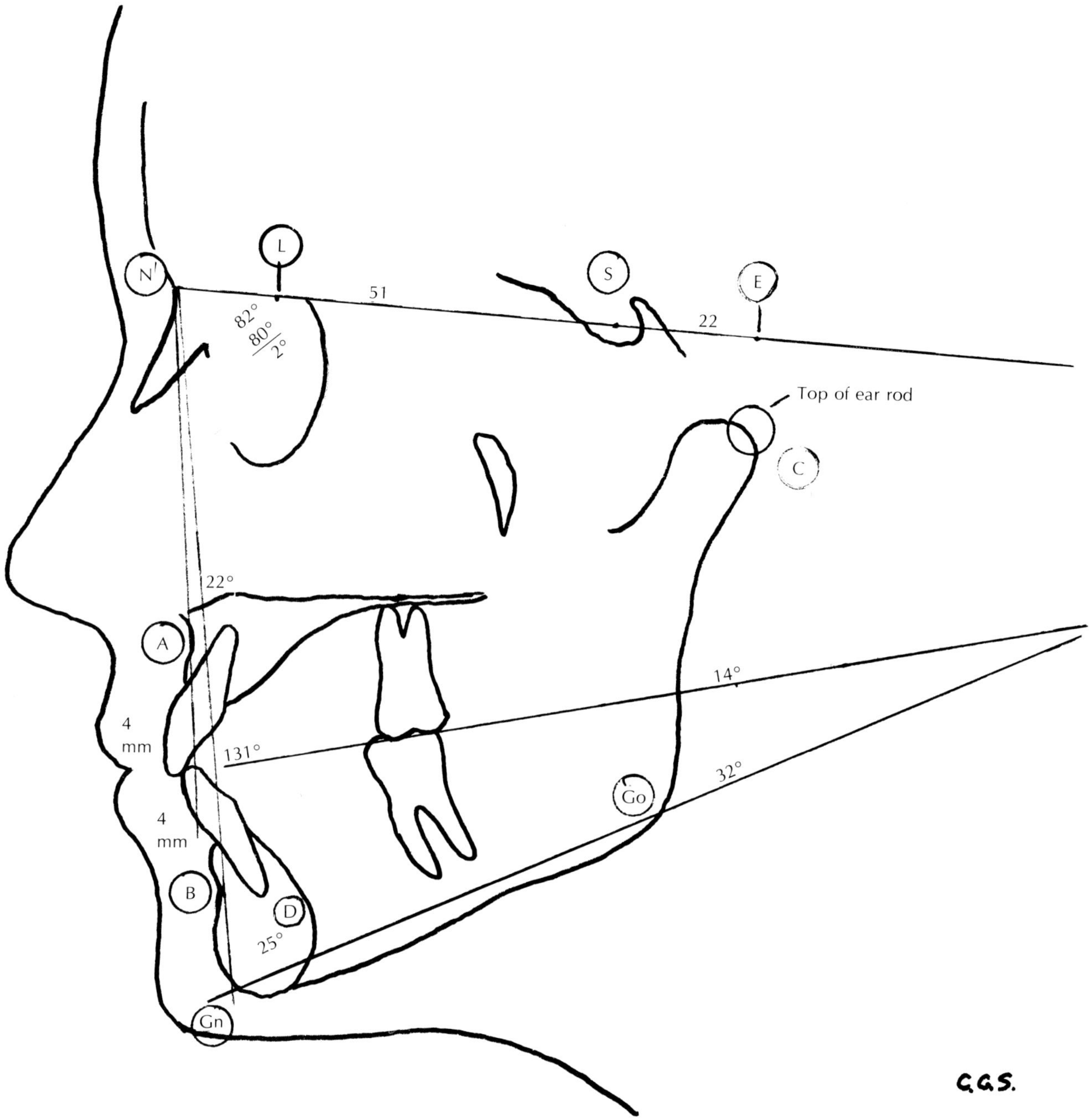

Fig. 27-7. Some of Steiner's more commonly used average norms.[16] By giving a visual image of the relationship of the teeth to bony landmarks, cephalometric tracing allows us to compare faces. Extreme open and closed bites seem to be more prone to TMJ problems. Normal faces may vary from these norms (for example, racial differences), but extreme deviations can be easily recognized. (From Steiner, C.C.: Angle Orthod. **29:**22, 1959.)

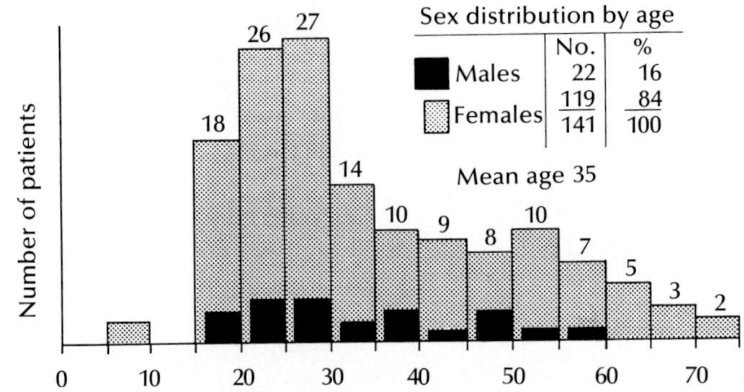

Fig. 27-8. Sex and age distribution of 141 TMJ patients in 5-year increments.

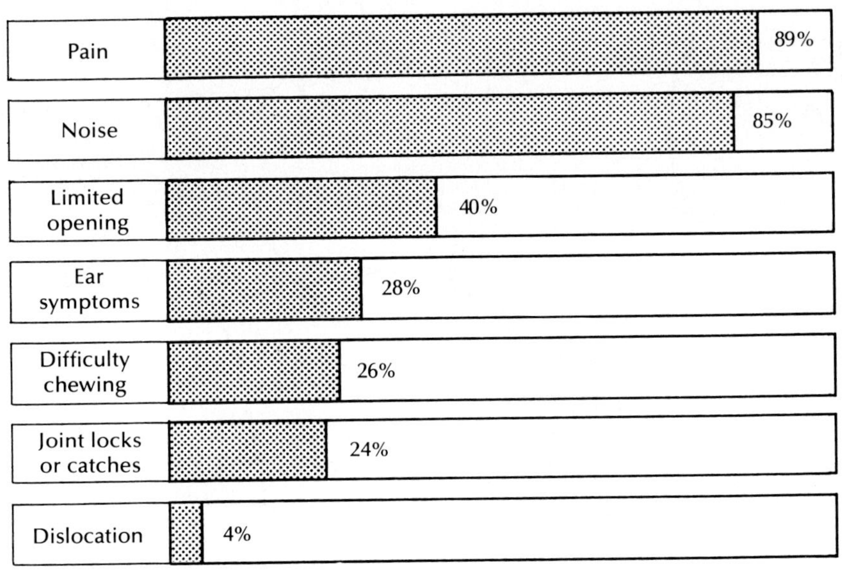

Fig. 27-9. Presenting symptoms in TMJ patients.

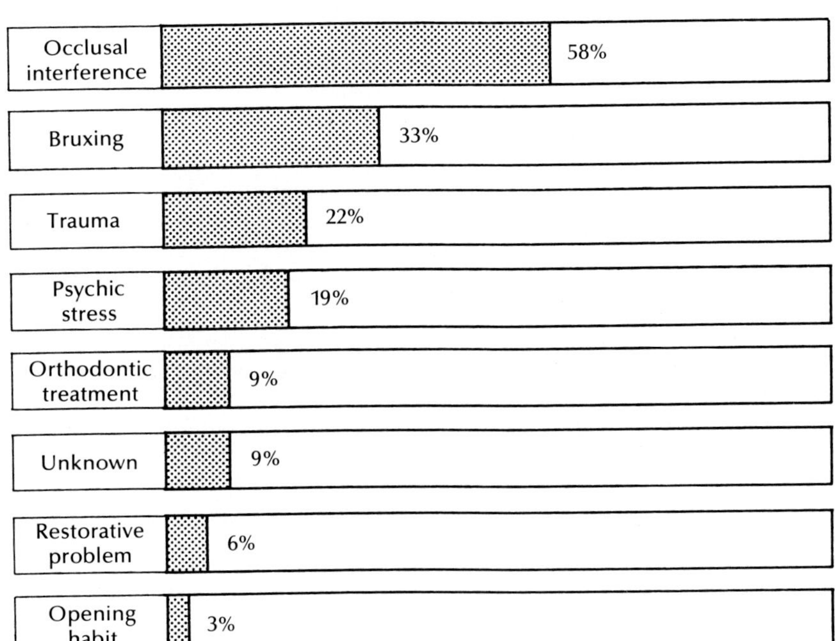

Fig. 27-10. Causative factors for 141 TMJ patients. Other causes, one each: staphylococcal infection as infant, surgery at early age, repeated cortisone shots, faulty night guard, faulty dentures.

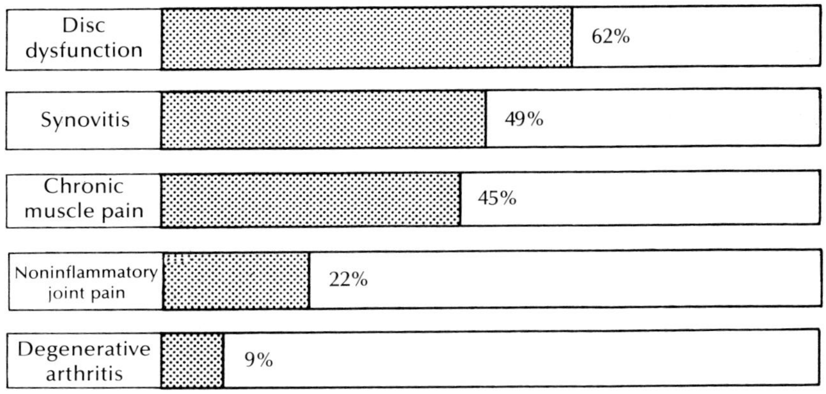

Fig. 27-11. Diagnosis of problem in 141 TMJ patients. Other diagnoses: fibrous ankylosis, 2%; early disc degeneration, 1%; perforated disc from trauma, 1%; no diagnosis, 4%.

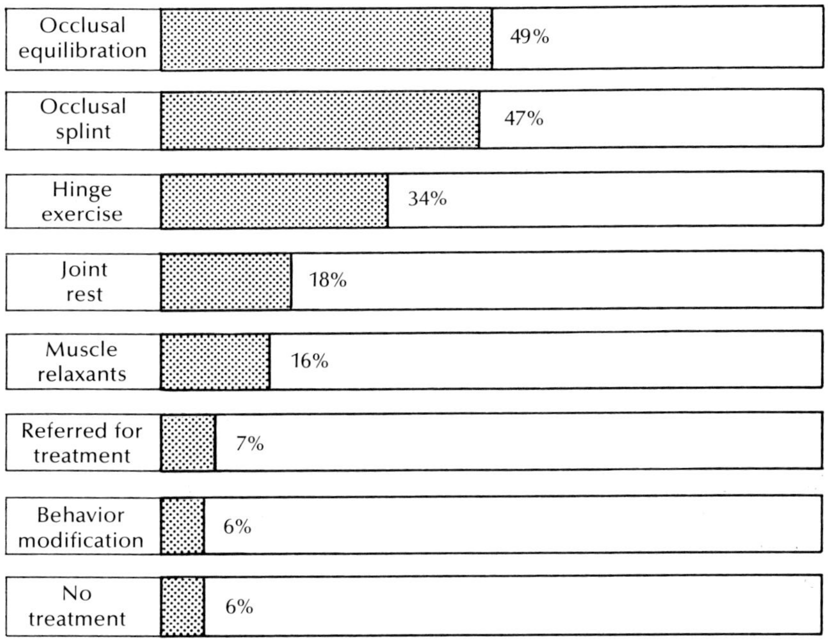

Fig. 27-12. Type of treatment used for 141 TMJ patients. Other treatments: local anesthetic to muscle or joint, 4%; surgery, 4%; cortisone injection to joint, 2%; other, 2%.

also showed that of a random sample of the public, 27% had received orthodontic treatment. It was their conclusion that there is no statistical correlation between TMJ problems and orthodontic therapy.

SUMMARY

The preceding review has attempted to show how a knowledge of orthodontics can help the clinician more fully understand the causes, methods of treatment, and prevention of the TMJ pain-dysfunction syndrome. The following outline summarizes the signs and symptoms, causes, diagnoses, and treatment modalities. The information has been gathered from many sources. Figs. 27-8 to 27-12 are from a study of 141 TMJ patients over a 5-year period by Moffett and Teel[6] at the University of Washington (Seattle). This work was particularly interesting because it put actual numbers on age, sex distribution, symptoms, causes, diagnoses, treatment methods, etc.

Much of the following outline is from a course given at the University of Southern California by Schireson and Mintzer.[14]

1. Signs and symptoms
   a. Pain—usually unilateral, a dull ache in the area that may radiate to
      (1) Angle of the mandibule
      (2) Temporal area
      (3) Lateral cervical area
   b. Muscle tenderness—may palpate
      (1) Over the neck of the mandible
      (2) Distal and superior to the maxillary tuberosity
      (3) Mandibular angle
      (4) Temporal crest
      (5) Lateral throat wall
   c. Clicking or popping noise—probably spasm of external pterygoid muscle causing disc to slip over condylar head (forward or backward) (this symptom alone does not indicate TMJ syndrome)
   d. Limitation of jaw function
      (1) Inability to open as wide as usual (4 to 5 cm is normal)
      (2) Deviation of mandible on opening
      (3) Incoordination of mandible on opening (asynchronous gait)
      (4) NOTE: These patients rarely have clicking now but may have had it in the past
2. Causes—a masticatory muscle spasm may be caused by the following
   a. Interferences
      (1) Centric
      (2) Eccentric
   b. Muscle fatigue because of tension-relieving oral habits (bruxing and clenching) (the emotional vector is high; the hostile, angry, frustrated person is more prone, but anxiety alone seldom causes bruxing or clenching)
   c. Muscle overextension
      (1) Fixed or removable prostheses that encroach on the intermaxillary space
      (2) Class II, division 1 malocclusion in which the person must reach excessively for an incisal bite
   d. Muscle overcontraction—loss of posterior support
      (1) Bilateral loss of posterior teeth
      (2) Settling of partial dentures
      (3) Excessive alveolar resorption under full dentures
      (4) Periodontal disease and/or excessive clenching
   e. Posterior displacement
      (1) Class II, division 2—linguoversion of the upper incisors guides mandible too far posteriorly
      (2) Klinorhynchy—excessive distal position of the maxilla, changing normal masticatory muscle vectors so this component force will tend to compress the condyle backward and upward into the fossa[12]
   f. Trauma (external)
   g. Excessive opening
3. Diagnosis and treatment
   a. Proper radiographs are essential to rule out joint damage
      (1) Cephalometric laminagraphy
      (2) Transcranial lateral oblique radiographs
      (3) Panorex radiographs
   b. If the radiographs are negative, then c through g are indicated
   c. Rest joint with soft diet, no gum chewing, and limited chewing and opening
   d. Use hot wet packs (or hydrocollator) 1/2 hour in the morning and 1/2 hour at night with gentle stretch opening exercise after heat; this must be followed rigidly for 3 weeks; 50% to 75% of patients show improvement
   e. If needed, a night guard (a splint to hold teeth at rest with a flat plane) may be used; some clinicians do this first
   f. Extreme cases may require diazepam (Valium) (2, 5, or 10 mg, two, three, or four times per day); sometimes 10 grains of aspirin every 3 hours is helpful; cortisone is usually not indicated, since inflammation is seldom involved; lidocaine (Xylocaine) into the joint area may help reduce a dislocation; trigger areas may be identified with procaine or ethyl chloride spray
   g. Occlusal spot grinding should be done carefully and *after* most of treatment items c through f; some clinicians grind obvious prematurities sooner
   h. Treatment of patients with irreparably damaged periarticular and intraarticular structures may require surgical intervention; however, surgery should be considered as a last resort
      (1) Reversible surgery[7]
      (2) Irreversible surgery[3]

The work of many authors has been referred to in an attempt to tie together pertinent information. May the future further enlighten us in this multifaceted field.

> And one might therefore say of me that in the book I have only made up a bunch of other people's flowers, and that of my own I have only provided the string that ties them together (M.E. de Montaigne).

REFERENCES

1. Bell, W.H.: Nonsurgical management of the pain-dysfunction syndrome, J. Am. Dent. Assoc. **79**:161, 1969.
2. Dorph, G., Solow, B., and Carlsen, O.: Masticatory dysfunction after orthodontic treatment? Tandlaegebladet **79**:789, 1975.
3. Henny, F.A.: Surgical treatment of the painful temporomandibular joint, J. Am. Dent. Assoc. **79**:171, 1969.
4. Liddle, D.W.: Second molar extraction in orthodontic treatment, Am. J. Orthod. **72**:599, 1977.
5. Mann, G.: Personal communication, 1979.
6. Moffett, B.C., and Teel, S.: A biologic approach to TMJ diagnosis and treatment planning, presented to the Northern Section of the Pacific Coast Society of Orthodontists, Feb. 7-8, 1975, Seattle, Wash.
7. Morgan, D.H.: Dysfunction, pain, tinnitus, vertigo corrected by mandibular joint surgery, J. South. Calif. State Dent. Assoc. **39**:505, 1971.
8. Morgan, D.H.: Personal communication, 1979.
9. Perry, H.T., Jr.: Relation of occlusion to temporomandibular joint dysfunction: the orthodontic viewpoint, J. Am. Dent. Assoc. **79**:137, 1969.
10. Ricketts, R.M.: Abnormal function of the temporomandibular joint, Am. J. Orthod. **41**:435, 1955.
11. Ricketts, R.M.: A foundation for cephalometric communication, Am. J. Orthod. **46**:330, 1960.
12. Roberts, D.: The etiology of the temporomandibular joint dysfunction syndrome, Am. J. Orthod. **66**:498, 1974.
13. Roth, R.H.: Temporomandibular pain-dysfunction and occlusal relationships, Angle Orthod. **43**:136, 1973.
14. Schireson, S., and Mintzer, H.: The temporomandibular joint and perioral pain, Course at University of Southern California, Los Angeles, Feb. 25-26, 1972.
15. Solberg, W.K.: Clinical dentistry, vol. 2, New York, 1976, Harper & Row, Publishers.
16. Steiner, C.C.: Cephalometrics for you and me, Am. J. Orthod. **39**:729, 1953.
17. Steiner, C.C.: Cephalometrics in clinical practice, Angle Orthod. **29**:22, 1959.
18. Williamson, E.H.: Temporomandibular dysfunction in pretreatment adolescent patients, Am. J. Orthod. **72**:429, 1977.

28 Interrelationship of myofacial pain syndrome, temporomandibular joint dysfunction, and orthodontics

MARTIN E. FRANKEL, D.M.D., M.D.S.

In the beginning there was Costen's syndrome. Since the 1930s when Costen originally published his work, many descriptive terms such as *temporomandibular joint dysfunction, myofacial pain syndrome, masticatory pain-dysfunction syndrome, craniomandibular pain* and *craniofacial pain,* have been used to describe what is in reality a multifaceted problem, endured by millions of patients. There is in actuality no one pathological entity that is truly descriptive of the syndrome. Its interrelationship with neural pathways, osseous structures, fascial spaces, and the head and neck musculature demands that any valid approach to these problems be multidisciplinary. Although a great number of these problems are of dental or occlusal origin, it is mandatory that the otolaryngologist, the neurologist, psychiatrist, physical therapist, oral surgeon, and orthodontist be involved in total overall care of the patient.

This chapter concentrates on the role of orthodontic care, both prophylactically and therapeutically. It has been estimated that approximately 20% of the population suffer from some form of craniofacial dysfunction. Unfortunately many of these individuals have suffered for such a prolonged period without help that they have been forced to adapt to living with their pain. One is reminded of times in England during the reign of Henry VIII when prisoners were trapped in the Tower of London, with no escape possible. Without question, this is the feeling related by most of these patients. It is as though they were doomed to constant suffering, with no solution in sight. Since many of these problems are occlusally related, the orthodontist well trained in head and neck pain and dysfunction is in a primary position to help many patients. It must not be forgotten, however, that this job cannot be done alone but requires the coordination of all the disciplines involved.

CASE HISTORY AND EXAMINATION

Of primary importance to the treatment of any patient suffering from head and neck pain is a thorough and complete case history of the patient. Fig. 28-1 shows the case history form used in my own office. As can be seen, it is a combination of various history forms in common use in the field. Fig. 28-2 shows the clinical examination form used. The procedure for complete history taking and thorough clinical examination is covered in Chapters 5 and 6.

THE NEUROMUSCULAR OCCLUSION

Until the advent of the Mandibular Kinesiograph (Jankelson) and the use of transcutaneous electrical neural stimulation to the facial nerve and the mandibular branch of the fifth nerve (Jankelson), all other means of establishing a mandibular relationship to the cranium were done on an arbitrary static basis without any regard to the musculature that controlled movement of the osseous structures. Except in the presence of pathological conditions of the components of the temporomandibular joint itself or traumatic injury to the joint, movement of the mandible is controlled primarily by the musculature, tendons, and ligaments. Except with the previously mentioned osseous defects of the temporomandibular joint and congenital osseous defects, the dentition itself controls the mandibular position and thereby can readily intitiate spasm of the controlling masticatory muscles with frequent referred or radiated pain. Exact condylar position is not critical. What is important is that the condyle, eminence, and glenoid fossa morphology be normal and that normal translation of the condyle be allowable without trauma against the fossa or excessive compression of the articular disc. In many instances it has been shown (using the Mandibular Kinesiograph) that the neuromuscular

Text continued on p. 520.

MARTIN E. FRANKEL, D.M.D., M.D.S., P.C.
Practice Limited to Dento-Facial Orthopedics

MYOFACIAL PAIN SYNDROME AND TEMPOROMANDIBULAR JOINT CASE HISTORY

Date ______________________ Case No. ____________
Patient's Name ______________________ Sex ____________
Age _____ Date of Birth ______________ Birthplace ____________
Responsible Party ______________________
Home Address ______________________ Home Tel. No. ____________
Business Address ______________________ Business Tel. No. ____________
Occupation ______________________
Employed by ______________________
Family Dentist ______________________
Family Physician ______________________
Referred By ______________________

1. Do symptoms affect one or both joints? right ( ) left ( ) both ( )
(If both joints, also mark which joint seems most affected.)

2. What symptoms do you have? (Please check appropriate areas. R=right, L=left.)

a. Pain in joint R( ) L( )
b. Pain in ear R( ) L( )
c. Pain around eyes R( ) L( )
d. Pain in lower jaw R( ) L( )
e. Pain in upper jaw R( ) L( )
f. Pain in neck R( ) L( )
g. Stiffness in neck R( ) L( )
h. Pain in shoulder R( ) L( )
i. Pain in forehead R( ) L( )
j. Pain in facial muscles (cheek area) R( ) L( )
k. Grating sound in joint R( ) L( )
l. Subjective hearing loss R( ) L( )
m. Clicking, snapping or popping sound in joint. (underline which sounds most descriptive.) If present, is it in R( ) L( )
n. Dizziness ("vertigo") ( )
o. Upset stomach - nausea ( )
p. Ringing sound in ears ("tinnitus") R( ) L( )
q. Headache ( )
r. Fullness, pressure, or blockage in ear R( ) L( )
s. Pain in tongue R( ) L( )
t. Duration of above symptoms (use specific letters which describe problem)
1. Constant ____________
2. Sporadic ____________
u. Facial twitch R( ) L( )
v. Tic or tic-like pain R( ) L( )
w. Total inability to open mouth ( )
If yes, is it:
1. Constant ( )
2. Sporadic ( )
x. Partial inability to open mouth (
If yes, is it:
1. Constant ( )
2. Sporadic ( )

y. Other symptoms: (please write in) ____________
____

3. Is there a trigger area which initiates the pain? Yes ( ) No ( )
(If yes, please describe) ______________________

4. How long have you been bothered by this problem?
(a) _____ years (b) _____ months (c) _____ weeks (d) _____ days

5. Have you had any injury to the jaw or face? Yes ( ) No ( )
(If yes, please explain) ______________________

Date: ______________ ______________________
signature of patient or guardian

Fig. 28-1. A, Case history form.

Continued.

MPDS AND TMJ DYSFUNCTION CASE HISTORY - PAGE 2 Patient ____________

6. Do you have arthritis? Yes ( ) No ( )

7. Have you ever had cervical traction? Yes ( ) No ( )

8. Have you had any other treatment for this problem? Yes ( ) No ( )
(If yes, explain -- medicine, exercise, dental appliance, etc.)

____

9. Have you had your teeth straightened (orthodontics)? Yes ( ) No ( )

10. Are you sensitive to metal rings or ear rings? Yes ( ) No ( )

11. Have you had your bite adjusted by your dentist? Yes ( ) No ( )
(If yes, please explain when)

____

12. Do you attribute the symptoms to any one incident? Yes ( ) No ( )
(If yes, explain)

____

13. Have you had cortisone injected into the joint? Yes ( ) No ( )
If yes, when? ____________ How many injections? ____________
By whom? ______________________________

14. Are you now on pain medication? Yes ( ) No ( )
If yes, what kind and how much? ______________________________

____

15. Do you know if you clench your teeth? Yes ( ) No ( )

16. Has anyone mentioned you grind your teeth ("brux")
at night during sleep? Yes ( ) No ( )

17. Do your jaws ache when chewing hard or tough foods? Yes ( ) No ( )

18. Do you chew gum? Frequently ( ) Moderately ( )
Infrequently ( ) Never ( )

19. Is there anyone else in your family with a similar
problem? (If yes, explain.) Yes ( ) No ( )

____

20. Do you have any orthopedic (bone) problems? Yes ( ) No ( )
(If yes, please describe.) ______________________________

21. Do you wear special shoes (lifts, etc.) Yes ( ) No ( )
(If yes, please describe.) ______________________________

22. Do you have any ear, nose, throat, or sinus problems
not already mentioned? Yes ( ) No ( )
(If yes, please describe.) ______________________________

____

Date: ____________ ______________________________
signature of patient or guardian

Fig. 28-1, cont'd. B, Page 2.

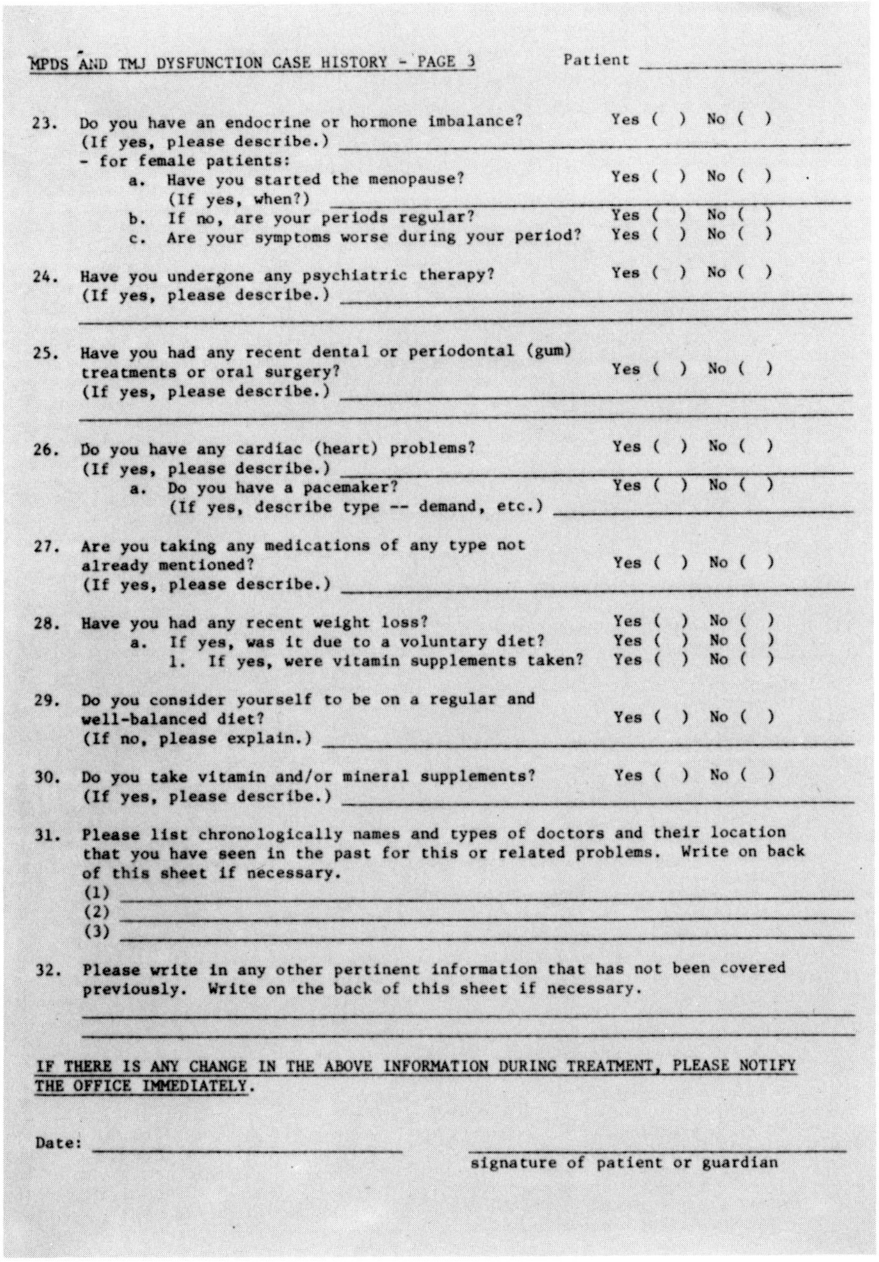

MPDS AND TMJ DYSFUNCTION CASE HISTORY - PAGE 3 Patient ____________

23. Do you have an endocrine or hormone imbalance? Yes ( ) No ( )
(If yes, please describe.) ____________
- for female patients:
a. Have you started the menopause? Yes ( ) No ( )
(If yes, when?) ____________
b. If no, are your periods regular? Yes ( ) No ( )
c. Are your symptoms worse during your period? Yes ( ) No ( )

24. Have you undergone any psychiatric therapy? Yes ( ) No ( )
(If yes, please describe.) ____________

25. Have you had any recent dental or periodontal (gum) treatments or oral surgery? Yes ( ) No ( )
(If yes, please describe.) ____________

26. Do you have any cardiac (heart) problems? Yes ( ) No ( )
(If yes, please describe.) ____________
a. Do you have a pacemaker? Yes ( ) No ( )
(If yes, describe type -- demand, etc.) ____________

27. Are you taking any medications of any type not already mentioned? Yes ( ) No ( )
(If yes, please describe.) ____________

28. Have you had any recent weight loss? Yes ( ) No ( )
a. If yes, was it due to a voluntary diet? Yes ( ) No ( )
1. If yes, were vitamin supplements taken? Yes ( ) No ( )

29. Do you consider yourself to be on a regular and well-balanced diet? Yes ( ) No ( )
(If no, please explain.) ____________

30. Do you take vitamin and/or mineral supplements? Yes ( ) No ( )
(If yes, please describe.) ____________

31. Please list chronologically names and types of doctors and their location that you have seen in the past for this or related problems. Write on back of this sheet if necessary.
(1) ____________
(2) ____________
(3) ____________

32. Please write in any other pertinent information that has not been covered previously. Write on the back of this sheet if necessary.
____

IF THERE IS ANY CHANGE IN THE ABOVE INFORMATION DURING TREATMENT, PLEASE NOTIFY THE OFFICE IMMEDIATELY.

Date: ____________ ____________
signature of patient or guardian

Fig. 28-1, cont'd. C, Page 3.

MARTIN E. FRANKEL, D.M.D., M.D.S., P.C.
Practice Limited to Dento-Facial Orthopedics

MYOFACIAL PAIN SYNDROME AND TMJ DYSFUNCTION CLINICAL EXAMINATION FORM

1. Facial Asymmetry:
   a. None
   b. Perceptible, Obvious, Gross asymmetry in the Right, Left ______________________ area.

2. Palpation Of The Joints:
   a. pain on TMJ palpation (teeth in rest position) - Right, Left, No.
   b. pain on TMJ palpation (teeth in C.O.) - Right, Left, No.
   c. pain during protrusive movements - Right, Left, No.
   d. translation of the condyle is Smooth, Grating, Asynchronous.
   e. digital examination of the external auditory canal discloses translation of the condyle on the - Right, Left, Both
   f. pain on palpation of the external auditory meatus - Right, Left, No

3. Ausculation Of The Joints:
   a. click: Left - open, close, none
      Right - open, close, none
   b. crepitus: Left - open, close, none
      Right - open, close, none

4. Palpation Of The Musculature (Pain - indicate origin, insertion, body)
   a. Masseter - right ________, left ________, no
   b. Internal Pterygoids - right ________, left ________, no
   c. External Pterygoids - right ________, left ________, no
   d. Temporalis - right ________, left ________, no
   e. Buccinator - right ________, left ________, no
   f. Digastrics - right ________, left ________, no
   g. Occipital - right ________, left ________, no
   h. Sternocleidomastoid - right ________, left ________, no
   i. Trapezius - right ________, left ________, no
   j. Scalenes - right ________, left ________, no
   k. other ______________________________________

5. Palpation Of The Cervical Lymph Nodes
   a. pain - Right, Left, No.

6. Opening Movement:
   a. Synchronous or Asynchronous
   b. Maximum Opening Without Pain ________ mm.
   c. Lateral Deviation On Opening - Right, Left, No
   d. Deviation first to the Right then Left - Yes, No
   e. Deviation first to the Left then Right - Yes, No.
   f. Deviation of about ________ mm.
   g. Can demonstrate a left lateral excursion - Yes, No
   h. Can demonstrate a right lateral excursion - Yes, No.

7. Examination of the Soft Tissues:
   a. External: skin of the face, lymph chains, lips ______________
   b. Vestibule and Tongue: vestibule, cheeks, mucosa, gingiva, tongue ______________________________________

Fig. 28-2. A, Clinical examination form.

MPDS AND TMJ DYSFUNCTION CLINICAL EXAMINATION FORM - PAGE 2

Patient: ______________________ Date: ______________

c. Tongue and Floor of the Mouth: floor of the mouth, the base, lateral borders, and ventral surfaces of the tongue ______________

d. Palate: hard palate, soft palate, uvula ______________

e. Fauces and Pharynx: tonsils, anterior and posterior palatine arches, nasopharynx ______________

8. Dental Examination (Radiographic):
   a. caries requiring immediate attention ______________
   b. pathology (exposures, abscesses, cysts) ______________
   c. periodontal pathology (alveolar bone loss, periodontal space) ______________
   d. impactions ______________

9. Dental Examination (Clinical):
   a. areas requiring immediate attention: i.e. deep caries, severe periodontal involvement, extractions, etc.
      1. ______________
      2. ______________
   b. absent teeth ______________
      1. reason for tooth loss ______________
      2. approximate date of tooth loss ______________
   c. prosthetic replacements and date ______________
      1. ______________
      2. ______________
      3. ______________
      4. ______________
   d. abrasion ______________
   e. incisal and occlusal wear facets ______________
   f. mobility ______________

10. Examination of the Occlusion (Clinical):
   a. malocclusion in C.O. (Angle Classification) ______________
   b. satisfactory prosthesis - Yes ( ) No ( ) ______________
   c. firm posterior support in C.O. - Yes ( ) No ( ) ______________
   d. cuspid protected occlusion
      1. right side - Yes ( ) No ( ) ______________
      2. left side - Yes ( ) No ( ) ______________
   e. balancing cusp interferences
      1. right side - Yes ( ) No ( ) ______________
      2. left side - Yes ( ) No ( ) ______________
   f. working cusp interferences
      1. right side - Yes ( ) No ( ) ______________
      2. left side - Yes ( ) No ( ) ______________
   g. fremitus of the teeth on closure into C.O. - Yes ( ) No ( )
   h. repeatability of C.O. - yes ( ) No ( )
   i. vertical overbite in C.O. ________ mm.
   j. horizontal overjet in C.O. ________ mm.

11. Radiographic Examination of the TMJ:
   a. condyle morphology
      1. right - Normal, Abnormal ______________
      2. left - Normal, Abnormal ______________

Fig. 28-2, cont'd. B, Page 2.

MPDS AND TMJ DYSFUNCTION CLINICAL EXAMINATION FORM - PAGE 3

Patient: ______________________ Date: ______________

b. fossa morphology
   1. right - Normal, Abnormal ______________________
   2. left - Normal, Abnormal ______________________
c. eminentia morphology
   1. right - Normal, Abnormal ______________________
   2. left - Normal, Abnormal ______________________
d. posture of condyle in fossa
   1. right - Normal, Abnormal ______________________
   2. left - Normal, Abnormal ______________________
   (The average measurements from the condyle to the eminence = 1.5mm., to the top of the fossa = 2.5mm., to the center of the auditory canal = 7.5mm.)
e. condyle translation
   1. right - Yes ( ) No ( )
   2. left - Yes ( ) No ( )
f. evidence of neoplasms
   1. right - Yes ( ) No ( )
   2. left - Yes ( ) No ( )
g. evidence of osteo-arthritic changes
   1. right - Yes ( ) No ( )
   2. left - Yes ( ) No ( )

12. Habits Noted During Examination:
   a. ______________________
   b. ______________________

13. Standing Postural Evaluation:
   a. head tilt ______________________
   b. shoulder height ______________________
   c. hip height ______________________
   d. leg length ______________________

14. Emotional Factors: (sample questions)
   a. Do you have children? ______________________
   b. Do you sleep well? ______________________
   c. Does your spouse help you? ______________________
   d. Does your job satisfy you? ______________________
   e. Do you have house guests (in-laws)? ______________________
   f. Are you nervous? ______________________
   g. Are you depressed? ______________________
   - notes on first impression of patient: ______________________
   ____
   - Should patient have M.M.P.I. test or Cornell Medical Index Test?
   Yes ( ) No ( )

15. Mandibular Kineseograph Findings: see separate diagnostic workup

16. Diagnosis:
   ____
   ____

Fig. 28-2, cont'd. C, Page 3.

MPDS AND TMJ DYSFUNCTION CLINICAL EXAMINATION FORM - Page 4

Patient: ______________________ Date: ______________

17. Treatment Plan (number in order of importance):

( ) no treatment	( ) orthopedic occlusal splint
( ) vapocoolant spray	( ) coronoplasty
( ) moist heat	( ) dietary counseling
( ) muscle exercises	( ) preventive counseling (habits)
( ) soft diet	( ) ENT consultation
( ) drug therapy	( ) medical consultation
( ) biofeedback	( ) neurological consultation
( ) myofunctional therapy	( ) psychiatric consultation
( ) removal of gross prematurities	( ) orthodontic consultation
( ) transcutaneous electrical neural stimulation	( ) prosthetic consultation
( ) plain occlusal splint	( ) surgical consultation

18. Prognosis:

____

19. Post-Treatment Requirements:
   a. ______________________________________
   b. ______________________________________
   c. ______________________________________

Additional Notes:

____

____

____

____

____

Post-Treatment Evaluation: Date: ______________

____

____

____

____

____

____

Fig. 28-2, cont'd. D, Page 4.

path of closure of the mandible is anterior to the centric-occlusion position. Closure into centric occlusion therefore causes retrusion of the mandible and stretching of the attached muscles, ligaments, and tendons, resulting in pain. An understanding of the Christenson phenomenon whereby protrusion of the mandible results in posterior disocclusion helps to further explain this phenomenon. This is not to state that all patients showing a large freeway space should have their vertical dimension altered, since the range of adaptability of the human is quite large, and inadequate data are available at this time as to what a normal freeway space is. It is therefore important to differentiate during orthodontic therapy between the symptomatic patient and the asymptomatic patient. Even with the absence of pain there are certain types of malocclusion where the Mandibular Kinesiograph would be of aid as a prophylactic measure toward preventing future temporomandibular joint dysfunctions or myofacial pain syndrome. These are discussed later in this chapter.

STANDARD ORTHODONTIC DIAGNOSTIC PROCEDURES (FOR ASYMPTOMATIC PATIENTS)

Routine diagnostic techniques include the following:

1. Study casts in centric occlusion
2. Panoramic radiograph (orthopantograph)
3. Bite-wing radiographs
4. Facial photographs (frontal and lateral)
5. Lateral cephalogram and analysis
6. Posteroanterior radiograph
7. Miscellaneous procedures, such as
   a. Bolten Index analysis
   b. Peck analysis
   c. Holdaway facial profile analysis

The results of these techinques are based on well-established criteria for classic orthodontic therapy and the correction of malocclusions. What has not been considered to date, however, is the position of the mandibular condyle and its relationship to future temporomandibular joint dysfunction and/or myofacial pain-dysfunction syndrome.

Unfortunately little data are available concerning growth of the mandible and more specifically condylar growth changes that occur with age. Although condylar morphological changes can occur through remodeling even after the age of approximately 21, the problems facing most orthodontists today are still found in patients ranging from 8 to 16 years old, where rapid growth is occurring. The determination of "normal" freeway space or vertical dimension is still an arbitrary one, however, and until an adequate serial study is done to determine the optimum vertical dimension (if one exists), clinicians will have to be satisfied with using an arbitrary measurement. A freeway space of approximately 1.5 to 2.0 mm has been considered normal, since this allows for cuspal disocclusion without undue use of the masticatory muscles. The orthodontic patient who exhibits no symptoms of myofacial pain or temporomandibular joint dysfunction should be treated at this time using the classic and well-established diagnostic criteria. There are certain exceptions, such as patients exhibiting a dual bite, a severely deep overbite that may be inhibiting normal forward movement of the mandible, a Class II, division 2 (angle) malocclusion, which may exhibit the same postlocked mandibular phenomenon, and a Class I (angle) malocclusion where there is a family predispostion toward a Class III (angle) malocclusion. The patient exhibiting a lateral tongue thrust in contrast to an anterior tongue thrust also should be examined using additional criteria, as described in the next section.

Although the concept of increasing vertical dimension would lead one to believe that an increase in arch length would occur, it should be remembered that this is in reality the same premise on which leveling of the curve of Spee is based, and it is tolerable as long as the anterior teeth are not moved so far anteriorly that they cause damage to the labial plate of alveolar bone and the attached gingiva.

ORTHODONTIC DIAGNOSTIC PROCEDURES USING NEUROMUSCULAR CONCEPTS AND TECHNIQUES

1. Study casts mounted in myocentric relation versus centric occlusion
2. Panoramic radiograph (orthopantograph)
3. Bite-wing radiographs
4. Facial photographs (frontal and lateral)
   a. Centric occlusion
   b. With myoprint registration in place
5. Lateral cephalogram and analysis
   a. Centric occlusion
   b. With myoprint registration in place
6. Posteroanterior radiograph
   a. Centric occlusion
   b. With myoprint registration in place
7. Posteroanterior radiograph (transorbital view)
   a. Centric occlusion
   b. With myoprint registration in place
8. Miscellaneous procedures (where indicated), such as
   a. Mandibular Kinesiograph analysis
   b. Bolten Index analysis
   c. Peck analysis
   d. Holdaway facial profile analysis

These diagnostic techniques are used therapeutically on those patients exhibiting either some form of temporomandibular joint dysfunction or myofacial pain syndrome or prophylactically on those orthodontic patients who exhibit the proper criteria, as stated in the previous section. Although the quantitative establishment of vertical dimension or freeway space would be arbitrary, these patients exhibit occlusions outside the normal range of mandibular movement or have inhibiting anatomical or genetic patterns that would lead one to believe that their centric occlusion is not allowing a free neuromuscular path of closure of the mandible.

There are certain possible sequelae of not obtaining a myocentric relationship and neuromuscular occlusion during orthodontic therapy. These are as follows:

1. TMJ dysfunction
2. Myofacial pain syndrome
3. Instability of results
   a. Mandibular anterior crowding
   b. Maxillary anterior crowding
   c. Incisal abrasion and/or occlusal wear facets
   d. Deepening of overbite
   e. Maxillary central incisor diastemata
   f. Myofunctional problems such as tongue thrust or reverse swallow
4. Periodontal pathological conditions

The first and second conditions are caused primarily by the patient's mandible being forced posteriorly into centric occlusion, causing disharmony of either the temporomandibular joint components or related musculature. Instability of the orthodontic result and periodontal pathosis would be a result of the neuromuscular tendency of the mandible to try to close in a more anterior postion while the mandible is being held posteriorly by the centric occlusal relationship.

Orthodontic treatment procedures

Removable biofunctional appliances have been used in Europe for many years. These include the Anderson, Schwartz, Bimler, Frankel, and the many modifications of these appliances which occur in the literature quite frequently. The concept of their use is to inhibit growth of the maxilla, but primarily to stimulate growth of the mandible and mandibular condyles, as well as to achieve vertical changes through normal growth and positive pressures. Although there are without question definite benefits in the use of such appliances, there are many negative aspects of their use that must be resolved. Primarily, one must be concerned with once again the arbitrary determination of anteroposterior relationships and vertical height. There have been numerous instances seen clinically where the use of such appliances has actually created TMJ dysfunctions or myofacial pain syndrome because of excessive pressues or improperly directed forces. Extraoral therapy such as maxillary face-bows, high-pull headgears, and cervicooccipital headgears are well established in the orthodontic armamentarium. They serve to inhibit anterior growth of the maxilla while allowing anterior growth of the mandible as well as cause actual distal movement of the maxillary buccal segments. Mandibular extraoral appliances such as chin cups have certain value when used at a very early age in Class III (angle) malocclusions, although no definitive study has been done to determine the effect of the posterior pressure on the posterosuperior surface of the mandibular condyle, glenoid fossa, or articular disc.

Fixed orthodontic appliances are most common and require no detailed explanation. They allow complete three-dimensional control of tooth movement. It must be stressed, however, that the main criterion must be not the mechanics of how the teeth should be moved or the jaws repositioned but to what position they should be moved.

Orthopedic repositioning splints placed on the mandible are a great adjunct either at the initiation of treatment or during treatment. Their use requires utilization of the Mandibular Kinesiograph to determine three-dimensional mandibular positioning on a neuromuscular basis. This splint is fabricated of acrylic and built up to a preestablished vertical dimension, giving the patient full cuspal anatomy with centric stops and freedom from lateral interferences. It can be used on a patient exhibiting symptoms prior to placement of orthodontic appliances, or it can be used over the orthodontic appliances themselves. The use of thin fiberglass-mesh inserts in the acrylic can help prevent breakage of the acrylic from occlusal forces. The purpose of the splint is to obtain a position of the mandible in relation to the maxilla that is within a tolerable range for the patient and to create a relaxed masticatory musculature. In the child exhibiting craniofacial dysfunction without the existence of malocclusion the splint can be used alone, and, quite frequently by initially removing acrylic over the first permanent molars, supraeruption of the dentition will occur. The second premolar acrylic is then removed, followed by the first premolar acrylic, and finally followed by elimination of the splint. This allows eruption of the dentition to the same vertical level as the original splint without orthodontic intervention. It is important that after this procedure the patient's dentition be equilibrated with an occusal indicator wax (Kerr) and transcutaneous electrical neural stimulation such as with the Myo-Monitor to ensure full centric stops and freedom from lateral interferences. There are instances with children and most specifically with adults whereby eruption of the teeth will not occur without assistance. In these cases orthodontic brackets can be bonded to the opposing teeth where movement is required, and vertical elastic bands can be worn for extrusion. The only teeth that will move are the mandibular teeth as they are pulled through the slot in the acrylic, since the normal occlusal relationship of the maxillary dentition into the mandibular splint will prevent extrusion of the maxillary dentition.

The controversy regarding extraction versus nonextraction in orthodontic therapy is no longer quite the debate it once was. Adequate criteria have been established for determining arch length, tooth size, and growth projections of the maxilla and mandible. Suffice it to say that if there is no arch length to tooth size discrepancy, no extractions are indicated, and if there is a discrepancy involved, then it must be up to the clinician's judgment whether the amount of discrepancy warrants the extraction of permanent tooth units. In situations with mandibular crowding where the second deciduous molar leeway space or interproximal stripping will be inadequate to allow for good arch alignment, there is no alternative to extractions. This does not, however, mandate the extraction of only the first premolars, since various combinations of premolars can be extracted by the clinician to result in the desired space, and proper control of the appliances can eliminate the problem of overreducing the facial profile. One important criteron is leveling of the curve of Spee for correction of deep overbites, and this unfortunately results in further decrease in arch length unless the lower incisors are to be thrown forward against the labial plate of bone. This same premise holds true in those instances where patients exhibiting TMJ dysfunction or myofacial pain syndrome have been made comfortable and stablized with an orthopedic repositioning splint, which mandates an increase in vertical dimension. There is no significant increase in arch length that can be tolerated by the periodontal tissues by increasing the vertical dimension. In those cases which show discrepancies of tooth size to arch length in excess of 5 mm, extractions are almost mandatory. Therefore, although establishing the correct neuromuscular pathway is vital in many patients undergoing orthodontic therapy or in those symptomatic patients who require orthodontic treatment, it should not be assumed that by increasing the vertical dimension the extraction of permanent tooth units will be elimated except in those instances of very minor discrepancies.

CASE HISTORIES

Case 1

This 13-year-old girl, with no previous orthodontic treatment, presented with the chief complaint of severe headaches over a 3- to 4-month period. Her clinical symptoms were spasmodic and severe occipital headaches. During clinical examination the palpation of the temporomandibular joints revealed slight tenderness and centric occlusion and protrusive movements. Translation of the condyle was smooth, and auscultation of the joints revealed slight crepitus on both the left and right sides. Palpation of the musculature revealed severe pain of the internal and external pterygoid muscles and slight tenderness of the central body of the temporal muscles. Mandibular opening movement was synchronous although limited, and the patient was able to demonstrate a left and right lateral excursion. Examination of the soft tissue was inconsequential, as was dental examination.

Radiographic findings showed no pathological conditions of the osseous structures of the temporomandibular joints. Mandibular Kinesiograph findings included vertical-velocity tracings indicating dyskinesia and bradykinesia on closing as well as a definite click on closure. There was a marked deviation of the patient's mandible to her left; the anterior-vertical ratio of closure was normal, although her vertical dimension was excessive, and there was a deviation of the mandible to her left side, indicative of external pterygoid dysfunction. The mandible was overclosed, posteriorly displaced because of anterior tooth interference, laterally displaced, and not on a relaxed neuromuscular trajectory; the patient also swallowed with her tongue between her teeth, which is quite common with an excessive freeway space. There was no associated history.

The diagnosis was dysfunctional temporomandibular joint arthritis with resultant myofacial spasm. The treatment plan was transcutaneous electrical neural stimulation and placement of a mandibular orthopedic repositioning splint to allow closure of the mandible into a correct neuromuscular path, thereby eliminating muscle dysfunction. This will be accomplished by decreasing the patient's freeway space and eliminating the lateral excursion. Follow-up therapy will consist of allowing orthodontic movement of the teeth into a correct neuromuscular position once the patient has become asymptomatic and this position is determined.

The study casts of the patient in centric occlusion and mounted in myocentric relation are shown in Figs. 28-3 and 28-4. Note the excessive freeway space present. An orthopedic repositioning splint was placed, and the patient showed a dramatic relief of symptoms within 72 hours. After approximately 3 months of no recurrences of pain, holes were cut into the acrylic splint, as shown in Fig. 28-5, to allow eruption of the posterior teeth. This is as described earlier in the chapter. Within a period of 4 months the patient was able to eliminate the splint, a full occlusal equilibration was performed, and no further therapy was required.

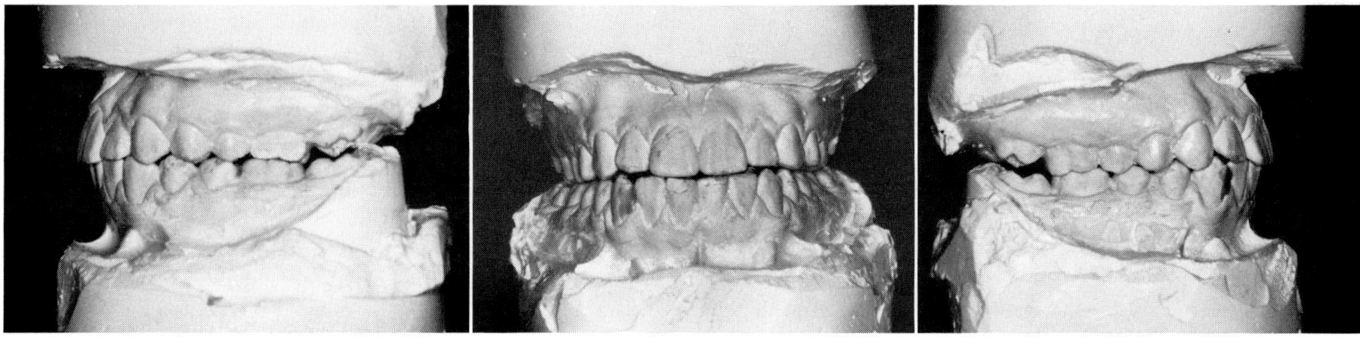

Fig. 28-3. Study casts of patient in case 1 in centric occlusion.

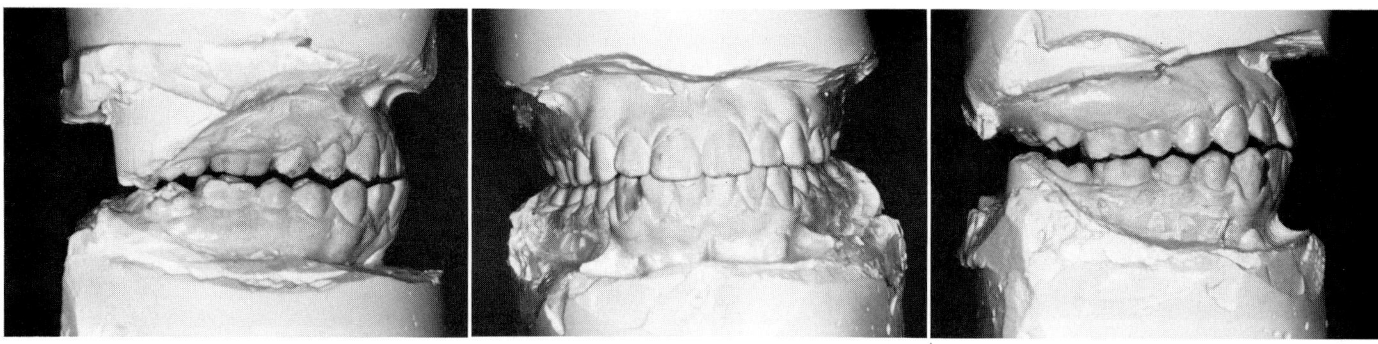

Fig. 28-4. Study casts of patient in case 1 mounted in myocentric relation.

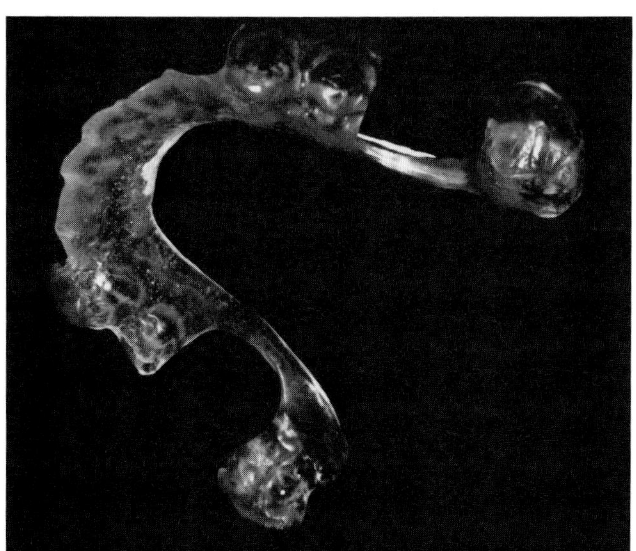

Fig. 28-5. Holes cut into acrylic splint to allow eruption of posterior teeth.

Case 2

This 15 year-old-girl, with previous orthodontic therapy, had a chief complaint of limited intraoral opening and pain in left temporomandibular joint area (both of which became apparent in approximately February 1979). Her clinical symptoms were pain in left temporomandibular joint area, frontal and left temporal headaches, an occasional audible click in the left temporomandibular joint, pain during mastication of hard foods and gum, and generalized facial pain in the area of the left zygoma.

During the clinical examination manual palpation of the musculature revealed tenderness of the left masseter in the region of the gonial angle, tenderness of the middle body of the left temporal, and tenderness of the left sternocleidomastoid muscle from the origin to the middle of the body. Interincisal opening was limited to 20 mm, and there was a lateral deviation of the mandible on opening to her right and on closing to her left. Auscultation of the temporomandibular joints revealed a click of the left one. Dental examination revealed wear facets of the incisal edges of the mandibular central incisor teeth.

Radiographically, no significant abnormalities of either the mandibular condyles, fossae, or eminences were found. With the Mandibular Kinesiograph the sagittal tracing showed a cross-over pattern, which is indicative of a forced posterior closure of the mandible, and the frontal tracing showed a deviation to the patient's right. Vertical-velocity tracings indicated both bradykinesia and dyskinesia. The anterior-vertical ratio of closure was negative, with an excessive interocclusal space and a lateral deviation to the patient's right side, indicative of external pterygoid dysfunction. An oscilloscope tracing of the neuromuscular path of closure indicated overclosing of the mandible, posterior displacement of the mandible because of anterior tooth interference, and lateral displacement. Closure of the mandible definitely was not on a relaxed trajectory.

Associated history included past complaints of swelling of her hands, although medical evaluation indicated no arthritis. It is assumed that both blood serum and fixation studies were done, together with radiographs. Her menses were also irregular (every 6 to 8 weeks).

The diagnosis was dysfunctional osteoarthritis of the temporomandibular joint with concurrent myofacial pain syndrome. It was quite apparent after seeing the patient's father that mandibular prognathism exists as a familial trait, and most likely she had attempted since about the age of 5 to overcome the cosmetic disfigurement of this prognathism by intentional retrusion of her mandible. Probably she exceeded her depth of capacity for this retrusion, resulting in the current findings.

The treatment plan was transcutaneous electrical neural stimulation in conjunction with an orthopedic repositioning splint. It is interesting to note from the original occlusion shown in Fig. 28-6 that the original orthodontist who treated the patient and eventually referred her to my office had every right to believe that the centric occlusal relationship presented was valid. Intraoral views of the patient with a mandibular orthopedic repositioning splint in place show the presence of a Class III (angle) prognathism. Relief from symptoms was obtained within a period of approximately 3 months; in this instance, however, it was necessary to place orthodontic brackets on the buccal surfaces of the posterior teeth to use vertical elastics to extrude the posterior teeth through the holes made in the acrylic. A simple removable appliance was used in the maxillary arch to correct the anterior cross-bite relationship. As of this date, she has reached the point of being totally asymptomatic, and it will be necessary shortly to refer her back to her orthodontist for correction of the Class III (angle) mandible prognathism.

Case 3

This 13-year-old girl was under orthodontic therapy for approximately 18 months for the correction of a Class I (angle) malocclusion complicated by a bimaxillary protrusion with a superimposed premaxillary protrusion. Initial routine orthodontic diagnosis called for the case to be treated with full edgewise appliances and maximum anchorage mechanics without extractions. The patient came into the office for a routine adjustment visit and complained of myofacial pain and discomfort. A Mandibular Kinesiograph procedure was performed with the following results: a sagittal tracing indicated a crossover pattern. The vertical-velocity tracing showed dyskinesia on opening and closing and a click on closing. The anterior-vertical ratio of closure was negative (the mandible

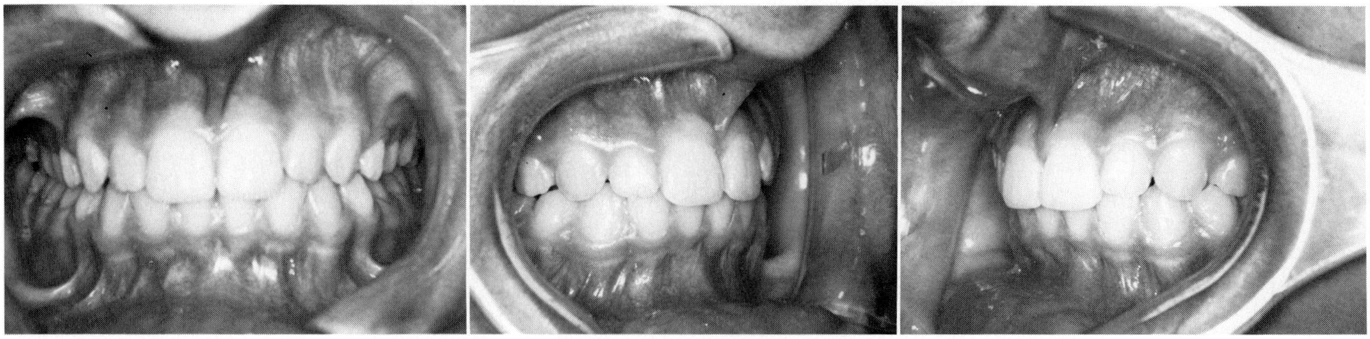

Fig. 28-6. Original occlusion of patient in case 2.

moving posteriorly during closure), the interocclusal space was excessive, and there was a lateral deviation of the mandible to the patient's left. Evaluation of the occlusal relationship indicated overclosure of the mandible, posterior displacement because of anterior interference, lateral displacement of the mandible, and a failure to achieve a relaxed trajectory on closure of the mandible. Since the parents had been divorced recently and the mother was a terminal cancer patient, the girl has a number of psychological problems that delayed resolution of the myofacial pain problem. An orthopedic repositioning splint was fabricated to fit over the present fixed orthodontic appliances. After approximately 5 months of transcutaneous electrical neural stimulation and repeated adjustments of the splint, the patient became asymptomatic. Holes were then cut into the acrylic splint, and vertical elastics were worn to decrease the freeway space to that present with the splint in place.

CONCLUSION

Although the brevity of this chapter does not allow detailed discussion of the various techniques available for orthodontic movement of teeth, it should be realized that the problems in the three simplistic examples given have occurred with great frequency in adults and with the same basic results. This is not meant in any way to negate the value of dental prostheses in the treatment of temporomandibular joint or myofacial pain problems, since many patients are treated with a combination of prosthesis and orthodontics. There are many instances, however, where orthodontics is the treatment of choice. It is difficult to conceive that a patient who presents with full permanent dentition, no edentulous areas, and relatively no caries would be subjected to full-mouth rehabilitation via prosthetic means when orthodontic tooth movement would prevent destruction of the tooth integrity. Much credit is due to Bernard Jankelson for his many years of work on neuromuscular occlusion and his development of techniques and instrumentation for clinical use. It is now our task to take this information and broaden our base of knowledge for treatment.

29 Orthognathic surgery

CHARLES D. HASSE, D.D.S., and DOUGLAS H. MORGAN, D.D.S.

Orthognathic (Greek *orthos,* straight; *gnathos,* jaw) surgery may be defined as the surgical management and treatment of malposition of the bones of the jaws.[6] Historically, the first type of procedure to correct skeletal malrelations was reported in 1849 by Hullihen.[9] In the ensuing 100 years numerous surgical techniques were discovered as the science of correcting jaw deformities began to take shape. The work of surgeons such as Blair,[2] Babcock,[1] Kostecka,[10] Wassmund,[20] and Schuchardt[17] comes to the forefront as that of the leaders of these initial endeavors.

In 1966 Hugo Obwegeser[13] of Zurich, Switzerland, presented a program before the American Society of Oral Surgeons that marked the American birth of the modern science of orthognathic surgery. The key point of his presentation was the utilization of new intraoral techniques for the correction of skeletal and dental malrelationships. Prior to his address most major osseous surgery was performed extraorally to eliminate the possibility of contamination with oral secretions and the resultant sequela of severe infection. Obwegeser's presentation reversed this thinking to the extent that oral and maxillofacial surgeons today routinely use intraoral approaches for correcting dentofacial deformities.

In the 1970s tremendous advances were made as the science of orthognathic surgery came of age. Numerous new procedures were developed, and many of the older procedures were refined. The biological basis for various maxillary and mandibular techniques was established, favorable long-term stability results were reported, and the incidence of postoperative complications was minimized. The excellent working relationships between general dentists, orthodontists, and the oral and maxillofacial surgeons have significantly improved diagnosis and treatment planning and ultimately patient results.

In our work helping individuals suffering from abnormalities of the temporomandibular apparatus we have agonized over the complexity of problems and the myriad of etiological factors inherent in TMJ disease. The preceding chapters have discussed numerous causes: trauma (dislocation, fracture), neoplasia (benign and malignant disease, ameloblastoma, osteochondroma), arthritis (infectious, rheumatoid, degenerative, traumatic), infection (osteomyelitis), inflammation (meniscitis, capsulitis, synovitis), iatrogenic (poor dental care, prolonged or unsuccessful dental procedures), dental (bruxism, occlusal interferences, partial edentulism), congenital (aplasia, hypoplasia or hyperplasia of the condyles, bifid condyle), and myofascial. An additional cause that is most significant in contributing to jaw joint problems is skeletal malrelationships of the maxilla and mandible.

The purpose of this chapter is, first, to briefly discuss the role skeletal disharmony of the upper and lower jaws plays in TMJ disorders and, second, to demonstrate how orthognathic surgery can eliminate some of these problems. Six case histories are presented at the end of the chapter to illustrate basic surgical orthognathic management of dentofacial abnormalities.

MANDIBULAR ADVANCEMENT

Patients requiring mandibular advancement show a wide spectrum of abnormal skeletal, neuromuscular, esthetic, and growth patterns. *Mandibular deficiency syndrome* (types I and II), *mandibular retrusion, mandibular retrognathism,* and *short-face syndrome* are some of the terms that describe the typical "Andy Gump" character in gross clinical form. The term *mandibular micrognathism* is usually associated with congenital syndromes, such as Pierre Robin's syndrome, mandibulofacial dysostosis, hemifacial microsomia, and Turner's syndrome, in patients who concomitantly exhibit other facial abnormalities. Rare anomalies such as condylar agenesis, condylar hypoplasia, and infantile apertognathia are other conditions that warrant mandibular advancement for correction.

In general, Class II dental malocclusions with a severe overjet and the usual deep bite present marked functional limitations that create a predisposing situation for TMJ disturbances (Fig. 29-1). The overjet makes incisal function possible only in a position of ex-

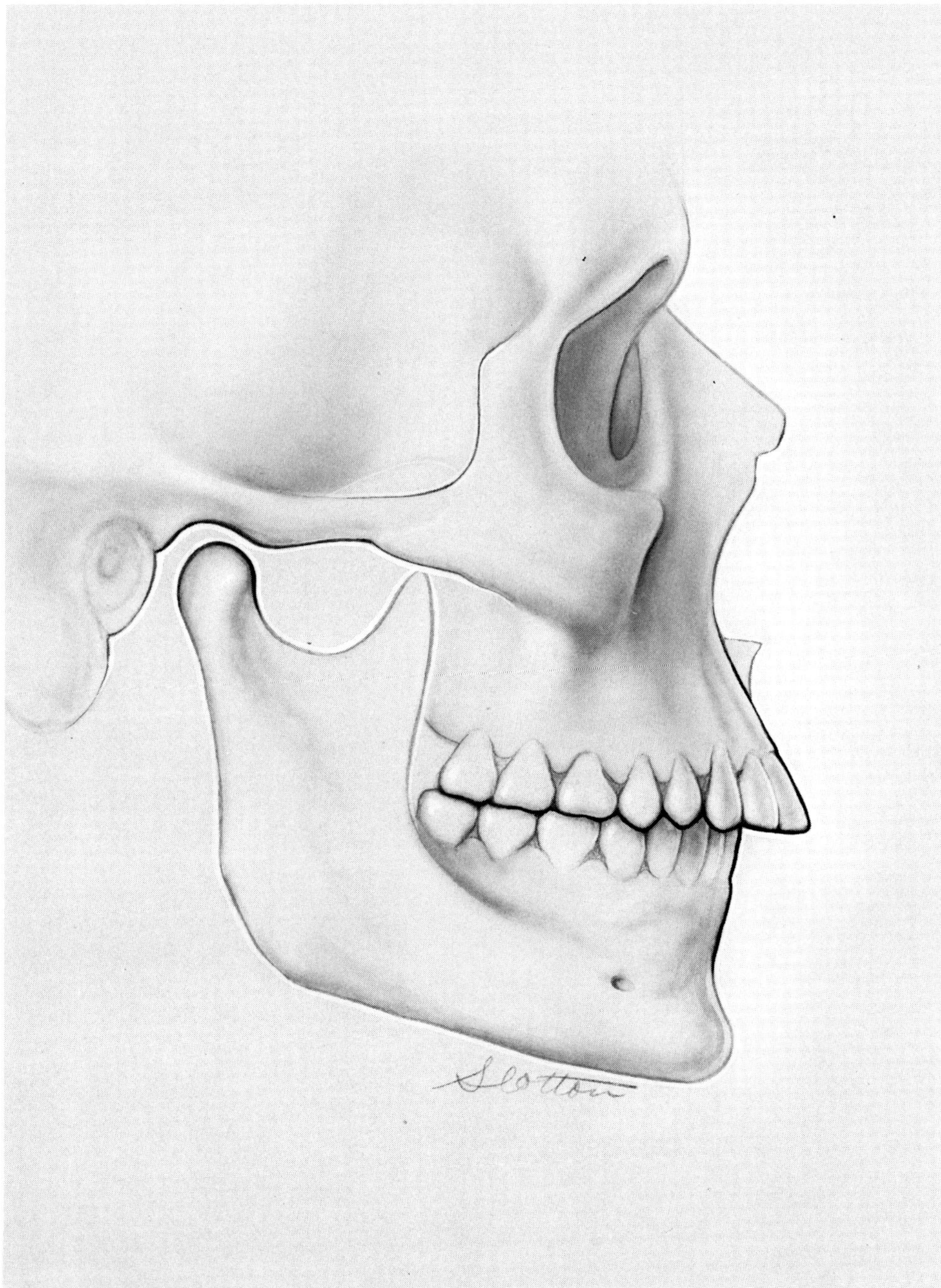

Fig. 29-1. Class II malocclusion of mandible with severe overjet involving maxillary teeth.

treme mandibular protrusion (Fig. 29-2). Thus, to incise food, the individual must constantly posture the mandible considerably more forward than does the person with a more normal bite. Through the years this continual excessive movement will put too much wear and tear on the anterior head of the condyle, disc, and slopes of the eminences, and eventually it can bring about a serious dysfunction and/or disease within the joint and muscles. Further destruction can be caused by the deep-bite tendency, which results in displacement of the condyle in a posterior position within the fossa. This has the effect of causing a remodeling of the

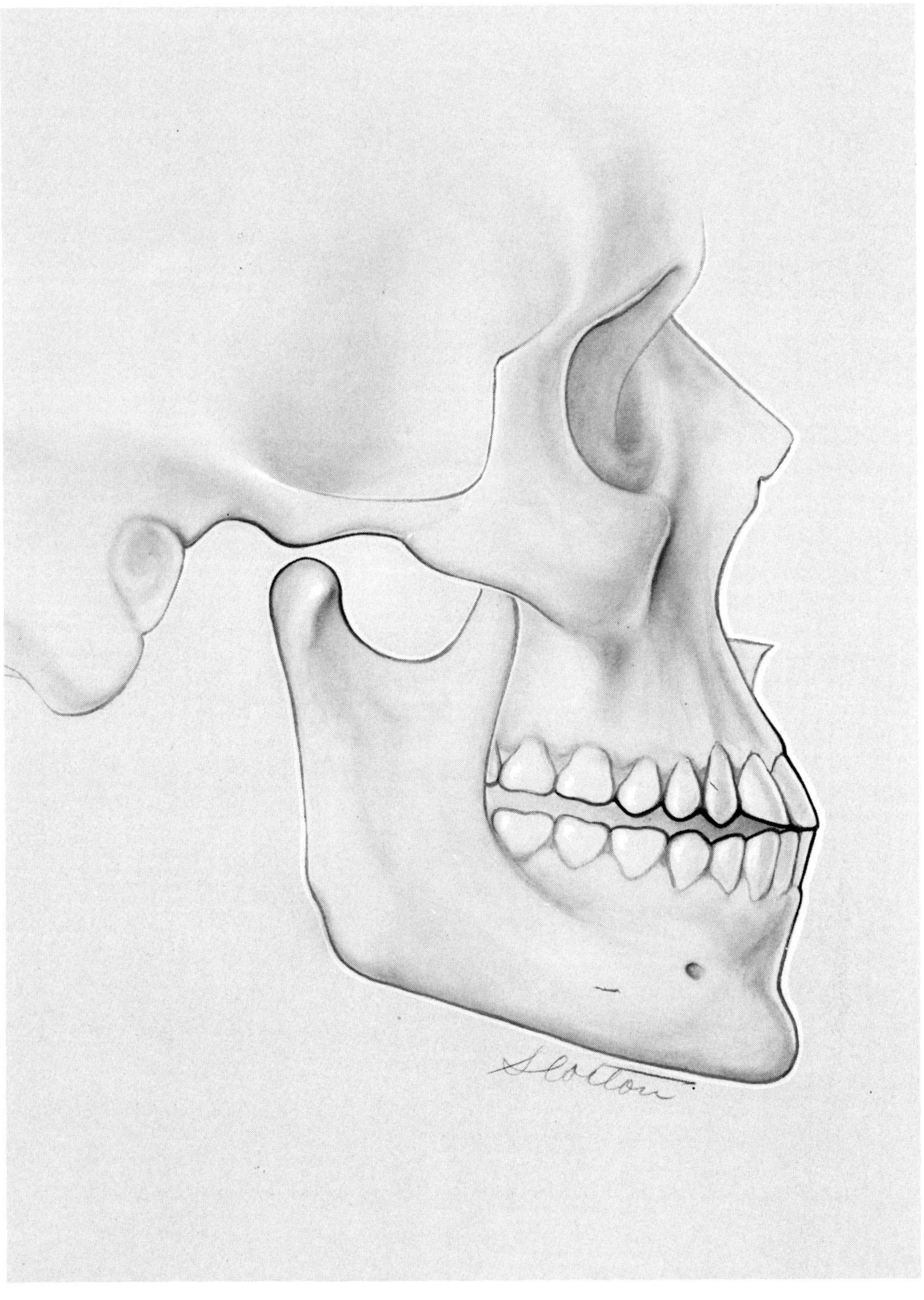

Fig. 29-2. Incisal teeth together, creating extreme mandibular protrusion and also placing condyle in abnormally forward position over ascending slope of eminence.

posterior head of the condyle and the posterior wall of the glenoid fossa (Figs. 29-3 and 29-4).

In most instances of mandibular advancement we prefer the modified sagittal split osteotomy of the mandibular ramus.[3] It has been our experience that, provided the rami have adequate dimension and form for sectioning and preserving a sufficient area of contact between the cut surface, a very stable and predictable result can be achieved using this approach. Furthermore, Schendel, Wolford, and Epker[16] have demonstrated that the modified sagittal split osteotomy can safely and predictably be done in most growing chil-

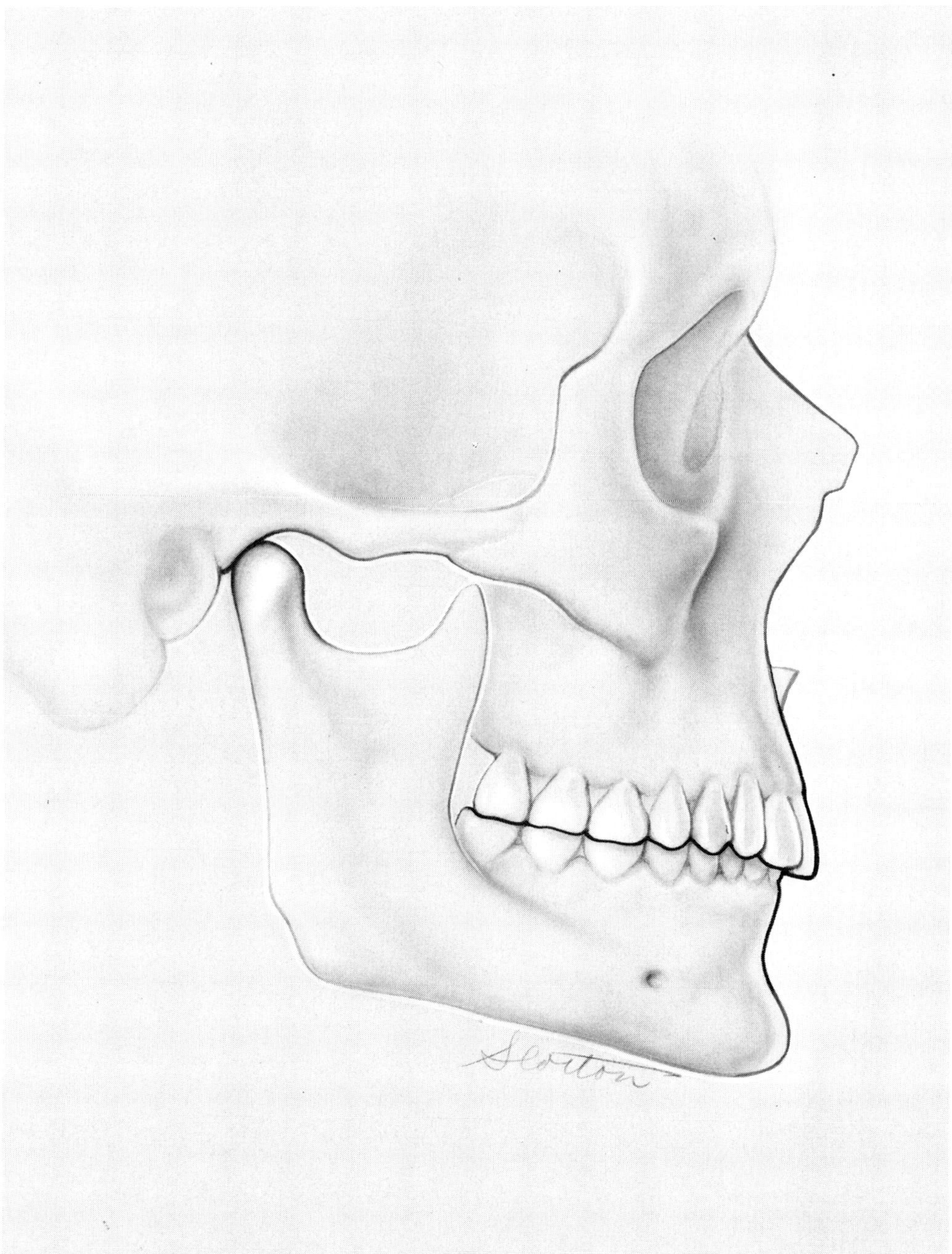

Fig. 29-3. Extreme overbite (closed bite), which tends to displace condyle into posterior position in fossa, causing damage to posterior head of condyle and posterior wall of fossa.

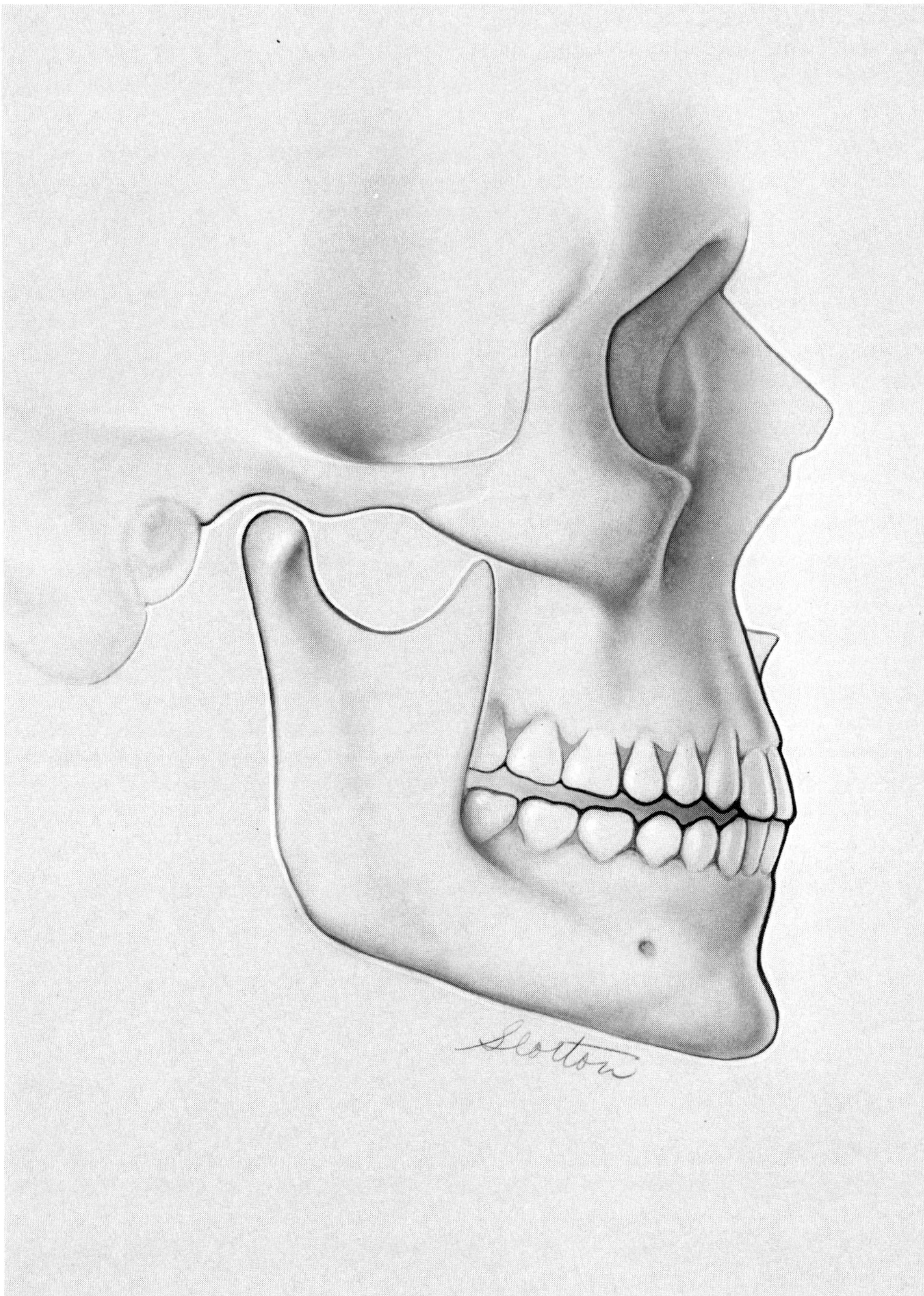

Fig. 29-4. Incisal bite does not create problem with condyle moving too far forward, as it does with other skeletal malrelationships.

dren after the age of 9. Of course proper case preparation and execution of the surgical procedure are essential to minimize complications or relapse and to optimize results.

We reserve the vertical oblique osteotomy of the ascending ramus[15] for cases in which there is extreme shortening of the ascending rami from bony hypodevelopment with an associated micrognathia or in instances in which there is a concomitant hypotrophy of the ramus with TMJ ankylosis (Fig. 29-5). Bone grafting may be required depending on the amount of space created between the proximal and distal segments by the advancement. We use a wedge of corticocancellous bone from the iliac crest in these situations. It should be noted that in cases of ankylosis the orthognathic surgery is performed secondary to, or in combination with, an arthroplasty and/or placement of a TMJ prosthesis.

MacIntosh[11] has used a total mandibular alveolar osteotomy to correct cases of infantile apertognathia (open bite from the molars forward that develops early in childhood) and condylar hypoplasia (Fig. 29-6). The major disadvantage of this technique lies in controlled management of the inferior dental nerve. We advocate complete exposure of the nerve by decortication of the buccal plate prior to completion of the medial horizontal bone cuts. After mobilization of the entire mandibular alveolar process has been completed and wired to place, the deshelved buccal plate is then particulated and placed as an autologous bone graft. With this approach, duration of postsurgical neurosensory change is significantly reduced. So too, this procedure then may be safely used in a wider spectrum of situations requiring advancement than the selected rare anomalies cited by MacIntosh.

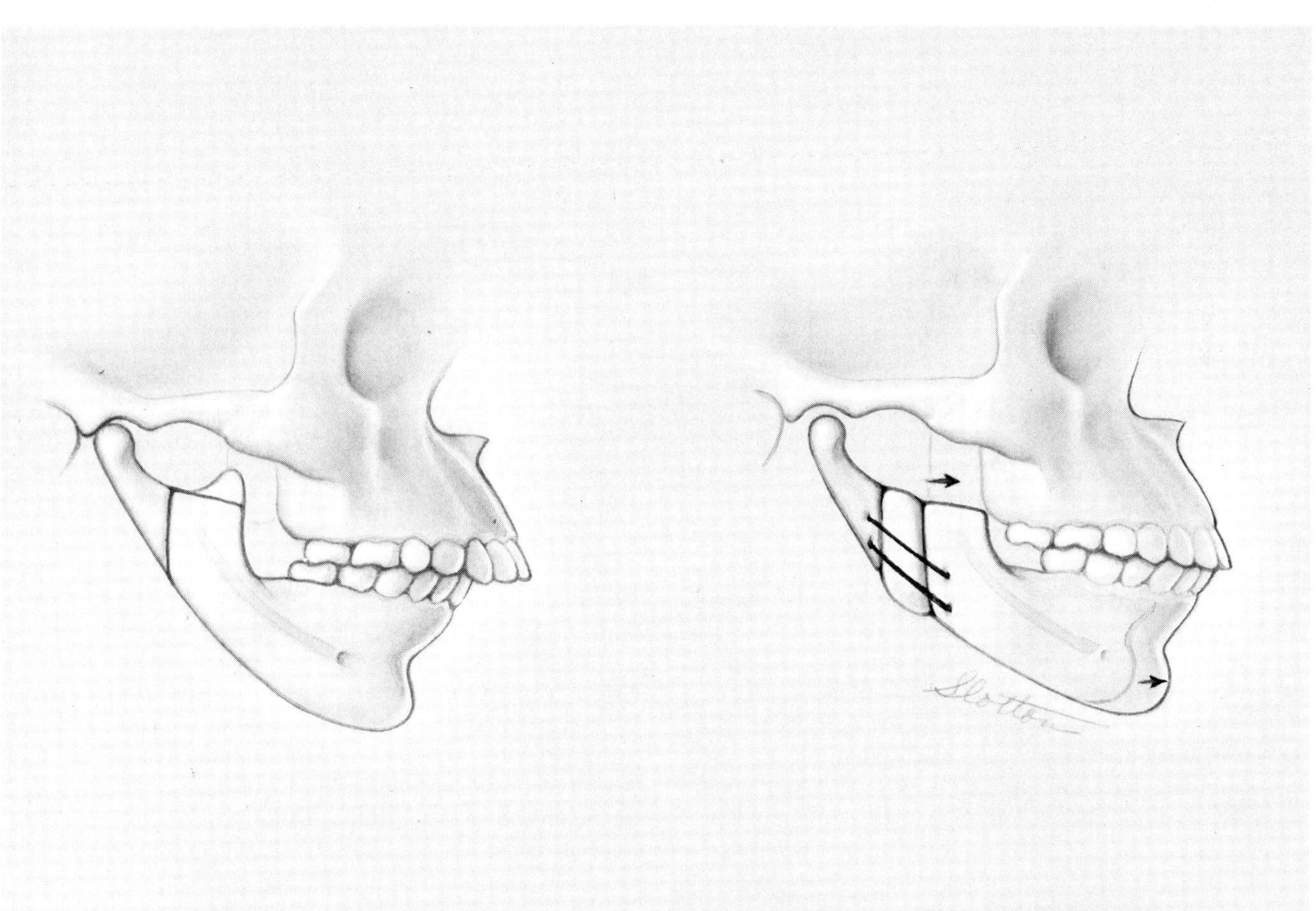

Fig. 29-5. Extreme shortening of ascending rami from bony hypodevelopment with associated micrognathia. Surgical correction requires advancement of mandible, coronoidectomy, and placement of corticocancellous bone graft.

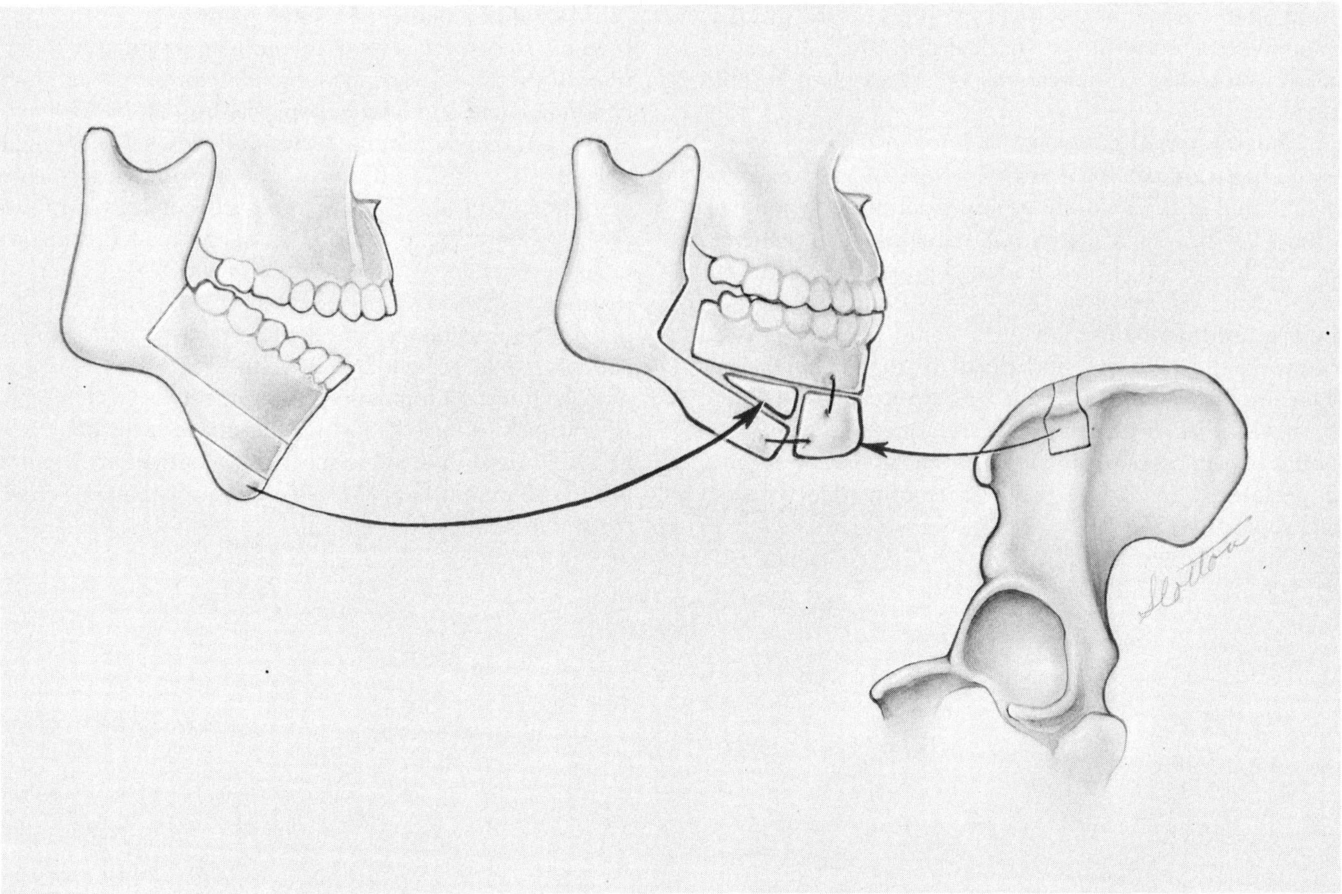

Fig. 29-6. Total mandibular alveolar osteotomy for correction of infantile apertognathism or condylar agenesis, as described by MacIntosh.[11]

MANDIBULAR SETBACK

One of the jaw deformities that comes to the attention of the oral and maxillofacial surgeon most often is mandibular prognathism, or the overdeveloped lower jaw. Besides the deformity of the lower third of the face because of the prominent mandible, a Class III dental malocclusion is almost always present. Frequently cross-bite and open bite accompany this condition. Other problems such as occlusal discrepancies with masticatory insufficiency, periodontal disease, poor speech, interferences with construction of satisfactory dental prostheses, unattractive facial esthetics, and temporomandibular joint dysfunction complete the picture. Such a condition cannot be treated satisfactorily solely by orthodontic therapy, and thus orthognathic surgery alone or in combination with orthodontics is necessary to correct the deformity.

Numerous clinicians have observed that patients with prognathic conditions are more susceptible to damage of the TMJ. Hovell[8] asserts that TMJ dysfunction occurs only in mild cases of prognathism when there is an end-to-end bite. Hinds and Kent[7] have reported obviation of temporomandibular joint pain following orthognathic surgery. Although this has been our experience, others have said that they have rarely seen a prognathic individual with a TMJ dysfunction.

Morgan has presented two cases in which individuals with mandibular prognathism had degenerative changes of the temporomandibular joint. In one of these cases the patient's articular eminences contained good cortical bone, but the prominences were extremely flattened. Morgan theorized that the hypodevelopment of the eminences was a result of lack of osteogenic stimulation during growth of the condylar head in translating over the bony eminences. This aberrant growth pattern led to disharmony of the excursive action of the disc, which resulted in bilateral tearing and subsequent clicking and pain.

In the other instance of prognathism leading to degenerative TMJ disease the eminences were developed but were worn and eroded. The patient was distressed by her unsightly facial profile and accordingly at-

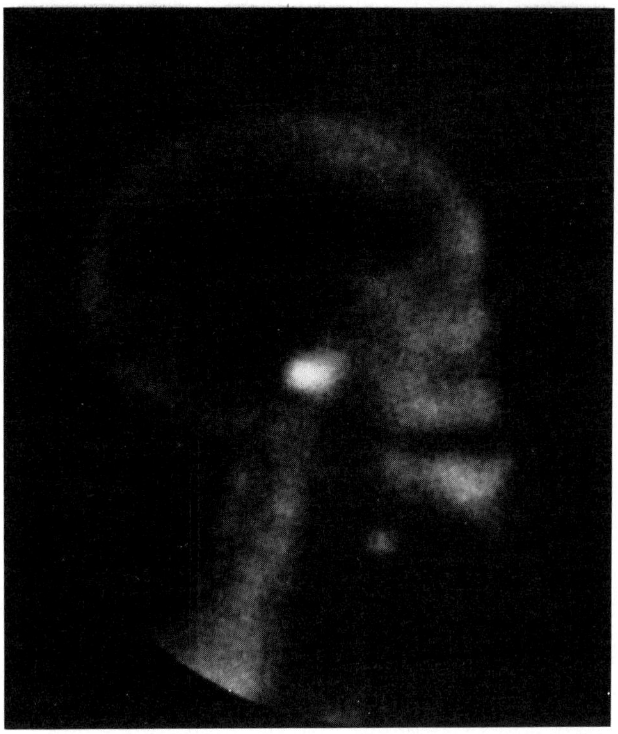

Fig. 29-7. Positive technetium 99m bone scan of patient (Case 2) with hyperplastic condyle.

tempted to manipulate her jaw backward. This unnatural action actually created pathological pressures on the joint surfaces and the condylar head. It has been our observation that the bony anatomy of the temporomandibular joint has the capacity to remodel to adapt as much as possible to the external pressures being applied to it. This remodeling, however, is determined by the functional adaptive capacity of the individual's stomatognathic system. Once the physiological limits of this system are exceeded, functional remodeling ceases, and a true pathosis (osteoarthritis) develops within the jaw joint.

Finally, in cases of prognathism in which there is extreme overclosure, it is not uncommon to find osteogenic changes in the postglenoid area. These subtle changes are readily demonstrable with radionuclide bone scans (technetium 99m) of the TMJ (Fig. 29-7). This may account for some of the hearing problems that have puzzled ENT specialists, since if the changes progress to the stage of erosion, they may affect the chain of ossicles and interfere with the transmission of sound from the middle ear to the inner ear. We suspect that future research efforts will show that the wide spectrum of symptoms associated with temporomandibular joint dysfunction in fact may be secondary to skeletal malrelationships of the upper and lower jaws.

Numerous procedures have been described for the correction of mandibular prognathism. Probably the most commonly used procedures today are the extraoral vertical oblique osteotomy, the intraoral vertical oblique osteotomy, the modified sagittal split osteotomy, the body ostectomy, and the subapical osteotomy. The latter two procedures bear consideration only in instances when the correction for mandibular excess is slight (less than 5 mm). Historically, the extraoral vertical oblique osteotomy has been a time-honored procedure that has yielded excellent results. We feel that it is the procedure of choice for cases in which the repositioning of the mandible is extreme (greater than 14 mm). This approach is most satisfactory for correcting deviate prognathisms or in conjunction with reconstructive bone graft procedures for the correction of unilateral disarticulation or discontinuity defects.

Probably the procedure generating the greatest popularity in the early 1970s was the intraoral vertical oblique osteotomy. Hinds and Kent[7] demonstrated that with the appropriate armamentarium and surgical technique the intraoral approach could be performed with considerable success. The major drawback to this approach remains restricted access and visibility. Some clinicians do not favor this approach because they feel that it is difficult to reliably control the position of the condylar head. We advocate notching the anterior segments and placement of a 0-chromic gut suture to

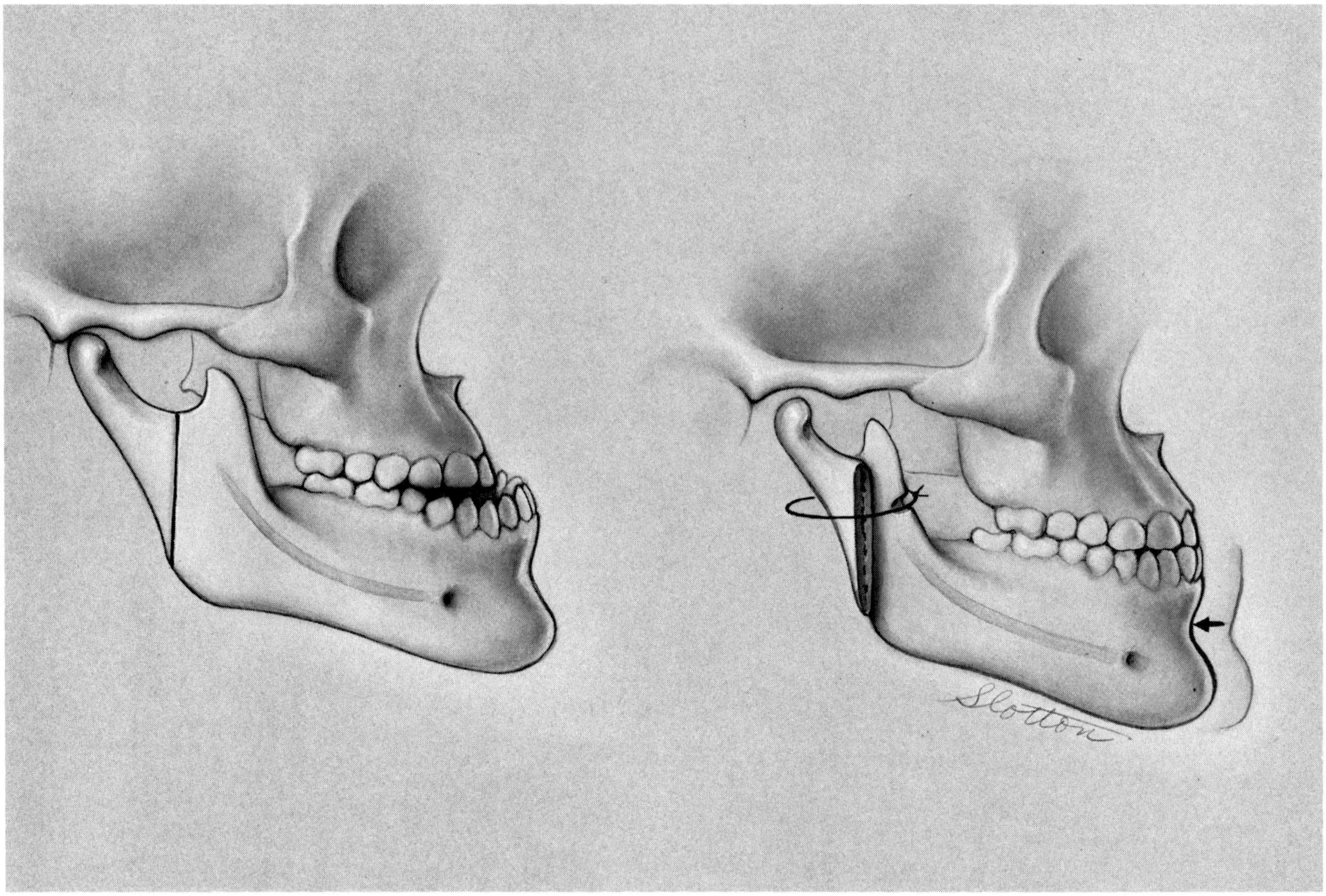

Fig. 29-8. Mandibular prognathism corrected by bilateral intraoral vertical oblique osteotomies of the mandibular rami. Note 0-chromic gut suture affixed around proximal and distal ramal segments to maintain contact but allow dynamic remodeling and repositioning of condyles within fossae.

maintain the desired close bony contact but allow dynamic remodeling of the condyle during the fixation period. With this modification relapse has been minimized (Fig. 29-8).

We favor the modified sagittal split osteotomy[3] for most cases of mandibular prognathism (less than a 14-mm setback). With slight overcorrection the surgeon can achieve a very predictable and stable result. Unlike with the mandibular deficiency patients, correction of mandibular prognathism prior to cessation of growth has met with relapse and redevelopment of the Class III dental malocclusion. Accordingly, it appears ill advised to operate on children until proportionate growth of the maxilla and mandible can be demonstrated by serial cephalometric radiographs or the growth spurt has been concluded as evidenced by hand-wrist radiographs.

MAXILLARY REPOSITIONING

Wassmund[20] introduced a surgical procedure for moving the entire maxilla. The operation, which has subsequently been called the Le Fort I osteotomy or total maxillary osteotomy, was first used to correct an anterior open bite. As anesthesia and surgical techniques became more sophisticated, European oral and maxillofacial surgeons developed segmental surgical osteotomies to correct maxillary alveolar deformities. In the past 5 years the art of surgical orthodontics has advanced significantly in this country, and numerous variations and refinements of the Le Fort I osteotomy have evolved. The surgeon now has the capabilities for superior repositioning, advancement or retrusion of the maxilla, inferior repositioning, and leveling of the total maxilla.

Surgery consists of separating the entire alveolar portion of the maxilla, usually including the palate, and repositioning it in the desired spatial position as predicated on clinical, esthetic, cephalometric, and model analysis. Deformities that may be corrected by this procedure are *maxillary retrusion* or *mandibular pseudoprognathism, maxillary protrusion, maxillary deficiency, long-face syndrome, apertognathia,* and *maxillary*

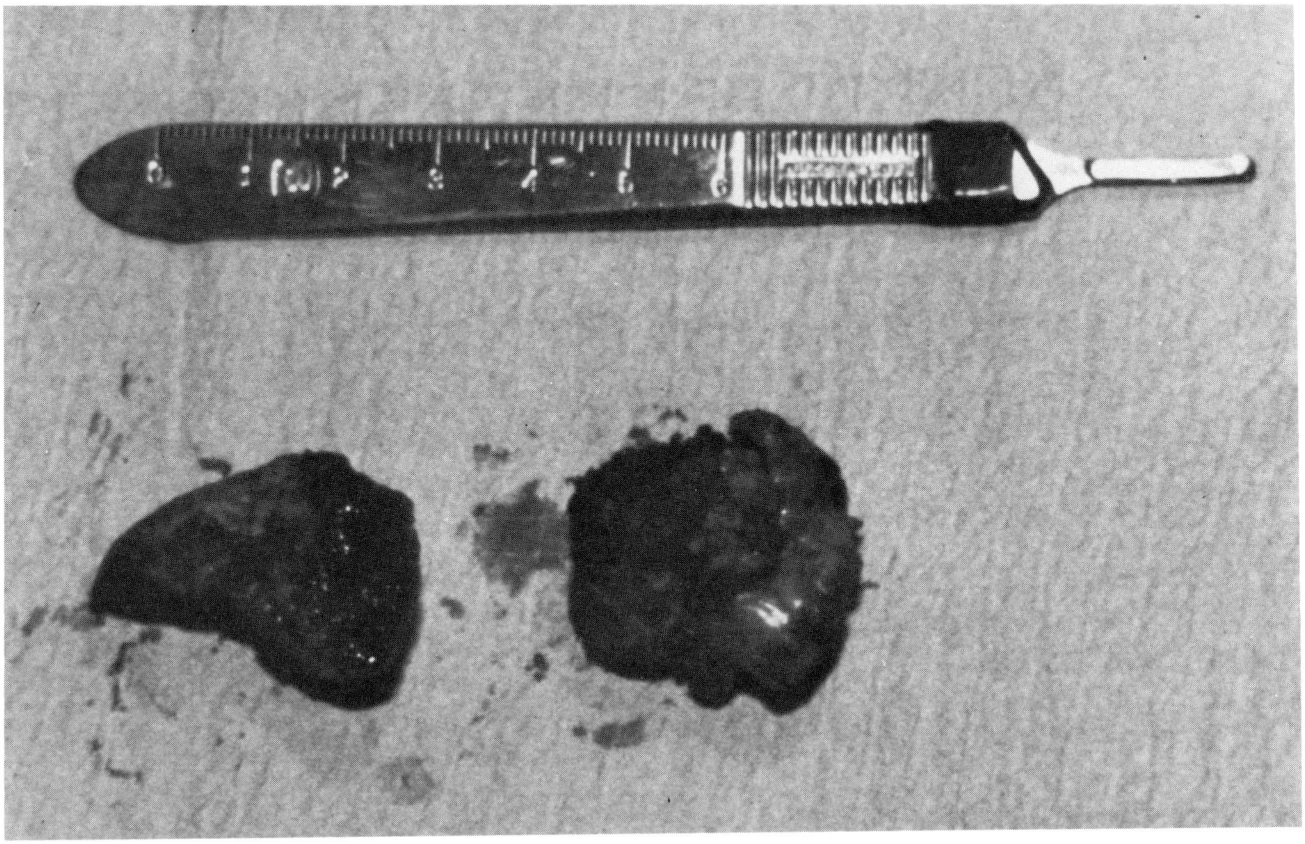

Fig. 29-9. Osteochondroma of condyle (surgical specimen) requiring use of costochondral bone graft for reconstruction.

alveolar hypoplasia or *hyperplasia* with abnormal vertical facial height. Thus any condition requiring the surgical repositioning of the maxilla superiorly, inferiorly, anteriorly, and posteriorly or the simultaneous segmentalizing of it to widen, narrow, level, or improve arch symmetry may be treated by maxillary repositioning.

The world literature contains few case reports linking skeletal maxillary discrepancies with temporomandibular joint dysfunction. Possibly this is because of a lack of recognition on the part of dentists and physicians of the true causative factor. Nevertheless, if one subscribes to the philosophy that disharmony between the upper and lower jaws can result in undue stress within the stomatognathic system, which can predispose a person to TMJ symptoms then any of the dentofacial deformities previously mentioned may be implicated. It remains the challenge and responsibility of the various dental specialists to recognize these conditions and to implement corrective therapy prior to the development of irreversible TMJ damage.

COSTOCHONDRAL GRAFTS

One final orthognathic technique that deserves comment is the use of costochondral grafts for reconstruction of the temporomandibular joint. Ware and Taylor[19] have demonstrated experimentally in growing animals that it is desirable after condylectomy to transplant bone with some inherent potential for continued growth. Thus this approach has particular application in the pediatric patient, since maintenance of some semblance of skeletal and dental harmony is desired during growth and development. MacIntosh and Henny[12] have used this approach in treating condylar hypoplasia and aplasia, TMJ ankylosis, and osteoarthritis and for reconstruction following neoplastic disease and trauma (Figs. 29-9 to 29-11).

Costochondral strut grafts from the sixth and seventh ribs can be carved and inserted with the cartilaginous end fitting into the glenoid fossa and the bony end inlayed and affixed to the outer surface of the ramus of the mandible. In unilateral cases it is usually necessary to perform a ramal osteotomy on the contralateral side to permit ideal positioning of the mandible. Bilateral ankylosis cases require that two ribs be taken. Prefabricated custom occlusal splints are necessary to help stabilize the occlusion in the corrected position during healing.

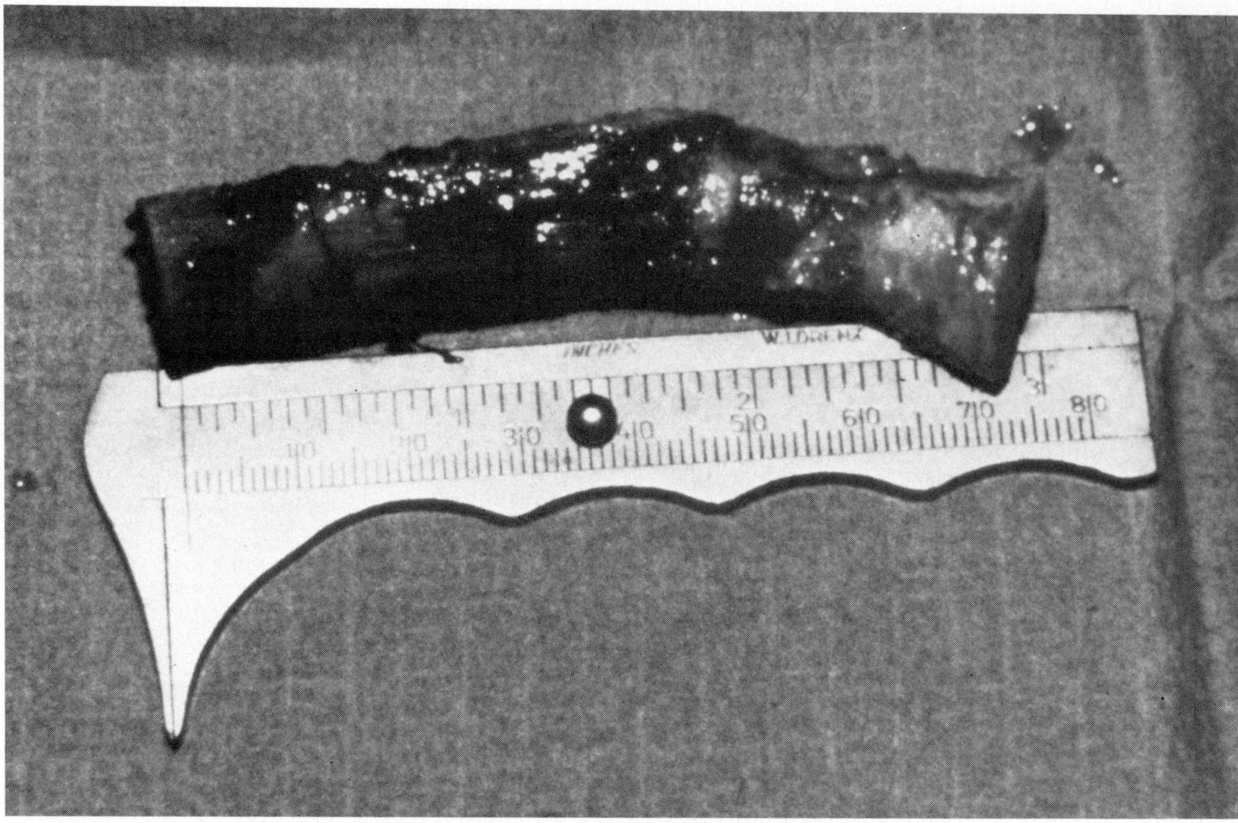

Fig. 29-10. Costochondral strut graft prior to insertion.

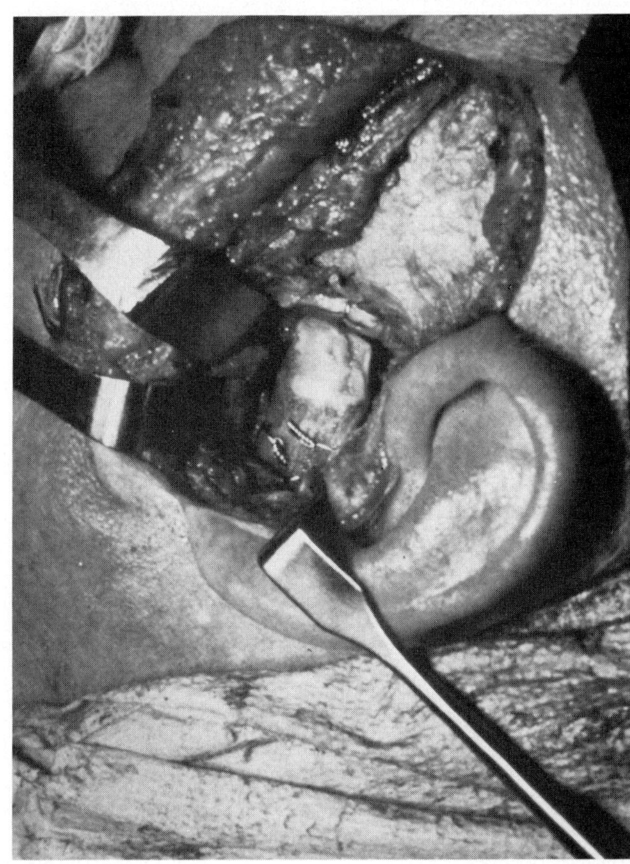

Fig. 29-11. Costochondral graft contoured to shape and inserted with cartilaginous end fitting into glenoid fossa. Note Silastic implant affixed to fossa.

CASE HISTORIES

Case 1

J.A., a 28-year-old Mexican American laborer, was first seen on February 3, 1981, for evaluation of his complaints of jaw pain, inability to chew food well, and pronounced facial asymmetry. The patient gave a history of sustaining trauma to the jaws (from fistfights) in two separate incidents several years prior to the onset of his symptoms. During the past $2^1/_2$ years the patient had sought treatment from various medical specialists for evaluation of his worsening jaw protrusion and progressive deviation of the chin toward the right side (Fig. 29-12). In addition, a severe malocclusion developed, necessitating dietary restrictions because of J.A.'s inability to properly masticate without extreme discomfort.

Clinical examination revealed the following: a palpable left condylar head that was considerably enlarged, bulging in the left preauricular area accompanying opening and closing of the jaws, shifting of the mandibular midline approximately 1 cm to the right side, drifting of the maxillary arch, Class III dental malocclusion with a prognathic facial appearance, overclosure of the occlusion into a telescopic bite whereby the maxillary teeth fit inside of the mandibular teeth, and elongation of the face with deviation of the chin away from the affected left side.

Radiographic studies (pantographic, TMJ tomograms, and anteroposterior facial bone) demonstrated extensive enlargement of the left condylar head and ramal area. The left condylar head protruded out of the glenoid fossa beyond the articular eminence. The cause of the deformity was hyperplasia of the left mandibular condyle, which was thought to have been induced by trauma. (See Fig. 8-50.) The past medical history was significant only for gallstones in 1976. There were no other serious illnesses, injuries, or allergies.

Restorative general dentistry and dental prophylaxis were accomplished to correct the patient's immediate dental problems.

After completion of the dental treatment, preoperative orthognathic surgery workup was instituted consisting of dental study models, clinical photographs, radiographs (cephalometric, periapical, and submentovertex), and technetium 99m bone scans of the TMJ. The radionuclide scans of the left side were extremely "hot," indicating that osteogenic activity was still taking place. (See Figs. 8-48 and 8-49, *B*.) Cephalometric analysis,[15] facial profile analysis,[5] and model surgery demon-

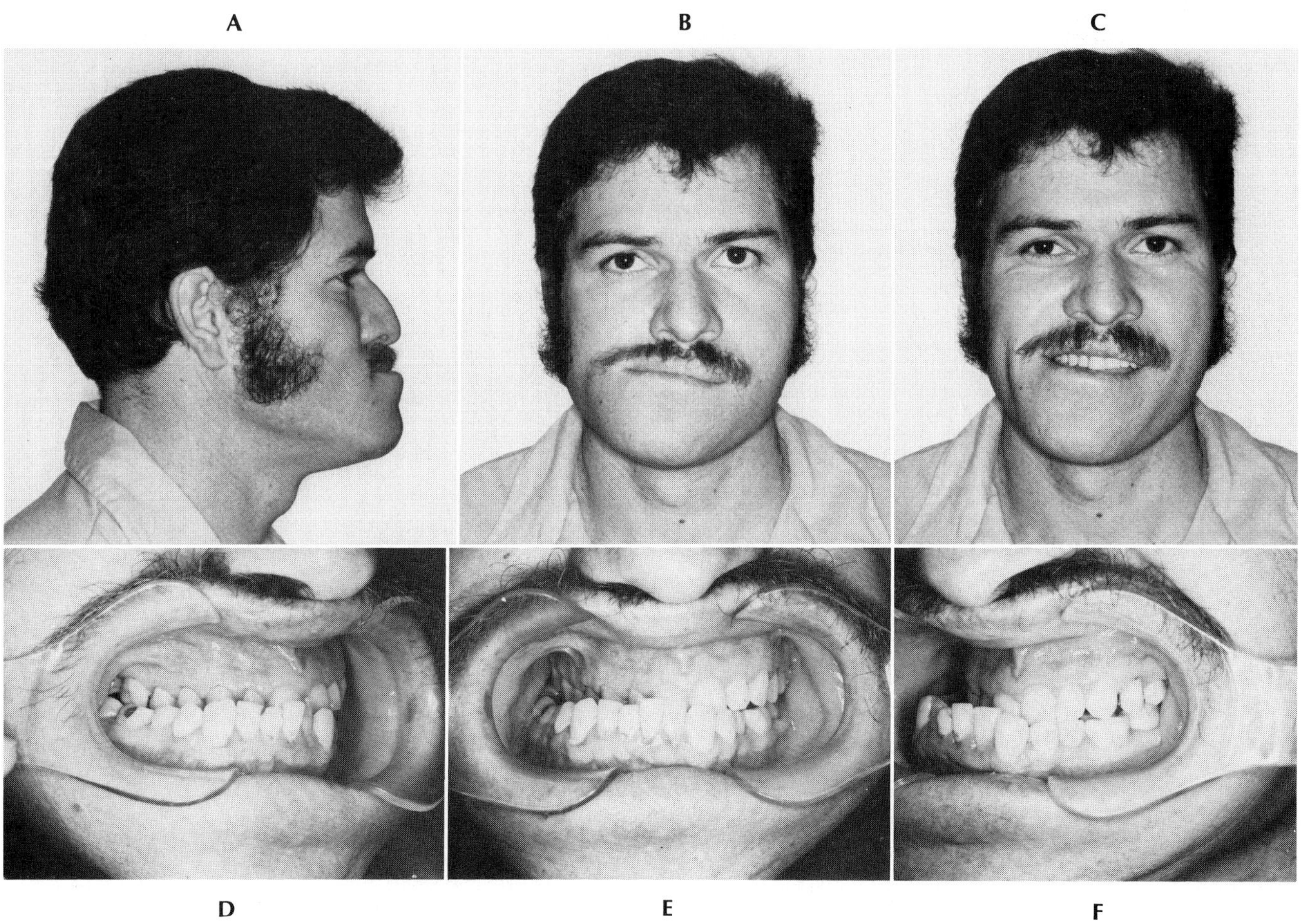

Fig. 29-12. Preoperative profile **(A),** full-face **(B** and **C),** and dental **(D** to **F)** views of J.A. demonstrating deviation of chin toward right side and Class III dental malocclusion.

strated that corrective surgery was necessary in both the maxilla and mandible to eliminate the cause of the deformity (the hyperplasia of the left condyle) and to correct the sequelae (malpositioning of the maxilla, mandible, and dentition). Only by realignment of both jaws could proper function and facial esthetics be restored.

Orthognathic surgery was performed on May 19, 1981, at the Western Medical Center. A modified Le Fort I maxillary osteotomy with segmentalization, a sagittal split osteotomy (Epker[3] modification) of the right mandibular ramus, and an extraoral vertical subcondylar oblique osteotomy with condylotomy were accomplished without incident with the patient under general nasal endotracheal anesthesia. (See Fig. 8-50.) Recovery was uneventful, and the patient was discharged 4 days postoperatively. Intermaxillary fixation was maintained for 8 weeks, and selective occlusal equilibration was used postsurgically to ensure maximum intercuspation of teeth without occlusal interferences.

One year after surgery J.A. demonstrates a stable, functional occlusion. He is asymptomatic for TMJ pain, and his facial deformity has been corrected (Fig. 29-13). The patient has been advised that future temporomandibular reconstruction (condylar replacement) may be necessary for the left side if there is any change in his occlusion or symptoms, but such surgery is unwarranted at this time given his excellent condition.

A B C

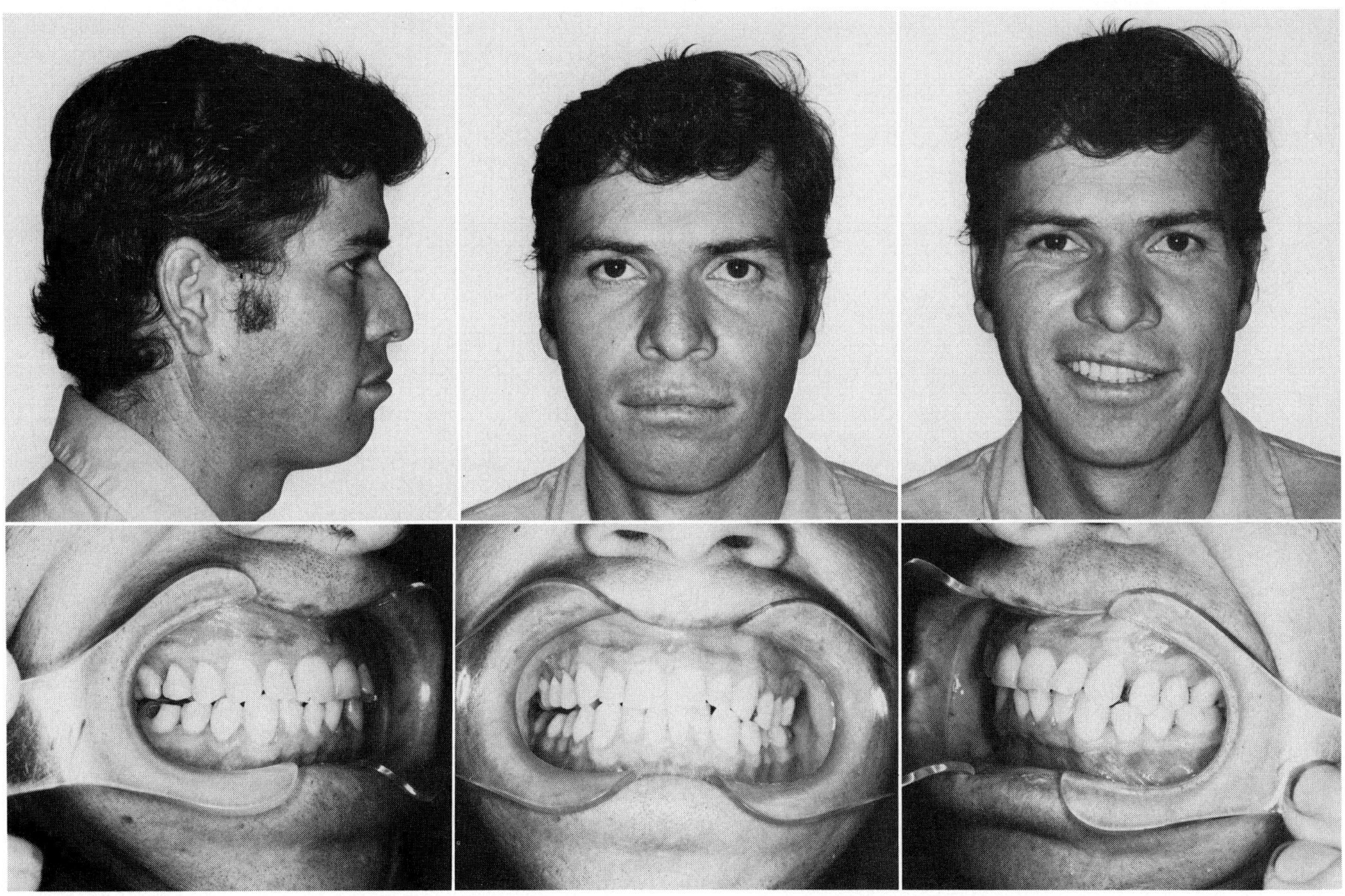

D E F

Fig. 29-13. Postoperative profile **(A)**, full-face **(B** and **C)**, and dental **(D** to **F)** photographs of J.A. showing correction of facial deformity and reestablishment of stable, functional occlusion.

Case 2

R.B., a 29-year-old white electrician, was referred to the Long Beach Veterans Administration Medical Center Oral and Maxillofacial Surgery Section in December 1979 for evaluation of a pronounced facial asymmetry (Fig. 29-14). The patient stated that he first began to notice that his jaw was enlarging to the right side in 1977. During the next $1^1/_2$ years the abnormal growth process accelerated, finally prompting R.B. to seek medical attention. (A later review of family photographs of R.B. revealed a moderate amount of deviation as early as 1971.)

Clinical examination revealed the following: shifting of the mandibular midline to the right side with an accompanying dental compensation (splaying) of the maxillary and mandibular teeth, end-to-end occlusion of the maxillary and mandibular incisor teeth, a dental cross-bite from the molars forward to the canine on the right side, left-sided lingual displacement of the mandibular arch with a significant maxillary overjet, heavy wear faceting and interferences in lateral and protrusive excursions, and loss of tooth no. 30.

Radiographic studies established the cause of the deformity as hyperplasia of the left mandibular condyle (Figs. 29-15 and 29-16). The cause of the hyperplasia is unknown. The past medical history was significant only for pulmonary coccidioidomycosis in 1972. There were no other serious illnesses, traumas or allergies.

In addition to his unpleasing facial appearance, the patient's concerns centered on a left-sided TMJ pain while chewing food, which limited masticatory function to one side only.

Preoperative orthognathic surgery workup was initiated consisting of dental study models, clinical photographs, radiographs (pantographic, cephalometric, TMJ tomograms, periapical, and anteroposterior facial bone), and technetium 99m bone scans of the TMJ. (See Fig. 29-7.) Cephalometric analysis,[18] facial profile analysis,[4] and further clinical examination revealed that corrective surgery was necessary in both the maxilla and mandible to align the arches at the midline, eliminate the cause of the deformity, that is, the hyperplasia of

A B C

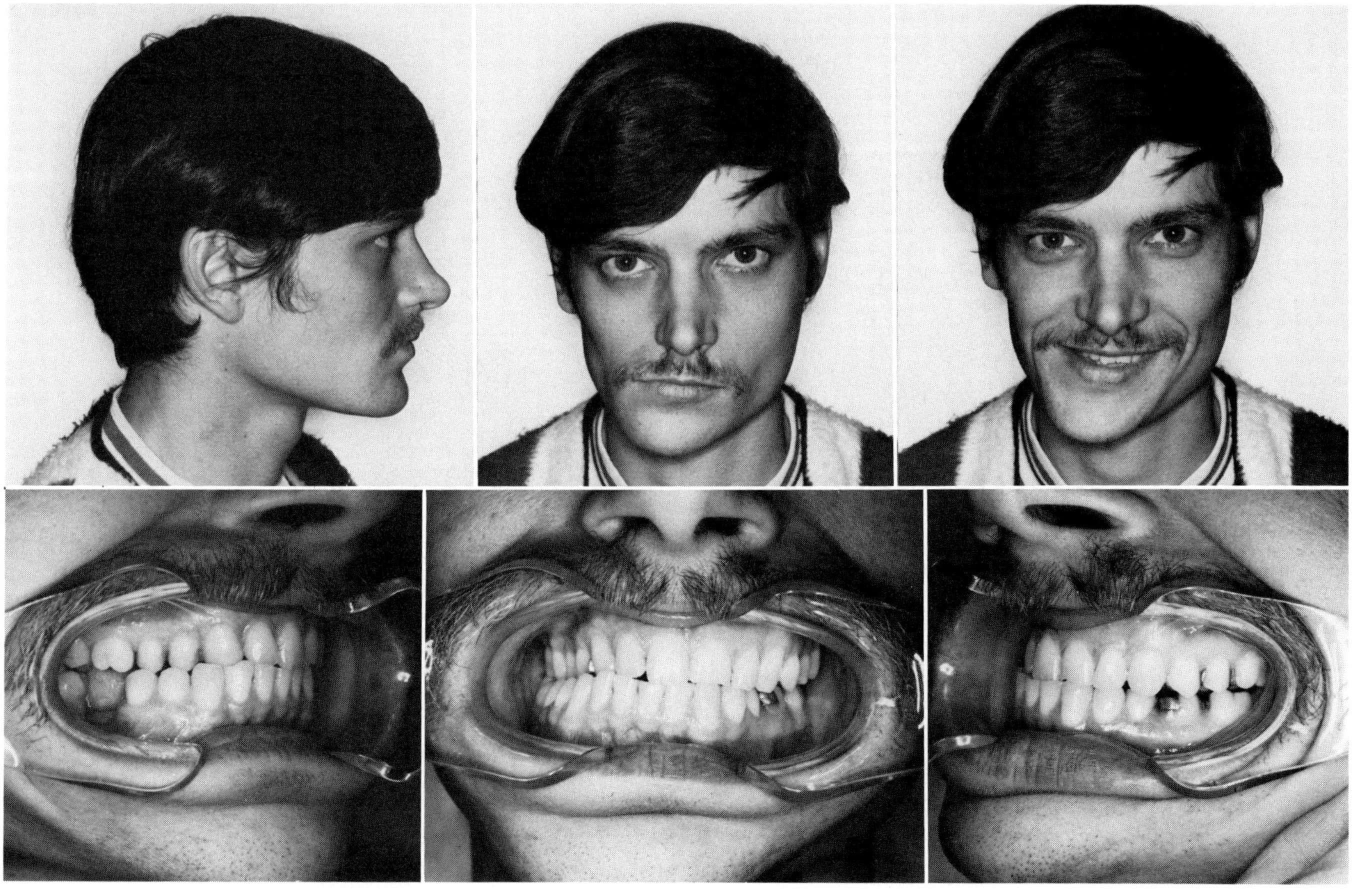

D E F

Fig. 29-14. Preoperative profile **(A)**, full-face **(B** and **C)**, and dental **(D** to **F)** views of R.B. demonstrating gross facial asymmetry and dental malocclusion.

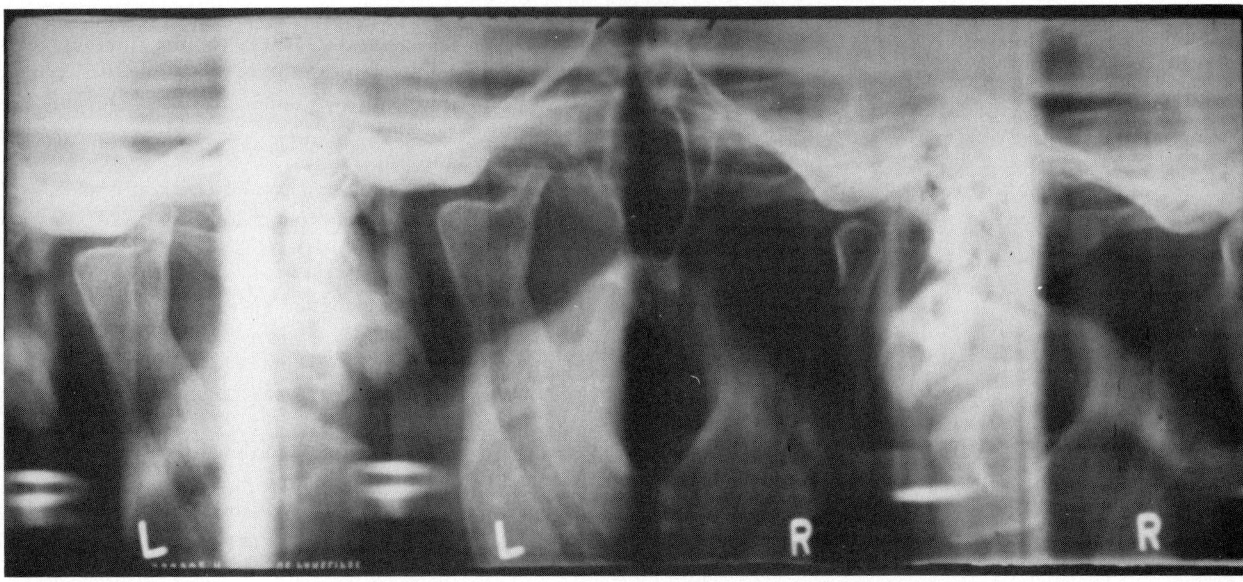

Fig. 29-15. Modified TMJ pantographic view.

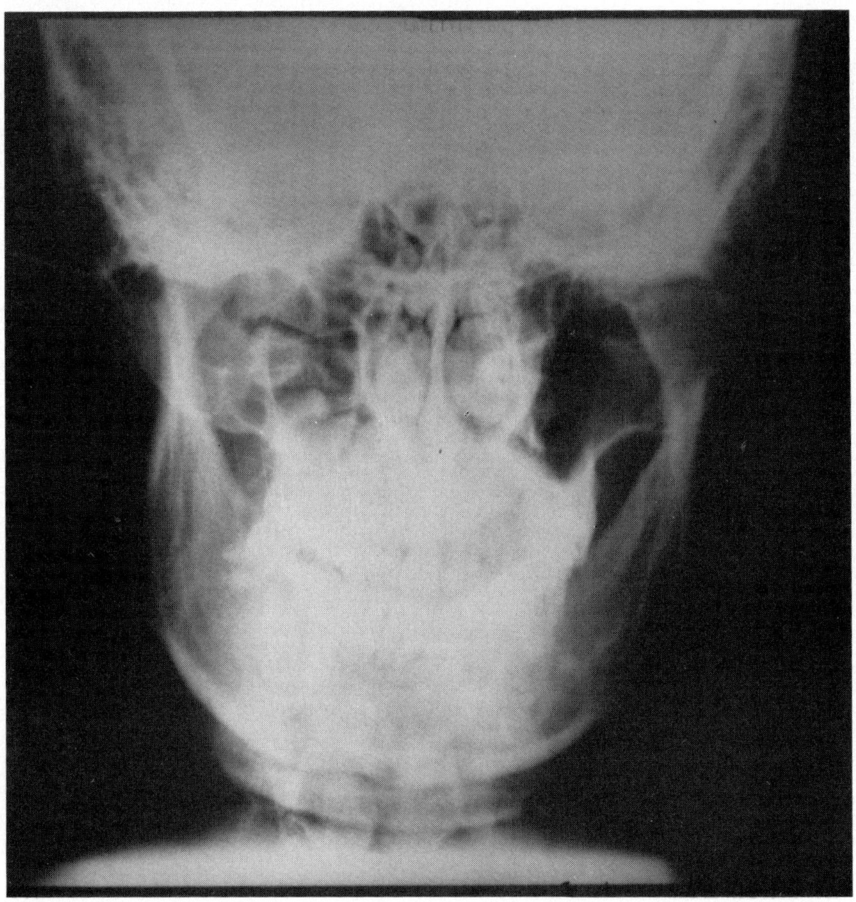

Fig. 29-16. Anteroposterior facial radiograph showing extreme left-sided condylar hyperplasia with bony exostosis.

the left condyle (Fig. 29-17), and to reestablish a functional occlusion with an esthetically pleasing result. Although adjunctive orthodontic therapy was desired (the patient declined for financial reasons), model surgery demonstrated that a satisfactory result could be achieved by surgery alone.

Orthognathic surgery was performed on June 13, 1980. A Le Fort I maxillary osteotomy with segmentalization (Fig. 29-18), a sagittal split osteotomy (Epker[3] modification) of the right mandibular ramus, and an extraoral vertical subcondylar oblique osteotomy of the left ramus with condylotomy were accomplished without incident with the patient under general anesthesia (Fig. 29-19). Intermaxillary fixation was maintained for approximately 7 weeks, after which time nighttime elastic traction was employed for an additional month. Selective occlusal equilibration was used to ensure maximum intercuspation without occlusal interferences. The patient experienced some intermittent paresthesia in the maxilla postoperatively.

As in case 1, the pretreatment surgical objectives were accomplished. Specifically the patient's occlusion was normalized, the facial asymmetry was corrected (Fig. 29-20), and R.B. has been asymptomatic for jaw and TMJ pain for $1^1/_2$ years. It is doubtful that further surgical intervention will be necessary, but reconstruction of the left temporomandibular joint and condylar replacement with a metal prosthesis or costochondral graft are surgical options available if needed.

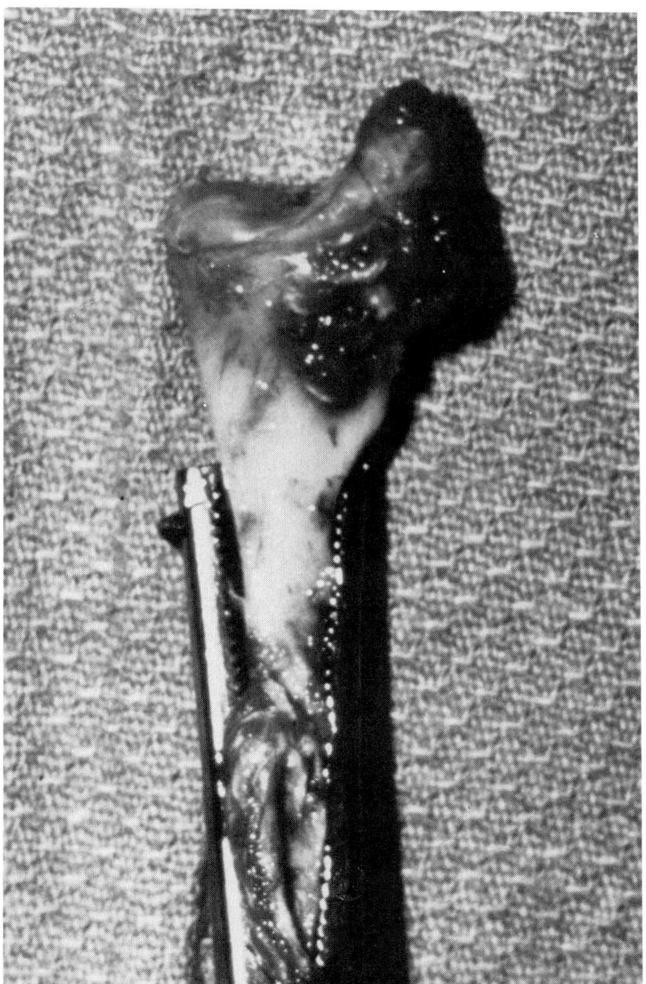

Fig. 29-17. Specimen of hyperplastic condyle after removal via extraoral vertical oblique osteotomy.

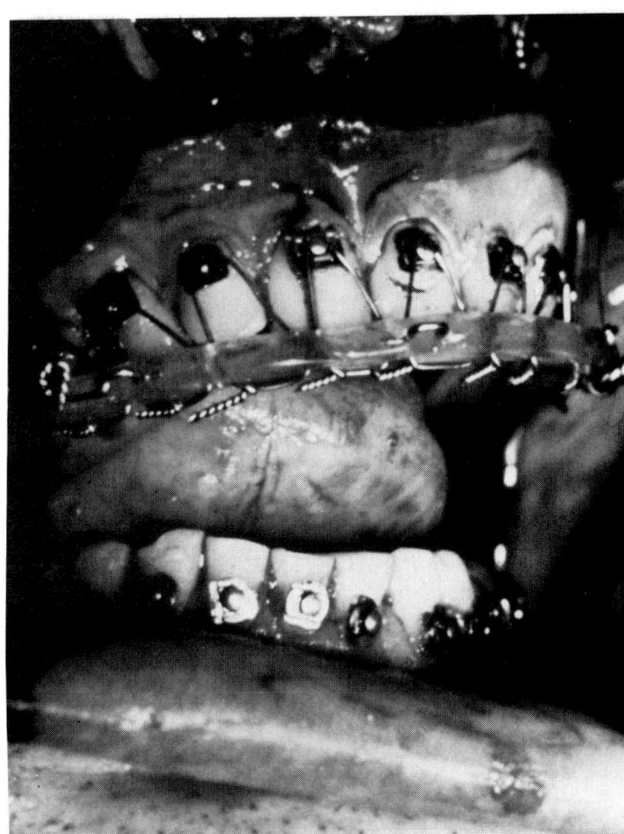

Fig. 29-18. Le Fort I osteotomy completed with teeth positioned in surgical splint.

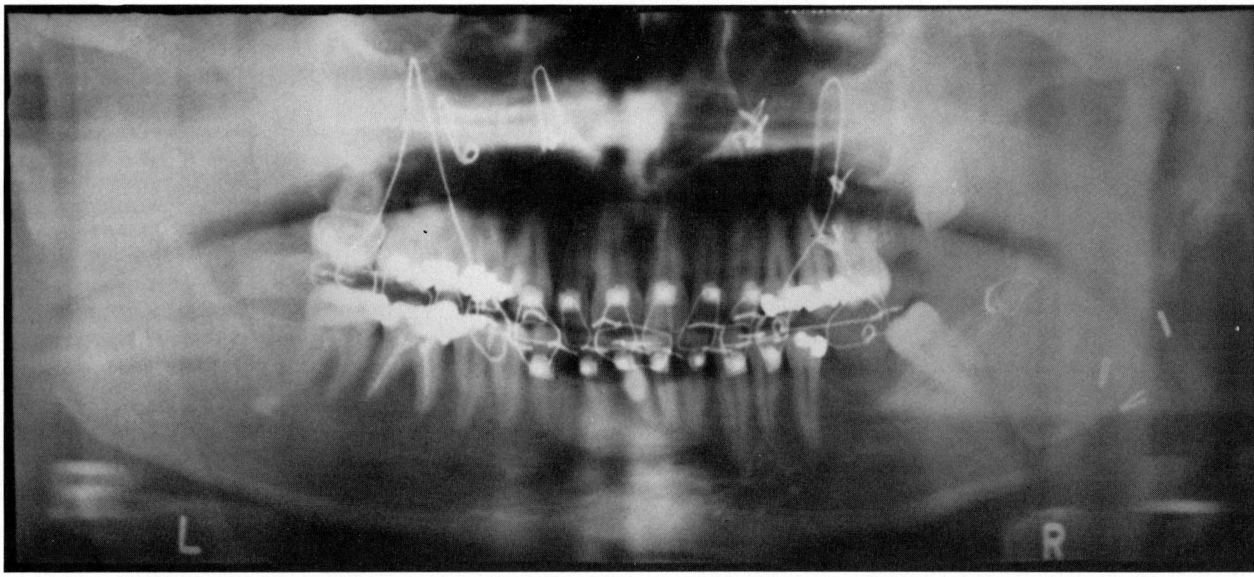

Fig. 29-19. Postoperative pantographic radiograph after Le Fort I maxillary osteotomy with segmentalization, sagittal split osteotomy of right mandibular ramus, and extraoral vertical subcondylar oblique osteotomy of left ramus with condylotomy.

A B C

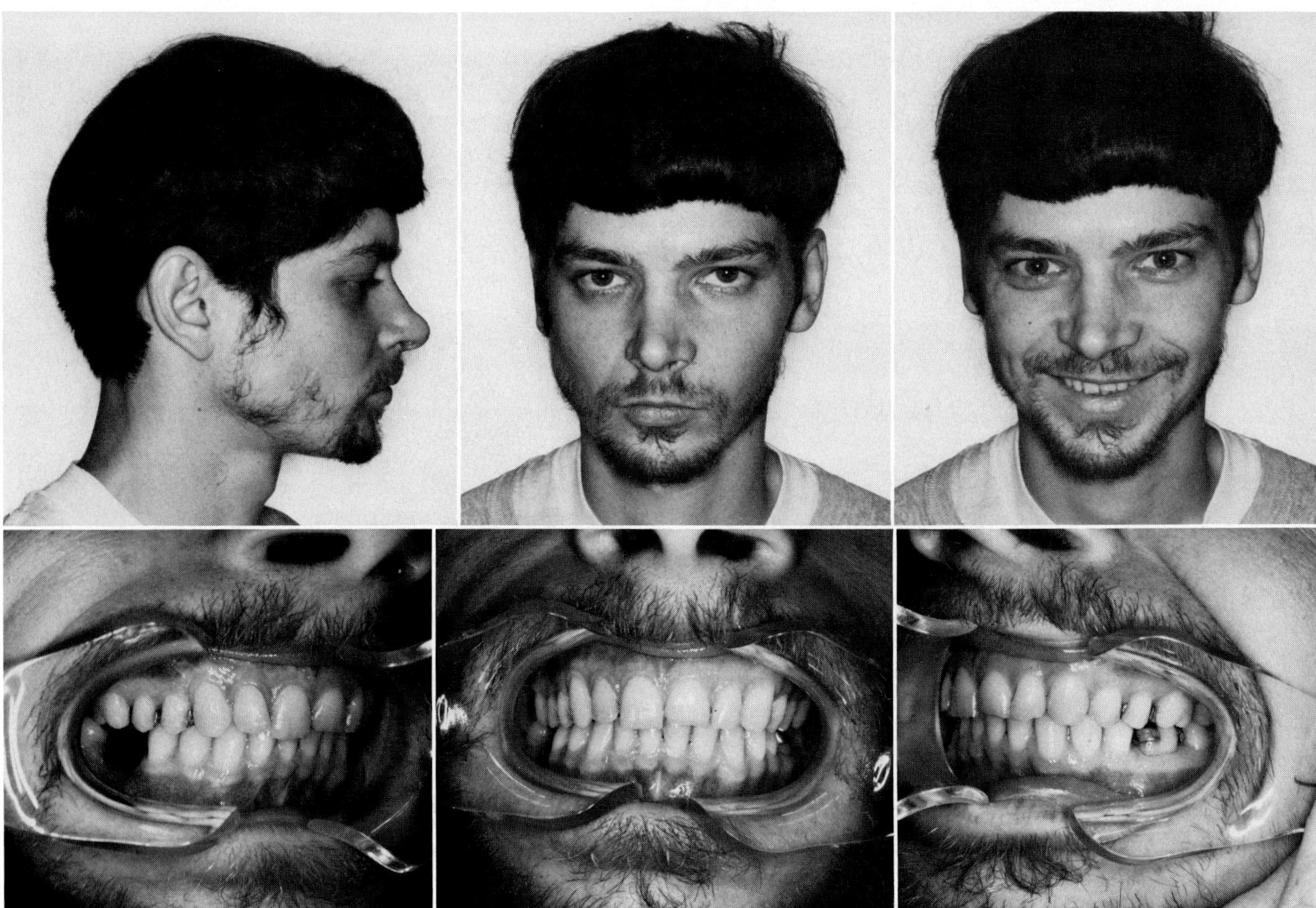

D E F

Fig 29-20. Postoperative profile **(A)**, full-face **(B** and **C)**, and dental **(D** to **F)** photographs of R.B. showing reestablishment of normal facial esthetics and occlusion.

Case 3

R.Y., a 21-year-old white college student, was referred to the Long Beach Veterans Administration Medical Center Dental Clinic in May 1979 for removal of his four third molar teeth. The patient had experienced generalized jaw and head pain for several months, and his private dentist thought that the patient's partially erupted third molars were the source of his discomfort. Clinical examination at the time of referral revealed that in addition to the painful third molar teeth, the patient had developed an end-to-end Class III dental occlusion with an accompanying slightly prognathic facial appearance and a mild asymmetry of the chin (Fig. 29-21).

The dental history showed that the patient had undergone previous orthodontic therapy at age 17 with a subsequent premature removal of his bands at age 18½. Consultation with the orthodontist revealed that at the time of band removal R.Y. had a functional Class I occlusion, but that he had apparently undergone a final growth spurt in which the mandible outgrew the maxilla.

The patient's medical history was significant only for bronchial pneumonia as a child.

Following removal of the third molar teeth as prescribed, preoperative orthognathic surgery workup was initiated consisting of dental study models, clinical photographs, radiographs (pantographic, cephalometric, TMJ tomograms, periapical, and anteroposterior facial bone), and technetium 99m bone scans of the TMJ. Cephalometric analysis,[18] facial profile analysis[4] (Fig. 29-22), and further clinical examination established that the patient's mild prognathic appearance was actually a pseudoprognathism, caused not by excessive mandibular anterior and posterior growth but rather by maxillary retrusion.

Model surgery demonstrated that correction was feasible. Accordingly, surgical treatment was directed toward correction of the maxillary retrusion, by forward and upward advancement of the maxilla, and correction of the asymmetry by a combined reduction sliding genioplasty with lateral repositioning and centering of the chin.

A B C

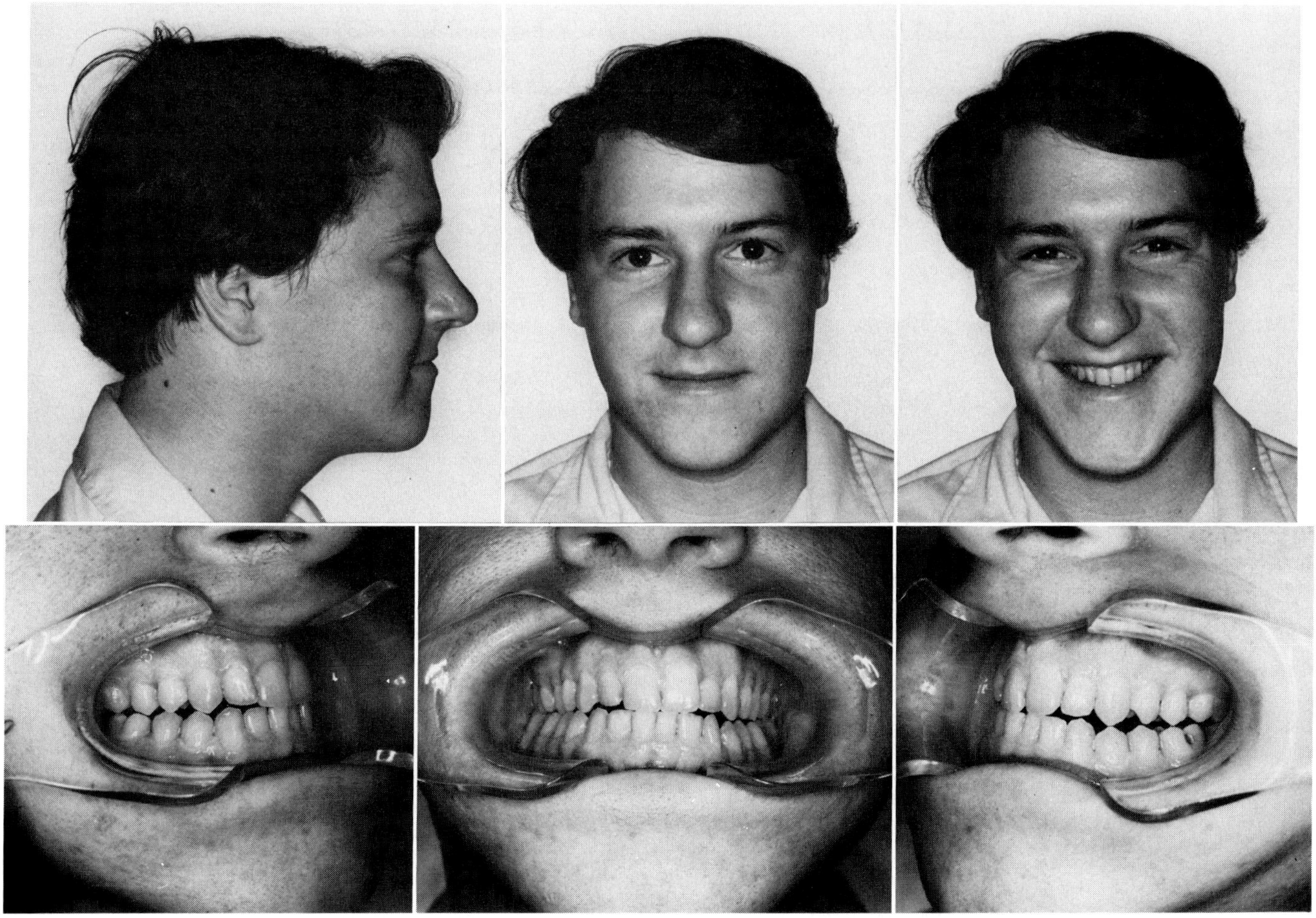

D E F

Fig. 29-21. Preoperative profile **(A)**, full-face **(B** and **C)**, and dental **(D** to **F)** views of R.Y. showing maxillary retrusive appearance and end-to-end dental malocclusion, which resulted in TMJ pain.

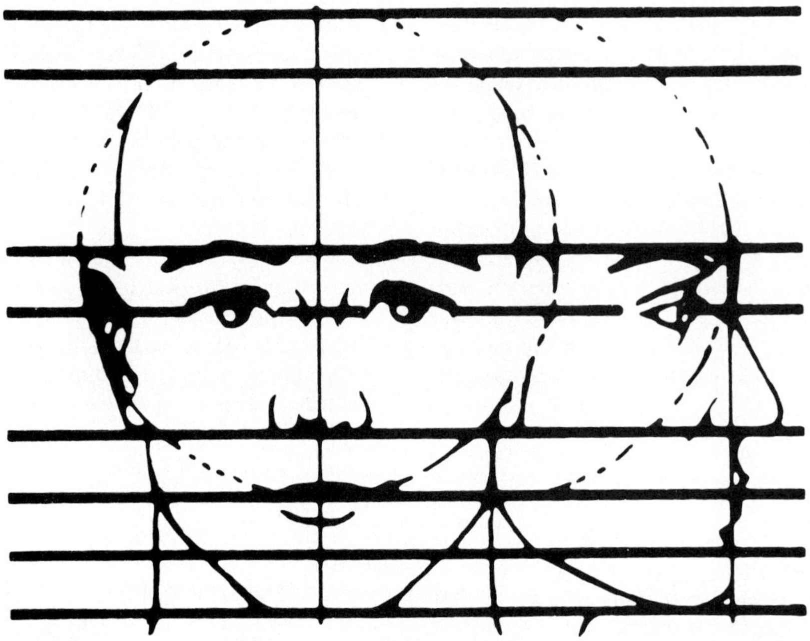

Fig. 29-22. Hasse[5] facial profile analysis used in preoperative orthognathic surgery workup to obtain optimum postsurgical facial proportion.

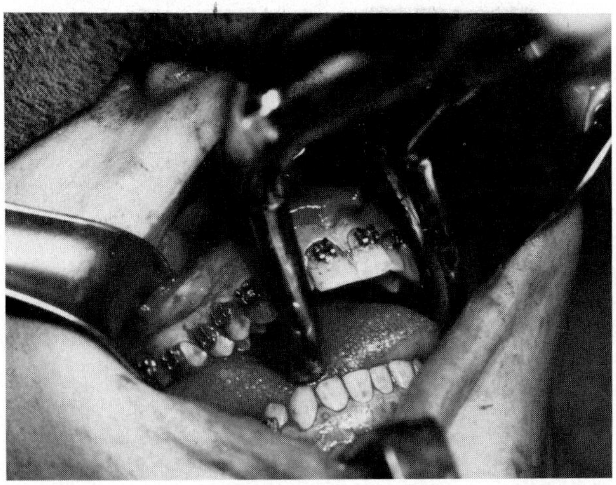

Fig. 29-23. Disimpaction forceps positioned prior to downfracturing of maxilla in Le Fort I operation.

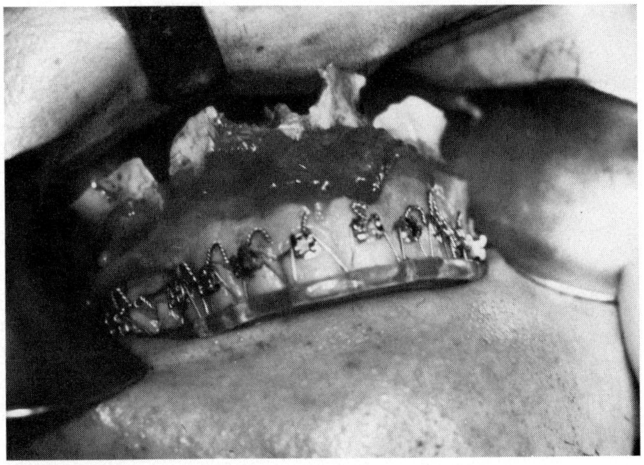

Fig. 29-24. Maxilla downfractured, segmentalized, and wired into surgical splint.

Orthognathic surgery was scheduled on August 13, 1979. A Le Fort I osteotomy with segmentalization and a genioplasty were accomplished without incident with the patient under general anesthesia (Figs. 29-23 and 29-24). Recovery was uneventful, and the patient was discharged 3 days postoperatively. The patient was not placed into intermaxillary fixation, but rather the maxilla was stabilized by combined direct interosseous wiring and infraorbital suspension wires directed to a dental splint.

Postsurgically, nighttime training elastics were used for several months to ensure optimum intercuspation of teeth and to prevent relapse. On November 28, 1979, the patient, under local standby anesthesia, underwent a tip rhinoplasty and narrowing of the alar base by a plastic surgeon.

Postsurgical follow-up appointments during the past 2 years have demonstrated that all presurgical treatment objectives have been accomplished. Namely, the patient's occlusion was normalized, his facial asymmetry was corrected, and most important, complete obviation of his headaches and jaw pain was achieved (Fig. 29-25).

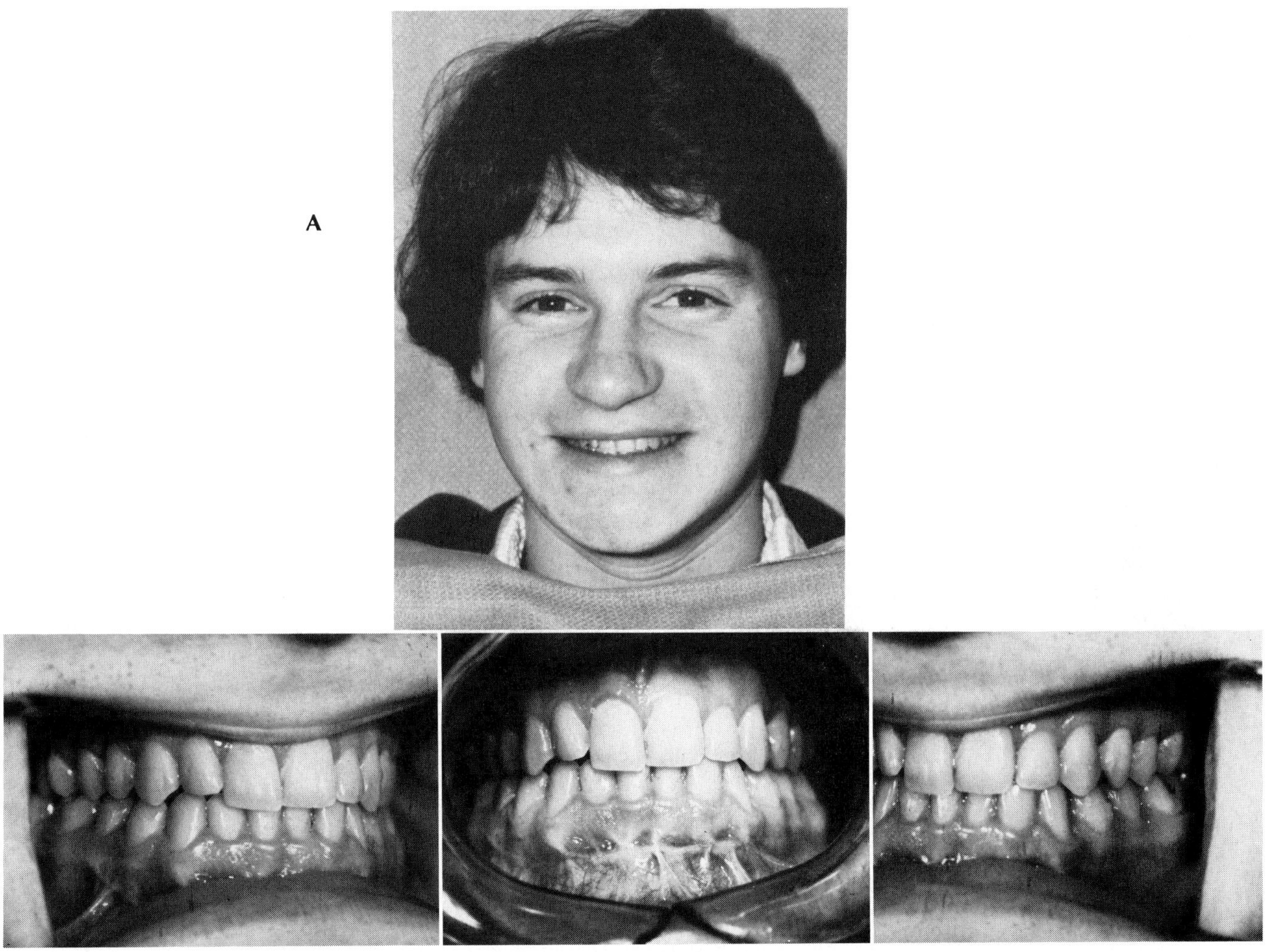

A

B C D

Fig. 29-25. Postoperative photographs of R.Y. demonstrating in full-face view **(A)** and dental views **(B** to **D)** the correction of traumatic end-to-end bite.

Case 4

P.P., a 46-year-old naval aviator, was referred to the Long Beach Veterans Administration Medical Center Oral and Maxillofacial Surgery Section in January 1980 for orthognathic surgery evaluation (Fig. 29-26). During the previous 2 years the patient had consulted with numerous medical and dental specialists for treatment of the following chief complaints:

1. Frontal, occipital, and preauricular head pain; generalized jaw pain
2. Bite off and inability to chew food properly or phonate without a lisp
3. Muscle pain in the base of the neck, upper back, and both arms
4. Ringing and buzzing in the ears

P.P. stated that these symptoms began in December 1977 after a severe case of the flu. Initially he began to awaken at night with pain in the left temple, which progressed to a state of blinding headaches by March 1978. Accompanying these headaches was the development of tinnitus. The patient was admitted to a naval hospital for extensive testing, including ENT consultation and examination, ophthalmological evaluation, neurological evaluation, brain scans, and subsequently EMI scans. The only positive finding was said to be that the patient needed glasses for distant vision.

The patient's symptoms persisted, and, in addition, he began to develop trismus from severe muscle spasms. The patient was referred from a private dentist in August 1978 to the University of California at Los Angeles Temporomandibular and Facial Pain Clinic. Examination at that time confirmed that P.P. had TMJ syndrome with an extensive myofascial component. The patient's dental history revealed a history of bruxism when doing heavy work and during periods of intense mental concentration (particularly flying jet aircraft).

Physical examination revealed TMJ pain bilaterally, greater on the right side than on the left; muscle tenderness and spasms, particularly of the left temporal and masseter muscles; a mild scoliosis of the back in the standing position; Class II dental and skeletal malocclusion with moderate overjet and deep bite; and trismus with limited interincisal

A B C

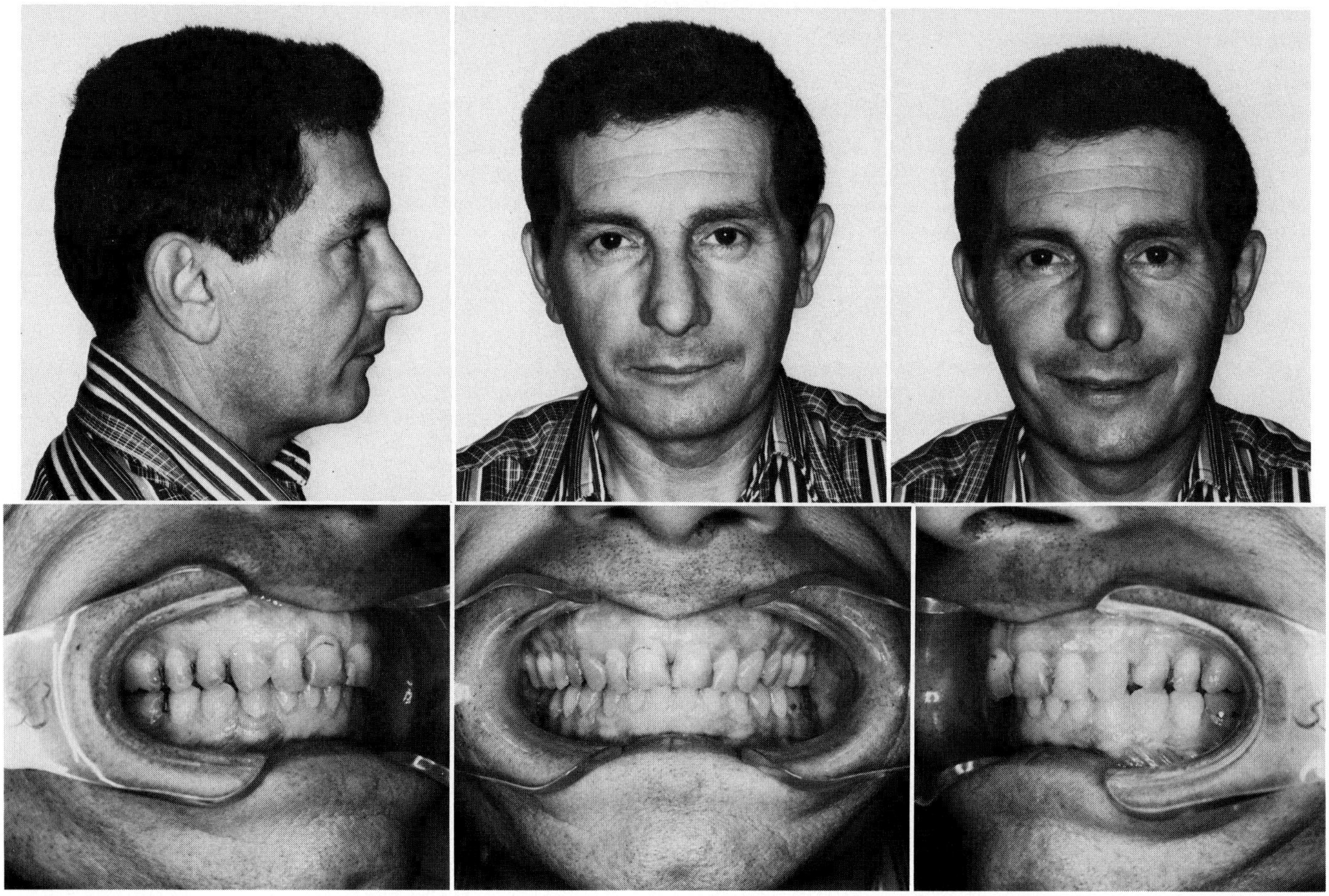

D E F

Fig. 29-26. Preoperative profile **(A)**, full-face **(B** and **C)**, and dental **(D** to **F)** views of P.P. demonstrating moderate mandibular retrognathic facial appearance and typical Class II configuration.

opening to approximately 26 mm. It also was noted during evaluation that the patient had an unconscious habit of protruding his mandible forward to achieve a more comfortable and stable occlusion.

Pantographic and dental radiography was unremarkable for additional causative factors of the patient's jaw pain. TMJ tomography demonstrated retropositioning of the condyles and loss of concentricity within the fossa.

Appropriate conservative treatment was immediately instituted, consisting of occlusal splint therapy, physical and muscle therapy, the use of vapocoolant spray with stretching techniques, soft diet, hydrocollator and ultrasound therapy, and the use of pharmacological muscle relaxants as needed. These conservative therapeutic measures achieved relaxation of the muscles and almost complete resolution of the patient's jaw and head pain and increased the interincisal opening to about 41 mm. There was, however, no alteration in his tinnitus.

Although significant improvement was realized, the splint therapy resulted in a worsening of the bite relationship. That is, the Class II malocclusion became more extreme as a result of normalizing TMJ and muscle relationships. Accordingly, the patient was referred for orthodontic and orthognathic surgery consultations.

Cephalometric analysis,[14] facial profile analysis[5] (see Fig. 29-22), clinical evaluation, and model surgery confirmed that it was feasible and advisable to advance the mandible to move the body forward and allow the teeth to more completely come into occlusion, while keeping the condyles fully seated in the fossae.

Orthognathic surgery was scheduled on February 1, 1980. A bilateral sagittal split osteotomy (Epker modification)[3] of the mandibular rami with advancement of the mandible was performed using general nasal endotracheal anesthesia (Fig. 29-27). Recovery was uneventful, and the patient was discharged 3 days postoperatively. The patient was maintained in intermaxillary fixation for 6 weeks, at which time he was referred to the orthodontist for postsurgical finishing of the case.

Final orthodontic completion of the case was achieved in February 1981. The patient's retrognathism with its associ-

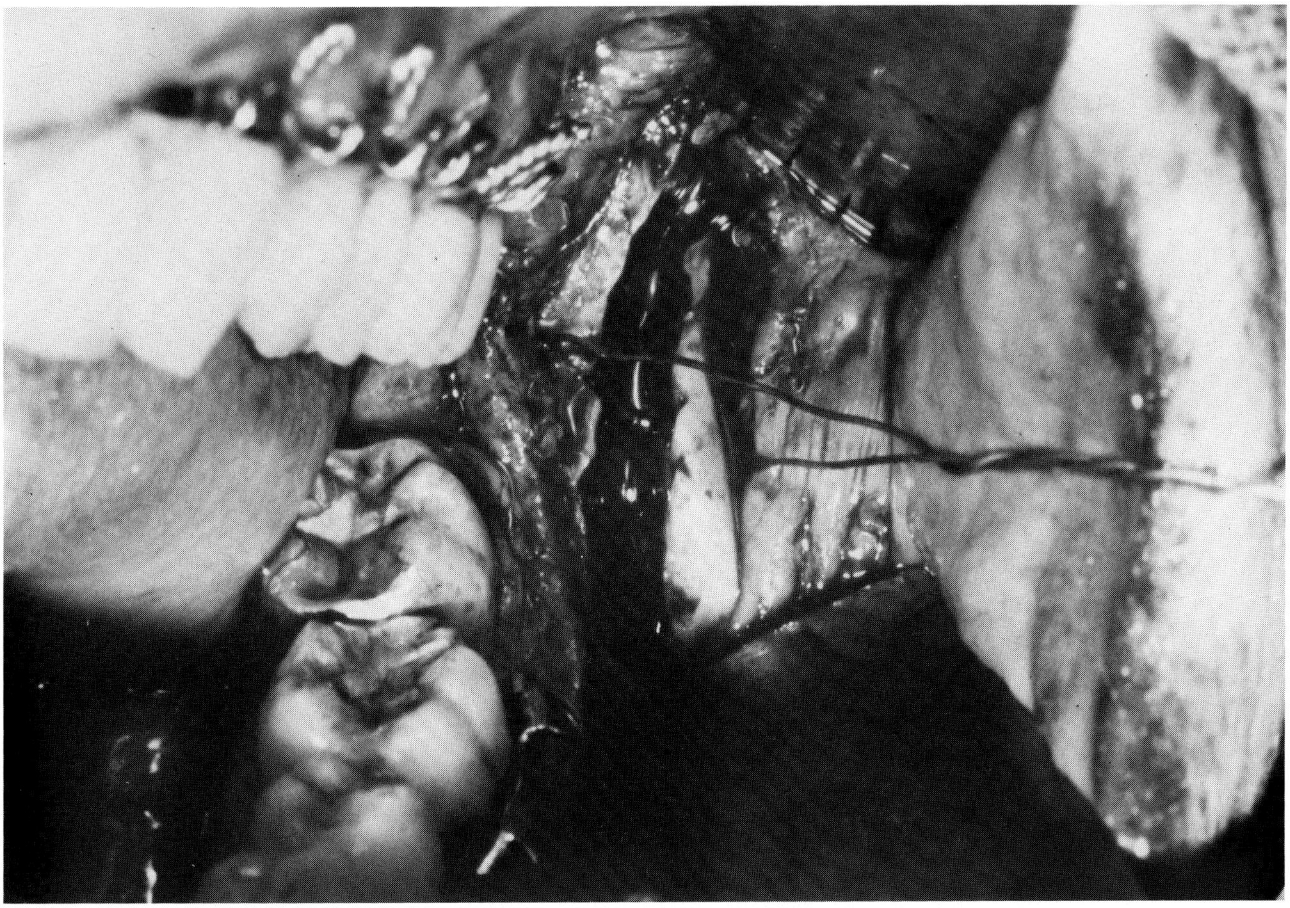

Fig. 29-27. Wiring together of proximal and distal segments in Case 4 after sagittal split osteotomy for mandibular advancement to correct retrognathism with associated TMJ pain.

ated Class II dental problems has been eliminated (Fig. 29-28). Postoperative TMJ films demonstrated proper condyle-to-fossa concentricity. Most important, however, the patient is symptom free with complete obviation of jaw, TMJ, and head pain. Remarkably, the tinnitus has resolved, suggesting perhaps that sustained proper positioning of the condyles within the fossae was responsible for the elimination of this phenomenon.

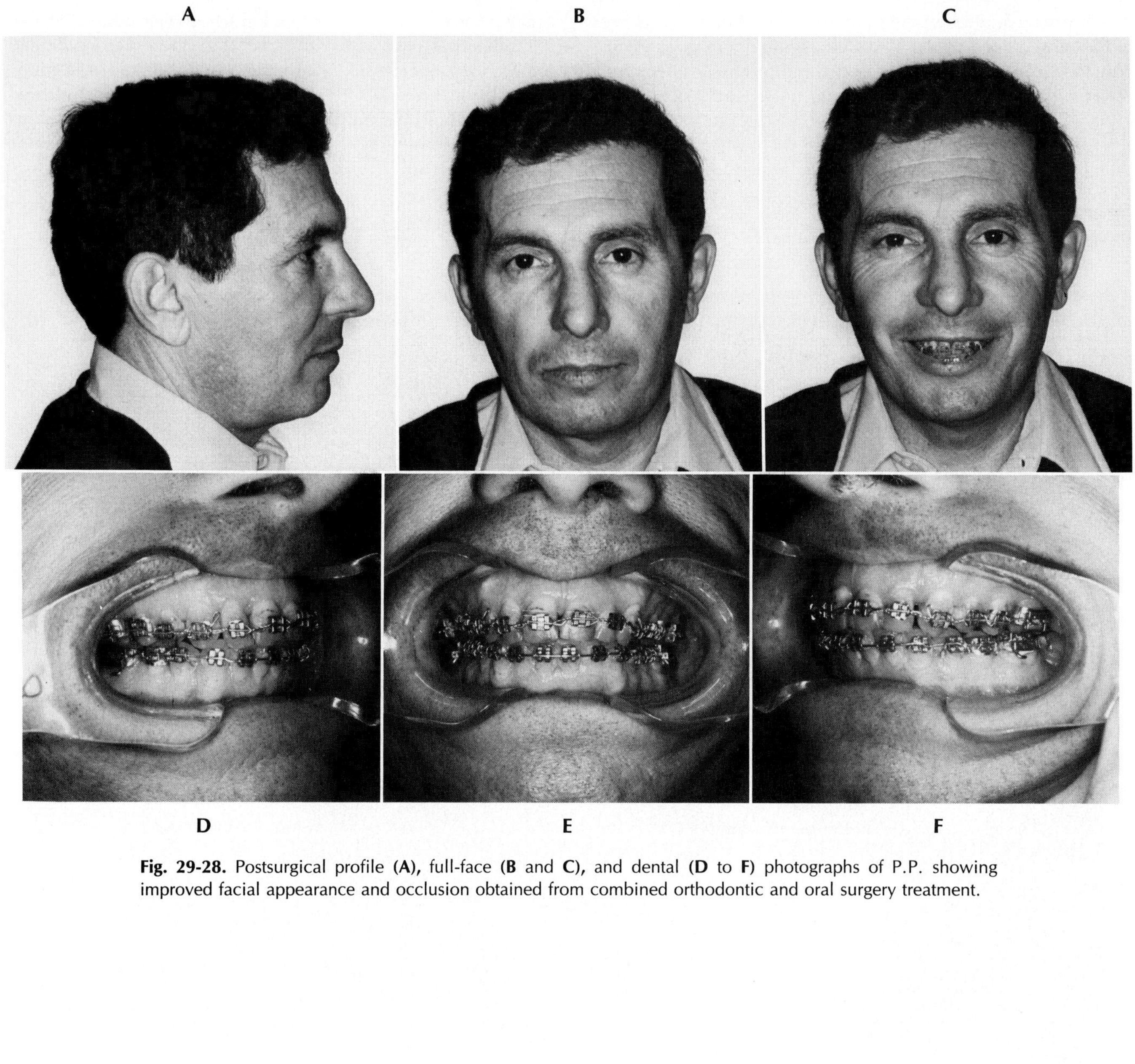

Fig. 29-28. Postsurgical profile **(A)**, full-face **(B** and **C)**, and dental **(D** to **F)** photographs of P.P. showing improved facial appearance and occlusion obtained from combined orthodontic and oral surgery treatment.

Case 5

K.B., a 25-year-old black hospital employee, sought treatment at the Long Beach Veterans Administration Medical Center Dental Clinic in December 1979 for a toothache. The patient had experienced intermittent right-sided mandibular discomfort for several months. In addition, a review of symptoms revealed that K.B. had occasional extreme head and TMJ pain, generalized fatigue and muscle ache, and tooth sensitivity on routine mastication.

Clinical examination demonstrated several obvious dental problems, including advanced dental caries with pulpal involvement for teeth nos. 4, 28, and 29, an unstable dental occlusion with loss of posterior teeth on the left side, heavy wear faceting with numerous excursive interferences, a prognathic facial appearance with an accompanying Class III dental malocclusion, and anterior overclosure with complete anterior telescoping of the maxillary dentition within the mandibular arch (Fig. 29-29).

The patient's medical history was noncontributory, with no previous severe illnesses, allergies, or injuries.

Routine general dentistry and endodontic therapy were accomplished to correct the patient's immediate dental problems. An orthodontic consultation was recommended, but the patient declined because of financial difficulties.

After completion of the dental treatment, preoperative orthognathic surgery workup was instituted, consisting of dental study models, clinical photographs, radiographs (pantographic, cephalometric, submental vertex, and TMJ tomograms), and technetium 99m bone scans of the TMJ. Cephalometric analysis,[14] facial profile analysis,[5] and further clinical examination confirmed that corrective surgery should be directed toward the mandible to eliminate K.B.'s true prognathism.

Model surgery showed that correction was feasible. Although orthodontic treatment presurgically was desired for optimum results, the model surgery demonstrated that a

A B C

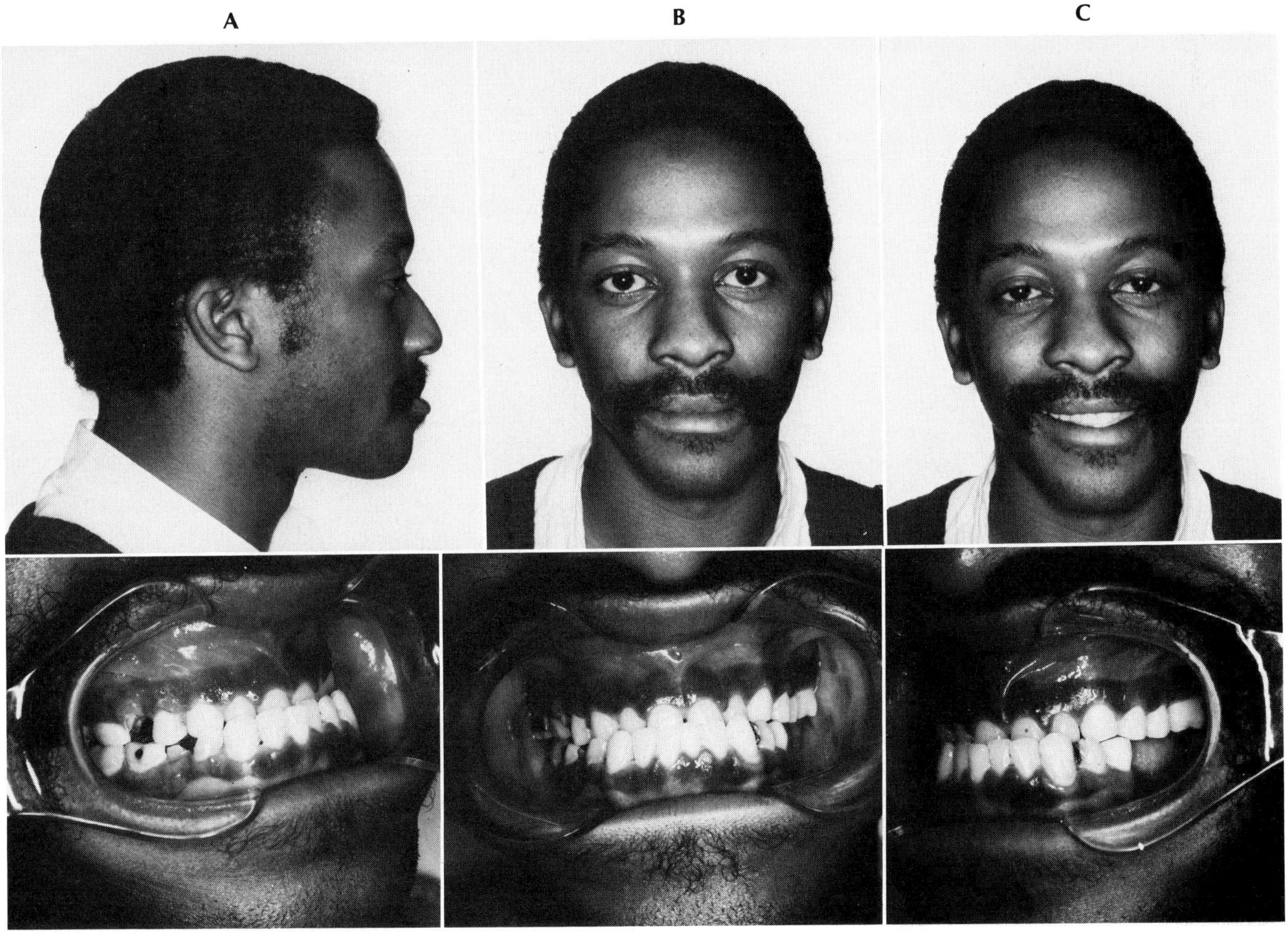

D E F

Fig. 29-29. Preoperative profile (A), full-face (B and C), and dental (D to F) views of K.B. demonstrating unpleasing prognathic appearance and Class III dental malocclusion with complete telescoping of anterior upper dentition.

functionally stable occlusion could be obtained with the use of presurgical and postsurgical occlusal equilibration. TMJ tomograms revealed that the condyles were positioned against the posterior aspect of the fossae. However, the technetium 99m bone scans were cold, suggesting that degenerative TMJ changes had not yet taken place.

Orthognathic surgery was performed on February 8, 1980. Bilateral intraoral vertical oblique osteotomies of the mandibular rami with an 8-mm setback were accomplished with the patient under general anesthesia. An O-chromic gut suture was affixed around the proximal and distal ramal segments during surgery to maintain bony contact and to allow dynamic remodeling and repositioning of the condyles within the fossae (Figs. 29-8 and 29-30). Postoperative TMJ films confirmed that the condyles had reseated and assumed a concentric position.

The patient's postoperative recovery was uneventful. Intermaxillary fixation was maintained for 7 weeks. Nighttime elastic traction (3 weeks) and selective occlusal equilibration were used as needed. The patient was referred to a prosthodontist for fabrication of a mandibular partial denture to further stabilize the bite on the left side and to prevent supraeruption of the maxillary posterior teeth.

As in the previous cases presented, the pretreatment objectives were accomplished. Specifically, the patient's occlusion was normalized, his prognathism was corrected, and he has been asymptomatic for jaw, TMJ, and head pain during the past year (Fig. 29-31).

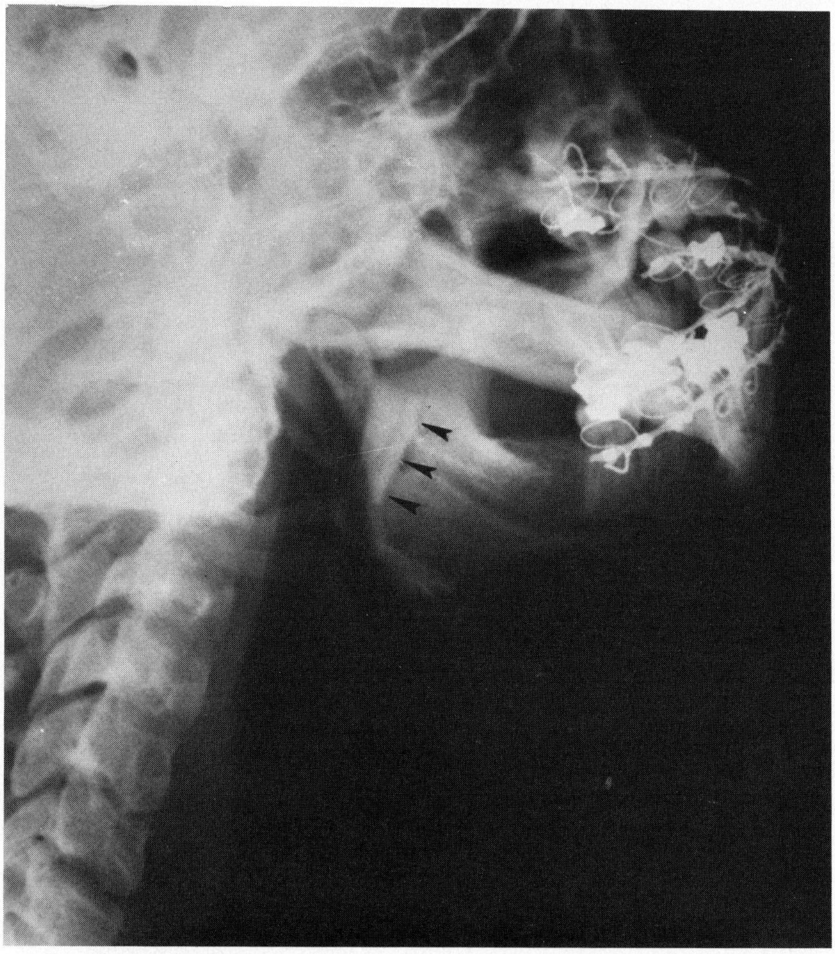

Fig. 29-30. Lateral oblique jaw film demonstrating overlapping of proximal and distal segments *(arrows)* and proper postoperative condylar positioning within fossa.

A B C

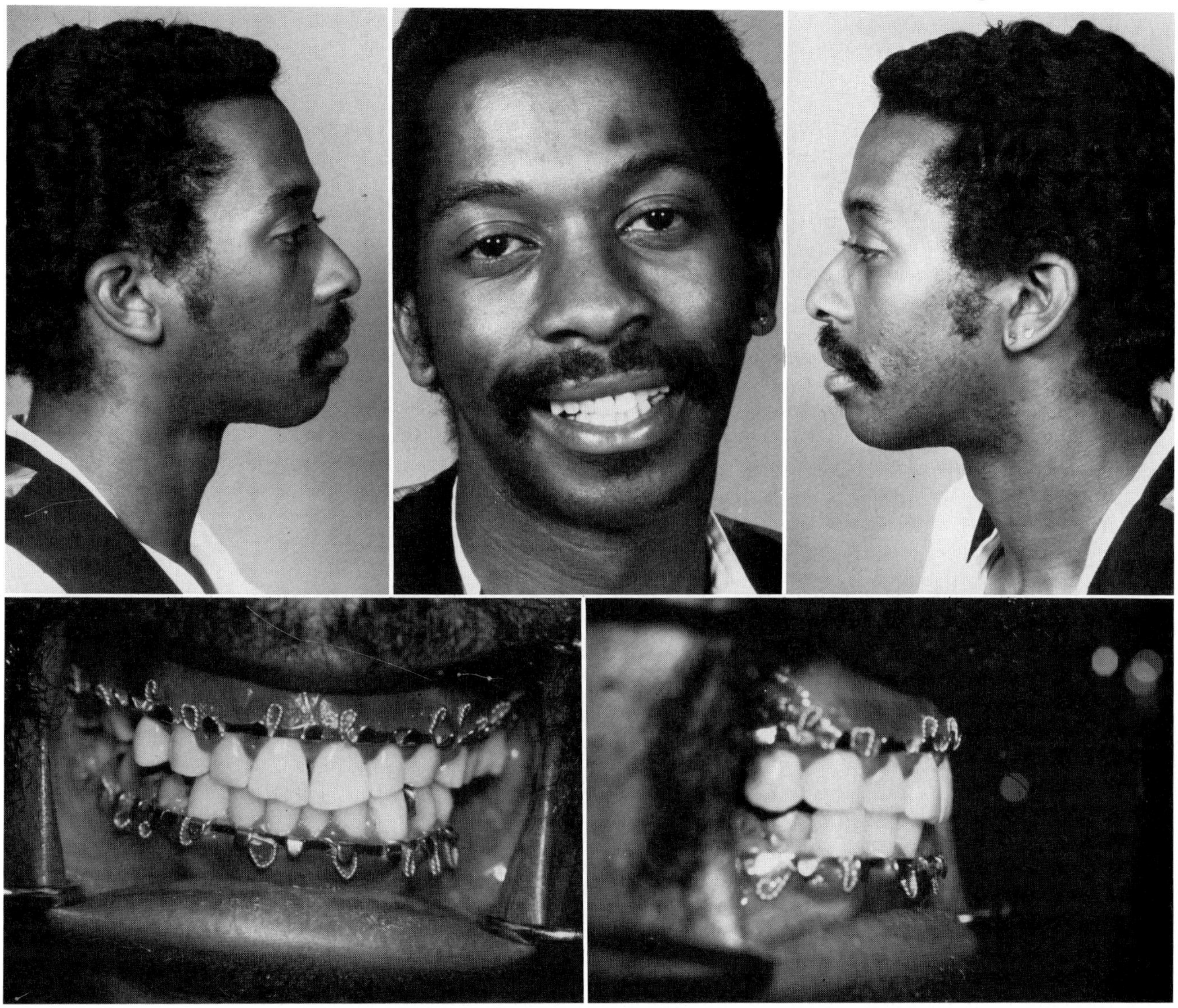

D E

Fig. 29-31. Postoperative profile (**A** and **C**), full-face (**B**), and dental (**D** and **E**) photographs of K.B. showing normal facial profile. View of immediate postoperative occlusion shows correction of Class III malocclusion. Nighttime elastic traction was used to help establish optimum bite.

Case 6

R.B. was referred in May 1972 for removal of her four third molars. She had headaches, and it was thought that if these teeth were removed, the head pains might be helped. The procedure was accomplished the month of referral in the office with the patient under methohexital sodium (Brevital Sodium). The patient still complained after 3 months of the same type of headaches. She had had orthodontic appliances from the age of 12, applied at a Midwestern dental school. The bands were eventually removed. Her teeth were in better alignment, but there was no improvement in her Class II relationship.

In August 1972 TMJ cephalometric radiographs and full-face films were taken. The TMJ films revealed erosion of the cortical layer of bone over both eminences, more severe on the left side (Fig. 29-32). There was also a significant widening of the disc-space relationship on the left side. Cephalometric, full-face, and profile films revealed a Class II relationship (Figs. 29-33 and 29-34). This was confirmed by Steiner[18] analysis. It was decided to institute orthodontic treatment. This involved removal of four first premolars.

Orthognathic surgery was scheduled for July 26, 1976. It was decided to perform a sagittal split osteotomy and advance the mandible. This was accomplished without incident. There was no paresthesia. She had an uneventful recovery.

Postoperative films were taken September 14, 1976. The TMJ films (Fig. 29-35) showed the condyles in good relationship to the fossae. On the left side the erosion of the eminences and the diminished disc space were noted. The right side showed less change over the eminence and a normal disc-space relationship. Cephalometric films showed the condyle in good relationship to the maxilla and mandible (Fig. 29-36). The posterior open bite was closed orthodontically over the ensuing $1\frac{1}{2}$ years of treatment (Fig. 29-37).

The patient has since stated that her headaches have been less severe. There is the possibility that the combined orthognathic surgery and orthodontics will prevent the necessity of surgery, even though there is significant organic change in the joint. The patient has been advised of the possible need for temporomandibular joint surgery if complete obviation of her pain is not realized.

It is probable that the damage to her temporomandibular joints would not have occurred had interceptive orthodontics and surgery been instituted earlier. The symptoms that caused much suffering later would not have developed. This clearly points out the relationship between the developmental skeletal malrelationships of the maxilla/mandible and abnormal stresses and strains on the temporomandibular joint. Ultimately these stresses and strains can lead to serious organic damage to the temporomandibular apparatus.

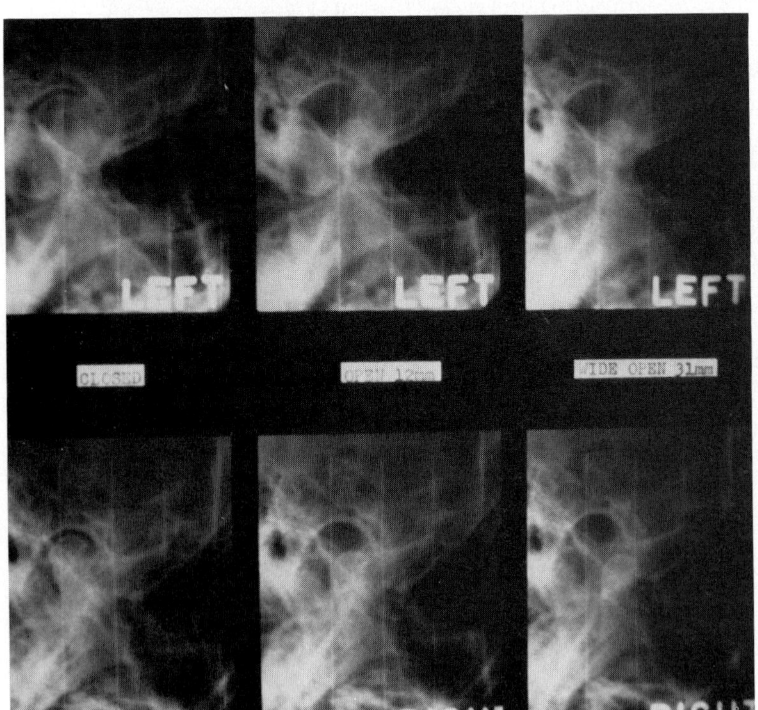

Fig. 29-32. *Left,* Specialized TMJ radiograph showing compression of disc space in left joint in closed view and erosion of cortical layer of bone over descending and ascending slopes of eminences. In functional views there is increased disc space. *Right,* In right joint some compression of disc space and some beginning erosion of eminences are evident. This is more normal functional movement.

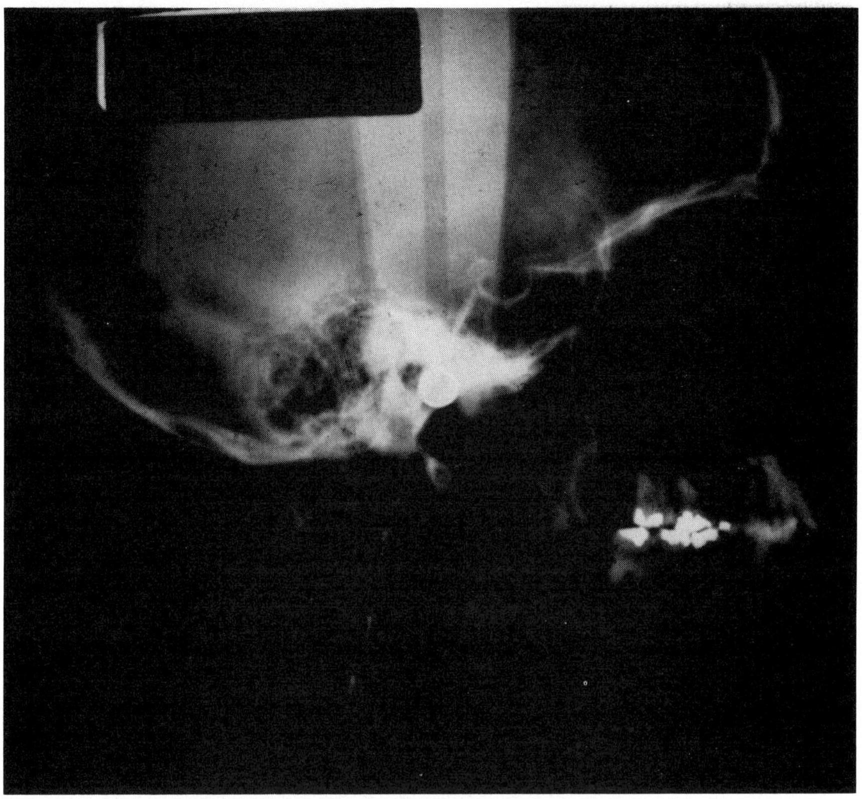

Fig. 29-33. Cephalometric profile showing typical Class II relationship and flaring of anterior teeth.

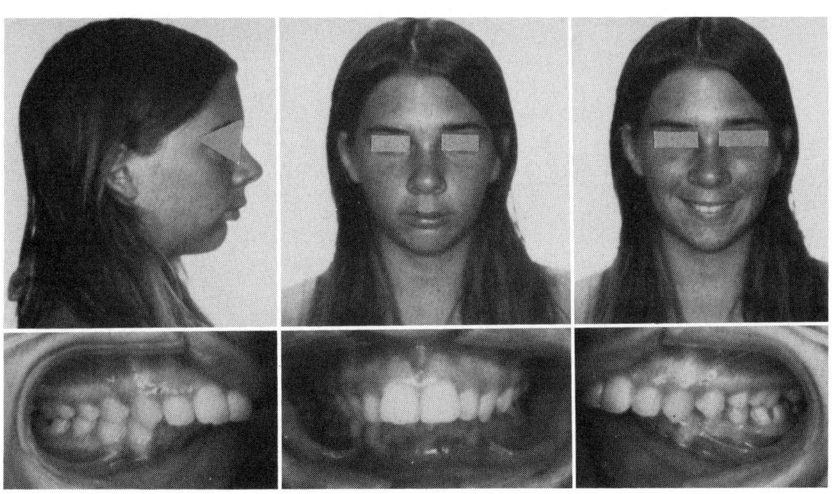

Fig. 29-34. Full-face, profile, and dental views of R.B. showing typical Class II configuration.

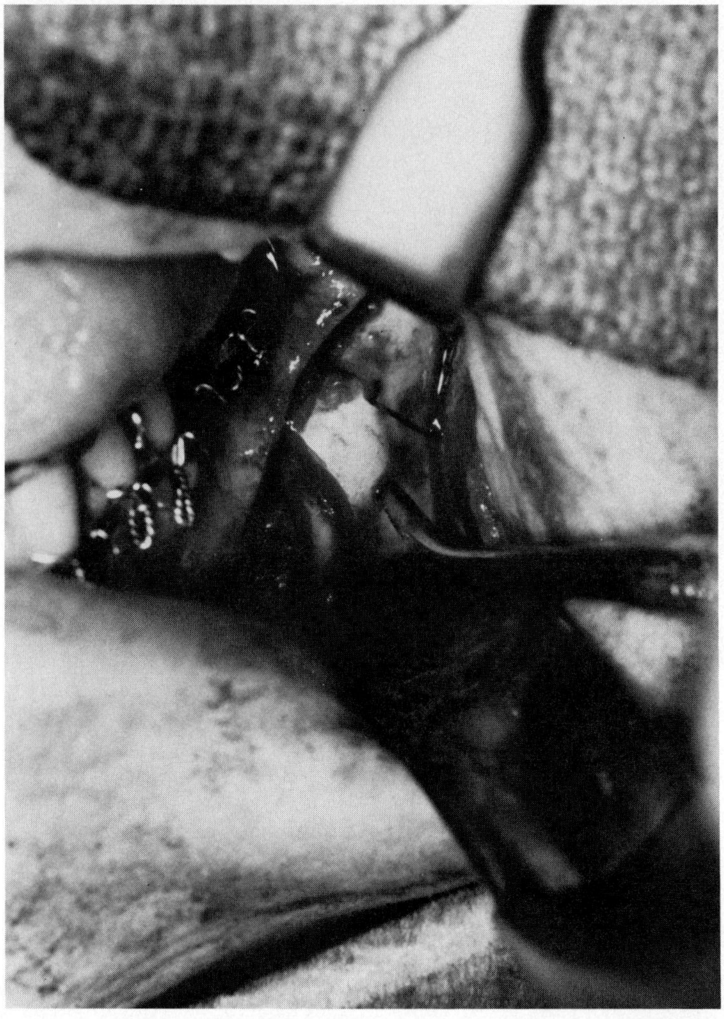

Fig. 29-35. During wiring of distal and proximal segments in modified sagittal ramus osteotomy,[3] Crane-Pick elevator is positioned in proximal piece. This technical approach ensures proper seating of condyles in glenoid fossae and prevents relapse and postsurgical TMJ problems.

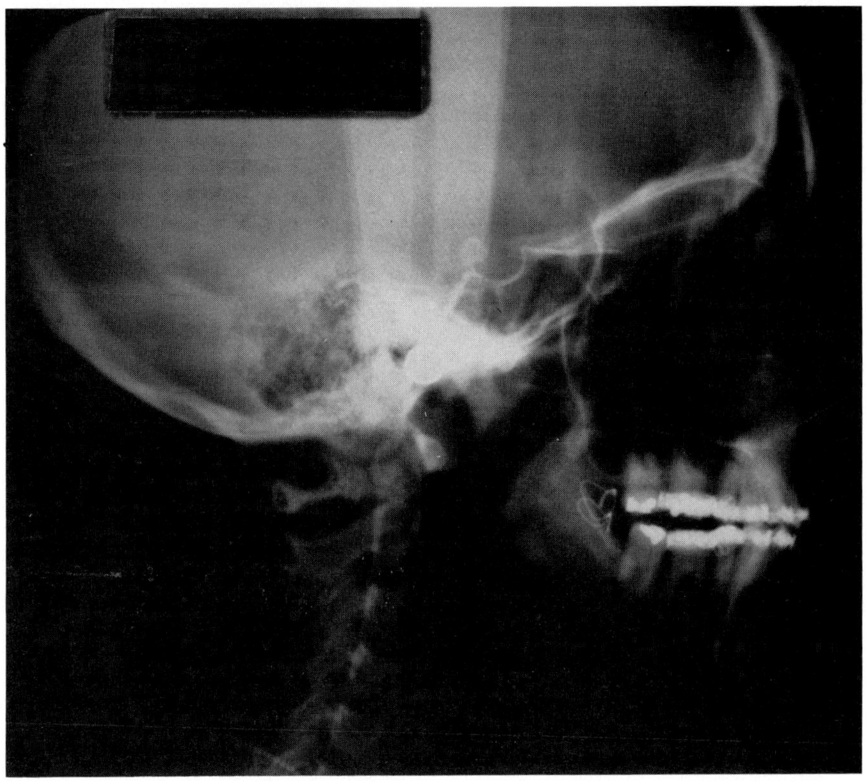

Fig. 29-36. Postoperative cephalometric views showing advanced mandible and interosseous wires from sagittal split osteotomy.

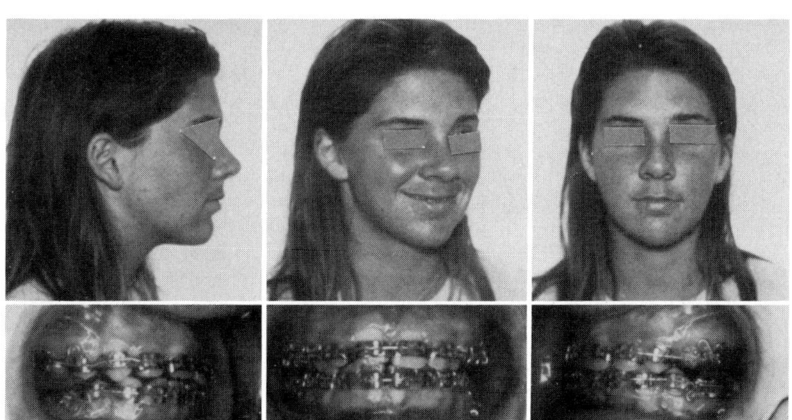

Fig. 29-37. Full-face, profile, and dental views showing results of combined orthodontic and orthognathic treatment.

ACKNOWLEDGMENT

Dr. Hasse would like to acknowledge the residents and staff of the Veterans Administration Medical Center, Long Beach, California, who assisted in the surgeries and medical management of some of the cases presented in this chapter. In particular, a specially deserved thanks is owed Drs. Dean L. Duncan, Jeff J. Pulver, and Sam J. Poidmore.

REFERENCES

1. Babcock, W.W.: Surgical treatment of certain deformities of the jaw associated with malocclusions of the teeth, J.A.M.A. **53**:833, 1909.
2. Blair, V.P.: Operations on jaw bones and face: study of etiology and pathological anatomy of developmental malrelations of maxilla and mandible to each other and to facial outline and to operative treatment, Surg. Gynecol. Obstet. **4**:67, 1907.
3. Epker, B.N.: Modifications in the sagittal osteotomy of the mandible, J. Oral Surg. **35**:157, 1977.
4. Gonzales-Ulloa, M., and Stevens, E.: Role of chin correction in profileplasty, Plast. Reconstr. Surg. **41**:477, 1968.
5. Hasse, C.D.: A facial profile analysis for orthognathic and craniofacial surgery, Unpublished paper, 1980.
6. Hasse, C.D.: Orthognathic surgery and the TMJ: transactions of the conference on diseases of the temporomandibular apparatus, Los Angeles, April 27-29, 1980.
7. Hinds, E.C., and Kent, J.N.: Surgical treatment of developmental jaw deformities, St. Louis, 1972, The C.V. Mosby Co.
8. Hovell, J.H.: Surgical treatment of mandibular prognathism, Ann. R. Coll. Surg. **27**:388, 1960.
9. Hullihen, S.P.: A case of elongation of the under jaw and distortion of face and neck, caused by burn, sucessfully treated, Am. J. Dent. Surg. **9**:157, 1849.
10. Kostecka, F.: Die Chirurgische Therapie der Progenie, Zahnärztl. Rundschaw. **40**:669, 1931.
11. MacIntosh, R.B.: Total mandibular alveolar osteotomy, J. Maxillofac. Surg. **2**:210, 1974.
12. MacIntosh, R.B., and Henny, F.A.: A spectrum of application of autogenous costochondral grafts, J. Maxillofac. Surg. **5**:257, 1977.
13. Obwegeser, H.L.: Transactions of the conference on comprehensive oral surgery, Washington, D.C., Walter Reed Army Medical Center, June 20-22, 1966.
14. Ricketts, R.M.: Cephalometrics synthesis, Am. J. Orthod. **46**:647, 1960.
15. Robinson, M., and Lytle, J.J.: Micrognathism corrected by vertical osteotomies of the rami without bone grafts, Oral Surg. **15**:641, 1962.
16. Schendel, S.A., Wolford, L.M., and Epker, B.N.: Mandibular deficiency syndrome. III. Surgical advancement of the deficient mandible in growing children: treatment results in 12 patients, Oral Surg. **45**:364, 1978.
17. Schuchardt, K.: Ein Beitrag zur Chirurgischen Keiferorthapadie unter Berucksichtigung ihrer Bedeutung fur die Behandlung Angeborener und Erworbener Kieferdeformitaten bie Soldaten, Dt. Zahn-Mud-Kieferhk **9**:73, 1942.
18. Steiner, C.C.: Cephalometrics in clinical practice, Angle Orthod. **29**:8, 1959.
19. Ware, W.H., and Taylor, R.C.: Cartilaginous growth centers transplanted to replace mandibular condyle in monkeys, J. Oral Surg. **24**:33, 1966.
20. Wassmund, M.: Lehrbuch der Praktischen Chirurgie des Mundes und der Kiefer, Bd. I. Leipzig, 1935, Meusser.

30 Neurosurgical treatment of facial pain

J. RONALD RICH, M.D., F.A.C.S.

The fifth cranial nerve, the trigeminal, has the important function of conveying sensation from the face. The dense population of cutaneous sensory receptors in the face, the fact that the trigeminal ganglion is the largest sensory ganglion in humans, and the complexity of the cerebral connections of the trigeminal sensory system all demonstrate the functional significance of this nerve. Acute pain transmission in this system serves an important warning function, protecting a person from potential harm. When this function has been served and pain becomes persistent and severe, it becomes deleterious and is no longer useful. Acute pain is treated by analgesic medications and specific therapy directed toward correcting the causative pathological process. If these measures fail and the pain passes into the chronic stage at a level that is intolerable to the patient, surgical treatment becomes a consideration. At present, with the exception of the microvascular decompressive operation used to treat certain forms of facial pain, the surgical treatment of chronic facial pain consists of partial or total ablation of some part of the trigeminal sensory system. One unsophisticated in the surgical treatment of facial pain might assume that any pain in the trigeminal nerve distribution would be controlled by proximal trigeminal destruction, but this unfortunately is not so. There are but a few types of facial pain that can be treated surgically with reliably acceptable rates of relief and complication. These are the trigeminal neuralgias of a primary or idiopathic nature (tic douloureux) and those secondary to demyelinating disease, some form of vascular compression, or invasion or compression by neoplasm.[90] Although there are other types of pain that may respond to surgical treatment, the evaluation and selection of such patients is probably best left to those who have knowledge and experience in dealing with patients complaining of facial pain. This is so because the majority of such patients will not be benefited by surgical treatment. These patients are infrequently tolerant of the subsequent facial sensory loss that ensues and often develop discomforting sensory aberrations while their initial pain continues, is improved but still intolerable, or worsens. The selection of nontrigeminal neuralgia patients likely to benefit from an operative procedure is an extremely difficult and, at times, impossible task. Above all, one must remember that surgery is not indicated simply because nothing else can be done.

PSYCHODYNAMICS OF FACIAL PAIN

Sherrington[125] described physical pain as "the psychic adjunct of an imperative protective reflex." The experience of pain is a unified blend of the pain sensation, the unpleasant affective component, and the reaction to the pain stimulus. Thus the perception of pain is a subjective experience influenced by psychic as well as physiological factors. Both must be considered if optimum surgical results are to be attained. Pain, whether from a primary psychogenic or physiological cause, is perceived by the patient similarly. The patient with psychogenic pain hurts just as much as the patient with pain caused by an invasive malignancy. Malingering is to be differentiated as deliberate deceit. Here the patient is not in pain or consciously overreacts to pain for some form of secondary gain. Such people are usually apparent to those experienced in dealing with chronic pain patients.

In the clinical analysis and therefore the management of facial pain it is of great importance to have knowledge of not only the physiological cause but also the presence of magnifying or reducing quantities of the pain experience brought about by the patient's feeling or behavior toward the pain and its influences on the patient's life. The patient is not benefited by a surgical procedure that relieves the trigeminal neuralgic pain but leaves an intolerable facial numbness or burning pain. Nor is a patient with psychogenic pain benefited by the performance of a surgical procedure that not only does not relieve the primary pain but additionally leaves troublesome numbness and sensory aberrations. If these problems are to be avoided, one must evaluate both the physiological and psychological implications of pain. Not infrequently, the latter requires detailed psychological testing and evaluation by a psychiatrist or psychologist knowledgeable about pain and patients having chronic pain. This should be carried out before consideration of a surgical procedure to relieve pain, not after, when the pain persists or other complaints appear.

ACUPUNCTURE

The origin of acupuncture therapy is unknown, although it is believed to date to the Stone Age in China. The earliest known medical text on the subject is ascribed to the Yellow Emperor Huang Ti, who lived from 2697 to 2596 BC.[2,150] Thereafter it remained primarily in the chests of those practicing traditional Chinese medicine. Recently the Chinese have begun to combine their traditional medicine with Western medicine, and in 1958 acupuncture was being used for surgical anesthesia. The advantages of no mortality, virtually no morbidity, lack of associated nausea and vomiting, and the prolongation of analgesia into the postoperative period resulted in widespread interest in the technique. Acupuncture has been used with varying success in the treatment of facial pain, especially trigeminal neuralgia.[105] The cyclical nature of trigeminal neuralgia with frequent long-term pain-free intervals precludes judgment of the effectiveness of acupuncture, since the patient follow-up studies in reported series are too brief to yield meaningful data. Leung, Fan, and Sechzer[87] encountered persistent pain in 20 of 22 treated patients, casting doubt on the efficacy of acupuncture in trigeminal neuralgia.

BASIS OF SURGICAL TREATMENT

The basis of essentially all forms of accepted surgical treatment of facial pain is denervation of the painful area. Since the pathophysiology of idiopathic and the secondary forms of trigeminal neuralgia in demyelinating disease and some forms of vascular compression is unproved, the fact that sensory denervation of the face cures them is unexplained. Nonetheless, it is a generally accepted fact that the efficacy of a surgical procedure in relieving pain in these patients is directly related to the degree and permanency of the facial sensory loss produced in the painful area. Permanent sensory loss follows interruption of the trigeminal pathways at or central to the ganglion cells of the gasserian ganglion. With such lesions, axonal regeneration does not take place because of the absence of necessary Schwann cells. Denervation by destruction of the peripheral branches and divisions of the trigeminal nerve obviously constitutes a much simpler procedure. At such levels, however, Schwann cells are present, and the regenerative powers are excellent. With regeneration comes return of sensory function and pain. Thus surgical treatments can be categorized into peripheral procedures (usually temporary) and intracranial or central procedures (usually permanent). The more proximal the peripheral lesion, the longer the regeneration time required for return of function and thus the longer the duration of pain relief.

PERIPHERAL PROCEDURES

Historical background

Nicolaus André[4] apparently perfomed the first successful surgical procedure for relieving trigeminal neuralgia in 1756 by cauterizing the infraorbital nerve. Marechal, the personal physician of King Louis XIV, had previously failed with an attempt at an infraorbital neurectomy and subsequently outlined the treatment for André. After Mayo's demonstration[91] in 1822 that the trigeminus was the sensory nerve of the face, section of its peripheral branches became the standard treatment for trigeminal neuralgia. Treatment by injection of neurolytic substances awaited the technical development of adequate instrumentation to instill such substances. Chloroform was recommended for injection by Bartholow[6] in 1876 and osmic acid by Neuber[94] in 1883. Although ethyl alcohol was advocated by Abadie[1] in 1902, it was not until 1918, when Sicard[126] demonstrated its superiority over many other agents, that it became the neurolytic agent of choice. With growing experience it became apparent that the excellent regenerative powers of the peripheral portions of the trigeminal nerve caused denervation at this level to result only in temporary relief. Thus the search for methods of more proximal and therefore longer-lasting approaches grew. Schloesser[119] in 1903 approached the mandibular division at the foramen ovale with an angulated needle, transorally. Ostwalt[99] in 1906 reported the lateral approach to injection of the maxillary and mandibular divisions near their respective foramina. Taptas[140,141] appears to have been the first to carry out a successful, albeit accidental, neurolytic injection of the gasserian ganglion, using a lateral approach to the foramen ovale. Harris[48] subsequently carried out a purposeful injection of the intracranial portion of the trigeminal nerve, using this approach. The more effective anterior percutaneous approach by a cheek puncture was demonstrated by Härtel[50] in 1912. He[51] again made a significant contribution to the efficacy and safety of intracranial injections by using radiographic control in 1935. Although further modifications and improvements were introduced by Ecker and Perl[24] in 1965, the usefulness of intracranial injection techniques appears limited. Frequent extratrigeminal complications resulting from the diffusibility of alcohol and other neurolytic substances in the cerebrospinal fluid surrounding the ganglion and root appear unacceptable in view of newer techniques offering less risk. Although acceptable results may be obtained by those with experience in microinjection or other intracranial injection techniques, this is not to be expected generally.[24,49,107]

Indications

The indications for the use of alcohol neurolysis have dramatically changed with the recent refinements of the percutaneous trigeminal rhizolysis technique. Previous indications have included (1) intolerable and medically intractable trigeminal neuralgia in the ophthalmic division but not involving the eye (to avoid corneal anesthesia), (2) cases in which the diagnosis was ill defined, (3) cases in which age or debilitation contraindicated craniotomy, (4) patients with bilateral pain or in whom it was thought likely to occur, that is, patients having multiple sclerosis, and (5) as a preliminary operation to allow the patient to become familiar with the effects of facial anesthesia on a temporary basis. Arguments against peripheral alcohol injections include that they are essentially always temporary and may delay a necessary, more permanent procedure until the patient is at a higher risk because of the general physical condition. This appears to be a minor argument in view of the little additional stress associated with the electrocoagulation technique. However, the dense sensory loss associated with alcohol neurolysis is not similar to that produced by the electrocoagulation method, in which touch is relatively spared, and thus it does not allow familiarization with the degree of sensory loss expected using the latter technique. This same argument carries for bilateral facial pain, where in fact the percutaneous rhizolysis with its relative sparing of touch sensation may be the procedure of choice. The exception to this is the use of the microvascular decompressive procedure in those patients presenting an acceptable operative risk for major open intracranial procedures and who are accepting of the procedure. Alcohol injection carries a significant risk with each injection of discomforting sensory aberrations, including anesthesia dolorosa, that frequently do not abate with nerve regeneration. Injections carry a high failure rate, especially with subsequent procedures.[3] Frequently after repeated alcohol injections pain recurs, and a significant sensory loss persists, making the performance of a percutaneous electrocoagulation lesion extremely difficult, since there is relatively little sensation in the painful area to monitor during lesion making. This does not interfere with localization of the electrode by stimulatory techniques. One also should not forget that alcohol injections are usually excruciatingly painful, albeit transiently so. Many patients do not desire subsequent procedures for this reason.

Peripheral neurectomy has generally been shown to be a more effective and safer method of palliative treatment.[43,117] Neurectomy tends to give more prolonged relief and is less frequently attendant with discomforting sensory aberrations. Palliative procedures appear extremely limited at present except in cases of diagnostic difficulty. However, they do seem to offer a method of testing the responsiveness of a pain syndrome to denervation and yield an excellent chance of sensory recovery should it not be successful. Neurectomy appears to be the procedure of choice, and if carried out with the patient under local anesthesia with brief unconsciousness produced by intravenous methohexital (Brevital) at the actual time of avulsion, it is a safe, essentially painless procedure. On occasion, when neurectomy is not feasible, for example, in pain states other than typical trigeminal neuralgia involving the deeper maxillary or mandibular division innervated structures, peripheral radiofrequency coagulation has been carried out using the lateral subzygomatic approach, coagulating the maxillary or mandibular division as it exits from the foramen rotundum or ovale.[114] Local anesthetic nerve blocks are notoriously poor in predicting the long-term effectiveness of denervation in patients having nontrigeminal neuralgia pain.

Techniques

Detailed techniques of alcohol injections and peripheral neurectomies are beyond the scope of this chapter. Excellent reviews are available in the books of Moore,[92] White and Sweet,[153] and Stookey and Ransohoff.[132] Similarly, techniques of peripheral neurectomy are reviewed by Thoma,[146] Quinn,[110] Ginwalla,[37] and Poppen.[109]

Results of alcohol blocks

Fairly consistent results have been demonstrated in large series of patients undergoing alcohol block as treatment for trigeminal neuralgia. When used as the initial treatment, approximately 20% to 30% fail, and the incidence of failure rises rapidly with each subsequent injection in those previously responding.[39] The average duration of pain relief in the combined series of Patrick,[100] Grant,[39] Horrax and Poppen,[59] and Peet and Schneider,[103] totaling over 1500 patients undergoing various successful alcohol blocks, was as follows:

Nerve injected	*Duration of relief*
Supraorbital-supratrochlear	8 1/2 months
Infraorbital	12 months
Maxillary division	12 months
Mandibular division	16 months

In the present series alcohol blocks were used as initial surgical therapy in 151 patients (Table 30-1). In

TABLE 30-1. Alcohol blocks: duration of relief with primary injections

	Supraorbital-supratrochlear	Infraorbital	Mental	Inferior alveolar	Maxillary	Mandibular
Failures	4	9	2	2	7	6
<3 months		9	1	1		
3 to 6 months		8	4	1	2	3
6 to 12 months	9	16	3	1	13	18
1 to 2 years	3	8		1	2	12
>2 years		3		1		2
TOTAL	16	53	10	7	24	41
Permanent	—	—	—	—	—	—
Mean (months)	11	9	4	9	12	17

Table 30-2. Alcohol blocks: duration of relief with secondary injections

	Supraorbital-supratrochlear	Infraorbital	Mental	Inferior alveolar	Maxillary	Mandibular
Failures	2	18	2	6	3	13
<3 months	2	10	1	3	1	2
3 to 6 months	1	7	1	4	2	4
6 to 12 months		7		2	1	4
1 to 2 years		4				2
>2 years				1		1
TOTALS	5	46	4	16	7	26
Permanent	—	—	—	—	—	—
Mean (months)	3	6	3	7.5	6	10

30 patients (20%) no relief was obtained, usually despite achievement of some degree of sensory loss. Of the 121 patients experiencing relief, the results were as follows: the infraorbital or inferior alveolar nerve was successfully blocked in 49 instances, with durations of relief ranging from less than 3 months to 3 years with a mean, in each case, of 9 months; the supraorbital-supratrochlear nerve blocks had a subsequent mean duration of relief of 11 months; and mental nerve blocks averaged a duration of relief of 4 months. More proximal blocking at the foramen rotundum or ovale yielded the expected longer durations of relief, approaching means of 12 to 17 months, respectively.

Repeated alcohol injections were doomed to failure in approximately 42% of the 104 patients who received them (Table 30-2). When effective, the duration was brief, usually less than 6 months. Although rare patients have reportedly had as much as 25 years of relief after alcohol injections, this is distinctly unusual and not to be expected. In the present series in no case did an alcohol block result in relief from pain for more than 3 1/2 years.

Complications of alcohol injections

Complications from peripheral alcohol blocks, although infrequent, are often troublesome. Discomforting sensory aberrations, anesthesia dolorosa, facial palsy, paralysis of extraocular movements, trigeminal motor paralysis, deafness resulting from injection into the eustachian tube, blindness, corneal anesthesia, and slough, ulceration, or gangrene of the skin are the most frequently reported complications.* In the present series approximately 35% complained of mild to moderate sensory aberrations such as crawling, itching, burning, or a sensation of swelling in the affected area. Although such sensations were discomforting, they were not incapacitating. Thirteen of the patients (5%) complained of severe dysesthesias or burning (anesthesia dolorosa). This occurred, in all but two patients, in blocking the infraorbital nerve or maxillary division. Both patients had burning dysesthesias in the tongue after mandibular division block. Subsequent retrogasserian rhizotomy or percutaneous rhizolysis failed to relieve the burning

*References 10, 43, 103, 117, and 155.

Table 30-3. Neurectomies: duration of relief with primary procedures

	Supraorbital-supratrochlear	Infraorbital	Mental	Inferior alveolar
Failures	1	2	2	
<3 months		1	1	
3 to 6 months	2	4	5	
6 to 12 months	2	12	17	3
1 to 2 years	4	20	12	5
>2 years	3	2	1	2
TOTAL	12	41	38	10
Permanent	—	—	—	—
Mean (months)	21	20	19	24

Table 30-4. Neurectomies: duration of relief with secondary procedures

	Supraorbital-supratrochlear	Infraorbital	Mental	Inferior alveolar
Failures	3	6	2	2
<3 months	1	4	2	1
3 to 6 months	2	4	6	2
6 to 12 months		4		1
1 to 2 years		5		
TOTAL	6	23	10	6
Permanent	—	—	—	—
Mean (months)	5	12	5	7

in approximately 50% of the patients. The majority of these, however, responded dramatically to a regimen of perphenazine (Trilafon) and amitriptyline (Elavil), as suggested by Taub[142] to treat postherpetic neuralgia. The only other complications were two instances each of Horner's syndrome and corneal anesthesia after mandibular division block at the foramen ovale.

Results of neurectomy

Despite repeated studies demonstrating that neurectomy is a more effective and longer lasting method of palliative treatment in patients having facial pain, alcohol injections have remained in the forefront.[43,110] The reasons for this superiority are readily apparent. First, the nerve is isolated and identified before neurectomy rather than depending on radiographic or even less effective methods of positioning the needles for alcohol injection. Second, one is assured of total destruction of the nerve at the isolated level rather than depending on alcohol diffusion for total neurolysis. Third, usually a proximal segment of nerve can be avulsed or cauterized and the canal occluded by various materials, thus delaying regeneration. Last, avulsion or neurectomy, in contrast to alcohol neurolysis, disrupts the continuity of the nerve, thus further impairing regeneration. Despite all these apparent advantages, regeneration takes place, and pain recurs. Although Quinn[110] states that he has been able to keep patients pain free using repeated neurectomies, others have not been so fortunate. As with neurolytic destruction, subsequent neurectomy procedures carry an increasingly high failure rate.

The present series included 101 patients in whom peripheral neurectomy was used as the initial form of surgical treatment (Table 30-3). Failure to relieve the pain occurred in only five patients (5%), and no complications ensued, not even a minor wound infection. The mean duration of relief was more prolonged than that obtained with alcohol blocks. The mean durations of relief when neurectomy was used as the initial surgical procedure were as follows: supraorbital-supratrochlear, 21 months; infraorbital, 20 months; mental, 19 months; and inferior alveolar, 24 months. With repeat neurectomy (45 instances) results were similar to those obtained with alcohol blocks, in that a higher failure rate (29%) and a shorter mean duration of relief (5 to 12 months) were achieved than with the primary procedures (Table 30-4). Likewise, similar to the alcohol blocks, peripheral neurectomy did not yield a single case of permanent relief.

INTRACRANIAL PROCEDURES

Indications

The primary indication for treating a patient using an intracranial surgical procedure is the presence of trigeminal neuralgia that is intolerable to the patient and not satisfactorily relieved by tolerable dosages of medication, primarily phenytoin (Dilantin) and carbamazepine (Tegretol). Narcotics generally should be avoided in treating patients with chronic pain syndromes. Carbamazepine, especially, has proved extremely effective in treating trigeminal neuralgia.[13,91] However, somewhere between 20% and 30% of patients develop complicating side effects, necessitating a discontinuation or decrease in dosage to the point that it no longer affords satisfactory relief. Also, although carbamazepine is initially effective, with time it ceases to be effective at maximum tolerated levels in a significant number of patients. Since the population at risk is composed primarily of elderly patients (the average age of patients coming to surgery in this series being 64 years), many with complicating medical disorders, any procedure requiring craniotomy is attended by a significant risk of mortality and morbidity. Such procedures may be contraindicated in or not acceptable to many patients. Contrarily, it is rare to find a patient so debilitated as to contraindicate a percutaneous procedure, since it does not require general anesthesia, and it is not extremely stressful to the patient. It would appear that either the translabyrinthine or the percutaneous descending trigeminal tractotomy could be used in treating those patients with pain caused by malignancy where the appropriate treatment would necessitate the production of anesthesia over the distributions of cranial nerves V, VII, IX, and X. If denervation of the ipsilateral upper cervical roots is necessary in addition, a suboccipital approach to sever these same cranial nerves with laminectomies of the upper cervical segments to perform posterior cervical rhizotomies would seem to be indicated. Any procedure producing permanent sensory loss would appear to be contraindicated in a patient with an ill-defined facial pain syndrome unless a temporary denervation procedure had demonstrated prolonged relief without disturbing side effects.

Techniques

A discussion of the now infrequently used techniques, including those requiring craniotomy and the percutaneous trigeminal tractotomy, is beyond the scope of this chapter. The subtemporal extradural trigeminal rhizotomy has been reviewed by Stookey and Ransohoff,[132] White and Sweet,[153] Peet and Echols,[102] and Kahn[70]; the subtemporal intradural trigeminal rhizotomy by Wilkins[154] and Henderson[54]; the decompression procedure by Taarnhøj[138]; the compression procedure by Shelden[123]; the suboccipital descending trigeminal tractotomy by Stookey and Ransohoff and by White and Sweet; the percutaneous descending trigeminal tractotomy by Crue and associates[14-16] and Fox[27]; the subtemporal transtentorial rhizotomy by Jannetta and Rand[68] and by Yaşargil[156]; the retrolabyrinthine trigeminal rhizotomy by Hitselberger and Pulec[58]; and the microvascular decompressive procedure by Janetta in Chapter 31.

SUBTEMPORAL EXTRADURAL TRIGEMINAL RHIZOTOMY

After the early development of peripheral palliative treatment of trigeminal neuralgia, direct operative approach to the intracranial portion of the trigeminal nerve and thus cure was dependent on the development of adequate anesthesia and aseptic techniques. Rose[116] was probably the first to permanently relieve a patient of trigeminal neuralgia. He used a lateral approach, transected the zygoma, trephined the sphenoid bone about the foramen ovale, and removed a portion of the gasserian ganglion. Horsley[61] carried out a similar approach, trephining the bone between the foramen ovale and foramen rotundum to sever the maxillary and mandibular divisions extradurally (but intracranially) and then avulsing the distal stumps. Shortly thereafter, using the same initial approach, he trephined the temporal bone, opened the dura mater beneath the temporal lobe and over Meckel's cave, and avulsed the trigeminal root from the pons. Hartley[52] followed with a transtemporal extradural approach in which he severed the maxillary and mandibular divisions at their respective foramina and excised the proximal stumps and the adjacent ganglion. Tiffany[147] suggested that attempts be made to spare the motor root in carrying out ganglionectomy and carried out selective ganglionectomies sparing the ophthalmic division, thus avoiding the frequent complication of neuroparalytic keratitis. The first subtemporal extradural rhizotomy, which later was to become the standard operative treatment for many years, was performed by Frazier in 1901.[129] It had developed in progressive fashion built on the framework laid before, with the addition of sparing of the gasserian ganglion as previously advocated by Horsley[60] and by Spiller and Frazier.[129] Subtotal section sparing the ophthalmic division was added by Frazier in 1915,[30,31] and a section sparing the motor root was added in 1919,[29,31] although Peet[101] had made a practice of the latter in 1918. By 1943 Frazier, Grant, and their colleagues had performed over 1100 such procedures.[41] Until the relatively recent modifications of the percutaneous trigeminal rhizolysis technique, only the standard Frazier subtemporal approach had withstood the test of time.

RESULTS AND COMPLICATIONS

The following represents an analysis of 10 large series of cases reported over the past 50 years, encompassing a total of 5274 patients.* Immediate pain relief occurred in over 95% of patients, with a long-term relapse rate varying from 1.1% with a total rhizotomy to 12.6% to 15% with fractional root sections.[54,117,153] Approximately 50% of these occurred in nontreated divisions. The other recurrences probably are the result of anatomical variation resulting in only partial sections of the affected divisions or operative difficulties preventing optimum performance of the proposed section. The operative mortality varies from 0.82% to 2.5%, with improved techniques in recent years lessening it to a general rate of about 1%.[112] Most of the deaths are associated with postoperative intracranial hematoma or cerebral infarction. The incidence of unintended corneal anesthesia is not available; however, neuroparalytic keratitis is seen in 0.9% to 15%.[103,132] Some degree of postoperative facial weakness is seen in from 3% to 8% and usually clears within a few months, although some series report a 2% incidence of permanency.[40,103,132] The combination of corneal anesthesia and a facial paresis carries an extreme risk of keratitis, and such patients should be treated with tarsorrhaphy. The incidence of paresis of extraocular movements, in some series, has been reported as high as 4%, although again it is usually temporary.[153] Some form of sensory aberration probably occurs in the anesthetic area in the majority of patients and proves troublesome in 15% to 29%. The usual description of the mild forms of these is a sensation of swelling, tightness, or tingling. In the more discomforting form they are usually described as a crawling, itching, or burning sensation. The severe form seen in approximately 5% to 26% of patients is called *anesthesia dolorosa*.[117,153] It can be as discomforting as or more severe than the patient's initial pain and usually is described as a severe constant burning, itching, or tearing pain. Further denervation procedures usually are not helpful in treating such symptoms. Again the use of psychotropic agents, as described by Taub[142] for postherpetic neuralgia, has frequently been helpful in my experience.

SUBTEMPORAL INTRADURAL TRIGEMINAL RHIZOTOMY

Herrmann[56] first advocated this approach in 1940 in an attempt to avoid troublesome extradural bleeding and the complication of a facial palsy, both seemingly related to the elevation of the dura from the floor of the middle cranial fossa. The latter is believed by some to be caused by coagulation to control the bleeding. Although others championed the cause, it proved to be a more complicated procedure than the standard extradural approach as result of trauma to the exposed temporal lobe and its vessels.[93,154] The increased incidence of complications, primarily aphasia and weakness, precluded widespread acceptance. Otherwise, the results and complication rate would seem to parallel the extradural approach. It would appear indicated only when the subtemporal dura is thin, adherent, and friable, thus complicating the extradural route.

SUBOCCIPITAL TRIGEMINAL RHIZOTOMY

Ramonède[111] developed the suboccipital trigeminal rhizotomy, apparently at the urging of Spiller, to section the root as close to the pons as possible.[33] It was thought that this would prevent regeneration, which it was believed might ensue if any Schwann cells were left on the proximal stump. Dandy[18-21] was a strong advocate of this approach, claiming it was fast and easy, cured with little or no sensory loss because of ability to selectively cut pain fibers and thus prevent keratitis, avoided facial palsy, and preserved the trigeminal motor root. Olivecrona[96] carried out a comparison study and was unable to substantiate Dandy's claims, stating that the suboccipital route should be used only if one was suspicious that a tumor in the cerebellopontine angle was the underlying cause of the pain.

In an analysis of four large series containing a total of 716 patients the mortality ranged from 2% to 4.5%.[19,28,97,151] The recurrence rate in most hands was higher than that in the subtemporal approach; in the series of Walker, Miles, and Simpon[151] it was 30%. This probably is a reflection of the technical difficulty in visualizing the trigeminal root from the suboccipital approach. The incidence of sensory aberrations, keratitis, and, unexpectedly, facial weakness is no better, even in experienced hands, than in the subtemporal approach.

Jannetta and Rand[67] have strongly supported Dandy's original premise[22] that vascular compression is the primary cause of trigeminal neuralgia. Jannetta[65,66] advocates this approach for mobilizing and displacing such vessels from the trigeminal root, thus curing without associated sensory loss. Although Jannetta finds the microvascular decompressive approach safe in his hands, the approach is attended by serious potential complications, including an approximate 1% mortality.[5,12,47,155] It would seem a rather radical approach in the elderly population, primarily at risk, even if it proved curative without the production of facial sensory loss. In contrast, the

*References 17, 32, 40, 54, 71, 81, 103, 116, 132, and 153.

microvascular decompressive procedure can be considered in those patients having ophthalmic division trigeminal neuralgia or those strongly desirous of having facial sensory loss, if they are accepting of the significant increase in morbidity and mortality compared with the percutaneous rhizolysis procedure, and if they present an acceptable risk for a major surgical procedure.

SUBTEMPORAL DECOMPRESSION AND COMPRESSION PROCEDURES

In 1952 Taarnhøj[138,139] introduced the subtemporal decompression procedure. The theory had been earlier advocated by Dandy[21,22] Gardner and colleagues,[34-36] and others[9] that compression of the trigeminal sensory root by abnormally placed vessels, a high petrous bone causing angulation of the root, or neoplasm could result in typical trigeminal neuralgia. Taarnhøj thought that the dural canal through which the root passes to Meckel's cave could be the constrictive force responsible. After his success by opening the dural canal and Meckel's cave, others followed, initially obtaining pain relief without the associated sensory loss that had previously been thought necessary for pain relief.[35,88,89,130] With more prolonged follow-up studies it became readily apparent that the recurrence rate in such procedures was an unexpectedly high 33% to 75%.[46,131,135] The long-term effectiveness of the decompression procedure, with detailed sensory testing, was found to be directly related to the amount of unexpected facial sensory loss resulting from operative manipulation. Because of this finding in their patients, Shelden and coworkers[122-124] advocated the production of additional sensory loss by "compression" of the gasserian ganglion and the trigeminal root by a small dental roll and later a blunt dissection. They believed that as little sensory loss "as perhaps 25%" would be adequate to relieve the pain of trigeminal neuralgia. Shelden[123] in 1964 reported on the results of 200 compression procedures. Pain recurred in 25% of the patients. Minimum sensory loss ensued in most, and no patient had severe sensory aberrations. Although the incidence of corneal anesthesia and therefore keratitis appears lower than is seen with rhizotomy, the rates of other complications are similar. Others reporting on the technique have had extremely high recurrence rates, from 24% to 70%. This is a major operative procedure, and the excessive recurrence rate is a distinct disadvantage not to be lightly considered.[26,38] Clinical observation has appeared to demonstrate that the efficacy and permanency of any surgical procedure in treating trigeminal neuralgia is directly related to the degree of pain sensation loss induced in the painful area. Any procedure sparing facial pain sensation is likely to have a high recurrence rate of pain.

MEDULLARY DESCENDING TRIGEMINAL TRACTOTOMY

Sjöqvist[128] first carried out a medullary tractotomy after it was suggested by Riley[115] and Kuntz[85] that in doing so only pain and temperature sensory loss would result, sparing touch and thus corneal sensation. It proved to be attended by high mortality, complication, and recurrence rates and thus fell into disrepute.* More recently Crue and associates,[14-16] Fox,[27] and others[57] have advocated techniques for performing percutaneous radiofrequency descending trigeminal tractotomies. The usefulness of this operation appears limited in that the procedure is more difficult and complicated than the present percutaneous trigeminal rhizolysis procedure. Furthermore, there is no reason to believe that this method will improve the high recurrence rates seen with medullary tractotomy performed by craniotomy. A possible advantage of such procedures is the production of complete analgesia in the distribution of cranial nerves V, VII, and X in some patients.[27] It may therefore prove of value in treating patients having facial pain caused by malignant tumors in an area of overlapping distribution by these nerves. Additionally, the rare patient presenting with bilateral trigeminal neuralgia or both trigeminal and glossopharyngeal neuralgia could be treated in such a fashion. Either procedure, however, is associated with technical complexity and a high incidence of complication, including ipsilateral cerebellar limb ataxia, contralateral hemisensory loss in the body, and laryngeal palsy. Refinement of both the open and percutaneous techniques is ongoing, and perhaps they may prove of future value in treating the aforementioned pain syndromes.[26,84]

SUBTEMPORAL TRANSTENTORIAL RHIZOTOMY

Jannetta and Rand[67,68] in 1966 reintroduced the subtemporal transtentorial retrogasserian rhizotomy. The procedure was based on Dandy's earlier theory[20, 21] that the trigeminal root was divided into three segments: the portio major (conveying pain and temperature sensation), the portio minor (the motor root), and the accessory fibers, or the portio intermedius (conveying touch and "automatic functions of the skin of the face"). It was believed that with the operating microscope the portio minor and portio intermedius could be spared while severing the portio major. Thus it was thought possible to control facial pain, sparing the touch fibers and therefore corneal sensitivity.[67,68] Dollinger[13] in 1908 used this route in three patients, in whom ganglionectomy proved impossible because of excessive bleeding. However, only with the aid of mag-

*References 9, 42, 45-47, 106, and 132.

nification and lighting by the operating microscope was recognition of these divisions believed possible by this approach.[68] Anatomical studies have failed to confirm the sensory specificity of the portio major and the portio intermedius fibers.[25,44,104,118] The procedure proved to have a relatively high complication rate, and clinically the patients did not demonstrate specific preservation of touch sensation.[113] The procedure has now been abandoned by both authors.[64]

TRANSLABYRINTHINE TRIGEMINAL RHIZOTOMY

Hitselberger and Pulec[58] in 1972 introduced a retrolabyrinthine approach to the trigeminal root using a microsurgical technique. They reported on eight patients undergoing the rhizotomy. Three had pain associated with acoustic neurinomas that were removed at the same time, three had idiopathic trigeminal neuralgia, and two had atypical facial pain. The results were excellent in all except one patient who had atypical facial pain. Like Dandy and Jannetta, they report preservation of light touch sensation. Although they advocate this transmastoid approach for sectioning the trigeminal root for trigeminal neuralgia, in view of the safer percutaneous approach, its use appears limited. It may prove useful for pain syndromes requiring sectioning of cranial nerve V, the sensory cranial nerve VII nervus intermedius), cranial nerve IX, and the upper roots of cranial nerve X or for glossopharyngeal neuralgia. It should enable displacement of compressing vessels from the trigeminal root should this be proved to be a cause of trigeminal neuralgia. An insufficient number of patients and the brief follow-up in this report do not allow adequate evaluation of the procedure at present.

PERCUTANEOUS TRIGEMINAL RHIZOLYSIS

Kirschner,[73] in 1931 introduced the technique of percutaneous electrocoagulation of the gasserian ganglion and trigeminal root using Härtel's anterior approach.[50] Its speed and simplicity soon led to widespread use in Europe.* However, inability to accurately control the location and extent of the lesions resulted in complication rates and mortality that led Tönnis and Kreissel[148] to caution against its use and precluded its acceptance in the United States. Others were able to attain improved results,† but it remained for White and Sweet[153] to modify the procedure before acceptable results could generally be obtained. Their modifications consisted of low-voltage pulse stimulation to localize the electrode, a thermistor to monitor tip temperature, a graded coagulation technique to control the lesions, and the use of an intravenous ultrashort-acting barbiturate to allow brief periods of unconsciousness during the painful portions of the procedure. Their excellent results have been substantiated by others.* This combined series totals 1648 procedures in 1614 patients. There was but one death, this being an 87-year-old patient who died of postoperative pneumonia.[95] The recurrence rates ranged from 5% to 28%; however, there was wide variation in the duration of follow-up monitoring.[120,136] Permanent complications outside the trigeminal system did not occur, although rare instances of carotid artery puncture, seizure, aseptic meningitis, temporal lobe abscess, extraocular palsies, and angina occurred.[95,98,136,137] Corneal anesthesia was seen in from 4.2% to 20% of the patients; however, keratitis was infrequent.[145,149] Severe sensory aberrations occurred in 0.4% to 4.6%.[95,120] Minor aberrations occurred in 10% to 45%.[120,149] Significant trigeminal motor weakness occurred in 11% to 53%, but in essentially all it was temporary.[95,137] The superiority of the procedure over the open surgical procedures has been demonstrated, and this procedure is now accepted as the surgical treatment of choice in the treatment of trigeminal neuralgia.[113,136]

Preparation

The patient is not premedicated, since full cooperation is necessary throughout the procedure. It is important that a thorough discussion take place the night before, so that the patient is reassured and knows what to expect and what is expected of him or her at each step in the procedure. If this is done, the patient will have no difficulty in carrying out the part. The patient is awake during the procedure except for brief periods of unconsciousness, induced by the administration of an ultrashort-acting barbiturate, methohexital (Brevital), during the painful aspects.

The patient is placed in the supine position on a fluoroscopy table in the radiology department. The shoulders, torso, and lower extremities rest on a 5-inch pad in such fashion that the head and neck may be hyperextended to obtain a basal view of the skull. A C-arm portable fluoroscopic unit with television monitor and disc image recorder is used for radiographic control. Since the unit may be angulated, only mild hyperextension is necessary to obtain proper positioning (Fig. 30-1). The basal projection is needed only during the passage of the electrode through the foramen ovale; at all other times the patient is maintained in a neutral position. If the patient has cervical spondylosis limiting

*References 7, 8, 55, 62, 74-78, 82, 108, 134, and 157.
†References 79, 80, 83, 121, 133, and 144.

*References 95, 98, 120, 127, 136, 137, 143, 145, and 149.

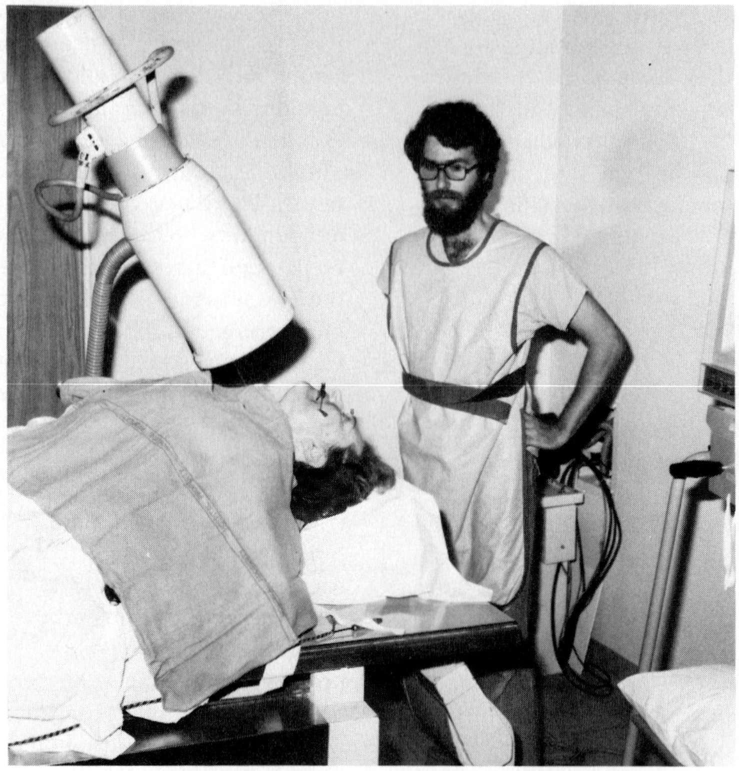

Fig. 30-1. Patient and fluoroscopic positioning for submentovertex (basal) view of skull for electrode placement. Radiographic technician assists throughout procedure. Additional angulation of C-arm is possible if needed because of limited extension of head and neck.

extension, oblique positioning as suggested by Whisler and Hill[152] and by Onofrio[98] may be used. The basal projection is easier to use. Triangulation from bony and dental landmarks on the basal view of the routine skull series has allowed proper placement of the electrode in two patients where the foramen ovale and adjacent bone had been totally destroyed by malignant neoplasma. Although plain or Polaroid radiographs will yield better bony definition than does fluoroscopy, they are more time consuming and are rarely necessary. Freehand passage of the electrode through the foramen ovale is easy with experience; however, some form of radiographic monitoring is necessary if one is to avoid the occasional entry into the foramen rotundum, foramen lacerum, pharyngotympanic canal, petrous bone, or jugular foramen.

Anesthesia

Preoperative medications or neuroleptic agents are not administered. They are not necessary for patient comfort if methohexital is given during the painful portions of the procedure, and they interfere with brisk awakening of the patient to an alert state. Accurate interpretation of stimuli is necessary for optimum results, and a patient depressed from the combined effects of cumulative dosages of methohexital and preoperative medication is unable to give optimum cooperation.

The initial dose of methohexital, necessary for satisfactory anesthesia, varies from patient to patient, ranging from 30 to 80 mg and averaging 50 mg. With the cumulative effect of the barbiturate and progressive coagulation, the requirement decreases for each subsequent dose. It must be given rapidly as a single bolus through at least an 18-gauge needle. Since the barbiturate will cause severe tissue reaction if extravasated, it should be given through a large Intracath placed in a large proximal vein. Methohexital is used to produce unconsciousness during the passage of the electrode through the foramen ovale and thus the mandibular division and during the periods of actual coagulation of the nerve. It acts rapidly to produce a brief 2- to 3-minute period of unconsciousness, after which the patient is fully responsive. The patients usually do not realize they have been unconscious and frequently ask when they are going to be "put to sleep." Additionally, most patients experience amnesia for the entire procedure that follows that administration of the local anesthesia. No patient has complained of severe pain during the procedure or refused a second procedure, if it be-

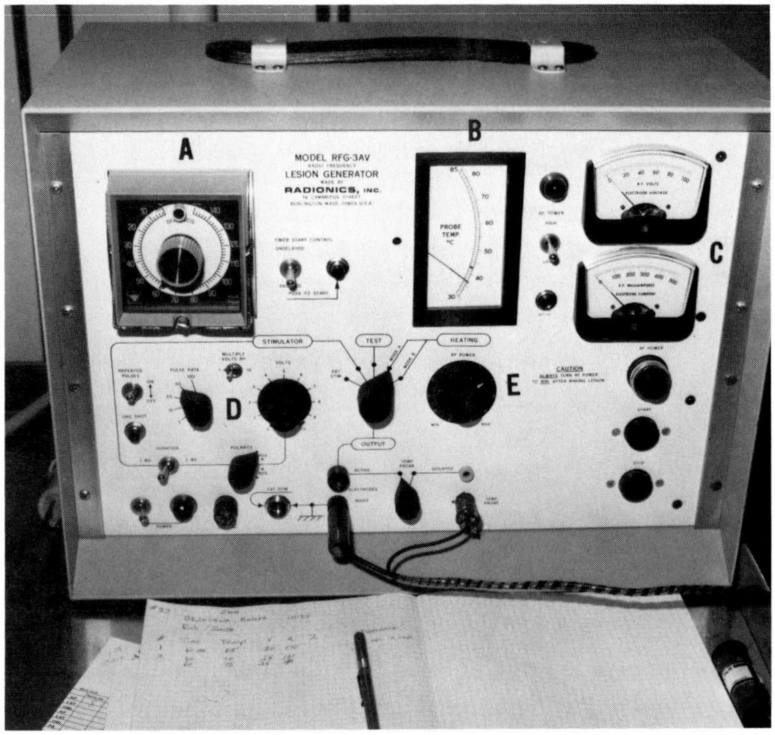

Fig. 30-2. Model RFG-3AV Radiofrequency Lesion Generator made by Radionics, Inc. *A,* Automatic lesion timer; *B,* probe temperature readout; *C,* electrode voltage and current meters; *D,* stimulator with variable pulse rate and voltage; *E,* rf power switch.

came necessary, because of pain. The surgeon is occupied with other duties during the procedure, and an anesthesiologist is used to administer the anesthetic agent and monitor the patient intraoperatively. Except for an occasional patient who develops the hiccups or shivers during the procedure, no anesthetic complications have been encountered in over 450 various procedures using this agent.

After the skin of the cheek, ipsilateral to the pain, and the contralateral frontal area are prepared with an aqueous iodine-complex solution, the patient is lightly draped with sterile towels. A solution of 50 ml of lidocaine 1%, to which 0.3 ml of 1:1000 aqueous epinephrine is added, is used to infiltrate the cheek and the frontal area. The injection should begin in line with the labial commissure, 2.5 cm lateral to it for the mandibular divisions and 3 cm lateral to it for the opthalmic and/or maxillary divisions or if all divisions are involved. The subcutaneous line through which the electrode will pass is infiltrated, and the oral mucosa is slightly ballooned from the coronoid process of the mandible. Infiltration should not be carried beyond here lest one block the inferior alveolar nerve, resulting in misleading sensory loss in its distribution. This same local anesthetic solution is infiltrated in the contralateral frontal area, and the 18-gauge stainless steel spinal needle used to inject it is left to serve as an electrical ground. This is easily accomplished if the needle is bent to conform with the convex shape of the cranium before insertion. It should be placed to a minimum depth of 2 cm to avoid burning the adjacent skin during the coagulation process.

Equipment

A radiofrequency (rf) lesion generator with metered rf voltage, current, and temperature readouts is used (Fig. 30-2). Since temperature is the basic lesioning parameter, its control is crucial for the desired, graded, and relatively select destruction of pain fibers. The voltage and current necessary to produce a given tip temperature may vary widely, depending on the conductivity of the tissue and fluid adjacent to the electrode tip. Since localization of the electrode is dependent on stimulation, a stimulator of variable voltage and frequency is essential. Although percutaneous cordotomy or other insulated electrodes may be used,[95] a commercially available electrode kit with varying tip exposure of 2, 5, 7, and 10 mm to achieve different lesion sizes is most useful (Fig. 30-3). The kit contains a temperature-monitoring electrode that passes through the center of the active electrode to monitor tip temperature, which is then relayed to the readout on the

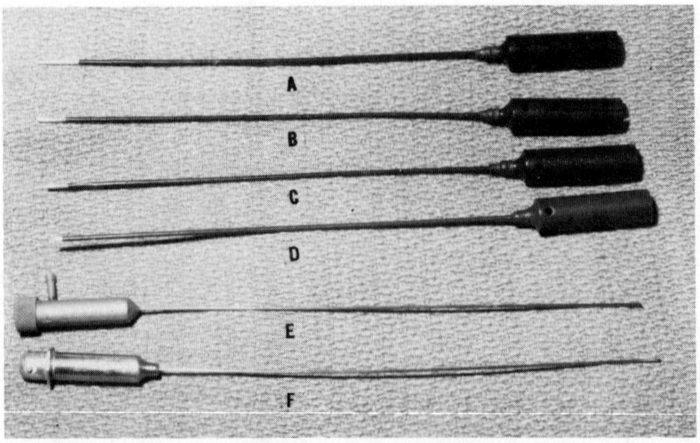

Fig. 30-3. Trigeminal electrodes consisting of 19-gauge cannulas with hard Teflon insulation. *A,* 10-mm tip; *B,* 7-mm tip; *C,* 5-mm tip; *D,* 2-mm tip; *E,* solid stylet; *F,* temperature-monitoring electrode.

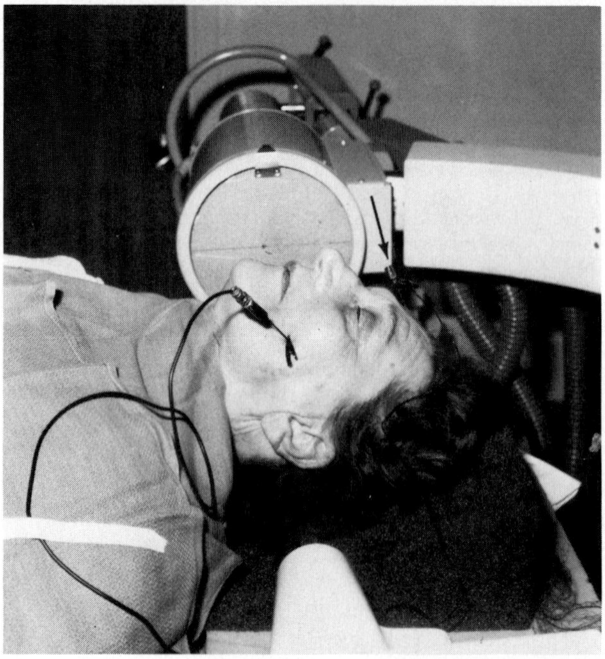

Fig. 30-4. Patient and fluoroscopic positioning for lateral view of skull. Electrode and thermistor probe are in position for selective maxillary division lesion. Note indifferent electrode in right frontal *(arrow).*

lesion generator. For convenience, a technician is used to run the stimulator and lesion generator, and the surgeon monitors the patient during the actual coagulation process.

Procedure

The appropriate electrode is selected: the 2-mm tip for selective second division, the 5-mm tip for selective third division, the 7-mm tip for combined second and third divisions, and the 10-mm tip for three divisions or for patients having pain resulting from neoplasm. It is inserted at the predetermined site relative to the labial commissure. The lateral view of the skull will help determine whether the electrode should be inserted above or below the commissure because of anatomical variation in the height of the petrous bone. If the superior portion of the petrous bone is rather low set from the sella turcica, the entrance should be 1 cm above the commissure; if it is high set, it should be 1 cm below. Further corrections can be made after the electrode approaches the foramen ovale. A gloved finger is placed inside the patient's mouth to guide the electrode

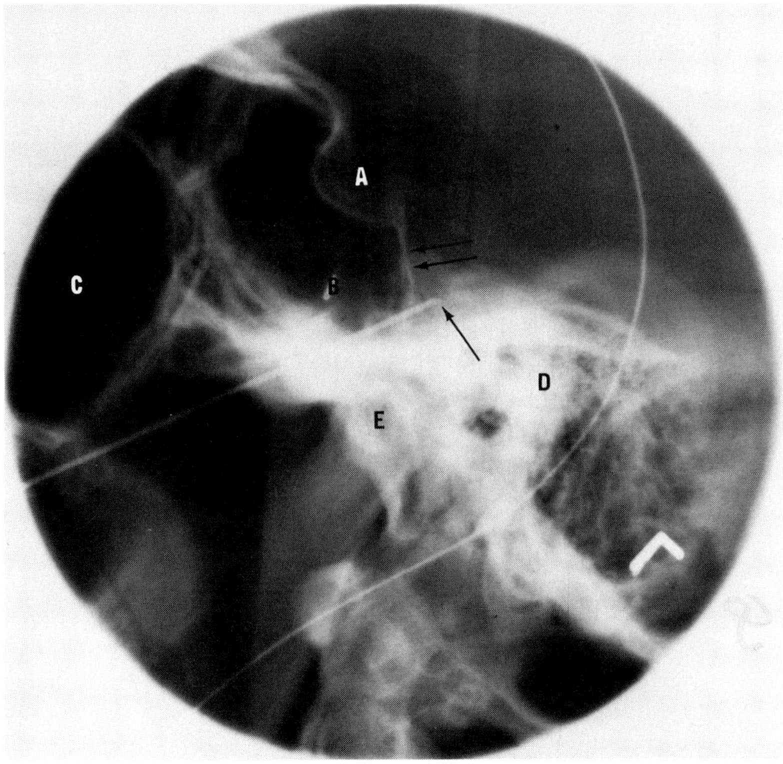

Fig. 30-5. Lateral radiograph (coned down) of skull. Electrode (↑) projecting 4 mm beyond clivus (↑↑). Craniectomy defect is result of previous subtemporal rhizotomy, which failed. *A,* Sella turcica; *B,* sphenoid sinus; *C,* maxillary sinus; *D,* petrous bone; *E,* head of mandible.

medial to the coronoid process and to prevent accidental penetration through the oral mucosa. The electrode should be directed on a trajectory bisecting the lateral aspect of the lacrimal caruncle in the coronal plane and passing through a point 3 cm anterior to the external auditory meatus in the sagittal plane. As the center of the foramen ovale is approached, lateral fluoroscopy is used to ensure the trajectory for optimum placement at a point just above the junction of the clivus and superior portion of the temporal bone. Appropriate corrections are made; if necessary, unconsciousness is produced with intravenous methohexital and the tip of the electrode inserted to the level of the clivus (Figs. 30-4 and 30-5). Occasionally a pterygo-alar bar will prevent penetration of the foramen ovale by the normal approach. Chouké and Hodes[11] have described this bony variation in approximately 7% of skulls. This barrier usually can be overcome by making the initial cheek puncture quite inferiorly. This allows a more direct, rather than oblique, entrance into the foramen. In this case the electrode tip will probably come to rest in the ganglion rather than the root; however, the results appear similar. This alternative should be carefully monitored radiographically as well as by stimulation and removal of the thermistor or stylet before lesion making. Lateral or medial deviation may cause placement of the electrode in the cavernous sinus or medial temporal lobe.

In contrast to Sweet and Wepsic[137] and Jefferson,[69] my patients have not found the passage of the 19-gauge electrode through the mandibular division at the foramen ovale particularly painless. This part of the procedure is therefore accomplished with the patient under methohexital anesthesia. It is important to enter the center of the foramen, and appropriate adjustments should be made to do so (Fig. 30-6). This ensures that with final positioning the electrode will remain within the root during its intracranial passage (Fig. 30-7). A more posterolateral placement allows the electrode to come to rest lateral to the dural sheath of the trigeminal nerve.[53,69,137] Thus it may not move medially enough with deeper placement to encounter the mandibular division rootlets, let alone those of maxillary and ophthalmic divisions. More posterior placement may cause the electrode to encounter the petrous bone, preventing advancement. Anteromedial placement also risks puncture of the carotid artery or the lateral wall of the cavernous sinus. As the electrode is inserted through the foramen, there is a sensation, although of lesser intensity, similar to that felt at lumbar puncture

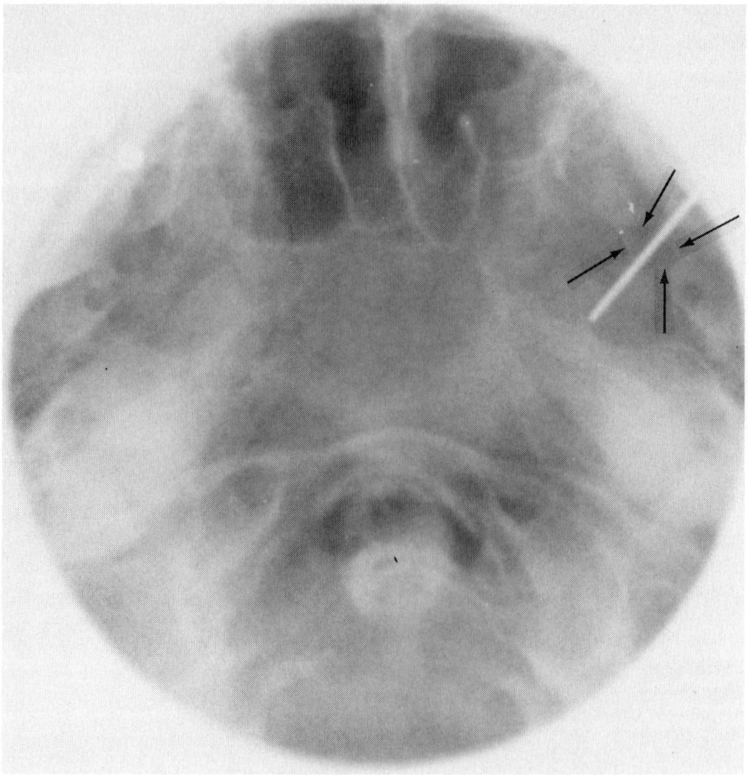

Fig. 30-6. Basal radiograph (coned down) of skull demonstrating passage of electrode through center of foramen ovale. Foramen is outlined by arrows.

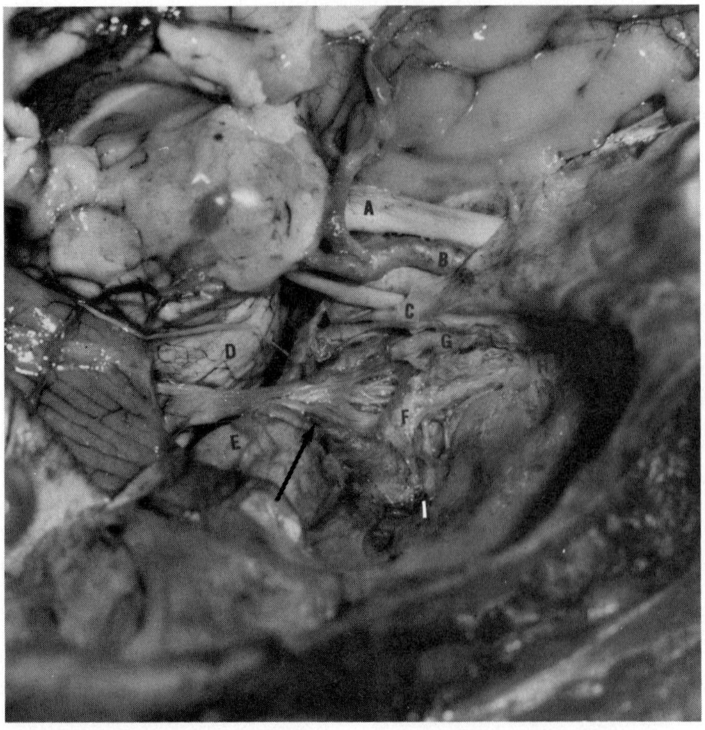

Fig. 30-7. Anatomical dissection with electrode placed for mandibular division lesion. Tip *(arrow)* has been placed outside trigeminal root for demonstration purposes. *A,* Optic nerve; *B,* internal carotid artery; *C,* oculomotor nerve; *D,* pons; *E,* superior aspect of petrous bone; *F,* gasserian ganglion; *G,* ophthalmic division; *H,* maxillary division at foramen rotundum; *I,* mandibular division at foramen ovale.

when the needle pierces the dura. There should be no resistance to further passage of the electrode. Because of this, there is a tendency for the electrode to drift deeper. A retaining clip therefore should be placed on the electrode flush with the skin to prevent this. Any resistance to further passage of the electrode requires electrode adjustment, since most likely the dura of the lateral wall of the cavernous sinus or the petrous bone is responsible. When the patient awakens, there will be a mild, dull, aching pain, usually in the preauricular area of the ipsilateral side of the face because of the presence of the electrode. The stylet is removed from the electrode, and cerebrospinal fluid usually flows freely. Occasionally no flow is forthcoming if the tip is located in the middle of the root. This does not contraindicate a lesion, although the return of blood at any time does. The temperature-monitoring probe should be removed and a check for bleeding made before each and every lesion. Again, the return of blood contraindicates a lesion at that location.

Final positioning of the electrode is determined by pulse and thermal stimulation techniques. Although multiple attempts have been made to find precise measurements localizing the various divisional fibers in relation to the foramen ovale and clivus, all have been remarkable for the anatomical variability found.[53,95,137] Thus analgesia in the opthalmic division has been obtained from 8 mm anterior to the clivus to 13 mm posterior to it, as seen on lateral radiographs.[137] Mandibular division analgesia has occurred from 12 mm anterior to 15 mm posterior.[137] Similar variation has been found when related to the posteromedial aspect of the foramen ovale and the lateral wall of the internal auditory meatus.[95] There is only a general relationship of passing from the mandibular division to the ophthalmic division as the electrode traverses from lateral to medial and anterior to posterior. The most reliable localizing methods are pulse and thermal stimulation with response from the awakened patient. A 50-cps pulse of 1-msec duration and radiofrequency heating of the electrode are used with reliable but not absolute accuracy. In the majority of patients threshold voltage is less than 0.2 V. At threshold the patient describes a sensation of buzzing, vibrating, or tingling and, infrequently, touching, moving, crawling, or pressing in the division being stimulated. The sensation is not painful. Only occasionally will the threshold be higher than 1.5 V unless prior lesions have been made at the location. Above this level, stimulation has proven unreliable, with frequent inability to produce an adequate lesion. In about 10% of cases coagulation will produce sensory loss in a division other than that stimulted. By gradually heating the tip of the electrode, thermal stimulation will occur. Heating has a much more reliable threshold of about 48° ± 2°C. With this, the patient will perceive a burning pain in the distribution of the stimulated fibers, which subsides with immediate shutoff of the current. Together both techniques yield excellent but not absolute reliability. When two different divisions are stimulated using these techniques, with further heating lesions may be produced in either or both in an unpredictable fashion. When attempting to produce sensory loss in the maxillary division and to spare the ophthalmic, a more satisfactory result will occur with placement of the tip to a position where stimulation produces effects in the lower portion of the maxillary division, that is, the upper lip, rather than higher.

Because of this lack of absolute predictability, several techniques may be used to avoid sensory loss in undesired areas. First, one should carefully monitor the sensory loss before and after each lesion. Second, if a skin or conjunctival flush occurs where sensory loss is not desired, immediately stop the heating, and make appropriate electrode placement corrections. Third, monitor the cilial (blink, lash) reflex continuously during the lesion, immediately shutting the current off if the reflex diminishes or disappears. If the level of consciousness is depressed to a point at which the reflex disappears, allow the patient to lighten until it reappears before beginning the lesion. An occasional patient will not have this reflex at any level of barbiturate depression, and thus its usefulness will be lost. In almost all patients it appears to be a sensitive indicator of ophthalmic divisional sensory loss and usually disappears before corneal anesthesia appears. It is also a valuable aid when one is attempting to produce hypalgesia in the ophthalmic division and still retain some protective corneal sensitivity. One can frequently heat the electrode until the cilial reflex is diminished over that contralaterally and find that a point of hypalgesia, but not anesthesia, has been reached with corneal sensitivity remaining. A neurotrophic or exposure keratitis is extremely unlikely if even minimum corneal sensation is retained. Corneal sensation is extremely delicate, and at times, with minimum change in temperature from the previous lesion, after only several seconds' duration, the cilial reflex is abruptly lost and, with it, corneal sensitivity. However, in approximately 80% of patients with ophthalmic division trigeminal neuralgia, hypalgesia can be produced while retaining some corneal sensation. When a patient presents with ophthalmic division pain, a discussion of the situation should be carried out, making no guarantee that corneal sensitivity can be spared. The surgeon and the patient should decide whether an attempt should be made to do so. The patient should understand that although retention of some corneal sensitivity lessens the risk of developing disturbing sensory aberrations and keratitis, it does so at a higher risk of failure to relieve pain and risk of recurrence of pain. With corneal anesthesia there is a definite risk of troublesome keratitis and subsequent loss of vision or even the eye. However, the risk is relatively low with proper precautions, even in the face of total corneal sensory loss. Conversely, the procedure can always be repeated if it fails, but the sensory loss, once produced, is not reversible.

Just as variable as the anatomical location of the different divisions relative to bony landmarks is the final electrode-tip temperature required to produce a lesion yielding appropriate sensory loss. Sweet and Wepsic[137] found this temperature to vary from 47° to 108°C. In the present series it has varied from 60° to 90°C. If one is attempting to produce total sensory loss as, for example, in trigeminal distribution pain resulting from malignant neoplasm, an initial high temperature of 85° to 90°C is acceptable. When treating idiopathic trigeminal neuralgia, where it is desirable to do a differential coagulation, one should use lower initial temperatures of 50° to 55°C for 1 minute with appropriate sensory testing of between 5°C or less stepwise incremental increasęs to tip temperature. This will result in a relative sparing of the larger, more heavily myelinated, alpha-beta nerve fibers and thus a preferential retention of touch sensation.[86] This is desirable in that it increases patient acceptance of the sensory loss and lowers the incidence of troublesome sensory aberrations, both of which are directly related to the degree of sensory loss produced.

The sensory end point must be individualized for the cause of the pain and the personality of the patient. In pain resulting from malignant neoplasms, adequate relief will ensue only with total anesthesia and analgesia. In trigeminal neuraliga the rate of success in permanently relieving the pain is directly related to the degree of pain sensation loss. The occurrence of trigeminal neuralgic pain in a trigeminal division distribution that is analgesic must be rare. In over 400 surgically treated patients I have seen only one that had pain in an analgesic division. This patient had typical neuralgic pain and trigger points only in the maxillary division. A percutaneous trigeminal rhizolysis yielded analgesia with hypesthesia estimated at 50% of normal and, initially, complete and total cessation of pain. She returned 3 months later with typical neuralgic pain in the same area without triggering points. She remained analgesic throughout the maxillary division, including its nasal and oral mucosal distributions. Local anesthetic block of the maxillary division at the foramen rotundum using fluoroscopic control yielded additional anesthesia but no pain relief. The following day local anesthetic block of the mandibular division at the foramen ovale yielded appropriate sensory loss and complete and total cessation of her pain. Subsequent electrocoagulation of the mandibular division resulted in analgesia with hypesthesia estimated at 50% of normal and pain relief. No change in the maxillary division hypesthesia resulted. She has now remained pain free for over 7 years.

With experience one can identify most of but not all the patients who will complain of disturbing numbness or sensory aberrations after a trigeminal destructive procedure. In these patients and those with pain in the ophthalmic distribution who so desire, the sensory loss is attempted to be limited to hypalgesia with the perception of single pinpricks estimated by the patient at about 50% as intense as those on the contralateral side. Frequently, at this level, touch sensation is normal or near normal. If the pain is not improved or recurs, and if the patient did not find the sensory loss disturbing, then the procedure can be repeated and further sensory loss produced. When the desired end point has been attained, a 20-minute period is always allowed before final sensory testing and removal of the electrode. Not infrequently an apparent fading occurs because of a more alert state resulting from the metabolism of the methohexital, necessitating the need for further lesions. The delay before final testing significantly decreases the failure and recurrence rates. Rarely during the procedure will a patient continue to have neuralgic pain after the electrode has been inserted. Three patients have had continued neuralgic pain, in the ophthalmic division in two and the mandibular division in one, for 3 to 4 days after the production of appropriate analgesia. In all of them the paroxysms abruptly ceased and have not recurred in periods of 8, 6, and 1 year, respectively. Similar delayed improvement has been reported by others after percutaneous trigeminal rhizolysis and trigeminal rhizotomy.[137]

COMPARISON OF INTRACRANIAL PROCEDURES

The following discussion covers a retrospective study of 106 patients undergoing craniotomy for surgical treatment of trigeminal neuralgia at the University of California at Los Angeles Medical Center between January 1956 and June 1972. I have treated an additional 393 patients with 409 percutaneous trigeminal rhizolyses at UCLA and at the Santa Monica Hospital Medical Center from November 1969 to October 1980. The patients undergoing craniotomy at UCLA were treated by the full-time faculty and neurosurgical residents under their supervision. Other procedures requiring craniotomy occasionally have been carried out; however, the number of patients involved is too small to allow meaningful interpretation of results. These patients are not reported here except for the posterior fossa rhizotomy group. Of the rhizolysis group, 381 pa-

Table 30-5. Results of intracranial procedures in patients followed up at least 2 years after operation.

	Excellent		Fair		Poor	
	Number	(%)	Number	(%)	Number	(%)
Posterior fossa rhizotomy	2	(50)	1	(25)	1	(25)
Subtemporal compression	8	(50)	1	(6)	7	(44)
Subtemporal extradural rhizotomy	55	(87)	1	(2)	7	(11)
Transtentorial rhizotomy	9	(64)	1	(7)	4	(29)
Percutaneous rhizolysis	293	(91)	6	(2)	21	(7)

Table 30-6. Complication rate of intracranial procedures

	Number	Complicated	(%)
Posterior fossa rhizotomy	4	3	(75)
Compression procedure	17	10	(59)
Middle fossa rhizotomy	70	50	(71)
Transtentorial rhizotomy	15	7	(47)
Percutaneous rhizolysis	409	57	(14)

tients with idiopathic trigeminal neuralgia and 12 patients with trigeminal neuralgia secondary to multiple sclerosis had but one procedure. Fourteen patients with idiopathic trigeminal neuralgia underwent a second procedure after failure of the first, and one patient has undergone three procedures. One patient in the idiopathic group and two in the multiple sclerosis group had a second procedure for bilateral neuralgic pain. Since the results are similar in the idiopathic and multiple sclerosis groups, they were combined for this analysis. In all craniotomy patients the diagnosis was idiopathic trigeminal neuralgia.

The five approaches used were posterior fossa rhizotomy (4), subtemporal compression (17), subtemporal extradural differential rhizotomy (70), subtemporal transtentorial rhizotomy (15), and percutaneous radiofrequency rhizolysis (409). Approximately 61% of the patients were 60 years old or older at the time of their surgical procedure. The mean age at operation, approximately 57 years, was similar for the various procedures, except that the transtentorial group tended to be younger (54 years) and the percutaneous rhizolysis group older (66 years).

Results

The percutaneous radiofrequency rhizolysis has large numbers of patients with shorter periods of follow-up monitoring because it is in current use, whereas none of the other methods has been used in over 9 years. To obtain adequate comparisons, measurement of the efficacy of the various procedures was based only on the results after 2 years, or less if pain recurred before that time. The results were graded as excellent (complete and total relief of pain), good (occasional or mild recurrent pain not requiring further treatment), and poor (recurrence of pain necessitating return to drugs or other therapeutic measures). The procedure was not judged a failure when there was recurrence in a division previously not affected and toward which the surgeon had not directed treatment. Failure rates of 25% for the posterior fossa rhizotomy, 44% for the compression procedure, and 29% for the transtentorial procedure appear unacceptably high for major operative procedures (Table 30-5). The standard subtemporal rhizotomy and the percutaneous rhizolysis yielded excellent results in approximately 90% of cases. Of all failures, 57% had persistent pain immediately after operation, and 83% had failure within 3 months. No correlation could be made between pain recurrence and age, sex, division involved, or duration of pain before the operation.

Complications

The complication rate for all procedures was high, ranging from 14% for the percutaneous route to 75% for the posterior fossa rhizotomies (Table 30-6). The apparently high complication rate in this series reflects the inclusion of corneal anesthesia and trigeminal motor weakness as complications. In contrast, few reported series have given specific information concerning the incidence of these complications; apparently the view was taken that they represented an inherent risk of the procedure. Generally, the tendency has been to consider that a complication has occurred only when keratitis ensues. Most of the complications were not serious and involved unintentional injury to the ophthalmic division, trigeminal motor root, or the facial nerve (Table 30-7). The transtentorial approach, however, produced an unusually high rate of serious cerebral dysfunction manifested by seizures, dysphasia, confusion, disorientation, and memory defect; all eventually resolved. Two additional patients who underwent transtentorial procedures had immediate postoperative cerebral infarctions, discovered at reexploration, which were apparently the result of coagulation and sectioning of drain-

Table 30-7. Complications of intracranial procedures

	Posterior fossa rhizotomy		Compression procedure		Subtemporal rhizotomy		Transtentorial rhizotomy		Percutaneous rhizolysis	
	No.	(%)	No.	(%)	No.	(%)	No.	(%)	No.	(%)
Procedures	4		17		70		15		409	
Death					1	(1)	1	(7)		
Infection					1	(1)				
Aseptic meningitis									2	(0.5)
CFS fistula							1	(7)		
Myocardial infarction					1	(1)				
Subdural hematoma					1	(1)				
Cerebral infarction							2	(13)		
Confusion, disorientation, memory defect	1	(25)	3	(18)	2	(3)	2	(13)		
Dysphasia					1	(1)	2	(13)		
Seizure							3	(20)		
Corneal anesthesia	3	(75)	1	(6)	22	(31)	5	(33)	21	(5)
Keratitis	1	(25)			3	(4)			4	(11)
Trigeminal motor paralysis or paresis			8	(47)	37	(53)	2	(13)	69	(17)
Facial paralysis or paresis	2	(50)	3	(18)	14	(20)				
Extraocular palsies	1	(25)	1	(6)	4	(6)			5	(1)
Hematotympanum			4	(24)	10	(14)	1	(7)		
Hearing loss, permanent					2	(3)	1	(7)		
Moderate sensory aberration	1	(25)	1	(6)	5	(7)	1	(7)	20	(5)
Anesthesia dolorosa			1	(6)	1	(1)			2	(0.5)

ing cortical veins. However, other than corneal anesthesia (33%) and motor root dysfunction (13%), no other cranial nerve injuries occurred. The standard middle fossa rhizotomy approach yielded extremely high complication rates of corneal sensory loss (31%), trigeminal motor weakness (53%), and facial nerve paresis or paralysis (20%). The compression procedure had an exceedingly low incidence of corneal anesthesia (6%); however, the frequency of other complications paralleled that resulting from the standard rhizotomy. A few instances of paresis of extraocular movement were seen: with the posterior fossa approach, one bilateral cranial nerve VI palsy; with the compression procedure, one cranial nerve III palsy; and with the middle fossa rhizotomy, one cranial nerve III palsy, two cranial nerve VI palsies, and one total ophthalmoplegia. Hematotympanum occurred in 15 patients undergoing a subtemporal approach to the trigeminal nerve. Extravasation of blood into the middle ear may occur after either the opening of mastoid or zygomatic air cells or fracture of the tegmen tympani (the thin, bony roof of the middle ear and associated air cells, forming the posterior floor of the middle cranial fossa). Subsequent serous otitis media resulted in significant permanent hearing loss in two patients. Complaints of bothersome mild-to-moderate sensory aberrations (crawling, itching, or burning) occurred in approximately 7% of the patients treated using root compression or rhizotomy by either the middle fossa or transtentorial approach. One of the four patients who underwent posterior fossa rhizotomy experienced this degree of abnormal sensation. Anesthesia dolorosa with severe burning dysesthetic pain occurred in one patient after a compression procedure and in one patient treated by middle fossa rhizotomy. The complications of the percutaneous radiofrequency technique were unintended corneal anesthesia in 21 patients (5%), keratitis in four patients (1%), cranial nerve VI paresis in four multiple sclerosis patients, cranial nerve IV paresis in one other patient (1%), moderate sensory aberration, including poor tolerance of facial sensory loss, in 20 patients (5%), anesthesia dolorosa in three patients (0.7%), trigeminal motor weakness in 69 patients (17%), and aseptic meningitis in two patients (0.5%).

All complications cleared completely except corneal anesthesia, the trigeminal motor paralysis in one compression patient and 29 middle fossa rhizotomy patients, the facial paresis in two middle fossa rhizotomy patients, the hearing loss in one middle fossa and one transtentorial rhizotomy patient, and the sensory aberrations.

One death occurred in the middle fossa rhizotomy group (1.4%) as a result of a postoperative subdural hematoma and cerebral infarction, and one death oc-

Table 30-8. Postoperative sensory patterns

	Analgesia and anesthesia	Analgesia and hypesthesia	Hypalgesia and hypesthesia	Only hypalgesia	Minimum to none
Posterior fossa rhizotomy	3				1
Compression procedure	4		8		5
Middle fossa rhizotomy	67		24		
Transtentorial rhizotomy		7	2		2
Percutaneous rhizolysis	20	212	133	37	7

curred in the transtentorial group (6.7%), also a result of cerebral infarction. The other procedures carried no mortality.

Postoperative sensory patterns

The sensory pattern in the area primarily affected, as recorded at the time of discharge from the hospital, varied greatly among the procedures (Table 30-8). Trigeminal rhizotomy from either the middle or posterior fossa approach infrequently yielded anything other than analgesia and anesthesia. The compression procedure resulted in hypalgesia and hypesthesia in about 50% of the patients, with the remainder evenly divided between total and minimum-to-no sensory loss. The majority of patients treated with either the transtentorial or percutaneous approach were analgesic with light touch preservation approximating 50% of that on the nonoperated side. The permanence of pain relief resulting from an intracranial procedure was directly related to the degree of pain sensation loss. In no case did pain recur in an analgesic area except in the unique case described under the percutaneous rhizolysis procedure. Failure most frequently resulted when only mild or no hypalgesia was present.

Duration of hospitalization

The duration of hospitalization, as measured from the day before operation through the day of discharge, would appear to serve as an indicator of the general morbidity associated with the different procedures. Posterior fossa and transtentorial rhizotomies resulted in average hospitalization periods of 19 and 16 days, respectively. Both the middle fossa rhizotomy and compression procedures had a mean duration of stay of 8 days. The briefest mean stay of 3 days was accorded the percutaneous radiofrequency rhizolysis group.

DISCUSSION

Permanent relief of medically intractable trigeminal neuralgia can be achieved only by surgical attack on some portion of the intracranial trigeminal complex. Peripheral procedures give only temporary relief and carry a risk, albeit low, of serious sensory aberration. Furthermore, the accompanying sensory loss could potentially interfere with accurate control of radiofrequency lesions and yields little information as to the patient's tolerance of the sensory loss accompanying an intracranial procedure, especially those which primarily affect only pain sensation. These disadvantages tend to limit their use primarily to patients who are severely debilitated or to assist in the evaluation of patients in whom the diagnosis is unclear. When a peripheral procedure appears to be indicated, neurectomy would seem to be the choice because of a lower failure rate, a longer duration of pain relief, and a lower complication rate.

Posterior fossa rhizotomy has drifted into disuse in view of the high mortality, morbidity, and recurrence rates attendant with its use. Up to the present only the standard Spiller-Frazier middle fossa extradural, differential, retrogasserian rhizotomy has withstood the test of time. Its failure and serious complication rates are low, and the relatively high incidence of corneal anesthesia, trigeminal motor paralysis, facial paralysis, and discomforting paresthesias, as well as total sensory loss in the affected area, have been accepted to attain pain relief. Trigeminal root compression, although likely to avoid corneal anesthesia and preserve some degree of sensation, has such a high pain recurrence rate as to preclude its use in most instances. The transtentorial microsurgical approach was introduced in an attempt to maintain light touch sensation and thereby avoid the sensory aberrations and disturbing numbness that frequently accompany total sensory loss. With this route it is also possible to lessen the frequency of complications involving the trigeminal motor root and other adjacent cranial nerves. To this end, it was a success; however, the serious cerebral dysfunction produced by necessary sacrifice of bridging cortical veins and elevation of the brain for intradural exposure presented formidable risk that resulted in its abandonment.

Microvascular decompression of the trigeminal nerve would appear to have a place in treating certain selected patients with medically intractable idiopathic trigeminal neuralgia. The procedure has a significant advantage of avoiding facial sensory loss and with it the risk of troublesome sensory aberrations. One must always remember that the patient population at risk is generally elderly, and a posterior fossa open surgical procedure in such patients carries significant risk. It should be performed only by those neurosurgeons skilled in microsurgical posterior fossa surgery. Even in the best of hands the procedure would appear to have not only the morbidity associated with the posterior fossa approach but also mortality approximating 1%.

The percutaneous radiofrequency technique significantly improves or alleviates the risks and complications associated with the other intracranial procedures. It presents minimum operative risk to the patient and has a low rate of complication. Since the surgeon is able to control the extent of the lesion using a graded technique with intermittent sensory testing, it is possible to produce only the degree of sensory loss necessary for permanent pain relief, usually analgesia with hypesthesia estimated at 50% of normal. In similar fashion, use of this graded method with the addition of radiographic control and stimulating techniques allows accurate control of the location of the lesion. It may be localized to a single division of the trigeminal nerve or extended to involve all three, as warranted. Because of this control, one should expect a high rate of success and at the same time fewer complications. The complications of sensory aberration and anesthesia dolorosa, which appear most frequently when total sensory loss is present, should be minimized. An added advantage is the relative lack of general morbidity that enables the patient to be ambulatory and eating on the evening of operation, discharged from the hospital the day after, and back to full-time employment or usual activities within several days.

ACKNOWLEDGMENTS

I wish to thank Dr. W. Eugene Stern and the other members of the faculty and resident staff of the Division of Neurosurgy of UCLA for kindly allowing me to include their cases in this study.

REFERENCES

1. Abadie, J.: Névralgie faciale: présentation de malade, Mém. Soc. Méd. Chir. Bordeaux, p. 59, 1902.
2. Acupuncture anesthesia (chen chu ma chueh), Hong Kong, 1973, Commercial Press Co.
3. Adson, A.W.: The diagnosis and treatment of trigeminal neuralgia, Ann. Otol. Rhinol. Laryngol. **35**:601, 1926.
4. André, N.A.: Observations pratiques sur les maladies de l'uréthre et sur plusieurs fait convulsifs, Paris, 1756, Delaquette, Imprimeur de College et de L'Academie Royale de Chirurgie.
5. Apfelbaum, R.: Microvascular decompression of the trigeminal nerve for tic douloureux, Presented to the American Association of Neurological Surgeons, Los Angeles, April 1979.
6. Bartholow, R.: A practical treatise on materia medica and therapeutics, New York, 1876, Appleton.
7. Bauer, K.H.: Unsere Technik der Koagulation des Ganglion Gasseri, Zentralbl. Chir. **14**:816, 1939.
8. Bauer, K.H.: Die Elektrokoagulation des Ganglion Gasseri, Chirugia **16**:1, 1944.
9. Brodal, A.: Central course of afferent fibers for pain in facial glossopharyngeal and vagus nerves, Arch. Neurol. Psychiatr. **57**:292, 1947.
10. Chakravorty, B.: Visual disturbance following fifth nerve ganglion injection: report of two cases, J. Neurosurg. **23**:354, 1965.
11. Chouké, K.S., and Hodes, P.J.: Pterygo-alar bar and recognition by roentgen methods in trigeminal neuralgia, Am. J. Roentgenol. **65**:180, 1951.
12. Craigmile, T.K.: Complications of the posterior fossa section of the trigeminal sensory root, Presented to the Western Neurosurgical Society, Pebble Beach, Calif. Nov. 5, 1969.
13. Crill, W.E.: Carbamazepine: drugs five years later, Ann. Intern. Med. **79**:844, 1973.
14. Crue, B.L., Jr., Todd, E.M., and Carregal, E.J.A.: Percutaneous trigeminal tractotomy, Excerpta Med. Int. Congr. Series **193**:564, 1969.
15. Crue, B.L., Jr., Todd, E.M., and Carregal, E.J.A.: Percutaneous radiofrequency stereotaxic trigeminal, tractotomy. In Crue, B.L., Jr., editor: Pain and suffering: selected aspects, Springfield, Ill., 1970, Charles C Thomas, Publisher.
16. Crue, B.L., Jr., Todd, E.M., Carregal, E.J.A., and Kilham, O.: Percutaneous trigeminal tractotomy, case report—utilizing stereotactic radiofrequency lesion, Bull. Los Angeles Neurol. Soc. **32**:86, 1967.
17. Cushing, H.W.: The major trigeminal neuralgias and their surgical treatment based on experiences with 332 Gasserian operations; varieties of facial neuralgia, Am. J. Med. Sci. **160**:157, 1920.
18. Dandy, W.E.: Section of the sensory root of the trigeminal nerve at the pons, Bull. Johns Hopkins Hosp. **36**:105, 1925.
19. Dandy, W.E.: An operation for cure of tic douloureux; partial section of the sensory root at the pons, Arch. Surg. **18**:687, 1929.
20. Dandy, W.E.: Certain functions of roots and ganglia of the cranial sensory nerves, Arch. Neurol. Psychiatry **27**:22, 1932.
21. Dandy, W.E.: Treatment of trigeminal neuralgia by the cerebellar route, Ann. Surg. **96**:787, 1932.
22. Dandy, W.E.: Concerning the cause of trigeminal neuralgia, Am. J. Surg. **24**:447, 1934.
23. Dollinger, J.: L'extraction des racines du trigumineau, remplaçant l'extirpation du ganglion de Gasser, dans le traitement des névralgies faciales graves, Assoc. Française de Chirurgie **21**:751, 1908.
24. Ecker, A., and Perl, T.: Precise alcoholic Gasserian injection for tic douloureux, J. Neurol. Neurosurg. Psychiatry **28**:65, 1965.
25. Emmons, W.F., and Rhoton, A.L.: Subdivision of the trigeminal sensory root: experimental study in the monkey, J. Neurosurg. **35**:585, 1971.
26. Falconer, M.A., and Harris, L.: Surgical treatment of the cranial neuralgias. In Vinken, P.J., and Bruyn, G.W., editors: Handbook of clinical neurology, vol. 5, Amsterdam, 1968, North-Holland Publishing Co.
27. Fox, J.L.: Delineation of the obex by contrast radiography during percutaneous trigeminal tractotomy: technical note, J. Neurosurg. **36**:107, 1972.
28. François, J., Hoffman, G., and Solemé, J.: La Kératite neuroparalytique et sa frequence après les différentes neurotomies pour névralgie essentielle du trijumineau, Neurochirgurgie **9**:81, 1966.
29. Frazier, C.H.: A refinement in the radical operation for trigeminal neuralgia, J.A.M.A. **76**:107, 1921.

30. Frazier, C.H.: Subtotal resection of sensory root for relief of major trigeminal neuralgia, Arch. Neurol. Psychiatry **13**:378, 1925.
31. Frazier, C.H.: Operation for the radical cure of trigeminal neuralgia; analysis of 500 cases, Ann. Surg. **88**:534, 1928.
32. Frazier, C.H., and Russell, E.C.: Neuralgia of the face: an analysis of 754 cases with relation to pain and other sensory phenomena before and after operation, Arch. Neurol. Psychiatry **11**:557, 1924.
33. Frazier, C.H., and Spiller, W.G.: A further report upon the treatment of tic douloureux by division of the sensory root of the Gasserian ganglion, Philadelphia Med. J. **10**:594, 1902.
34. Gardner, W.J.: Trigeminal neuralgia, Clin. Neurosurg. (Proc. Cong. Neurol. Surg.) **15**:1, 1968.
35. Gardner, W.J., and Pinto, J.P.: Taarnhøj operation: relief of trigeminal neuralgia without numbness, Cleve. Clin. Q. **20**:364, 1953.
36. Gardner, W.J., Todd, E.M., and Pinto, J.P.: Roentgenographic findings in trigeminal neuralgia, Am. J. Roentgenol. **76**:346, 1956.
37. Ginwalla, M.S.: Surgical treatment of trigeminal neuralgia of third division, Oral Surg. **14**:1300, 1961.
38. Graf, C.J.: Trigeminal compression for tic douloureux: an evaluation, J. Neurosurg. **20**:1029, 1963.
39. Grant, F.C.: Alcohol injections in the treatment of major trigeminal neuralgia, J.A.M.A. **107**:771, 1936.
40. Grant, F.C.: Results in the operative treatment of major trigeminal neuralgia, Ann. Surg. **107**:14, 1938.
41. Grant, F.C.: Surgical methods for relief of pain in the head and neck, Res. Publ. Ass. Res. Neur. Ment. Dis. **23**:408, 1943.
42. Grant, F.C., and Weinberger, L.M.: Experiences with intramedullary tractotomy: relief of facial pain and summary of operative results, Arch. Surg. **42**:681, 1941.
43. Grantham, E.G., and Segerberg, L.H.: An evaluation of palliative surgical procedures in trigeminal neuralgia, J. Neurosurg. **9**:390, 1952.
44. Gudmundsson, K., Rhoton, A.L., and Rushton, J.G.: Detailed anatomy of the intracranial portion of the trigeminal nerve, J. Neurosurg. **35**:592, 1971.
45. Guidetti, B.: Tractotomy for the relief of trigeminal neuralgia; observations in 124 cases, J. Neurosurg. **7**:499, 1950.
46. Hamby, W.B.: Effectiveness of various operations for trigeminal neuralgia, J. Neurosurg. **17**:1039, 1960.
47. Hamby, W.B., Shinners, B.M., and Marsh, I.A.: Trigeminal tractotomy; observations in 48 cases, Arch. Surg. **57**:171, 1948.
48. Harris, W.: Alcohol injection of the Gasserian ganglion for trigeminal neuralgia, Lancet **1**:218, 1912.
49. Harris, W.: An analysis of 1433 cases of paroxysmal trigeminal neuralgia (trigeminal tic) and the end results of Gasserian alcohol injection, Brain **63**:209, 1940.
50. Härtel, F.: Die Leitungsanästhesia und Injektionsbehandlung des Ganglion Gasseri und der Trigeminusstamme, Arch. Klin. Chir. **100**:193, 1912.
51. Härtel, F.: Röntgenologische Darstellung des Foramen ovale des Schadels und ihre Bedeutung für de Behandlung Trigeminusneuralgie, Dtsch. Med. Wochenschr. **61**:1069, 1935.
52. Hartley, F.: Intercranial neurectomy of the second and third divisions of the fifth nerve, N.Y. J. Med. **55**:317, 1892.
53. Henderson, W.R.: The anatomy of the gasserian ganglion and the distribution of pain in relation to injections and operations for trigeminal neuralgia, Ann. R. Coll. Surg. Engl. **37**:346, 1965.
54. Henderson, W.R.: Trigeminal neuralgia: the pain and its treatment, Br. Med. J. **1**:7, 1967.
55. Hensell, V.: Ist die Elektrokoagulation des Ganglion Gasseri auch heute noch berechtigt? Chirurgia **28**:544, 1957.
56. Herrmann, J.D.: Transdural temporal approach to the posterior root for rhizotomy, Presented to the American Academy of Neurological Surgery, Cleveland, Nov. 1940.
57. Hitchcock, E.: Stereotactic trigeminal tractotomy, Ann. Clin. Res. **2**:131, 1970.
58. Hitselberger, W.E., and Pulec, J.L.: Trigeminal nerve (posterior root) retrolabyrinthine selective section: operative procedure for intractable pain, Arch. Otolaryngol. **96**:412, 1972.
59. Horrax, G., and Poppen, J.L.: Trigeminal neuralgia: experiences with and treatment employed in 468 patients during the past ten years, Surg. Gynecol. Obstet. **61**:394, 1935.
60. Horsley, V.: An address on the surgical treatment of trigeminal neuralgia, Practitioner **65**:251, 1900.
61. Horsley, V., Taylor, J., and Coleman, W.S.: The various surgical procedures devised for the relief or cure of trigeminal neuralgia (tic douloureux), Br. Med. J. **1**:1139, 1191, 1249, 1891.
62. Hübner, B.: Ist die Elektrokoagulation des Ganglion Gasseri bei der Trigeminusneuralgie noch zeitgemäss? Bericht über 524 Operationen an 372 Patienten von 1952-1967, Langenbecks Arch. Chir. **322**:577, 1968.
63. Jannetta, P.J.: Arterial compression of the trigeminal nerve at the pons in patients with trigeminal neuralgia, J. Neurosurg. **26**:159, 1967.
64. Jannetta, P.J.: Complications from microsurgical treatment of tic douloureux: letter to the editor, J. Neurosurg. **40**:675, 1974.
65. Jannetta, P.J.: Personal communication, 1974.
66. Jannetta, P.J.: Microsurgical relief of neurovascular trigeminal nerve compression in tic douloureux: abstracts of the First World Congress on Pain, International Association for the Study of Pain, Florence, Italy, 1975.
67. Jannetta, P.J., and Rand, R.W.: Transtentorial retrogasserian rhizotomy in trigeminal neuralgia by microsurgical technique, Bull. Los Angeles Neurol. Soc. **31**:93, 1966.
68. Jannetta, P.J., and Rand, R.W.: Transtentorial retrogasserian rhizotomy in trigeminal neuralgia. In Rand, R.W., editor: Microneurosurgery, St. Louis, 1969, The C.V. Mosby Co.
69. Jefferson, A.: Trigeminal root and ganglion injections using phenol in glycerine for the relief of trigeminal neuralgia, J. Neurol. Neurosurg. Psychiatry **26**:345, 1963.
70. Kahn, E.A.: Trigeminal rhizotomy: the temporal approach, J. Neurosurgery **25**:242, 1966.
71. Kalyanaraman, S., and Ramamurthi, B.: Trigeminal neuralgia—a review of 331 cases, Neurol. India **18**(Suppl. 1):100, 1970.
72. Killian, J.M., and Fromm, G.H.: Carbamazepine in treatment of neuralgia: use and side effects, Arch. Neurol. **19**:129, 1968.
73. Kirschner, M.: Zur elektrochirurgie, Arch. Klin. Chir. **167**:761, 1931.
74. Kirschner, M.: Zur electrokoagulation des Ganglion Gasseri, Zentralbl. Chir. **47**:2841, 1932.
75. Kirschner, M.: Die Punktionstechnik und die Elektrokoagulation des Ganglion Gasseri: über gezielte Operationen, Langenbecks Arch. Chir. **176**:581, 1933.
76. Kirschner, M.: Zur Behandlung der Trigeminusneuralgie, Erfahrungen an 250 Fällen, Arch. Klin. Chir. **186**:325, 1936.
77. Kirschner, M.: Die Behandlung der Trigeminusneuralgie (nach Erfahrungen an 1113 Kranken), Munch. Med. Wochenschr. **89**:235, 263, 1942.
78. Kirschner, M.: Zur Behandlung der Trigeminusneuralgie, Munch. Med. Wochenschr. **89**:235, 1974.
79. Klar, E.: Uber Erfahrungen mit Elektrokoagulation bei Trigeminusneuralgie an der Heidelberger Universitätsklinik, Langenbecks Arch. Chir. **294**:713, 1960.
80. Klar, E., and Piotrowski, W.: Die Electrokoagulation des Ganglion Gassen im Greisenalter. In Proceedings of the International Association of Gerontology, Vienna, 1966.

81. Krayenbühl, H.: Idiopathic trigeminal neuralgia, acta clinica no. 9, Documenta Geigy, Basel, Switzerland, 1969, J.R. Geigy S.A.
82. Kubanyi, E.: Sur le traitement de la névralgie du nerf trijumeau par l'électro-coagulation intracranienne dur ganglion de Gasser (d'après 301 cas), Lyon Chir. **41**:681, 1946.
83. Kubanyi, E.: Trigeminusneuralgie: die Differentialdiagnose und Therapie der Gesichtsschmerzen, Vienna, 1956, Verlag Urban & Schwartzenberg.
84. Kunc, Z.: Tractus spinalis nervi trigemini; fresh anatomic data and their significance for surgery, Prague, Rozpravy Ceskoslovenskě Academie Věd., 1964.
85. Kuntz, A.: Discussion of paper by Ranson, S.W.: Cutaneous sensory fibers and sensory conduction, Arch. Neurol. Psychiatry **26**:1140, 1931.
86. Letcher, F.S., and Goldring, S.: The effect of radiofrequency current and heat on peripheral nerve action potential in the cat, J. Neurosurg. **29**:42, 1968.
87. Leung, S.J., Fan, C., and Sechzer, P.H.: Acupuncture therapeutics, Anesth. Analg. (Cleve.) **53**:942, 1974.
88. Love, J.G.: Decompression of the gasserian ganglion and its posterior root: a new treatment for trigeminal neuralgia (preliminary report), Proc. Staff Meet. Mayo Clin. **27**:257, 1952.
89. Love, J.G.: The surgical treatment of trigeminal and glossopharyngeal neuralgia: decompression of the gasserian ganglion and its root for trigeminal pain, J. Int. Coll. Surg. **21**:1, 1954.
90. Mahoney, W.: Die Epidermoide des Zentralnervensystems, Z. Neurol. Psychiat. **155**:416, 1936.
91. Mayo, H.: Experiments to determine the influence of the portio dura of the seventh and of the facial branches of the fifth pair of nerves, Anat. Physiol. Comment. **1**:107, 1822.
92. Moore, D.: Regional block, ed. 3, Springfield, Ill., 1961, Charles C Thomas, Publisher.
93. Morello, G., Bianchi, M., and Migliavicca, F.: Combined extra-intradural temporal rhizotomy for treatment of trigeminal neuralgia: results in 409 patients, J. Neurosurg. **34**:372, 1971.
94. Neuber, G.: Eine neue Amputationsmethode. Ueber Osmiumsäure—Injektionen bei peripheren Neuralgien, Kiel, Germany, 1883, Lipsius & Tischer.
95. Nugent, G.R., and Berry, B.: Trigeminal neuralgia treated with percutaneous radiofrequency lesions, J. Neurosurg. **40**:517, 1974.
96. Olivecrona, H.: The surgery of pain, Acta Psychiatr. Scand. (Suppl.) **46**:268, 1947.
97. Olivecrona, H.: Trigeminal neuralgia, Triangle **5**:60, 1961.
98. Onofrio, B.M.: Radiofrequency percutaneous Gasserian ganglion lesions: results in 140 patients with trigeminal pain, J. Neurosurg. **42**:132, 1975.
99. Ostwalt, F.: Ueber tiefe alkohol-cocain-oder alkohol-stovain-injektionen bei trigeminus-und anderen neuralgien, Berl. Klin. Wochenschr. **43**:10, 1906.
100. Patrick, H.T.: The technic and results of deep injections of alcohol for trifacial neuralgia, J.A.M.A. **58**:150, 1912.
101. Peet, M.M.: Tic douloureux and its treatment with a review of the cases operated upon at the University Hospital in 1917, J. Mich. Med. Soc. **17**:91, 1918.
102. Peet, M.M., and Echols, D.H.: Surgery of disorders of cranial nerves. In Bancroft, F.W., and Pilcher, C., editors: Surgical treatment of the nervous system, Philadelphia, 1946, J.B. Lippincott Co.
103. Peet, M.M., and Schneider, R.C.: Trigeminal neuralgia: a review of 689 cases with a follow-up study of sixty-five percent of the group, J. Neurosurg. **9**:367, 1952.
104. Pelletier, V.A., Poulos, D.A., and Lende, R.A.: Functional localization in the trigeminal root, J. Neurosurg. **40**:504, 1974.
105. Peng, A.T.C., et al.: Acupuncture for relief of chronic pain and surgical analgesia, Am. Surg. **40**:50, 1974.
106. Penman, J.: The differential diagnosis and treatment of tic douloureux, Postgrad. Med. J. **26**:627, 1950.
107. Penman, J.: Trigeminal sensory root injection. In Rob, C., and Smith, R., editors: Operative surgery, vol. 8, Philadelphia, 1958, F.A. Davis Co.
108. Piotrowski, W.: Derzeitiger Standpunkt zur Elektrokoagulation des Ganglion Gasseri beim Gesichtsschmerz, Langenbecks Arch. Chir. **322**:573, 1968.
109. Poppen, J.L.: An atlas of neurosurgical techniques, Philadelphia, 1960, W.B. Saunders Co.
110. Quinn, J.H.: Repetitive peripheral neurectomies for neuralgia of second and third divisions of trigeminal nerve, J. Oral Surg. **23**:600, 1965.
111. Ramonède, L.: Exérèse du trijumeau, Presse Méd. **11**:789, 1903.
112. Rasmussen, P.P.: Facial pain: a clinical study with special reference to the symptomatology, aetiology and surgical therapy, Copenhagen, 1965, Munksgaard.
113. Rich, J.R.: Trigeminal neuralgia: a comparison of surgical methods of treatment, Presented to the American Association of Neurological Surgeons, Los Angeles, April 1973.
114. Rich, J.R.: Unpublished data, 1975.
115. Riley, W.H.: Discussion of Frazier, C.H.: Trigeminal neuralgia: 14 years experience with fractional section of the sensory root as the major operation, J.A.M.A. **89**:1742, 1927.
116. Rose, W.: Removal of the gasserian ganglion for severe neuralgia, Lancet **2**:914, 1890.
117. Ruge, D., Brochner, R., and Davis, L.: A study of the treatment of 637 patients with trigeminal neuralgia, J. Neurosurg. **15**:528, 1958.
118. Saunders, R.L., and Sachs, E.: Relation of the accessory rootlets of the trigeminal nerve to its motor root: a microsurgical autopsy study, J. Neurosurg. **33**:317, 1970.
119. Schloesser, C.: Heilung peripherer Reizzustärge sensibler und motorischer, Nerven. Ber. Ophthal. Ges. **31**:84, 1903.
120. Schürman, M., Butz, M., and Brock, M.: Temporal retrogasserian resection of trigeminal root versus controlled elective percutaneous electrocoagulation of the ganglion of Gasser in the treatment of trigeminal neuralgia: report on a series of 531 cases, Acta Neurochir. (Wien) **26**:33, 1972.
121. Schürmann, K., and Butz, M.: Retroganglionare Trigeminuswurzelresektion durch temporal Schädeleröffnung oder kontrollierte partiele Elektroverödung des Ganglion Gasseri in der operativen Behandlung der idiopathischen Trigeminusneuralgie, Zentralbl. Neurochir. **29**:139, 1968.
122. Shelden, C.H.: Compression procedure for trigeminal neuralgia: review and clinical appraisal of 10 years' experience, Presented to American Academy of Neurological Surgery, Key Biscayne, Fla., Nov. 1964.
123. Shelden, C.H.: Compression procedure for trigeminal neuralgia, J. Neurosurg. **25**:374, 1966.
124. Shelden, C.H., Pudenz, R.H., Freshwater, D.B., and Crue, B.L.: Compression rather than decompression for trigeminal neuralgia, J. Neurosurg. **12**:123, 1955.
125. Sherrington, C.: The integrative action of the nervous system, London, 1947, Cambridge University Press.
126. Sicard, J.A.: Treatment of "essential" facial neuralgia by local alcoholisation, Med. Presse **106**:60, 1918.
127. Siegfried, J.: Un nouveau traitement neurochirurgical de la névralgie du trijumeau: analgésie sans anesthésie, Neurochirurgie **19**:585, 1973.
128. Sjöqvist, O.: Eine neue Operationsmethode bei Trigeminusneuralgie; Durchschneidung des Tractus spinalis trigemini, Zentralbl. Neurochir. **2**:247, 1937.
129. Spiller, W.C., and Frazier, C.H.: The division of the sensory root of the trigeminus for relief of tic douloureux; an experimen-

tal, pathological and clinical study with a preliminary report of one surgically successful case, Philadelphia Med. J. **8**:1039, 1901.
130. Stender, A.: "Gangliolysis" for the surgical treatment of trigeminal neuralgia, J. Neurosurg. **11**:333, 1964.
131. Stender, A., and Grumme, T.: Late results of gangliolysis as a treatment for trigeminal neuralgia, J. Neurosurg. **31**:21, 1969.
132. Stookey, B.P., and Ransohoff, J.: Trigeminal neuralgia: its history and treatment, Springfield, Ill., 1959, Charles C Thomas, Publisher.
133. Stöwsand, D., Markakis, E., and Laubner, P.: Zur Elektrokoagulation des Ganglion Gasseri bei der idiopathischen Trigeminus-Neuralgie, Nervenarzt **44**:44, 1973.
134. Sunder-Plassmann, P.: Ergebnisse der Elektrokoagulation des Ganglion Gasseri bei Trigeminusneuralgie, Zentralbl. Chir. **66**:2234, 1939.
135. Svien, H.J., and Love, J.G.: Results of decompression operation for trigeminal neuralgia 4 years plus after operation, J. Neurosurg. **16**:653, 1959.
136. Sweet, W.H.: Percutaneous differential thermal trigeminal rhizotomy for the management of facial pain. In Penzholz, H., Brock, M., Hamer, J., Klinger, M., and Spoerri, O., editors: Advances in neurosurgery: brain hypoxia-pain, vol. 3, Berlin, 1975, Springer-Verlag.
137. Sweet, W.H., and Wepsic, J.G.: Controlled thermocoagulation of trigeminal ganglion and rootlets for differential destruction of pain fibers. I. Trigeminal neuralgia, J. Neurosurg. **40**:143, 1974.
138. Taarnhøj, P.: Decompression of the trigeminal root and the posterior part of the ganglion as a treatment in trigeminal neuralgia; preliminary communication, J. Neurosurg. **9**:288, 1952.
139. Taarnhøj, P.: Decompression of trigeminal root, J. Neurosurg. **11**:299, 1954.
140. Taptas, N.: Les injections d'alcool dans le ganglion de Gasser à travers le trou ovale, Presse Med. **19**:798, 1911.
141. Taptas, N.: De l'injection d'alcool dans le ganglion de Gasser à travers le trou ovale; injection dans le trou grand rond, Arch. Int. Laryngol. **36**:423, 1913.
142. Taub, A.: Relief of post herpetic neuralgia with psychotrophic drugs, J. Neurosurg. **39**:235, 1969.
143. Tew, J., and Mayfield, F.: Trigeminal neuralgia: a new surgical approach (percutaneous electrocoagulation of the trigeminal nerve), Laryngoscope **83**:1096, 1973.
144. Thiry, S.: Expérience personnelle basée sur 225 cas de névralgie essentielle dur trijumeau traités par électrocoagulation stéreotaxique du ganglion de Gasser entre 1950 et 1960, Neurochirurgie **8**:86, 1962.
145. Thiry, S., and Hotermans, J.M.: Traitement la névralgie essentielle du trijumeau par stéreotaxie et electrocoagulation partielle sélective du ganglion de Gasser: expérience portant sur 365 cas traités entre 1950 et 1970, Neurochirurgie **20**:55, 1974.
146. Thoma, K.H.: Oral surgery, ed. 5, St. Louis, 1969, The C.V. Mosby Co.
147. Tiffany, L. McL: Intracranial neurectomy and removal of the gasserian ganglion, Ann. Surg. **19**:47, 1894.
148. Tönnis, W., and Kreissel, H.: Die Bedeutung einer sorgfältigen Differential-diagnose für die chirurgische Behandlung der Trigeminusneuralgie, Dtsch. Med. Wochenschr. **76**:1202, 1951.
149. Turnbull, I.: Percutaneous rhizotomy for trigeminal neuralgia, Surg. Neurol. **2**:385, 1974.
150. Veith, I.: The Yellow Emperor's classic of internal medicine, Berkeley, Calif., 1972, University of California Press.
151. Walker, E., Miles, F.C., and Simpson, J.R.: Partial trigeminal rhizotomy using suboccipital approach, Arch. Neurol. Psychiatry **75**:514, 1956.
152. Whisler, W., and Hill, B.J.: A simplified technique for injection of the Gasserian ganglion, using the fluoroscope for localization, Neurochirurgie **15**:167, 1972.
153. White, J.C., and Sweet, W.H.: Pain and the neurosurgeon, a 40-year experience, Springfield, Ill., 1969, Charles C Thomas, Publisher.
154. Wilkins, H.: The treatment of trigeminal neuralgia by section of the posterior sensory fibers using the transdural temporal approach, J. Neurosurg. **25**:370, 1966.
155. Wilkins, R.H.: Comments on treatment of tic douloureux, Neurosurgery **1**:21, 1977.
156. Yaşargil, M.G.: Trigeminal neuralgia: transtentorial approach. In Yaşargil, M.G., editor: Microsurgery applied to neurosurgery, Stuttgart, W. Germany, 1969, Georg Thieme Verlag.
157. Zenker, R.: Die Behandlung der Trigeminusneuralgie unter besonderer Berücksichtigung der Grundlagen, der Ausführung und der Ergebnisse der Punktion und Elektrokoagulation des Ganglion Gasseri nach Kirschner, Ergeb. Chir. Orthop. **31**:1, 1939.

31 Microvascular decompression in the treatment of trigeminal neuralgia

PETER J. JANNETTA, M.D.

Trigeminal neuralgia (tic douloureux, trifacial neuralgia) is lancinating face pain that is more common in midlife and later, but the age distribution follows the usual gaussian bell-shaped curve. It is more common on the right side than on the left, more common in the maxillary and mandibular distribution (V_2, V_3, $V_{2\text{-}3}$), and uncommon in V_1. It is seen more frequently in women than in men. The pain is of sudden onset and offset. Attacks are commonly precipitated by talking, eating, shaving, washing the face, drafts of cold air, etc. Variable trigger points, where a light touch will precipitate an attack, are frequent. They are evanescent, variable, and usually located around the snout but rarely are located outside the distribution of the pain. The pain is described as like electrical shocks or a hot poker and universally as the worst pain the patient has ever had. It usually lasts from seconds to a few minutes but may go on for up to an hour. The characteristics of the first 411 patients operated on by me and my colleagues at the University of Pittsburgh, all of whom underwent microvascular decompression of the trigeminal nerve root entry zone, are described later.

In reviewing our patient material regarding trigeminal neuralgia we found that 80% of our patients were initially seen by a dentist rather than a physician.[11] Further, the diagnosis was uncommonly established early on: patients had teeth extracted without relief of their pain. This occasionally was done at the insistence of the patient, but more frequently because the dentist had not made the proper diagnosis. Indeed, early in our series our patients had seen more than two dentists and usually more than one physician before the diagnosis was first considered. This chapter therefore includes a rather detailed description of the clinical syndrome of trigeminal neuralgia in addition to a description of the anatomical relationships of the trigeminal nerve, a review of the evidence for trigeminal nerve root entry zone abnormality (usually vascular compression distortion) as the cause of trigeminal neuralgia, a discussion of the preoperative evaluation of a patient with trigeminal neuralgia intractable to medication, a brief survey of the indications for operation, and a description of microvascular decompression with findings and results in our series of patients.

The initial onset of trigeminal neuralgia is characteristically very memorable to the patient.[11] No matter how many years ago the first attack occurred, the patient will remember minute details about the time of day, where the pain was, what it felt like, how long it lasted, etc. This is in sharp contrast to other face pain problems where the onset is mild, gradual, and not memorable. Occasionally a patient will have a prodrome of paresthesia and dysesthesia in the area of the future tic. These episodes are mild, brief, and may be separated from a first bout of true tic by some time. Some patients will have relatively long pain-free intervals, up to many months after the first attack, before the pain becomes established.

Most tic patients can give a history of present illness in which it can be considered that positional changes have an influence on the pain. It has long been known that tic patients usually do not have many attacks at night. It has been hypothesized that this is because the sleeping brain is not susceptible to the tic, and those attacks which do occur have been blamed on stimulation of a trigger point by bed clothing and so forth. I have observed at operation that the vessels of the brain and the brain stem appear to move differentially with changes in the position of the head. This is so whether the arachnoid has been opened or not, but of course the presence of a craniectomy, no matter how small, may have some distorting influence. With the patient in the sitting position the artery or vein is universally seen to be compressing, notching, and grooving the root entry zone of the nerve. But when the patient is in the lateral position, such that the ipsilateral side is the up side, the blood vessel may be a millimeter or 2 away from the root entry zone. The groove in the nerve is usually seen, however, and the vessel can be moved back to the point of the groove very easily. The converse should be true, that is, with a patient on the contralateral side the differential movement may impact the vessel against the root entry zone more significantly. On questioning, it can be found that frequently the patient gets into a position of comfort when going to bed at night so that the pain settles down before sleep. The patient is usually supine or lies in the contralateral-lateral decubitus position for relief from pain. At my request five patients in this series, all of whom were having severe tic, were asked to go to bed, lie in their position of comfort, and stay that way through the night without going to sleep. In doing this the patients found that their tic quieted down only to recur if they got out of bed again. Unfortunately they were not asked to lie in the contralateral decubitus position. This will be done in another group. It may be of significance that many patients with hyperactive disorders of the other cranial nerves which are caused by neurovascular compression, (that is, facial, acoustic, and glossopharyngeal nerves), also may have the same kind of positional history, perhaps not as frequently as with cranial nerve V problems except for those with nerve VIII problems.

Patients in this series with tumors as the cause of their trigeminal neuralgia appear to have a history and physical findings that are no different from the classic tic history. Indeed, only those patients who did have a classic history are included in this series.

The chronic, all-pervading worry and frequent panic over the threat of the next attack of pain in this patient population cannot be overemphasized. The patient who suffers from trigeminal neuralgia for a prolonged period may develop some element of constant burning pain in the face, a symptom that is rarely discussed in the literature. This type of pain may rarely supervene totally. Carbamazepine (Tegretol) in many of our patients has abolished trigeminal neuralgia only to bring about constant burning pain, which then regressed with concomitant recurrence of tic after cessation of the drug.

When there is a family history of trigeminal neuralgia, the patients in the second generation of tic may be younger than those in the first generation at age of onset. The side of the pain appears to be the same as that of the parent who had tic. This has certainly not been validated statistically at this point but may be of interest. I recently treated a woman with right-sided trigeminal neuralgia that developed at age 48, whose sister developed right-sided trigeminal neuralgia at age 37, and whose mother and great-uncle both had right-sided trigeminal neuralgia starting in their 60s.

Patients with trigeminal neuralgia frequently have mild sensory loss in the pure trigeminal distribution. This was first noted by Lewy and Grant[16] in 25% of their patients with trigeminal neuralgia. On careful testing we have noted it in about one third of our patients who had not undergone a prior operative procedure. It must be emphasized that these are mild changes. Only one of these patients had a tumor as the cause of the neurovascular compression. Two principles must be adhered to if one is to find these abnormalities: the first is that the pure trigeminal distribution must be tested, that is, the nose and the area around the eyes, including the corneal reflex; the second is that the examiner must follow routine neurological practice for tracing sensory abnormality by starting from the abnormal and going to the normal. The abnormal area is usually around the nasolabial fold region over the upper lip. It consists of mild hypalgesia, frequently with associated hypesthesia. Mild repetitive pinprick stimulus is used starting in this area and going in every direction from it and then evaluating it against the opposite side. The corneal reflex may be decreased, especially in first division trigeminal neuralgia, and this may be true in only part of the cornea, especially the upper half. These changes will revert to normal gradually after microvascular decompression of the nerve.

Trigger points are found most commonly in the area of the snout and around the eyes, which is the area of pure distribution of the trigeminal nerve. Trigger points are evanescent and move about over a time, implying a dynamic changing process, which is reasonable if one considers the electron microscopic changes noted in trigeminal neuralgia.[23]

Jaw opening is frequently uneven in patients with trigeminal neuralgia, as though there were some lag on the side of the pain. This may be simply because the patient will guard against an attack of tic, but since we know that the motor-proprioceptive fascicles are frequently denervated in trigeminal neuralgia,[25] it is possible that some of this abnormal movement is a result of unilateral motor trigeminal denervation or disordered proprioception. These changes of denervation in the temporal and/or masseter muscles revert gradually to normal after microvascular decompression.[10,11]

The patient having severe attacks of pain will hold the face quite still with minimum mobility of the muscles of facial expression and will talk with a "stiff upper (and lower) lip." During an attack, although it occurs rapidly, jaw clenching is quite commonly seen. It is not known whether this is a response to the pain by the subject, something automatic that happens in the disordered physiology of the trigeminal nerve precipitating the attack, or a sequence of the same abnormal impulses that are extant at the time of the attack. Neurophysiological studies may clarify this point. The unshaved and unwashed face, the unbrushed teeth, and the unmade-up face are not seen as frequently as previously, since the newer medications have certainly helped diminish acute exacerbations of pain. However, periodontitis and dental caries are common when a patient has been suffering for a long time because he or she cannot tolerate dental care. Patients should be reassured that they may go to the dentist soon after discharge from the hospital.

THE ANATOMY OF THE TRIGEMINAL NERVE

The trigeminal nerve is located high and anteromedial in the posterior fossa. It arises from the lateral pons just medial to the ala of the cerebellum and courses in a generally horizontal anterolateral direction between the pons and Meckel's cave. The diameter of the nerve is surprisingly variable, and there is some variability in relationships of the roots. But in general, the 100 or more fascicles making up the dorsal root in Meckel's cave ramify widely and decrease in number, so that as the nerve approaches the brain stem, there are about 65 fascicles that can usually be counted. Fascicles coalesce into a somewhat gelatinous area surrounded by tough pia mater within 1 to 1.5 cm of the brain stem. This is the so-called fibrous cone, as described by Dandy.[3-5] Two motor-proprioceptive fascicles exit the pons on the supermedial side of the portio major. They arise as a spray of fascicles that fuse within a centimeter or so into two distinctly separate but contiguous structures. Some connections are seen between motor-proprioceptive and sensory roots, variable in number, with connections all the way to and including the gasserian ganglion. The motor-proprioceptive fascicles, after fusing, course on the medial side of the sensory root. They then cross under the gasserian ganglion and exit the intracranial cavity under the third division at the foramen ovale.

The fibrous cone region is truly an internal as well as external cone, as seen in multiple serial histological sections of the trigeminal nerve. It is seen, in such tissue sections, that the various fascicles of the dorsal root enter a truncated area of tissue that is widest at the brain stem and contains central nervous system myelin. Each axis cylinder peripheral to this point in the dorsal root is covered by Schwann cell myelin. A good percentage, perhaps 20% of the fascicles do not enter this fibrous cone but instead separately enter the pons between the motor-proprioceptive fascicles and the portio major. Physiological studies in Lende's laboratory,[20a] verified in our laboratory,[10] have shown that the "motor" fascicles are indeed motor proprioceptive. The coalescent portio major at the brain stem, or fibrous cone, is surrounded by pia-arachnoid separate from all other fascicles. This can be transected in its entirety, preserving not only the motor-proprioceptive fibers but also the "accessory" fascicles (intermediate fascicles) that have arisen from the dorsal root at variable distances from the brain stem.[8,10,11,22] The latter fascicles have a separate pial covering to the brain stem. If selective section of the portio major is carried out truly at the brain stem, considerable light touch preservation is obtained with preservation of the corneal reflex, although it may be somewhat diminished. Histological studies by Vidic and Stefanotas[27] of the trigeminal nerve in several species have verified the presence of three groups of fascicles at the brain stem. Electrophysiological studies in humans, done by Ley and Bacci[17] after selective portio major section, have verified such a realignment of functional distribution involving concentration of pain pathways in the portio major.

Some variations do exist in the relationships of the various fascicles of the trigeminal nerve root entry zone.[8] It has been shown that the entry zone may be more or less obliquely horizontal or vertical. The relationships remain the same with the exception of an occasional aberrant fascicle found in large cadaver series. Such fascicles and such variations have not caused any difficulty in aligning oneself to the nerve properly at operation. Provost and Hardy[22] have verified the presence of "accessory" or "intermediate" fascicles of the trigeminal nerve and have described three variations in the anatomy. They state that "As the intermediate fibers mediate the tactile sensations and major portion mediates thermoalgesic sensations, a selective rhizotomy of the major portion resulted in a complete relief of trigeminal pain with preservation of normal tactile sensations." However, Pertuiset and colleagues[21] have been able to identify intermediate fascicles at operation in only one out of two cases.

As discussed, the trigeminal nerve is located high, anterior, and medial in the posterior fossa. Considerable dissection is necessary to elevate the cerebellum from the lower cranial nerves to visualize the trigeminal nerve clearly from a low suboccipital craniectomy. It is practically impossible to see the trigeminal nerve root entry zone from this approach unless the cerebellum has already been hollowed out by a cerebellopontile angle tumor, such as an acoustic neuroma or a cholesteatoma. In Dandy's approach to the nerve[3-5] dissection is carried around the cerebellum, rather like opening the pages of a book, with the anterior surface of the cerebellum acting as one page and the petrous bone as the other. In this approach the trigeminal nerve is seen well at Meckel's cave and posteriorly, but visualization of the true root entry zone may be difficult, although much easier than from underneath the cerebellum. However, if the superior surface of the cerebellum is exposed and the lateral sinus and adjacent tentorium are elevated slightly with stay sutures, one can achieve an excellent appreciation of the trigeminal nerve in situ.

One must appreciate that the angle of the entry zone of the trigeminal nerve in relation to the plane of the surface of the pons is a very acute angle. The nerve here may be nearly parallel to the plane of the pons, much like the angle of a flagpole to the plane of the abdomen of a flag bearer. The portio major side of the entry zone thus spreads posteriorly for a considerable distance. Minimum to essentially no cerebellar retraction is necessary to expose the nerve except for the posterolateral region of the portio major, which is covered by the ala of the cerebellum. The superior petrosal vein, which usually blocks the view, originates in cerebellar transcortical venous structures over the anterosuperior and anterior surface of the cerebellum, with generally two major branches coalescing to form an inverted Y of variable length, which enters the superior petrosal sinus. The structure is encased in arachnoid, often all the way up to the superior petrosal sinus. The trigeminal nerve is seen just medial and anterior to this vein, usually in the same field at 10 times magnification as the trochlear nerve coursing around the brain stem.

In the normal situation the horizontal loop of the superior cerebellar artery parallels the trochlear nerve just below it. This vessel usually bifurcates quite proximally such that there are two and rarely three loops coming around the midbrain-pons junction to course posteromedially to the superior cerebellar surface and adjacent brain stem. In elderly patients this loop is seen to be quite elongated, but it still remains generally horizontal. The cephalad-caudad angle at which the trigeminal nerve enters and exits the brain stem also varies. The trigeminal nerve can be vertical or horizontal at the brain stem. Meckel's cave is anterolateral to the root entry zone but at the same cephalad-caudad level in younger people, and the nerve has a generally horizontal course. However, in elderly patients the brain may sag, and the trigeminal nerve can be seen to course cephalad at a fairly high angle before entering Meckel's cave.

In dolichocephalic patients the angle between the two petrous ridges is quite acute, and the nerve may not enter Meckel's cave at a right angle to the petrous bone. In more brachycephalic patients the angle between the petrous bones is closer to 90 degrees, and the trigeminal nerve enters Meckel's cave at more of a right angle to the petrous bone. The nerve runs in a more directly anteroposterior direction and is more parallel and directly adjacent to the pons in the dolichocephalic group. Exposure of the nerve and vascular micromanipulation may be more difficult in the dolichocephalic patients because superolateral exposure is limited.

If the surgeon is to view these structures with ease and clarity, several considerations must be observed. First, the neck must be in traction and slightly flexed using a pin-fixation head holder. Second, the bony dissection of the suboccipital craniectomy should be carried over the lateral sinus and should be lateral enough to expose the initial portion of the descending limb of the sigmoid sinus. High lateral exposure is critical for easy visualization of the trigeminal nerve. Third, magnification is necessary to see normal structures as well as abnormalities in the trigeminal root entry zone.

REVIEW OF THE EVIDENCE REGARDING THE ETIOLOGY OF TRIGEMINAL NEURALGIA

Various theories, frequently speculative, have been proposed regarding the etiology of trigeminal neuralgia. The literature is large, and the ideas of many serious investigators who have considered aspects of the etiology cannot be included in this brief review. Until recently no one other than Dandy[3-5] has found a reasonably consistent abnormality in trigeminal neuralgia. Dandy described abnormalities, usually vascular, about the dorsal root of the trigeminal nerve in the posterior fossa in over 40% of patients, with other questionable abnormalities. Dandy apparently never attempted to move vessels away from the nerve but avulsed the nerve with a hook. He therefore could not state to the satisfaction of others that the vessels were causative factors, but he did treat trigeminal neuralgia effectively by tumor resection in those cases where a tumor was present. Dandy found tumors in 5.6% of his 215 cases, an ectatic basilar artery pressing on the sensory root in 2.8%, cavernous angiomas in 2.3%, an artery compressing the root in 30.7%, and a branch of the petrosal vein crossing the sensory root passing directly through it in another 14%. He was less convinced about the etiological relationship of the veins. In another 1% of the cases he found congenital malformations at the base of the skull, and in seven cases the sensory root was tightly adherent to the brain stem. He saw no gross abnormalities of any kind in 40% of his cases.

Revilla[24] studied 473 patients from the Johns Hopkins Hospital who were operated on by a cerebellar approach between 1925 and 1945. Among these patients were found 24 tumors of the posterior fossa producing trigeminal neuralgia: eleven were neurilemmas, nine were epidermoid cysts, and four were meningiomas. Gardner[6] explored the trigeminal nerve in the posterior fossa in 18 patients with recurrent trigeminal neuralgia. He found an arterial loop compressing the nerve in six, an acoustic tumor in two, a crowded posterior fossa because of basilar impression in one, a "cirsoid aneurysm" (ectatic artery) of the basilar artery in one, and homolateral dislocation of the pons that was compressing the nerve in two cases. He found no explanation for the trigeminal neuralgia in the remaining six cases.

Knight[13] in 1954 studied the incidence of herpes simplex virus in patients with tic douloureux, and although all his patients had high antibody titers for herpes simplex, no control group unaffected with tic douloureux was similarly studied. Recent studies of herpes simplex virus cultures in the trigeminal ganglion[2] would appear to corroborate other impressions that the virus is endemic to human ganglia in general and that vescicles may appear with any nonspecific trauma. Such would appear to be the case in our series of retromastoid craniectomies.[10,11]

Lee,[15] Taarnøj,[26] and Olivecrona[20] described sagging of the hindbrain in elderly patients and suggested that this would cause traction of the trigeminal nerve at the petrous ridge. Gardner, Todd, and Pinto[7] stated that the demineralization of the base of the skull in aging results in an upward tilt of the petrous pyramid, and the consequent angulation of the sensory root over the petrous ridge would produce "short circuiting" and cause trigeminal neuralgia. They noted that trigeminal neuralgia was three times as common on the side of the higher petrous ridge, if asymmetry of the ridges was noted radiographically, than on the side of the lower ridge. Others have found that this is not statistically significant. Malis[18] modified Taarnhøj's technique of middle fossa decompression by opening the dura propria and crossing bands of fibers to mobilize the trigeminal nerve. Forty-four operations were done on 43 patients with delayed relief of 4 or 5 days in eight of the patients, the only procedure other than in the present series with this sequence of pain relief. It is of interest in our cadaver studies that opening the dura propria allows considerable lateral mobility of the trigeminal roots in the posterior fossa, conjecturally allowing the nerve to "escape" a blood vessel.

Lewy and Grant[16] noted in patients with trigeminal neuralgia that there was a 50% incidence of cardiomegaly, angina pectoris, and heart murmurs and an extremely high incidence of arteriosclerotic vascular disease, and he built a superb case for arteriosclerosis as a cause of trigeminal neuralgia but then concluded that trigeminal neuralgia was a manifestation of a thalamic dysfunction, limited to the face in general but associated with other somatic complaints. It is of interest that 80% of their patients had signs of pyramidal or extrapyramidal disease. Sixty percent had evidence of renal dysfunction, and 20% had a family or personal history of migraine.

Kerr[12] has proposed that there may be a defect in the floor of the middle fossa under the gasserian ganglion, especially in elderly patients. The carotid artery thus may pulsate against the ganglion. He proposed that "The carotid acts as a traumatic agent impinging on the ganglion root, thus promoting a more severe breakdown of myelin sheath in older individuals . . . or the carotid pulsation may act simply as an additional irritative factor in a primarily degenerate disease of the nerve." Kerr proposed this as a theory and clearly affirmed that he had no evidence that the bony defect was pertinent to the clinical situation.

Until recently the operative procedures for trigeminal neuralgia were done without magnification. The situation can be somewhat likened to the evaluation of disease in the era before introduction of light or electron microscopy: abnormalities were present all the time that could not be appreciated with extant technology. In many instances a gross abnormality, such as an acoustic neuroma, arteriovenous malformation, or aneurysm, was noted in the posterior fossa during operations for trigeminal neuralgia. In such cases the diagnosis of idiopathic or cryptogenic trigeminal neuralgia was quickly changed to the primary diagnosis of acoustic neuroma, and the trigeminal neuralgia therefore was, called *symptomatic*. With the magnification and lighting afforded by the binocular surgical microscope, in concert with an operative procedure directed at the brain stem area of the trigeminal nerve, it appears that all trigeminal neuralgia is symptomatic. Only gross lesions could be appreciated in the past, but now we can see and treat subtle situations of disordered, hyperactive sensory function.

Primary first division trigeminal neuralgia is rare. Correlation in the present series of face-pain location with the direction from which neurovascular compression takes place shows that the 4% of patients with primary first division trigeminal neuralgia all had trigeminal root entry zone compression-distortion by an arterial loop compressing the caudad-lateral portio major. The loop appeared to be the anteroinferior cerebellar artery or a branch of the same in more patients. The direct correlation of superomedial compression by the superior cerebellar artery in lower facial tic and a laterally compressing vessel in isolated V_2 trigeminal neuralgia has been astonishingly clear in the series, so the operative exposure can be planned rather precisely.

Trigeminal neuralgia is found predominantly in middle and older age persons. The correlation of trigeminal neuralgia with arteriosclerosis was nicely described by Lewy and Grant[16] in 1938. This correlates with arteriosclerotic tortuous elongation of arteries such that vascular loops may impinge on cranial nerves. The reason for the predominance in females is not clear to me. It may be explained by the fact that the posterior fossa may be smaller in women than in men, and a horizontal looping of the superior cerebellar artery may not be able to continue to develop laterally but instead is caught by arachnoid, perhaps impinged by the tentorium and by the petrous bone, and slides along the belly of the pons rather than out into the cerebellopontile angle. This is conjectural, and better information is needed. The reflections of several observers[7,18] of demineralized soft bone and sagging brain in the elderly person may also be contributory. The presence of mild, real, sensory, and electromyographic motor deficit after prolonged trigeminal neuralgia, all of which are reversible after neurovascular decompression, belies other impressions of lack of neurological deficit.

The tendency to progression in frequency and severity of the episodes may correlate with progressive elongation of a vascular loop. Waning of pain can be explained by neural accommodation and electron microscopic evidence that has shown simultaneous denervation and reinnervation such that "short circuits" may be obliterated only for others to re-form. Treatment with some antiepileptic drugs does help some patients with tic douloureux. These are drugs which cut down neuronal transmission, normal or abnormal. It would appear by electron microscopic studies and early electrophysiological studies that there must be abnormal neuronal transmission in the trigeminal nerve of a patient with trigeminal neuralgia.

The occasional bilateral cases would appear to be more than just coincidence. We have seen and relieved bilateral neurovascular compression by the superior cerebellar arteries in a recent sequential bilateral case. A 67-year-old man developed unilateral right-sided V_2-V_3 tic and was successfully operated on 6 years later. Pain began in the left V_3 distribution 6 months later, and he was operated on shortly thereafter with consequent relief. Multiple sclerosis patients have been shown at postmortem examination to have a demyelinated plaque at the root entry zone.[19] We have now shown this in operative patients, as has Lazar,[14] and the clinical correlation is agreeable with the hypothesis. Operative findings of abnormality of the trigeminal nerve root entry zone in trigeminal neuralgia, usually vascular, serve as key evidence implicating such abnormality as a causative factor. These findings are reviewed later in this chapter. The postoperative course following decompression of the nerve at the pons is also illuminating in that mobilizaton of a vessel off the nerve without nerve trauma frequently leaves the patient with trigeminal neuralgia in the immediate postoperative period. The pain gradually becomes less frequent and severe and then disappears. This temporary pain is usually relieved by phenytoin therapy even when this same medication did not help preoperatively. The subtle sensory abnormalities found in long-standing trigeminal neuralgia revert to normal postoperatively, with improvement usually beginning immediately. The area of facial numbness following recurrence after other destructive operative procedures may shrink significantly after vascular decompression and has disappeared entirely in a few patients in whom it was mild.

Vascular compression-distortion of the nerve root entry zone has been noted by me in two brains at postmortem examination. These patients had unilateral tic douloureux on the appropriate side. Photographs of the second specimen have bee published.[14] Such specific changes have not been noted in a large number of brains at operation and at postmortem examination in those without trigeminal neuralgia, although vascular approximation is seen in about 20% of cadaver brains. It is conceivable that such changes will be further clarified later, since the duration and degree of vascular compression-distortion necessary to cause trigeminal neuralgia are not currently known.

INDICATIONS FOR OPERATION

The procedure described here appears to be indicated in patients with intractable trigeminal neuralgia who are in reasonably good health and who are not responding to medical therapy. Most of our patients have had therapy of phenytoin and carbamazepine, which was stopped for reasons of failure, toxicity to necessary dosage, or other untoward reactions. It is unfortunate that the elderly frail patients appear to be more sensitive to the side effects and complications of carbamazepine. Microvascular decompression is contraindicated in the very elderly and in those who are in poor health, but the usual older person in generally good health appears to tolerate the procedure easily. Many of our patients come to us with recurrent trigeminal neuralgia after a prior operative procedure. A prior unsuccessful procedure, or a recurrence, is no contraindication to operation. In our institution we limit radiofrequency rhizotomy to those patients who are elderly, frail, or ill, with an estimated life expectancy of less than 5 years.

The quality of life appears to differ if one has been made numb in the face versus no numbness, as with microvascular decompression, which I believe to be the procedure of choice. Others, without personal interest or bias, feel the same.[1,28] Radiofrequency lesion and microvascular decompression are compared in Table 31-1.

Table 31-1. Comparison of radio frequency rhizotomy (RF) and microvascular decompression (MVD) in the therapy of intractable trigeminal neuralgia

	RF	MVD
Pain relief		
Early	Excellent	Excellent
Late	Good	Excellent
Morbidity/mortality	Minimum	Moderate
Late problems	Sensory aberrations	None

OPERATIVE TECHNIQUE

The patient is prepared 12 hours preoperatively with dexamethasone, 10 mg intramuscularly. This is continued postoperatively in a dosage of 4 mg every 6 hours for 48 hours and then discontinued. The patient is anesthetized, intubated, and placed in the contralateral-lateral decubitus position (Fig. 31-1) using a pin-fixation head holder. A Doppler ultrasonic flowmeter is then positioned over the right atrium, and cardiac sounds are monitored throughout the operation for sounds of air emboli and changes in cardiac rate and rhythm. The neck is flexed to the point where the chin is one to two finger breadths from the sternum and the head rotated slightly to the ipsilateral side. In older patients the cerebellum appears to be comparatively smaller in the posterior fossa than in younger patients, perhaps because the brain has "sagged" and there is some atrophy.

The ipsilateral posterior side of the head from the midline to the ear and from just below the vertex to the hairline is shaved in the operating room. A vertical incision approximately 6 to 7 cm long is made, 2 cm medial to the mastoid process, with about one third of the incision above the superior nuchal line (Fig. 31-2). The incision is placed lateral enough to avoid the greater occipital nerve. The incision is carried directly to the calvaria except caudally where further dissection of the deeper muscles is performed with the electrocautery. Periosteal elevators are used to separate the nuchal muscles, fascia, and pericranium away from the calvaria. A self-retaining angulated retractor is placed (Fig. 31-3). The posterior aspect of the mastoid eminence is partially cleared. The electrocautery blade on cutting current is helpful in separating the attachments of the nuchal line to the calvaria.

A craniectomy about 3.5 or 4.0 cm in diameter is performed high and lateral in the posterior fossa, exposing the horizontal portion of the lateral sinus and extending to the sigmoid sinus laterally. The dura mater is incised about 3 or 4 mm under the lateral sinus and extending inferolaterally for several centimeters. The supralateral dura mater flap is incised to the lateral sinus and the dura sutured to the galea, tenting the lateral sinus up and away. More bone may be rongeured supralaterally at this point if exposure is not adequate. It is important to achieve this supralateral ex-

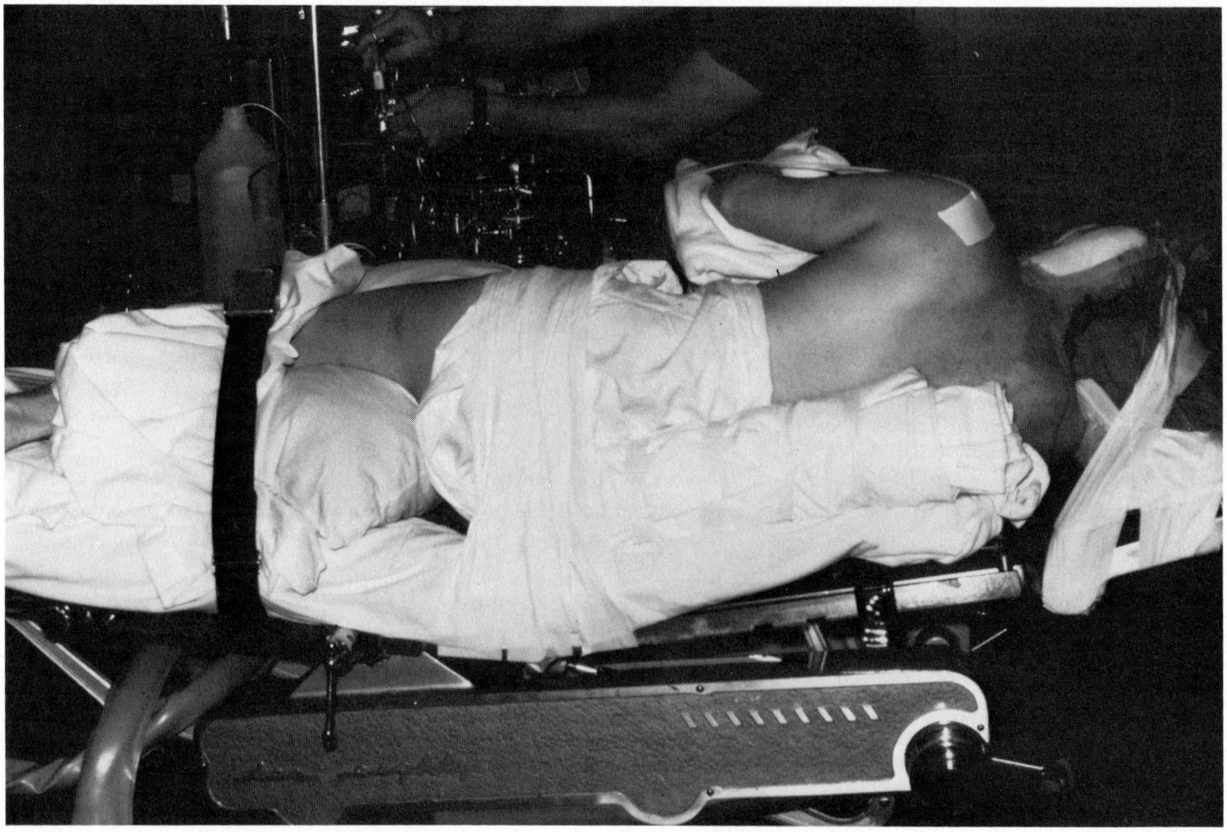

Fig. 31-1. Contralateral-lateral decubitus position for retromastoid craniectomy and microvascular decompression of cranial nerves. Excessive flexion or lateral turning of head is unnecessary.

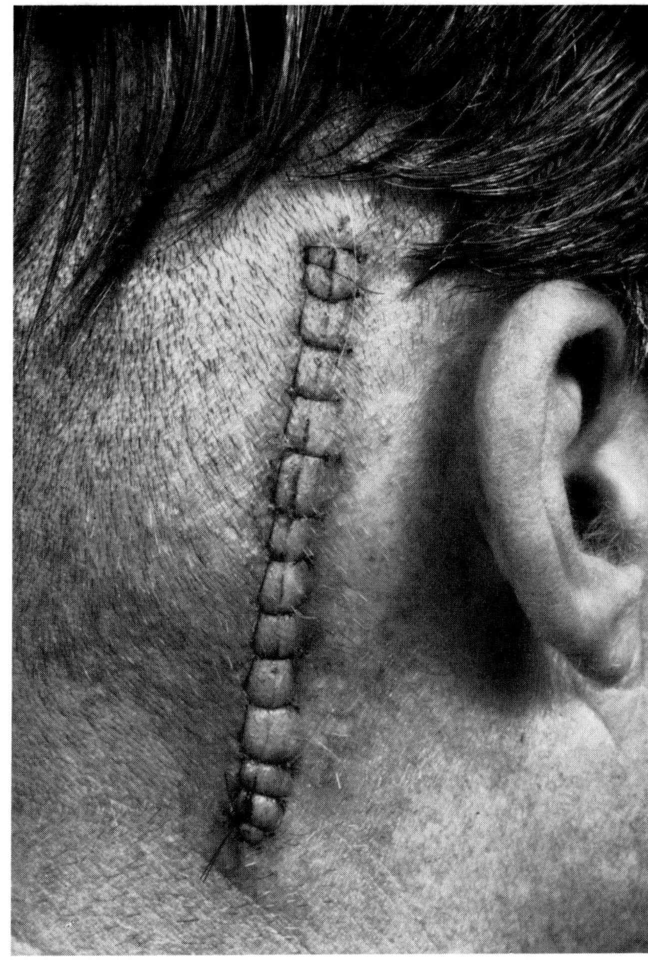

Fig. 31-2. Incision for retromastoid craniectomy is placed one finger breadth medial to the mastoid eminence and generally parallel to hairline.

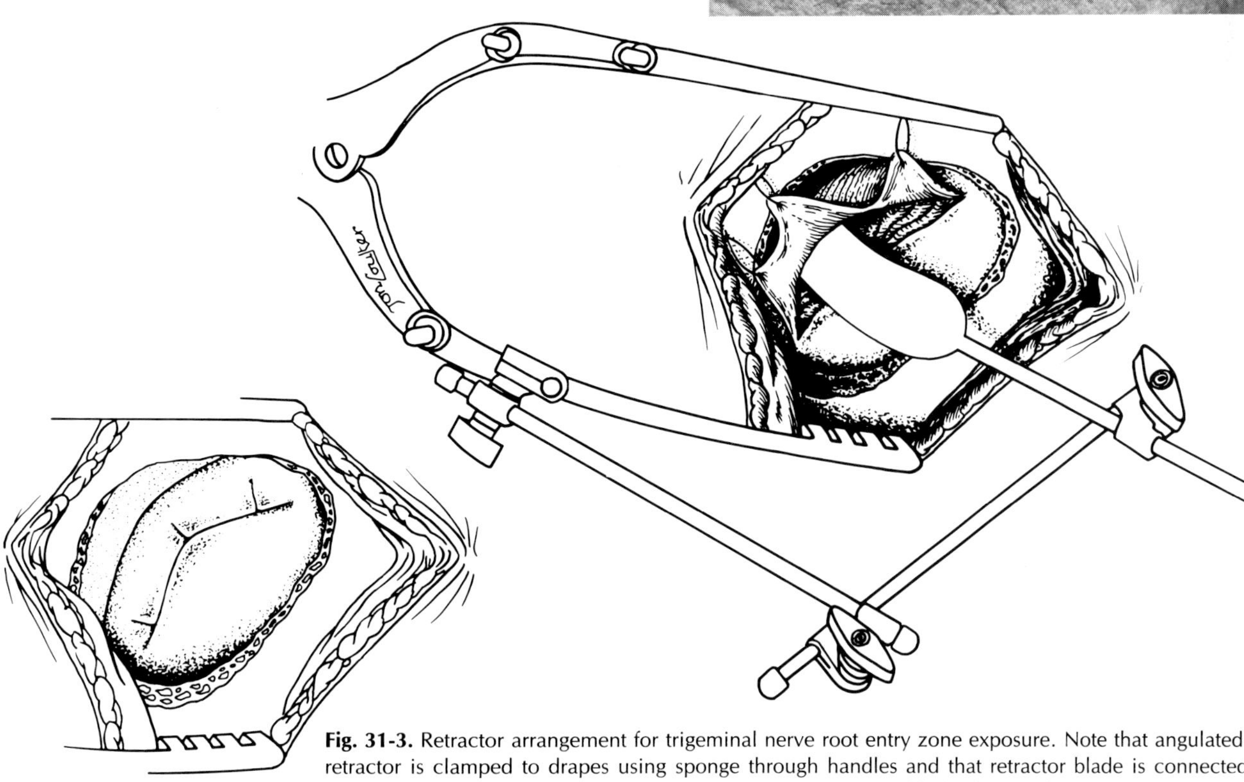

Fig. 31-3. Retractor arrangement for trigeminal nerve root entry zone exposure. Note that angulated Weitlaner retractor is clamped to drapes using sponge through handles and that retractor blade is connected with two connecting rods to post of Weitlaner. We now use narrower blade than is shown. Blade is bent proximally and not curved at all. Cerebellum is protected with piece of rubber dam and small cottonoid.

posure, and the short time necessary to obtain the exposure is well worth it. A microsurgical retractor blade, attached to a post on the angulated retractor, is then put into place over a piece of rubber dam from a piece of rubber glove cut to size. A relatively narrow blade is used, and no cerebellar retraction is done at this point. The retractor is placed superficially over the lateral aspect of the superior surface of the cerebellum.

The Zeiss surgical microscope with a 250-mm focal length objective is then used for the remainder of the procedure. Minimum retraction is necessary to find the superior petrosal vein, which is shaped like an inverted Y. The arachnoid is opened, using sharp dissection, over the vein, which is then coagulated with bipolar coagulation. A set of microsurgical instruments with bayonet-shaped handles is used for this and the remainder of the intracranial dissection. The Valsalva maneuver is performed after partial and after complete section of the vein, since it is easy to miss some of the anterior limb of the Y in coagulating.

After the superior petrosal vein is divided, the retractor is placed more deeply, again over the rubber dam, which prevents trauma to the cerebellum. The arachnoid is opened anteromedial to the vein, giving an excellent view of the trigeminal nerve. The trochlear nerve is usually seen before the trigeminal nerve is clearly visualized and is easily avoided. The dissection is too cephalad if the trochlear nerve is in the center of the field. The trigeminal nerve lies obliquely, coursing from Meckel's cave to the pons just anteromedial to the superior petrosal vein. A variable degree of sideward tilt of the operating table may be necessary at this point and subsequently to give a good line of sight to the trigeminal nerve. The retractor, with joints only partially tightened, can be moved about gently and gradually as dissection continues. The retractor must not be allowed to slip down over the side of the cerebellum onto the seventh and eighth cranial nerves or to significantly compress the cerebellum. The arachnoid is next dissected from the trigeminal nerve. It may be adherent both to the nerve and to the artery compressing the distorting nerve. The arachnoid must be separated from the trigeminal nerve for most of the length of the posterior roots. After the clinician gains some experience, the artery–trigeminal nerve relationship can usually be appreciated before the arachnoid is opened.

The usual situation in lower facial tic douloureux is that the superior cerebellar artery is found coursing cephalad around the pons and then bifurcating, with the medial and lateral branches impinging on the anterosuperior aspect of the entry zone of the nerve, the motor-proprioceptive fascicle side, as it loops back to the brain stem and cerebellum (Fig. 31-4). After sharp and blunt dissection of the widely opened arachnoid from the nerve and the visible part of the artery, the

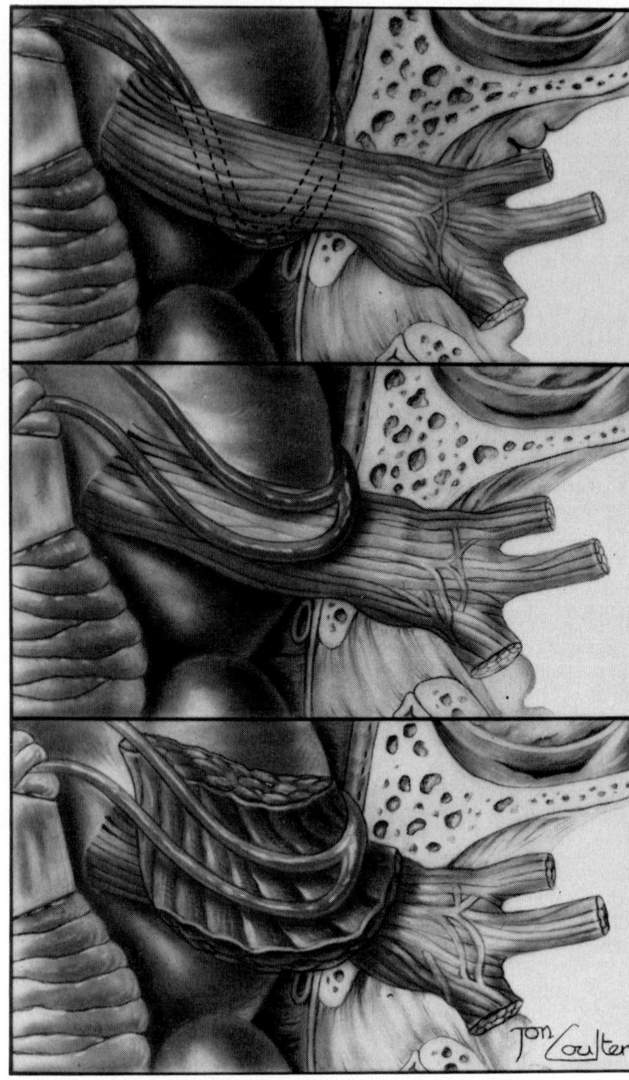

Fig. 31-4. Representation of vascular compression of right trigeminal nerve by superior cerebellar artery *(top)*, mobilization of artery *(middle)*, and interposition of implant *(bottom)*.

arterial loops are gently teased out from between the trigeminal nerve and the pons. The loops are usually longer in older patients and especially in those with long-standing trigeminal neuralgia. They must be manipulated carefully. The arterial loops may be quite adherent to the nerve or easily separable. Perforating branches to the pons have accommodated in length to the loop and will not tear with gentle manipulation of the vessel over the trigeminal nerve. The vascular loops may be too long to move safely, especially in older patients. In this case selective section of the portio major is preferable (although rarely necessary).

In first division tic douloureux the anteroinferior cerebellar artery is seen compressing the inferolateral portion of the trigeminal nerve entry zone at the pons at the portio major side. The superior cerebellar artery has a normal horizontal loop in this case. Multiple vessels are not uncommon.

A small implant of Teflon felt, plastic sponge, or muscle from the incision is placed between the brain stem and nerve on one side and the artery on the other. The implant is placed between the artery and the nerve at the brain stem. The Valsalva maneuver is performed several times under control of the anesthetist to see if the relationships are stable.

A piece of absorbable gelatin sponge (Gelfoam) is placed over the arachnoid opening. The retractor is removed and the dura closed with interrupted and running sutures of silk. The incision is closed in layers and a small dry dressing applied. Postoperatively, the head of the bed is kept elevated about 10 degrees. The patient is usually able to return from the neurosurgical continuous care unit to his or her room on the morning of the first postoperative day. Postoperative care is routine, as for any intracranial neurosurgical procedure.

If the trigeminal nerve is manipulated at operation, the patient awakens pain free. If the nerve is not traumatized during the dissection, the patient will probably have trigeminal neuralgia for a few to several days postoperatively. The attacks may not begin for several days after operation if trauma to the nerve has been minimal. The pain is usually well controlled with small doses of phenytoin. Such gradually decreasing postoperative trigeminal neuralgia has been seen in about one fourth of our patients. The postoperative trigeminal neuralgia gradually decreases in frequency and severity and disappears, not to recur. Common self-limited postoperative morbidity has consisted of temporary postoperative headaches. Operative results are collated in Table 31-2. Generally, if a patient remains free from pain for 1 year postoperatively, there will be no recurrence. We have now operated on over 600 patients with primary vascular compression, with two operative deaths, none in over 4 years. In 25 patients with tumors as the cause of their tic we have had two operative deaths, again none in over 4 years. Some patients have some occasional pain with or without medication. These patients are well and were having severe pain despite larger doses of stronger medications preoperatively. To date, we have lost just one patient to follow-up.

Microvascular decompression appears to be a safe, effective treatment for trigeminal neuralgia. It is definitive, since the cause of the pain is relieved without causing numbness, paresthesia, or anesthesia dolorosa. The patient has therefore no reminder of the past pain. It is indicated in patients with intractable trigeminal neuralgia who are in reasonably good health.

Patient series

This group consisted of 411 patients with classic trigeminal neuralgia, 239 women and 172 men age 19 to 76, with a median decade of 50 to 60 years old. The pain was located on the right side in 246 patients, on the left side in 153 patients, and bilaterally in 12 patients. The pain usually had a lower and/or central facial location, with 40 patients having pain over the entire $V_{1\text{-}2\text{-}3}$ distribution and only eight patients having pure V_1 pain. Seventy-five patients suffered from V_2 pain, 67 from V_3, 65 from $V_{1\text{-}2}$, and 159 from $V_{2\text{-}3}$. The duration ranged from less than 1 to 67 years.

Table 31-2. Microvascular decompression (MVD) in trigeminal neuralgia

Result of operation	Number	Percent	
Well after MVD*	343	83.5	83.5
No pain, taking medication	38	9.3	92.8
Occasional mild pain, no medication	2	0.5	93.3
Frank recurrence	22		
Relief after RFL†	17	4.1	97.4
Persistent severe pain	5	1.2	98.6
Deceased	5	1.2	99.8
Postoperatively (3)			
Suicide (1)			
Accident (1)			
Status unknown	1	0.2	100.0
TOTAL	411	100.0	

*Repeat operation necessary in 15 patients.
†Radiofrequency lesion.

Operative findings

Abnormalities of the root entry zone of the trigeminal nerve in these 411 patients are as follows:

Arterial	242
Aneurysm	1
Venous	57
Ateriovenous malformation	1
Mixed arterial/venous	96
Tumor	15
No pathosis	1
Unrecorded	1

Several points can be made about the clinical-pathological correlation:

1. These abnormalities are quite specific and can be correlated with the location and type of symptom, that is, lower facial trigeminal neuralgia is usually caused by a blood vessel (most commonly superior cerebellar artery on the rostral side of the nerve), V_1 tic by a vessel on the caudal aspect of the root entry zone, and isolated V_2 tic by a vessel on the side of the nerve. Similar correlations are seen in hemifacial spasm and in

cochlear and/or vestibular symptoms in the eighth nerve.
2. Multiple vessels are commonly found and were frequently missed early in this series.
3. Veins that have been coagulated and divided may recollateralize, causing recurrence of symptoms.
4. Blood vessels are uncommonly seen cross-compressing the root entry zone of an asymptomatic cranial nerve inspected at operation when another nerve is being operated on. I do not know why some vascular cross-compression, like much cervical and lumbar disc disease and spondylosis, produces no symptoms.
5. Root entry zone vascular compression is frequently subtle. Well-trained microsurgeons may not appreciate up to 30% of the abnormalities early in their experience with these procedures. These are "unforgiving procedures,"[9] which demand petty attention to detail if one is to make valid observations and operate safely.

Operative results and complications

Several points of interest should be briefly discussed. Repeat operations were sometimes necessary to decompress the nerve satisfactorily. The most common reason for lack of response was a missed blood vessel or vessel that had not been properly decompressed; next was a recollateralized vein, and last, new late vascular compression caused by continuing arterial elongation. Thirty-eight patients take some medication, usually small doses of phenytoin, to remain pain free. Two have occasional discomfort without medication. These groups together (with total or significant relief) constitute 92.8% of the patients.

Operative deaths in the entire series were from stroke (two patients) and brain stem infarction (two patients); one was a 79-year-old woman, and two were patients with tumors (one, a leukemic patient, was admitted for a radiofrequency rhizotomy and had a 4-cm diameter acoustic neuroma; one had a large undiagnosed angioma). We have now had no operative deaths in over 350 consecutive patients.

REFERENCES

1. Apfelbaum, R.I.: A comparison of percutaneous radiofrequency trigeminal neurolysis and microvascular decompression of the trigeminal nerve for the treatment of tic douloureux, Neurosurgery **1**:16, 1977.
2. Baringer, J.R., and Swoveland, P.: Recovery of herpes-simplex virus from human trigeminal ganglions, N. Engl. J. Med. **288**:648, 1973.
3. Dandy, W.E.: Section of the sensory root of the trigeminal nerve at the pons, Bull. Johns Hopkins Hosp. **36**:105, 1925.
4. Dandy, W.E.: Operation for cure of tic douloureux; partial section of the sensory root at the pons, Arch. Surg. **18**:687, 1929.
5. Dandy, W.E.: Treatment of trigeminal neuralgia by the cerebellar route, Ann. Surg. **96**:787, 1932.
6. Gardner, W.J.: Concerning the mechanism of trigeminal neuralgia and hemifacial spasm, J. Neurosurg. **19**:947, 1962.
7. Gardner, W.J., Todd, E.M., and Pinto, J.P.: Roentgenographic findings in trigeminal neuralgia, Am. J. Roentgenol. **76**:346, 1956.
8. Gudmundsson, K., Rhoton, A.L., and Rushton, J.G.: Detailed anatomy of the intracranial portion of the trigeminal nerve, J. Neurosurg. **35**:592, 1971.
9. Haines, S.J., Martinez, J.A., and Jannetta, P.J.: Arterial cross-compression of the trigeminal nerve at the pons in trigeminal neuralgia, J. Neurosurg. **50**:257, 1979.
10. Jannetta, P.J.: Microsurgical approach to the trigeminal nerve for tic douloureux. In Krayenbuhl, H., Maspes, P.E., and Sweet, W.H., (editors): Progress in neurological surgery, vol. 7, Pain—its neurosurgical management, Basel, Switzerland, 1976, S. Karger GA.
11. Jannetta, P.J.: Treatment of trigeminal neuralgia by suboccipital and transtentorial cranial operations, Clin. Neurosurg. **24**:538, 1977.
12. Kerr, F.W.L.: Evidence for a peripheral etiology of trigeminal neuralgia, J. Neurosurg. **26**:168, 1967.
13. Knight, G.: Herpes simplex and trigeminal neuralgia, Proc. R. Soc. Med. **47**:788, 1954.
14. Lazar, M.: Trigeminal neuralgia: recent advances in management, Tex. Med. **75**:45, 1978.
15. Lee, F.C.: Trigeminal neuralgia, J. Med. Assoc. Ga. **26**:431, 1937.
16. Lewy, F.H., and Grant, F.C.: Physiopathologic and pathoanatomic anatomic aspects of major trigeminal neuralgia, Arch. Neurol. Psychiatr. **40**:1126, 1938.
17. Ley, A., and Bacci, F.: Trigeminal neuralgia: sensory defects and clinical results after selective division of the fifth nerve root by the suboccipital approach, using microsurgical technique. Excerpta Medica Fifth International Congress Neurological Surgery, Tokyo, 1973, p. 123.
18. Malis, L.I.: Petrous ridge compression and its surgical correction, J. Neurosurg. **26**:163, 1967.
19. Olafson, R.A., Rushton, J.G., and Sayre, G.P.: Trigeminal neuralgia in a patient with multiple sclerosis: an autopsy report, J. Neurosurg. **24**:755, 1966.
20. Olivecrona, H.: La cirugia del dolor, Arch. Neurochir. **4**:1, 1947.
20a. Pelletier, V.A., Poulos, D.A., and Lende, R.A.: Functional localization in the trigeminal root, J. Neurosurg. **40**:504, 1974.
21. Pertuiset, B., Philippon, J., Fohanno, D., and Khalil, M.: Traitement microchirurgical de la névralgie Laciale essentielle par neurotomie rétrogassérienne sélective transtentorielle, Rev. Neurol. **126**:97, 1972.
22. Provost, J., and Hardy, J.: Microchirurgie du trijumeau: anatomie fonctionnelle, Neurochirurgie **16**:459, 1970.
23. Reaves, D.L., Moses, H.L., and Ganote, C.E.: Electron microscopy of the trigeminal ganglion: trigeminal neuralgia, Arch Pathol. **79**:571, 1965.
24. Revilla, A.G.: Tic douloureux and its relationship to tumors of the posterior fossa, J. Neurosurg. **4**:233, 1947.
25. Saunders, R.L., Krout, R., and Sachs, E., Jr.: Masticator electromyography in trigeminal neuralgia, Neurology (Minneap.) **21**:1221, 1971.
26. Taarnhøj, P.: Decompression of the trigeminal root and the posterior part of the ganglion as treatment of trigeminal neuralgia, J. Neurosurg. **9**:288, 1952.
27. Vidic, B., and Stefanotas, J.: The roots of the trigeminal nerves and their fiber components, Anat. Rec. **163**:330, 1969.
28. Voorhies, R., and Patterson, R.H.: Management of trigeminal neuralgia, J.A.M.A. **245**:2521, 1981.

32 Modern diagnosis and management of musculoskeletal dysfunctions of the head and neck

BERNARD JANKELSON, D.M.D.

Diversity of opinion has long characterized the approach to the etiology and treatment of the various manifestations of mandibular dysfunction. By the latter part of the nineteenth century there was a distinct awareness of the disturbance and speculation as to its nature. That speculation has continued throughout the past century.

The ailment became known as the temporomandibular joint (TMJ) syndrome, perhaps because the physical manifestations, such as grinding noises, clicking, and pain, were most obvious in the joint. The search for causality soon centered on the occlusion of the teeth, since they shared articulation of the mandible to the skull with the affected temporomandibular joints. Alteration of the occlusion by grinding became the most common method of treatment.[1]

In the early part of this century the concept that generalized, emotionally induced muscle tension initiated, perpetuated, and was responsible for the dysfunction attained considerable acceptance.[18,19,23-25] Proponents of this theory, although largely discounting the role of occlusion, consider generalized muscle tension the primary cause. Their theory led to the descriptive designation of myofascial pain-dysfunction (MPD) syndrome.[23,24]

ADVANCES IN ELECTRONIC DIAGNOSTIC AND TREATMENT INSTRUMENTATION

In other areas of body dysfunction the advent of electronic diagnostic and treatment instrumentation has literally revolutionized the clinical approach. Examples in the field of cardiovascular dysfunction are the electrocardiogram (ECG), which has long been used to retrieve and display diagnostic information, and the cardiac pacemaker, which was designed to control and monitor muscle contraction. In the diagnosis and monitoring of neurological dysfunction the electroencephalogram (EEG) electrically provides previously unattainable diagnostic data. In the field of neuromuscular dysfunction the electromyogram (EMG) generally provides similar capability.

In the field of craniomandibular dysfunction no comparable instrumentation has been available to the clinician. The ability to electronically retrieve diagnostic data and to control and monitor craniomandibular muscle contraction until recently had not kept pace with progress in the management of other specialized body areas. Comparable instrumentation for diagnosis and treatment of musculoskeletal dysfunctions of the head and neck had to await the development of today's electronic and computer capability. High-technology instrumentation for the routine diagnosis and treatment of craniomandibular dysfunction in everyday practice has now become a reality.[15,16]

The Myo-Monitor

The Myo-Monitor* (Fig. 32-1), specifically designed to accomplish relaxation of the mandibular musculature by stimulation of the fifth and seventh nerves,[15,20] simultaneously relaxes the various mandibular muscles to their resting lengths. The resulting physiological rest position provides the indispensable reference from which to attain a neuromuscular (myocentric) occlusal position.[6-10,14]

Uses of the Myo-Monitor

To propel the mandible from rest position through the interocclusal (freeway) space to the position of myocentric occlusion. At intervals of $1^1/_2$ seconds, in response to the Myo-Monitor stimulus, the muscles con-

*Myo-Tronics Research, Inc., Seattle, Wash.

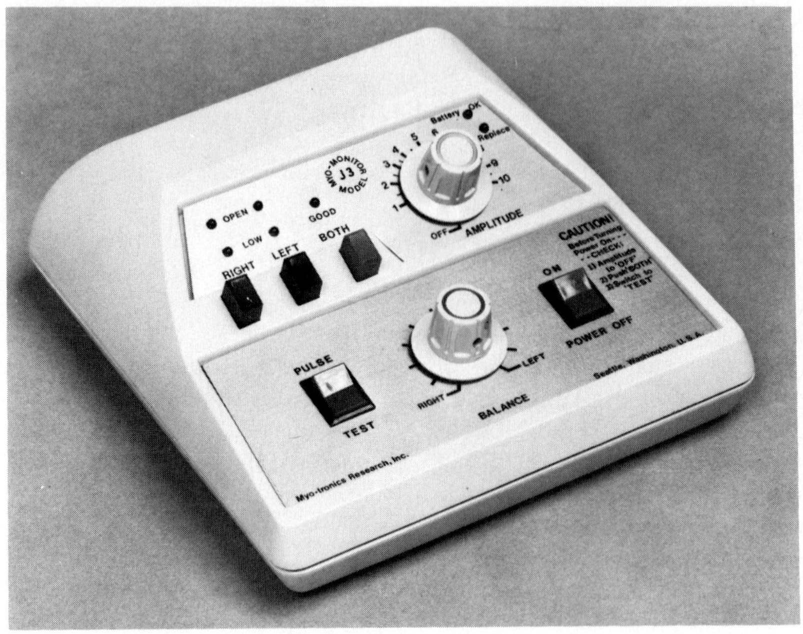

Fig. 32-1. J3 Myo-Monitor.

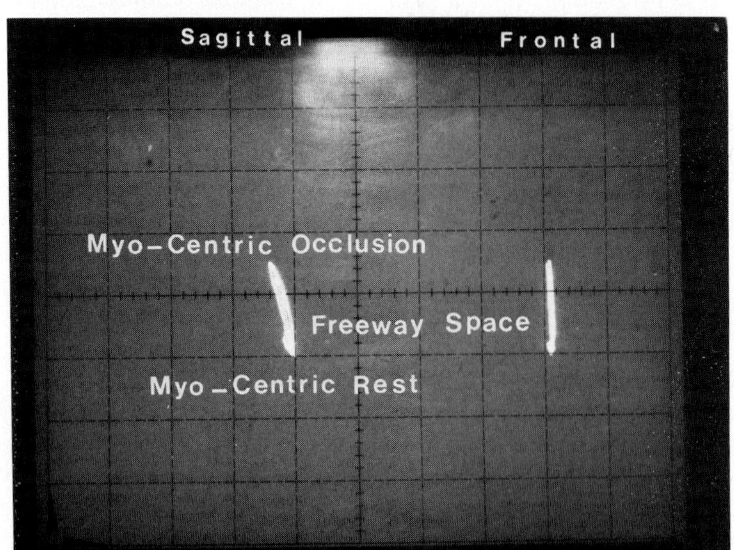

Fig. 32-2. Electronically induced isotonic trajectory of closure from rest to position of myocentric occlusion.

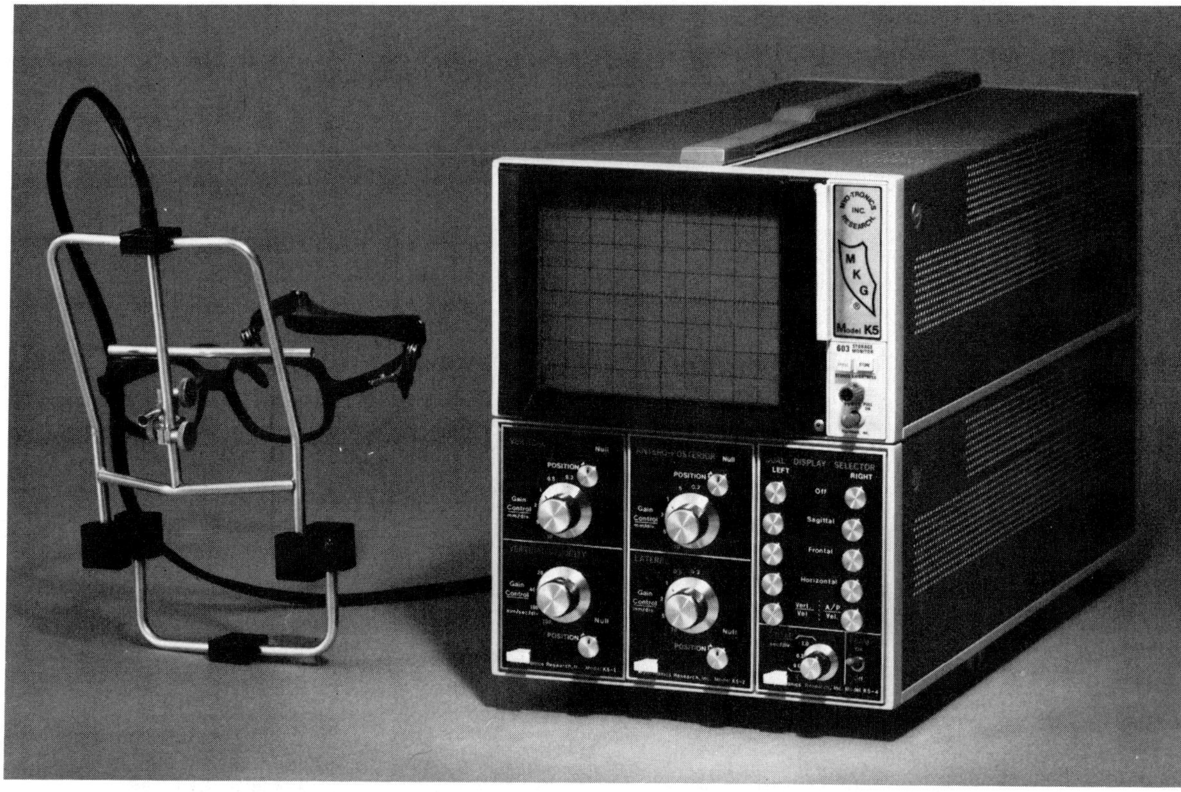

Fig. 32-3. Mandibular Kinesiograph for tracking mandibular movement and skeletal relation to skull.

tract and propel the mandible on a relaxed isotonic trajectory through the freeway space to the position at which occlusion would be most favorable to the perpetuation of a relaxed neuromusculature[7,8] (Fig. 32-2). Propelling the mandible from rest position to occlusion under the influence of balanced, programmed stimuli bypasses the disruptive influence of proprioception that is present in central nervous system–directed closure and eliminates variables induced by manipulation imposed on the mandible by the practitioner. *The resulting myocentric occlusal position is a result of decisions made by the relaxed musculature itself.*

To relieve facial pain. Transcutaneous electrical neural stimulation (TENS) is being increasingly used in various areas of the body for relief from pain. A rationale for this procedure was suggested by the gate control theory of Melzak and Wall[8] and now by the data regarding the excretion of endorphins—large polypeptide opiate molecules—which appear in the bloodstream following electrical stimulation. The Myo-Monitor is being used effectively as a palliative modality and an adjunct to the overall treatment of atypical facial neuralgia, headache, earache, ticlike pain, and tic douloureux.[9]

To record skeletal relation at various degrees of mouth opening. The Mandibular Kinesiograph* (MKG)[6-12,16] was developed to electronically track mandibular movement and to record the skeletal relation of the mandible to the skull in three spatial dimensions, plus the fourth dimension of time (Figs. 32-3 and 32-4). The additional capability to track vertical velocity of the mandible during opening and closing movements[12-16] not only provides an overall assessment of the functional status of the musculature but also diagnostically records and displays the presence of joint dysfunction, which occurs as interarticular disc displacement that interferes with untrammeled muscle movement[5] (Fig. 32-5).

Computerization of the data. The MKG Data Analyzer* (Fig. 32-6) is a dedicated, microprocessor-based minicomputer that interfaces with the MKG. It refines linearization accuracy of the MKG data, cancels 60-cycle electrical noise interference, and provides an alphabetical-numeric display on the MKG screen.[12]

---

*Myo-Tronics Research, Inc., Seattle, Wash.

A

B

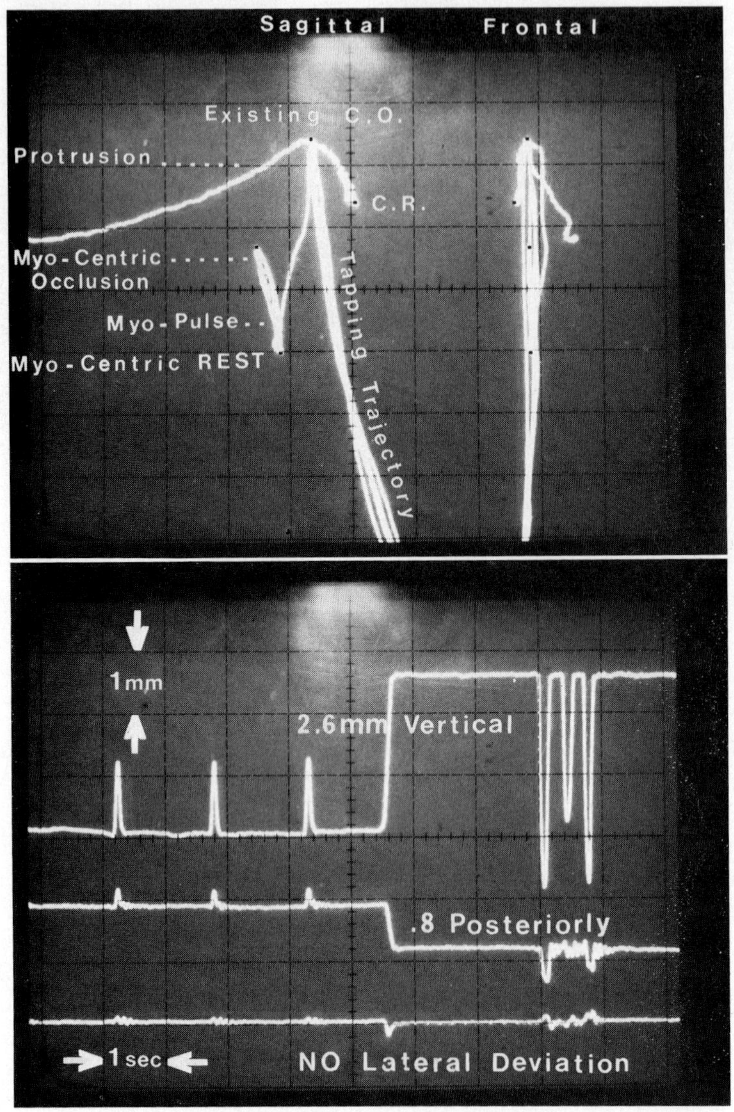

Fig. 32-4. A, Polaroid photograph of MKG display (1 mm per division). Centric occlusion *(C.O.)* position is posterior and vertical to myocentric position. A single closure to the malpositioned C.O. programs a chronic malpositioned (tapping) trajectory. **B,** Simultaneous three-channel (vertical, anteroposterior, lateral) sweep mode display on Kinesiograph CRT screen shows periodic mandibular movement and relaxation phase in response to Myo-Monitor stimuli, followed by voluntary closure, then several taps to occlusion.

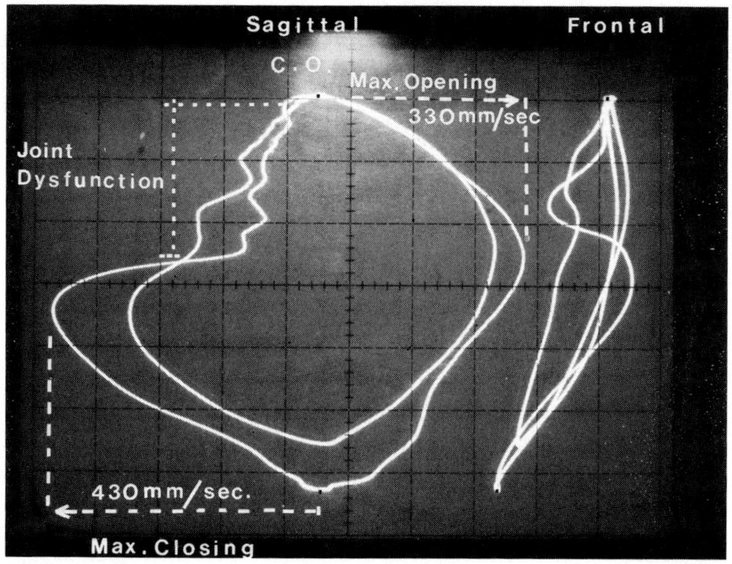

Fig. 32-5. Simultaneous (MKG) display of vertical velocity and frontal view of lateral deviation. Note "click points" as mandible closes to occlusion.

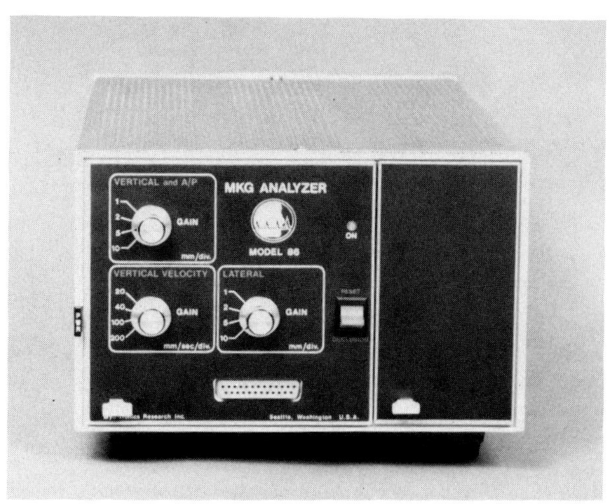

Fig. 32-6. Dedicated microprocessor-based data analyzer (minicomputer).

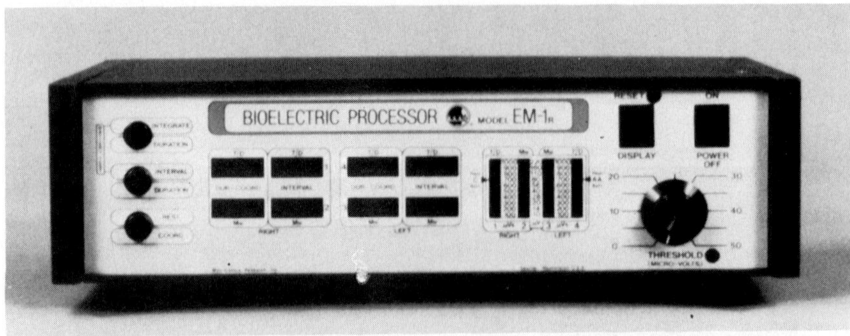

Fig. 32-7. High-sensitivity four-channel portable solid-state EMG, which operates in everyday clinical environment and provides raw, filtered, or integrated data.

A

B

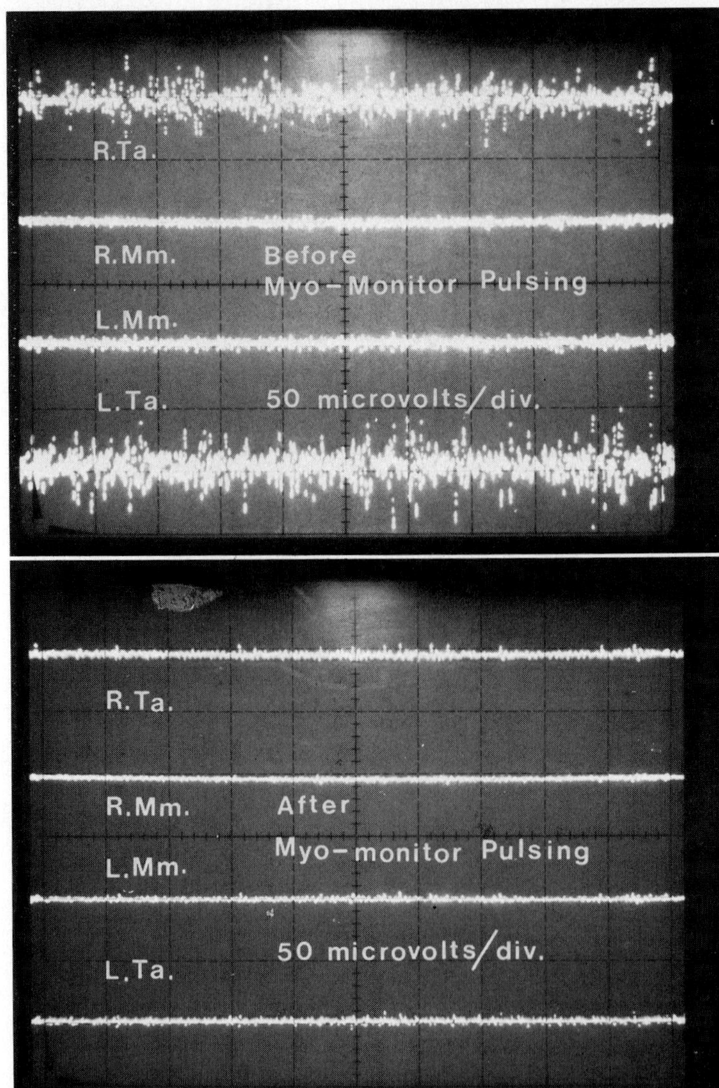

Fig. 32-8. A, Before Myo-Monitor relaxation. **B,** After 40 minutes of Myo-Monitor relaxation.

To measure electrical activity of specific muscles. The Myo-Tronics EMG Bioelectric Processor (Fig. 32-7) is a compact, solid-state EMG. It eliminates the need for shielded rooms and advances electromyography into the everyday office environment. The Myo-Tronics EMG is used to diagnostically assess the degree of activity in individual muscles before treatment (Fig. 32-8, *A*) and to monitor the response of the various muscles during treatment. Since the relaxation response to stimulation is influenced by factors such as variations in muscle metabolism and existing energy reserves in different individuals and the chronicity and duration of muscle tension,[4,22] the EMG enables the clinician to determine whether after using the Myo-Monitor the muscles have relaxed fully in the usual 40 minutes of pulsing (Fig. 32-8, *B*), or whether more time is still required for further relaxation before proceeding with the maxillomandibular record.[3]

SPECIFIC CAUSES OF MUSCULOSKELETAL DYSFUNCTION OF THE HEAD AND NECK

Aside from conditions such as accidental injury, rheumatoid arthritis, neoplasms, metastatic gonorrheal infection, rickets, scurvy, acromegaly, and cretinism, derangements of the temporomandibular joints most commonly seen by the dentist are a result of trauma stemming from excessive and prolonged torquing forces exerted on the articular structures by chronically hyperactive mandibular musculature.[10] Subjected to such repeated trauma, interarticular discs become thin, perforated, and/or displaced from the head of the condyle. Sustained muscle pressures acting on the bony structures cause disc disruption and remodeling of condylar heads and articular eminences. The resulting osteoarthrosis is usually accompanied by some degree of osteoarthritis and fibrositis.

CLUSTER SYMPTOMS OF MUSCULOSKELETAL DYSFUNCTION OF THE HEAD AND NECK

In the past decade it has become generally recognized that the syndrome is not only a dysfunction of the TMJ complex but also that a *cluster* of symptoms going beyond that of joint pain and dysfunction characterize the condition. In addition to TMJ involvement, other manifestations of the syndrome might include acute and chronic tension headaches, neck and shoulder stiffness, earache, eustachian tube dysfunction and ear stuffiness, tinnitus, vertigo, atypical facial neuralgia, tic douloureux, and ticlike pain.[2a]

Any of these symptoms may exist alone or in combination with any of the others. Because of the varied and often opposing concepts of diagnosis and treatment, mandibular dysfunction is commonly regarded as a disturbance with multiple causes.[18,19,23-25] Now, however, modern electronic computer science has uncovered a common cause for this cluster of symptoms, establishing them as variations of response to a common underlying factor.

Nature of the musculoskeletal head and neck syndrome

The data clearly identify a classifiable disease entity and establish two basic aspects of the disease:

1. There is a skeletal malrelation of the mandible to the skull, mandated by proprioceptive dictation that the muscles hold the mandible on a distorted trajectory to accomplish closure to a malpositioned occlusion. The resulting distorted position of the mandible, held by the muscles under tension, now malposes the condyles in the joint space.[13]
2. Neuromuscular hyperfunction, spasm, and myostatic contracture induced by the proprioceptive dictation hold the mandible on a deflected, mucularly unbalanced trajectory to accomplish intercuspation to a three-dimensionally malpositioned occlusion. (See Fig. 32-4.)

In summary in the syndrome of musculoskeletal dysfunctions of the head and neck: (1) the soft tissue disturbance lies primarily in the neuromusculature, ligaments, and tendons of the area, and (2) the bony, skeletal malrelationships, stemming from neuromuscular adaptation to malpositioned dental occlusion, change the relationships of the temporomandibular joints and their articular components.

How malpositioned occlusion creates malpositioning of the condyles within the joint space

When a malpositioned occlusion induces sustained muscle contracture, condylar structures are pulled out of their relaxed position in the glenoid fossae. They then impinge against the pain and pressure nerve receptors located at the borders of the joint space. The most common cause of condylar dysfunction in the components of the temporomandibular joint is trauma from sustained contraction of a deranged craniomandibular musculature.

The mandibular muscles are endowed with significantly more muscle spindles than are any other muscles of the body.[17] The unique proprioceptive mechanism in the oral cavity operates to program the muscles to close the mouth to the existing intercuspal position. If the occlusion of the teeth occurs at the most neuromuscularly quiet position, the musculature carries the mandible to this myocentric occlusal position with unstrained muscle contraction. On the other hand, for example, if occlusion is positioned posterior to the myocentric relationship, the temporal and digastric muscles particularly are programmed to chronically contract so that occlusion of the teeth can be accomplished. These muscles will then be in a state of chronic shortening.[7,8] Another complication is that their antagonists, the external pterygoids, will be in a state of myostatic stretch. If the occlusion is malpositioned lateral to the right or left, the opposite external pterygoids are chronically contracted to bring the teeth to occlusion.

The data derived from MKG recordings establish clearly and consistently that it only requires a single closure to a malpositioned occlusion to program the craniomandibular muscles into the unremitting myostatic contracture mandated proprioceptively by the occlusion. (See Fig. 32-4, *A*.) The frequency of closure to occlusion during acts such as swallowing continually reinforces the dictum to the musculature to hold the mandible on the strained trajectory required to close to occlusion.

TREATMENT OF THE DERANGED TEMPOROMANDIBULAR JOINT

Realigning the occlusion so the teeth intercuspate as the mouth closes through the freeway space on the neuromuscular trajectory from myocentric rest position also provides the most favorable environment for the temporomandibular joints to repair the damage caused by persistent muscle-induced trauma. The rapidity with which symptoms such as restricted opening, clicking, crepitus, and pain subside will depend on the degree of damage within the joint.

The myocentric position of occlusion

The myocentric position is characteristically anterior to the conventional retruded centric-relation position, so the condyles are situated more anteriorly in the joint space. In addition, the three-dimensional myocentric position is frequently more open vertically compared with the existing occlusion, further contributing to anterior positioning of the condyles, which provides a more favorable environment for a displaced disc to be repositioned and reattached to the head of the condyle.[5]

Joint surgery

If the joint, given time, does not respond to the conservative noninvasive therapy of relaxing the muscles and then repositioning the mandible orthopedically, it may be assumed that the damage within the joint is irreparable with noninvasive treatment and that surgical intervention may be necessary.[17] *It is important that after surgery attention be given to reconciliation of the occlusion to the new skeletal relation resulting from the joint surgery.*

Diagnostic and treatment procedures

Conventional procedures, such as TMJ radiographs and muscle palpation, are carried out as usual. However, today's instrumental capability to retrieve and quantify data goes considerably beyond these conventional procedures. The first step in diagnosis is to obtain the Kinesiograph data as to the extent of skeletal malrelation and muscle hyperactivity. Additional information as to the status of various individual muscles may be obtained with the Myo-Tronics EMG.

Relaxation of the mandibular musculature

The next step in diagnosis is to relax the mandibular musculature by pulsing with the Myo-Monitor for approximately 40 minutes, or more if indicated by EMG recordings. The mandible should then be lying suspended at neuromuscular rest position.

Registration of myocentric occlusal position

To *register* the myocentric maxillomandibular relation, one must propel the mandible from rest position on a tension-free, isotonic trajectory through the interocclusal (freeway) space to the muscularly quiet myocentric occlusal position.

Because the sudden introduction of any registration material alters the muscle response, it is important to first determine the myocentric "empty mouth" relation of the mandible to the skull, either by placing adhesive tape on the nose and chin as a reference, then adjusting a pair of inside calipers to the inside vertical position, or, preferably, by electronically monitoring the empty-mouth position of the mandible on the MKG screen. Then, when the myoprint* registration is being taken, either of these references can be used to monitor and correct mandibular position during registration. Electronically monitoring the position of the mandible on the MKG screen under great magnification further ensures the precision of the registration.

The casts are mounted on the Myo-Tronics Terminus Articulator* using the myoprint registration. If indicated, a Myo-Tronics repositioning appliance[11] (splint) is fabricated and equilibrated using the Myo-Monitor. When, under the influence of the more neuromuscularly favorable jaw position, the symptoms subside, and the corrected maxillomandibular skeletal relation is then used as the reference for orthodontic treatment, using recently developed orthodontic techniques and appliances that treat the case three dimensionally. When, with the casts mounted on the Myo-Tronics Terminus Articulator to the corrected myocen-

*Myo-Tronics Research, Inc., Seattle, Wash.

tric relation, freeway space is so excessive that prosthetic reconstruction cannot be done without excessive crown length, vertical dimension should first be corrected by orthodontic eruption of the posterior teeth. New orthodontic techniques make this a very practical procedure. The determination of whether prosthodontic full-mouth reconstruction is indicated depends on the extent to which the cuspal anatomy has been destroyed and whether it must be restored to achieve a cusp-to-fossa occlusion.

SUMMARY

The diagnosis and treatment of musculoskeletal dysfunctions of the head and neck enter a new phase with the availability of high-technology electronic instrumentation. It enables the practitioner to derive objective, electronically measured data on which to base the diagnosis and by which to monitor progress of treatment. The data shed new light on the nature of the disturbance.

The new findings establish the nature and the specificity of the craniomandibular TMJ syndrome. The *skeletal malrelationships* here described affect the articular components, consisting of the occlusion and the temporomandibular joints. The *soft tissue disturbance* lies primarily in the neuromusculature.

REFERENCES

1. Dawson, P.E.: Evaluation, diagnosis and treatment of occlusal problems, St. Louis, 1974, The C.V. Mosby Co.
2. DeSteno, C.V.: The pathophysiology of TMJ dysfunction and related pain: clinical management of head, neck and TMJ pain and dysfunction, Philadelphia, 1977, W.B. Saunders Co.

2a. Dinham, R.: Treatment of tic douloureux with Jankelson Myo-Monitor, J. Hawaii Dent. Assoc., vol. III, 1970.

3. Dixon, H.H., and Dickel, H.A.: Tension headache, Northwest Med. **66**:817, 1967.
4. Dixon, H.H., O'Hara, M., and Peterson, R.D.: Fatigue contracture of skeletal muscle, Northwest Med. **66**:813, 1967.
5. Farrar, W.B., and McCarty, W.L., Jr.: Inferior joint space arthrography and characteristics of condylar paths in internal derangements of the TMJ, J. Prosthet. Dent. **41**:548, 1979.
6. George, J.P., and Boone, M.E.: A clinical study of rest position using the Kinesiograph and Myo-Monitor, J. Prosthet. Dent. **41**:456, 1979.
7. Jankelson, B.: Functional positions of occlusion, J. Prosthet. Dent. **30**:559, 1973.
8. Jankelson, B.: Neuromuscular aspects of occlusion, Dent. Clin. North Am. **23**:157, 1979.
9. Jankelson, B.: Neuromuscular technology for complete dentures. In Proceedings of the Second International Prosthodontic Congress, St. Louis, 1979, The C.V. Mosby Co.
10. Jankelson, B.: Research findings and resultant management of craniomandibular (TMJ) symptom cluster syndrome. In Proceedings of the Second International Prosthodontic Congress, St. Louis, 1979, The C.V. Mosby Co.
11. Jankelson, B.: A manual—The Myo-Tronic orthopedic splint, Seattle, Wash., 1980, Myo-Tronics Research, Inc.
12. Jankelson, B.: Measurement accuracy of the Mandibular Kinesiograph—a computerized study, J. Prosthet. Dent. **44**:656, 1980.
13. Jankelson, B.: The effect of the Myo-Monitor on relaxation of the craniomandibular musculature, Unpublished manuscript, 1981.
14. Jankelson, B., and Radke, J.C.: The Myo-Monitor: its use and abuse (2 parts), Quint. Int., Feb. 1978; March 1978.
15. Jankelson, B., Sparks, S., Crane, P.F., and Radke, J.C.: Neural conduction of the Myo-Monitor stimulus: a quantitive analysis, J. Prosthet. Dent. **34**:245, 1975.
16. Jankelson, B., Swain, C.W., Crane, P.F., and Radke, J.C.: Kinesiometric instrumentation: a new technology, J. Am. Dent. Assoc. **90**:834, 1975.
17. Kubota, K., and Masegi, T.: Muscle spindle supply to human jaw muscle, J. Dent. Res. **56L**:901, 1977.
18. Laskin, D.M.: Etiology of the pain dysfunction syndrome, J. Am. Dent. Assoc. **79**:144, 1969.
19. Lupton, D.E.: Psychological aspects of temporomandibular joint dysfunction, J. Am. Dent. Assoc. **79**:131, 1969.
20. Martinis, A.J., Jankelson, B., Radke, J.C., and Adib, F.: Effects of the Myo-Monitor on cardiac pacemakers, J. Am. Dent. Assoc. **100**:203, 1980.
21. McCarty, W.L., Jr., and Farrar, W.B.: Surgery for internal derangements of the temporomandibular joint, J. Prosthet. Dent. **42**:191, 1979.
22. Myo-Tronics Research, Inc.: Interpretation of the MKG tracings, a manual, Seattle, Wash., 1981, Myo-Tronics Research, Inc.
23. Schwartz, L.: Pain associated with the temporomandibular joint, J. Am. Dent. Assoc. **51**:394, 1955.
24. Schwartz, L.: Disorders of the temporomandibular joint, Philadelphia, 1959, W.B., Saunders Co.
25. Sutcher, H., et al.: Comparison of responses to pharmacological and physical placebo therapy in TMJ dysfunction patients, IADR Abstracts, p. 243, 1966.

33 Legal aspects

EDWIN J. ZINMAN, D.D.S., J.D.

ELEMENTS OF A SUIT FOR PROFESSIONAL NEGLIGENCE

Tort law defined

A *tort* is a civil wrong independent of contract. *Guilt* applies to criminal offenses that are inapplicable to the civil law. Accordingly, "guilty of malpractice" is a nonsequitur. Money damages rather than punishment of fine and/or imprisonment distinguish the tort remedy from criminal law penalties.

Negligent conduct

Malpractice is one variant of tortious conduct when the term is applied to carelessness or negligence of professional persons, such as physicians, dentists, attorneys, architects, engineers, or accountants. As applied to medicine and dentistry, it is the failure to treat a patient in accordance with proper, accepted practice, called *due care,* resulting in harm to the patient.

Burden of proof

In a malpractice suit the plaintiff has the burden of proof and must show a preponderance of evidence to sustain the plaintiff's verdict. Essential elements of proof are (1) a doctor-patient relationship (a fiduciary obligation of trust and fair dealings thereby results), (2) breach of the practitioner's fiduciary duty owed to the patient, and (3) injuries or damages proximately resulting from breach of this duty.

LEGAL CAUSES OF ACTION FOR PROFESSIONAL MALPRACTICE

Warranty of cure

Under the Code of Hammurabi a physician was responsible for a cure, and if the patient suffered loss of an eye, authorities removed the treating physician's eye. Presumably, justice was blind in those days, along with some of the medical practitioners. Over time the emphasis has shifted from responsibility based on an untoward result to a system in which fault must be proved. Under modern law no liability results from honest errors of judgment, so long as the judgment appeared reasonable in foresight, even though in hindsight a different judgment would seem better.

Breach of warranty and/or contract

Ordinarily a physician or dentist is not a guarantor or an insurer of successful TMJ therapy nor of a particular method of treatment. Failure, relapse, or poor results may occur despite the best of care, and this is ordinarily not actionable, provided that standard therapeutic methods are followed and the patient is warned in advance of likely untoward results.[1]

An exception to this general rule permits recovery if the therapist warrants a cure or promises improvement and the warranted cure fails to materialize or less than the promised result occurs.[2] If the clinician is foolish enough to guarantee services in a manner totally satisfactory to the patient or to guarantee that the patient will be "as good as new" or that a particular appliance will fit perfectly, then the patient may sue for breach of contract and/or warranty.

In *Coleman v. Garrison,* 349 A. 2d 8 (Del. 1975) the court refused to enforce a warranty promise of 100% success in the absence of an express agreement supported by consideration separate from the surgical fee. Separate consideration, however, is not required under the majority rule.

In *Cirafici v.* ______, Ill. Appl. 407 N.E. 2d 633, (1980) the following occurred:

Illinois appellate court rules that patient is entitled to a trial on her claim of breach of contract and warranty by dentist. The dentist-defendant replaced the plaintiff's partial dentures with dental implants. According to the patient the dentist allegedly induced her to have the implant procedure by assuring her that the implants would permit her to "eat corn on the cob and other foods for which natural teeth are particularly suitable." After 2 years the dentist removed the implants, acknowledging their failure. The trial court dismissed the plaintiff's claim of breach of contract and warranty. The appellate court reversed, ruling that the plaintiff alleged an express warranty to achieve a specific result and not a mere implied warranty; plaintiff, therefore, deserved an opportunity to prove her claim at trial.

Battery

Injury resulting from unconsented treatment may result in suit under the legal theory of battery, regardless of how skillful the treatment or well meaning the therapist and even though due care is observed in treatment.[3] Except in the event of an emergency under circumstances where it is not reasonably possible to obtain consent in advance, the physician or dentist may not lawfully extend treatment or an operation beyond the area of consent given. In the absence of an emergency the practitioner has committed a battery on the patient, regardless of due care in the performance of the unconsented therapy.

For instance, a patient's consent to TMJ surgery for one condyle does not grant the surgeon the right to operate on both condyles. A patient's consent to spot occlusal grinding does not confer consent to performance of full-mouth reconstruction. Both spot grinding and reconstruction are aimed at the correction of occlusal discrepancies. However, spot grinding limits occlusal adjustment to a select area of the teeth through nonrestorative means, whereas reconstruction encompasses occlusal correction of all teeth in conjunction with placement of new restorations. Thus the scope of consent would be exceeded unless the patient is advised of the restorative means employed to correct the occlusion in advance.

Informed consent

Patient's right to know. The legal doctrine of informed consent in most jurisdictions is considered to be a variant of negligence. However, if the scope of the consent is exceeded, then the proper cause of action is battery rather than negligence.

A fundamental distinction between battery and negligence is that in the case of battery an intentional element is present, whereas negligence is unintentional. For this reason lay testimony is sufficient to prove battery, whereas expert testimony may be required under a negligence action.

The present trend among the various states affirms patients' right to know the treatment to which they subject themselves, independent of the clinician's judgment of the patients' best interest or high-minded purpose of treatment.[4] Inherent in the judicial thinking is the concept that all adults of sound mind have an absolute right to determine for themselves what shall be done to their person or body.[5]

A patient has the right to refuse treatment, even if death is the inevitable consequence of the refusal, a so-called right to die, judicially recognized in the celebrated case of comatose Karen Ann Quinlan.[6]

A significant number of jurisdictions limit disclosure to what a reasonable practitioner would inform his patient under the same or similar circumstances, rather than an absolute right of the patient to be fully informed.[7]

Expert testimony, under the present trend of informed consent decisions, is not necessary, since the "duty to disclose all risks is one imposed by law because of the fiduciary relationship between the physician and his patient."[8]

The essence of a professional relationship is based on the professional's position of superior knowledge. This fiduciary relationship requires full disclosure of the practitioner's special knowledge to the patient, so that the patient will be capable of making an intelligent and fully informed consent to treatment. Accordingly, an uninformed consent vitiates apparent consent without full disclosure.

Disclosure of general versus specific risk. Disclosure of general risks does not discharge the duty to disclose substantial or specific risks.[9] The doctrine of informed consent imposes on a physician or dentist the duty to disclose to the patient all relevant information concerning a proposed treatment, including the collateral hazards attendant thereto, so that the patient's consent to treatment would be an intelligent choice based on complete information.[10,11]

General consent versus specific consent. General consent forms, which contain language in which the patient agrees to "all treatment deemed advisable or necessary" by the treating practitioner, often carry no more legal weight than the printer's ink on the paper. Such forms should be used only for routine tasks and not for specific surgical procedures. Valid consent necessitates that a patient be fully informed of the specific material risks of treatment, considering the likelihood of injury and its seriousness.[12] If the potential injury is slight, a patient need not be informed even though the risk may materialize, since there is no duty to inform of relatively minor risks in common procedures.[12,13]

A physician or dentist may withhold disclosure of untoward consequences of treatment if it would unduly alarm the patient[13] and if full disclosure would be detrimental to the patient's total care and best interests.[14] Disclosure of a lesser included risk may suffice if the greater and more serious risk is discussed.[15]

An intelligent discussion of proposed treatment with patients necessary for informed consent includes the following:

1. Diagnosis
2. Reason for treatment

TORT GENERAL HOSPITAL
Informed consent (surgical)

Patient ____

Date ______________________________ Time ______________ AM / PM

This consent is given on the basis of the information set forth below, which I represent and acknowledge has been explained to me to my satisfaction.

1. Dr. ______________________ (the "Doctor") has explained to me that I suffer from the following condition:

____

2. The Doctor has explained to me that the likely risks to my health if the condition remains untreated are as follows:

____

3. The Doctor has explained to me that he or she recommends the following procedure (hereinafter sometimes called the "Procedure") to treat the above-described condition:

____

4. The Doctor has explained to me that the inherent and potential risks of the Procedure are as follows:

____

I am also aware that there are certain risks attendant to the performance of any surgical procedure, such as severe loss of blood, infection, and cardiac arrest, and that other unforeseeable risks may exist.

5. The Doctor has explained to me that the likely results from the proposed Procedure, if successful, are as follows:

____

6. The Doctor has explained to me that instead of the recommended Procedure, the following alternative procedures are available for the treatment of my condition:

____

7. The Doctor has explained to me that after commencing the proposed Procedure, he or she may find that some other procedure is preferable. The Doctor also has explained to me that during the course of an operation there are sometimes disclosed theretofore unknown conditions that good surgical procedure indicates should be remedied so as to avoid the necessity of a further operation.

8. The Doctor has explained to me that my consent to the procedures herein described may be withdrawn at any time prior to performance thereof, either verbally or in writing.

9. I acknowledge that neither the Doctor nor the Hospital nor any of its officers, agents, employees, or servants have made any promises to me, oral or written, in connection with the procedures described herein. I recognize that every such procedure involves some uncertainty and that no result can ever be guaranteed.

10. Other: ____

11. I understand that the scope of the consent that I am asked to give can, at my option, take one of the three following forms, and I hereby elect to authorize the Doctor and/or any assistants that may be selected (the patient should cross out two of the following three paragraphs that are not applicable):

a. To perform the following operation and no other:

____
Technical name

In the event that the authorized procedure cannot be carried out, I am fully aware that by so limiting the Doctor's authority, he or she will be precluded from treating my condition by any other procedure.

b. To perform the following operation:

____
Technical name

and, because I realize that the Doctor may find, after the commencement of the operation, that some other procedure is preferable to remedy my condition, I hereby also authorize the Doctor and/or said assistants to use such other procedure.

TORT GENERAL HOSPITAL
Informed consent (surgical)—cont'd

c. To perform the following operation:

____
Technical name

and, because I realize that the Doctor may find, after the commencement of the operation, that some other procedure is preferable to remedy my condition, I hereby also authorize the and/or said assistants to use such other procedure; and, in addition, if he or she discovers any heretofore unknown conditions, I authorize the Doctor and/or said assistants to take such steps as in his or her professional judgment are necessary to remedy such conditions; but this authorization does not include the removal of any reproductive organs or any procedure that would be likely to result in sterility

unless I sign here (____)
as well as below.

I represent that I have read and understand the foregoing.

____
Patient or authorized representative Date

____
Witness Date

____
Physician making disclosures Date

____
Spouse Date

(If patient is unable to sign or is a minor, complete the following):

Patient is unable to sign because ____

____
Authorized representative Date

GENERAL CONSENT FORM

I hereby consent to the performance of treatment on ________________________
Myself or name of patient

by Dr.________________________. Such treatment will consist of________________________

____

____
Description in general terms

The nature and purpose of the treatment rendered, the possible hazards, and alternative methods of treatment have been fully explained to me. No guarantee, warranty, or assurance has been given to me that the treatment will be successful or to my complete satisfaction.

In accordance with preoperative instructions given to me by Dr.________________________, if sedative or general anesthetic drugs are to be administered, I have not consumed any food or liquids during the 12 hours preceding my scheduled surgery.

____
Name of patient or legal guardian Date

____
Witness Date

CONSENT
Temporomandibular (jaw joint) surgery

I hereby authorize Dr._______________________________ and whomever he or she may designate as assistants to perform on ___________________________________ the following operation:
Name of patient or myself

____

and if any unforeseen condition should arise in the course of the operation, calling for the Doctor's judgment or for procedures in addition to or different from those now contemplated, I further request and authorize the Doctor to do whatever he or she deems advisable.

I have been informed that the purpose of the operation is an attempt to treat and possibly correct my temporomandibular joint (jaw joint) on the _______________________ side(s).
Right, left, both

Furthermore, I have been informed that other possible alternative methods of treatment include:

____

Risks of the operation include but are not limited to postoperative swelling, pain, inability to open my mouth for several days, weeks, or longer, and paresthesia (numbness) of the nerves of the jaw, which may persist for several weeks, months, or, in rare occasions, permanently.

I acknowledge that no guarantee, warranty, or assurance of success has been made as to the results that may be obtained from the operation, and a risk of failure, relapse, or worsening of my present condition exists.

I further understand that if no treatment is rendered, the present condition of my jaw joint(s) will probably worsen in time, but it may possibly remain the same or improve without the proposed operation.

I consent to the disposal of tissue, to photographs of operative parts, and to admission to the operating room personnel or persons deemed necessary by the attending surgeon.

I certify that I have read fully and understand the above consent to the operation and the explanation therein referred to or made, that all blanks or statements requiring insertion or completion were filled in, and that inapplicable paragraphs, if any, were stricken before I signed.

____
Name of patient or legal guardian — Date

____
Witness — Date

3. Nature of care and treatment explained in layman's terms
4. Alternatives to treatment, if any, including prognosis if proposed care is not followed or performed
5. Prospects of success weighed against risk of failure, relapse, or a poor result
6. Likely substantial inherent and collateral risks or complications of treatment
7. Consequences of not accepting proposed treatment[16]

No reported appellate court decision has required that disclosure and consent be in written form.[17,18] Although oral disclosure and consent are legally sufficient, a written consent, such as the accompanying example signed by the patient has greater probative value a practical matter.

Experimental procedures

The highest degree of disclosure for informed consent is required with unproved methods and with experimental or research studies. Human subjects must be given full and complete information under the Nuremberg Code,[19] the World Medical Association and American Medical Association Guidelines,[20] and the regulations of the Food and Drug Administration,[21] National Institutes of Health,[22] and state drug laws.[23] Editors of distinguished scientific journals have rejected otherwise competent articles if the experimental subjects were not provided the opportunity for informed consent, particularly if the procedures performed were of no therapeutic benefit to the human volunteer.[24,25]

Some state statutes prohibit certain categories of experimental research as criminal acts, subjecting the researcher to felony prosecution.[26]

In the event that experimental drugs, devices, or treatment is prescribed, add the following paragraph to the consent form:

> I fully understand that the *(procedure, treatment, drug,* or *device)* to be used is experimental in nature and not necessarily accepted by medical or dental science at the present time and that the consequences cannot be predicted.

Invalid consent

Misrepresentation. In all jurisdictions consent to an operation is invalidated if it is obtained by representations that are false to the knowledge of the surgeon making them.[27,28] Misrepresentations that amount to fraud carry the additional liability of a separate action for punitive damages, which are not covered by insurance. The surgeon should refrain from giving the patient the wrong impression,[28] telling the patient that which is positively misleading, or minimizing the known danger to induce the patient's consent.[29]

Although a physician or dentist might resent the obligation of informing before performing because he or she "knows best," most professional liability suits are brought by disappointed patients. A frank disclosure in advance reduces a patient's expectancy of a perfect result.

It is the experience of myself and others,[30] in preparing informed consent forms for the practitioner, that the patients appreciate the practitioner's thoroughness and gratefully sign the consent form. Should the patient not sign, it may be in everyone's interest that the proposed surgery not proceed, since the cure might be worse than the disease for that particular patient.

Delegation of disclosure. Disclosure is a nondelegable duty, which cannot be assigned to auxiliary personnel or pamphlets. Office staff and literature may supplement but not replace the surgeon's direct disclosure statements to the patient. In the case of mental incompetents or children, disclosure must be made to the parents or legal guardian.[31]

Disclosure to sedated patients. Sedative drugs should not be administered contemporaneously when obtaining the patient's consent, since the patient's diminished capacity to comprehend and understand militates against any intelligently given consent.

Minor's consent. A minor child, unless emancipated, requires the consent of the parent or legal guardian, which is binding even though the minor may object. Failure to obtain consent for nonemergency treatment is a technical battery, since in theory the minor is legally incompetent to judge his or her best interests in the absence of parental consultation. Thus a minor's consent is vitiated without the concurrence of the parent or legal guardian.

Although emergency treatment of children does not require parental consent, if the parents are readily available, it would be prudent to obtain their consent in advance of treatment.

Parental consent may be omitted if the patient is of the age of discretion, that is, 15 years or older.[32] In most states, courts now hold that the older emancipated minor possesses the right to consent to treatment without parental consent.[33] No reported recent cases have held a physician liable for treatment of a minor of 14 years or older for lack of parental consent where the minor has consented and treatment was given with beneficial intent.[34]

Negligence

Skill, care, and judgment. The practitioner must possess and apply with reasonable diligence the knowledge, skill, care, and judgment that is ordinarily exercised by practitioners of similar training under similar circumstances and in the same or similar communities.[35] The law requires neither perfection nor that the practitioner possess the highest degree of skill possible. Ordinary care under the circumstances is all that the law requires. Conduct above and beyond the standard of care is clearly praiseworthy but not mandatory. On the other hand, conduct that falls short of the minimum standards of due care constitutes professional negligence.

In determining whether a breach of duty in any negligence action has occurred, courts apply the standard of the "reasonable man." If the reasonable, prudent person would have avoided the difficulty, the defendant will be held to have been negligent. On the other hand, if the "reasonable man" would have acted similar to the defendant, no negligence can exist. By way of analogy, in an automobile accident on a wet and slippery road the defendant may be negligent even if he or she was driving at the posted speed at the time of collision with the plaintiff, since the reasonable, prudent driver would have slowed down and proceeded more cautiously under the circumstances.

The aforestated principle of negligence law is applied to situations wherein a patient alleges that a practitioner has been negligent in diagnosing, caring for, or treating the patient's malady; that is, the "reasonable man" standard is that of the duly careful member of the profession.

Duty to refer. One who undertakes to treat assumes the responsibility of possessing those skills ordinarily required to adequately care for the patient's illness or disease.[36] It is the practitioner's further duty to refer the patient to those physicians, dentists, or facilities with specialized knowledge, if such specialized knowledge or skill is required and/or the diagnosis is uncertain.*[37] Moreover, it is no defense that the defendant used the best equipment and supplies possessed, when due care dictated treatment with better equipment, instruments,[38] or facilities.[39] Thus if the practitioner lacks equipment for proper TMJ radiography, a referral to those institutions or specialists with such equipment is in order. In instances in which a cervical collar is instituted as part of therapy, it is advisable for the physician to refer the patient to a dentist for construction of a bite plate or occlusal guard to protect the condyles from degenerative changes, particularly in cases of collapsed posterior occlusion.[40]

In *Clark*[41] an orthodontist diagnosed a TMJ syndrome and referred the patient to a so-called TMJ specialist. Although the patient, a minor, failed her consultation appointment with the TMJ specialist, the jury rendered a substantial plaintiff verdict for the orthodontist's failure to treat the TMJ condition with the methods of the TMJ specialist, rather than with conventional orthodontics.

Duty to consult. In select cases the physician or dentist is obligated to consult with the referring practitioner or with prior treating practitioners.[42] If the defendant has knowledge or notice of prior treatment that is likely to increase the risks of future treatment, a duty arises to consult with the previous practitioners. Should lack of knowledge result from failure to obtain an adequate medical or dental history from a patient, liability would result.

Knowledge of prior TMJ surgery or treatment, history of head trauma, previous wearing of an orthopedic collar,[40] or drugs prescribed by other practitioners could influence current TMJ therapy. Such information may be generally known only by the patient, with the specific details lacking. In such an instance consultation with prior practitioners would be appropriate.

Specialty care. One practicing as a "specialist" must possess and exercise that degree of competence held by other specialists in the treatment of such an organ, disease, or injury.[43] A different and higher standard of care is expected of a specialist. Because of the differing standards, in a given situation a specialist may be negligent, although a general practitioner would not be under the same circumstances.[44]

TMJ therapy often necessitates a multidisciplinary approach. Thus in an appropriate case a specialist in one field of medicine or dentistry is obligated to consult with other specialists in allied health care fields to rule out underlying occult organic diseases or tumors that mimic,[45] coexist with, aggravate, or become manifested as a TMJ dysfunction.[46]

Duty to maintain professional skills and knowledge. Some states require continuing education as a condition of license renewal,[47] but no specific course content is required. Nonetheless a clinician must have due regard for the advances in medical or surgical science at the time of treatment.[48] Thus it is no defense to a claim of professional negligence that a particular technique or disease entity was not taught at the time of the defendant's training in the field, if such information later becomes available and recognized.[49] In accord, the Vermont Supreme Court has stated: "What was proper two years ago may be malpractice today."[50]

Negligent custom versus standard of care. Customary practice in the community may be evidence of the standard of care but is not conclusive. Slipshod or careless practices cannot be justified on the basis that others are equally as careless, nor can a negligent custom be defended on the basis that it is widespread.[51] For example, jaywalking or speeding over 55 mph may be customary practices, although neither is legal or laudable. Moreover, even if the majority of practitioners do not customarily take radiographs of adequate diagnostic quality, this does not transform such negligent custom into acceptable practice.[52]

At the turn of the century the U.S. Supreme Court[53] held, "What usually is done may be evidence of what ought to be done, but what ought to be done is fixed by a standard of reasonable prudence, whether it usually is complied with or not."

In *Hooper*[54] Justic Hand noted:

> [I]n most cases reasonable prudence is in fact common prudence; but strictly it is never its measure; a whole calling may have unduly lagged in the adoption of new and available devices. It never may set its own tests, however persuasive be its usages. Courts must in the end say what is required; there are precautions so imperative that even their universal disregard will not excuse their omission.

The standard of due care remains inviolate irrespective of how many practitioners conform to or deviate from its principle. In *Helling*[55] virtually none of the ophthalmologists in the state performed glaucoma examinations for patients under the age of 40. Despite the prevailing customary practice, the Supreme Court of Washington held that, as a matter of law, the standard of care required glaucoma testing. Strong in the Court's consideration was that the test was simple, relatively inexpensive, well known, and harmless.* Finally, the

*A.M.A.'s *Principle of Medical Ethics* suggests: "A physician should seek consultation upon request; in doubtful or difficult cases; or whenever it appears that the quality of medical service may be enhanced thereby."

*The Schultz Tonometer and the Goldman Applanometer were the testing devices referred to by the Court.

Court viewed the benefit of preventing irreversible ocular damage as outweighing the slight burden of an additional ophthalmological test, although the incidence of glaucoma approximated only 1 in 25,000 for individuals under age 40.

Assuming, *arguendo* (in the course of the argument), a customary practice among some practitioners to not examine or test for TMJ symptoms,a court might determine such a practice to be a negligent custom in violation of the standard of care. By analogy, obtaining clinical history of TMJ signs and symptoms is relatively simple, inexpensive, and harmless, and the existence of TMJ disease is well known. Where a TMJ syndrome is included in a differential diagnosis, reasonable and prudent practice in conformance with the standard of care necessitates ruling out the TMJ diagnosis, and, if present, treatment or referral should follow.

Res ipsa loquitur. When an instrumentality that causes an injury, without any fault of the injured person, is under the exclusive control of the defendant at the time of injury, and the injury is such that in the ordinary course of events it does not occur if the one having such control uses proper care, the law infers negligence on the part of the one in control as the cause of the injury.[56] The negligent inference arises from a doctrine of common knowledge called *res ipsa loquitur*, in Latin, "the thing speaks for itself," which simply means that the event would not have happened unless someone was negligent.

Specific acts of negligence need not be proved because the facts relating to the injury are in the exclusive control of the defendant.

Where TMJ complications occur as a nonnegligently induced inherent risk of dental treatment or independent of therapy, the res ipsa loquitur doctrine does not apply. Failure to advise of the substantial risk of such an occurrence, where reasonably foreseeable as in select types of orthodontic treatment,[56] constitutes negligent lack of informed consent, particularly since most orthodontic treatment is wholly elective.

Specific acts of negligence with casual relationships to injury render the doctrine inapplicable. An example is when TMJ symptoms are aggravated by failure to perform occlusal adjustment or equilibration where the dentist knew in the exercise of reasonable diligence, or should have known, of the presence of TMJ complications proximately related to hyperoccluding restorations.

Abandonment. Abandonment of a patient, in which no reasonable alternative for required care is available, referred, or provided, constitutes a negligent breach of the practitioner's duty to the patient. Abandonment can occur either by the practitioner's express withdrawal or by his or her failure to continue treatment. Failure to follow through with full treatment or to advise the patient of the need for postoperative care or visits if required are examples of negligent abandonment of the patient.[57] Postoperative care may require additional radiographs, follow-up monitoring with specific instructions to the patient,[58] further treatment, or surgery. A change of circumstances, such as a deteriorating or worsening condition of the patient, may require altering the postoperative care and reevaluation as to the proper course to be followed. However, in an emergency situation the mere rendering of treatment does not by itself establish a doctor-patient relationship that continues beyond the immediate needs of an emergency situation.[59]

Since a reciprocal relationship exists between practitioner and patient, it continues unless terminated by mutual consent of the parties or revoked by unilateral dismissal. In instances in which dismissal of a patient is appropriate, reasonable notice must be given. A registered letter addressed to the patient advising him or her of the dismissal and providing the names of substitute practitioners or other facilities would be helpful safeguard when patients do not return for follow-up care.

Subsequent treating practitioners. Subsequent treating or examining dentists or physicians are liable should they negligently aggravate any injuries that arose from the first practitioner or tortfeasor's lack of due care.[60] Malpractice in treating a patient injured by another is judged to be reasonably foreseeable. Accordingly, subsequent or additional malpractice does not exculpate the original tortfeasor.

Vicarious liability. When the physician or dentist possesses the right of control over associates[61] or assistants,[62] regardless of actual exercise of that control, the physician or dentist is liable for their negligent conduct performed in the course and scope of employment. Control and not compensation is the test for imposition of liability. The right of supervision and direction distinguish the master from the servant, regardless of whether the servant is temporarily borrowed[63] or is paid as an independent contractor.

Unnecessary surgery. It is axiomatic that surgery of the temporomandibular apparatus should only be conducted when nonsurgical conservative therapeutic modalities have not proved successful.

Certain types of temporomandibular surgery previously acceptable, such as bilateral condylectomies, are now outmoded for the chronic sufferer of a myofascial pain-dysfunction syndrome. Nevertheless, such unnecessary surgery persists because of a diversity of reasons.

Unnecessary surgery has resulted in punitive damage awards in both medicine[64] and dentistry[65] and in license revocation.

A recent study[66] at Cornell University Medical College has revealed that as many as 13% of persons who are advised to undergo surgery may not require the surgery at all. In those hospitals with effective tissue committees there has been a steady decrease of unwarranted surgery.[67]

Partnership liability. Each partner is liable for the professional negligence of another partner, performed within the scope of the partnership's business. By virtue of the joint nature of the liability, and irrespective of whether the action is brought against the partnership in its own name or in the names of the individual members as copartners, statutory authority permits a plaintiff who is entitled to recover to enter judgment against all the partners even though only one, or less than all of them, has been served. Execution on such judgment is limited to the partnership property and the real and personal property of the partners summoned.[68]

A professional corporation is also liable for the torts committed by its agents or servants under the legal doctrine of respondeat superior.[69] The corporation shareholders are not personally liable, whereas in the partnerhip entity each partner's personal assets may be executed on in satisfaction of a judgment for damages.

DEFENSES

Alternative treatment

If there are several alternative treatment modalities available to a practitioner and not all are universally employed by all practitioners of good standing, it is not a negligent error of judgment for a practitioner to elect in his or her best judgment one of the less favored, but otherwise acceptable, methods of treatment.[70] However, if a physician or dentist, when confronted with alternative means of treatment, elects to follow none of them, then this defense is inapplicable.[71]

Thus grave diagnostic errors by practitioners can be of two kinds: negligent or blameless. A physician or dentist cannot be held liable for an exercise of medical judgment if he or she has used proper and adequate diagnostic methods. Simply put, a practitioner cannot be liable for an exercise of *good* judgment. It is fully as possible in the dental profession as elsewhere to employ good judgment in reaching what ultimately proves to be a wrong answer. Equally clearly, however, diagnostic errors will sound in tort if made without careful examination, including customarily used clinical examinations and laboratory tests.

For example, a dentist who extracts a tooth, failing to remove all of it, may commit a diagnostic error in failure to use x-ray examinations for initial or follow-up procedures when a tooth fragment is left in the jaw. This was the case in *Butts v. Watts*, 290 S.W. 2d 777, 781 (Ky. App. 1956), where the jury also inferred negligence from the fact that physicians in subsequent attendance were able to clear up the plaintiff's condition quickly when the treatment was changed. When another dentist did perform an x-ray examination, he discovered the fragment of tooth. In the circumstances shown the jury could well believe that there was a factor to be taken into account on the overall question of postoperative negligence without having an expert tell them so. Thus res ipsa loquitur was applicable because a commonly known diagnostic procedure—x-ray examinations—was ignored.

Prosser[72] states the dispositive point with confidence and precision: "[T]he physican is required to exercise reasonable care in ascertaining the operational facts upon which his diagnosis is based, and will be liable if he fails to do so." Even a faulty diagnosis may not of itself constitute negligence, but failure to use all reasonable means of collecting the best factual data to arrive at the proper diagnosis may be evidence of negligence.[73]

Untoward result

An untoward or poor result does not by its mere occurrence constitute negligent conduct, provided that such occurrence may be an unavoidable or inherent risk of the procedure.[74] Unless a complication is negligently induced, there exists no provable professional liability.

TMJ therapeutic modalities, although myriad, report varying degrees of success,[75] including effectiveness of placebo therapy.[76] A clinician who proceeds with one method that, in hindsight, was not as efficient or beneficial as another choice may nonetheless be exculpated, provided the approach selected appeared reasonably prudent in foresight and was an otherwise professionally acceptable treatment.

Gratuitous service

Performance of professional services without a fee is no defense to a malpractice allegation[77] and does not diminish the obligation to exercise reasonable care and diligence.[78]

No duty to treat

A doctor-patient relationship cannot be unilaterally created but must be mutually consented to. A physician or dentist's right to select patients necessarily includes the right to refuse treatment, even in an emergency. One is not legally required to be one's brother's keeper.[79]

Patient's obligations

The patient owes a duty to the dentist or physician to follow instructions, which may include the necessity for further treatment. Thus, if appliances are constructed, the dentist is entitled to a reasonable opportunity to make necessary adjustments and may not be held liable if failure of the treatment is caused solely by lack of patient cooperation.[80]

Statute of limitations

All states limit the period in which a suit may be brought either by a fixed number of years from the date of the alleged negligence, from the time of the last treatment, or from the time when the patient discovered the negligent cause of the injuries or in the exercise of reasonable diligence should have discovered same. Statutes of limitations were enacted for reasons of fairness, so that suits can be pursued when memories are freshest and before material witnesses die or evidence disappears.

Under the majority rule a suit is barred unless filed within a specified time from the alleged negligent treatment. However, discovery statutes represent a growing trend in the law by extending the filing date from the time of treatment until the patient's discovery of the negligence.[81] Foreign objects discovered many years after surgery or cases of continuing and repeated acts of negligence extending over many years of treatment justify such statutes based on delayed discovery.

In *Arnold*,[82] under a discovery statute enacted long after treatment had been terminated for the patient, suit was timely filed for injuries that allegedly occurred some 15 years after the physician treated the patient. The defendant could not recall having ever treated the patient, nor did he maintain records of patients extending as far back as the date of treatment alleged by the plaintiff. Thus records should be preserved in all instances in which latent injuries might later be claimed.

If the defendant assures the patient that "you will be all right in time" and actively dissuades the patient from consulting others, these may be facts that a jury could consider as bearing on the question of the defendant knowing of the negligence and concealing that fact from the patient. Such conduct constitutes fraudulent concealment and extends the statute of limitations period until the patient discovers the truth.[83]

If, however, the defendant has made an honest mistake and did not realize the nature of the patient's problems, the statute of limitations might be strictly construed, and the suit could be barred as an untimely assertion of a stale claim.

Locality rule

An expert witness who is to be judged competent by the court must be familiar with the standard of practice in the community. Originally, and currently in a small minority of jurisdictions, the locality rule required an expert witness to be familiar with the standard practice in the specific local community in which treatment occurred. Initial modifications of the rule eventually expanded the geographical limits beyond the "same locality" to a "same or similar locality," which is the present majority rule.[84] At least eleven states have broadened the locality rule to a national standard of care or standard of practice.[85] Thus the place where professional care is provided becomes another circumstance to be considered or ignored. Remaining intact, however, is the rule that the requisite degree of care rendered must conform to what a class of reasonable and prudent practitioners would possess and exercise under the same or similar circumstances.

Initially the rule protected practitioners in rural or small towns who had limited access to modern facilities and continuing education compared with their urban peers. As transportation and communication methods improved, the reason for the rule eroded along with the courts' decisions to impose a double standard of care in the smaller community. Nationally distributed journals, taped presentations, clinical courses, and wide availability of professional society meetings with national speakers provide a country-wide flow of current clinical information, which justifies a national standard of care.

Proof of damages

Even if consent to a procedure is legally void, the patient must prove damages as a proximate result of the unconsented surgery. In *Garzione*[86] a $150,000 jury verdict in favor of a plaintiff nurse who suffered a leg amputation was reduced on appeal to $1. Although liability for assault and battery was sustained, the appellate court reduced the amount of damages, since uncontradicted medical testimony showed the amputation had been necessary, and there was no competent evidence that the leg could have been successfully treated.

Contributory negligence

Under the doctrine of pure contributory negligence the fault of the plaintiff operates as a complete bar to his or her recovery, provided that such negligence has in any degree contributed as a proximate cause of the damaging act.[87] If the patient can be said to be at fault to any appreciable extent, recovery is precluded, and contributory negligence forms a complete defense. Thus, in states that have pure contributory negligence, the plaintiff who has contributed, no matter how slightly, to his or her own injury may not recover for such injuries, regardless of how negligent the defendant may have been.

The harshness of this defense doctrine is gradually being supplanted by an increasing number of states adopting comparative negligence rules, whereby the negligence of the plaintiff serves as an offset to the amount of recovery but does not bar recovery. Under pure comparative negligence rules the plaintiff can recover even when relatively more negligent than the defendant.[88] A few states require that the plaintiff be no greater than 50% negligent in causing the accident, as compared with the defendants.[89] Thirteen states bar a plaintiff's claim if his or her contributory negligence is equal to or greater than the defendant's negligence.*

Expert witness testimony required

Only an expert witness is entitled to present opinion testimony in professional liability suits, whereas nonexpert witnesses may only give factual testimony. Thus a witness to an incident must state only what he or she saw or did but may not give an opinion as to the cause of the accident unless such opinions are within the common knowledge and experience of laymen. Because a physician or dentist is an expert in the field, he or she is qualified to state an opinion that establishes a causal relationship between the trauma and the injury or pathological condition that he or she diagnosed or treated.

Expert witnesses are of two basic types: the percipient factual witness who rendered treatment or the nontreating expert witness who bases the opinion on the hypothetical questions posed at the trial. The treating practitioner is a factual or percipient witness and may also testify as an expert by stating his or her opinion in such matters as the cause of a TMJ syndrome. By contrast, the expert witness who never examined or treated the patient is permitted only to testify from the hypothetical questions based on the evidence presented at the trial and on hearsay information, provided that such information is the type of hearsay on which experts reasonably rely.[90]

Courts have ruled expert witnesses as competent to testify in matters outside their particular field of specialty.[91] Qualified specialists have been judged competent to testify regarding the standard of care of a general practitioner,[91] the standard of care prior to the practitioner's beginning practice,[92] and the standard of care of a general surgeon regarding orthopedic surgery.[93] Health professionals performing similar types of procedures will be held to the same standard of care.[94] Consequently, a plastic surgeon, otolaryngologist, and oral surgeon are each competent as to the applicable standard of care in performing surgery of the temporomandibular apparatus.

Textbooks as evidence

The Federal Rules of Evidence (Rule 803 [18]) now provide that statements contained in published treatises and periodicals on the subject of medicine may be read as evidence during the direct examination of the plaintiff's expert if such writings are called to the expert's attention and he or she states that they were relied on in the testimony. Thus, as stated in *Moore's Federal Practice*,[94a] the treatise is established as reliable "whenever the expert witness testifies on direct examination . . . that he relied upon the treatise in his testimony." In such a case the statements from the treatise may be read as evidence for their full substantive value. Most state evidentiary rules permit textbooks to be introduced solely for impeachment purposes rather than as substantive evidence.

Proximate cause

To prevail at trial, a plaintiff must prove that the defendant's alleged negligent error or omission was a substantial contributing factor to the plaintiff's injury.[95] If the answer to the following question is negative, then the defendant proximately caused the injury: "But for the defendant's negligence, would the injury have occurred?" For example, a patient with a history of smoking complains to Dr. *A* of chest pain. Dr. *A* takes radiographs and diagnoses the condition as pleurisy. The patient's symptoms continue, and shortly thereafter he consults Dr. *B*, who diagnoses his condition as terminal metastatic lung cancer. In reviewing Dr. *A's* radiographs of 6 weeks ago, Dr. *B* determines that Dr. *A* misdiagnosed the plaintiff's condition. However, since the cancer had already metastasized at the earlier date, earlier diagnosis would not have affected the plaintiff's prognosis.[96]

Thus the practical approach emerges that from a mix of circumstantial evidence, expert testimony, and common knowledge, a basis emerges to infer a causal linkage or relation between the defendant's culpable acts or omissions and the plaintiff's harm, and this renders legitimate the inference that such misconduct is a necessary antecedent and, thus a cause of the harm.[97]

Good Samaritan exemption

In 1959 California became the first state to enact legislation protecting Good Samaritans from tort liability.[98] Prior to this enactment a Good Samaritan rendering aid in an emergency could be held liable only if he or she acted unreasonably or negligently.[99] Thus individuals might be apt to refrain from giving emergency aid for fear of being subject to legal action.

Currently there exist Good Samaritan statutes in all 50 states, the District of Columbia, and the Virgin Islands. These statutes range from very general[100] to very specific,[101] and each is designed to protect the Good Samaritan from frivolous litigation.[102]

A Good Samaritan statute which states that no licensed physician who in good faith renders emergency

*These states are Arkansas, Colorado, Georgia, Idaho, Hawaii, North Dakota, Maine, Massachusetts, Minnesota, Oklahoma, Oregon, Utah, and Wyoming.

care at the scene of an emergency shall be liable for any civil damages as a result of any negligent emergency care has been ruled applicable to certain hospital emergencies. For instance, a chief resident physician was not held to be an ex officio member of the hospital emergency team and therefore was exempt from liability under the Good Samaritan statute after responding to a code blue cardiac-pulmonary alert.[103]

There are no reported cases in which a patient has ever obtained a judgment against a physician who rendered emergency treatment while acting as a gratuitous Good Samaritan.[104,105] Thus the fear of rendering emergency aid because it is thought to invite litigation appears unfounded. Nearly all states have enacted Good Samaritan statutes that relieve legal liability for ordinary negligence when the Good Samaritan physician or other member of the healing arts rendered emergency care outside the hospital or office.[99,106]

PROPHYLACTIC MEASURES

Record keeping

A surgeon has a legal obligation to prepare an acceptable operative report.[107] Failure to maintain and retain accurate and complete records is often strictly construed against the defendant. As memories dim in time, the patient's records may become the most important evidence in a professional liability suit, regardless of the factual issues. Certainty that all necessary TMJ tests were performed as evidenced by detailed records, contemporaneously recorded, is preferable to testimony of the defendant's usual practice.

Alteration of records may be viewed with distrust as evidence of a guilty conscience. If records are materially altered after the passage of time, the record should clearly show the later entry as a subsequent addition, the reason for the record correction, and the initials of the person changing the record. In *Thor*[108] the original records were missing at the time of deposition and trial, having been recopied earlier. Although the recopied records were alleged to be an accurate facsimile of the original ones, nonetheless the appellate court held that an inference of negligence resulted and shifted the burden of proof to the defendant to come forward and reasonably explain the absence of the original records.

Defense malpractice attorneys prefer poor records to none at all. Accordingly, patients' records should be maintained indefinitely and either placed in storage or preserved on microfilm.[109]

Radiographs

Examination. Complete testing for the clinician to arrive at a reasonably certain TMJ diagnosis often includes appropriate radiographic examination. Radiographs must be not only adequate in number but also diagnostic in quality. Advances in TMJ radiography, such as duplicable transcranial lateral oblique radiographs with functional views and duplicable cephalometric tomograms, may render other TMJ film techniques obsolete. Accordingly, reliance on outmoded or outdated radiographic techniques poses an area of negligent diagnosis, since better or more reliable testing methods are readily available.

Ownership. If radiographs represent a portion of the practitioner's clinical records, the original films belong to the physician or dentist who ordered their taking to form a basis for rendering a diagnostic opinion or judgment. Duplicating film copies should be made available to a patient or the patient's attorney on request.* The original radiographic films can remain as a permanent part of the patient's medical or dental record without risk of loss or alteration should their production be required later. However, the original radiographs are subject to release pursuant to a valid subpoena. Moreover, reasonably clear copies must be provided to another practitioner when authorized by the patient, since there is a legal duty to provide all reasonable information concerning a patient's condition.

History and examination

Other chapters in this book deal with the recommended methods of history taking (Chapter 5) and adequate examination (Chapter 6). It is axiomatic that TMJ treatment in the absence of a detailed history and examination is not good practice. A practitioner undertaking treatment of the TMJ should first consider or rule out tumors, neoplasms, aural disease, nasal and pharyngeal disorders, other medications, psychosomatic illnesses, and other systemic complications.

Prescribing central nervous system depressants

Liability has been imposed on physicians for prescribing or dispensing drowsiness-producing medica-

---

*California Evidence Code 1158 provides: "Whenever, prior to the filing of any action or the appearance of a defendant in an action, an attorney at law presents a written authorization theretofor signed by an adult patient, by the guardian or conservator of his person or estate, or, in the case of a minor, by a parent or guardian of such minor, or by the personal representative or an heir of a deceased patient, *or a copy thereof,* a physician and surgeon, dentist, registered nurse, dispensing optician, registered physical therapist, podiatrist, licensed psychologist, osteopath, chiropractor, clinical laboratory bioanalyst, clinical laboratory technologist, *or pharmacist or pharmacy,* duly licensed as such under the laws of the state, or a licensed hospital, shall make all of the patient's records under his or its custody or control available for inspection and copying by such attorney at law or his representative, promptly upon the presentation of the written authorization.

"Failure to make such records available, during business hours, within 5 days after the presentation of the written authorization, may subject the person or entity having custody or control of the records to liability for all reasonable expenses, including attorney's fees, incurred in any proceeding to enforce the provisions of this section."

tions when the physician has failed to warn the patient not to drive while under the influence of these drugs. In one case a bus driver along with his injured passengers were all awarded damages against a physician who prescribed an antihistamine to the bus-driver patient without warning him of the side effect of drowsiness, which occurred while at the wheel of this bus.[110] When sedative-hypnotics, that is, tranquilizers, barbiturates, muscle relaxants, and/or potent analgesics, including propoxyphene,[111] are prescribed in conjunction with TMJ therapy, central nervous system depression may occur, either singly or in combination with other depressant drugs. Where consistent with the drug manufacturer's package insert, add the following to the patient's prescription to warn of additive soporific effects of central nervous system depressive drugs:

Caution: Medication produces drowsiness, either alone or in combination with other sedative drugs or alcohol. *Do not* drive or operate dangerous machinery within four (4) hours of taking medication.

Rapport

The expanding use of auxiliary personnel may increase office efficiency at the expense of depersonalizing the doctor-patient relationship. Discontinuity resulting from frequent staff turnover can further contribute to interpersonal communication breakdown with a patient.

Patients suffering from temporomandibular joint disorders are frequently shunted from specialist to specialist with little time devoted to in-depth understanding of the multiple manifestations of the syndrome. A succession of therapeutic personnel tends to weaken any doctor-patient rapport that otherwise would become annealed by the bonds of time.

Most patients are reluctant to sue a well-meaning practitioner, regardless of underlying negligence, if the clinician nurtured a solid patient relationship through long-term empathetic concern. Providing understanding for the patient's TMJ problems at the chair is far less time consuming than listening to the patient's complaints of negligent treatment in a courtroom.

Disparagement

Criticism of a patient's former practitioner's treatment methods or results is the genesis of more professional malpractice suits than any other single factor. Should questionable prior therapy be adduced at the time of the original consultation with a new patient suffering from temporomandibular joint complaints, it is advisable to communicate directly with the earlier treating clinician. A more nearly objective evaluation of prior treatment will result, along with an appreciation of the totality of circumstances under which the previous treatment occurred; additionally, the clinician will obtain a greater understanding of the patient's tolerance and response to treatment and/or prior significant medical or dental history.

Medical practitioners have long been called to task for their conspiracy of silence in failing to testify against negligent peers.[112] This occurs despite the fact that many states exempt from discovery any statements or testimony arising from proceedings of peer review committees concerned with quality of care.[113] Additionally, peer review and hospital staff committee members may be exempt from personal liability in the absence of malice.[114] Professional licensing boards have been traditionally lax in self-policing the health professions through license suspension and/or revocation, although there have been a few recent notable exceptions.[115]

Dentistry apparently has recognized the moral bankruptcy of any self-serving conspiratorial attempts and affirmatively requires members to report faulty treatment to the local peer review committee of the dental society. The American Dental Association's Code of Professional Conduct, Section I to G, provides, "A dentist has an obligation to report to the appropriate reviewing agency of his state or constituent dental society instances of gross and/or continual faulty treatment by other dentists." Also, California's Board of Dental Examiners requires similar reporting. Any attempted intimidation of the plaintiff's expert witnesses may shift the burden of proof to the defendant as evidence of consciousness of the defendant's guilt.[116] Furthermore, it may subject any conspiring intimidators to license discipline for unprofessional conduct.[117]

REFERENCES

1. *Canterbury v. Spence,* 464 F.2d 772, 1972.
2. *Depenbrok v. Kaiser Foundation Health Plan, Inc.,* 144 Cal. Rptr. 724, 79 Cal.App.3d 167, 1978.
3. *Corn v. French,* 289 P.2d 173, 71 Nev. 280, 1955.
4. *Petterson v. Lynch,* 299 N.Y.S.2d 244, N.Y. 1969; *Sauro v. Shea,* 390 A.2d 259, Penn. 1978.
5. *Schloendorff v. Society of New York Hospital,* 211 N.Y. 125, 129, 105 N.E. 92, 93, 1914.
6. *Matter of Quinlan,* 348 A.2d 801, N.J. 1975, Modified and remanded, 70 N.J. 10, 355 A.2d 647, 1976.
7. *Getchell v. Mansfield,* 489 P.2d 953, 957, 1971; *Di Filippo v. Preston,* 53 Del. 539, 173 A.2d 333, 1960; *Roberts v. Young,* 369 Mich. 133, 119 N.W.2d 627, 1963; *Williams v. Menehan,* 191 Kan. 6, 379 P.2d 292, 1963; *Govin v. Hunter,* 374 P.2d 421, Wyo. 1962; *ZeBarth v. Swedish Hosp. Medical Center,* 81 Wash. 2d 12, 499 P.2d 1, 1972; *Negaard v. Estate of Fedâ,* 152 Mont. 47, 446 P.2d 436, 1968; *Green v. Hussey,* 127 Ill.App.2d 174, 262 N.E.2d 156, 1970.
8. *Watkins v. Parpala,* 2 Wash.App.2848, 469 P.2d 974, 1970.
9. *Mallet v. Pirkey,* 171 Colo. 271, 466 P.2d 466, 1970.
10. *Birnbaum v. Seigler,* 273 App. Div. 817, 76 N.Y.S.2d 173, 1948.
11. *Martin v. Baillar,* 540 P. 2d 118.
12. *Holland v. Sisters of Joseph Peace,* 522 P.2d 208.

13. *Cobbs v. Grant,* 502 P.2d 1, 104 Cal. Rptr. 505, 8 Cal.3d 299, 1972.
14. *Watson v. Clutts,* 262 N.C. 153, 136 S.E.2d 617, 1964.
15. *Nishi v. Hartwell,* 473 P.2d 116, Hawaii 1970; see also *Morgenroth v. Pacific Medical Center, Inc.*, 126 Cal.Rptr. 681, 1976.
16. *Truman v. Thomas,* 165 Cal.Rptr. 308, 1980.
17. Simonaitis, J.E.: Written disclosure not necessary, J.A.M.A. **231:**1391, 1975.
18. *Kelly v. Gershkoff,* 312 A.2d 211, R.I. 1973.
19. Beecher, H.K.: Research and the individual, Boston, 1970, Little, Brown & Co.
20. Frost, N.: A surrogate system for informed consent, J.A.M.A. **233:**800, 1975.
21. Federal Food, Drug and Cosmetic Act, Section 505, as amended 1976; 21 U.S.C. § 355.
22. Institutional Guide to DHEW Policy on Protection of Human Subjects, publication No. NIH 72-102, Department of Health, Education, and Welfare, Dec. 1971.
23. California Sherman Food, Drug and Cosmetic Law, Article 4, §26668-26670, as amended 1974.
24. Woodford, F.P.: Ethical experimentation and the editor, N. Engl. J. Med. **286:**892, 1972.
25. Laforet, E.: The fiction of informed consent, J.A.M.A. **235:**1579, 1976.
26. Massachusetts General Laws: Chapter 112, Section 12J. See also Public Law 93-348, in which Congress established the National Commission for the Protection of Human Subjects of Biomedical and Behavioral Research.
27. *Birnbaum v. Seigler,* 273 App. Div. 817, 76 N.Y.S.2d, 1973.
28. *Funke v. Fieldman,* 512 P.2d 539, Kan. 1973.
29. *Salgo v. Leland Stanford, etc. Bd. of Trustees,* 317, P.2d 170, 154 Cal. App.2d 560, 1957.
30. Alfidi, R.J.: Informed consent, a study of patient reaction, J.A.M.A., **216:**1325, 1971.
31. *Darrah v. Kite,* 301 N.Y.S. 201, 286, 1969.
32. Shartel, B., and Plant, M.: The law of medical practice, Springfield, Ill., 1959, Charles C Thomas, Publisher.
33. *Smith v. Seibly,* 431 P.2d 719, Wash. 1967.
34. Holder, A.: Medical malpractice law, New York, 1975, John Wiley & Sons, Inc.; Holoweiki, J.: Do you need parental consent to treat a minor? Med. Econ., Sept. 17, 1979 p. 218; Zinman, E.: Emergency care—some legal implications, Dent. Surv. **55:**46, 1979.
35. *Deveraux v. Smith,* 213 S.W.3d 170, Tex. Civ. App. 1948.
36. *Butler v. Louisiana St. Bd. of Education,* 331 So.2d 192, La. App. 1976.
37. *Steeves v. U.S.*, 294 F. Supp. 446, D.C., S.C. 1968.
38. *Smith v. Mallinckrodt Chem. Works,* 251 S.W.155, Mo. 1923.
39. *Wilson v. Corbin,* 41 N.W.2d 702, Iowa 1950.
40. Shore, N.A.: Cervical traction and temporomandibular joint dysfunction: report of a case, J. Am. Dent. Assoc. **68:**4, 1964.
41. *Clark v. Laughlin,* 68 Cal.App.3d 506, 137 Cal.Rptr, 354, 1977.
42. *Langford v. Kosterlitz,* 280 P. 80, Cal. 1930.
43. *Belk v. Schweizer,* 149 S.E.2d 565, N.C. 1966.
44. *Toth v. Community Hospital at Glen Cove,* 239 N.E.2d 368, N.Y. 1968.
45. Greene, C.: The temporomandibular syndrome, J.A.M.A. **224:**622, 1973.
46. *Graham v. Roberts,* 142 App. D.C. 305, 441 F.2d 995, 1970.
47. Cal. Bus. & Prof. Code § 1645.
48. *Goheen v. Graber,* 181 Kan. 197, 309 P.2d 636, 1957; *Collins v. Meeker,* 424 P.2d 488, 198 Kan. 390, 1967; *Adkins v. Rapp,* 14 N.E.2d 727, Ind. 1938.
49. *Funke v. Fieldman,* 512 P.3d 539, Kan. 1973.
50. Wood, B.: Handbook of dental malpractice, Springfield, Ill., 1967, Charles C Thomas, Publisher.
51. *Lundahl v. Rockford Memorial Hospital Association,* 235 N.E. 671, Ill. 1968; *Incolingo v. Ewing,* 282 A.2d 206, Penn. 1971.
52. Biedeman, R.W., Johnson, O.N., and Alcox, R.W.: A study to develop a rating system and evaluate dental radiographs submitted to a third party carrier, J. Am. Dent. Assoc. **93:**1010, 1976; Zinman, E: Usual and customary versus prudent practice, J. Tenn. Dent. Assoc. **60**(3):9, 1980.
53. *Texas & Pac. Ry. v. Behymer,* 189 U.S. 468, 470, 23 S.Ct. 622, 623, 47 L.Ed. 905, 1903.
54. *The T.J. Hooper,* 60 F.2d 740, 2d Cir. 1932.
55. *Helling v. Carey,* 519 P.2d 98, 83 Wash. 2d 514, 1974; *Gates v. Jensen,* 595 P.2d 919, 1979; *Morgan v. Sheppard,* 188 N.E.2d 808, 1963; *Lundahl v. Rockford Memorial Hospital Assoc.*, 235 N.E.2d 671, 1968; but see *Barton v. Owen,* 71 Cal.App.3d 471, 139 Cal.Rptr. 494, 1977.
56. *Negaard v. Estate of Feda,* 152 Mont. 43, 446 P.2d 636, 1968; *Fortner v. Koch,* 261 N.W.273, Mich. 1935.
57. *Butts v. Watts,* 290 S.W.2d 777, Ky. 1956; *Donathan v. McConnell,* 121 Mont. 230, 193 P.2d 819, 1948.
58. *Largess v. Tatem,* 291 A.3d 398, Vt. 1972.
59. *Crosby v. Grandview Nursing Home,* 290 A.2d 375, Me. 1972.
60. *Becker v. Walthers,* 541 P.2d 523, Nev. 1975.
61. *Heimlich v. Harvey,* 255 Wis. 471, 39 N.W.2d 394, 1949.
62. *Huss v. Vande Hey,* 29 Wis.2d 34, 138 N.W.2d 192, 197, 1965; *Mullins v. DuVall,* 25 Ga.App.690, 104 S.I.513, 1920.
63. *Ardehold v. Bishop,* 94 Okla. 203, 221 P.752, 1923.
64. *Gonzales v. Nork and Mercy Hospital of Sacramento,* Case no. 228566 Sacramento Superior Court, Nov. 19, 1973.
65. *Sinopoli v. Issvoran,* Alameda County Superior Court, Docket no. H-43098-0, Cal., April 17, 1979.
66. Conason, R.L., editor: Medical Malpractice Litigation, New York, 1978, Practicing Law Institute.
67. Effect of a tissue committee on appendectomy in a general hospital, Wisc. Med. J., p. 137, 1960.
68. *Martinoff v. Triboro,* 228 N.Y.S.2d 139, 141-142, and New York Partnership Law Section 24.
69. *National Bank of California v. Miner,* 167 C. 532, 140 P.27, 1914.
70. *Scarano v. Schnoor,* 158 Cal.App.2d 612, 323 P.2d 178, 1958, 68 A.L.E.2d 416; *McHugh v. Audet,* 72 F.Supp. 394, C.C.Pa. 1974. *Clemens v. Regents of the University of Cal.*, 1970, 8 Cal.App.3d 1, 87 Cal.Rptr. 108, appeal after remand, 1971, 20 Cal.App.3d 356, 97 Cal.Rptr. 589; *Majetich v. Westin,* 276 Cal.App.2d 216, 80 Cal.Rptr. 787; 4 Witkin, Summary of California Law, ed. 8, Torts §515.
71. *Spadaccini v. Dolan,* A.D.2d, 407 N.Y.S.2d-840; *Toth v. Community Hospital,* 22 N.Y.2d 255 at 264 fr 2.
72. Prosser, W.L.: Law of torts, ed. 4, 1971, West Publishing Co., p. 163.
73. *Clark v. United States,* 402 F.2d 950, C.C.A.4, 1968.
74. *Germann v. Matriss,* 55 N.J. 193, 260 A.2d 825, 1970.
75. Carlsson, S., Gale, E., and Ohman, A.: Treatment of temporomandibular joint syndrome with biofeedback training, J. Am. Dent. Assoc. **91:**602, 1975.
76. Goodman, P., Greene, C., and Laskin, D.: Response of patients with myofascial pain dysfunction syndrome to mock equilibration, J. Am. Dent. Assoc. **92:**755, 1976.
77. *Robbins v. Parker,* 8 P.2d 908, 1932.
78. *Dubois v. Decker,* 130 N.Y. 325, 23 N.E. 313, 1891.
79. *Findlay v. Board of Supervisors,* 72 Ariz. 58, 230 P.2d 526 (1951); *Rice v. Rinaldo,* 147 Cal.App.2d 833, 835, 305 P.2d 1020, 1022, 1957.

80. *Chubb v. Holmes,* 150 A. 516, Conn. 1930; *Wemett v. Mount,* 292 P.93, Ore. 1930.
81. *Sanchez v. South Hoover Hospital,* 18 Cal.3d 93, 126 Cal.Rptr. 617, 1976; *Munoz v. Purdy,* 91 Cal.3d 942, 154 Cal.Rptr. 472, 1979.
82. *Arnold v. Wolley,* 514 P.2d 599, Idaho 1973.
83. *Swope v. Printz,* 468 S.W.2d 34, Mo. 1971.
84. *Dickens v. Everhart,* 199 S.E.2d 440, N.C. 1973.
85. *Shire v. Freedman,* 206 N.W.2d 166, Wis. S. Ct. 1973; 49 Wis.2d 41, 58 Wis.2d 269; 181 N.W.2d; 208 N.W.2d 328; *Shildret v. Annapolis Emergency Hospital Association,* 349 A.2d 245, Md. Ct. App. 1975, 276 Md.187.
86. *Garzione v. Vassar Brothers Hospital,* 320 N.Y.2d 830, 286, N.E.2d 731, N.Y. 1972.
87. *Ray v. Wagner,* 286 Minn.354, 176 N.W.2d 101, 1970.
88. *Li v. Yellow Cab,* 119 Cal.Rptr. 858, 13 Cal.3d 804, 532 P.2d 1226, 1975.
89. Schwartz V.: Comparative negligence, Indianapolis, 1974, Allen Smith Co.; Conn. Public Act No. 73-622; Nev. Laws 1973, Ch. 787; N.H. Rev. Stat. Ann., § 507:7-a; N.J. Rev. Stat. Ann., §§ 2A:15-5.1 to 2A:15-5.5; Tex. Vernon's Civ. Stat., Art. 2212a, § 1.2; Vt. Stat. Ann. 1959, tit. 12, § 1036; Wis. Stat. Ann., §§ 895.045; *Nimmer v. Purtell,* 69 Wisc.2d 21, 230 N.W.2d 258, 1975.
90. *Luque v. McLean,* 8 Cal.App.3d 136, 104 Cal.Rptr. 443, 1972.
91. *Evans v. Ohanesian,* 39 Cal.App.3d 121, 112 Cal.Rptr. 236, 1974.
92. *Cline v. Lund,* 31 Cal.App.3d 755, 107 Cal.Rptr. 629, 1973.
93. *Benzmiller v. Swanson,* 117 N.W.2d, N.D. 1962.
94. *Chadock v. Cotton,* 157 Cal.Rptr. 640, 1979.
94a. Moore's federal practice, ed. 2, vol. 11, §803, subsection 18, Learned treatises, subsection 3.
95. Proximate cause in malpractice cases, 13 ALR 2d 11; *Foley v. Bishop Clarkson Memorial Hospital,* 173 N.W.2d 881, Neb. 1970.
96. Cancer: malpractice in connection with diagnosis of cancer, ALR 3d 915.
97. Prosser, D.: Torts 241-244 ed. 4th, 1971; Small, Gaffing at a thing called cause, Tex. Law Rev. **31**:630, 1953; *Stone v. Foster,* 106 Cal.App.3d 344, App., 164 Cal.Rptr. 901, 1980.
98. *Colby v. Schwartz,* 144 Cal.Rptr. 624, 1978; Comment, first aid to passengers: Good Samaritan statutes and contractual releases from liability, S.W. Law J. **31**:695, 1977.
99. Luke **10**:33.
100. Releases from liability, S.W. Law J. **31**:695, 1977; Thirty states have statutes that protect "any person" who gives emergency assistance: ALASKA STAT. §09.65.090 (Supp. 1976); ARIZ. REV. STAT. ANN. §32-1471 (West Supp. 1975); ARK. STAT. ANN. §72-624 (Supp. 1975); DEL. CODE tit. 16 §6801 (Supp. 1976); FLA. STAT. ANN. §768.13 (West Supp. 1976); GA. CODE ANN. §84-930 (1975); HAWAII REV. STAT. §663-1.5 (Supp. 1975); IDAHO CODE §5-330 (Supp. 1976); IND. CODE ANN. §34-4-12-1 (Burns 1973); IOWA CODE ANN. §613.17 (West Supp. 1977); ME. REV. STAT. ANN. tit. 14 §613.17 (West Supp. 1977); MD. ANN. CODE art. 43,§132 (Supp. 1977); MINN. STAT. ANN. §604.05 (West Supp. 1976); MONT. REV. CODES ANN. §17-410 (1967); NEV. REV. STAT. §41.500 (1975); N.H. REV. STAT. §508.12 (1973); N.J. STAT. ANN. §2A:62A-1 (West Supp. 1977); N.M. STAT. ANN. §12-25-3 (1976); N.C. GEN. STAT. §§20-166(d), 8-95 (1975); OHIO REV. CODE ANN. §2305.23 (Page Supp. 1977); OKLA. STAT. ANN. tit. 76, §5 (West 1976); S.C. CODE §15-1-310 (Supp. 1976); S.D. CODE §20-9-4.1 (1970); TENN. CODE §63-622 (1976); TEX. REV. CIV. STAT. ANN. art. 1a (Vernon 1977); VT. STAT. ANN. tit. 12, §517 (1973); VA. CODE §54-276.9 (Supp. 1977); WASH. REV. CODE ANN. §4.24.300 (Supp. 1976); W.VA. CODE §55-7-15 (1976); WYO. STAT. §33-343.1 (Supp. 1975).
101. Twenty States, the District of Columbia and the Virgin Islands have statutes that protect only medical or licensed personnel: ALA. CODE ANN. tit. 7,§121(1) (Supp. 1975); CAL. BUS. & PROF. CODE §§2144, 2727.5 (West Supp. 1976); COLO. REV. STAT. §13-21-108 (Supp. 1976); CONN. GEN. STAT. §52-557b (1977); D.C. CODE §2-142 (1973); ILL. ANN. STAT. ch. 91, §2a (Smith-Hurd Supp. 1976); KAN. STAT. §65-2891 (Supp. 1977); KY. REV. STAT. §411.148 (Supp. 1974); LA. REV. STAT. ANN. §§37:1731-:1732 (West 1974); MASS. ANN. LAWS ch. 112§12B (Michie/Law Co-op 1975); MICH. COMP. LAWS ANN. §14.563 (1976) §691.1501 (1976); MO. STAT. ANN. §190.195 (1976); MISS. CODE ANN. §73-25-37 (Supp. 1976); NEB. REV. STAT. §25-1152 (1975); N.Y. EDUC. LAW §6527 (McKinney Supp. 1977); N.D. CENT. CODE §§43-17-37-38 (Supp. 1975); ORE. REV. STAT. §30.800 (1975); PA. STAT. ANN. tit. 12 § 1641-1643 (Purdon Supp. 1977); R.I. GEN. LAWS §5-37-14 (1975); UTAH CODE ANN. §58-12-23 (1974); V.I. STAT. ANN. tit. 27 §42 (1970); WIS. STAT. ANN. §448.03 (West Supp. 1976).
102. For example, the stated purpose of the Alaskan Good Samaritan statute is to "induce voluntary rescue by removing the fear of potential liability which acts as an impediment to such rescue." ALASKA STAT §09.65.090 (Supp. 1976). See also, Zaremski, M.J.: The "Good Samaritan" goes to court—does the law protect him? J. Legal Med. vol. 1, 1979; Norris, J.: The current status and utility of American emergency medical care liability law, Committee on Medicine and Law of the Insurance, Negligence and Compensation Law Section of the American Bar Association, 1979.
103. *McKenna v. Cedars of Lebanon Hospital,* 155 Cal.Rptr. 631, 93 Cal.App.3d 282, 1979.
104. Harney, D.: Medical malpractice, Indianapolis, 1973, Allen Smith Co.
105. To my knowledge, the only state appellate cases with discussions on the Good Samaritan statutes are *Colby v. Schwartz,* 144 Cal.Rptr. 624, 1978; *Guerrero v. Copper Queen Hospital,* 112 Ariz. 104, 537 P.2d 1329 1975; *Barnum v. Rural Fire Protection Company,* 24 Ariz. App. 233, 537 P.2d 618, 1975; *Markman v. Kotler,* 52 A.D.2d 579, 382 N.Y.S.2d 522, 1976; *Dreibelbis v. Bennett,* (Ind.) 319 N.E.2d 634 , 1974; *Lee v. State,* (Alaska) 490 P.2d 1206, 1971; *Dahl v. Turner,* 80 N.M. 564, 458 P.2d 816, 1969.
106. Cal. Bus. & Prof. Code § 2144. See statutes summarized in Harney, D.: Medical malpractice, Appendix A., Indianapolis, 1973, Allen Smith Co.
107. *Patrick v. Sedgewick,* 413 P.2d 169, Alaska 1966.
108. *Thor v. Boska,* 113 Cal.Rptr. 296, 38 Cal.App.3d 358, 1974.
109. Zinman, E.J.: How long to hold patient records, Dent. Management, p. 29, Oct. 1979.
110. *Kaiser v. Suburban Transportation System,* 398 P.2d 14, Wash. 1965; see also *Wilson v. Hungate,* 434 S.W.2d 580, Mo. 1968; *Whitfield v. Daniel Construction Co.,* 83 S.E.2d 460, S.C. 1954.
111. Bennett, I.: Misuse of propoxyphene, J.A.M.A. **235**:1986, 1976.
112. *Graham v. Sisco,* 248 Ark. 6, 449 S.W.2d 949, 1970.
113. California Evidence Code 1157, 40 Am. Jur. 2d Hospitals and Asylums § 43.
114. California Evidence Code 1156; Discovery of Hospital's internal records of communication as to qualifications or evaluations of individual physicians, 81 ALR 3d 944. See also Limited immu-

nity for acts performed by persons participating in peer review committees composed chiefly of physicians and surgeons or dentists, or both, Cal. Health and Safety Code, section 1370. Re: Absolute privileges of statements made to peer review committees: See Cal. Civil Code 43.7 (Immunity of Members of professional society, hospital staff, and peer review committees) and Civil Code Section 47 (Privileged publication or broadcast: what constitutes) as amended in 1979. See also, *Hackathal v. Weissbein,* 24 Cal.3d 55, 154 Cal.Rptr. 423, 592 P.2d 1175, 1979.

115. Zinman, E.: Toxicity and mepivacaine, J. Am. Dent. Assoc. **92:**858, 1976.
116. *Meyer v. McDonnell,* 392 A.2d 1129, 1978.
117. Cal. Bus. & Prof. Code Section 1680(§) of the Dental Practice Act.

34 Prevention of disease

NORMAN M. POKRAS, D.D.S., M.S.D.

We in the medical and allied professions have been uniquely successful in the past 100 years. Dramatic and sophisticated systems have been devised for the recognition, treatment, and prevention of disease. These systems are based on a rather complete understanding of the causes of specific disease states and on their physiological effects. Enormous strides have been made with the use of these systems. Degenerative diseases, however, have resisted efforts at prevention, control, and treatment.

Many explanations have been offered for our failure with this group of diseases, including that an elongated life span and modern life-style, which increase wear and tear, will favor these diseases. It is also said that treatment of degenerative diseases is not as glamorous as that of other diseases and that patients generally resist preventive measures. The latent period is many years for these diseases; disease recognition therefore may be too late. One reason that has not been investigated well is our preoccupation with disease states and our failure to really define *good health*. We offer a patient precious little unless abnormalities are revealed that we have been preconditioned to recognize. In short, we have defined *good disease* but not *good health*. The importance of this failing is that many diseases are not preventable through our present modus operandi and may require, in addition, preventive measures aimed at arming the subject with a higher health index. For this category of illness we will have to finally learn how to improve the state of health of those people who are supposedly disease free in an effort to make them less disease prone. Joint diseases, in general, and temporomandibular joint disease, in particular, are in this category.

The TMJ apparatus acts as a lightning rod, absorbing adverse stimuli from oral and extraoral foci. Diseases here result from a culmination of those abnormal stresses which often predate the overt disease by months or even years. These etiological factors actually may be absent by the time the familiar signs and symptoms appear, the disease itself being only the debris of these often forgotten underlying factors.

Prevention of TMJ disease therefore involves a thorough understanding of not only its many etiological factors but also of those factors which may gird this structure against them. In other words, we must learn how to make the TMJ complex healthier.

Many years were required to convince ourselves that dental caries is a preventable disease. Convincing our colleagues (and ourselves) that the TMJ syndrome is preventable may present a more difficult problem; we have yet to convince many that it actually exists.

Green[8] received questionnaires from 1000 physicians and dentists. He asked them if they believed there actually was a syndrome consisting of pain around the TMJ, noises coming from the TMJ, subluxation, limitation of movement, deviation on opening, and difficulty on mastication. It was shocking that 50% of the physicians did not think there was such a syndrome and even more so that 35% of the dentists were equally skeptical! Interestingly enough, of the gnathological group that was queried, 88% were convinced of its existence. So, as a preliminary to the discussion of prevention, I might suggest that we all reinforce in our minds the entire concept of TMJ or myofunctional syndrome and review its pathophysiology.

PATHOLOGICAL PHYSIOLOGY OF THE TMJ SYNDROME

The difference between the TMJ and other joints in the body is the key to understanding the problems we are dealing with. As a free-gliding hinge joint, the TMJ functions with some structural instability. This is probably related to the fact that humans are in the midst of evolutionary change in which the development of the temporomandibular complex is not yet completely suitable to our present life-style. Lower animals can open widely; snakes can actually disarticulate their jaws to accommodate large food boluses. Nonfusion of the cranium in lower animals aids in this movement, but the

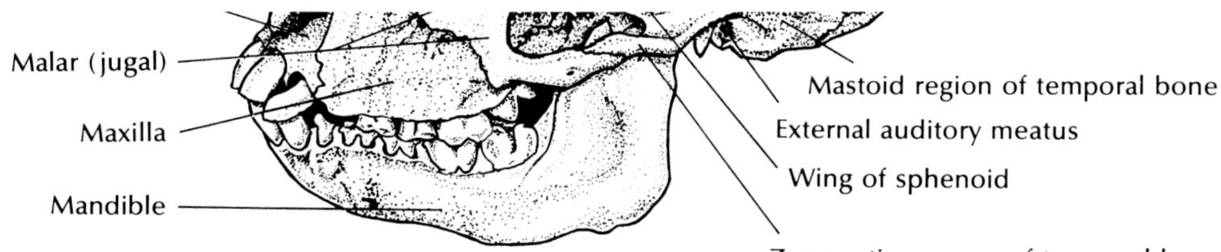

Fig. 34-1. Lateral view of skull of monkey showing lack of articular eminence. (From Weichert, C.K.: The anatomy of chordates, ed. 4, New York, 1970, McGraw-Hill Book Co. Used with permission of McGraw-Hill Book Co.)

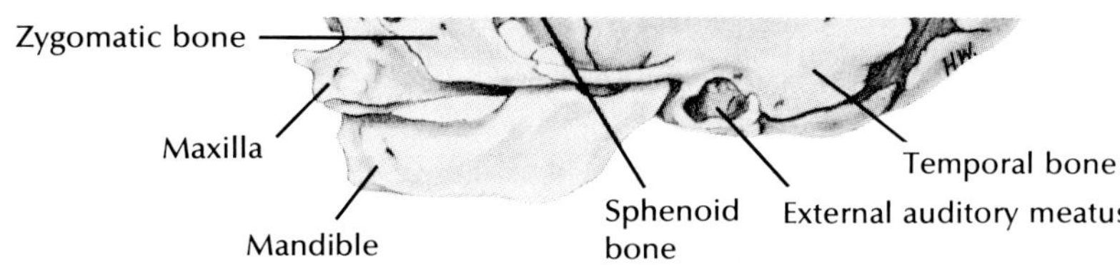

Fig. 34-2. Skull of term fetus showing lack of articular eminence. (From Francis, C.C.: Introduction to human anatomy, ed. 6, St. Louis, 1968, The C.V. Mosby Co.)

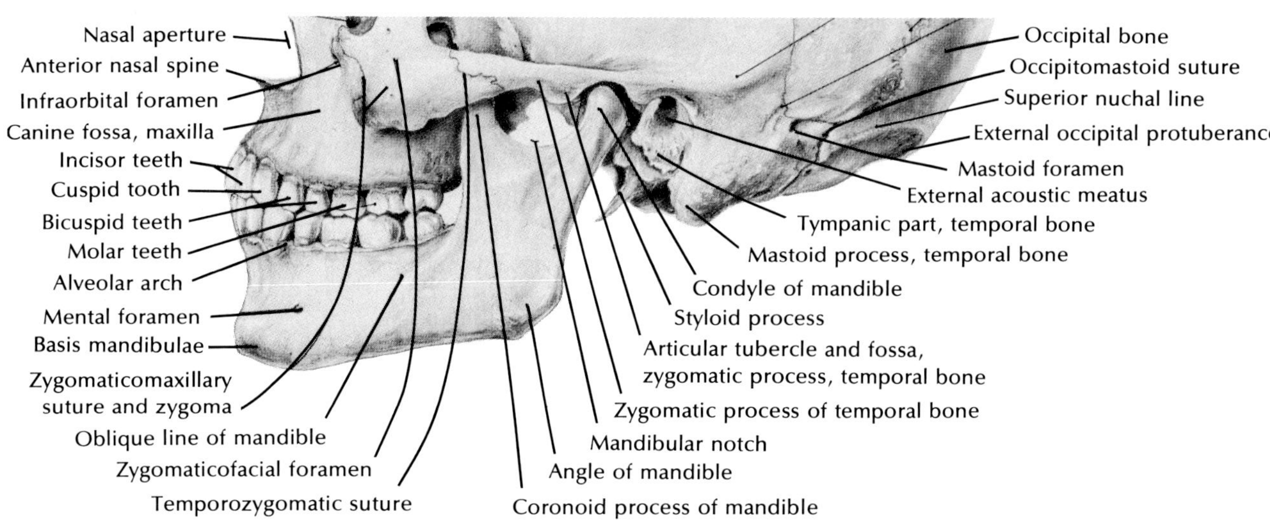

Fig. 34-3. Lateral view of adult human skull showing normal articular eminence. (From Woodburne, R.T.: Essentials of human anatomy, ed. 5, New York, 1973, Oxford University Press.)

mobility of the mandible in animals even to the highest anthropoid apes is a *pure hinge movement*.[13] The hinge sliding movement, then, is a uniquely human trait. It evolved as a response to the assumption of an upright posture and the development of changes in the base of the skull, restricting posterior movement of the condyles. All this is generally accepted by the profession. The development of a prominent articular eminence seems to restrict anterior movement and makes a complicated and unstable maneuver necessary for wide opening. Figs. 34-1 to 34-4 reveal development of the articular eminence in the monkey and modern humans.[2,3] As a matter of fact, lower animals have little antecedent for this structure, and its evolution has not been dealt with in any substantial study. If we can believe Haeckel's famous biogenetic law that animals tend

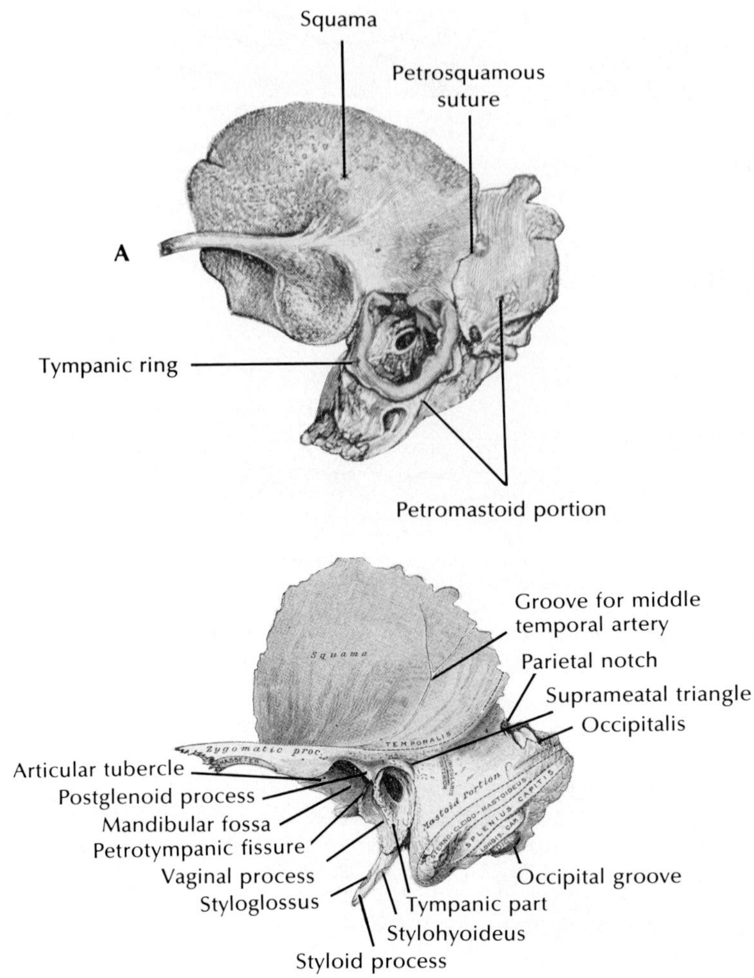

Fig. 34-4. A, Temporal bone at birth (no eminence). **B,** Temporal bone of human adult showing normal eminence. (From Goss, C.M.: Gray's anatomy, ed. 29, Philadelphia, 1973, Lea & Febiger.)

to repeat evolutionary development during their own development,[5] the fact that the articular tubercle is almost nonexistent in the newborn[13] has much significance here (Fig. 34-4). It seems to further suggest the evolution of this structure. Extremely wide opening, then, is made much more complicated in the human being by this anterior eminence and certainly puts an additional strain on those muscles which must guide the disc and condyle anteriorly. As a matter of fact, pathological conditions of the TMJ generally occur with a more prominent eminence or a steeper anterior slope.[1]

The temporomandibular joint is what Sicher and DuBrul[13] describe as a hinge joint in a moving socket. We all know that what stability it does have depends on the equilibrium of the many muscles that are attached to it. In fact the joint is most vulnerable when it is undergoing translatory (anteroposterior) movements. These movements are mostly present during extreme opening, which, by the way, we all force patients to perform. The muscles involved in translatory movements are those most often involved in spasms (external pterygoid muscle, anterior and posterior fibers of the temporal muscle, and the deep portion of the masseter muscle). It is interesting to note that these muscles have an action similar to that of the antigravity muscles of the body, which are also among those most prone to spasm.[11] All this seems to strongly suggest that wide opening is not a physiological movement in man.

Thus to a symptom complex that begins insidiously with muscle spasms related to the instability of the anatomical structure are added iatrogenic, psychological, physical, and structural insults. If this happens long enough in a susceptible individual, the result is degenerative joint disease, but on the way the joint passes through the entire gamut of joint pathosis.

RECOGNITION OF THE TMJ SYNDROME–PRONE INDIVIDUAL

It was shown by Rosenbaum[12] that a 3-minute screening examination could accurately turn up 95% of the patients who have the TMJ syndrome. He found that by simply palpating the muscles of mastication and the TMJ and forcefully retruding the jaw he could discover these patients. Furthermore, he found that there was a simple question that could be asked, which was almost definitive: "Does your jaw ever feel tired?" From the point of view of prevention the practitioner is not looking for those patients who have the syndrome but rather for those who are predisposed to it. The following examinations are useful for this purpose:

1. Measure and record interincisal distance at maximum opening.
2. Record structural anomalies such as retrognathism, prognathism, or other obvious asymmetry.
3. Record obvious emotional illness as evidenced by dress, makeup, expression, and patient reaction. Overt depressive states are suggestive of predisposition and make the TMJ syndrome more difficult to treat.
4. Observe opening movement for smoothness; auscultate the TMJ for area sounds.
5. Palpate muscles of mastication and accessory muscles for tenderness.
6. Forcefully retrude the mandible.
7. Note missing and unreplaced posterior teeth.
8. Check condylar position for concentricity if TMJ radiographs are available. Asymmetrical joint spaces have been associated with dysfunction.[14]
9. Check Panorex or TMJ radiographs for steep eminence.
10. Ask the patient
    a. Have you ever had cervical traction?
    b. Do your jaws ever feel tired?
11. Check obvious occlusal disharmonies.
12. Recognize that this is a disease primarily of women and that it is especially likely to be exacerbated during menses.

I believe the emphasis on what my recommendations are for prevention will depend on how positive this screening turns out. Admittedly these patients are not the easiest to motivate, but it is far easier to mention to them briefly that you are attempting to prevent this complication than to have the patient raise questions on a subsequent appointment about a trismus, clicking, or pain that appeared directly after therapy.

THE THREE CATEGORIES OF DISEASE PREVENTION

Management of the immediate, acute, stressful situation

The acute or stressful situation includes not only the fractured mandible with a contused TMJ or acute whiplash injuries, which are so prevalent, but also the TMJ trauma associated with impacted third molar surgery or long dental appointments with wide opening for prolonged periods. It also includes the immediate postoperative period after placement of multiple restorations or a new partial denture. When I recognize a patient who is especially prone to developing this syndrome and I know that I must submit this patient to additional stresses such as those which are most likely to have adverse effects (stretching, pain production, occlusal disruption, or actual needle trauma to one of the masticatory muscles), I take several precautionary measures.

First, I inform the patient about TMJ physiology and possible postoperative TMJ symptoms. I then explain the transitory nature of the condition so that additional psychological trauma can be avoided.

Second, I advise the patient to perform a variation of physiotherapy on the muscles that I believe will be most traumatized and thrown into spasm. This consists of performing protrusive movements of the mandible against firm fist pressure and slowly relaxing while the pressure is maintained. Variations of this can be done; either left or right lateral protrusive excursions may be added and the patient advised that these excursions must be performed six, eight, or ten times a day for approximately 1 minute. The teeth are separated just enough to disengage the occlusion, but the patient is told *not* to open the mouth widely as part of the exercise. This exercise requires that all the masticatory muscles contract to stabilize the mandible out of occlusion, and then the muscles that move the mandible in a horizontal position do the work of placing the mandible in protrusive relationship. These are the muscles most likely to be in spasm. This exercise, which was presented by Dr. Sanford Moose at a meeting in San Francisco in 1961, will force the external pterygoid muscle, anterior and posterior fibers of the temporal muscle, and deep portion of the masseter muscle to work in unison and, hopefully, relax their spasms in unison as well. The patient is advised absolutely not to open widely until the mouth opens of its own volition. This exercise will tend to prevent the early signs of this syndrome because they are associated with those conditions which result from spasm. Spasms arise because of overexertion, which leads to localized ischemia, pain, and greater reflex motor activity. Greater motor activity creates greater local muscle tension and ischemia, and so on; this cycle may be prevented by stretching (warm-up) exercises before and directly after surgery.[4] The exercise described does this and secondarily teaches tension control.[7] Exercise is my main preventive therapy before surgery.

Third, I believe that 5 or 10 mg of diazepam (Valium) the night after a stressful situation or intramuscularly at the time of appointment will be helpful. Amitriptyline,[6] a tricyclic antidepressant, has also been found to be effective.

Fourth, dexamethasone (Decadron) given intramuscularly at the time of appointment will tend to act as a deterrent to or equalizer for inflammatory changes caused by excessive myositis. Although dosage and contraindications must be carefully reviewed, a dosage of 8 mg has proved effective for the average adult. Additional and diminishing dosages may be continued for several days for additional benefit and to avoid adrenal depression.

Fifth, meperidine (Demerol) and hydroxyzine pamoate (Vistaril) or another similar tranquilizer, in varying strengths of each, are recommended for severe pain. *Milder synthetics should never be substituted for meperidine or codeine when there is a question of effectiveness*. Remember, the object is to break the cycle of hyperactivity-spasm-ischemia-pain.

Sixth, hot wet packs to the right and left TMJ areas are always recommmended.

Seventh, a diet of soft foods cut into small pieces is always suggested for varying periods after the appointment.

Eighth, patients are advised to avoid opening wide at all costs.

Management of specific causative factors before they manifest themselves in overt disease

Occlusal disharmony, structural disharmony, abusive use, emotional factors, and infections must be corrected. This is well-known preventive therapy.

Recommendations for increasing the level of health of the TMJ

I have separate recommendations for making the TMJ healthier. These involve strengthing the muscles involved in maintaining the position of the disc and bones involved (the hard and soft tissues).

1. Specific TMJ cervical exercises, as previously explained, which have been shown to be effective in preventing and treating spasm[9]
2. Jogging
3. Weight lifting with barbells (patient may follow any acceptable manner and concentrate on shoulders and back)
4. Yoga or other tension-relieving programs such as Transcendental Meditation (TM)
5. Other specific tension-relieving programs such as those advocated by Jacobson[9] or Kraus[10]
6. Instructions concerning avoidance of wide opening

CONCLUSION

The temporomandibular joint syndrome can be prevented only if we understand the multifaceted nature of the disease and of the anatomical structure itself.

Prevention must involve primarily an effort on behalf of our professions to *improve the health* of this structure. It must be approached as part of the treatment of the entire patient and not only from the point of view of a diseased and separate entity. It is of the utmost importance to view the structure not as a diseased or well structure but as a structure in transition.

Second, this complex structure must be girded against the shocks of obvious chronic causative factors, including occlusal and structural disharmonies, abusive use, emotional factors, and infections.

Third, the unavoidable immediate trauma to the temporomandibular joint complex must be treated, and the patient must be aided in understanding this potential problem.

REFERENCES

1. Bell, W.E.: Synopsis—oral and facial pain and the temporomandibular joint, Dallas, 1967, Egen Co., Weldon E. Bell, publisher.
2. Buettner-Janusch, J.: Origins of man: physical anthropology, New York, 1966, John Wiley & Sons, Inc.
3. Clark, W.E.LeG.: Antecedents of man: an introduction to the evolution of the primates, Chicago, 1960, Quadrangle Books.
4. DeVries, H.A.: Physiology of exercise for physical education and athletics, Dubuque, Iowa, 1966, William C. Brown Co., Publishers.
5. Eaton, T.J., Jr.: Comparative anatomy of the vertebrates, New York, 1951, Harper & Row, Publishers.
6. Gessel, A.H.: Electromyographic biofeedback and tricyclic antidepressants in myo-fascial pain dysfunction syndrome: psychological predictors of outcome, J. Am. Dent. Assoc. **91**:1049, 1975.
7. Gessel, A.H., and Alderman, M.M.: Management of myofascial pain dysfunction with tension control training, Psychosomatics **12**:302, 1971.
8. Green, C.S.: A survey of current concepts and opinions about the myo-fascial pain dysfunction (MPD) syndrome, J. Am. Dent. Assoc. **86**:128, 1973.
9. Jacobson, E.: Anxiety and tension control, Philadelphia, 1964, J.B. Lippincott Co.
10. Kraus, H.: Therapeutic exercises, ed. 2, Springfield, Ill., 1962, Charles C Thomas, Publisher.
11. Moulton, R.E.: Emotional factors in non-organic temporomandibular joint pain, Dent. Clin. North Am., p. 609, Nov. 1966.
12. Rosenbaum, M.: The feasibility of a screening procedure regarding temporomandibular joint dysfunction, Oral Surg. **39**:382, 1975.
13. Sicher, H., and DuBrul, E.L.: Oral anatomy, ed. 6, St. Louis, 1975, The C.V. Mosby Co.
14. Weinberg, L.A.: TMJ function and its effect on centric relation, J. Prosthet. Dent. **30**:182, 1973.

Epilogue

The temporomandibular joints in dentistry and dental medicine

DAVID J. GOODFRIEND, D.D.S.

As a pioneer in the discovery of the role of the temporomandibular joint[2] in dentistry and dental medicine, I wish to present its history, its present status, and its probable role in the future of these disciplines.

My initial acquaintance with the temporomandibular joint occurred in 1922 as the result of meeting Dr. Edward C. Kirk, Emeritus Dean of the University of Pennsylvania Dental School and editor of the *Dental Cosmos*. I had established a dental clinic at the Graduate School of Medicine of the University of Pennsylvania. Since I was the only dentist on the staff, Dr. John Kolmer asked me to cooperate in the research of bacterial selective pathogenicity. Although my role was limited to removal of infected teeth and inoculation of periodontal granulomas in test tubes, I also learned research procedures.

At that time Dr. Greenbaum, a dermatologist, asked me to participate in the treatment of a case of pemphigus, the symptoms of which started in the oral cavity. I wrote an article[1] that included a table that differentiated the blebs of pemphigus from those of other lesions that occur in the mouth. Kirk provided colored illustrations by an anatomical artist and published the article in the *Dental Cosmos*.

Kirk then suggested that I devote my career to research. He called to my attention his article[4] on the pathology of abnormal dental occlusion and the articles by Wright[6] on hearing loss and by Monson[5] on "Impaired Function as Result of Closed Bite."

In 1922 Kirk influenced my appointment by Dean Turner as official researcher of the Dental School of the University of Pennsylvania. Turner suggested that I dissect the temporomandibular joint and study the anatomy. He referred me to Professor Eliot R. Clark, Head of Anatomy at the University's Medical School. I explained to Dr. Clark that my purpose was the correlation of data regarding normal and abnormal dental bites or occlusions with normal and abnormal anatomy of the temporomandibular joint. Thus in 1922 I began my studies of the temporomandibular joint.

Dr. Clark accompanied me in examining the dental occlusions of cadavers. I selected those which had normal, adequate dentitions and occlusions and those with varied abnormal occlusions consisting of loss, breakdown, attrition, and other abnormalities. The selected specimens were decapitated, and the heads were placed in a large container in a separate room for my studies.

I dissected away tissue to expose the dental occlusion and the lateral aspect of the temporomandibular joints. The teeth and jaws were wired into the presenting occlusal and maxillomandibular relationships. The heads were then frozen. Sections of the frozen specimens were made through temporomandibular joints and adjacent structures by means of a band saw to show the normal and abnormal anatomical form and relationship of the temporomandibular joints and their relationships with other structures.

The dissections showed that normal adequate dentition and occlusal relationships were associated with normal TMJ anatomy, and the mandibular condyles were olive shaped with smooth surfaces and were located in the center of the temporal fossae in the closed posture of the jaws. There was adequate space between the condyles and adjacent structures.

The dissections of the heads with abnormalities of the dental bite showed the abnormal form and anatomical malrelationships of the rough-surfaced mandibular condyles. The malrelationships involved the displaced discs, erosions of the temporal fossa, the petrotympanic fissure, reduced lumen of the auditory canal, and distortion of the drum, middle ear, and eustachian tube. The assumption may be made that these abnormalities were pathognomonic of symptoms and dysfunctions of TMJ syndromes (Figs. 1 to 3).

In 1927 the University of Pennsylvania established

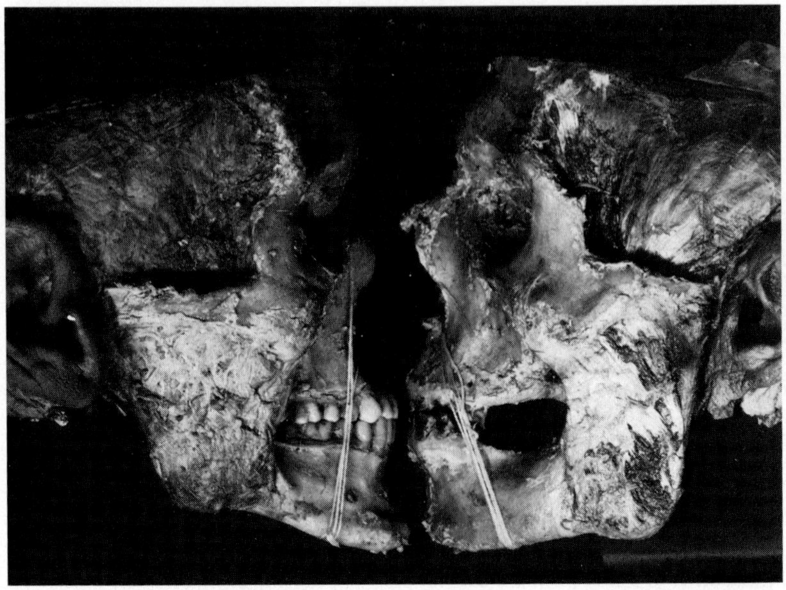

Fig. 1. Dissections of temporomandibular joints with normal *(left)* and abnormal *(right)* dental bites and occlusion.

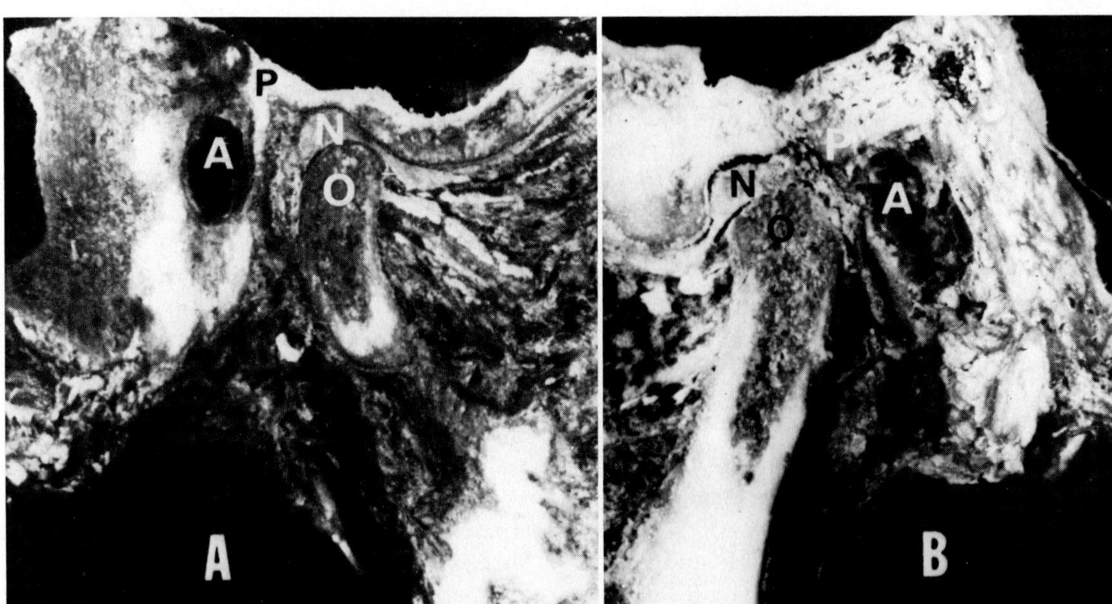

Fig. 2. A, Normal temporomandibular joint: ear anatomy with normal dental occlusion. **B,** Abnormal anatomy with abnormal dental occlusion. *A,* Auditory canal; *P,* petrotympanic fissure; *O,* TMJ condyle; *N,* TMJ disc.

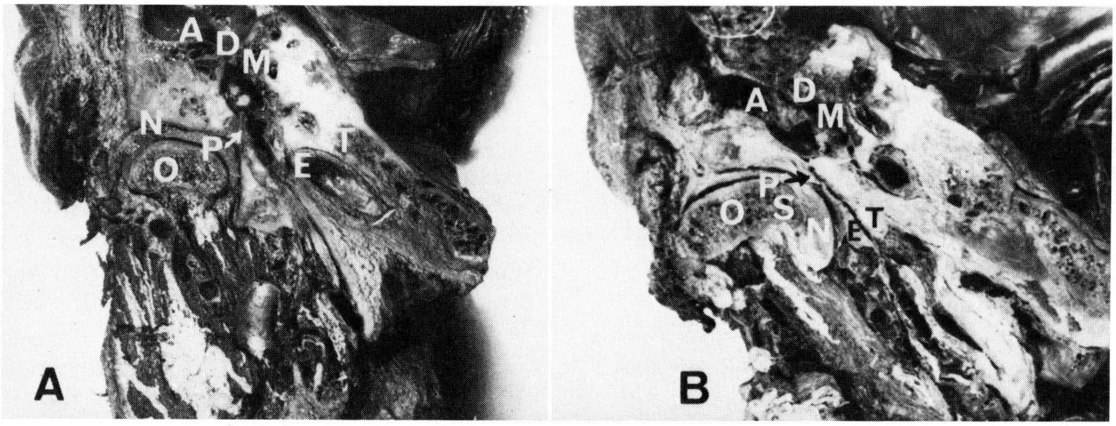

Fig. 3. A, Normal anatomy with normal dental occlusion. **B,** Abnormal anatomy with abnormal dental occlusion. *A,* Auditory canal; *D,* drum; *ET,* eustachian tube; *O,* TMJ condyle; *N,* TMJ disc; *M,* middle ear; *P,* petrotympanic fissure.

the Edward C. Kirk Dental Research, including Professor Clark, Head of Anatomy, Professor Coates, Head of Otolaryngology, Professor Pancoast, Head of Radiology, Professor Twitmeyer, Head of Psychology and Ear Clinic, and me as Director.

Professor Coates set up a special ear clinic to which he referred the first 25 negative objective ear cases. I studied their dental occlusion and temporomandibular joints and found abnormalities in 22 of the 25 patients. Professor Pancoast provided x-ray studies of these patients' temporomandibular joints in accordance with the 20-degree, sagittal, closed- and open-jaw technique that I formulated with Drs. Kornblum and Hoedes. These showed radiographic correlation with the anatomical abnormalities of the joints and dental occlusion with otological findings and vestibular symptoms and dysfunctions.

Two of these patients were selected for dental treatment because they had undergone thorough medical studies. The diagnosis of both was Meniere's disease. One of the patient's Meniere's disease was attributed to incurable infected labyrinthitis. The cause of the other patient's Meniere's disease was vascular tumor on both sides of his brain stem. My treatment of both patients was entirely dental-orthopedic correction of traumatic, inadequate malocclusions. Both patients had complete relief of the Meniere's disease and prevention of recurrences during 5- to 7-year postoperative reviews.

My work in cooperation with Professor Edwin B. Twitmeyer and Dr. Yales S. Nathanson from 1927 to 1948 included the diagnosis and treatment of patients of the speech clinic whose symptoms included deafness and disordered speech kinesthesia. The treatment of these patients included correction of dental occlusal abnormalities and modification of deleterious habits.

The Edward C. Kirk Dental Research was liquidated in 1948, and my findings had been published in many issues of the *Journal of Prosthetic Dentistry*, the *Journal of the American Dental Association*, and the *Archives of Otolaryngology*. The latter article was a 35-page report under the auspices of the American Medical Association. From 1948 to the present I have diagnosed and treated many patients with temporomandibular and related syndromes and have continued studies of the work of others in the field. This represents my 56 years as a practicing dentist. My experience has convinced me that temporomandibular syndromes and related disorders are predisposed, exacerbated, and caused by abnormalities of the dental occlusion. Also, the responsibilities for prevention, diagnosis, and treatment are those of the practicing dentists and cooperating physicians who first see these patients.

Muscle spasms, external injuries, deleterious habits, and stressful life situations unquestionably play an important role in the predisposition and exacerbation of craniomandibular disorders, but the bottom line of therapy consists of the reestablishment of a harmonious balanced dental occlusion that supports adequate maxillomandibular relationships and positions the closed-jaw condyle in the forecenter of the temporal fossa.

The outstanding contribution to my work in this field has been the cooperation with Herbert T. Kelly, M.D., F.A.C.P. This was initiated by his personal experience, just as divine guidance or serendipity aided me in the progress of my work in temporomandibular joint studies. This factor resulted in my fortuitous relationship in 1954 with Dr. Kelly. I happened to enter the hospital and was guided by his nurse into the room where he was being prepared for cranial surgery. As I entered his room, the attending neurologist (whom I didn't know but who probably was familiar with my work in the Pennsylvania Medical School) greeted me with the statement, "This isn't one of your cases, Dr. Goodfriend." I then asked him, "How do you know?" He answered, "He has no ear symptoms." I replied that I had met Dr. Kelly only once, and he seemed to be favoring his right ear. Kelly, who was lying in bed with his eyes closed, opened them and said, "Goodfriend is right, my ear is closed with a loud tinnitus." With that Mrs. Kelly aksed me what my treatment was. I explained that the same symptoms in other patients had been caused by disorders of the dental bite and were relieved by bite correction. With that, the attending internist said, "I have never heard anything so stupid," and walked out of the room.

The neurologist then suggested that I examine Dr. Kelly's bite. I found a serious traumatic occlusal abnormality and a locked bite. I asked the neurologist if he would agree to postpone the surgical operation for 2 to 4 weeks to allow time for my diagnosis and therapeutic test; he agreed.

My diagnostic procedures included the first stage of a two-stage procedure. This consisted of cast overlays of the upper and lower premolar and molar occlusal surfaces. The occlusal curvatures were plotted in harmony with the temporomandibular joints at a height that corrected the occlusal trauma and provided lateral clearance. These factors repositioned the temporomandibular joint to normal relationships in accordance with radiographic criteria. The cast overlays were cemented in place temporarily with the understanding that they would be worn and adjusted to harmonious occlusion for 2 to 4 months, during which time the patient would continue to test subjective responses.

Dr. Kelly wore the overlays for 4 months without recurrence of previous attacks of dizziness, nausea, vomiting, or loss of consciousness. The ear blocking and tinnitus cleared, and he resumed practice and normal activities.

The temporary overlays were replaced one segment at a time by permanent dentistry. This permitted equilibration of each segment before proceeding with the next. There were no recurrences of previous symptoms during the period of traumatic procedures of permanent dentistry, and there have been no recurrences of Meniere's disease and related symptoms during the past 27 years.

We have cooperated in the treatment of over 200 patients with varying symptoms, the most devastating of which were episodes of dizziness and related vestibular and auditory symptoms and dysfunctions (deafness). These included chronic pain of the head, face, neck, and other regions of distribution of the auriculotemporal, trifacial, facial digastric, and palatal nerves. These symptoms involve the broad spectrum of temporomandibular, auditory vertigo, and Meniere's disease syndromes, which are frequently confronted in medicine and dentistry.

All these 200 patients were initially and accurately diagnosed by Dr. Kelly. Protocols were maintained in 105 patients who cooperated to completion of our cooperative therapy. The findings of the medically controlled and medicodental therapy are recorded in the following article by Dr. Kelly and myself.

REFERENCES

1. Goodfriend, D.J.: Pemphigus, Dent. Cosmos, p. 2, Oct. 1924.
2. Goodfriend, D.J.: Dysarthrosis and subarthrosis of mandibular articulation, Dent. Cosmos **74**:523, 1932.
3. Goodfriend, D.J.: Symptomatology and treatment of abnormalities of mandibular articulations, Dent. Cosmos **75**:844, 1933.
4. Kirk, E.C.: Malocclusion as a problem in pathology, Pacific Dent. Gaz. **25**:654, 1917.
5. Monson, G.S.: Impaired function as a result of closed bite, J. Nat. Dent. Assoc. **8**:833, 1921.
6. Wright, W.H.: Deafness influenced by malposition of jaw, J. Nat. Dent. Assoc. **7**:979, 1920.

Vertigo attributable to dental and temporomandibular joint causes*

HERBERT T. KELLY M.D., F.A.C.P., and **DAVID J. GOODFRIEND, D.D.S.**

The relationship of dental occlusal defects to temporomandibular joint abnormalities is well established. The temporomandibular joints are situated in a dynamic region of the head where abnormalities can cause moderate to serious disabling dysfunctions and diseases (Fig. 4). These include blurring of vision, otalgia or ear pain, tinnitus or ear noise, hyperacusis or senstitivity to sound, aerotitis media or ear block, deafness, and vertigo.

Since these symptoms may be caused by traumatic dental malocclusion, medical recognition of this cause and its dental orthopedic correction can make a significant contribution to their prevention and treatment. This has been shown by our medicodental study of the dental causes of vertigo.

Vertigo and dizziness is a common disabling and frightening symptom-complex which is frequently encountered in medical practice. It is a false sense of motion experienced by an individual within himself or of his environment. Alpers[1] listed 73 causes of vertigo including: ear, eye, systemic, gastrointestinal, neurologic, psychogenic, vascular, infectious, metabolic, and degenerative diseases. Gowers[2] found that 89 per cent of patients with vertigo has associated ear symptoms. Cawthorne[3] found that 1,349 of 1,523 cases, or 88 per cent, of patients with vertigo were attributable to disorders of the ears. This is the type of vertigo which may be caused by dental occlusal-temporomandibular joint abnormalities (Figs. 5 and 6).

*Read before the American Equilibration Society in Chicago. Reprinted from J. Prosthet. Dent. 14:159, 1964.

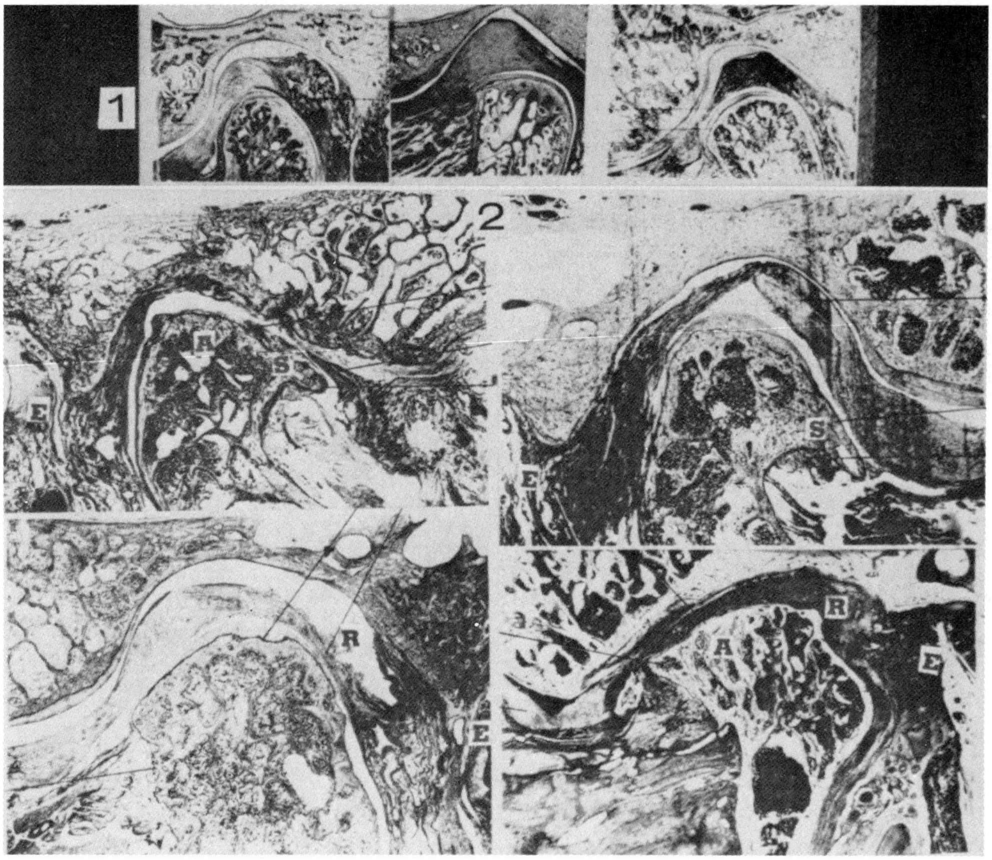

Fig. 4. *(Above, 1)* Three types of normal temporomandibular joints associated with normal adequate dental occlusions. *(Below, 2)* Temporomandibular joint degeneration caused by deterioration of dental occlusions. *A,* Erosion of the condyle surface. *R,* Degeneration and displacement of meniscuses. *S,* Spur formations. *E,* Auditory meatuses.

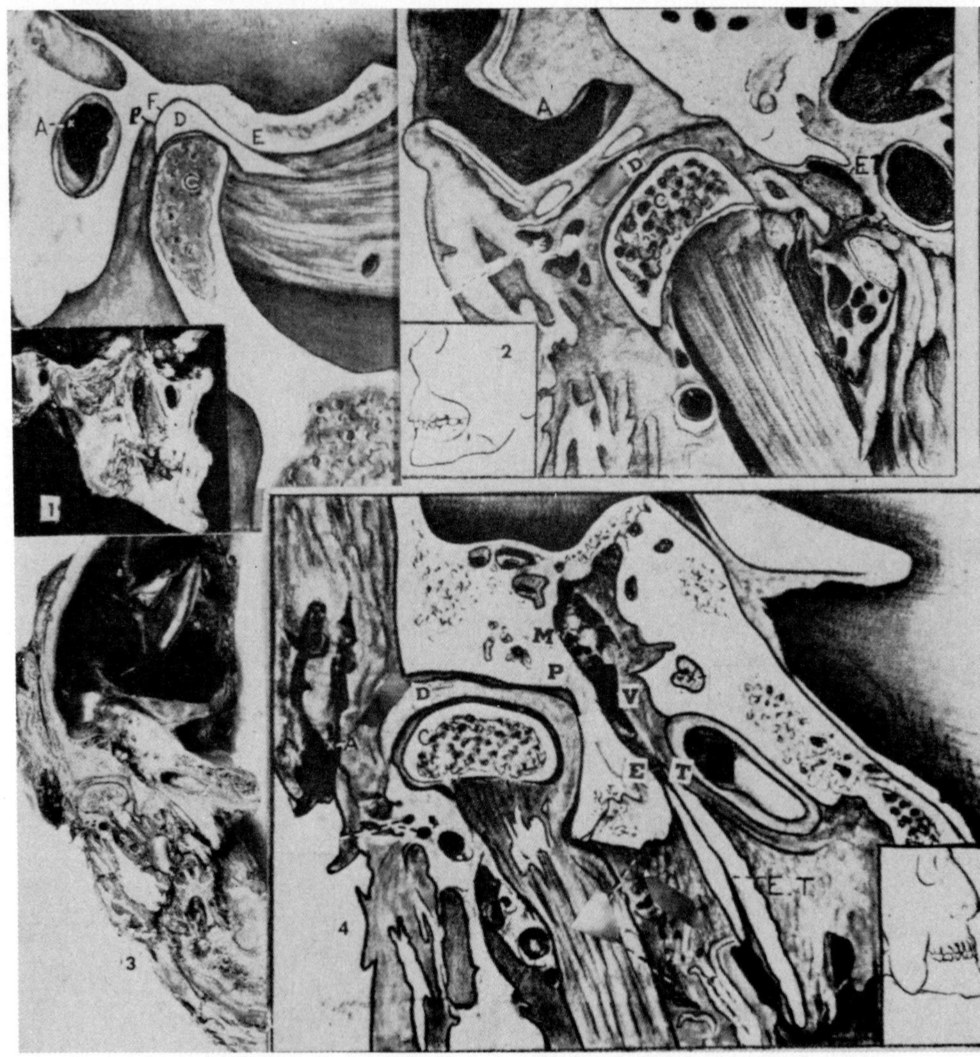

Fig. 5. Sections of temporomandibular joint-ear regions associated with normal adequate dental occlusions. *C,* The rounded form of condyles. *D,* The meniscuses. *F. and E.,* Smooth fossa-eminence surfaces. *A,* Auditory meatuses. *P,* Petrotympanic fissures. *M,* Middle ears. *V,* Vestibules. *E.T.,* Eustachian tubes.

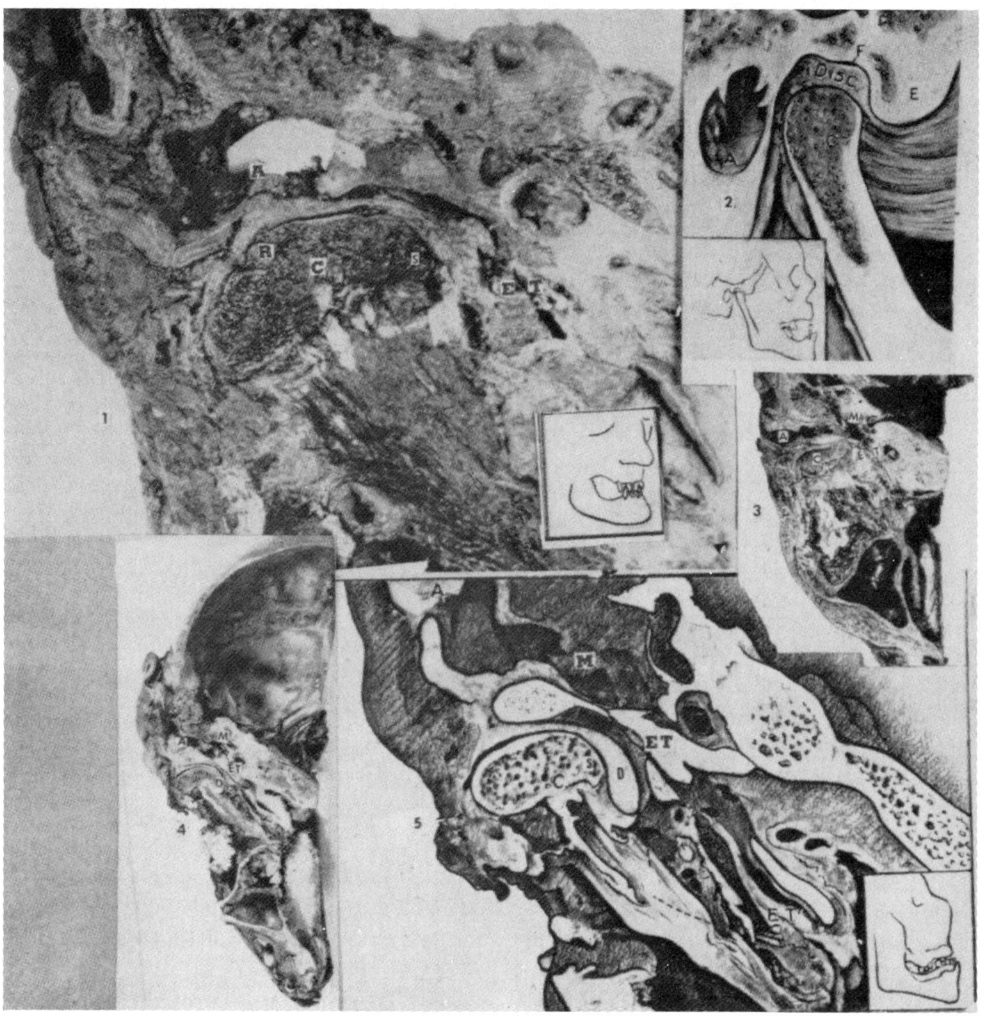

Fig. 6. Sections of temporomandibular joint-ear regions associated with deteriorated dental occlusions which show: *C,* Displaced condyles. *D,* Displaced and degenerated meniscuses. *S,* Spur formations and deformity of condyles. *R,* The rough surface of a condyle and perforation of the meatus. *A,* Auditory meatuses. *M,* The ear drum and middle ear. *E.T.,* A deformity of the Eustachian tubes.

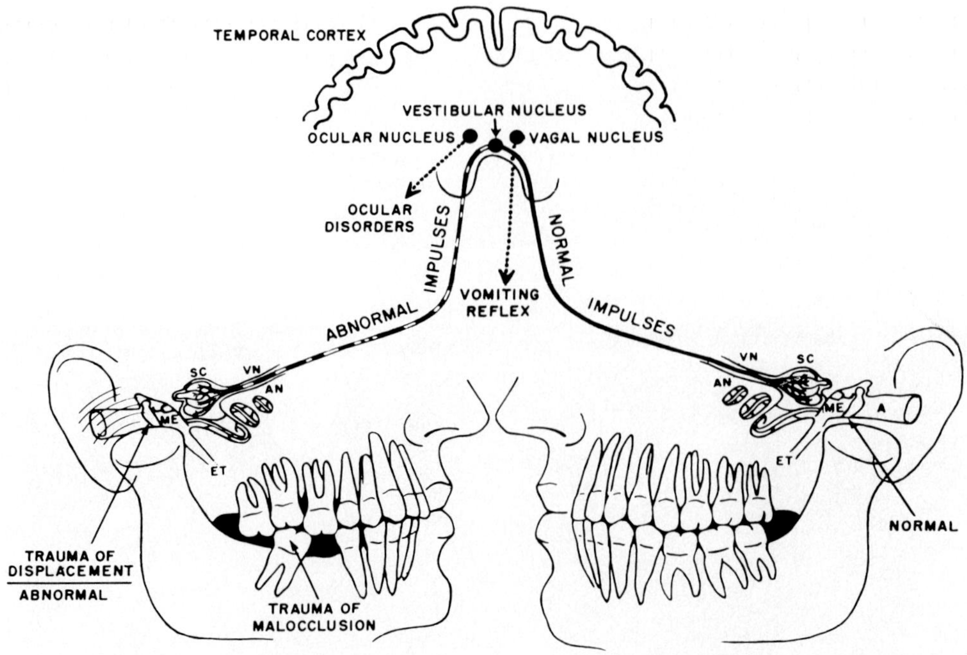

Fig. 7. A diagram which shows unilateral occlusal trauma resulting in abnormal vestibular impulses conveyed by one ear as compared with the other. Traumatic malocclusion of one side may cause abnormal pressure in that joint and traumatic movements of the other joint. Differences of vestibular impulses cause vertigo and associated symptoms. *A,* Auditory meatus. *ME,* Middle ears and ear drums. *ET,* Eustachian tubes. *SC,* Semicircular canals and vestibules. *VN,* Vestibular nerve. *AN,* Auditory nerve.

DENTAL CAUSES OF VERTIGO

Cawthorne[3] observed that vertigo may be caused by differences of the impulses which are conveyed to the vestibular center of the brain by one ear as compared with the other. Also, that the severity of the resultant vertigo is directly related to the degree of difference and the suddenness of its occurrence.

The conduction system of the ears which convey these impulses is situated in close relationship with the temporomandibular joints. Dental occlusal and temporomandibular joint abnormalities, which usually occur unilaterally, may irritate and injure the adjacent conduction system of one ear more than the other. This results in a difference or imbalance of vestibular impulses which cause vertigo (Fig. 7).

The dental causes of vertigo are exacerbated by clenching and bruxing of the teeth, by traumatic, compulsive mastication, and by dental or surgical trauma. Organic diseases, disturbed life situations, and fatigue lower the vestibular threshold and contribute to the causes of vertigo.

The dental occlusal abnormalities which may cause vertigo include developmental and retrogressive malocclusions of deciduous and permanent teeth, and inadequate dental treatment. It is important to emphasize that, in our experience, vertigo is a symptom which usually follows a sudden change in the dental status. Joint symptoms, tinnitus, deafness, and neuralgias may be found in patients in whom the dental abnormalities develop slowly as well as suddenly. Thus, if developmental malocclusions and attrition of teeth occur gradually they may not cause vertigo because the vestibular center adapts to the gradual changes in vestibular impulses. However, these dental conditions are potential etiologic factors which may become active causes of vertigo by the loss of teeth and traumatic dental surgical treatment.

The dental-temporomandibular joint causes of vertigo are "overclosed," traumatic dental occlusion, and traumatic malrelationships of the temporomandibular joints with the adjacent structures of the ear. These dental causes are activated by trauma, fatigue, intrapsychic strain, emotional stress, fingernail biting, cigar and pipe smoking, and organic diseases which lower the vestibular threshold.

CLINICAL MATERIAL AND DIAGNOSTIC PROCEDURES

We studied all vertigo patients during an 8 year period. The initial diagnostic procedures were medical.

They included case history, physical and neurologic examinations, laboratory tests, skull roentgenograms, and other studies. Dental diagnoses were made of patients whose eyeground and neurologic studies did not show evidence of abnormal intracranial pressure. This decision was based upon the fact that initial reversible dental procedures differentiated the cause of vertigo.

One hundred and twenty-eight patients were studied. One patient had a brain tumor and 2 had malignant hypertension. Twenty did not accept dental treatment. One hundred and five patients cooperated to completion of the dental treatment. Sixty-eight were women and thirty-seven were men. The ages ranged from 8 to 89 years, with an average of 55 years.

The dental diagnosis was made by the physician and the dentist. This included palpation of the temporomandibular joints during opening, closing, and lateral movements of the jaw, palpation of the muscles of mastication, examination of the occlusion, facial measurements, and temporomandibular joint roentgenograms.

CLINICAL FINDINGS

All patients in this study had previously received dental treatment which was acceptable to them and to their dentists. The patients and their previous dental and medical consultants were apparently unaware that occlusal defects could cause vertigo. Many patients said that their dentists had told them that they had "bad bites" but, despite histories of temporomandibular joint symptoms, treatment was not recommended.

In taking case histories, it was difficult for the physician to elicit dental complaints as well as for the dentist to secure history of ear and vertigo complaints. In many patients, the symptom-complex of vertigo had been attributed by previous diagnosticians to probable brain tumor, brain degeneration, hypertension, vestibular hydrops, Meniere's disease, abdominal epilepsy, cholecystitis, and psychoneuroses.

Case histories frequently correlated the onset of vertigo with dental treatments, such as the removal or replacement of teeth. In several patients, the onset of symptoms was correlated with traumatic, "overclosed" new dentures. This also occurred when old dentures were worn for too many years. Many patients associated vertigo attacks with eating tough foods and attributed the vertigo to an allergic reaction to those foods rather than to the trauma of mastication. Fingernail, pipe, and pencil biting were found to be triggering mechanisms, and unilateral chewing was frequently practiced by these patients. Vertigo frequently occurred upon awakening, and it could be correlated with clenching and bruxing during sleep. In many patients, it was not possible to correlate the vertigo with activities involving the jaws.

Pain and paresthesia of the regions over the joints, face and posterior part of the neck, and muscular spasm frequently were associated with vertigo. Patients occasionally complained of difficulty in swallowing. Fifty per cent of the patients had other ear symptoms including tinnitus, aerotitis media, and hearing disorders. Fifty-five per cent of the patients had a past or present history of clicking, noisy, and painful temporomandibular joints. Ten per cent complained of excessive, jerky jaw movements, and 7 per cent had limited jaw movements.

The characteristics of the vertigo of these patients were the same as those of vertigo which medical literature attributes to other causes. Patients described their vertigo symptoms as blurring of vision, dizziness, light-headedness, staggering gait, and fear of heights, platforms or stairs. The attacks were usually paroxysmal, lasting from a few minutes to 30 minutes or more. They became more frequent and severe during the course of the illness. Associated eye symptoms included difficulty in focusing and visual hallucinations. Vagal symptoms included pallor, perspiring, nausea, vomiting, diarrhea, epigastric pain, and syncope. Psychogenic symptoms were attributable to a feeling of insecurity, anxiety, and a fear of morbid causes of the vertigo, particularly brain tumor and cardiovascular disorders.

TREATMENT

The initial medical treatment was directed to achieve patient acceptance of the dental cause of vertigo and the indicated dental treatment. While it may be assumed that patients accept the physician's diagnosis and treatment, we found it was necessary to mobilize the patient. The anxiety characterized by helplessness and fear which is engendered by vertigo made this medical phase of treatment important and difficult. The paroxysmal overwhelming dizziness, blurring of vision, the nausea, vomiting and wretching, the turbulent eye movements, blackouts and loss of control have few parallels in the entire field of medicine. It was difficult to persuade the patient, his family, and his medical and dental consultants that these serious symptoms could be caused by dental occlusal defects and temporomandibular arthrosis.

Since this study was directed to test the dental causes of vertigo and the therapeutic effectiveness of dental corrective treatments, the physician's efforts were limited to psychotherapy, medical, and nutritional therapy before and concurrent with the dental treatments and to diagnostic procedure to check the results of the dental treatments.

The dental treatment of patients with natural teeth was a two-phase procedure. It was directed to establish

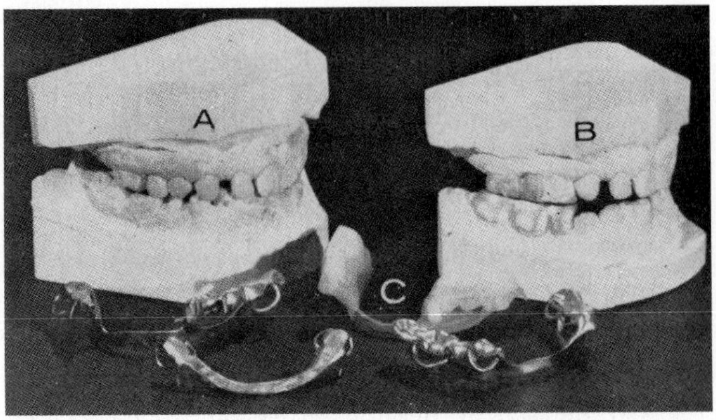

Fig. 8. *A,* A malocclusion exacerbated by removable appliances *(C)* which was associated with symptoms that progressed from a clicking joint to neuralgia and vertigo. *B,* Overlays of the unprepared teeth which temporarily reconstructed the upper and lower occlusal surfaces to a plotted curve of occlusion in harmony with the temporomandibular joints. These are worn until the symptoms are relieved and then they are reproduced by permanent restorations.

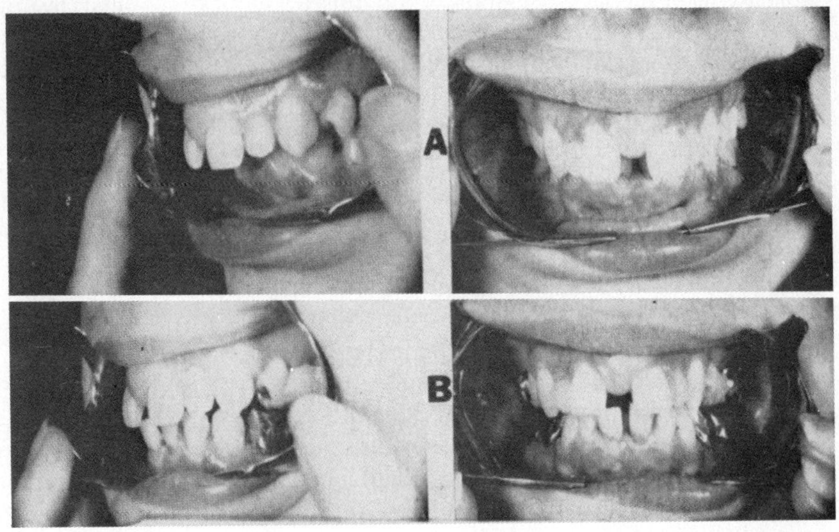

Fig. 9. *A,* The malocclusion that caused neuralgia, dizziness, nausea, vomiting, blackout, and loss of consciousness in a patient from age 12 years to 30 years. *B,* The overlays on the upper and lower right and left bicuspid and molar teeth completely relieved all symptoms.

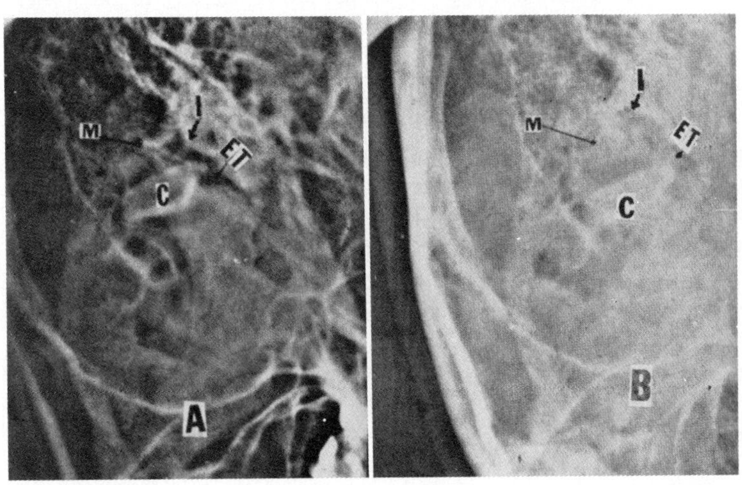

Fig. 10. Vertex roentgenograms of temporomandibular joint-ear regions. *A* shows: *(C)* the flat posterior surface of the condyle with a medial spur in the Eustachian tube *(ET).* The approximation of the condyle with malleus middle ear ossicle *(M)* and vestibular nerve *(I).* *B* shows: *(C)* a normal rounded condyle with the spur resorbed and the normal relation of the condyle with the malleus and middle ear *(M),* the vestibule *(I),* and the Eustachian tube *(ET)* resulting from the correction of the malocclusion by means of overlays and occlusal reconstructions.

a harmonious dental occlusion that adequately supported nonpathogenic relationships of the temporomandibular joints with the ears and Eustachian tubes. The first phase consisted of placing cast metal overlays on the unprepared upper and lower premolar and molar teeth. The occlusal surfaces were plotted as segments of spheres in harmony with the temporomandibular joints (Fig. 8). The overlays were cemented on the unprepared teeth and equilibrated to lateral occlusion in accordance with Schuyler's datum.[4] The selective equilibrating adjustments were repeated weekly for 3 or 4 weeks, because it was found that an altered occlusion is likely to continue to change for that length of time.

The patients wore the treatment overlays for periods of 2 months to 2 years. This is essential to test their therapeutic results because vertigo frequently has periods of remittance. If the overlays did not relieve the vertigo, they were either further equilibrated or remade, or finally removed. In the latter instances, it was assumed that the dental occlusion was not the cause of the vertigo and the patient's occlusion resumed its former status. In patients in whom the overlays relieved the vertigo, it usually relieved the crepitic and abnormal joint and jaw movements, and tinnitus and other ear symptoms. Acute deafness was relieved, but no improvement was observed in patients with deafness of long duration. The second phase of dental treatment consisted of placing permanent reconstructions of the premolar and molar teeth. One overlay was replaced at a time and the permanent reconstructions were equilibrated with the remaining overlays before replacing the next overlay.

In patients who required fixed prosthesis or removable appliances, the dental treatment consisted of procedures in which both the upper and lower occlusal surfaces were altered to establish a curve of occlusion in harmony with the temporomandibular joint surfaces. The harmonious occlusal surfaces were established by porcelain artificial teeth and metallic onlays of abutment teeth. There were no interlocking cusps or overlaps, and free lateral occlusion was equilibrated in accordance with Schuyler's[4] principles (see Figs. 9 and 10).

RESULTS

The results of the treatment of the 105 patients are tabulated in Tables 1 and 2. These show that in 94 of the 105, or 89 per cent, the vertigo and dizziness were relieved by the dental orthopedic and medical supportive treatments. Also, that this treatment relieved 83 per cent of associated symptoms of light-headedness, blurring of vision, staggering gait, uncertainty of heights, nausea, vomiting, blackouts, and loss of consciousness. Eighty-three per cent of ear disorders were cured or improved. All patients with temporomandibular joint dysfunctions received relief and 79 per cent were cured. Sixty-four per cent of the patients having neuralgia were cured or relieved by the dental-medical treatment.

Two years after the completion of this study, or 10 years after treating certain of the patients, questionnaires were sent to all patients. Since they were private patients who had paid substantial fees for dental treatment, it was assumed that those responding would in-

Table 1. Dental-medical treatment of patients with vertigo*

Symptoms	No. of symptoms	Results of treatment			
		Complete relief	Partial relief	No relief	Per cent complete relief
Dizziness	105	94	7	4	89
Visual disorders	97	85	7	5	83
Nausea	23	17	2	4	75
Vomiting	19	15	3	1	80
Blackouts	24	21		3	88
Loss of consciousness	20	17		3	87
Staggering gait	10	8	2		80
Uncertainty of heights	11	5	2	4	43
Diminished hearing	47	16	19	12	35
Ear noises	46	20	17	9	43
Sensitivity to noise	22	9	13	4	40
Ear blocking	32	19	9	4	59

*89 per cent received complete relief of vertigo; 45 per cent received complete relief of ear disorders.

Table 2. Dental-medical treatment of temporomandibular joint and neuralgia symptoms of 105 patients with vertigo*

Symptoms	No. of symptoms	Results of treatment: Complete relief No.	Complete relief Per cent	Partial relief	No relief
Joint					
Crepitus	32	27	84	5	0
Pain	16	11	70	5	0
Limited movement	10	8	80	2	0
Excessive movement	4	2	50	2	0
Neuralgia					
Facial pain	32	21	65	6	5
Head pain	26	17	65	6	3
Ear pain	26	16	62	8	2
Neck pain	40	26	65	10	4

*79 per cent received complete relief of temporomandibular joint symptoms; 64 per cent received complete relief of neuralgia symtpoms.

clude those with the worst results. Forty-four patients responded to the questionnaire. These corroborated the favorable findings of the original protocols which are tabulated in Table 1, and showed that 83 per cent of the vertigo of these patients was completely relieved by the medical-dental orthopedic treatment.

The therapeutic effectiveness of the corrective dental appliances was further tested by their removal in certain patients. Removal of the appliances returned the occlusions to their previous condition and usually resulted in recurrence of vertigo and other symptoms. These symptoms were relieved by replacing the appliances. This is illustrated by the experience of a woman 80 years of age who had had symptoms of progressive deafness and tinnitus of 30 years' duration. During the previous 2 years, she suffered with severe paroxysmal attacks of dizziness, nausea, vomiting, and blackouts. Her treatment consisted of maxillary and mandibular removable appliances. These relieved the vertigo and associated symptoms but failed to achieve patient acceptance. The appliances were then reinserted and adjusted. This relieved the vertigo and the patient was able to go home unaided. She continued to wear the appliances without recurrence of the attacks of vertigo.

Most of the patients who rejected dental treatment continued to suffer from vertigo and associated symptoms. Many patients whose vertigo was relieved by dental-medical treatment, but whose habits of bruxing and clenching continued, subsequently complained of slight disorders of equilibrium and feared a recurrence of vertigo. These were relieved by selective equilibration of occlusion which usually required one short dental appointment. The following cases were typical of this study.

CASE HISTORIES

Case 1

A boy, 8 years of age, had symptoms of severe vomiting following the eating of solid food. Previous medical and otologic studies failed to find an organic etiology. The vomiting was attributed to a behavior problem. Severe disciplinary measures, including whippings after each attack, did not improve the symptoms and resulted in an undernourished, maladjusted child. The diagnosis indicated vertigo attributable to a severe, "overclosed" Class 2 malocclusion. Correction of the maxillomandibular malrelationships and occlusion with overlays quickly enabled the boy to eat solid foods, eliminated the vomiting, and restored the child to normal behavior.

Case 2

A girl, 8 years of age, had symptoms of blackout and syncope. These had been previously diagnosed as "abdominal epilepsy." The diagnosis indicated that the vertigo was attributable to an "overclosed" Class 2 malocclusion with the loss of deciduous molar teeth. Overlays of the posterior teeth were constructed to establish normal maxillomandibular and temporomandibular joint-ear relationships. There were no blackouts or syncope during a 2 year period of wearing these temporary appliances.

Comment. Neither this child nor the first patient could describe the symptoms of vertigo but reported subjective clearing of their heads following the dental treatment.

Case 3

A single woman, 30 years of age, had paroxysmal attacks of dizziness, nausea, vomiting, and loss of consciousness. The attacks had begun when the patient was 11 years of age and had occurred 5 or 6 times yearly, usually after eating. Between attacks, she had continuous dull pain in the temporal regions which was worse on the left side. Her vision was distorted and she could not discern the source of sounds. She had received various medical and dental treatments during the past 20 years without relief. The attacks occurred at meals. The fear of confused hearing had made her completely dependent upon her mother. This dependency resulted in the previous diagnosis of psychogenic vertigo, but psychiatric therapy afforded no relief. In January, 1957, our diagnosis indicated that her symptoms were caused by traumatic dental occlusion (Fig. 9, *A*) and reflected trauma of the displaced left condyle in the middle ear and Eustachian tube. Malocclusion had been exacerbated by orthodontic treatment that interlocked her anterior teeth in occlusion. The loss of the lower left first molar tooth further exacerbated the malrelationships. This had resulted in a fanning out of the upper teeth and overgrowth of the upper central interdental (incisive) papilla. Temporomandibular joint roentgenograms showed posterior, superior displacement of the condyles into pathogenic relations with the adjacent structures of the ears. The left condyle was flattened as a result of pressure against the anterior wall of the ear. The medial surface had a sharp spur which had penetrated the middle ear and the Eustachian tube (Fig. 10, *A*). The dental treatment consisted of temporary overlays of the remaining upper and lower right and left premolar and molar teeth (Fig. 9, *B*). This established normal joint relations with the adjacent structures of the ears. This temporary and reversible occlusal correction completely relieved all symptoms within a period of 4 weeks. There were no recurrences during the next 3 months. The overlays were then replaced with permanent dental reconstructions. This was completed in October, 1957. Roentgenograms made upon completion of the dental treatment showed that the condyle spur had been absorbed, the surface rounded, and the relation of the condyle with the adjacent parts of the ear and Eustachian tube had been normalized (Fig. 10, *B*). There have been no recurrences of symptoms during the past 5 years. The patient quickly learned to discern the source direction of sound, could eat without fear of vomiting and syncope, and was without head pains. She emancipated herself from dependence on her mother and achieved a satisfactory social adjustment.

Case 4

A 62-year-old woman had suffered paroxysmal attacks of severe vertigo, violent vomiting, blackout, and loss of consciousness during a 14 year period. Her symptoms included severe limitaton of jaw movement, pain of the left temporomandibular joint region, and paresthesia in the left side of her face. Her teeth had been restored with inlays in a locked, traumatic occlusion which accommodated a diminished maxillomandibular dimension of occlusion and a missing lower right first molar. The lower incisor and canine teeth had worn depressions in the lingual surfaces of the upper anterior teeth. She had previously received extensive cranial surgery, and medical and psychiatric treatments which did not relieve the vertigo and associated symptoms. Reconstruction of the dental occlusion to establish harmonious occlusions of her teeth and normal temporomandibular joint-ear relations completely cured the vertigo and eliminated the vomiting and syncope. The painful mastication was relieved. Normal mandibular movements were gradually restored and sensation returned to the left side of her face. This patient has been observed every 3 months during the past 8 years. There have been no recurrences of any of these symptoms.

Case 5

A married woman, 67 years of age, had a previously diagnosed Meniere's disease of 17 years' duration. Her symptoms had included paroxysmal attacks of tinnitus, dizziness, violent vomiting, and syncope. The attacks occurred at irregular intervals without warning of pre-attack symptoms. Previous medical, neurologic, and otologic studies failed to indicate or show organic etiology. The lower right first molar had been lost and the opposing upper first molar had extruded. The anterior teeth were in deep interlocking and overlapping relationships. The temporomandibular joint-ear roentgenograms showed that the right mandibular condyle was displaced superoposteriorly into pathogenic contact with the auditory meatus and ear drum, and had penetrated the lateral wall of the Eustachian tube. The occlusal surfaces of the upper and lower, right and left bicuspid and molar teeth were reconstructed by equilibrated temporary overlays that established nonpathogenic temporomandibular joint relationships. These were worn for 2 years, during which time there were no recurrences of dizziness, nausea, vomiting, or syncope. Permanent crown that reproduced the occlusion of the temporary overlays were then constructed. There have been no recurrences of previous Meniere's symptoms during the past 5 years.

Comment. The pathologic condition of the dental occlusion-temporomandibular joint relationships of many patients was associated with inadequate complete dentures. These included prostheses with which the case histories correlated with the onset of vertigo, and dentures which had been worn for extensive periods that rendered them inadequate and pathogenic. The latter is illustrated by the following cases.

Case 6

A woman, 89 years of age, had worn the same dentures for over 50 years. She had Parkinson's disease and vertigo, and had fallen several times. It was decided that prevention of subsequent falls and likely bone fractures indicated the need for the construction of new dentures. These relieved the vertigo and prevented subsequent falls.

Case 7

A man, 87 years of age, had worn the same dentures for 47 years with complete dental comfort and function despite the fact that the occlusal vertical dimension was greatly reduced and a hole had been worn in the palate of the upper denture. His symptoms included recurrent severe attacks of vertigo associated with incoordination of the skeletal-muscular system which he interpreted as paralysis of his legs. These attacks occurred several times daily, especially after meals. As his history correlated the attacks with meals, the patient interpreted this as probable allergic food reaction or digestive disorders. New dentures which increased the occlusal vertical dimension by 25 mm. and established harmonious occlusion with normal temporomandibular joint-ear relations resulted in

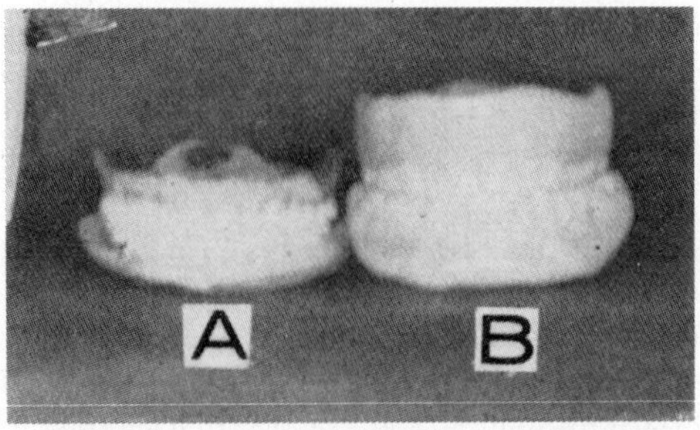

Fig. 11. *A,* The complete dentures have an inadequate vertical dimension and a hole in the palate of the upper denture. These were worn for 47 years with complete patient acceptance, and they resulted in severe vertigo and associated symptoms. *B,* The new dentures with a normal vertical dimension involving an opening of 25 mm. which the patient readily accommodated and which completely relieved all symptoms.

complete relief of the vertigo and elimination of the associated symptoms (Fig. 11).

DISCUSSION

Lesions of the aural vestibular system causing vertigo may result from trauma, infection, neuronitis, hydrops or other causes. At present, the most widely invoked cause is hydrops of the labyrinth. However, there has been no explanation for the cause of hydrops, or any correlation of its presence with, and its absence between, paroxysmal attacks of vertigo. The treatment for vertigo based upon this theory includes surgical destruction of the labyrinth. Cawthorne[3] examined the perilymph space and membranous labyrinth with a binocular microscope during 250 of these operations for vertigo. He said, "In none has there been any deviation from the normal appearance or rate of flow of the perilymph. The membranous canal and ampulla have in all cases been of normal size and normal translucency."[3]

Our findings have been reported in progress.[5-7] They corroborated those of Monson,[8] Wright,[9] Kirk,[10] Goodfriend,[11-15] Green,[16] Pippin,[17] Costen,[18-20] and Kelly.[21] Kelly[21] collaborated with Guild in the study of submarine candidates who developed ear symptoms following tests in the pressure chamber. All had adenoids, edema of the Eustachian tube, and stasis of tubal lymphatics. Correction of the dental occlusion-temporomandibular pathology relieved 46 of the 50 patients examined. These patients were then able to resume pressure tests and enter submarine service without recurrence of ear symptoms. Fifty controls underwent adenoidectomy, radiation, and other otolaryngolic treatment but were unable to resume pressure chamber work.

SUMMARY

1. An 8 year study of 105 patients with vertigo indicates that a surprisingly high percentage of vertigo associated ocular and vagal symptoms are caused by dental occlusal and temporomandibular joint abnormalities which irritate and injure the adjacent structures of the ears.
2. The symptoms of these patients included pain, blurring of vision, dizziness, staggering gait, light-headedness, nausea, vomiting, abdominal pain, blackouts, and loss of consciousness. These symptoms had resulted in previous inadequate diagnoses of Meniere's disease, brain tumor, brain degeneration, hypertension, athersclerosis, cholecystitis, abdominal epilepsy, and psychoneuroses.
3. Dental treatment that established a harmonious dental occlusion and nonpathogenic relationships of the temporomandibular joints, with the adjacent structures of the ear, resulted in complete relief of vertigo and associated symptoms in 89 per cent of the patients.

CONCLUSION

The findings of this study and of Goodfriend's[15] previous 10 year study indicate that physicians and dentists should give early consideration to dental-occlusal temporomandibular joint causes in the diagnosis of vertigo and associated pain, blurring of vision, disorders of hearing, nausea, vomiting, blackouts, and loss of consciousness.

REFERENCES

1. Alpers, B.J.: Vertigo and Dizziness, New York, 1954, Grune & Stratton, Inc.
2. Gowers, W.R.: Manual of the Nervous System, ed. 2, London, 1893, Macmillan Company.
3. Cawthorne, T.: Modern Trends in Diseases of the Ear, Nose and Throat, London, 1954, Butterworth & Co., Ltd.
4. Schuyler, C.H.: Correction of Occlusal Disharmony of the Natural Dentition, New York State D.J. **13**:445, 1947.
5. Kelly, H.T., and Goodfriend, D.J.: Vertigo Attributable to Mandibular Joint-Bite Abnormalities, J. Am. Coll. Dentists. **24**:182, 1957.
6. Goodfriend, D.J., and Kelly, H.T.: Medical Significance of Equilibration of the Masticating Mechanism, J. Pros. Den. **10**:496, 1960.
7. Goodfriend, D.J., and Kelly, H.T.: Temporomandibular Joint Criteria in Dentoprosthetic Rehabilitation, J. Am. Dent. A. **60**:197, 1960.
8. Monson, G.S.: Impaired Function as Result of Closed Bite, J. Nat. Dent. A. **8**:833, 1921.
9. Wright, W.H.: Deafness Influenced by Malposition of Jaw, J. Nat. Dent. A. **7**:979, 1920.
10. Kirk, E.C.: Malocclusion as a Problem in Pathology, Pacific D. Gaz. **25**:654, 1917.
11. Goodfriend, D.J.: Dysarthrosis and Subarthrosis of Mandibular

Articulation, Dental Cosmos **74:**523, 1932.

12. Goodfriend, D.J.: Symptomatology and Treatment of Abnormalities of Mandibular Articulation, Dental Cosmos **75:**844-1111, 1933.
13. Goodfriend, D.J.: Abnormalities of Mandibular Articulation, J. Am. Dent. A. **21:**204, 1934.
14. Goodfriend, D.J.: Role of Dental Factors in Cause and Treatment of Ear Symptoms and Diseases, Dental Cosmos **78:**1292, 1936.
15. Goodfriend, D.J.: Deafness, Tinnitus, Vertigo and Neuralgia, Arch. Otolaryng. **46:**1, 1947.
16. Pippin, B.N.: Treatment of Temporomandibular Joint Lesions Caused by Denture Mutilation, Washington Univ. D.J. **10:**77, 1944.
17. Costen, J.B.: Neuralgias and Ear Symptoms Associated With Disturbed Function of the Temporomandibular Joint, J.A.M.A. **107:**252, 1936.
18. Costen, J.B.: Correlation of X-Ray Findings in the Mandibular Joint With Clinical Signs, Especially Trismus, J. Am. Dent. A. **26:**405, 1939.
19. Costen, J.B., Clare, M.H., and Bishop, G.H.: The Transmission of Impulses via the Chorda Tympani Nerve, Ann. Otol. Rhin. & Laryng. **60:**591, 1951.
20. Costen, J.B.: Differential Diagnosis of Mandibular Joint Neuralgia, D. Abst. **3:**141, 1958.
21. Kelly, W.J.: Research Project X-434, Medical Research Dept. United States Submarine Base, New London, Conn., Jan. 21, 1946.

Index

A

Abandonment of patient, negligent, 607
Accu-O-Matic instrument, 341, 342, 345-348
Acetaminophen, analgesic action of, 351, 352
Acetyl coenzyme A, pyruvic acid conversion to, 31-32
Acetylsalicylic acid, 350-351, 352, 510
Acoustic neuroma in trigeminal neuralgia, 584, 590
Acquired occlusion, 253-254
  case history on treatment of, 414-417
  rationale for accepting, 254
Acrylic prosthesis, case histories on, 405-410
Actin as contractile protein in skeletal muscle, 27, 28-29, 30
Active exercise therapy, 320-321, 482-483
Activities and hobbies affecting muscular development, 463, 466
Acupoint therapy, electrical, 340-349, 481
Acupuncture, 335-339
  for anesthesia, 183
  in determining medication and nutritional needs, 481
  needles used for, 335, 341
    electrical stimulation of, 340-349, 481
    manual stimulation of, 335-336
  postoperative, 372
  results of treatment with, 338-339, 346, 348
  in trigeminal neuralgia, 558
Addiction to drugs in therapy for chronic pain, 198, 350, 352, 493
Adenoids; *see* Tonsil and adenoid enlargement
Adjustable articulator, technique for mounting casts on, 104-115, 129
Adrenocorticosteroid therapy, 353; *see also* Cortisone therapy
Advancement, mandibular, 526-531
Age of patients, 214-215, 505, 508
  and growth spurt affected by surgery, 534
  in myofunctional therapy, 466
  in orthodontics, 520
  in osteoarthritis, 216
  in rheumatoid arthritis, 216
  in trigeminal neuralgia, 562, 573, 576, 580, 584-585, 586, 589
Aggravating factors affecting course of symptoms, 76
Aggressive behavior of TMJ patients, 237, 241, 486, 487, 490, 493
Aglossia, 55
Alclofenac, 351
Alcohol injections in trigeminal neuralgia, 558, 559-561
Allergic reactions, 59-63
  biofeedback treatment of, 333
  and bruxism, 62-63
  to cow's milk, 43, 59
  to dental materials, 74, 375, 480
  diet modifications in, 462
  early signs of, 59-62
  history of, 74, 480
  homeopathic treatment of, 480
  mouth breathing in, 43, 59
  as muscle imbalance symptom, 465, 472, 478
Alternative treatments, legal aspects of, 608
Alveolar nerve, inferior
  alcohol blocks of, 560
  neurectomy of, 561
Alveolar osteotomy, mandibular, 531-532
Amitriptyline
  for postherpetic neuralgia, 561
  for prevention of TMJ disease, 620
Analgesics for pain in TMJ disease, 350-352
Ananase; *see* Bromelain
Anatomy
  of determinants of occlusion, 119
  of ear, nose, and throat structures, 224-225
  of TMJ, 4, 8-25
  of trigeminal nerve, 582-583
Anderson appliances, 521
Anderson pins for fixation of fractures, 447
Anectine; *see* Succinylcholine for muscle spasms
Anesthesia
  acupuncture for, 183
  alcohol nerve blocks for, 558, 559-561
  corneal, as complication of trigeminal neuralgia treatments, 560, 561, 563, 564, 571-572, 573, 574
  dolorosa, after trigeminal neuralgia treatments, 560, 563, 574, 576
  during percutaneous trigeminal rhizolysis, 565, 566-567
  general, TMJ trauma during, 65, 74, 124
  local, in muscle spasm therapy, 297-298, 319, 353
Anesthetic agents, local, intramuscular injection into trigger zones, 297-298, 319, 353
Anger of patients, 237, 238-239, 242, 486
Angiocatheter insertion for TMJ arthrography, 151-156, 157
Angiomas, cavernous, and trigeminal neuralgia, 583
Animal studies of biofeedback, 328
Ankyloglossia, 57-58, 480
Ankylosing spondylitis, case history on surgical treatment of, 436-438
Ankylosis of TMJ, 216, 443-460
  bony, 216, 368, 369, 451-452, 455-456
  case histories on, 448-452, 455-457
  fibrous, 216, 368, 448, 451-452, 455-456
  after fractures, 443, 445, 447, 448-452
  prosthesis for, 369, 447, 448-453, 455-457
  and pseudoankylosis, 368
  surgical treatment of, 355, 368, 369, 455-457, 531
Ankylotic tongue, 464-465, 469
  case history on treatment of, 472-473
Anterior bite plate appliance, 267
Anterior cross-bite, equilibration techniques for, 257
Anterior jaw programmer, construction of, 106-110
Anterior teeth
  in equilibration techniques, 257
  examination of, 312
  in guidance of mandibular movements, 246, 247
  restoration of, 260

Anthranilic acids, 351
Antianxiety drugs, 352-353
Antiepileptic drug therapy in trigeminal neuralgia, 585
Antihistamine therapy in vertigo, 353
Antiinflammatory agents for TMJ disease, 350-352
  nonsteroid, 350-351
Antinuclear factor as test in muscle spasms, 283
Antivert; *see* Meclizine
Antivertiginous drugs, 353
Anxiety of TMJ patients, 213-214, 510
  biofeedback treatment of, 328-333
  drug therapy in, 352-353
Apertognathia, surgical correction of, 531-532, 534
Appendage sucking, 35, 36-37, 38-40, 462, 470, 472-473
Appliances
  legal aspects in use of, 600, 608-609
  in muscle spasm treatment, 315
  Myo-Tronics repositioning, 598
  prosthetic, 365-378; *see also* Prosthetic replacements
  splints, 265-277; *see also* Splint therapy
  for tongue control, 482-483
  in vertigo treatment, 632
Arbitrary techniques of hinge-axis recording, 250-251
Arch
  dental, length of, in determining need for tooth extractions, 522
  palatal, width of, 465, 469
Arm exercises in spasm therapy, 321, 322, 323
Arteriosclerosis as cause of trigeminal neuralgia, 584
Arteritis, cervical, radiography in, 166-167
Arthralgia, 75, 357
Arthritis of TMJ, 139, 214-216, 233
  acute gouty, 217
  atrophic, 215; *see also* Rheumatoid arthritis
  biofeedback treatment in, 332
  condylectomy for, 365
  deformans, 215; *see also* Rheumatoid arthritis
  degenerative, 214; *see also* Osteoarthritis
  dysfunction and myofacial spasm in, case history on, 522-523
  history of, 73
  hypertrophic, 214; *see also* Osteoarthritis
  infectious, 216
    chronic, 215; *see also* Rheumatoid arthritis
  locations of pain in, 358
  radiographic examination in, 215, 283, 368-369
  rheumatoid, 215; *see also* Rheumatoid arthritis
Arthrography of TMJ, 151-156, 159-160
Arthroplasty, 365-378
  case histories on, 414-417, 436-438
  combined with meniscectomy, 377-378, 380
  preoperative evaluation in, 371
Arthroscopy, transcutaneous, 156-158
Arthrosis of TMJ, 214
  surgical treatment of, 368
Articular capsule of TMJ, 10, 212
Articular disc of TMJ
  anatomy of, 10, 212
  compression of, 214, 359, 448-449
  degeneration of, 168, 444
  function of, 212, 359, 365-368
    and bone-on-bone contact in disorders, 168-172, 189-191, 204-205, 359, 444
  microscopic examination of, 378-379
  perforation of, 168, 359, 444
    case histories on, 402-405, 418, 448-449
    surgery for, 402-405, 448-449
  radiographic examination of, 168, 208-209
Articular disc of TMJ—cont'd
  surgical removal of, 359, 360-364, 377-378, 380, 402-405
Articular eminence, 245
  anatomy of, 8, 10, 212
  angle of, 247-248
  evolutionary development of, 617-618
  flattening of, radiographic examination of, 202-203, 204-205
  prosthesis for, 360, 369-378
    for ankylosis, 369, 447, 448-453, 455-457
    case histories on, 196-197, 200-204, 382-436, 447-457, 491, 492
    insertion of, 372-373
    after meniscectomy, 364, 377-378, 380
    reactions to need for, 489
  relationship with condylar head, 359, 365-368
    disorders in, 168-172, 189-195, 200-201, 204-205, 359, 360, 444
    in rheumatoid arthritis, 382-389
    and stress impasse stage IV, 492
  surgical removal of, 360, 361, 414, 418
Articular meniscus; *see* Articular disc of TMJ
Articulator mounted casts, 88, 104-115, 123, 129-131
  advantages of, 254-255
  axis-orbital plane transferred to, 120-121
  centric relation mounting of, 120-121, 129-131
  clinical phase of mounting procedure for, 104-112
  in equilibration procedures, 125, 258-259, 263
  face-bow device for adjustment of, 104-106, 120-121, 251
  functional occlusal analysis of, 129-131
  hinge-axis transfer to, 250-252
  laboratory phase of mounting procedure for, 112-115
  myoprint registration of mandibular position for, 598
  on Myo-Tronics Terminus articulator, 598
  in orthodontic procedures, 520, 522-523
  pantographic recordings for adjustment of, 126
  quick mount procedure for, 129, 251
  in reconstruction process, 260
  recording mandibular excursions for, 252
  setting of, 114
  skull-fossa-condyle geometry transferred to, 120-121, 126
Aryl acetic acids in TMJ disorders, 351
Aryl propionic acids in TMJ disorders, 351
Aspirin therapy, 350-351, 352, 510
  side effects of, 350-351
Assistants of practitioner, negligent conduct of, 607
Associates of practitioner, negligent conduct of, 607
Asymmetry of face
  assessment of, 83, 91, 465
  in infants, 65
  myofunctional therapy for, 476, 478
  orthognathic surgery for, 537-545
Asymptomatic patients, orthodontic diagnostic procedures for, 520
Ativan; *see* Lorazepam in treatment of muscle spasms
Atlas, palpation of transverse process of, 313
ATP
  in energy metabolism, 30-32
  in genesis of myospasm, 32-34
Attachments of mandibular muscles, 19-20
Attitudes
  of patients; *see* Psychological considerations
  of practitioners
    in examination procedures, 82, 211, 238
    in prevention of negligence suits, 612
Audiometry, 227
Auditory nerve examination, 99
Auriculotemporal nerve, anatomy of, 24
Automobile accidents, case histories on surgery for trauma in, 396-401, 451-452

Autonomic nervous system, activities of, 87
Autoprogressive relaxation exercises in spasm therapy, 320-326
Autopsy material, TMJ analysis in, 378-379, 621
Axis-orbital plane, 120
  face-bow transfer of, 120-121, 251
  location and marking of, 120

B

Balance
  of oral musculature, 53-59, 234-235
    assessment of, 101, 103, 464-466
    biofeedback for restoration of, 330
    and effects of imbalance, 53-59
    and facial symmetry, 65, 83, 91, 461, 465, 476, 478
    factors affecting development of, 461-463
    infant feeding patterns affecting, 45, 48, 53-59, 462
    myofunctional therapy for restoration of, 53, 59, 88, 371-372, 461-485
    and swallowing patterns, 51-52
  postural; *see* Postural considerations
  in vertigo; *see* Vertigo
Balancing side of mandible, 247
Barbiturates in TMJ disease, 353
Basilar artery abnormalities in trigeminal neuralgia, 583-584
Battery, legal theory of, 601
  compared with negligence, 601
Behavior
  of patient; *see* Psychological considerations
  of practitioner, legal aspects of, 600-615
Bell's palsy
  ear pain in, 200
  electromyographic biofeedback treatment of, 330
Bennett movement of mandible, 247, 250
Benzodiazepines in spasm treatment, 352
Bimler appliances, 521
Biofeedback monitoring, 327-334
  advantages of, 328
  animal research on, 328
  applications of, 327-328, 329-330, 332-333
  case histories on, 331-332
  compared with hypnosis, 328-329
  home use of, 328, 331
  in muscle spasm treatment, 298-299, 327-334
  office procedures for, 330
  selection of candidates for, 330, 332
  steering wheel device for, 328, 331, 332
  for tongue movements, 483
Bionator, 499
Birth control pills, effects on TMJ of, 313
Birth trauma, 462, 479
  TMJ dysfunction related to, 65
Bite relationship; *see* Occlusion
Bite wing radiographs in orthodontic diagnostic procedures, 520
Biting habits affecting muscular development, 462, 463, 465, 470
Biting personality prototype, 237, 487
Bladder
  acupuncture point, electrical stimulation of, 341
  infection of, history of, 303
Blastemas, condylar and temporal, 4
Blocks, alcohol, 558, 559-561
Blood vessel disease, history of, 74
Body image in TMJ syndrome, 238, 239
Bolten Index analysis, 520
Bone cavities, maxillary or mandibular, and trigeminal or atypical facial neuralgias, 217-220
  surgical treatment of, 217, 220
Bone graft procedures
  costochondral, for TMJ reconstruction, 535-536
  for mandibular repositioning, 531, 533
Bone-on-bone contact in TMJ, 359
  radiographs of, 168-172, 189-191, 204-205
  after trauma, 444
Bone scanning, radionuclide, 161-165
  with technetium 99m, 161-164, 533, 537, 539, 543, 549, 550
Bonine; *see* Meclizine
Bony ankylosis of TMJ, 216
  case histories on, 451-452, 455-456
  surgical correction of, 368, 369, 455-456
Border movements of mandible, 125-126
  recording of, 126, 252
Brain structures
  controlling jaw movement, 25
  sagging in trigeminal neuralgia, 584-585, 586
Breach of contract or warranty in malpractice, 600-601
Breast feeding, 35, 40, 42-45
  and manual expression of milk, 45
  nipple substitutes for, 45, 48-50
  positioning infant for, 42
  preparation of expectant mothers for, 43-45
  swallowing pattern in, 42, 50
  value of, 42, 43
Breast shields, use of, 43-45
Breathing patterns
  in allergies, 43, 59
  assessment of, 124, 313, 465
  in chronic mouth breathing, 59
  device for changing, 483-484
  in exercises for spasms, 325
  in muscle imbalances, 464, 466, 478
Brevital; *see* Methohexital in percutaneous trigeminal rhizolysis
Broad occlusal contact areas, 258
Bromelain, 353
  postoperative use of, 372
Bruxism, 202, 214, 233, 359, 508, 510
  in allergic children, 62-63
  biofeedback treatment for, 330
  case histories on, 414-417, 490, 491
  drug therapy for, 353
  history of, 303, 305
  kinesiology in treatment of, 497
  in muscle imbalance, 465
  night guard for, 267-268
  psychological factors in, 214, 490, 491, 510
  radiographic examination in, 202-203
Bruxomania, 87
Buccinator mechanism, 53, 54
  tongue muscle balance with, 53
Business information in history taking, 301
Butazolidin; *see* Phenylbutazone

C

Caffeine intake, vascular effects of, 303
Calcium
  serum levels, laboratory tests for, 283
  supplemental, in spasm treatment, 354
Cancer, oral, examination for, 86; *see also* Neoplasms
Canines, maxillary, in equilibration procedures, 257
Capsular ligament of TMJ, 10, 212
Carbamazepine therapy
  side effects of, 585
  in trigeminal neuralgia, 562, 581, 585
Carbohydrate intake in nutritional evaluation, 317

Caries rate
and success of restorative procedures, 264
in trigeminal neuralgia patients, 582
Carisoprodol, 353
Carotid artery abnormalities in trigeminal neuralgia, 584
Case histories, 512
on articular eminence prostheses, 196-197, 200-204, 382-436, 447-457, 491, 492
on biofeedback monitoring, 331-332
on fractures, 447-458
on myofunctional therapy, 472-478
on orthodontic procedures, 522-525
psychological considerations in, 239-242, 487, 489, 490-492, 525
radiograph interpretations in, 166-210
on splint therapy, 276, 476, 522-525
on surgical procedures, 378-379, 382-441, 491, 492, 537-556
on vertigo, 620, 632-634
Casts
for occlusal study
hand-held, 88, 123
mounted, 88, 104-115, 129-131; *see also* Articulator mounted casts
restorative, 260-262, 624
compared with equilibration, 259
final, 261-262
provisional, 260-261
in vertigo treatment, 631, 633
for splint construction, 271
Cavities of maxillary or mandibular bones and trigeminal or atypical facial neuralgias, 217-220
Cementation of restorative castings, 261-262
Central nervous system depressants, legal aspects of prescribing, 611-612
Centric equilibration techniques, 255-258
Centric occlusion, 120-121, 266
acquired, 253-254
analysis of, 127-128
compared with centric relation, 254
compared with myocentric occlusion, 266
definition of, 253-254
habitual or customary, 253-254
long, 253
marking location of interferences in, 128, 130
Centric relation position, 254
analysis of, 127-128
broad contact areas in, 258
compared with centric occlusion, 254
definitions of, 265-266
in equilibration procedures, 255-258
of mounted diagnostic casts, 120-121, 129-131
occlusion built to, 266
testing for interferences in, 128
Centric slide, 121
Cephalometric radiographs, 132, 133, 135, 136, 146, 510
of closed bite, 173
compared with transcranial lateral oblique views, 173
interpretation of, 173, 174, 176
in orthodontic procedures, 505, 507, 520
of prognathic mandible, 179, 180
Cerebellar arteries in trigeminal neuralgia, 584, 588-589
Cervical arteritis, radiography in, 166-167
Cervical traction, TMJ trauma in, 65, 76, 213
biofeedback treatment of, 331
surgical correction of, 455-456
Cervicooccipital headgears, 521
Cervi-Pillow, 303, 317
Chewing habits affecting muscular development, 463
Chief complaint of patient, 74-75
Childhood of TMJ patients, 488, 490, 491, 493
Children and infants, 35-69
allergies of, 43, 59-63
breast feeding of, 35, 40, 42-45
bruxism in, 62-63
condylar displacement in, 66-68, 445
degenerative TMJ in, 68
legal aspects in treatment of, 605
mouth breathing in, 43, 59
muscle imbalance in, 53-59, 462
prevention of TMJ dysfunction in, 68
rheumatoid arthritis in, 216
sucking reflex of, 35-41
swallowing patterns of, 45-51, 53
trauma of TMJ in, 65-66
at birth, 65, 462, 479
Chin cups, 521
Chin depression exercise, 324, 325
Chlordiazepoxide, 352
Chloride ion concentrations, 30
Chlorzoxazone, 353
Chorda tympani nerve, 225
Christenson phenomenon, 520
Chymotrypsin, 353
Cigarette smoking
history of, 303
teeth grinding after ending habit of, 491
Cilial reflex during percutaneous trigeminal rhizolysis, 571
Citric acid cycle, 32
Class I malocclusion, 520
case history on orthodontic treatment of, 524-525
Class II malocclusion; *see* Retrognathism, mandibular
Class III malocclusion; *see* Prognathism
Clenching of teeth
history of, 303
radiographic examination in, 202-203
Clicking sounds; *see* Noises in joint
Clinical examination form, 91-103
Clinical phase of cast mounting procedure, 104-112
Clinoril; *see* Sulindac
Clofenamic acid, 351
Clorazepate dipotassium in treatment of muscle spasms, 352
Closed reduction of condylar fractures, 446
case histories on, 448-449
Closed-bite condition, orthodontic treatment of, 505
Closing movements
examination of, 279, 498
muscle group actions for, 17, 25, 59, 211
sounds heard in, 356-357
Cluster symptoms of musculoskeletal dysfunction in head and neck, 597-598
Coagulation technique for trigeminal neuralgia treatment, 565-572
Cochlea of ear, 224
Codeine, 352
Coffee intake, excessive, history of, 303
Compound movement of pivoting condyle, 249-250
Compression
of articular disc, 214, 359, 448-449
of gasserian ganglion in trigeminal neuralgia treatment, 562, 564
vascular, as cause of trigeminal neuralgia and decompression technique for treatment, 580-590
Compression procedures for trigeminal neuralgia, 562, 564
compared with other procedures, 572-575
Computerization of data from Mandibular Kinesiograph, 593

Condylectomy, 361, 364-365
case histories on, 390-395, 402-405, 414, 418
high, 363, 364, 402-405, 414, 418
Condyles, mandibular
articular disc spatial relationship disorders, 212, 214
articular eminence relationship to, 359, 365-368
disturbed, 168-172, 189-195, 200-201, 204-205, 359, 360, 444
bone scans of, 161-163, 164
congenital absence of, Panorex of, 178
dislocation of; *see* Dislocation or displacement of condyles
embryological development of, 4-5
excessive function of, 500, 502
fossa relationship to, 119-121, 124, 126, 245-250, 500, 501
fractures of, 216-217, 233, 443-460
hyperplasia of, 68, 162
case histories on surgical treatment of, 429-436, 537-538, 539-542
hypoplasia of, 526, 531
intercondylar distance as determinant of mandibular movements, 248-249
malpositioned occlusion affecting position of, 597-598
palpation of, 83, 91, 251, 279, 444
penetrating eustachian tube, 633
pivoting, 247, 249-250
radiographic examination of, 161-163, 164, 196, 202-209
surface of head of, 212
surgical reduction of, case history on, 429-436
surgical removal of, 361, 363, 364-365, 390-395, 402-405, 414, 418
surgical repositioning of, 364
trauma to, in dental procedures, 66
Condyloramal fractures, open reduction of, 446
Condylotomy, 361
Congenital disorders
mandibular advancement in correction of, 526
in missing condyles, Panorex of, 178
in origin of TMJ syndrome, 124, 233
in trigeminal neuralgia, 583
Congestion, nasal, 59, 62, 331, 333, 472, 478
Consent to procedures, 601-605
in experimental procedures, 604-605
forms for, 602-604
general and specific, 601-604
informed, 375, 601-605
invalid, 605
preoperative, 375
Consultations with previous practitioners, legal aspects of, 606
Contact areas, occlusal
broad, 258
premature, 258, 314-315; *see also* Interferences, occlusal
three-point, 262-263
Continuing education of practitioner, legal aspects of, 606
Contraceptives, oral, effects on TMJ, 313
Contract breach in malpractice, 600-601
Contractile tissues, 26
Contractions, muscular, 26
in genesis of myospasms, 22-24; *see also* Spasms, muscular
protein interactions in, 27, 28-30
ratchet theory of, 27
Contracture of muscles
onset of, 76
physiological (hemostatic), 33
symptoms of, 77
Contralateral side of mandible, 247
Contrast medium
iodine containing, in arthrography, 151-156, 158
radiopaque, interpretation of results with, 198-199
Contributory negligence, 609-610
Corneal anesthesia as complication of trigeminal neuralgia treatments, 560, 561, 563, 564, 571-572, 573, 574
Corneal reflex testing in trigeminal neuralgia, 581
Coronoplasty, 68; *see also* Equilibration
Corrective exercises for muscle spasms, 319, 320-326
Cortisone therapy, 402, 510
case histories on, 490, 491
Costen's syndrome, 232
tinnitus in, 332
Costochondral grafts for TMJ reconstruction, 535-536
Costs of procedures
for chronic pain, 493
for reconstruction, 264
with Weiss appliance, 276
Counterirritation in muscle spasm treatment, 298
Counting technique in relaxation exercises, 323-326
Course of patient symptoms, 76-77
in trigeminal neuralgia, 580-582
Cow's milk
allergy to, and mouth breathing in, 43, 59
compared with human milk, 42, 43
Cranial bones
birth trauma of, 479
correction of malalignment of, prior to myofunctional therapy, 479-480
Cranial faults, 479-480
Cranial nerves
fifth; *see* Trigeminal nerve
ninth, neuralgia of, 564
second, examination of, 99
seventh; *see* Facial nerve
Craniectomy for microvascular decompression of trigeminal nerve, 586-587
Crepitation in joint, 357; *see also* Noises in joint
Cross-bite
anterior, equilibration techniques for, 257
condylar displacement in, 67-68
Cure warranty, legal aspects of, 600
Cusp-fossa relationship
in functional occlusion, 118-119
tripodization in, 262-263
Customary centric occlusion, 253
Cyclizine, 353
Cyclobenzaprine, 353
Cyclooxygenase system, antiinflammatory agents inhibiting, 350, 351
Cysts, epidermoid, in trigeminal neuralgia, 583

D

Dalmane; *see* Flurazepam
Darvon; *see* Dextropropoxyphene, analgesic action of
Decadron; *see* Dexamethasone in prevention of TMJ syndrome
Decision making on treatment plan, 260
Decompression procedures for trigeminal neuralgia, 562, 563-564, 580-590
Decongestant spray in intranasal examination, 229
Defensive behavior of TMJ patients, 236, 237, 238, 240, 241, 486, 490
Deflected jaw movements as chief complaint of patient, 75
Degenerative changes of TMJ
in children, 68
detection of, 161, 168
microscopic examination of, 378-379
in osteoarthritis, 214-215, 359-360; *see also* Osteoarthritis
after trauma, 215, 359-360, 444

Deltoid muscle function testing, 497
Demerol; *see* Meperidine
Denar Corporation transcranial lateral oblique system, 144-146, 147
Dental floss in interference testing, 129
Dental procedures
  for headaches, inappropriate, 235
  historical perspective on role of TMJ in, 621-624
  history of, 77
  kinesiology techniques in, 497-499
  legal aspects of, 600-612
  occlusion modified by, 253
  postoperative, 371, 372
  preoperative, 371
  TMJ trauma in, 66, 76, 232, 233
    biofeedback treatment of, 330, 331-332
    case histories on, 393, 405-410
    legal aspects of, 607
    surgical correction of, 405-410
  in vertigo treatment, 625-635
Dentition; *see* Teeth
Dentonamics instrument for recording mandibular excursions, 252
Dentures, 315
  biofeedback for adjustment to, 332
  occlusion modified by, 253
  spasms caused by, 510
  vertigo associated with, 633
Dependent behavior of TMJ patients, 237, 239, 240, 486, 487, 490, 493
Depressant drug therapy
  legal aspects of, 611-612
  in prevention of TMJ syndrome, 620
Depressor muscles for jaw opening, 24, 59, 211, 212
Dermatron instrument in homeopathic treatments, 480-481
Determinants of occlusion, 119-120, 247-250
  transferred to articulator, 126
Development and growth, 1-69; *see also* Growth and development
Deviate swallow, 53
Deviations in jaw movements, measurement of, 85-86, 95, 127
Dexamethasone in prevention of TMJ syndrome, 620
Dextropropoxyphene, analgesic action of, 351
Diabetes, biofeedback treatment in, 333
Diagnostic procedures, 71-242, 508-509
  attitude of examiner in, 82
  casts in, 88, 104-115; *see also* Articulator mounted casts
  in differential diagnosis of TMJ disease, 211-223
  ear, nose, and throat considerations in, 224-231
  electronic instrumentation in, 512, 520, 591-597
  forms used in, 91-103, 308-309. 513-519
  in fractures, 444-445
  history taking in, 73-81; *see also* History taking
  and informing patient about results of, 601
  initial examination in, 82-116, 278-283, 296
  kinesiology techniques in, 497, 498
  legal aspects of, 265, 608, 611
  localization of dysfunctioning muscles in, 497, 498
  in muscle imbalance, 464-466
  in muscle spasms, 278-296, 300, 301-315
  occlusal analysis in, 117-131
  in oral cancer, 86
  orthodontic, 520-521, 522-525
  orthopedic considerations in, 232-235
  in osteoarthritis, 215
  outline of, 510
  preoperative, 356-360
  psychogenic considerations in, 236-242
  radiographic, 132-210; *see also* Radiographic examinations
Diagnostic procedures—cont'd
  for recognition of individuals prone to TMJ syndrome, 619
  prior to splint therapy, 265
  in trigeminal neuralgia, 580
  in vertigo, 628-629
  waxing up in, 260
Diazepam therapy, 510, 620
  in muscle spasms, 298, 352
  postoperative, 372
Diclofenac, 351
Diet; *see* Nutrition
Differential diagnosis of TMJ disease, 211-223
Diffunisal, 351
Digastric muscle, 211
  anatomy of, 17, 21
  functions of, 17, 211, 212
  in malpositioned occlusion, 597-598
  palpation of, 93, 96, 498
Dilantin; *see* Phenytoin in trigeminal neuralgia
Dilaudid; *see* Hydromorphone
Dimenhydrinate, 353
Disc; *see* Articular disc of TMJ
Disclosure of information on treatment procedures, legal aspects of, 601, 604, 605
Discovery statutes on negligent treatments, 609
Dislocation or displacement of condyles
  biofeedback treatment of, 330
  case histories on, 405-410, 438-441
  in children, 66-68
  chronic, 196-197, 214, 360, 438-441
  distal, 66, 500, 503
  in fractures, 444, 445-446
  pain in, 214
  prosthesis inserted for, 202
  radiographic examination of, 196, 202-205
  restrictive device for, 438-441
  surgical treatment of, 202, 360, 362, 405-410, 438-441, 455-456
Dizziness, patient complaint of, 227, 307
Doctor-patient interactions; *see* Patient-doctor interactions
Dolorology, 493
Dramamine; *see* Dimenhydrinate
Dream analysis, 492
Drowning phenomenon of infants with use of conventional nipples, 45
Drug therapy, 350-354, 510
  addiction to, 198, 350, 352, 493
  biofeedback affecting need for, 333
  Dermatron instrument in evaluation of, 480-481
  headaches resistant to, and neurotic behavior, 232
  history of, 74
  homeopathic approach to, 480-481
  legal aspects of, 605, 611-612
  for muscle spasms, 187, 298, 319, 352-353
  for osteoarthritis, 351
  in prevention of TMJ syndrome, 620
  for trigeminal neuralgia, 562, 581, 585, 589, 590
Dry needling technique in muscle spasms, 298
  postoperative, 371
Due care, legal aspects of, 600
Duties of practitioner, legal aspects of, 605-606, 608
Dysfunctions, muscular; *see* Myofunctional considerations
Dyskinesia, orofacial
  psychological effects of, 240
  in violinist, 463
Dysmasesis, 357
Dysponetic signaling in muscle dysfunction, 498

E

Eagle's syndrome, 220-222
Ears, 224-231
  acupuncture points on, 336, 337, 340
    diagram of, 343
    electrical stimulation of, 341-349
    peripheral, 345-346
    procedure for locating, 345-346
  of allergic children, 63
  anatomy of, 224-225
  examination of, 228-230
    in muscle spasms, 282
    preoperative, 371
  in hearing disorders, 227, 533, 623, 631, 633
  history of infections in, 73-74
  muscle imbalance affecting, 465, 476
  nerves of, 225
  pain in, 227-228
    in Bell's palsy, 200
    biofeedback treatment of, 331, 332
    in prognathism, 179
    radiographic examination in, 200-201
  relationship of TMJ to, 5-6, 224-228, 623-624
  sensation of fullness in, 225, 227, 381
  tinnitus in, 194, 226-227; *see also* Tinnitus
Edema, proteolytic enzyme therapy for, 353
Education
  of patients
    in myospasm treatment, 296
    and right-to-know policy, 601
  of practitioner, legal aspects of, 606
Ego of TMJ syndrome patients, 237, 238, 242
Elavil; *see* Amitriptyline
Elbow in exercises for spasms, 320, 321, 322, 323
Electrical acupoint therapy, 340-349, 481
Electrical stimulation
  of acupuncture points, 340-349, 481
  trancutaneous neural
    Myo-Monitor instrument for, 270-271, 272, 372, 521, 591-593, 597, 598
    in orthodontic procedures, 521, 522, 524, 525
    for pain relief, 593
  of trigger areas in spasm therapy, 318, 319, 325, 339
Electroacupuncture, 340-349, 481
Electrocoagulation method in trigeminal neuralgia, 565-572
Electrodes
  for Myo-Monitor, 270-271
  for percutaneous trigeminal rhizolysis, 565-571
Electroencephalographic biofeedback, 327
Electrogalvanic stimulation in spasm therapy, 318, 325
Electromyographic recordings
  in biofeedback technique, 327-334
  Myo-Tronics Bioelectric Processor for, 597, 598
Electronic diagnostic and treatment instrumentation, 591-597
  for hinge-axis recording, 251
  Myo-Monitor, 270-271, 272, 372, 521, 591-593, 597, 598
  for recording mandibular excursions, 252
Electronystagmography, 227
Elevator muscles for jaw closing, 17, 24, 59, 211
Embryological development
  muscle imbalance related to, 462, 466, 479
  of sucking reflex, 35, 36-37
  of TMJ, 4-7
Emergency procedures
  legal aspects of, 601, 605, 607, 610-611
  in reconstruction process, 260
Emergency procedures—cont'd
  for spasms, 276
Eminectomies, 360, 361
  case histories on, 414, 418
Eminence, articular; *see* Articular eminence
Emotional factors; *see* Psychological considerations
Employment of patient; *see* Occupation of patient
Endolymph of ear, 224
End-plate myoneural junction, 27
Energy metabolism, 30-32
Enolic acids, 351
Environmental conditions
  adverse reactions to, 480
  affecting muscular development, 462-463
Enzymes, proteolytic, therapeutic use of, 353
Epinephrine in local anesthetic solution, 567
Equanil; *see* Meprobamate therapy
Equilibration, 68, 253-259
  advantages of, 259
  on articulated diagnostic casts, 254-255, 259
  centric, 255-258
  contraindications to, 263
  equipment for, 255
  finishing of, 259
  after fractures, 446
  indications for, 258
  legal aspects of, 607
  limitations of, 263, 264
  for minimal occlusal deviation, 263
  orthodontic treatment prior to, 521
  postoperative, 371
  reconstruction procedures after, 260
  in splint adjustment, 271
  therapeutic appliance for, 315
  in vertigo treatment, 631, 632
Ethnic background of TMJ patients, 217
Ethyl chloride spray, 510
  for muscle spasms, 298
Eustachian tube of ear, 224
  condyle trauma to, 633
Evidence of negligence, textbooks and witnesses as, 610
Evolutionary development of TMJ, 3, 5-7, 616-618
Examination procedures; *see* Diagnostic procedures
Excursions; *see* Movements, mandibular
Exercise therapy, 482, 483
  active and passive types of, 320-326, 482-483
  after condylar fractures, postoperative, 453
  in muscle spasms, 297, 319, 320-326
  in prevention of TMJ syndrome, 619-620
Exhaustion, biofeedback treatment of, 333
Experimental procedures, informed consent to, 604-605
Expert witness testimony in liability suits, 610
External fixation of fractures
  with open reduction, 446
  pins for, 446, 447, 453
Extractions of teeth, 217-220, 505
  legal aspects of, 608
  in orthodontic procedures, 522
Extradural trigeminal rhizotomy, subtemporal, 562-563
  compared with other procedures, 572-575
Extraoral examination of fractures, 444
Extraoral vertical oblique osteotomy, 533, 538
Extraskeletal pin fixation, 446, 447, 453
Eye(s)
  of allergic children, 59
  contact by TMJ patients, 238
  questions for assessment of, 303, 307

F

Face pack for application of wet heat, 317
Face-bow device, 104-106, 521
 in axis-orbital plane transfer, 120-121
 in hinge-axis recording, 251
Facial asymmetry
 assessment of, 83, 91, 465
 in infants, 65
 myofunctional therapy for, 476, 478
 orthognathic surgery for, 537-545
Facial expression
 in muscle imbalances, 464, 474-475
 in TMJ syndrome, 238, 239
 in trigeminal neuralgia, 581-582
Facial nerve, 225
 atypical neuralgia of, 217-220
  Myo-Monitor for relief of, 593
  personality of patients with, 486
 examination of, 99
 trauma in surgery, 445
Facial pain
 Myo-Monitor for relief of, 593
 neurosurgical treatment of, 557-579
 psychodynamics of, 557-558
 in trigeminal neuralgia, 580
Facial photographs in orthodontic diagnostic procedures, 520
Facial profile analysis
 in orthodontic diagnostic procedures, 520
 prior to orthognathic surgery, 543, 544, 547
Faciliatory exercises in spasm therapy, 325
Family relationships of TMJ syndrome patients, 238, 239-242
Fascia lata function testing, 497
Fauces
 initial examination of, 86, 95
 in oral cancer examination, 86
Fears of patients, 237, 238
Fence appliances, 482, 483
Fenclogic acid, 351
Fenoprofen, 351
Fetal development
 muscle imbalance related to, 462, 466, 479
 of sucking reflex, 35, 36-37
 of TMJ, 4-7
Fibers, muscle, 26-27
Fibrocartilage of TMJ, 8-10; *see also* Articular disc of TMJ
Fibrositis of masticatory muscles, 213
Fibrous ankylosis of TMJ, 216
 after fractures, case histories on, 448, 451-452, 455-456
 surgical correction of, 368, 455-456
Fifth cranial nerve; *see* Trigeminal nerve
Fight or flight response, 498
 inhibition of, 300-301
 sympathetic nervous system in, 87
Final cast restorations, 261-262
Finger sucking, 35, 36-37, 38-40, 462, 470, 472-473
Fixation of condylar fractures, 443, 445
 with open reduction, 446
 pins for, 446, 447, 453
Flat occlusion, 253
Flexeril; *see* Cyclobenzaprine
Floor of mouth, examination of, 86, 95
Flufenamic acid, 351
Fluid-filled splints, 268
Fluori-Methane spray
 interincisal opening measured after, 313
 in muscle spasm therapy, 298, 315-316, 319, 353
Flurazepam, 352
Flutist, oral muscular development of, 463
Foot
 acupuncture points on, 340
  diagram of, 344
  electrical stimulation of, 341
 examination of, 279
Forceps delivery, TMJ trauma in, 65
Forearm muscles, biofeedback monitoring of, 330
Forehead antiheadache acupuncture point, 348-349
Forehead resistive exercise, 324, 325
Fossa, glenoid; *see* Glenoid fossa
Fractures, condylar, 216-217, 443-460
 ankylosis after, 443, 445, 447, 448-452
  articular eminence prosthesis for prevention of, 447, 448-452, 455-457
 case histories on, 447-458
 classification of, 444
 clinical examination of, 444-445
 closed treatment of, 446, 448-449
 open reduction of, 445-446, 447, 448-449, 453
 in origin of TMJ syndrome, 233
 other mandibular fractures with, 446
 pin fixation of, 446, 447, 453
 signs and symptoms of, 444-445
Frankel appliances, 521
Frontal muscles, biofeedback monitoring of, 330, 331-332
Frontoplateau splint, 267
Fullness in ear, sensation of, 225, 227
 patient evaluation of surgery for, 381
Functional analysis of masticatory system, 10, 123, 233, 616-618
 muscular; *see* Myofunctional considerations
 occlusal, 121-131

G

Gag reflex, kinesiology in control of, 497
Gait of opening movement, examination of, 84-85
Gallbladder acupuncture points, 337
 electrical stimulation of, 341, 346
Gallium bone scans, 161
Gargle exercise, 325
Gasserian ganglion, 564, 565
 carotid artery impinging on, 584
GE Panelipse, 139
Genetic factors
 in mandibular prognathism, 524
 in muscular development, 462
 in predisposition to malocclusion, 520, 521
Geniohyoid muscle, action and nerves of, 17
Genioplasty, 545
Geometry of mandibular movement, 119-120, 124, 245-250
 transferred to articulator, 120-121, 126
Glenoid fossa
 anatomy of, 8, 10
 congenital malposition of, 479
 in cusp-fossa relationship, 118-121, 126, 262-263
 prosthesis covering, 369
 surface of, 10, 212
Glossopharyngeal neuralgia with trigeminal neuralgia, 564
Glossoptosis, 63-64
Glucose in energy metabolism, 31-32
Glycolysis and pyruvic acid formation, 31
Gnathological treatment, 245-264
 equilibration in, 253-259
 limitations of, 263-264
 reconstruction in, 259-262
Gnathostomatic system, 117-119; *see also* Masticatory system
Golgi organ electroacupuncture treatment, 346, 347

Good Samaritan exemption in negligence law, 610-611
Goodfriend, David J., 621-635
Gouty arthritis, acute, 217
Gradual onset of dysfunction and pain, 76
Grafts, bone
  costochondral, 535-536
  in mandibular repositioning, 531, 533
Grating sound in joint; *see* Noises in joint
Gratuitous service, negligence in, 608
Greenstick fractures of condyles, 444
Grinding of teeth
  habitual; *see* Bruxism
  selective, for occlusal adjustment, 125, 255-259, 500, 505, 510, 601
Group actions of muscles, 17-24
Growth and development, 1-69
  evolutionary, 3, 5-7, 616-618
  of muscular system, factors affecting, 461-463
  in prenatal period, 4-7, 35, 36-37, 462, 466, 479
  radiographic assessment of, 534
Gum chewing, 463, 510
Gunshot wounds, surgical procedures for, 373

H

Habits of patient
  and articular eminence flattening, 202
  assessment of, in initial examination, 103
  history of, 77
  in muscle imbalances, 462, 463, 465, 466, 470, 478
  in muscle spasms, suggestions for correction of, 317
  postoperative elimination of, 372
  and postural problems, 303
  questions for assessment of, 303
  sucking, 35, 36-37, 38-40, 462, 465, 470, 472-473
  in telephone use, 303, 463
  in vertigo, 628, 629, 632
Habitual occlusion, 253; *see also* Centric occlusion
Hair care, questions for assessment of, 307
Hand
  acupuncture points on, 336, 338, 340, 345
    electrical stimulation of, 341
  radiographic examination of, for growth assessment, 534
Hand-held occlusal study models, 88, 123
Hand-to-nose gestures of patient in initial examination, 82
Head and neck musculoskeletal dysfunctions, 234, 312, 591-599
  cluster symptoms of, 597-598
  soft tissue disturbance in, 597, 599
  specific causes of, 597
Headaches
  biofeedback treatment of tension in, 329
  drug therapy for
    narcotic addiction after, 198
    and neurotic behavior in drug resistance, 232
  electroacupuncture treatment of, 348-349
  history of, 74, 302, 304, 306
  initial examination in, 93-95
  mechanical, 235
  misdiagnosis of cause of, 235
  psychogenic, 332
  radiographic examination in, 168-172, 189-191, 198-199
  tension, 329, 333
Health of TMJ
  concept of, 616
  increasing level of, 620
Hearing
  in occlusion abnormalities, 623, 631, 633
  in TMJ dysfunction, 227, 533
Heat therapy, 510, 620
  in muscle spasms, 297, 317
  postoperative, 372
Helplessness of patients, 236, 237
Hemostatic contractures of muscles, 33
Hering-Breuer reflex, 331
Herpes simplex virus
  and drug therapy for postherpetic neuralgia, 561, 563
  incidence in trigeminal neuralgia, 584
High-pull headgears, 521
Hindbrain sag of trigeminal neuralgia patients, 584-586
Hinge axis, 245, 246
  and axis-orbital plane, 120-121, 251
  location and marking of, 120
  terminal position, 106, 120, 251
  transferred to articulators, 120-121, 250-252
    arbitrary techniques for, 250-251
    rotational techniques for, 251
  true, establishment of, 129
Hinged-sliding movement of TMJ, 10, 119, 616-617
Hip height determination, 279, 307
Historical background
  of TMJ in dentistry and dental medicine, 621-624
  of TMJ surgery, 355-356
  of trigeminal neuralgia treatment, 558-559
History taking, 73-81, 83, 278, 512-515
  on chief complaint, 74-75
  on course of symptoms, 76-77
  dental, 77
  on environmental factors, 462-463, 480
  forms for, 78-81, 83, 302-306, 480, 513-515
  importance of, 73
  legal considerations in, 307, 611
  listening to patient during, 211
  on location of symptoms, 75
  medical, 73-74
  in muscle imbalance, 462-463, 466
  in muscle spasms, 278, 301-307
  in occlusal analysis, 77, 123
  on onset of symptoms, 76
  patient reactions to, 237-238
  on previous care, 73
  on psychological factors, 74, 302, 510
  of symptom patterns, 75-77
  tape recording of, 301-302
  in trigeminal neuralgia, 580-581
Hobbies affecting muscular development, 463, 466
  assessment of, in initial examination, 103
Holdaway facial profile analysis, 520
Home use of biofeedback, 328
Homeopathic treatment, 480-481
Hopelessness felt by TMJ patients, 236, 237, 239, 240, 242
Hospitalization for intracranial procedures in trigeminal neuralgia, duration of, 575, 576
Hydrocollator treatment, 510
Hydrogen atoms
  in energy metabolism, 32, 33
  oxidation by enzymes, 32, 33
Hydromorphone, 352
Hydrops of labyrinth; *see* Meniere's disease
Hydrostatic splints, 268
Hydroxyzine pamoate, 620
Hygiene, oral
  affecting success of restorative procedures, 264
  in trigeminal neuralgia patients, 582
Hyperalgesia, secondary, 75

Hypermobility of condylar head, surgical treatment of, 360
Hyperplasia, condylar, 68
  bone scans of, 162
  case histories on surgical treatment of, 429-436, 537-538, 539-542
Hypertension, biofeedback treatment of, 333
Hyperthyroidism
  biofeedback treatment in, 333
  muscle spasms in, 296
Hypertrophic arthritis, 214; *see also* Osteoarthritis
Hyperuricemia and myospasms, 296
Hypnosis, compared with biofeedback, 328-329
Hypnotic drugs, 352, 353
Hypocalcemia, 283
Hypokinetic disease, 296
Hypoplasia of condyle, orthognathic surgery for, 526, 531
Hypotension acupuncture point, 348, 349
Hypothyroidism, biofeedback treatment in, 333
Hypovitaminosis, 283

I

Iatrogenic TMJ dysfunctions, 35-69
Ibuprofen, 351
Ice massage in spasm therapy, 324, 325
Idling side of mandible, 247
Iliac crest observation in examination procedures, 279, 307
Imbalance, muscular; *see* Balance of oral musculature
Immobilization after muscle spasms, 296
Implants, dental
  allergic reactions to, 74, 375, 480
  malpractice suit regarding, 600-601
Impressions of teeth, technique for obtaining model of, 104-106
Incorporative personality prototype, 487
Indene acetic acids, 351
Indocin; *see* Indomethacin
Indoleacetic acids, 351
Indomethacin, 351
Infants; *see* Children and infants
Infections
  history of, 73-74
  postoperative, 375
Infectious arthritis, 216
  chronic, 215
Inflammation
  antiinflammatory agents for, 350-352
  bone scans of, 161, 163
  deep pain and myospasms in, 77
  prevention of, 620
  proteolytic enzyme therapy for, 353
Informed consent, 375, 601-605
Infrahyoid muscles, 17, 211, 212
Infraorbital nerve
  alcohol blocks of, 559-560
  neurectomy of, 561
Initial examination of patient, 82-116, 278-283, 296
Initial location of symptoms, 75
Injections
  of alcohol in trigeminal neuralgia, 558, 559-561
  of anesthetic agents for muscle spasms, 297-298, 319, 353
  of steroids, 353
Interarticular fibrocartilage of TMJ; *see* Articular disc of TMJ
Intercondylar distance as determinant of mandibular movements, 248-249
Interferences, occlusal, 122, 509
  centric, 128, 130, 258
  indications for elimination of, 213
  marking location of, 128-129, 130-131, 314-315
Interferences, occlusal—cont'd
  marking location of—cont'd
    on mounted diagnostic casts, 130-131
    Mylar tape for, 128
  protrustive, 128, 130, 258
  reduction of, 125, 255-259, 500, 505, 510, 601
    sequence for, 258-259
  working and nonworking, 128, 130, 259
Interincisal opening measurements, 310-312
  after vapocoolant spray, 313
Intermaxillary fixation of condylar fractures, 443, 445
  active and passive, 445
  amount of time on, 445, 446
  elastic, 445, 446
Internal lateral ligament, 13, 212
Interpersonal relationships of TMJ patients, 487, 488, 490-491, 493
Interpretation of radiographs, 166-210
Intracanthus view of TMJ, 132-137
Intracapsular condylar head fractures, 444
Intracranial procedures for trigeminal neuralgia, 562-576
  comparison of, 572-575
  complications of, 573-575, 576
  indications for, 562
Intradural trigeminal rhizotomy, subtemporal, 562, 563
Intramuscular injections of anesthetic agents for muscle spasms, 297-298, 319, 353
Intraoral vertical oblique osteotomy, 533-534, 550
Iodine-containing contrast medium for arthrography, 151-156, 158
Ischemia, muscle, spasms from, 33, 74
Isometric muscle contraction, 303
Isotonic muscle contraction, 303

J

Jankelson Splints, 270-273
  construction of, 271-273
Jaw deviation exercise, 325
Jaw jut exercise, 324, 325
Jaw programmer, anterior, construction of, 106-110
Jogging, recommendation for, 620
Juvenile rheumatoid arthritis, 65, 216

K

Kent TMJ appliance, case history on use of, 457-458
Keratitis after trigeminal neuralgia treatments, 563, 564, 571-572, 573, 574
Ketoprofen, 351
Keypunch operators, muscle pains of, 317
Kidney
  acupuncture point, electrical stimulation of, 341
  infection of, history of, 303
Kinesiology, 497-499
  applications of, 497
  concepts of, 498
  definition of, 497
  muscle testing techniques of, 480, 481, 497, 498
  other treatment procedures used with, 499
Klinorhynchy, 510
Knots of muscles, rolling of, 316-317
Krebs cycle, 32

L

Labial frenum in muscle imbalances, 464, 474
Laboratory phase
  of cast mounting procedure, 112-115
  of muscle spasm studies, 283, 296
Labyrinth, hydrops of; *see* Meniere's disease

- Laminagraphy, 137-138, 146
  - cephalometric, 510
- Large intestine acupuncture point, 336, 338, 339, 345
  - electrical stimulation of, 341
- Laryngoscopy, indirect, 231
- Larynx, inspection of, 229, 231, 282
- Lateral ligament, 13, 212
- Lateral movements of mandible
  - Bennett movement in, 247
  - condylar displacement in, 67-68
  - examination of, 86
    - in muscle spasms, 279
  - interferences to
    - marking location of, 130
    - removal of, 259
  - muscles for, 211, 212
  - recording of, 252
  - rotational center of, 245-247
  - sounds heard in, 357
- Lateral side of mandible, 247, 249-250
- Laterodetrusion of condyle, 250
- Lateroprotrusion of condyle, 250
- Lateroretrusion of condyle, 250
- Laterosurtrusion of condyle, 250
- Laterotrusion of mandible, 247, 250
- Latex fixation studies in muscle spasms, 283
- Le Fort I osteotomy, 534, 538, 541, 545
- Leaning habits affecting muscular development, 463
- Leg length determination, 279, 303, 307
- Legal aspects, 600-615
  - in consent to procedures, 375, 601-605
  - of drug therapy, 605, 611-612
  - in history taking, 307, 611
  - of negligence, 605-608
- Liability
  - partnership, 608
  - vicarious, 607
- Librium; *see* Chlordiazepoxide
- Lidocaine, 510
  - for anesthesia during percutaneous trigeminal rhizolysis, 567
  - in muscle spasm therapy, 297, 353
  - in tinnitus, 353-354
- Ligamentous structures of TMJ, 10-14, 212
- Limb length determination in examination procedures, 279, 303, 307
- Lips
  - examination of, 101, 464, 467
  - in muscle imbalance, 45, 464, 467
  - Piccard's, 45
- Listening to patient, by examiner, 82, 211, 238
- Liver acupuncture point, electrical stimulation of, 341
- Locality rule on standards of practice, 609
- Location of symptoms, initial and secondary, 75
- Lockjaw, 266-267, 339
- Long centric occlusion, 253
- Long-face syndrome, surgical correction of, 534
- Longissimus cervicis muscle, palpation of, 312-313
- Longus colli muscle, palpation of, 312-313
- Lorazepam in treatment of muscle spasms, 352
- Lucia jig, 266-267

M

- McCormack temporomandibular joint board, 140-141
- Macroglossia, 59
- Magnification radiography, 150-151, 152-155
- Malignant lesions, bone scans of, 161
- Malocclusion, definition of, 117-118; *see also* Occlusion
- Malpractice suits, 600-612
- Mandible
  - balancing side of, 247
  - cavities in, and trigeminal or atypical facial neuralgias, 217-220
  - as chief complaint of patient, 75
  - condylar process of; *see* Condyles, mandibular
  - congenital displacement of, 479
  - deficiency syndrome of, 526
  - embryological development of, 4-5
  - evolutionary development of, 3
  - malposture of, 233, 234
  - in micrognathism, 526, 531
  - movements of, 119-120; *see also* Movements, mandibular
  - muscles of, 14-24, 58-59, 211-212, 270-271
  - osteotomies of
    - alveolar, 531-532
    - modified sagittal split, 529-531, 533, 534, 538, 541, 547
    - vertical oblique, 531, 533-534, 538, 541, 550
  - in prognathism; *see* Prognathism
  - repositioning of
    - appliances for, 265-276, 498-499; *see also* Splint therapy
    - prior to myofunctional therapy, 480
    - surgical, 429-436, 526-534
  - rest position of, 265, 598
  - in retrognathism; *see* Retrognathism, mandibular
  - surgical reconstruction of, 373, 375
  - trauma of, 429-436
    - in children, 65-66
    - in fractures, 216-217, 233, 443-460
- Mandibular division of trigeminal nerve
  - alcohol blocks of, 559-560, 561
  - percutaneous rhizolysis of, 570, 571, 572
  - radiofrequency coagulation of, 559
- Mandibular fossa; *see* Glenoid fossa
- Mandibular Kinesiograph recordings, 512, 520, 593-595, 598
  - of centric-relation occlusion, 266
  - computerization of, 593
  - of malpositioned occlusion, 266, 598
  - of myocentric occlusion, 598
  - in orthodontic procedures, 521, 522, 524
  - in preoperative evaluation, 371, 405
- Mandibular-malleolar ligament, 13-14, 225
- Mandibular notch, acupuncture point in, 338
- Mandibular pain-dysfunction syndrome, psychological factors in, 213-214
- Marezine; *see* Cyclizine
- Marital relations of TMJ patients, 490-491
- Marking ribbon for identifying occlusal interferences, 128
  - on mounted diagnostic casts, 130
- Masseter muscle
  - action and nerves of, 17, 211, 212
  - acupuncture points in, 337
    - electrical stimulation of, 346, 348
  - anatomy of, 14-17, 211, 212, 281, 290, 292
  - biofeedback monitoring of, 330, 331
  - deep layer of, 292-293
  - examination of, 310, 311
  - imbalanced, 464
  - oxygen consumption of, 211
  - pain referral patterns of, 281, 291, 293
  - painful, 83-84
  - palpation of, 83-84, 89, 91, 498
  - rolling knots of, 316, 317
  - spasms of, 618
  - stretch and spray of, 314
  - superficial layer of, 290-291

Masseteric nerve, 24
Masticatory system, 117-119, 233
functions of, 123, 233
mandibular movements in, 119
muscles of, 14-24, 58-59, 211-212, 214
accessory, 17
palpation of, 83-84, 89-90, 91-94
primary, 14-17
pain in, 74-75
teeth in, 118-119
Mastoid bone, palpation of, 229
Maxilla
cavities in, and trigeminal or atypical facial neuralgias, 217-220
deficiency of, surgical correction of, 534
Le Fort I osteotomy of, 534, 538, 541, 545
multiple fractures of, case history on, 451-452
surgical repositioning of, 534-535
total osteotomy of, 534
Maxillary arch correction prior to myofunctional therapy, 480
Maxillary artery, internal, surgical trauma of, 445
Maxillary division of trigeminal nerve
alcohol blocks of, 559-560
percutaneous rhizolysis of, 571
radiofrequency coagulation of, 559
Maxillary face-bows, 521
Mechanical headaches, 235
Meckel's cartilage, 4, 5, 6
Meclizine, 353
Meclofenamic acid, 351
Medical Systems Group of Vishay Company, 314-315
Medications; *see* Drug therapy
Medullary descending trigeminal tractotomy, 564
Mefanamic acid, 351
Megavitamin therapy, 354
Membranes of muscle cells, 30
Meniere's disease, 623, 624, 634
case history on treatment of, 633
tinnitus in, 226
Meningiomas in trigeminal neuralgia, 583
Meniscectomy, 359, 360-364
with articular eminence prosthesis placement, 377-378, 380, 402-405
Meniscus, articular, of TMJ; *see* Articular disc of TMJ
Mental nerve
alcohol blocks of, 560
neurectomy of, 561
Mentalis muscle activity in swallowing, 464, 468
Mentally incompetent patients, legal aspects in treatment of, 605
Meperidine, 352, 620
Meprobamate therapy
for anxiety and muscle spasms, 352-353
postoperative, 372
Meridian points for acupuncture, 335, 336-338, 340
Dermatron instrument using, 481
electrical stimulation of, 340-349
Metabolism
ATP synthesis in, 30-32
history of disturbances in, 74
Metallic prostheses
allergy to, 74, 375
case histories on, 393, 398
Methocarbamol in muscle spasm treatment, 353
Methohexital in percutaneous trigeminal rhizolysis, 565, 566-567, 569, 572
Micrognathia, mandibular, 526
surgical correction of, 531
Microscopic studies of pathological TMJ conditions, 378-379
Microstomia, 55
Microvascular decompression in trigeminal neuralgia treatment, 580-590
compared with radiofrequency rhizotomy, 585
indications for, 585
operative technique for, 586-590
positioning patient for, 586
results of, 589
Midcondylar neck fractures, 444
Middle fossa rhizotomy for trigeminal neuralgia compared with other procedures, 572-575
Milk
allergy to, mouth breathing in, 43, 59
comparison of human and cow, 42, 43
Miltown; *see* Meprobamate therapy
Minerals, supplemental, 354
Minimal occlusal deviation, treatment of, 263
Mini-O-Matic instrument for electroacupuncture, 341, 343
Minnesota Multiphasic Personality Inventory, 74, 283
Minor patients, legal aspects in treatment of, 605; *see also* Children and infants
Mirrors for inspection of nasopharynx and larynx, 229, 231
Misrepresentation, invalidating consent, 605
Mogodon; *see* Nitrazepam
Moist heat applications, 510, 620
in muscle spasm treatment, 297, 317
postoperative, 372
Molars
extraction of, 505
in interference during chewing, 500
Morphine, action of, 352
Motivation for therapy
and lack of cooperation, legal aspects of, 608-609
in myofunctional therapy, 466, 482, 483
Motor unit, 26
Motorcycle accidents, case histories on surgery for trauma in, 448-449, 453
Motrin; *see* Ibuprofen
Mounted study casts; *see* Articulator mounted casts
Mouth
breathing through
in allergies, 43, 59
chronic, 59
in dysmasesis, 357
examination of, 229-230
for cancer, 86
initial, 86-87, 95
floor of, 86, 95
in microstomia, 55
procedures for occlusal analysis in, 127-129
restricted opening of, 75, 85, 187-188, 241-242, 357, 455-456
vestibule of, 86, 95
Movements, mandibular, 119-120, 212-213
Bennett, 247, 250
border, 125-126, 252
broad contact areas in, 258
closing, 17, 23, 59, 279, 356-357, 498
condylar displacement in, 66-68
examination of, 84-86, 95, 127, 279, 498
geometry of, 119-121, 124, 126, 245-250
lateral; *see* Lateral movements of mandible
in muscle spasms, 279
muscles for, 14-24, 58-59, 211-212, 270-271
normal, 85, 127, 212
occlusal interferences during; *see* Interferences, occlusal

Movements—cont'd
  opening; *see* Opening movements
  protrusive; *see* Protrusion, mandibular
  recording of, 252, 260
    Mandibular Kinesiograph in, 593; *see also* Mandibular Kinesiograph recordings
    pantographic, 125-126, 129
  reflex, 24-25, 119
  restricted, 75, 85, 187-188, 241-242, 357
    in trismus, 266-267, 339
  retrusive, 24, 211, 212, 357, 524
  rotational, 58, 119, 245-247, 251
  sounds heard in; *see* Noises in joint
  translational, 58, 119, 168, 618
Multidisciplinary care, legal aspects of, 605-606
Multiple sclerosis, trigeminal nerve in, 559, 573, 585
Muscles, 14-34; *see also* specific muscles
  balance of; *see* Balance of oral musculature
  biofeedback monitoring of, 327-334
  buccinator mechanism of, 53
  contractile tissues of, 26
  drug therapy for relaxation of, 352-353
  in dysponetic cycle, 498
  electrical activity of, 597
  exercises for relaxation of, in spasm therapy, 320-326
  factors affecting development of, 461-463
  fibers of, 26-27
  functional considerations of; *see* Myofunctional considerations
  group actions of, 17-24
  of head and neck, diagnosis and management of dysfunctions in, 591-599
  kinesiology in analysis of, 480, 481, 497-499
  mandibular, 14-24, 211-212, 270-271
    depressor, 24, 25, 211, 212
    elevator, 17, 24, 59, 211
  of mastication, 14-24, 58-59, 211-212, 214
    accessory, 17
    palpation of, 83-84, 89-94
    primary, 14-17
  oral myofunctional therapy for, 461-485
  in origin of TMJ syndrome, 211-212, 233-235
  pain in, 211-212, 357
    in myofascial pain-dysfunction syndrome, 76-77; *see also* Myofascial pain-dysfunction syndrome (MFPD)
    prolonged, 234
  physiological (hemostatic) contracture of, 33
  reflex system of, 24-25
  rolling knots of, 316-317
  spasms of; *see* Spasms, muscular
  stress resistance testing of, 497, 498
  of tongue, 53-57
Musical instrument use affecting muscular development, 463, 471
Mutually protected occlusion, 253
Myalgia, 75, 211-212, 234, 357
Myelography in head and neck pains, 198
Mylar tape for interference testing, 128
  on mounted diagnostic casts, 130
Mylohyoid muscle, action and nerves of, 17
Myocentric occlusion, 265
  compared with centric occlusion, 266
  complications from disharmony in, 521
  Myo-Monitor used for, 591-593
  registration of, 598-599
Myofascial pain-dysfunction syndrome (MFPD), 211, 591
  dental history in, 77
  electrical acupoint therapy for, 340-349
Myofascial pain-dysfunction syndrome (MFPD)—cont'd
  interrelationships of treatments for, 506
  irritation of trigger areas in, 213
  progression of symptoms in, 76-77
  Weiss appliance for, 273-276
Myofibrils of skeletal muscle, 27, 28
Myofilaments of skeletal muscle, 27, 28
Myofunctional considerations
  in biofeedback, 327-334
  in chief complaint of patient, 75, 76-77
  in dental kinesiology, 497-499
  in examination of patient, 88, 101, 103, 464-466
  in head and neck musculoskeletal dysfunctions, 591-599
  in muscle imbalances, 53-59, 234-235, 461-485
  in muscle spasms; *see* Spasms, muscular
  in oral myofunctional therapy, 461-485
    active and passive types of, 320-326, 482-483
    case histories on, 472-478
    sequence of treatments in, 479-484
    structural considerations in, 479-480
  in postoperative management, 371-372, 453
  in preoperative management, 371
  in prevention of TMJ syndrome, 619-620
  in sucking and biting habits, 45, 462, 472-473
Myo-Monitor, 591-593, 597, 598
  in orthodontic procedures, 521
  postoperative use of, 372
  used prior to splint prescription, 270-271, 272
Myoneural (end-plate) junction, 27
Myosin, 27, 28-29, 30
Myositis of masticatory muscles, 214
Myospasms; *see* Spasms, muscular
Myo-Tronics EMG Bioelectric Processor, 597, 598
Myo-Tronics repositioning appliance, 598
Myo-Tronics Terminus Articulator, 598

N

Nalbuphine, 352
Nalfon; *see* Fenoprofen
Narcotic drug therapy, 351-352
  addiction to, 198, 352, 493
  in trigeminal neuralgia, 562
Nasal conditions; *see* Nose
Nasopharynx, inspection of, 229, 231
Neck
  exercises in spasm therapy, 321, 325, 326
  muscles of, 234, 312, 591-599
    moist heat applied to, 317
    stress resistance testing of, 498
    stretch and spray of, 315
    in torticollis, 307
  pains in, 312
    initial examination of, 93-95
    narcotic addiction in, 198
    radiographic examination in, 198-199
  palpation of, 230, 312-313
Needles for acupuncture, 335-336, 341; *see also* Acupuncture
Negligent conduct, 600-612
  compared with battery, 601
  contributory, 609-610
  in customary practices, 606-607
  discovery statutes on, 609
  expert witness testimony on, 610
  Good Samaritan exemption in, 610-611
  locality rule on, 609
  partnership liability for, 608

Negligent conduct—cont'd
  peer review of, 612
  proof of damages in, 609
  statute of limitations on, 609
  textbooks as evidence of, 610
  vicarious liability for, 607
Neonatal sucking reflex, 35-41, 462
  in breast feeding, 42-45
Neoplasms
  diagnosis of, 161, 217
  oral examination for, 86, 229-230
  surgical procedures for, 373
  TMJ disease misdiagnosed as, 192-193
  in trigeminal neuralgia, 564, 572, 581, 583, 584, 589, 590
Neo-Synephrine; *see* Phenylephrine in intranasal examination
Nerves, 24-25, 358
  alcohol blocks of, 558, 559-561
  dysponetic signaling of, 498
  of ear, 225
  embryological development of, 5-6
  evaluation of, 87, 99, 307, 310
    preoperative, 371
  facial; *see* Facial nerve
  of mandibular musculature, 14, 16-17
  pain in; *see* Neuralgia
  trigeminal; *see* Trigeminal nerve
Neuralgia
  atypical facial, 217-220, 486, 593
  postherpetic, 561, 563
  trifacial; *see* Trigeminal nerve, neuralgia of
  trigeminal; *see* Trigeminal nerve, neuralgia of
Neurectomy, peripheral, for trigeminal neuralgia, 559, 561-562, 575
Neurilemmas in trigeminal neuralgia, 583
Neurolytic agents in trigeminal neuralgia treatment, 558
  alcohol injections in, 558, 559-561
Neuroma, acoustic, in trigeminal neuralgia, 584, 590
Neuromuscular mandibular repositioner
  for children, 67, 68, 69
  Weiss appliance for, 273-276
Neuromuscular occlusion, 512, 520, 521
Neuronal transmission in trigeminal neuralgia, 585
Neuropathy, peripheral entrapment, 313
Neurosis, occlusal, 233
Neurosurgical treatment of facial pain, 557-579
Neurotic behavior in drug-resistant headaches, 232
Nicotinic acid in tinnitus treatment, 353
Night guard splints, 267-268
Nipples of human breast, 45, 47, 48
  artificial substitutes for, 45, 48-50
Nitrazepam, 352
Nitrites, dietary, 317
Noises in joint, 356-357, 358
  of children, 66, 68
  in external pterygoid muscle disturbances, 212, 510
  in fractures, 444
  in muscle spasms, 279, 510
  prior to painful limitation, 75
  patient evaluation of surgery for, 381
  in prognathism, 179
  stethoscope detection of, 83, 227, 279, 312
Nonmasticatory mandibular movement, 119
Nonsteroid antiinflammatory drugs (NSAIDS), 350-351
  side effects of, 351
Nonverbal communication during examination of patient, 82, 238, 302
Nonworking interferences, marking location of, 128, 130
Nose, 224-231
  congestion of, 331
    in allergic children, 59-62
    biofeedback treatment of, 333
    in muscle imbalances, 472, 478
  examination of, 229, 231
  pains in, 227-228
  septum deviation correction prior to myofunctional therapy, 480
  in tension nose, 229
Nubain; *see* Nalbuphine
Nuk exerciser, 39-41
Nuk Sager nipple, 45
Nursing infants
  artificial nipples for, 45, 48-50
  breast feeding for, 35, 40, 42-45
Nutrition, 354, 478, 510
  in acupuncture treatment, 341, 345, 348, 349
  affecting muscular development, 462, 465
  allergic reactions to diet in, 43, 59, 462, 480
  in biofeedback treatment, 331
  after condylar fractures, 446
  dysponetic signaling in improper, 498
  evaluation of, 87, 317, 341, 465
    Dermatron instrument in, 480-481
    in history taking, 74, 303
  infant feeding patterns in, 35-50, 462
  in kinesiology, 499
  in mandibular muscle myopathy, 74
  in muscle spasms, 299, 317
  in myofunctional therapy, 478, 480
  in prevention of TMJ syndrome, 620
  soft diet for, 357
  in tinnitus, 353
Nystagmus in vertigo, 227

O

Obligations of patient, legal aspects of, 608-609
Oboe player, muscular imbalance of, 463
Occlusal neurosis, 233
Occlusal slide, 121
Occlusion, 117-131, 252-253
  acquired, 253-254, 414-417
  affecting condylar position, 597-598
  casts in study of, 88, 104-115; *see also* Articulator mounted casts
  centric, 120-121, 266; *see also* Centric occlusion
  in chief complaint of patient, 75
  Class I, 520, 524-525
  Class II; *see* Retrognathism, mandibular
  Class III; *see* Prognathism
  contact areas in, 258, 262-263, 314-315
  criteria for assessment of, 121-129
  deep overbite in, 122
  definition of, 117
  determinants of, 119-120, 126, 247-250
  in ear disorders, 623-624, 631
  equilibration techniques for adjustment of, 255-259; *see also* Equilibration
  family predisposition to malocclusion, 520, 521
  functional analysis of, 118-119, 123
    on mounted diagnostic casts, 129-131
  in head and neck syndrome, 597-598
  history taking about, 77, 123
  ideal, 252, 265
  infant feeding affecting, 35-50, 462
  initial examination of, 87, 97
  interferences to, 122; *see also* Interferences, occlusal

Occlusion—cont'd
kinesiology in treatment of, 497, 498-499
large overjet in, 122
limitations in treatment of, 263-264
Mandibular Kinesiograph assessment of, 512, 520; *see also* Mandibular Kinesiograph recordings
minimal deviation of, 263
in muscle imbalance, 466
in muscle spasms, 282
myocentric position of, 265, 266, 521, 591-593, 598-599
new system for checking and recording, 314-315
orthodontic treatment of, 253, 500, 504, 505
and pain in TMJ region, 124, 213, 591
periodontal complications in hyperfunction of, 254
posterior bite collapse in, 122
procedures for analysis of, 127-129
reconstruction techniques for, 259-263, 508, 510, 601, 631, 633
sources of wear in, 254
splints for adjustment of, 265-277; *see also* Splint therapy
types of, 253
in vertigo, 75, 625-635
Occupation of patient
history taking about, 303, 307
muscle spasms related to, 317
postural problems related to, 303
stress in, 489, 491, 492
Onset of symptoms, 76
in trigeminal neuralgia, 580
Open reduction of condylar fractures, 445-446
ankylosis after, 447
case histories on, 447, 448-449, 453
internal or external fixation in, 446
Open-bite occlusion, 253
Opening movements, 127
deviation of, 85-86, 95
examination of, 84-86, 95, 127, 279, 498
in muscle spasms, 279, 297
muscles for, 24, 59, 211, 212
normal amount of, 85, 127
in origin of TMJ syndrome, 508, 510, 618-619, 620
protrusive and lateral excursions in, 86
restriction of, 75, 85
in dysmasesis, 357
psychological and physical factors in, 241-242
radiographic examination of, 187-188
surgical treatment of, 187-188, 455-456
in trismus, 266-267, 339
sounds heard during, 356-357; *see also* Noises in joint
symptomatic of TMJ disorder, 508, 510
in trigeminal neuralgia, 581
voluntary resistance, 297
wide, prevention of, 620
Ophthalmic division trigeminal neuralgia, 564, 571, 572
Opioid analgesics, 352
Opium, 352
Opposite lateral excursion, removal of interferences to, 259
Optic nerve examination, 99
Oral examination, 229-230
in fractures, 444-445
in muscle spasms, 282
for neoplasm detection, 86, 229-230
in occlusal analysis, 123
Oral myofunctional therapy, 461-485
Orbiting side of mandible, 247
Orofacial muscle imbalance; *see* Balance of oral musculature
Orthodontic procedures, 500-525
appliances used in, 521
case histories on, 522-525
diagnostic, 520-521
legal aspects of, 606, 607
occlusion adjustment in, 253, 500, 504, 505
review of literature on, 500-505
and temporomandibular joint syndrome, 505-509
Orthognathic surgery, 526-556
case histories on, 537-556
costochondral grafts in, 535-536
mandibular repositioning in, 526-534
maxillary repositioning in, 534-535
Orthopantograph, 520
Orthopantomyograph, 139
Orthopedic influences in TMJ syndrome, 87, 99, 232-235; *see also* Postural considerations
Orudis; *see* Ketoprofen
Os-Cal Forte, 354
Os-Cal 40 tablets, postoperative, 372
Ossicles of middle ear, 224
Ostectomy for mandibular setback, 533
Osteoarthritis, 73, 214-215, 359-360
compared with rheumatoid arthritis, 216, 368
drug therapy for, 351
history suggesting, 76
orthodontic treatment of, 524
surgical treatment of, 368-369
case histories on, 402-405, 421-424,
symptoms of, 214-215
Osteoarthrotomy for bony ankylosis, case history on, 455-456
Osteoblastic activity, bone scans in assessment of, 161, 162
Osteogenic activity, bone scans in assessment of, 162, 164, 165
Osteomas
causing limitation of movement, 217
radiographic examination of, 183-186
Osteoporosis in prolonged muscle pain, 234
Osteotomy
mandibular
alveolar, 531-532
modified sagittal split, 529-531, 533, 534, 538, 541, 547
for setback, 533-534
subapical, 533
vertical oblique, 531, 533-534, 538, 541, 550
maxillary
Le Fort I, 534, 538, 541, 545
total, 534
Otic ganglion, 24
Otoscopy, 229
Overbite
deep, 122
measurement of, 127
Overjet
large, 122
measurement of, 127
Overlap in occlusion
horizontal, 122
vertical, 122
Overlays, dental, in vertigo treatment, 631, 633; *see also* Reconstruction procedures, occlusal
Oxazepam, 352
Oxidative enzymes, oxidation of hydrogen atoms by, 32, 33
Oxidative phosphorylation, 32, 33
Oxycodone, 352
Oxyphenbutazone, 351
Ozopropazone, 351

P

Pacifers, malocclusion from, 38, 40
Pain
acupuncture for relief from, 335-349
analgesic agents in, 350-352
arthralgic, 75, 357
biofeedback treatment in, 330, 331
chronic, behavioral effects of, 236-239, 300, 350, 493, 557
in ear, 179, 200-201, 227-228, 331, 332
facial
neurosurgical treatment of, 557-579
psychodynamics of, 557-558
in head; *see* Headaches
initial and secondary locations of, 75
kinesiology in treatment of, 497
in muscle imbalance, 465, 476
of muscle spasms, 74, 276, 278, 300
and pain-spasm-pain cycle, 34, 234, 330, 331
myalgic, 75, 357
and atrophy of affected muscle, 234
myofascial, 76-77, 211-212, 213, 273-276, 340-349, 506, 591
Myo-Monitor used for relief of, 593
in neck, 93-95, 198-199, 312
in nose, 227-228
patient description of, 74-76, 498
postoperative, 380
psychogenic, 557
questions for assessment of, 302-303, 304-305, 306
referred, 34; *see also* Referred pain
source of, 358
splints for, 266
surgical treatments for, 377, 380, 557-579
in TMJ region, 75-77, 83, 357, 358, 508, 510
factors causing, 76, 360
occlusal considerations in, 124, 213, 591
symptoms of, 123-124
treatment centers for, 493
trigeminal sensory system transmission of, 557; *see also* Trigeminal nerve, neuralgia of
Palatal arch width, measurement of, 465, 469
Palate, examination of, 86, 95, 465
Palpation
of condyles, 83, 91
in fractures, 444
for hinge-axis recording, 251
in muscle spasms, 279
of mastoid bone, 229
of muscles, 83-84, 89-94, 498, 510, 598
digastric, 93, 96, 498
in individuals prone to TMJ syndrome, 619
masseter, 83-84, 89, 91, 498
pterygoid, 90, 91-92
sternocleidomastoid, 93, 98, 498
temporal, 93, 94, 310, 311, 498
trapezius, 93, 100, 310, 311, 498
in vertigo, 629
of neck, 230, 312-313
of tongue, 229
Palsy, facial
Bell's, 200, 330
after trigeminal neuralgia treatment, 560, 563
Panographic or panoramic radiographs, 138-139
in Eagle's syndrome, 220-222
machines for, 139
in orthodontic procedures, 520
Panorex film for, 139, 178, 510
Panorex radiographs, 139, 178, 510
Pantographic recording of mandibular movement, 125-126, 129
Papain, 353
Papase, 353
Paraaminophenol derivatives, analgesic action of, 351
Paraflex; *see* Chlorzoxazone
Paralysis
as complication of trigeminal neuralgia treatment, 560, 563
electromyographic biofeedback treatment of, 329-330
Parents of TMJ patients, 487, 488, 490-491, 493
consenting to treatment of children, 605
Parotid tumor, TMJ disease misdiagnosed as, 192-193
Partnership liability, 608
Pascal's law, 268
Passive exercise therapy, 325, 482-483
Pathological conditions in TMJ, 233, 616-619
microscopic studies of, 378-379
Pathological occlusion, criteria for, 121-129
Patient-doctor interactions, 236-238
in history taking, 211, 301-302
in initial examination, 82
legal aspects of, 600-612
listening in, 82, 211, 238
in myospasm treatment, 296-297
nonverbal communication in, 82, 238, 302
and stress impasse stage IV, 492
Peck analysis, 520
Pediatric patients; *see* Children and infants
Peer review of negligence, 612
Pentazocine, 352
Percodan; *see* Oxycodone
Perforation of articular disc, 168, 359, 444
case histories on, 402-405, 418, 448-449
surgery for, 402-405, 448-449
Perilymph of ear, 224
Periodontal involvement
affecting restorative procedures, 264
in muscle imbalance, 465, 471, 474-475
in occlusal hyperfunction, 254
Peripheral entrapment neuropathy, 313
Peripheral procedures for trigeminal neuralgia, 558-562, 575
alcohol injections, 558, 559-561
neurectomy, 559, 561-562, 575
Perphenazine for postherpetic neuralgia, 561
Personality of TMJ patients, 237-239, 486-487, 488, 493, 510
Peshek antiheadache acupuncture point, 348-349
Petrosal vein abnormalities in trigeminal neuralgia, 583
Petrous ridge of trigeminal neuralgia patients, 584
Pharmacological methods; *see* Drug therapy
Pharynx, examination of, 86, 95, 229
Phenacetin, analgesic action of, 351
Phenaphen; *see* Acetaminophen, analgesic action of
Phenazocine, 352
Phenothiazines, 353
Phenylbutazone, 351
Phenylephrine in intranasal examination, 229
Phenytoin in trigeminal neuralgia, 562, 585, 589, 590
Phosphorylation, oxidative, 32, 33
Photographs, facial, in orthodontic diagnostic procedures, 520
Physical examination of patient
initial, 82-116
in muscle spasms, 278-296, 307-315
oral cavity in; *see* Oral examination
palpation of muscles and joints in; *see* Palpation
Physiological (hemostatic) contracture of muscle, 33
Physiological occlusion, criteria for, 121-129

Physiotherapy
postoperative, 372
preoperative, 371
Piccard's lip, 45
Pierre Robin's syndrome, 63
Pin fixation of fractures, 446, 447
case histories on, 453
Pituitary forehead acupuncture point, 348-349
Pivoting condyle, 247, 250
compound movement of, 249-250
Planography, 137-138; *see also* Tomography
Platysma muscle, anatomy of, 17
Pointer-reference methods for hinge-axis recording, 251
Pollution, environmental, adverse reactions to, 480
Popping sounds; *see* Noises in joint
Portio divisions of trigeminal nerve
intermedius, 564-565
major, 564-565, 582, 588
minor, 564-565
Posterior bite collapse, 122
Posterior fossa rhizotomy for trigeminal neuralgia compared with other procedures, 572-575, 576
Posterior pivot splint appliance, 268
Posterior tooth loss, effects of, 500, 510
Posteroanterior radiographs in orthodontic diagnostic procedures, 520
Postherpetic neuralgia, 561, 563
Postnasal drip, biofeedback treatment of, 333
Postoperative period
care of patient during, 371-372, 377
negligent, 607
patient evaluation of surgery in, 380-381
Postorthodontic patients, TMJ syndrome in, 505-509
Postural considerations, 63-65, 87, 99, 232-235
in examination procedures, 307
head and neck position in, 234, 312, 597
in history taking, 303
leg length determination in, 279, 303, 307
in muscle spasms, 278-279
Potassium ion concentrations, 30
Pregnancy
affecting TMJ, 313
fetal development in; *see* Fetal development
Premature occlusal contacts, 255-256, 314-315; *see also* Interferences, occlusal
Premolar teeth
in chewing interference, 500
extraction of, 505
Prenatal period
muscle imbalance related to, 462, 466, 479
sucking reflex in, 35, 36-37
TMJ in, 4-7
Preoperative evaluation procedures, 371
Prevention
of negligence suits, 611-612
of TMJ disease, 68, 616-620
Prinadol; *see* Phenazocine
Problem-solving behavior of TMJ patients, 488-489, 492
Procaine, 353, 510
for muscle spasms, 297, 319
Profile analysis, facial, 520, 543, 544, 547
Prognathism, 520, 521, 532-534
case histories on, 524, 537-538, 543-545, 549-551
ear pain in, 179
familial trait of, 524
and pseudoprognathism, 533
Prognathism—cont'd
radiographic examination of, 176-177, 179-182
surgical correction of, 182, 537-538, 543-545, 549-551
TMJ changes in, 532-533
Programmer, anterior jaw, construction of, 106-110
Progression of symptoms, 76
Progressive relaxation exercises in spasm therapy, 320-326
Prophylactic measures
legal, 611-612
in maintaining TMJ health, 68, 616-620
Prostaglandin synthesis, antiinflammatory agents inhibiting, 350, 351
Prosthetic replacements, 365-378
allergic reactions to, 74, 375, 480
for articular eminence; *see* Articular eminence, prosthesis for
complications of, 375, 380
customized, case history on, 436-438
difficult adjustment to, in muscle imbalance, 465, 471
hinge-axis, 457
muscle spasm caused by, 375, 510
right-angle, 455
selection of, 373
for teeth; *see* Dentures
for total TMJ replacement, 373, 375, 380-382, 396-410
Proteins
contractile, 27, 28-30
in nutritional evaluation, 317
Proteolytic enzyme therapy, 353
Protrusion
mandibular
anterior guidance of, 247
determinants of, 247-248
eminence angle affecting, 247-248
examination of, 86, 279
interferences to, 128, 130, 258-259
in muscle spasms, 279
muscles for, 24, 211
in prognathism; *see* Prognathism
recording of, 110-112, 252
sounds heard in, 357
maxillary, surgical correction of, 534
Provisional castings, restorative, 260-261
placement of, 260-261
remounting of, 261
Proxemics in initial examination of patient, 82
Proximate cause in negligence law, 610
Pseudoankylosis, 368
Pseudoprognathism, mandibular, surgical correction of, 534
Psychological considerations, 124, 236-242, 486-494, 557
affecting course of symptoms, 76
in behavior modification techniques, 483
in bruxism, 214, 490, 491, 510
in case histories, 239-242, 487, 489, 490-492, 525
in chronic pain, 236-239, 300, 350, 493, 557-558
diagnostic tools for assessment of, 283
in early childhood dynamics, 488, 490, 491, 493
in facial pain, 557-558
in headaches, 232, 332
history taking about, 74, 302, 510
in initial examination of patient, 88, 101
in mandibular pain-dysfunction syndrome, 213-214
in motivation for therapy, 466, 482, 483, 608-609
in muscle spasms, 276, 296-297, 315
in origin of TMJ syndrome, 76, 213-214, 591
in orthodontic treatments, 525
in prevention of negligence suits, 612
in reconstruction procedures, 263-264

Psychological considerations—cont'd
research on, 486-487
in stress impasse stages, 487-490, 492, 493
in stress management programs, 493, 619-620
in surgical procedures, 375
in postoperative management, 372
in preoperative evaluation, 371
in vertigo, 227
Pterygoid muscles
external, 211
anatomy of, 17, 18, 281-282, 294
compensatory changes after condylar fractures, 445, 447
functions of, 17, 211, 212
in malpositioned occlusion, 598
in mechanical headaches, 235
pain referral patterns of, 281-282, 295
painful, 84
palpation of, 91-92
spasms of, 202, 212, 438, 618
noises due to, 510
postoperative, 375
internal, 211
anatomy of, 17, 18
functions of, 17, 211, 212
pain referral patterns of, 281
palpation of, 90, 91
Pyruvic acid
conversion to acetyl coenzyme A, 31-32
glycolysis in formation of, 31

Q

Quick mount of diagnostic casts, 129, 251

R

Radiation exposure
in magnification radiography, 150-151
in xeroradiography, 148
Radiofrequency coagulation for pain relief, 559
Radiofrequency rhizolysis, percutaneous, in trigeminal neuralgia, 565-572
compared with other procedures, 572-575, 576
Radiofrequency rhizotomy in trigeminal neuralgia, 585, 590
Radiographic examinations, 132-210, 315, 510, 598
in arthritis, 215, 283, 368-369
arthrography, 151-156, 159-160
cephalometric, 132, 133, 135, 136, 146; *see also* Cephalometric radiographs
comparison of, 160-161
contrast medium used in, 151-156, 158
in Eagle's syndrome, 220-222
of hand-wrist, 534
in headaches, 168-172, 189-191, 198-199
in hinge-axis recording, 251
in initial examination, 87, 97, 99
interpretation of, 166-210
intracanthus view in, 132-137
legal aspects of, 606, 608, 611
magnification in, 150-151, 152-155
of mandibular or maxillary bone cavities, 217-220
in muscle spasms, 279, 282-283
of normal TMJ, 159
for occlusal analysis, 123, 131
in orthodontic procedures, 520
panographic, 138-139, 178, 220-222, 510, 520
of pelvic girdle, 307
postoperative, 372
Radiographic examinations—cont'd
preoperative, 371, 537, 539, 543, 547, 549
in prognathism, 176-177, 179-182
of prosthesis, 405
radiation exposure during, 150-151
radionuclide bone scanning, 161-165
with technetium 99m, 161-164, 533, 537, 539, 543, 549, 550
in splint therapy, 273
tomographic, 137-138, 146
compared with other procedures, 160-161
of osteoma, 183, 185-186
transcranial lateral oblique views in, 140-146, 147; *see also* Transcranial lateral oblique views
transcutaneous arthroscopy, 156-158
in trigeminal neuralgia, 217-220, 565-566, 569
and views obscured by radiopaque material, 198-199
xeroradiographic method of, 148-150, 183, 185-186
Radionuclide bone scanning, 161-165
of hyperplastic condyle, 533
with technetium 99m, 161-164, 533, 537, 539, 543, 549, 550
Raggedy Ann/Andy exercise in spasm therapy, 321, 323
Rake appliances, 482, 483
Rapport in doctor-patient relationship, 612
Ratchet theory of muscular contraction. 27
Reality perception in chronic pain, 236
Reasonable man standard in negligence law, 605
Reassurance of patient in myospasm treatment, 296
Reciprocal muscle inhibition, 297
Reconstruction procedures, occlusal, 259-263
advantages of, 263
compared with equilibration, 259
complications of, 508, 510
final, 261-262
legal aspects of, 601
limitations of, 263-264
for minimal occlusal deviation, 263
provisional, 260-261
recall of patient after, 262
treatments recommended prior to, 260
in vertigo treatment, 631, 633
Record keeping, legal aspects of, 611
Reduction of condylar fractures
closed, 446, 448-449
open, 445-446, 447, 448-449, 453
Reduction techniques for occlusal adjustment, 125, 255-259, 500, 501, 505, 510
Referral of patient, legal aspects of, 605-606
Referred pain, 34, 75
arising from myofascial trigger areas, 213
to ear, 227
of muscle spasms, 300
patterns of, 281-282, 301
questions for assessment of, 303
radiographic examination in, 168-172
Reflexes
gag, 497
Hering-Breuer, 331
inhibition of, in spasm therapy, 297, 298
in mandibular movement, 24-25, 119
rooting, of infants, 38, 50
sucking, 35-41; *see also* Sucking reflex
Reflexology, 489
Regressive behavior of TMJ patients, 488-489, 490, 493
Rela; *see* Carisoprodol
Relaxation techniques
biofeedback for, 327-334

Relaxation techniques—cont'd
drug therapy for, 352-353
exercises for, in muscle spasm therapy, 320-326
interrelationship of, 506
Myo-Monitor for, 598
Relieving factors affecting course of symptoms, 76
Removable mandibular repositioner, Weiss appliance as, 273-276
Repositioning of mandible
appliances for, 265-276, 498-499; *see also* Splint therapy
prior to myofunctional therapy, 480
surgical, 429-436, 526-534
Repression of thoughts and impulses by TMJ patients, 240, 241
Reptile jaw joint, 3, 616
Resilient splints, 267-268
Resistive exercises in spasm therapy, 325
Respiratory tract allergies, 59-62
Rest position of mandible, 265
Myo-Monitor for achievement of, 598; *see also* Myo-Monitor
Restoration procedures, 259-263; *see also* Reconstruction procedures, occlusal
Restriction of opening movement, 75, 85, 187-188, 241-242, 357, 455-456
in trismus, 266-267, 339
Restrictive device for treatment of chronic dislocation, 438-441
Retained infantile swallow, 51, 53
Retainer, orthodontic, for tooth migration, 477
Retrognathism, mandibular, 526-528
case histories on, 414-417, 546-548, 552-555, 632
division 1 of, 500, 502, 510
division 2 of, 500, 503, 510, 520
orthognathic surgery for, 546-548, 552-555
Retromaxillary venous plexus, surgical trauma of, 445
Retrusion
mandibular
intentional, in prognathism, 524
muscles for, 24, 211, 212
in retrognathism; *see* Retrognathism, mandibular
sounds heard in, 357
maxillary, surgical correction of, 534
Rheumatic fever, 215-216
Rheumatoid arthritis, 73, 215
articular eminence prosthesis in, 382-389
drug therapy in, 351
juvenile, 65, 216
laboratory studies in, 283
predisposing causes of, 215
surgical treatment of, 368-369
symptoms of, 215, 216, 368
total TMJ replacement in, 382
Rhinoscopy, 229
Rhizolysis, percutaneous trigeminal, 565-572
compared with other procedures, 572-575, 576
Rhizotomy for trigeminal neuralgia
middle fossa, 572-575
posterior fossa, 572-575, 576
radiofrequency, 585, 590
suboccipital, 563-564
subtemporal
extradural, 562-563, 572-575
intradural, 562, 563
transtentorial, 562, 564-565, 572-575
translabyrinthine, 565
Rhomboid muscle, 211
Rights of patients, legal aspects of, 600-612
to die, 601
to know about procedures, 601
Ringing sounds in ear; *see* Tinnitus
Rinn Corporation transcranial lateral oblique system, 144-146
Rinne's test, 229
Risks of procedures disclosed to patients, 601, 604, 605
Robaxin; *see* Methocarbamol in muscle spasm treatment
Rooting reflex of infants, 38, 50
Rotation of mandible, 58, 119, 245-247, 251

S

Sadistic impulses, oral, of TMJ patients, 237, 239
Sagittal split osteotomy
case histories on, 552
modified, 533, 534, 538, 541, 547
Salicylic acid therapy, 350-351, 352, 510
side effects of, 350-351
Sarcolemma, 28
Sarcomeres, 27
Saxophone player, oral muscular development of, 463
Scalenus muscle, 211
Scanning, radionuclide, of bone, 161-165
with technetium 99m, 161-164, 533, 537, 539, 543, 549, 550
Schwartz appliances, 521
Sclerosis, multiple, trigeminal nerve in, 559, 573, 585
Scopolamine, 353
Screening for TMJ syndrome, 619
Secondary location of symptoms, 75
Sectography, 146
Sedated patients, legal aspects of disclosure statements to, 605
Sedimentation rate in osteodegenerative processes, 283
Selection of patients
for biofeedback training, 330, 332
legal aspects of, 608
Self-image of TMJ patients, 236-242
Semicircular canals of ear, 224
Sensory patterns, postoperative, in trigeminal neuralgia, 575, 576, 585
Serax; *see* Oxazepam
Setback, mandibular, 532-534
Sex of TMJ patients, 508
Sexual behavior of TMJ patient, case history on, 490-491
Shiners, allergic, 59
Shore appliance, 268-270
case history on, 276
construction of, 268-270
Short-face syndrome, 526
Side shift of mandible, 247, 250
immediate, 247, 250
Silastic inserts, 382
allergic reactions to, 375
in articular eminence prosthesis, 369, 371; *see also* Articular eminence, prosthesis for
after high condylectomy, 363, 364
Sinus headaches, 227
Sinusitis, chronic, treatment of, 331
Skeletal muscle, 26-34
Skull-fossa-condyle geometry, 119-120, 124, 245-250
transferred to articulator, 120-121, 126
Sleeping patterns
biofeedback training affecting, 333
bruxism in, 62
Cervi-Pillow affecting, 303, 317
history taking about, 302-303
and muscle imbalances, 463, 473, 478
in muscle spasms, suggestions for correction of, 317
and stiffness on awakening, 76
in trigeminal neuralgia, 580-581

Slide of mandible, 120-121
elimination of, 256, 257
in premature occlusal contacts, 255-256
Small intestine acupuncture points, 336, 339
electrical stimulation of, 341
Smell, sense of, of allergic children, 63
Snapping sounds, 356-357; *see also* Noises in joint
Sodium ion concentrations, 30
Soft splints, 267-268
Soft tissues
in head and neck musculoskeletal dysfunction, 597, 599
xeroradiography of, 148
Solacen; *see* Tybamate
Soma; *see* Carisoprodol
Sounds
of allergic child, 63
in jaw movements, 356-357; *see also* Noises in joint
Spasms, muscular, 32-34, 300-326, 357, 618
agents inducing, production and accumulation of, 34
biofeedback treatment of, 298-299, 327-334
causes of, 32-34, 213, 510
in children, 67, 68
diagnosis of, 278-296, 300, 301-315
drug therapy for, 187, 298, 319, 352-353
emergency procedures for, 276
exercise therapy for, 297, 319, 320-326
history taking on, 278, 301-307
kinesiology treatment of, 497, 498
orthodontic treatment of, 522
pain of, 74, 276, 278, 300
and pain-spasm-pain cycle, 34, 234, 330, 331
physical examination in, 278-296, 307-315
prevention of, 619-620
psychological considerations in, 276, 296-297, 315
of pterygoid muscle, external, 202, 212, 375, 438, 510, 618
splint therapy for, 266
trigger zones in, 34, 213, 281-282, 297-298, 300-301, 318, 319, 353
ultrasound therapy for, 319, 325
Speciality care, legal aspects of, 606
Speculum, nasal, for intranasal examination, 229
Speech disorders
in muscle imbalances, 234, 465, 472-473, 478
in occlusion abnormalities, 623
in osteoarthritis of TMJ, 421-422
psychological effects of, 240
Sphenomandibular ligament, 13, 212
Spinal column, tongue pressure on, in glossoptosis, 63-64
Spindle cell electroacupuncture treatment, 346, 347
Splenius capitus muscle, 93, 102
Splint therapy, 263, 264, 265-277, 498-499, 510, 521
case histories on, 276, 476, 522-525
for children, 67, 68, 69
in combination with myofunctional therapy, 476
compared with equilibration procedures, 259
construction of splints for, 271-273
counterproductive use of, 176
effects of, 266
in fractures, 446
for muscle spasms, 266
Myo-Tronics repositioning appliances in, 598
for neck pain, 166
postoperative, 371
prior to reconstruction, 260
in retrognathism, 547
Spondylitis, ankylosing, case history on surgery in, 436-438
SS White Panorex Unit, 139
Standard of care in negligence law, 606-607
locality rule on, 609
witness testimony on, 610
Statute of limitations, 609
Steering wheel biofeedback device, 328, 331, 332
Sternocleidomastoid muscle, 211
anatomy of, 281, 286
electrical stimulation of, 318, 348
in mechanical headaches, 235
pain referred from, 281, 287
palpation of, 93, 98, 498
rolling knots of, 316, 317
stress resistance testing of, 498
Steroid therapy, 353; *see also* Cortisone therapy
Stiffness on awakening, history of, 76
Still's disease, 65, 216
Stomach acupuncture points, 337-338
electrical stimulation of, 341
Stress
of muscles, and resistance testing of, 497, 498
of TMJ patients; *see* Psychological considerations
Stretching of muscles
excessive, 213
therapeutic, 315-316
Stroke, electromyographic biofeedback treatment of, 329
Stuart technique for recording mandibular excursions, 252
Study casts, 88, 104-115; *see also* Articulator mounted casts
Stylohyoid muscle, action and nerves of, 17
Styloid process of temporal bone, elongation of, 229
in Eagle's syndrome, 220-222
Stylomandibular ligament, 13, 212
Subapical osteotomy, 533
Subcondylar fractures, 444
open reduction of, 446
Subluxation of condyles; *see* Dislocation or displacement of condyles
Suboccipital trigeminal rhizotomy, 563-564
Subtemporal decompression and compression procedures for trigeminal neuralgia, 564
Subtemporal trigeminal rhizotomy
extradural, 562-563, 572-575
intradural, 562, 563
transtentorial, 562, 564-565, 572-575
Subtractive equilibration procedures, 125, 255-259, 500, 501, 505, 510
contraindications for, 257
Succinylcholine for muscle spasms, 187
Sucking habits, 35, 36-37, 38-40, 462, 465, 470, 472-473
Sucking reflex, 35-41
and effects of appendage sucking, 35, 36-37, 38-40, 462, 470, 472-473
and breast feeding, 35, 40, 42-45
Nuk exerciser for, 39-41
prenatal, 35, 36-37
Sudden onset of pain and dysfunction, 76-77
Suicidal behavior in chronic pain, 490
Sulindac, 351
Sunday bite, 83
Suprahyoid muscles, 17, 211, 212
Supraorbital nerve
alcohol blocks of, 559-560
neurectomy of, 561
Supratrochlear nerve
alcohol blocks of, 559-560
neurectomy of, 561
Surgical procedures, 355-442, 510, 598
acupuncture anesthesia in, 183

Surgical procedures—cont'd
- case histories on, 378-379, 382-441, 491, 492, 537-556
- diagnostic criteria for, 356-360
- for facial pain, 557-579
- for fracture reduction, 445-446, 447, 448-449, 453
- historical background of, 355-356, 558-559
- informed consent to, 375, 601-605,
- legal aspects of, 375, 601-605, 607-608
- for mandibular or maxillary bone cavities, 217, 220
- for mandibular repositioning, 429-436, 526-534
- for maxillary repositioning, 534-535
- microscopic examinations in, 378-379
- orthognathic, 526-556
- patient evaluation of, 380-381
- postoperative management in, 371-372, 377, 607
- in prognathism, 182, 537-538, 543-545, 549-551
- proof of damages from, 609
- for restricted opening movements, 187-188, 455-456
- and stress impasse stage IV, 492
- TMJ pain after, 124, 213, 619-620
- total TMJ restoration in, 373, 375, 380-382
- for trigeminal neuralgia, 557-590
- unnecessary, 607-608

Swallowing patterns, 45-52, 59
- abnormal, 51, 53
- appliances for retraining of, 482-483
- in breast feeding, 42, 50
- closure to occlusion during, 598
- deviate, 53
- head and neck position affecting, 312
- infantile, 45-51
  - retained, 51, 53
- initial examination of, 103
- mature, 51-52
- muscle functions in, 51-52
- in muscle imbalances, 464, 465, 467-468, 474, 476
- muscle spasms affecting, 234
- in prenatal period, 35
- transitional, 51

Symmetry of face
- assessment of, 83, 91, 465
- in infants, 65
- myofunctional therapy for imbalance of, 476, 478
- orthognathic surgery for imbalance of, 537-545

Symptoms of TMJ dysfunction, 83, 356-360, 597
- course of, 76-77
- history of, 75-77
- initial, 358
- location of, 75
- onset of, 76
- presenting, 508, 510

Synovial membranes of TMJ, 10

Synovitis in capsular ligament, 212

T

Talwin; *see* Pentazocine

Tandearil; *see* Oxyphenbutazone

Tape recording of patient history, 301-302

Taste, sense of
- of allergic children, 63
- prenatal development of, 35

Technetium 99m bone scans, 161-164
- of hyperplastic condyle, 533
- prior to orthognathic surgery, 537, 539, 543, 549, 550

Teeth
- anterior; *see* Anterior teeth
- clenching of, 202-203, 303

Teeth—cont'd
- dentures for replacement of; *see* Dentures
- in equilibration techniques, 68, 253-259; *see also* Equilibration
- examination of, 86-87, 95, 229, 313
- extraction of, 217-220, 505, 522, 608
- functions in gnathostomatic system, 118-119
- grinding of; *see* Bruxism
- migration of, 253, 465, 471, 474, 477
- in muscle imbalance, 53, 465, 471, 474, 477
- occlusion of; *see* Occlusion
- in orthodontic procedures, 500-525
- reconstruction procedures for; *see* Reconstruction procedures, occlusal
- tongue affecting position of, 55-57
- of trigeminal neuralgia patients, 582

Tegretol; *see* Carbamazepine therapy

Telephone habits affecting muscular development, 303, 463

Temperature biofeedback, 327, 328

Temple resistive exercise, 325

Temporal bone
- anatomy of, 224
- embryological development of, 4-5
- in rotated position, 479-480
- styloid process of, 220-222, 229

Temporal muscle
- anatomy of, 14, 15, 281, 284
- biofeedback monitoring of, 330
- functions of, 14, 211, 212
- imbalance of, 464
- in malpositoned occlusion, 597-598
- in mechanical headaches, 235
- pain referral patterns of, 281, 285
- painful, 83-84
- palpation of, 93, 94, 310, 311, 498
- spasms of, 618
- stretch and spray of, 314

Temporal nerve, posterior deep, 24

Temporomandibular joint
- ideal, 500, 501
- normal, 82-83, 159, 501

Temporomandibular joint instrument for recording mandibular excursions, 252

Temporomandibular joint syndrome
- definition of, 232
- origin of, 233, 591
- pathological physiology of, 616-619
- psychogenic factors in, 236-242
- recognition of individuals prone to, 619
- symptoms of, 75-77, 83, 232, 356-360, 508, 510, 597

Temporomandibular ligament, 13, 212

Tendons, prolonged pain in, 234

Tension headaches
- biofeedback treatment of, 329
- physical causes of, 333

Tension nose, 229

Tension of TMJ patients; *see* Psychological considerations

Tensor tympani muscle spasms, biofeedback relaxation of, 330

Terminal hinge-axis position, 106, 120, 251

Testimony of expert witnesses in liability suits, 610

Textbooks as evidence of negligence, 610

Therapy localization technique, 497, 498

Thiamine in tinnitus treatment, 353

Throat, 224-231
- examination of, 86, 95, 229, 231, 282

Thumb-sucking, 38-40, 462
- affecting muscular development, 462, 470
- controlling habit of, 38, 40

Thumb-sucking—cont'd
of older child, case history of, 472-473
prenatal, 35, 36-37
Thyroid disorders
biofeedback treatment in, 333
muscle spasms in, 296
Tic douloureux, 580; *see also* Trigeminal nerve, neuralgia of
Tinnitus, 194, 226-227, 377
biofeedback treatment of, 332
drug therapy for, 353-354
as initial symptom of TMJ dysfunction, 358
occlusion abnormalities in, 624
orthognathic surgery in, 546-548
TMJ; *see* Temporomandibular joint
Tocainide hydrochloride, in tinnitus treatment, 353-354
Tolectin; *see* Tolmetin
Tolmetin, 351
Tomography, 137-138, 146, 173, 174
compared with other radiographic procedures, 160-161
of osteoma, 183, 185-186
Tongue
affecting tooth position, 55-57
in aglossia, 55
in ankyloglossia, 57-58, 480
ankylotic, 464-465, 469, 472-473
appliances for training, 482-483
biofeedback monitoring of, 483
in breast feeding, 50
compared with artificial nipple sucking, 45, 48-49
cluck exercise of, 325
examination of, 86, 95, 101, 229, 313, 464, 466, 468-469
in glossoptosis, 63-64
hypotonic, 59
in macroglossia, 59
in muscle imbalance, 53, 464, 466, 468-469, 474
muscles of, 53-57
pains of, radiographic examination in, 196-197
palpation of, 229
scalloping of, 464, 468, 474
thrust of, 50, 53, 240, 462
Tonsil and adenoid enlargement
examination of, 229, 465, 469, 472
in mouth breathing, 59, 465
and removal prior to TMJ treatment, 57, 465, 472-473
Tonsillar fossa, palpation of, 229
Tooth conditions; *see* Teeth
Tort law defined, 600
Torticollis, history of, 307
Torus
mandibularis, 55-57
palatinus, 55
Total TMJ replacement, 373, 375, 380-382
case histories on, 396-410
Toxic conditions, evaluation of, prior to myofunctional therapy, 480-481
Traction
cervical, TMJ trauma in, 65, 76, 213, 331, 455-456
mandibular and maxillary, 448
Tractotomy, trigeminal
medullary descending, 564
percutaneous, 562
Tranquilizers, 352-353
in prevention of TMJ syndrome, 620
Transcendental Meditation (TM), 620
Transcranial lateral oblique views, 140-146, 510
compared with other procedures, 160-161, 173
of condylar position, 197, 206-207, 208-209
Transcranial lateral oblique views—cont'd
of diminished joint space, 189, 191, 192-193, 194-195, 200-201
of eminence flattening, 202-203
in head pain evaluation, 168, 169, 198-199
interpretation of, 176-177
McCormack temporomandibular joint board used for, 140-141
of osteoma, 183, 186
of prognathic mandible, 179, 181, 182
of restricted opening movements, 187-188
xeroradiography methods for, 148-150
Transcutaneous arthroscopy, 156-158
Transcutaneous electrical neural stimulation (TENS), 593
Myo-Monitor instrument for, 270-271, 272, 372, 521, 591-593, 597, 598
in orthodontic procedures, 521, 522, 524, 525
Transducers, electronic, in hinge-axis recording, 251
Translabyrinthine trigeminal rhizotomy, 565
Translational movements, 58, 119, 168, 618
Transtentorial rhizotomy, subtemporal, 562, 564-565
compared with other procedures, 572-575
Transverse process of atlas, palpation of, 313
Tranxene, 352
Trapezius muscle
anatomy of, 281, 288
in electroacupuncture treatment, 348
in mechanical headaches, 235
pain referral patterns of, 281, 287
palpation of, 93, 100, 310, 311, 498
rolling knots of, 316, 317
stress resistance testing of, 498
stretch and spray of, 315
wet heat applied to, 317
Trauma
affecting muscular development, 462
in automobile accidents, case histories on surgery for, 396-401, 451-452
biofeedback treatment of, 330, 331
in birth, 65, 462, 479
case histories on surgery for, 393, 396-401, 410-413, 425-436, 448-449, 451-452, 537-538
of cervical traction, 65, 76, 213, 331, 455-456
in children, 65-66
degenerative changes of TMJ after, 215, 359-360, 444
of dental procedures, 66, 76, 232, 233, 330, 331-332, 393, 405-410, 607
of eustachian tube from condyles, 633
in fractures of condyles, 216-217, 233, 443-460
of gunshot wounds, surgical treatment in, 373
head and musculoskeletal dysfunction after, 597
history of, 74, 303
in negligent conduct, 601, 607
in origin of TMJ disorders, 76, 124, 213, 233, 235, 509, 510
prevention of, 619-620
of whiplash, 213, 233, 235, 330
Treatment procedures, 245-494, 509; *see also* specific procedures
acupuncture in, 335-339
electrical, 340-349
in allergic and toxic conditions, 480-481
biofeedback in, 327-334
decision making in, 260
drug therapy in, 350-354
electronic instrumentation for, 591-597
equilibration in, 253-259
in fractures and ankylosis, 443-460
gnathological, 245-264
homeopathic, 480-481
interrelationships of, 479-484, 505, 506

Treatment procedures—cont'd
kinesiology in, 480, 481, 497-499
legal aspects of, 375, 600-615
for muscle spasms, 276, 278-326
Myo-Tronics EMG for monitoring of, 597
occlusal considerationsin, 117-131
oral myofunctional, 461-485
orthodontic, 500-525
outline of, 510
psychological, 486-494
reconstruction in, 259-262
selection of, 479-484
splints in, 265-277
and stress impasse stage IV, 492
structural considerations in, 479-480
surgical, 355-442
orthognathic, 526-556
in trigeminal neuralgia, 557-590
Tricarboxylic acid cycle, 32
Triceps muscles, testing function of, 497
Trifacial neuralgia; *see* Trigeminal nerve, neuralgia of
Trigeminal nerve
anatomy of, 24-25, 582-583
examination of, 99
in jaw reflex system, 24-25
mandibular division of, 559-560, 561, 570, 571, 572
maxillary division of, 559 560, 571
neuralgia of, 217-220, 557-590
acupuncture therapy for, 558
age of patients with, 580, 584-585, 586, 589
bilateral, 559, 564, 585
complications of treatments for, 573-575, 576
decompression and compression procedures for, 562, 563-564, 580-590
drug therapy for, 562, 581, 585, 589, 590
duration of hospitalization for, 575, 576
etiology of, 583-585, 589-590
glossopharyngeal neuralgia with, 564
historical background of surgery for, 558-559
indications for operation in, 585
initial onset of, 580
intracranial procedures for, 562-576
Myo-Monitor treatment of, 593
percutaneous rhizolysis in, 565-575, 576
peripheral surgical procedures for, 558-562, 575
postoperative sensory patterns in, 575, 576, 585
primary first division, 584, 588-589
radiographic examinations in, 217-220, 565-566, 569
rhizotomy in, 562-565, 572-575, 576, 585, 590
symptomatic, 584
tumors in, 581, 583, 589
vascular compression in, 580-581, 583, 585
ophthalmic division of, 564, 571, 572
pain transmission in, 557, 585
rhizolysis of, percutaneous, 565-575, 576
rhizotomy of, 562-565, 572-575, 576, 585, 590
root entry zone of, 582-583, 585, 589-590
tractotomy of
medullary descending, 564
percutaneous, 562
Trigger points in trigeminal neuralgia, 580, 581
Trigger zone of spastic muscle, 34, 213, 300-301
digital muscular examination for, 281-282
electrical stimulation of, 318, 319
heat applied to, 297
intramuscular anesthetic injections in, 297-298, 319, 353
Trilafon; *see* Perphenazine for postherapetic neuralgia
Triple warmer acupuncture point, 337
electrical stimulation of, 341
Tripodization of cusp-fossa relationship, 262-263
Trismus, 267
acupuncture treatment of, 339
splints for, 266-267
Tropomyosin, 29-30
Troponin, 29-30
Trypsin, 353
Tumors; *see* Neoplasms
Tybamate, 353
Tybatran; *see* Tybamate
Tylenol; *see* Acetaminophen, analgesic action of

U

Ultrasound therapy, 313
in muscle spasms, 319, 325
Unnecessary surgery, legal aspects of, 607-608
Uric acid levels in myospasms, 296

V

Valium; *see* Diazepam therapy
Vapocoolant spray
interincisal opening measured after, 313
in muscle spasm therapy, 298, 315-316, 319, 353
Vascular components, questions for assessment of, 302-303
Vascular compression in trigeminal neuralgia, 580-581, 583, 585
Vertical dimensions
in equilibration techniques, 257
in hinge-axis transfer to articulator, 251-252
improper, dysponetic signaling in, 498
kinesiology in determination of, 497, 499
normal, 520
in splint therapy, 499
and teeth extractions, 522
Vertical oblique osteotomy of mandibular ramus, 531, 533-534, 538, 541, 550
extraoral approach, 533, 538, 541
intraoral approach, 533-534, 550
Vertigo, 214, 227, 625-635
case histories on, 629, 632-634
diagnostic procedures in, 628-629
drug therapy for, 353
as initial symptom of TMJ dysfunction, 358
ocular symptoms of, 227, 629, 634
psychogenic, 227
surgical treatment of
patient evaluation of, 381
results of, 377
vagal symptoms of, 629, 634
Vestibule of mouth, 86, 95
Vicarious liability, 607
Victim role of patients, 236-237
Violinist, oral dyskinesia of, 463
Vision assessment, 307
Vistaril; *see* Hydroxyzine pamoate
Vitallium prosthesis, 369, 381
allergic reactions to, 375
case histories on, 405-410
for chronic dislocation, 438-441
for stabilization of fractures, 446
Vitamins
deficiency of, and malfunction of muscle systems, 283
therapy with, 354
in muscle spasms, 319

V.I.V. shrug, 317, 320, 322
Volterol 50; *see* Diclofenac
Vomiting, case history on treatment of, 632
Vulnerability of patients, 238, 239

W

Warranty of cure, legal aspects of, 600-601
Waxing up, diagnostic, in restorative process, 260
Weber's test of hearing, 229
Weight lifting with barbells, 620
Weiss neuromuscular removable mandibular repositioner, 273-276
Whiplash injury
  biofeedback treatment of, 330
  in origin of TMJ syndrome, 213, 233, 235
Witnesses in liability suits, 610
Work of patient; *see* Occupation of patient
Working interferences, 128, 130
Working side of mandible, 247, 249-250

X

Xeroradiography, 148-150
  of osteoma, 183, 185-186
  radiation exposure in, 148
Xylocaine; *see* Lidocaine

Y

Yawning and sudden onset of pain and dysfunction, 76
Yoga, 620

Z

Zomax; *see* Tolmetin
Zygomatic-frontal nerve weakness, informed consent concerning, 375
Zygomectomy, 360, 362